The Practice

of LARGE

ANIMAL

SURGERY

Volume I

PAUL B. JENNINGS, JR., V.M.D., M.Sc.

Diplomate, American College of Veterinary Surgeons

1984

W. B. SAUNDERS COMPANY • PHILADELPHIA • LONDON • TORONTO • MEXICO CITY • RIO DE JANEIRO • SYDNEY • TOKYO

W. B. Saunders Company: West Washington Square
Philadelphia, PA   19105

1 St. Anne's Road
Eastbourne, East Sussex BN21 3UN, England

1 Goldthorne Avenue
Toronto, Ontario M8Z 5T9, Canada

Apartado 26370—Cedro 512
Mexico 4, D.F., Mexico

Rua Coronel Cabrita, 8
Sao Cristovao Caixa Postal 21176
Rio de Janeiro, Brazil

9 Waltham Street
Artarmon, N.S.W. 2064, Australia

Ichibancho, Central Bldg., 22-1 Ichibancho
Chiyoda-Ku, Tokyo 102, Japan

Library of Congress Cataloging in Publication Data

Main entry under title:

The Practice of large animal surgery.

Includes bibliographical references.

1. Veterinary surgery.   I. Jennings, Paul B.   II. Title:
Large animal surgery. [DNLM: 1. Animals, Domestic—
Surgery. SF 911 J54p]

SF911.P7   636.089'7   81–40676
ISBN 0–7216–5118–6 Set   AACR2
ISBN 0–7216–1347–0 Vol I
ISBN 0–7216–1348–9 Vol II

Set ISBN   0-7216-5118-6
Vol I ISBN   0-7216-1347-0
The Practice of Large Animal Surgery   Vol II ISBN   0-7216-1348-9

Last digit is the print number: 9   8   7   6   5   4   3   2   1

CONTRIBUTORS

T. C. Amis, B.V.Sc., Ph.D.
Assistant Professor, School of Veterinary Medicine, University of California, Davis, California; Assistant Professor, Veterinary Medical Teaching Hospital, School of Veterinary Medicine, University of California, Davis, California

Don E. Bailey, D.V.M.
Visiting Professor, College of Veterinary Medicine, Oregon State University, Corvallis, Oregon; Private Practitioner, Rosebud, Oregon

William J. Donawick, D.V.M., Diplomate, American College of Veterinary Surgeons
Mark Whittier and Lila Griswold Allam Professor of Surgery, School of Veterinary Medicine, University of Pennsylvania, Philadelphia, Pennsylvania

G. E. Fackelman, D.V.M., Diplomate, American College of Veterinary Surgeons
Professor of Surgery, School of Veterinary Medicine, Tufts University, North Grafton, Massachusetts; Hospital Director, Tufts University Large Animal Hospital, North Grafton, Massachusetts

James G. Ferguson, B.Sc., D.V.M., M.Sc.
Associate Professor, Department of Veterinary Anesthesiology, Radiology, and Surgery, Western College of Veterinary Medicine, University of Saskatchewan, Saskatoon, Saskatchewan, Canada; Supervisor, Large Animal Surgery, Veterinary Teaching Hospital, Western College of Veterinary Medicine, University of Saskatchewan, Saskatoon, Saskatchewan, Canada

John F. Fessler, D.V.M., M.S., Diplomate, American College of Veterinary Surgeons
Professor of Large Animal Surgery, Department of Large Animal Clinics, School of Veterinary Medicine, Purdue University, West Lafayette, Indiana

**Murray E. Fowler, D.V.M., Diplomate, American College of
Veterinary Internal Medicine**

Professor of Veterinary Medicine, School of Veterinary Medicine,
University of California, Davis, California; Chief of Service, Zoolog-
ical Medicine, Veterinary Medical Teaching Hospital, School of
Veterinary Medicine, University of California, Davis, California

G. Frederick Fregin, V.M.D.

Professor, Virginia-Maryland Regional College of Veterinary Medi-
cine, Virginia Tech, Blacksburg, Virginia; Director, Marion duPont
Scott Equine Medical Center at Morven Park, Leesburg, Virginia;
Associate Director, Veterinary Medical Teaching Hospital, Virginia-
Maryland Regional College of Veterinary Medicine, Virginia Tech,
Blacksburg, Virginia

J. R. Gillespie, D.V.M., Ph.D.

Professor, School of Veterinary Medicine, University of California,
Davis, California; Professor, Veterinary Teaching Hospital, School
of Veterinary Medicine, University of California, Davis, California

**Peter F. Haynes, D.V.M., M.S., Diplomate, American College of
Veterinary Surgeons**

Professor of Veterinary Surgery, School of Veterinary Medicine,
Louisiana State University, Baton Rouge, Louisiana; Section Chief,
Large Animal Clinic, Louisiana State University Veterinary Teach-
ing Hospital and Clinics, Baton Rouge, Louisiana

**R. B. Heath, D.V.M., M.S., Diplomate, American College of Veterinary
Anesthesiologists**

Professor of Clinical Anesthesia, College of Veterinary Medicine,
Colorado State University, Fort Collins, Colorado; Staff Member,
Colorado State University Veterinary Teaching Hospital, Fort Col-
lins, Colorado

John P. Heggers, Ph.D.

Research Associate Professor of Surgery, Plastic and Reconstructive, University of Chicago, Chicago, Illinois; Director, Research
and Laboratories, University of Chicago Burn Center and the Section of Plastic and Reconstructive Surgery, University of Chicago,
Chicago, Illinois

**F. D. Horney, D.V.M., Diplomate, American College.of Veterinary
Surgeons**

Professor of Large Animal Surgery, Ontario Veterinary College,
University of Guelph, Guelph, Ontario, Canada; Large Animal Sur-
geon, Teaching Hospital, Ontario Veterinary College, University of
Guelph, Guelph, Ontario, Canada

**Bruce L. Hull, D.V.M., M.S., Diplomate, American College of
Veterinary Surgeons**

Professor of Surgery, College of Veterinary Medicine, Ohio State
University, Columbus, Ohio

Paul B. Jennings, Jr., V.M.D., M.S., Diplomate, American College of Veterinary Surgeons

Robert F. Jochen, V.M.D.
Manager, Professional Services, Pitman-Moore, Inc., Washington Crossing, New Jersey

Carleton L. Lohse, D.V.M.
Associate Professor, Department of Anatomy, School of Veterinary Medicine, University of California, Davis, California

I. G. Mayhew, B.V.Sc., Ph.D., Diplomate, American College of Veterinary Medicine (Specialties of Internal Medicine and Neurology)
Associate Professor, Department of Medical Sciences, College of Veterinary Medicine, University of Florida, Gainesville, Florida; Chief, Large Animal Medicine Service, Veterinary Medical Teaching Hospital, University of Florida, Gainesville, Florida

C. Wayne McIlwraith, B.V.Sc., M.R.C.V.S., M.S., Ph.D., Diplomate, American College of Veterinary Surgeons
Associate Professor of Surgery, College of Veterinary Medicine and Biomedical Sciences, Colorado State University, Fort Collins, Colorado; Staff Member, Veterinary Teaching Hospital, Colorado State University, Fort Collins, Colorado

J. M. Naylor, B.Sc., B.V.Sc., M.R.C.V.S., Diplomate, American College of Veterinary Internal Medicine
Associate Professor, Department of Veterinary Internal Medicine, Western College of Veterinary Medicine, University of Saskatchewan, Saskatoon, Saskatchewan, Canada; Staff Member, Large Animal Medicine, Veterinary Teaching Hospital, Western College of Veterinary Medicine, University of Saskatchewan, Saskatoon, Saskatchewan, Canada

Victor Perman, D.V.M., Ph.D., Diplomate, American College of Veterinary Pathologists
Professor, Department of Veterinary Pathobiology, College of Veterinary Medicine, University of Minnesota, St. Paul, Minnesota; Clinical Pathologist, University Veterinary Hospital, College of Veterinary Medicine, University of Minnesota, St. Paul, Minnesota

Lionel F. Rubin, V.M.D., Diplomate, American College of Veterinary Ophthalmologists
Professor of Ophthalmology, School of Veterinary Medicine, University of Pennsylvania, Philadelphia, Pennsylvania

G. Michael Shires, B.V.Sc., M.R.C.V.S., Diplomate, American College of Veterinary Surgeons
Professor of Surgery and Hospital Director, Veterinary Teaching Hospital, College of Veterinary Medicine, Oregon State University, Corvallis, Oregon; Head of Surgery, Veterinary Teaching Hospital, Oregon State University, Corvallis, Oregon

Ted S. Stashak, D.V.M., M.S., Diplomate, American College of Veterinary Surgeons

Associate Professor of Surgery, College of Veterinary Medicine, Colorado State University, Fort Collins, Colorado

Michael A. Stedham, D.V.M., M.S., Diplomate, American College of Veterinary Pathologists

Formerly Chief, Division of Veterinary Pathology, Armed Forces Institute of Pathology, Washington, D.C.; Currently, Senior Scientist, Tracor Jitco Inc., Rockville, Maryland

E. P. Steffey, V.M.D., Ph.D., Diplomate, American College of Veterinary Anesthesiologists

Professor and Chairman, Department of Surgery, School of Veterinary Medicine, University of California, Davis, California; Chief, Anesthesia/Critical Patient Care Service, Veterinary Medical Teaching Hospital, School of Veterinary Medicine, University of California, Davis, California

A. Simon Turner, B.V.Sc., M.S., Diplomate, American College of Veterinary Surgeons

Associate Professor of Surgery, College of Veterinary Medicine, Colorado State University, Fort Collins, Colorado

J. T. Vaughan, D.V.M., M.S., Diplomate, American College of Veterinary Surgeons

Dean, School of Veterinary Medicine, Auburn University, Auburn, Alabama; Professor, Department of Large Animal Surgery and Medicine, School of Veterinary Medicine, Auburn University, Auburn, Alabama.

Donald F. Walker, D.V.M.

Professor and Department Head, Department of Large Animal Medicine, School of Veterinary Medicine, Auburn University, Auburn, Alabama

Charles E. Wallace, D.V.M., M.S., Diplomate, American College of Veterinary Surgeons

Associate Professor, Department of Large Animal Medicine, College of Veterinary Medicine, University of Georgia, Athens, Georgia; Staff Member, Veterinary Medical Teaching Hospital, University of Georgia, Athens, Georgia

PREFACE

The idea for this textbook arose from a conversation with a good friend on the future of veterinary medicine. With the diversity of the profession and the changing role of the veterinarian in the 20th century, a sudden change of specialty in mid-career is a distinct possibility. A primarily small animal clinician might be reluctant to perform large animal surgery unless he had a text that provided a brief review of anatomy and physiology plus the most current "how-to-do" techniques available. This text is intended to fill this need. In addition, we hope it is helpful to the large animal practitioner who wants a comprehensive surgical text with useable information.

My thanks to the contributing authors for their support and perseverance during the long days of this project. Mr. Carroll Cann of W. B. Saunders held my hand in the beginning, and Messrs. Ray Kersey and Sandy Reinhardt kept the project (and me) going through to its completion.

My sincerest appreciation to the fine ladies who deciphered my handwriting and edited and typed the manuscripts during this project: Mrs. Nancy G. Whitten of Tacoma, WA, and Ms. Ann Wilkinson of San Francisco, CA.

We welcome the readers' comments and suggestions for improvement of this work.

PAUL B. JENNINGS, JR., V.M.D.

CONTENTS

ix

CHAPTER 1

PREOPERATIVE EVALUATION

THE BOVINE SURGICAL PATIENT

F. D. HORNEY, D.V.M.

GENERAL EXAMINATION

There is a tendency for most young veterinary graduates to latch on to the obvious and disregard the less obvious or that which requires detailed examination. However, the economics of rural practice frequently do necessitate some compromise to avoid time-consuming and therefore expensive examination procedures. A systematic examination of the patient is essential, regardless of the need to first institute emergency treatment in life-threatening situations, e.g., bloat.

Show stock, which have had routine handling, present no difficulty in submitting to the physical examination. Such is not the case with range or feed lot animals, in which varying degrees of fractiousness will be encountered on handling. As a result of the exertion and anxiety of the animal during this period of confinement, plus the association of unpleasant if not painful procedures with previous confinements, the animal is in other than a normal resting state. The animal's vital signs will not fall within normal resting state ranges and

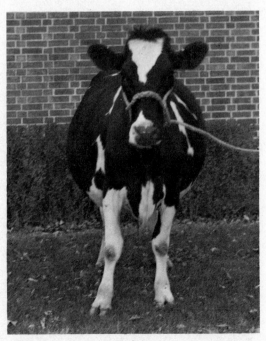

Figure 1–2 Alert response to examiner's approach.

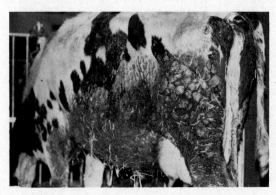

Figure 1–1 Soiling due to environment.

must be assessed in relation to the extent of handling and the individual animal's response to such handling.

General appearance of the animal may be impaired by environment. Extensive soiling, such as may be occasioned in feed lots or with intensive rearing, may make assessment of the integument difficult if not impossible (Fig. 1–1). It is necessary to take this into consideration when such adverse conditions exist. The animal should be alert and inquisitive in response to the approach of the examiner (Fig. 1–2). No discharges or soiling should be present around the eyes, nose, or genitals. Fecal soiling of the perineum and tail may be present.

This cursory examination will provide a starting point for the examinations, and while a thorough history is being obtained the vital signs can be assessed in more detail. Much of the interpretation is subjective and depends on the clinical acuity of the individual. However, recorded measurements will give objective evidence for comparison when repeat examinations are carried out. All systems are assessed on the general inspection, but not to the extent to which they will be assessed on thorough examination of each system individually.

If lying down, an animal will normally stand when approached, getting up on its hind legs first and then up on its front legs. The general examination is continued (after visual assessment) by taking the rectal temperature. In the time required for the temperature to register, the abdominal and chest contours can be visually assessed for symmetry (Fig. 1–3A and B). The character of the pulse can be noted using coccygeal or femoral arteries. The pliability and heat of the skin can be judged by palpating the hips and upper hind limbs. The external genitalia should also be inspected, as should the udder in the female. The thermometer is removed, and the character of the feces on the instrument is observed before reading.

The left side of the animal is then examined. Increased distension or a tucked up appearance, if present, will be obvious from the rear vantage point

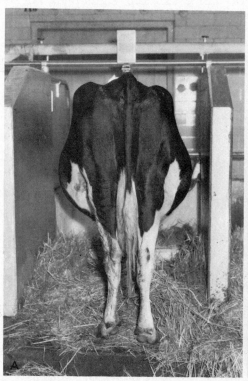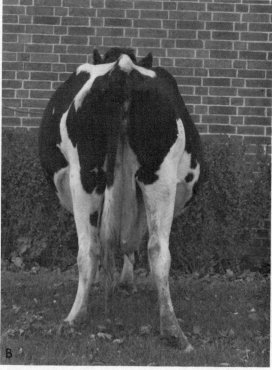

Figure 1–3 *A,* Pear-shaped abdominal contour. *B,* Asymmetrical abdominal contour.

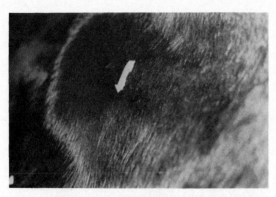

Figure 1-4 Hemolymph nodes.

while taking the temperature. Peripheral lymph nodes in the region may be assessed by palpation. The flank wall movement in response to underlying visceral activity will give some idea of rumen activity, which should also be assessed by palpation and auscultation through the flank wall. Hemolymph nodes may be enlarged in the region of the paralumbar fossa. One or two of these nodes may be present in normal animals (Fig. 1-4).

Auscultation of the left chest should be carried out over the lung field, assessing the character of respiratory sounds and confirming the rate previously recorded while taking the temperature. The rate, rhythm, and quality of the heart rate should also be noted. Lymph nodes in the area, specifically the prescapular nodes, should be palpated. The brisket should be examined for evidence of edema since, in cattle, ventral edema shows early in this site.

On moving from the left flank area, the cervical region should be observed for esophageal movements if the animal is ruminating or swallowing. The jugular furrow should be closely inspected for evidence of jugular engorgement. Laryngeal compression should be used to induce a cough, and regional lymph nodes and the thyroid gland should be checked by palpation.

With the examiner standing in front of the animal, the symmetry of the head should be noted. The alertness of the animal can be assessed by observing eye movement and the erectness of the ears. When concentrating on the eye, the adnexa (lids, conjunctiva, cornea, and sclera) and menace response can be assessed for normality. Mouth breathing should be noted if present, and any submandibular enlargement should be palpated to determine the cause (Fig. 1-5A and B).

With a strong light, visually inspect the oral cavity, remembering that proper protection should be available and used if the animal is from an area where endemic rabies is a problem. Then, move around to the right chest area and repeat the examination as carried out on the left chest.

The general inspection is continued by visually observing the right flank. A more detailed assessment is possible by percussion and auscultation. If there is abdominal distension, fluid, if present, can be detected by a light, sharp tap, which will set the wave in motion. In large animals, an assistant sharply taps the flank wall while the examiner carefully feels or observes the opposite wall for the fluid wave or undulation as the fluid contacts the flank wall. Repeated

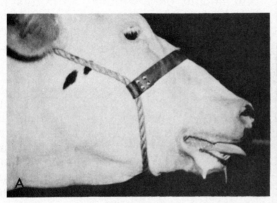
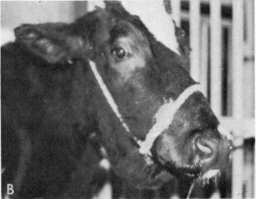

Figure 1-5 *A*, Mouth breathing. *B*, Submandibular edema.

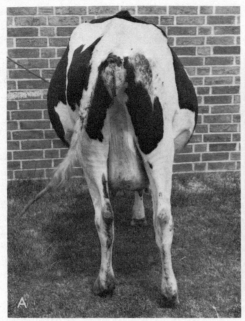
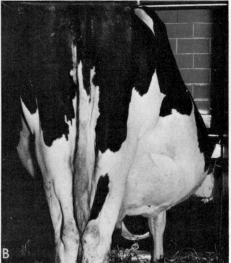

Figure 1–6 *A*, Fluid distension of abdomen. *B*, Abomasal impaction.

deep shaking motions (succussion) will result in splashing sounds if excess fluid is contained in organs such as the abomasum, where a mixture of gas and fluid is present. Percussion and auscultation will establish if abnormal gaseous distension is present. Deep palpation will pick up liver enlargement, since a normal liver should not be palpable behind the rib cage. Gaseous distension of the abomasum can usually be differentiated from that of the cecum by delineating the area of tympany. This will help establish the identity of the involved organs. Impactions are more difficult to identify, especially if they involve the abomasum or omasum (Fig. 1–6A and B).

Having completed the general inspection, one or more systems may be selected for closer examination, and additional diagnostic tests may be required. If all systems appear normal and the animal is a candidate for elective surgery, the surgical problem, e.g., hernia, neoplasm, and so on, will be assessed from a physiological or pathological viewpoint.

RESPIRATORY SYSTEM

Fortunately, the respiratory system is normal in most elective or clinical surgical cases. This should not give one a false sense of security, because iatrogenic mechanical pneumonia may have been caused by the owner administering treatment for suspected digestive disturbances. It is therefore advisable to inquire if anything has been given by mouth, mineral oil being the agent most frequently involved. Aspiration is also possible during the course of investigative tubing when the forestomach is excessively distended; pressure causes regurgitation of rumen contents around the tube, permitting ingesta to lie in the pharynx, where inspiratory efforts may permit aspiration of such contents.

Younger animals may have residual lung pathology from enzootic pneumonia and should be examined with this in mind. Sheep and cattle are also hosts to lungworm infestation, which may decrease the volume of the normal lung. These factors may affect the animal's ability to withstand surgery.

Having assessed the respiratory pattern, the nose should be checked for evidence of discharge. Uniformity of air flow through the nostrils should be determined, and the condition of the nasal mucous membrane should be assessed. Discharges should not be present, and the presence of blood or casts should be considered contraindications to surgery until fully investigated.

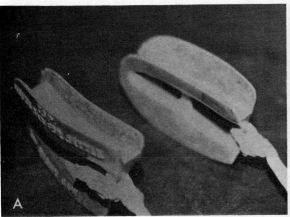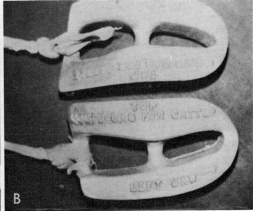

Figure 1–7   A and B, Drinkwater mouth gags.

Space-occupying lesions involving the pharynx or trachea may embarrass respiration; a manual inspection of the pharynx is necessary to avoid missing such a lesion. A Drinkwater mouth gag is an efficient and reliable instrument for use in adult cattle to avoid injury to the examiner (Fig. 1–7).

Lung auscultation requires constant practice and experience. It is also well established that clear-cut differentiation is not usually possible, even though specific adventitious sounds may be justifi-

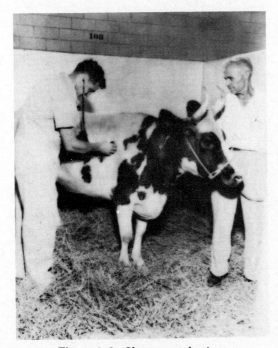

Figure 1–8   Chest auscultation.

ably associated with certain lung changes (Fig. 1–8).

CARDIOVASCULAR SYSTEM

A consistent routine procedure of visual observation and auscultation is, economically, the only possible approach to the examination of the cardiovascular system in most large animal practices. Some veterinarians suggest that an EKG should be an essential part of any cardiovascular examination; however, most agree that only when there is apparent abnormality on auscultation is an electrocardiogram necessary.

Jugular vein engorgement may be observed on initial inspection and should be re-examined in more detail (Fig. 1–9). A slight jugular pulse is normal in most ruminant animals, but a systolic pulse (exaggerated jugular pulse or pulsation during systole) is indicative of an insufficient tricuspid valve, permitting reflux of blood up the jugular vein. Repeated intravenous injections are occasionally given by owners and may result in venous thrombosis, perivascular cellulitis, and/or abscessation along the jugular furrow, all of which will distend the jugular furrow and must be differentiated from cardiovascular disease. Although most abnormalities will be detected by a stethoscopic examination, a hand placed flatly on the chest wall will detect thrills, and, occasionally in some

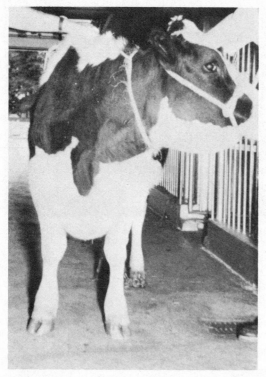

Figure 1-9 Jugular vein engorgement and brisket edema.

animals, a visible cardiac beat can be assessed by the impact the thrill causes against the chest wall. The character of the peripheral pulse will have been recorded or judged on initial inspection. Any abnormality of the heart should be considered a contraindication to surgery until the abnormality is defined and the risk of surgical intervention in the particular case explained to the owner. Abducted elbows may indicate that the animal is suffering from chest pain or may simply reflect an acquired stance owing to pressure against a stanchion bar (Fig. 1-10A and B). Additional information on preoperative evaluation of the cardiovascular system is presented later in this chapter.

DIGESTIVE SYSTEM

Historically, the digestive system in cattle has been the system most frequently requiring surgical intervention. The size and weight of the rumen makes it very difficult to surgically manipulate this organ. A fasting period of 36 to 48

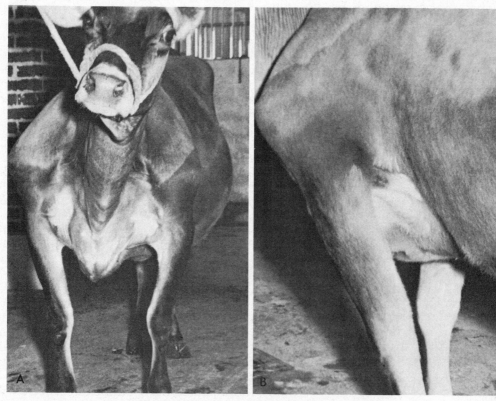

Figure 1-10 *A* and *B*, Abducted elbow stance.

hours reduces the volume of rumen content and thus eliminates a tendency for recumbent cattle to bloat during surgery. Excess bulk of ingesta or gaseous distension complicates the procedure regardless of whether the animal is under general anesthesia or is restrained in recumbency under local or regional anesthesia.

Animals suffering from surgical disorders of the digestive tract vary in appearance from extreme gauntness to gross distension. Varying degrees of weakness and dehydration with acid-base and electrolyte disturbances may also be present, especially when large volumes of fluid are sequestered in a static or obstructed alimentary tract. Dehydration states in abomasal torsion are virtually impossible to correct by fluid therapy prior to surgical intervention. The administration of general anesthetics or sedatives and even physical restraint in such animals may precipitate syncope and subsequent loss of the animal. It is therefore advisable to consider standing surgical intervention in such cases.

As mentioned earlier, there is frequently extensive caking of manure on the ventral abdomen, which defies even the most efficient clippers; such soiling might lead one to decide in favor of a flank approach, even though a more direct ventral approach would otherwise be preferred. The extent of the surgical intervention and the anticipated problems of adequate exposure will have to be weighed carefully against the risks involved in general anesthesia and a more direct ventral approach to the site. This is frequently the major decision to be made on pre-operative evaluation and, in spite of a careful work-up, the wrong approach may be selected.

In electing a flank approach, the procedure may be more involved than would be safe in the standing patient. In such instances, the operation should be stopped and regarded as a diagnostic or confirmatory procedure, since a weaving, treading patient is not conducive to successful surgery. Plans can then be made to complete the surgery through another more favorable approach and with more satisfactory immobilization of the patient (Fig. 1–11).

URINARY SYSTEM

The signs observed in urinary tract disturbances may mimic or at least suggest a digestive disturbance. Substantial renal damage may occur without pain; however, pyelonephritis in dairy cows may cause significant clinical manifestations of pain, including violent kicking and treading with occasionally violent thrashing. The animal may fall and stand, only to fall again. Treading from one hind foot to the other or kicking with the hind feet is more commonly observed than is violent thrashing in recumbency. Tail switching and pulsing of the urethra, owing to attempts to urinate, are fairly consistent in urethral obstruction due to calculi. Examination of the penis is hampered in young stock by the inability to expose the penis owing to the immature state of separation of penis and sheath.

Neonates suffering from omphalophlebitis may have infection or cystic distension of the urachus, causing persistent straining on urination. Usually there is evidence of a pervious urachus with urine dripping from the umbilicus when the animal strains.

Urine may be collected by manually stimulating the perineal region or by catheterization in the female. Catheterization is not possible in the immature steer or bull, and only after relaxing the penis by sedating the animal or by pu-

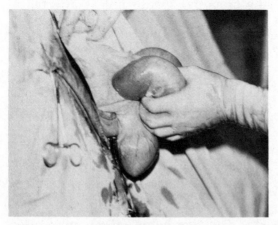

Figure 1–11 Intussusception of the jejunum. Surgery best performed with the animal recumbent.

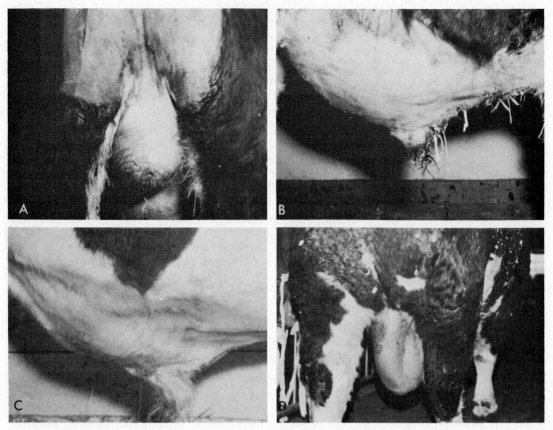

Figure 1–12 *A* and *B*, Urethral rupture. *C*, Hematoma of the penis. *D*, Indirect hernia.

dendal nerve block is it possible to catheterize mature male subjects.

Abnormal swellings in the region of the sheath orifice, sheath, and base of the scrotum must be assessed to differentiate such conditions as urethral rupture, hematoma of the penis, abscessation, and hernia (Fig. 1–12A, B, C, and D).

REPRODUCTIVE SYSTEM

In animal production, fertility and live vigorous progeny are necessary for economic survival. It is therefore important to assess the animal's latent ability to fulfill this function and to determine if congenital defects and/or hereditary traits exist that detract from the animal's reproductive value.

In the male, visual assessment of the scrotum and lower abdominal contour is an important part of the examination.

Although palpation of the scrotum is possible when the temperature is taken in the general inspection, more detailed palpation should be conducted during assessment of the reproductive system. The penis is normally contained within the preputial sheath unless affected by lesions such as penile fibropapillomata, in which case the weight of the lesion causes dropping and exposure of the penis. Immature bull calves have a natural adhesion between the penis and sheath, which makes it impossible to expose the penis for the first six to nine months of life, as indicated under the general examination. In beef bulls of Brahma or zebu crosses, preputial tissue may be exposed, and, therefore, these breeds are predisposed to balanitis when environmental factors permit abrasions. Viral infections, such as infectious bovine rhinotracheitis (IBR), may affect the genital mucosa.

Internal examination in mature males

should include palpation of the prostate, the seminal vesicles, and the ampulla. Seminal vesiculitis, if bilateral, may be difficult to identify since there is not a normal with which to compare the diseased gland. Congenital or acquired penile deviations may be present, but these would not be observed unless the animal was permitted to mount or was stimulated with the electroejaculator.

In the female, an internal examination will be required to adequately assess the ovaries, uterus, and cervix. If the animal was born twin to a bull calf (freemartin), the earlier development of the male gonads leads to suppression of the development of female genital organs, resulting in varying degrees of hypoplasia of the internal genitals (arrested development of müllerian ducts). Internal examination to specifically assess pregnancy is commonly carried out. It is the responsibility of the veterinarian to take precautions against spreading possible infection and/or damaging the rectal mucosa during such examinations.

INTEGUMENTARY SYSTEM

This outer covering with its hair coat is frequently an indication of the general health of the animal. The animal's environment, as indicated in general inspection, may obscure this organ because manure may be caked over a good portion of the body. Diseases of the skin are relatively common and may be generalized or localized, infectious, nutritional, hereditary, or allergic. Emphysema of the subcutaneous tissue is occasionally observed, and, while its origin may be obscure, it may simply be the result of a relatively innocuous hypodermic injection with improper technique or may follow emergency trocarization of the rumen.

The mucocutaneous junctions, skin folds, and contact surfaces, such as axilla and thigh, should be examined carefully for abnormal skin texture and/or lesions. Although many of the skin lesions would in no way interfere with surgical procedures, some are definitely public health hazards in that they are occasionally transmitted to the individuals handling the animal.

MUSCULOSKELETAL SYSTEM

Most veterinary students tend to link lameness examination with horses and not cattle. However, a definitive diagnosis of lameness is equally important in cattle in the pre-operative work-up to avoid attaching blame to a specific lesion, such as a small interdigital fibroma, when another cause of lameness is present. Subtle changes in gait are more difficult to detect in this species because many animals object to being led and therefore will have to be observed moving freely. A confined space should be available to avoid having the animal get too distant from the observer. A close-clipped paddock or cement-surfaced paddock also helps to avoid high grass obscuring lesions and/or limb placement that might provide clues to diagnosis. Good conformation and healthy feet are important to carry the animal's weight, particularly in beef breeds. The upright stance that appears to satisfy breeders tends to subject the limb to excessive concussion, with resulting disastrous wear and tear on joints and joint attachments.

Musculoskeletal trauma must be considered in downer animals (Fig. 1–13),

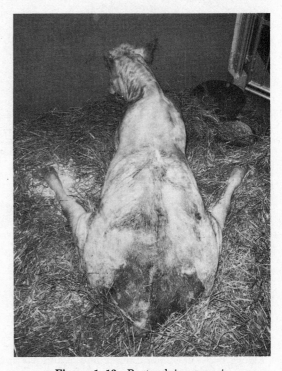

Figure 1–13 Post-calving paresis.

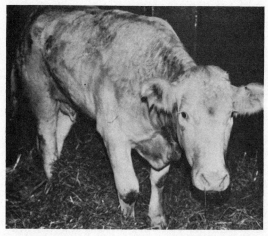

Figure 1–14 Same cow after a prolonged period of recumbency.

particularly in the upper hind limb where joint, nerve, or muscle damage may complicate metabolic disease and may cause animals to remain recumbent even after the metabolic disorder is corrected (Fig. 1–14). Mixed neuromuscular lesions are also a significant factor in ataxia and

paresis. These may be iatrogenic (traction delivery of the fetus), congenital (arthrogryposis), and/or hereditary (spastic paresis) in origin (Fig. 1–15A, B, C, and D).

NERVOUS SYSTEM

Organic disease, functional disturbances, and reflex stimulation account for most of the clinical manifestations of abnormal nervous system performance. There are also many metabolic diseases that present with signs of nervous system involvement. Having carried out a general inspection that has made possible an overall assessment of the various systems, the examiner should note variations from normal that may indicate central or peripheral nerve involvement. These may be in conjunction with other systems, such as drooling of saliva due to inability to swallow in listeriosis (Fig. 1–16), hyperesthesia due to meningitis in the septicemias of colibacillosis, locomotor disturbances in alert and normal-

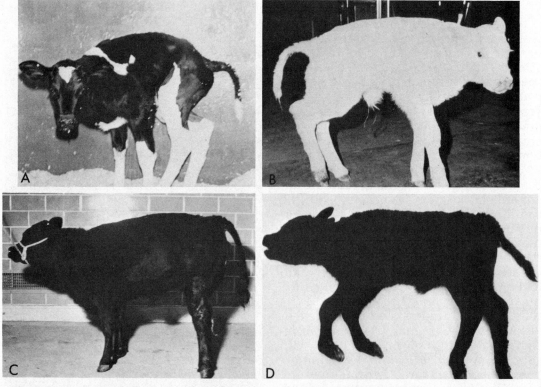

Figure 1–15 *A,* Femoral nerve and quadriceps muscle injury. *B,* Traction delivery injury. *C,* Spastic paresis. *D,* Arthrogryposis.

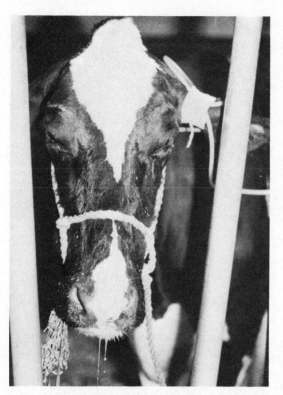

Figure 1–16 Dysphagia in listeriosis.

eating animals as seen in cerebellar hypoplasia. A detailed neurological examination is indicated whenever such unexplained signs present themselves on initial inspection. See Chapter 4 for additional information.

LYMPHATIC SYSTEM

The peripheral and visceral lymphatics vary in size but may generally be classed as larger in young animals than in mature subjects. An assessment of the peripheral nodes is important in a clinical examination and should be noted on initial inspection. Even when peripheral nodes appear to be within the normal size range, there may be sufficient swelling of retropharyngeal lymph nodes to interfere with swallowing. Enlarged mediastinal lymph nodes may interfere with normal eructation in the ruminant, resulting in rumen bloat. In any pathological process, regional lymph node reaction is observed and may in fact provide valuable information as to the cause of the problem.

OCULAR SYSTEM

Unless specific abnormalities or lesions are observed, a clear, bright, alert eye without evidence of discharge and a normal menace reflex should satisfy the examiner that the eye is relatively normal. Retraction or prominence of the globe may suggest dehydration or post-orbital pressure, respectively (Fig. 1–17A and B). There is, however, a wide variation of normal, and it is wise not to dwell on subtle differences, especially on initial examination of the surgical patient. See Chapter 20 for additional information.

SUMMARY OF PREOPERATIVE EVALUATION

A general inspection will have determined the current status of the patient and will therefore have provided a starting point from which to commence continuous care of the patient through the surgical intervention. Elective procedures will be the ones most commonly performed owing to the economics of food animal production. Farm surgery does not permit elaborate or sophisticated intensive care of the patient. Since, in most of these elective surgical cases, the patient is young and healthy, there will be little need for a vigorous preoperative treatment regimen. However, this should not lull one into a false sense of security, because the low risk patient is occasionally the one that ends up in difficulty or is actually lost. The owner of the animal should be informed of the risks attendant to the particular surgery contemplated for his animal. This is more easily done by the experienced practitioner than by the new graduate. Insurance companies may require an extra premium to continue the protection on the animal through the elective surgical procedure. The insurance company, therefore, should be notified before performing surgery to avoid having an insurance claim rejected.

There is nothing so disconcerting as to begin a surgical procedure and then realize that an essential piece of equipment is missing or that the restraint and

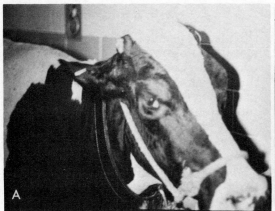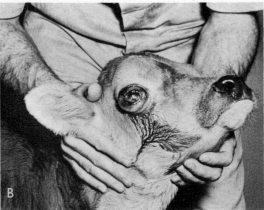

Figure 1–17 *A*, Severe dehydration. *B*, Post-orbital pressure.

facilities are less than optimal. Much of this can be avoided by careful planning, but situations will develop that try the patience of even well-seasoned practitioners. There is no point in operating if the patient is not likely to withstand the surgical stress. Such poor risk cases are frequently a complete write-off insofar as the owner is concerned. Veterinarians hope to avoid missing a surgical diagnosis, since extensive treatment may be given before surgery is deemed necessary. This places the owner in an unfavorable position because his investment in the animal may be greater than the future value he may obtain from the animal. Since many of these cases are uneconomical, the owner must be fully informed and must make the choice as to whether he wants to continue having the case treated.

Although most elective cases require little in the way of ancillary tests, base line data are essential for continuing care of the animal. The results of such tests should be on hand at the time the elective surgical procedure is carried out, and properly labeled radiographs should be available to avoid errors such as selecting the wrong limb. The minimum data base should include a white count, a packed cell volume (PCV), total solids, and a blood urea nitrogen (BUN) (see Chapter 3).

Although there are relatively few problems arising in bovine practice caused by drug incompatibility in the surgical patient, it is still advisable to have a thorough medical history on the animal insofar as this can be obtained from the owner or agent. If the animal is to be restrained in lateral or dorsal recumbency or is to be given a general anesthetic, it is best to avoid adding to the bulk of the digestive system. Attempt to decrease this bulk by keeping the animal off feed for a period of 24 to 36 hours prior to surgery. Water should be limited in the 12 hours immediately preceding the surgical intervention. In animals that are to be anesthetized or restrained in recumbency, particular attention should be paid to the amount of fluid sequestered in the abomasum in the case of torsion and/or volvulus because of the marked metabolic alkalosis that is usually present with such clinical cases. Many animals with simple left abomasal displacement may show cardiac irregularities and would respond adversely to restraint in recumbency. These cases should be handled by performing surgery under regional anesthesia with the animal standing and only after outlining the risks to the owner.

In conclusion, there is nothing more satisfying than to have accurately assessed the status of the animal and performed the proper surgical procedure that will restore the animal to a healthy and normal state. If the response is less than optimal, as long as the owner has been fully informed prior to the surgery, you will usually have a satisfied client.

THE EQUINE SURGICAL PATIENT

C. Wayne McIlwraith; B.V.Sc., M.R.C.V.S., M.S., Ph.D.

Preoperative evaluation and preparation of the patient are necessary to ensure the best possible safety index for a given procedure. Preoperative care is designed both to ensure that an elective patient is in good systemic condition for surgery and to assess the specific supportive needs of the compromised patient.

This statement should be qualified, however, because no given protocol guarantees that problems will not develop during or after surgery. Subjective assessments have to be made even when quantitative laboratory data are available. Although there is uniform agreement that a thorough physical examination is essential, there is tremendous variation among surgeons as to what constitutes a routine preoperative laboratory screen, particularly with regard to the elective patient. Is a complete blood count (CBC) adequate or should a blood chemistry profile also be run? If it is a question of economics should the choice of a laboratory test vary according to the value of the patient? In terms of potential litigation, what constitutes a normal preoperative laboratory profile has not been defined, and test cases are lacking. An individual surgeon has to reach his own decision on what should be standard for an elective patient. The choice always involves compromise, and occasionally this compromise may be challenged when a problem develops that could have been predicted by a test that was not part of the routine profile. In these cases the surgeon should re-assess his profile in terms of the probability or frequency with which such a problem might recur. For consistency, particularly in a large hospital, there has to be a protocol that is based on careful thought and experience; it should not be dictated by isolated disasters. It is better to have a protocol that everybody agrees on and can live with so that the routine is not ignored; a controversial or excessive protocol can breed contempt and disregard, which can only be corrected by a catastrophe.

DIAGNOSIS OF THE SURGICAL PROBLEM

The diagnosis of individual surgical problems is discussed elsewhere in this text and does not need review here. However, it is mentioned here because accurate diagnosis and the formulation of a correct treatment plan are integral parts of the preoperative assessment. If there is any doubt about the surgical diagnosis, a second opinion should be sought. Veterinarians should be selective in their use of surgery as a diagnostic procedure. Although exploratory laparotomy is a justified and necessary surgical procedure, the author is concerned about the number of medial patellar desmotomies, for instance, that are performed on horses with undefined hind limb lameness and prior to the administration of any nerve blocks to eliminate other problems in the differential diagnosis.

Once a definitive diagnosis is made, other problems should be ruled out. This is discussed under physical examination.

REASONS FOR PREOPERATIVE EVALUATION

As mentioned before, a preoperative evaluation is needed both to ensure normalcy in the elective patient and to recognize specific needs in the nonelective patient. Guidelines for the latter case are well established, and the surgeon should

13

not feel restrained in the tests he runs. However, guidelines for the elective patient are not well defined. Although it is possible to justify almost anything, the surgeon must reach a balance between the ideal, the practical, and the economical.

In an elective patient, thorough preoperative examination is needed to ensure that the patient is free of other systemic disease and to rule out anemia, dehydration, or cardiovascular problems; all these factors are relevant to the assessment of the anesthetic risk. The evaluation is also necessary to assess the potential for postsurgical problems and to predict wound healing. Factors of importance here include obesity, debilitation, parasitism, anemia, hypoproteinemia, and recumbency. Attention must also be paid to the local wound and to the presence and degree of phlegmon or cellulitis, findings that may dictate delay of surgery and initiation of treatment measures to improve the condition of the tissues prior to surgery.

If there are compromising problems, preoperative treatment and/or delay of surgery may be appropriate. In some instances of elective surgery, the need may not justify the risk. If surgery is going to be performed on a compromised patient, the owner should be fully informed of the situation. However, it is to be noted that this measure does not provide insurance and some owners have very short memories when a new problem develops. The surgeon should always remember that as soon as his scalpel touches an animal he seems to inherit responsibility for all of the patient's problems past, present, and future. Some of this must be accepted, but clinicians can help the situation with good communication with both clients and (in many cases) referring veterinarians. It should also be noted that the information communicated to the owner should be accurate; exaggerating the potential risk to protect oneself in case of a problem is unprofessional and unethical.

In the emergency patient or the patient in which surgery is essential, whether surgery is justifiable or safe is not the point in question. In these instances, the preoperative evaluation is designed to ensure the safest possible passage through anesthesia and surgery and to minimize postoperative problems. If possible, these compromises are minimized as much as possible prior to surgery.

The preoperative evaluation is also relevant to the formulation of a surgical plan. There may be specific requirements for anesthesia or surgical instrumentation. The nature of the problem may dictate whether the staff surgeon or the surgery resident acts as primary surgeon.

Good preoperative evaluation and assessment of the operative risk constitute central features of surgical judgment, that quality that is so necessary in a competent surgeon.

HISTORY

A complete history and physical examination are the central parts of the preoperative examination for *all* surgical patients. In many practice situations this may constitute the entire evaluation but it should never be compromised.

Age of the animal is significant. A young healthy foal has an advantage in terms of wound healing and bone remodeling following orthopedic surgery, for instance. On the other hand, immaturity of the hepatic microsomal system of foals decreases the anesthetic tolerance. Immunodeficiencies are also potential problems, and infectious diseases and parasitism are more likely to be present. Older horses may require more specific attention to liver and kidney function, but geriatric problems are not routinely present in the horse in the same fashion as in the dog.

Specific questions should include the feeding program, vaccination history, and any previous illnesses including coughing, nasal discharge, fever, and colic. The worming program should be noted as well as fecal consistency. Knowledge of the previous use of any medications is also important, particularly phenylbutazone, corticosteroids, and antibiotics. The deleterious side effects of phenylbutazone have been variously underestimated and exaggerated. In ponies, phenylbutazone can readily produce toxic effects characterized by a protein-losing gastroenteropathy (Snow et al. 1981). Marked losses can occur in the absence of ulceration, but massive ulceration is common and may cause fatalities. Horses seem relatively resistant to toxicity at therapeutic doses (Snow et al. 1981), but nephritis is being recognized at necropsy in horses that received significant amounts of phenylbutazone.

In horses presented for joint surgery it is important to know if corticosteroids have been injected into the joint previously. Poor communication between owners and trainers and ownership changes often make this assessment difficult. To safeguard against potential problems with infection or healing, joint surgery should not be performed within two months of injection. If the history is uncertain, a delay of surgery of at least two months is recommended until the history is certain. Previous antibiotic administration is not detrimental per se but can potentially contribute to induction of salmonellosis or other nosocomial infections in the patient undergoing major surgery.

Questioning of the feeding program is important to assess the amount of grain and concentrate the horse has been given. High grain intake is generally considered to potentially increase the risk of postanesthetic rhabdomyolysis. Although there may be no modification of the anesthetic regimen, it may dictate a change in the clinician's assessment of the operative risk. (If the author talks to owners prior to their bringing in horses for elective surgery, he requests decreasing or eliminating the grain ration for two weeks prior to surgery.) Similarly, a heavy, overweight (often related to a previous condition) horse or a horse with a previous history of rhabdomyolysis may dictate a change in the assessment of the surgical risk and/or the surgical plan.

The veterinarian also needs to know the insurance status of the horse. If the horse is insured, permission from the insurance company to operate is needed.

PHYSICAL EXAMINATION

A complete physical examination is a minimum requirement for any animal undergoing general anesthesia. An organized sequence to ensure assessment of all systems is assumed. Examination of the cardiovascular system is discussed in detail elsewhere. Elevated temperature and respiratory disease in young animals probably constitute the most common abnormalities found in horses presented as "normal" patients. If icterus is present, it must be assessed in relation to the animal's current feed consumption. Adjunctive tests, including CBC, chest radiographs, transtracheal washes, and immunocompetence tests, may be indicated before a decision to perform surgery is made. Elective surgery should be delayed on any animal that is suspected of having or developing systemic illness.

Other special diagnostic procedures, such as endoscopic examination and abdominal paracentesis, are used if there is a specific indication. A complete musculoskeletal examination is indicated prior to limb surgery to eliminate any other conditions that may alter the prognosis or even negate the usefulness of surgery. Rectal examination is useful in the preoperative assessment of cryptorchids to distinguish between abdominal and inguinal cryptorchids preoperatively (when the testes cannot be detected on external palpation). This distinction is based on palpation of the vas deferens passing through the vaginal ring, not on palpation of the testes (Adams 1964). Although useful, it is not essential to the preoperative plan, and if the clinician is inexperienced with the technique the horse is better left without the rectal examination. However, rectal examination is an important technique in the diagnosis of abdominal conditions (see Chapter 15).

LABORATORY TESTS

This is the most variable area in preoperative evaluation and necessarily so. What tests are run will depend on the condition the animal has. What tests are run on a "normal" elective patient is the most difficult area to define. The generalizations and guidelines that follow are the current opinions of the author. (The author does not guarantee to retain all of these as veterinarians continually learn and future catastrophes will probably dictate some changes.)

The use of minimal clinicopathological screening can be justified if a thorough history taking and physical examination are performed and no abnormalities are found. Although negligence is unacceptable, the author is equally skeptical of the routine running of panels of multiple tests in teaching institutions without even discussing with students any specific indications. Nowadays, a panel of 12 or more blood chemistry tests usually costs less than three to four individual bench tests, but some selectivity should be retained, at least at a theoretical level.

For short anesthetic or surgical outpatient procedures on healthy animals, such as normal castration or general anesthesia for pelvic radiographs, a packed cell volume (PCV) and total protein (TP) are considered sufficient. A PCV of less than 30 is viewed with concern and dictates at least adjunctive testing (CBC, fecal examination for parasites) to evaluate possible causes. Total protein is useful as a screen to evaluate the functional state of the liver, the nutritional state of the patient, and hydration in the presence of anemia (Fessler, 1975). Values of less than 5.5 g/dl or greater than 8 g/dl justify further investigation.

For elective surgery, the horse is hospitalized the night before surgery, and a CBC is performed. A PCV of less than 30, a TP of less than 5.5 mg/dl, or abnormalities in the leukogram are indications for further examination and possible postponement or cancellation of surgery. Variations in the CBC in association with travel, state of training, breed of horse, excitement, and previous drug therapy are acknowledged and allowances or repeat testing may be necessary, but as a primary screen the CBC is considered most useful. Serum enzymes (CPK and SGOT) should be evaluated if rhabdomyolysis is considered to be a potential problem. However, if these tests are used, flexibility in interpretation is necessary to allow for the increases that will develop in association with long-distance travel and other trauma including intramuscular injections. Liver specific enzyme tests, sorbital dehydrogenase and gamma-glutamyl transferase (SDH and GGT), are not routinely performed unless there are specific indications in the history or clinical examination. The significance of any degree of hepatitis in a horse undergoing general anesthesia has been emphasized (Moore et al. 1976). Most people agree that a BUN assay should be routinely performed in the candidate for major surgery. There are also valid arguments for measurement of urine specific gravity. The author has noted some kidney problems that were not apparent on initial clinical examination. Urinalysis is not generally indicated.

Electrolyte or blood gas evaluations are not considered necessary in "normal" horses if their hydration is apparently normal. Specific bleeding tests are not routinely performed unless there is suggestion of liver compromise. Bleeding disorders in the horse are very rare, but with the recent use of Panwarfarin in the treatment of navicular disease, clinicians need to be more aware of such conditions.

The screening of foals under two months of age for adequate immunoglobulin levels by the zinc sulfate turbidity test or direct immunoglobulin measurement by single radial immunodiffusion (McGuire, Poppie, and Banks 1975) is indicated, particularly if infectious disease is already present.

Nonelective and emergency surgeries require additional tests in the preoperative evaluation. The best example is the acute abdominal patient in which assessment of acid-base status in addition to hydration is important. The evaluation of these patients is discussed elsewhere. Electrolytes are more important postoperatively and are only assessed preoperatively in a few situations.

One other need for the collection of preoperative laboratory data that should be noted is to have a baseline from which to evaluate changes that may develop postoperatively.

TIMING OF SURGERY

With the exception of simple procedures such as castration, which is performed on an outpatient basis, elective surgery patients should be hospitalized the day prior to surgery. This allows the horse to become accustomed to the hospital environment and to recover from any effects incurred with long-distance travel. At the same time, long periods of hospitalization prior to surgery are inappropriate. Excessive hospitalization increases the risk of the horse acquiring nosocomial infection.

Acute abdominal patients are emergency surgeries and should be operated on as soon as they are stabilized systemically. Fractures are nonelective surgeries, but they are not necessarily emergencies. If the fracture can be immobilized sufficiently by external fixation, surgery does not have to be performed in the middle of the night. Surgery the following day when the horse has recovered somewhat from the trailer ride, a full team is on hand, and all instrumentation is available has many advantages. Some fractures, because of their locations, demand immediate attempts at internal fixation. The practice of purposefully delaying surgery and internal fixation on compound fractures to allow soft tissue "clean up" as is practiced in man is of questionable value in the horse. The degree of immobilization achieved with a cast is only relative even with a distal fracture; further soft tissue damage rather than improvement can be anticipated in many cases.

PATIENT PREPARATION

Nonemergency surgical patients should be held off feed; 12 hours is usually sufficient. In some special instances (nonemergency elective exploratory laparotomy) longer periods of feed deprivation are indicated to achieve emptying of the colon. However, routinely holding patients off feed for long periods is contraindicated because it constitutes another stress to the animal. Water is not withheld.

Depending on the condition and the preoperative evaluation, perioperative antibiotics may be used. This decision should be made at this stage so that administration is commenced one to six hours prior to surgery (Hurley, Howard, and Hahn 1979). Other medications may also be indicated preoperatively, such as phenylbutazone before surgery on the upper respiratory tract.

Overnight preparation of the surgical site is commonly performed. If possible, the surgical area should be clipped to minimize anesthetic time. With orthopedic surgery, subsequent scrubbing of the area with povidone-iodine (Betadine) and sterile bandaging of the limb are good practices as long as no nicks are made in the skin. The nicks may become pustules by the time surgery is performed. For this reason, shaving of the surgical site is not appropriate at this stage, and clipping and sterile preparation are only of benefit if there is no trauma to the skin. Alternatively, the procedures can be performed on the standing animal immediately prior to anesthetic induction.

Patients should be groomed (washed if necessary) to eliminate grass contamination and debris, the hooves cleaned out, and the mouth flushed prior to anesthesia. Patient preparation beyond this is covered in other areas of the text.

REFERENCES

Adams, O. R.: An improved method of diagnosis and castration of cryptorchid horses. J.A.V.M.A. 145:439, 1964.

Fessler, J. F.: Pre-surgical evaluation of the large animal patient—including the rationale for specific laboratory tests. Arch. A.C.V.S. 4:34, 1975.

Hurley, D. L., Howard, P., Hahn, H. H.: Perioperative prophylactic antibiotics in abdominal surgery. Surg. Clin. North Am. 59:919, 1979.

McGuire, T. C., Poppie, M. J., and Banks, K. L.: Hypogammaglobulinemia predisposing to infections in foals. J.A.V.M.A. 166:71, 1975.

Moore, J. N., Traver, D. S., and Coffman, J. R.: Large bowel obstruction and chronic active hepatitis in a horse. VM/SAC 71:1457, 1976.

Snow, D. H., Douglas, T. A., Thompson, H., Parkins, J. J., and Holmes, P. H.: Phenylbutazone toxicosis in equidae: A biochemical and pathophysiologic study. Am. J. Vet. Res. 42:1754, 1981.

PORCINE PREOPERATIVE EVALUATION

Bruce L. Hull, D.V.M., M.S.

Preoperative evaluation in the swine is probably more difficult to accomplish than in other species. Because of this difficulty, a complete history is important. This history should concern not only the individual animal involved but any herd history that could have a bearing on the case. Because general anesthesia may be used in some porcine surgical procedures, history of any respiratory problems or indications of porcine stress syndrome are very important. Halothane anesthesia accentuates signs of porcine stress syndrome and, therefore, should be used only after warning the owner, especially in herds where porcine stress syndrome is a known problem.

Handling pigs tends to cause undue excitement in these animals; therefore, observation from a distance will often reveal more than an evaluation with a stethoscope. One should observe respirations, hair coat, general appearance, and ability to move. After this observation one should take the patient's temperature.

If the surgery is an elective procedure, feed should be withheld for 24 hours before administering general anesthesia.

THE SHEEP AND GOAT

Don E. Bailey, D.V.M.

After a diagnosis is made, a preoperative examination of the animal is necessary. Elective surgery, such as castration and dehorning, does not require as complete an examination as does emergency surgery. The risk of surgery is evaluated on an economic scale in many cases, although some situations involve very valuable animals.

Before the preoperative examination is made, a history of the animal should be completed. The history should include vaccinations and wormings, the body condition, the feeding program, health of the other animals in the herd, and so on. A heavily parasitized, undernourished sheep or goat is a poor surgical risk.

After the history is reviewed, the physical examination of the patient should be completed. This starts with a recording of body temperature and pulse and respiration rates. Auscultation of the heart and lungs is also important. Observation of the lower conjunctiva of the eye will disclose anemia, if present. A fecal examination should be made if anemia is indicated. The wool and hair coat condition is an indicator of external parasites and general health. Foot diseases should be sought in cases of lameness. Any ocular or nasal discharge should be noted. The age of the animal should be recorded; it influences the economic decision whether surgery will be performed. If age is not known, the incisor teeth can give an estimate of age. A preoperative physical examination should also determine if the animal is anorectic. The degree of distension of the rumen is important to consider before giving anesthesia. The degree, if any, of dehydration of the animal is important. The more complicated the surgery contemplated, the more important the preoperative physical examination.

The cost of the operative procedure is sometimes the major deciding factor. After the veterinarian makes a diagnosis and performs a physical examination, the owner will make the decision whether to perform the surgery. This decision is based on the cost and the anticipated return of value.

THE CARDIOVASCULAR SYSTEM OF THE LARGE ANIMAL SURGICAL PATIENT

G. Frederick Fregin, V.M.D.

Evaluation of specific body systems does not exclude the necessity of a complete physical examination. The initial observations are made, when possible, with the animal at rest in a quiet environment, since exertion and anxiety alter most clinical measurements. The values obtained must be assessed in light of the animal's surgical problem, response to handling or shipping, and any emergency treatment that may have been instituted.

Anesthetic management of large animals with cardiopulmonary disease requires an understanding of respiratory and cardiovascular physiology and the pathophysiology of the condition for which they have been presented, and monitoring and support of vital functions. Particular attention should be paid to conditions that compromise oxygen delivery to tissue. Cardiovascular disorders, anemia, sepsis, toxemia, metabolic abnormalities, and hyper- or hypothermia must be corrected to maintain normal arterial blood O_2 and CO_2 (Himes et al. 1967; Short, Cuneio, and Cupp 1971; Adams, Teske, and Mercer 1976). Previous administration of medications such as organophosphate deworming preparations, phenothiazine-type drugs, aminoglycoside antibiotics, recent general anesthesia, and long-term systemic corticosteroids may influence the approach to preanesthetic preparation and supportive therapy (antibiotics, intravenous fluids and electrolytes, and so on) necessary to improve or stabilize the animal's physical status.

HISTORY

A thorough and comprehensive history should be obtained, although this often constitutes a challenge as great as diagnosing the abnormality with which the animal has been presented. Dyspnea on exertion, cough, epistaxis, incoordination, collapse, ventral pitting edema, venous distension, and cardiac murmurs or arrhythmias are common presenting signs in animals with primary or secondary cardiovascular abnormalities. The association of these findings with a history of recent systemic illness or recurrent illness and chronic weight loss is not uncommon (Fregin 1982; Raphel and Fregin 1980).

A major objective in the history taking should be to assess the degree and time of occurrence of the limitation to exercise tolerance and the onset of other clinical signs. This information is vital to the diagnosis, the approach to surgical and medical care, and the prognosis for recovery.

INSPECTION

Examination of the visible mucous membranes for capillary refill time and color and the peripheral veins for the amount of distension provides important information in assessing the functional status of the cardiovascular system. The level of filling of the jugular veins and their patency should also be determined. The jugular venous pulsations should be symmetrical and visible up to a height of approximately 10 cm above the level of the shoulder (i.e., right atrium). Special attention must be paid to the presence or absence of subcutaneous pitting edema along the ventral abdomen and sternum, below the ramus of the mandible, and over the pectoral muscles (brisket), since this is one of the earliest signs of right-sided congestive heart failure. Edema of the limbs may be a less reliable sign in the horse (i.e., "stocking up"), although it is frequently present in severe cardiac decompensation.

PALPATION

Palpation should be used to locate the position of the apex beat and the point of maximum intensity of cardiac murmurs (i.e., thrill). Displacement of the cardiac impulse and its intensity should also be noted. The cardiac impulse is usually most intense over the fourth and fifth left intercostal spaces at the level of the costochondral junction. The impulse may sometimes be felt to a lesser degree on the right side in the third and fourth intercostal spaces slightly above the sternal border. Displacement of the cardiac impulse has been noted in large animals with marked ascites, excessive tympany, hydrops amnii, twin pregnancy, and large abscesses or tumors within the thoracic cavity. The intensity of the cardiac impulse is diminished by heavy muscling, obesity, pleural or pericardial effusion, subcutaneous edema, and pulmonary emphysema. The strength of the impulse may be increased when the heart rate is elevated by excitement, exercise, or febrile diseases and with some cardiac arrhythmias.

A palpable thrill is always associated with a heart murmur and should not be confused with the coarse vibrations of the thoracic wall that may sometimes be produced by the heart sounds and by vigorous cardiac activity. A thrill usually indicates heart disease and is most reliable when accompanied by a heart murmur of grade 3 or greater. Thrills may be palpated over arteriovenous fistulas and during rectal examination over aneurysms (i.e., cranial mesenteric artery). Animals with pleuritis or pericarditis may show evidence of pain or increased sensitivity when pressure is applied over the third to fifth intercostal spaces in the lower third of the thorax.

PERCUSSION

Percussion of the thorax should follow a systematic pattern and is used to establish the area of cardiac dullness and the borders of the lung field. The use of a plexor and pleximeter or the fingers should be practiced until a satisfactory ability to percuss accurately has been developed. Thoracic radiographs may serve to verify the clinical findings; however, in the field, radiographic equipment is often not suitable for use on large domestic animals. Percussion should allow detection of gross changes in cardiac size, evidence of pleural or pericardial effusion, large thoracic masses, and changes in the size or density of the lung field.

In cattle, the foreleg should be moved forward to expose the area to be examined, since more than half of the heart lies beneath the triceps muscle. The normal area of cardiac dullness in the bovine extends from the caudal border of the second rib to the anterior edge of the sixth rib. The caudal border of the heart is separated from the thoracic wall by the thin ventral portion of the cardiac lung lobe; thus, percussion over this site elicits only relatively dull sounds. The area of cardiac dullness is approximately the size of the palm of the hand on the left side of the thorax in normal adult cattle, whereas on the right side it is smaller (Fig. 1–18) (Raphel and Fregin 1980).

In horses, the normal area of cardiac dullness is bounded over the left thoracic wall by the sternum ventrally and the caudal reflection of the triceps muscle craniad (third left intercostal space). The

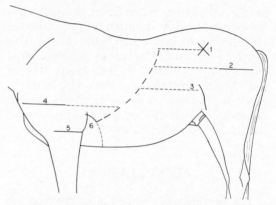

Figure 1–19 Normal equine lung fields and area of cardiac dullness as determined by percussion. 1 = tuber coxae (level of seventeenth rib), 2 = tuber ischii (level of fifteenth rib), 3 = middle of thorax (level of thirteenth rib), 4 = point of shoulder (level of eleventh rib), 5 = olecranon, 6 = area of cardiac dullness. (Adapted from Cook: Proceedings of the Annual Meeting of the British Equine Veterinary Association, 1964.)

dorsal limits extend 5 to 6 in above the left sternal border at the level of the fourth rib and then descend in an arc through the fifth intercostal space, 2 to 3 in dorsal to the sternal border, reaching the sternum at the sixth intercostal space (Fig. 1–19) (Cook 1964). The area of cardiac dullness on the right side extends from the third to fourth intercostal spaces 2 to 3 in dorsal to the right sternal border.

The areas previously defined are only approximations that vary with the shape of the thorax and the thickness of the chest wall. Changes in the area of cardiac dullness can be associated with pathological changes of the heart or lungs. The area of cardiac dullness is increased with the gross cardiac enlargement that might occur with cardiac dilation. Pericardial effusion produces a more extensive and pronounced dullness, whereas accumulated gas in the pericardial sac may change the dorsal percussion sounds from dull to tympanic. Pneumonia or pleural effusion may appear to cause a relative increase in the area of cardiac dullness. In the absence of other reliable signs of heart disease, the presence of dyspnea or abnormal sounds synchronous with respiration suggests that lung consolidation or pleural effusion is responsible for the increased area of dullness. The areas may be decreased with expanded lung

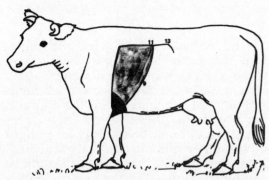

Figure 1–18 Lung field (gray shading) and area of cardiac dullness (black shading) as determined by percussion in the normal bovine. The numbers indicate the ribs used as landmarks. (Adapted from Raphel and Fregin: Comp. Cont. Ed. Pract. Vet. 2:S259, 1980.)

fields (i.e., pulmonary emphysema), disappearing first in the fifth left intercostal space, becoming more ventral in the third to fourth intercostal spaces, and even disappearing over the right side of the thorax. Percussion over the anteroventral thorax may demonstrate increased sensitivity or pain, suggesting traumatic or inflammatory lesions.

AUSCULTATION

The location of the areas suggested for cardiac auscultation are shown in Figures 1–20 and 1–21. The terms *mitral*,

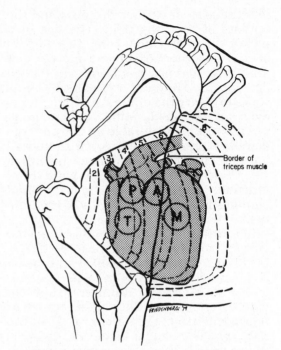

Figure 1–21 The areas of cardiac auscultation as viewed from the left side of the thorax in the equine. Mitral valve area (M): left fifth intercostal space just above a horizontal line drawn halfway between the point of the shoulder and the sternum. Aortic valve area (A): left fourth intercostal space slightly below a horizontal line drawn through the level of the point of the shoulder at the caudal border of the triceps brachii muscle. Pulmonic valve area (P): left third intercostal space just below the level of the point of the shoulder beneath the triceps brachii muscle. Tricuspid valve area (T): left third intercostal space just above a horizontal line drawn halfway between the point of the shoulder and the sternum, beneath the triceps brachii muscle. On the right side, the tricuspid valve is located in the area of the third to fourth intercostal spaces in the lower third of the thorax under the triceps brachii muscle.

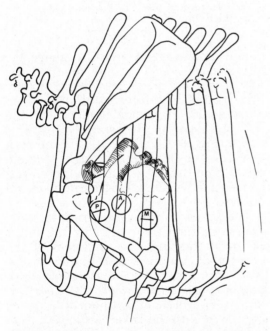

Figure 1–20 The areas of cardiac auscultation as viewed from the left side of the thorax in the bovine. Mitral valve area (M): left fourth intercostal space just above a horizontal line drawn halfway between the point of the shoulder and the sternum. Aortic valve area (A): left third intercostal space just below a horizontal line drawn through the point of the shoulder. Pulmonic valve area (P): left second intercostal space or third rib slightly below the aortic valve. Tricuspid valve area: left third rib just above a horizontal line drawn halfway between the point of the shoulder and the sternum, beneath the triceps brachii muscle. On the right side, the tricuspid valve is located in the second to third intercostal spaces just above a horizontal line drawn halfway between the point of the shoulder and the sternum. (Adapted from Raphel and Fregin: Comp. Cont. Ed. Pract. Vet. 2:S259, 1980.)

aortic, pulmonic, and *tricuspid* represent the general anatomic locations of these valves (Raphel and Fregin 1980; Fregin 1979). The projection of heart sounds and murmurs onto the thoracic surface from these areas may vary slightly and must be interpreted in light of the other clinical and physical findings. Auscultation of the heart should be combined with simultaneous palpation of the median artery or its continuation and should take place under quiet conditions. On the left side of the chest, the stethoscope should be placed on the thorax over the third or fourth intercostal space dorsal and medial to the olecranon. The first heart sound (S_1) is associated with the initial movements of the ventricles, closure of the atrioventricular valves, opening of the semilunar valves, and onset of ventricular ejection (Fregin 1979). It is longer, duller, and louder than the second heart sound. S_1 is usually best heard in the mitral and tricuspid valve areas or slightly lower toward the apex of the heart (Fregin 1979). Splitting or multiple components of the first heart sound may be heard in healthy cattle and horses. In the author's clinical experience, first heart sounds with multiple components have been detected more frequently in cows with lymphosarcoma than in normal cattle. The second heart sound is of higher frequency and shorter duration than S_1. It is associated with closure of the semilunar valves and opening of the atrioventricular valves and is best heard at the base of the heart. In adult cattle with low resting heart rates, the third and fourth heart sounds may occasionally be heard, although less frequently than in horses (Raphel and Fregin 1980). The third heart sound (S_3) consists of single or multiple low pitched, low amplitude vibrations, which when audible are best heard toward the apex of the heart below the mitral and tricuspid valve areas (Fregin 1979). The sounds are associated with the end of the period of rapid ventricular filling and are thought to result from the deceleration of the rapidly dilating ventricles as they reach their limit of distensibility. In heart failure with ventricular dilatation S_3 will frequently be accentuated (Fregin 1982).

The fourth heart sound (S_4) is a low frequency sound consisting of one or two groups of vibrations occurring just before the onset of S_1 and occasionally must be distinguished from splitting of the first heart sound. In incomplete atrioventricular block with dropped beats, S_4 may be heard in an isolated form without a ventricular beat (S_1–S_2) (Fregin 1979, 1982). During the intravenous administration of calcium solution in cattle, S_3 or S_4 may become accentuated and audible. A summation gallop S_3/S_4, as described in the horse, may be auscultated in some cattle with elevated heart rates.

Heart rate should coincide with pulse rate. A rate of over 90 beats/min in resting adult cattle, over 100 beats/min in young cattle, or over 125 beats/min in calves denotes tachycardia (Rosenberger 1979). A heart rate of less than 60 beats/min (bradycardia) is uncommon in normal cattle and may be caused by conditions that increase vagal tone or occasionally by cardiovascular disease.

Heart rhythm in cattle is usually regular, with no change in the intensity of the first or second heart sound. Irregularity of the heart rhythm or the intensity of the heart sounds is frequently associated with cardiac disease.

Cardiac rhythm originates from the sinoatrial node and is maintained within an optimal range by its pacemaker activity. Certain factors alter the automaticity of these nodal cells. Depression follows vagal stimulation, and acceleration of sinus impulse formation follows sympathetic stimulation. The range of normal sinus rhythm in mature horses at rest is 26 to 50 beats/min, with an average rate of 34 beats/min. The normal sinus rhythm of ponies is 44 beats/min and that of foals around 90 beats/min (Fregin 1982).

Sinus tachycardia and *bradycardia* are relative terms in that precise definition in horses is difficult owing to the normally wide variation in heart rates. The age, breed, and temperament of the animal appear to be important factors in determining the resting heart rate. Variations in autonomic nervous system tone of the heart are associated with the greatest fluctuations in resting heart rate in normal horses. Sinus tachycardia is probably present when the sinus rate exceeds 50 beats/min in mature horses, whereas rates of less than 26 beats/min represent sinus bradycardia.

Sinus tachycardia may accompany fever, anemia, hemorrhage, shock, colic, and congestive heart failure. In sinus bradycardia, the heart rate should increase as usual with exercise or excitement or after the administration of atropine. Sinus bradycardia may result from stimulation of the vagal nerve anywhere along its course, liver disease, increased CNS pressure, and malnutrition.

Cardiac murmurs and friction sounds consist of a longer series of vibrations than those described for the normal heart sounds. Cardiac murmurs in the bovine, as in other species, may be of pathological or occasionally of innocent origin (Fregin 1977). Murmurs may be associated with acquired heart disease (e.g., endocarditis) or congenital heart disease (e.g., ventricular septal defect). When systolic murmurs of grade 2 or less occur at the heart base without other reliable signs of cardiac disease, they may be of innocent origin. Determination of the point of maximum intensity of a murmur as well as the time of its occurrence during the cardiac cycle helps in defining the underlying cause.

ELECTROCARDIOGRAPHY

Electrocardiography may be beneficial in the diagnosis of cardiac disease. In cattle with traumatic pericarditis and advanced effusion, there is a generalized decrease in ECG amplitude in the limb leads (Fisher and Pirie 1965; Ettinger 1974). In early cases of pericardial effusion, there may be no decrease in the amplitude of the electrocardiogram, as has been reported in other species (Ettinger 1974). As the effusion increases in volume, a corresponding decrease in amplitude may occur. The presence of fibrinopurulent material surrounding the heart is frequently associated with an even greater decrease in ECG amplitude. In 22 cattle with traumatic pericarditis seen at the University of Pennsylvania, School of Veterinary Medicine (New Bolton Center), 21 had decreased ECG amplitudes in the limb leads. Following pericardiocentesis and removal of some of the exudate in several of these cows, the amplitude of electrocardiographic complexes increased, approaching normal values (Raphel and Fregin 1980).

ECG changes in cattle with endocarditis or lymphosarcoma of the heart are not specific for those diseases, but when considered in conjunction with other clinical findings they may aid in diagnosis (Lacuata et al. 1980; Marshak et al. 1962).

Cardiac arrhythmias can be confirmed by electrocardiography. An irregularity in heart rhythm accompanied by an increased heart rate and a difference in the intensity of heart sounds is highly suggestive of atrial fibrillation in the cow. Cardiovascular examination in horses with atrial fibrillation usually reveals an absolutely irregular ventricular rhythm, with a heart rate of 40 to 60 beats/min, although tachycardia and even bradycardia may occur. The diagnosis is based on the absence of P waves, the presence of fibrillation waves, and irregularly spaced QRS-T complexes (Fregin 1982). Atrial fibrillation, in the author's experience, has most commonly been seen in cattle with gastrointestinal distrubances. Digoxin may be used to slow the ventricular rate, and diuretics may be required if signs of congestive heart failure are present. If spontaneous reversion to a normal sinus rhythm does not occur following surgical and/or medical intervention, treatment with quinidine sulfate may be considered.

Atrial and ventricular ectopic contractions, varying degrees of heart block, atrial and ventricular tachycardia, and atrial flutter have been noted in horses with inflammatory or degenerative myocardial lesions, metabolic and electrolyte abnormalities, gastrointestinal disorders, and drug toxicities. Treatment should begin as soon as possible with correction of acid-base and electrolyte abnormalities and administration of digoxin if congestive heart failure is present. Antiarrhythmic drugs must be used with caution, since lidocaine may cause twitching and convulsions in unanesthetized horses and quinidine sulfate may further depress cardiac output (Fregin 1982).

REFERENCES

Adams, H. R., Teske, R. H., and Mercer, H. D.: Anesthetic antibiotic interrelationships. JAVMA 168:409, 1976.
Cook, W. R.: Proceedings of the Annual Meeting of the British Equine Veterinary Association, 1964, p. 18.
Ettinger, S. J.: Pericardiocentesis. Vet. Clin. North Am. 4:403, 1974.
Fisher, E. W., and Pirie, H. M.: Traumatic pericarditis in cattle: A clinical physiological study. Br. Vet. J. 121:552, 1965.
Fregin, G. F.: The Cardiovascular System. Equine Medicine and Surgery, Vol. 1, 3rd ed. Mansmann, R.A., McAlister, S., and Pratt, P.W.

(eds.): Santa Barbara: American Veterinary Publications, Inc. 1982, Chap. 14, pp. 645–701.

Fregin, G. F.: Cardiovascular sound and cardiac auscultation in the normal horse. Comp. Cont. Ed. Pract. Vet. 1:S28, 1979.

Fregin, G. F.: General guidelines for clinical examination of the cardiovascular system in large animals. In Current Veterinary Therapy VI. Kirk, R. W. (ed.) Philadelphia: W. B. Saunders, 1977, pp. 410–417.

Himes, J. A., Edds, G. R., Kirkham, W. W., and Neal, F. C.: Potentiation of succinylcholine by organophosphate compounds in horses. JAVMA 151:54, 1967.

Lacuata, A. Q., Vamada, H., et al.: Electrocardiographic and echocardiographic findings in four cases of bovine endocarditis. JAVMA 176:1355, 1980.

Marshak, R. R., Covell, L. L., et al.: Studies on bovine lymphosarcoma. I. Clinical aspects, pathological alterations, and herd studies. Cancer Res. 22:202, 1982.

Raphel, C. F., and Fregin, G. F.: Clinical examination of the cardiovascular system in cattle. Comp. Cont. Ed. Pract. Vet. 2:S259, 1980.

Rosenberger, G.: Clinical Examination of Cattle. Berlin: Verlag Paul Parey, 1979, pp. 101–114.

Short, C. E., Cuneio, J., and Cupp, D.: Organophate induced complications during anesthetic management in the horse. JAVMA 159:1319, 1971.

CHAPTER 2

NUTRITION, METABOLISM, AND THE SURGICAL PATIENT

J. M. NAYLOR, B.Sc., B.V.Sc., M.R.C.V.S.

The surgeon should be aware of the patient's nutrient requirements and its ability to meet these requirements through feed intake during the pre- and postoperative periods. Feed intake is often depressed during illness (when nutrient requirements are increased), and nutritional support is therefore particularly important at this time.

To support the patient it is important to know the normal nutrient requirements and how these are modified by illness. In this chapter factors that favor catabolism and loss of body tissues following surgery, sepsis, or trauma and the adverse effects of prolonged undernutrition and overnutrition are considered. Methods of evaluation and nutritional supportive therapy in animals are also described.

CATABOLIC RESPONSE TO INJURY

Nutritional requirements are increased by injury, infection, stress, and pain (Fleck 1980). Minor surgery has little effect on nutritional requirements in humans, but trauma and especially infection increase nutritional requirements. Elective abdominal surgery increases energy and protein requirements

The author wishes to acknowledge the helpful assistance given by Drs. D. S. Kronfeld, G. F. Hamilton, and P. Brightling.

by about 20 per cent (Spivey and Johnston 1972), infection and major injury increase requirements to a greater extent, and severe trauma can raise requirements by 200 to 400 per cent (Dudrick, Copeland, and MacFayden 1975). The catabolic effect of these changes is exacerbated by depressed food intake associated with both the primary illness and withdrawal of food prior to and following surgery.

In healthy animals, undernutrition results in glycogen catabolism. Glycogen stores are small and are utilized rapidly (McGarry, Meier, and Foster 1973), so that by 24 hours fat is the major fuel source (McGarry, Meier, and Foster 1973; Freminet et al. 1976). Adipose tissue triglycerides are broken down into free fatty acids and glycerol. Free fatty acid metabolism is variable; some are degraded by way of acetylcoenzyme A (acetyl-CoA) and are completely oxidized to provide energy for hepatic and muscle functioning. Fatty acids can also be converted to ketone bodies or can be reesterified to triglycerides, which can accumulate within the liver or return to the circulation. These pathways vary with the species; pregnant sheep and lactating cows are prone to ketonemia (Kronfeld 1972), whereas ponies (Wensing et al. 1973) and uremic horses (Naylor, Kronfeld, and Acland 1980) develop marked hypertriglyceridemia. The fasting animal has difficulty maintaining glucose supply for nervous tissue, red blood cells, and the renal medulla. Glucose turnover decreases (Freminet et al. 1976) as glucose utilization by muscle and brain is partially replaced by ketone body utilization. Glycerol from lipolysis and alanine from protein metabolism are used as substrates for hepatic and renal gluconeogenesis to meet obligatory glucose demands (Klain et al. 1977; Heard et al. 1977).

Fasting metabolism is more complex in the surgical patient. Moderate to severe injury is followed by an "ebb" or shock phase in which metabolic rate is depressed (Cuthbertson 1980) and then a flow phase of hypermetabolism and increased oxygen consumption. During hypermetabolism there is a simultaneous rise in urinary excretion of nitrogen, phosphate, sulfate, and potassium owing in part to protein catabolism. Hypercatabolism is greatest in patients in the best condition prior to injury and in those with the most severe tissue destruction (Cuthbertson 1980). Hypercatabolism is a generalized body response and cannot be attributed merely to the loss of body substance from the injury site alone (Cuthbertson 1980). In general, this hypercatabolic phase is greatest within three days after injury (Blackburn, Maini, and Pierce 1977); although nutritional support will ameliorate nitrogen and energy balance, it is difficult to get net storage and synthesis of extra body mass in this phase (Cuthbertson 1980). An adaptive phase follows in which the changes are reversed and the body slowly recovers (Blackburn, Maini, and Pierce 1977).

Injured patients show different patterns of protein catabolism as well as differences in metabolic rate. Comparison of experimentally injured and fasting healthy animals shows that liver (visceral) protein is preferentially conserved in the injured animal at the expense of muscle protein (Richard 1980). The net effect is catabolism of muscle protein to provide amino acids for hepatic synthesis (Blackburn, Maini, and Pierce 1977) of fibrinogen and other acute phase reactant proteins. In contrast, healthy fasted animals have similar losses of both liver and muscle protein (Richard 1980). Mobilization of depot lipid, typical of fasted healthy patients, may be suppressed in the sick patient. For example, some septic states are characterized by hyperinsulinemia (Richard 1980). Muscle can be resistant to the glucoregulatory effects of insulin, and glucose utilization is impaired (Richard 1980). The net effect of this insulin resistance is suppression of fat metabolism at the expense of increased protein catabolism (Richard 1980).

An awareness of the demand for energy, protein, and other nutrients following surgery has resulted in attempts to balance these with increased nutrient intake. In general, these studies have shown that additional feeding decreases the overall loss of body weight and protein stores (Voitk et al. 1972; Newton, Clark, and Woods 1980). However, it is often more difficult to achieve positive nutritional balance immediately postoperatively because the hormonal balance strongly favors catabolism. In spite of this, studies in humans have shown the beneficial effects of nutritional support, and enteral and intravenous alimentation are now accepted therapies in human medicine. Nutritional support has been particularly beneficial for premature infants of very low birth weight and patients with gastrointestinal fistulas and burns or other severe trauma (Dudrick, Copeland, and MacFayden 1975). For example, in patients with small intestinal fistulas, resting the gut by intravenous or enteral feeding through a tube passed distal to the fistula resulted in a high rate of spontaneous closure and an 8 per cent mortality compared with a 33 per cent mortality in patients not receiving nutritional support (Himal et al. 1974). Profiles for assessing the nutritional and metabolic status of patients are used to select people with protein or protein-calorie malnutrition for intensive nutritional support. The incidence of post-surgical complications is greatest in patients in poor nutritional condition preoperatively (Buzby et al. 1980). Postoperative complications, including severe sepsis, shock, and death, can be reduced by adequate preoperative nutritional support (Mullen et al. 1980). Preoperative nutritional support restores the body's protein reserves and immune function, enabling the patient to mobilize its defenses to fight the stresses of surgery. Veterinarians treating patients with debilitating illnesses should be aware of the risks involved in operating on animals in a poor nutritional state.

ADVERSE EFFECTS OF UNDERNUTRITION

Immune Function. Immunity and other host defense mechanisms are susceptible to nutritional manipulation. The types of malnutrition commonly seen in veterinary practice are deficiencies of protein and energy or protein alone. This chapter is concerned only with these types of malnutrition and does not consider the effects of specific vitamin or mineral deficiencies.

The effects of mild, short-term undernutrition are not well documented. Anorexia may be beneficial in the acute stages of infectious diseases. Force feeding mice infected with *Listeria monocytogenes* increased mortality (Murray and Murray 1976). The mechanism of this beneficial effect of hypophagia in acute infectious disease is unknown. Complete food deprivation in horses rapidly affects host defense. When horses were deprived of food but not water for five days, neutrophil phagocytosis fell from 97 to 78 per cent and Arthus-mediated immunity was only half as efficient as in the fed animals (Naylor and Kenyon 1981).

Long-term effects of protein and energy undernutrition include lymphoid hypoplasia, manifested as splenic and thymic atrophy with hypoplastic lymph nodes, and decreased body lymphocyte counts (Dionigi et al. 1977; Smythe et al. 1971; Chandra 1972; McFarlane and Hamid 1973; Asirvadham 1948; Law, Dudrick, and Abdou 1974). Cellular and humoral immunity, including antibody response to bacterial antigen, is depressed (Skinsnes and Woodridge 1948; Reddy et al. 1976; Keusch 1974). Defects in neutrophil function include decreases in bacteriodical activity (Palmblad 1976; Seth and Chandra 1972) and impairment of the leukocytic response to blood loss and inflammatory stimuli (Asirvadham 1948). There are also decreased serum concentrations of proteins, which facilitate the attraction, engulfment, and destruction of foreign antigens by phagocytes (Dionigi et al. 1977; Sirisinha et al. 1973; Keusch 1974).

The result of impairments in the host defense mechanism in chronically undernourished animals is a predisposition to bacterial infection, thereby making treatment of existing infections more difficult, i.e., greater amounts of antibiotic are required to cure bacterial infections in malnourished animals (Skinsnes and Woodridge 1948). Although severe undernutrition decreases antibody production to certain antigens, hypergammaglobulinemia is seen in malnourished patients as a result of chronic stimulation by infectious agents (Chandra 1972; Beisel 1974).

The response to some bacterial antigens has been unaffected by malnutrition (Reddy et al. 1976). There are also some reports of beneficial effects of protein or energy deprivation in certain diseases (Good et al. 1976).

Malnourished animals are more susceptible to parasitism than healthy animals. McCance (1960) observed that restricting feed intake prevented the growth of piglets but not their parasites; several animals died of roundworm infestations before routine deworming was instituted. This may reflect competition for available nutrients as well as decreased immune function. Comparison of high (18 per cent) and low (11 per cent) protein diets in lambs and pigs infected with nematodes revealed that low protein diets exacerbated the effects of parasitism; decreased feed intake, weight gain, more severe clinical signs, and larger worm burdens occurred in the low protein groups (Downey, Connolly, and O'Shea 1969; Stephenson et al. 1977).

Reproductive Performance. Nutrition and reproduction are often associated in the management of sheep. Sheep kept on subsistence diets on poor pastures are often given supplemental feed before mating. This process, known as flushing, substantially improves the number of ova ovulated and increases fertility (Robinson 1973). This effect is not produced when sheep already in good condition are supplemented (Bramley, Denehy, and Newton 1976; Robinson 1973). Underfeeding is less common in other species but can decrease fertility in cattle (Hill et al. 1970), pigs (McCance 1960; Lintern-Moore 1978), and horses, and this should be considered when managing reproductive problems. In cattle, the rapidity of uterine involution and the period to first heat are favorably influenced by both body condition at calving and the amount of feed provided during lactation.

Visceral wound healing is only affected in the most extreme cases of malnutrition, whereas abdominal wall and cutaneous wound healing are influenced by general nutritional status (Irving 1978).

Death can result from severe cachexia. Animals die when a loss of over 20 to 25 per cent of body weight occurs. Young animals are more sensitive and die following a smaller weight loss (Morrison 1944). Death may be due to respiratory muscle failure and is said to occur when one-half to one-third of protein mass is catabolyzed (Sandek and Felig 1976).

ADVERSE EFFECTS OF OVERNUTRITION

Paradoxically, obesity predisposes to metabolic disorders commonly associated with undernutrition. This can be understood with the aid of the following example. An obese sheep has excessive fat; this provides a reservoir of calories but also occupies abdominal space. The volume of the abdominal cavity available to the gut, and thus ingesta, is limited (Forbes 1969). When the animal is fed a high energy density diet or has little nutrient demands except those of maintenance, this is not important. However, a pregnant sheep that has become fat during the second trimester and is then maintained through the last trimester on poor pasture may develop problems. Limited abdominal space limits feed intake; a sheep in lean condition can eat more than a fat sheep (Forbes 1969). The fat animal mobilizes adipose tissue to meet the energy deficit and is prone to develop pregnancy toxemia.

A complex syndrome of diseases associated with obesity in cattle is described by the term "fat cow syndrome" (Fig. 2–1). This condition is encountered in cows overfed during the dry period and the latter part of lactation when the de-

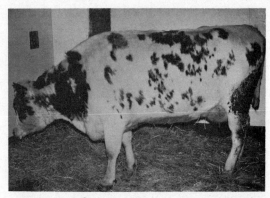

Figure 2–1 This cow became fat during a prolonged dry period (10-months). Following a difficult calving she went off feed, became ketotic, and developed a fatty liver. Response to therapy was poor, and the cow was sold for slaughter.

mands for milk production are small (Kronfeld 1980). Retained placenta and downer cow problems occur at parturition, whereas displaced abomasum, ketosis, and fatty liver are seen after parturition (Morrow 1976; Morrow et al. 1979). The recovery rate is poor, and the surgeon should remember this when advising the farmer.

Obesity is also thought to predispose to a number of other problems, including infertility (Witherspoon 1977) and dystocia in fat mares, and may aggravate lameness.

Obesity presents the surgeon with a special problem. Anesthesia is complicated because many anesthetic agents are lipid soluble. Drug dosages may have to be adjusted for obese patients, and recovery times may be prolonged. Obesity also interferes with the surgical approach. It is more difficult to find anatomic landmarks, and wound closure is complicated by the presence of excess adipose tissue.

Sudden increases in the amount of feed ingested or in the introduction of new feeds may result in digestive disturbances.

ASSESSMENT OF NUTRITIONAL STATUS

Clinical assessment of nutritional status is usually made based on body condition and feed intake; body weight and serum chemistry can also be useful in assessing physical condition.

Table 2–1 RELATIVE WEIGHT OF FEEDS*

Feed	Weight of 1 Liter (kg)	Weight of 1 US Quart (lb)
Alfalfa meal	.27	0.6
Barley	.68	1.5
Beet pulp	.27	0.6
Corn	.77	1.7
Cottonseed meal	.68	1.5
Linseed meal	.41	0.9
Molasses, cane	1.30	3.0
Oats†	.45	1.0
Rye	.77	1.7
Soybeans	.82	1.8
Wheat	.86	1.9
Wheat bran	.23	0.5

*Modified from Schryver and Hintz: Feeding Horses. Ithaca: Cornell University Press, 1975.

†Oats are very variable in their weight per unit volume.

Food Intake. When the history is taken, the attendant should be questioned about the amount of feed consumed. Grain intake is often reported in terms of volume. Table 2–1 can be used to convert volume measurements to weight. However, it should be remembered that these are only a guide; oats in particular can vary greatly in their weight per unit volume. The clinician can best assess how much is being fed by measuring out five scoops of grain into a bag for subsequent weighing on a scale. Owners do not usually know the amount of hay fed each day; an estimate can often be made by determining the time it takes to consume one bale knowing that rectangular bales often weigh 20 to 25 kg.

The amount of feed actually eaten should be assessed; the quantity of grain left in the manger and of hay trampled into the bedding should be evaluated. In group feeding situations dominant animals may force small or weak animals out of the feeding area, and sick animals may allow healthy mates to eat all the feed.

The quality of the feed is important, and feed should be inspected for dampness or mold. Spoiled feed is likely to be found at the edges of hay stacks and in silage pits and grain stores and may be rejected by animals and left in the manger. Hay is very variable in quality; good hay has a lot of leaves, very few coarse stems, a green color, a sweet smell, and no evidence of mold or dust.

Body Condition. A useful index of nutritional status is body condition. In mature animals extracellular compartments such as skeleton (Pomeroy 1941) and extracellular fluid (Barac-Neito 1978) are well preserved during energy malnutrition, whereas fat and muscle are extensively catabolized in undernutrition (Pomeroy 1941; Widdowson, Dickerson, and McCance 1960), giving rise to the phrase "flesh falls away from the bones." Energy undernutrition accentuates skeletal elements, whereas overnutrition results in fat accumulation, which smoothes the body contour. Early work with pigs suggested that growth spreads as a series of waves originating at the head, spreading to the extremities of the limb and tail, and meeting in the loins. The reverse occurs when mature animals are placed on submaintenance diets, with the rump and loins showing the first signs of undernutrition. Undernourished pigs become thinner with a shallower and a more angular body and a disproportionately large head and shoulders (Pomeroy 1941). Similarly, horses and cattle lose tissue over the rump and lumbar spine, which become more prominent; loss of tissue over the ribs is seen in the later stages of undernutrition. Systems of scoring the bodily condition of cattle have been developed based on body conformation at the base of the tail and over the hips and back (Fig. 2–2 and Table 2–2). Unshorn sheep are deceptive in appearance, and palpation is the only reliable method of assessing their body condition.

Nutritional restriction affects body weight in growing animals, but the proportions at a given weight are unaffected (Allen 1970). However, when growth ceases or when weight is lost, body composition is not related to weight. For example, in studies in pigs, the skeleton (Dickerson and McCance 1961) and brain (Pomeroy 1941; McCance, Ford, and Brown 1961) continued to increase in mass even though total body weight did not. This can give the animal the appearance of a body that is too small for its head. Body condition in young animals is assessed using expected

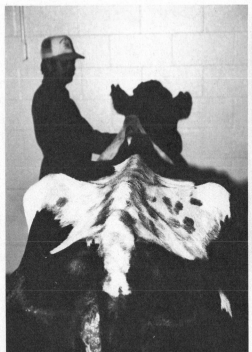
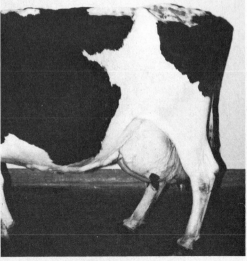

Score 1

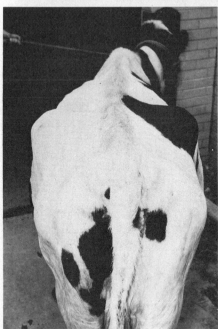
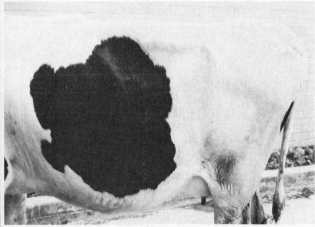

Score 2

Figure 2–2 Assessment of body condition of cows can be accomplished using a scoring system. This allows determination of body condition independent of effects of frame size. Holstein cows have mean scores of 2.5 in the first 80 days of lactation; low-producing cows put on condition during lactation, but high-producing cows do not. Dry cows have a mean body score of 3.5. Cows in condition 1 are too thin; cows in condition 5 are too fat. The condition 5 cow has a deformed tail head; she had been dry for over a year. Modified from Wildman et al.: J. Dairy Sci. *65*:495, 1982.

Illustration continued on following page

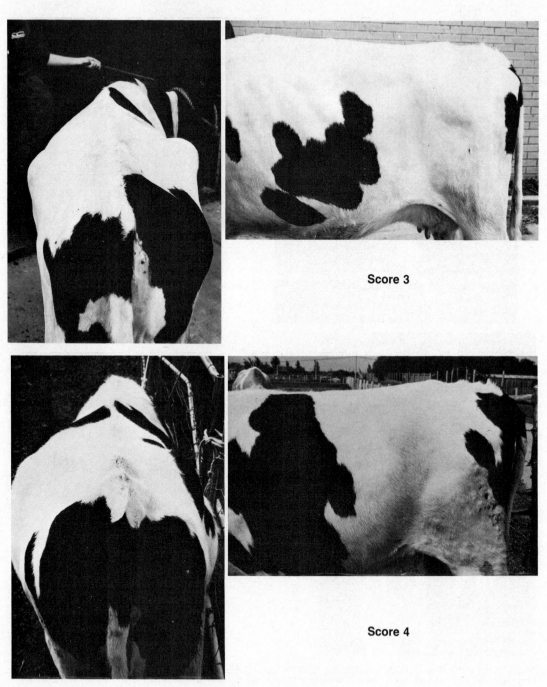

Score 3

Score 4

Figure 2–2 *Continued*

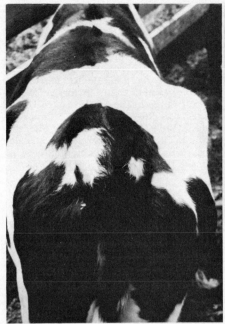
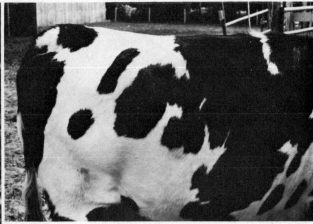

Score 5

Figure 2–2 *Continued*

Table 2–2 SCORING SYSTEM FOR BODY CONDITION OF COWS

	Score				
	1	2	3	4	5
Lumbar Transverse Processes	Limited flesh covering; sharp ends; overhang paralumbar fossa	Individual processes discernible but not prominent; do not overhang paralumbar fossa to a marked extent	Can feel processes with light pressure. Do not overhang paralumbar fossa	Processes palpable with firm touch. Skin covering lateral edge of processes is flat or rounded in contour	Bone structures not apparent
Spinous Processes of Thoracic and Lumbar Vertebrae	Individual processes are easily seen	Processes distinguishable by palpation but not visually	Processes are covered by a rounded ridge of flesh	Rounded and smooth	
Tuber Coxae and Tuber Ischii	Sharp, negligible flesh covering; major depression between them	Some flesh covering; small depression between them	Rounded and smooth	Span between tuber coxae is flat	
Area between Tail Head and Tuber Ischii	Severely depressed; bone structures appear sharp	Depressed; some flesh covering	Smooth, no signs of fat deposition	Rounded; fat deposition	Tail head buried in fat

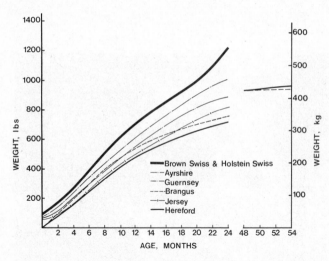

Figure 2–3 Stunting in young animals can result in a small animal of normal proportions. Growth curves are useful in determining whether an animal is small for its age. Stunting can be the result of disease or diet. Curves for Brown Swiss, Holstein Swiss, Ayrshire, Guernsey, and Jerseys are for dairy heifer; curves for Herefords and Brangus are for beef heifers kept at range in the southwestern United States. (Modified from de Torre and Rankins: J. Anim. Sci. 46:604, 1978; and from Hillman et al.: Cooperative Extension Service Bulletin 412, Michigan State University, 1982.)

weight and height for age growth curves (Figs. 2–3 and 2–4).

Undernourished cattle and horses often have dull, dry hair coats flecked with keratin. A variety of changes occur in the hair of undernourished pigs, and the skin tends to become hyperkeratotic (McCance 1960). Sheep lose their wool in times of nutritional stress and the fleece falls from the skin.

Necropsy. At necropsy there is loss of muscle and adipose tissue in undernourished animals, and fat deposits undergo serous atrophy. In pigs (Pomeroy 1941) and other large animals subcutaneous fat is lost before abdominal fat. Muscle mass should be assessed independently of fat stores. For example, cachectic sheep with Johnes' disease may have abdominal fat reserves, but severe muscle wasting occurs, which is presumably

responsible for the weakness and death in the late stages of this disease.

Blood Chemistry. Blood lipids are affected in severe cases of undernutrition; free fatty acid levels are greatly elevated during total anorexia in cattle (Baird, Heitzman, and Hibitt 1972), sheep (Kronfeld and Raggi 1966), pigs (Baetz and Mengeling 1971), and horses (Naylor, Kronfeld, and Acland 1980). Energy intake in cattle can be predicted from the serum free fatty acid concentration (Parker and Blowey 1976; Holmes and Lambourne 1970).

In lactating cows and pregnant sheep, severe energy imbalance resulting from the combination of poor feed intake and increased metabolic demands is accompanied by accumulation of ketone bodies in blood. In underfed equids a mild ketonemia may develop, but the remark-

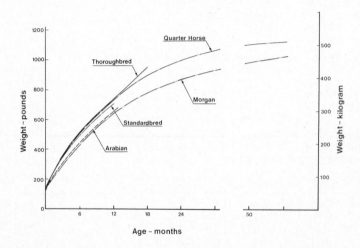

Figure 2–4 Growth curves for horses of different breeds. (Based on data from Hintz: Proceedings of the American Association of Equine Practitioners 24:455, 1978; and from Schryver and Hintz: Extension Information Bulletin 94, Cornell University, 1975.)

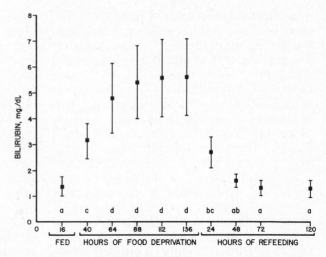

Figure 2–5 Food deprivation results in marked increases in unconjugated bilirubin in horses. This figure shows the responses of six horses to food deprivation. Values are means ± 1 standard deviation. Icterus in sick horses often represents a response to poor feed intake rather than liver disease. (Reproduced with permission from the Proceedings of the Society of Experimental Biology and Medicine 165:86, 1980.)

able change is hypertriglyceridemia (Naylor, Kronfeld, and Acland 1980). Normal triglyceride concentrations do not rule out poor feed intake in horses; there is much individual variation in the response to feed deprivation, and there is a 40-hour lag between withdrawal of feed and elevation of plasma triglyceride levels (Naylor, Kronfeld, and Acland 1980). Markedly elevated triglyceride concentrations make serum and plasma opaque and are described by the term "hyperlipemia." In ponies this occurs when poor feed intake is aggravated by the demands for pregnancy, lactation, or illness. Ponies with pituitary tumors can exhibit hyperlipemia even though feed intake is good, presumably as a result of hormonal imbalances (Naylor, Kronfeld, and Acland 1980). In horses hyperlipemia is often associated with the combination of poor feed intake and uremia.

Decreased blood glucose concentrations in undernutrition are too small to be useful on an individual basis. In horses the differences between fed and fasted values are mainly due to an alimentary glycemia in the fed state; this is especially noticeable if samples are taken within a few hours of grain feeding (Breukink 1974).

Protein intake and serum urea nitrogen concentrations tend to parallel each other (Manston et al. 1975). Fasting produces changes in serum urea nitrogen. In horses (Naylor 1982), ponies (Baetz and Pearson 1972), and pigs (Baetz and Mengeling 1971), serum urea nitrogen values range from 15 to 20 mg/dl during the fasting period. Blood albumin and

hemoglobin concentrations decline when diets are deficient in protein (Manston et al. 1975), but protein-losing conditions and toxic depression of the bone marrow are more common causes of low values in sick animals.

Fasting hyperbilirubinemia occurs in all the domestic species (Baetz and Mengeling 1971; Cakala and Bieniek 1975) but is only of importance in the horse (Naylor, Kronfeld, and Johnson 1980) and man. In horses, serum bilirubin may approach 9 mg/dl during fasting (Naylor, Kronfeld, and Johnson 1980) (Fig. 2–5); hyperbilirubinemia is less marked in ponies. Anorexia, rather than liver disease, is the common cause of jaundice in sick horses. Fasting hyperbilirubine-

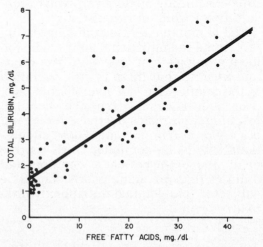

Figure 2–6 The hyperbilirubinemia of fasting is closely associated with the rise in nonesterified fatty acids. (Reproduced with permission from the Proceedings of the Society of Experimental Biology and Medicine 165:86, 1980.)

mia can be differentiated from liver disease because only unconjugated bilirubin moves out of the normal range during fasting. The rise in bilirubin is associated with increased plasma nonesterified fatty acid concentrations (Fig. 2–6), possibly because fatty acids compete with bilirubin for binding to ligandin, a hepatocyte-binding protein. The magnitude of fasting hyperbilirubinemia can be predicted from plasma nonesterified fatty acid concentrations, and this may prove useful in differentiating bilirubinemia caused by fasting from that induced by liver diseases (see Fig. 2–4). In horses, fasting alone does not elevate liver-derived serum enzyme concentrations (Naylor, Kronfeld, and Johnson 1980) unless hepatic damage develops secondary to fat infiltration in the hyperlipemia syndrome (Naylor, Kronfeld, and Acland 1980).

NUTRITIONAL GUIDELINES

The most exact method of feeding animals requires calculation of nutrient requirements and formulation of a ration to satisfy these needs within the limits of the animals' feed intake. Tables of feed composition and nutrient requirements can be found in the *Nutrient Requirements of Domestic Animals,* published by the National Research Council. A detailed analysis of nutrient intake is time-consuming and may involve consultation with a nutritionist.

The clinician can use guidelines to approximate the nutritional status. The following suggestions are approximations and assume that there is little variation in the composition of a given forage; age, poor preservation, excessive heating, leaching, and molds decrease forage energy and protein content. These suggestions should be combined with routine evaluation of the patient's condition, and animals that are doing poorly should be subjected to a detailed nutritional workup.

Maintenance

The nutrient requirements of herbivorous farm animals are usually satisfied with forages (i.e., pastures, hay, or silage) that contain 20 to 40 per cent crude fiber on a dry matter basis and that are known as roughages. The digestible energy requirements for maintenance of cattle and horses are identical and can be satisfied by feeding hay daily in an amount equal to 1.5 per cent of body weight. Alfalfa and timothy hay may contain 90 per cent dry matter and may have similar energy concentrations; good quality timothy hay contains less protein, but there is enough for maintenance purposes. The maintenance requirement for sheep expressed in terms of body weight is not linear; an 80 kg sheep requires 1.75 per cent of body weight of hay, whereas a 50-kg sheep requires 2.2 per cent.

Grass or alfalfa silage contains about 30 per cent dry matter and can be substituted for hay at the rate of 3 kg silage to 1 kg hay. Corn silage has a higher energy density, and 2.5 kg is equivalent to 1 kg hay. Silage is not usually fed to horses, partly because of the danger of forage poisoning, a botulism-like syndrome.

Production

Milk, gestation, work, cold, and any stress require additional nutrient requirements, which are often satisfied by feeding concentrates. Concentrate feeds are used when roughage has insufficient energy and protein density to satisfy requirements within the limits of feed intake. Dairy cows are often fed concentrate in the last six weeks of gestation in preparation for the high-grain diets necessary to support milk production in early lactation. Grain and grain products are energy concentrates; 2 kg of wheat grain is equivalent to 3 kg of good quality hay. Soybean meal is a common protein concentrate combining the advantages of low cost, a 44 per cent protein content, and a relatively balanced amino acid composition. Animal protein supplements, such as casein, often have a higher biological value than plant protein supplements, presumably because of the relative proportions of amino acids in the different supplements. The high cost of animal protein supplements tends to limit their use to young growing animals and sick patients. There is an inverse relationship between energy and fiber concentrations in feeds, with concentrates being low in fiber.

Dairy cows have increased dietary requirements for energy, protein, and fiber during lactation. Correct nutrition in late gestation and early lactation is important to avoid hypocalcemia and ketosis. Low-fiber diets depress milk butter fat and may predispose to indigestion, liver abscessation, and abomasal displacement. Hay or other roughage fed at the maintenance level may help prevent these problems. The energy requirements of milk production can be satisfied by feeding concentrate at the rate of 1 kg for every 2.5 to 3.5 kg of milk produced, depending on the energy density of the concentrate. High-producing cows are fed large amounts of grain in an attempt to meet nutritional requirements within the limits of feed intake, whereas low-producing animals can produce some of their milk from roughage alone. The protein content required from the concentrate in the ration depends on the level of production of the cow and whether corn silage or timothy or alfalfa hay is the principal roughage fed.

Pregnancy

Pregnancy does not increase nutrient requirements during the first two trimesters; overfeeding during these periods results in fat animals prone to dystocia and, in sheep, pregnancy toxemia. Most of the fetal growth occurs in the last trimester, and additional feeding is required during this period. Horses require 10 per cent more energy and 20 per cent more protein during the last 90 days of gestation. Cattle require a 30 per cent increase in energy for the last 60 days of gestation; the protein requirement is twice the maintenance level. Sheep have the largest increase in requirements, an additional 80 per cent of the maintenance energy. Protein and calcium are also required, and this helps explain the susceptibility of pregnant sheep to pregnancy toxemia and hypocalcemia. The nutrient demands of pregnancy can be met by increasing the amount of hay fed

in proportion to the increment in energy requirement above maintenance, e.g., cattle can be fed 2 per cent of body weight as hay. In practice, dairy cows are usually fed hay-grain or silage-grain mixes for the last six weeks of pregnancy to condition them for feeding during lactation. Alfalfa hay should not be fed to preparturient cows because it is calcium-rich and predisposes to milk fever; high calcium intake in late pregnancy dulls the homeostatic mechanisms needed to regulate blood calcium when the rapid loss of calcium into milk commences at lactation.

It is difficult to maintain pregnant sheep on roughage alone during the last trimester of gestation, particularly in sheep with twin pregnancies. The risk of developing problems is greater if there is severe competition at the feed rack, if hay quality is poor, or if feed intake is limited by excessive abdominal fat. Parasites, poor weather, and twinning also elevate nutrient demands and limit feed intake. To minimize the risk of pregnancy toxemia in sheep, grain feeding is recommended during the last trimester; grain can be introduced at the rate of 0.12 kg/head/day 60 days before parturition and slowly increased to 1 kg at parturition.

Disease

Febrile states elevate nutrient requirements by 13 per cent for every 1°C above normal. Elective abdominal surgery increases energy and protein requirements by 20 per cent, infection and major injury by 25 per cent, and severe sepsis by about 50 per cent. These increased demands, together with disease-induced hypophagia, make it particularly difficult to meet requirements through feed intake in surgical patients. This is of importance when predicting the outcome for patients in poor body condition faced with major surgery or long-term therapy.

Young Animals

Long-term survival of neonates born by caesarean section can be greatly enhanced by appropriate feeding practices.

Young animals are nutritionally vulnerable and require careful feeding during hospitalization.

Colostrum is especially important to help protect the young animal against both diarrhea and septicemia. Newborn animals should be kept with their dams for the first 24 hours of life to allow continuous access to colostrum and to improve absorption of immunoglobulin from the gut (Selman, McEwan, and Fisher 1971a; 1971b). The turgidity of the udder, the offspring's behavior, and belly fill can be used to gauge colostrum intake. Slippery floors, mismothering, mastitis, undernutrition of the dam (Logan 1977), and poor udder conformation (Selman, McEwan, and Fisher 1970a; 1970b) all contribute to inadequate colostrum intake by the calf. Beef-bred heifers may produce an insufficient volume of colostrum. Offspring born by caesarean section or following obstetrical intervention may obtain insufficient colostrum because either the dam or the offspring is too weak to allow nursing to take place. Colostrum is concentrated in the udder during the last five weeks of gestation (Brandon, Watson, and Lascelles 1971); therefore, premature animals may suckle low-immunoglobulin colostrum.

Following birth by caesarean section or when there is doubt about the sufficiency of voluntary colostrum intake, supplementary first-milking colostrum should be hand fed. A colostrum bank can be maintained for the offspring of those dams that produce insufficient colostrum. Up to 1 pint of colostrum from mares and 2 pints from dairy cows can be obtained within three to six hours after parturition when the offspring has had time to suckle. This should be labelled and can be stored in the frozen state for over a year. Calves, lambs, and foals should receive 5 per cent of body weight as colostrum within four hours of birth (Fig. 2–7); an additional 5 per cent of body weight should be given 6 to 12 hours later. The absorption of immunoglobulin decreases linearly from birth and ceases by 24 to 30 hours after parturition in calves, lambs, and foals. Keeping the offspring with its dam for the first 24 hours aids the absorption of immunoglobulin (Selman, McEwan, and Fisher 1971a; 1971b).

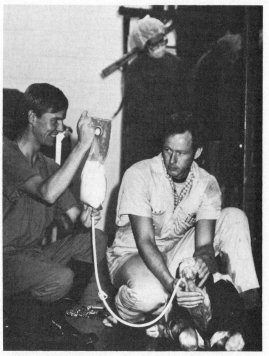

Figure 2–7 At the University of Saskatchewan, calves born by caesarian section are routinely fed 2 liters of colostrum as soon as possible after birth. Calves that have a poor suckling reflex can be tube fed.

Steroid preparations, which take one to three days to induce parturition, do not affect the excretion or absorption of immunoglobulin. A preparation marketed in Australia takes a number of weeks to induce parturition and inhibits the concentration of immunoglobulin in colostrum and its subsequent absorption by the calf (Brandon, Husband, and Lascelles 1975).

A number of simple tests are available to evaluate the colostrum status of the newborn animal. In healthy calves, the refractometer offers a simple and inexpensive method of estimating immunoglobulin concentrations. Calves with serum total proteins less than 5.5 gm/dl or plasma proteins less than 6.0 gm/dl are usually considered to be hypoimmunoglobulinemic and have an increased risk of disease (Naylor et al. 1977; Naylor 1979) (Fig. 2–8). Calves that have absorbed no colostral immunoglobulin have plasma total proteins of less than 5.0 gm/dl. The refractometer test is used on calves one to eight days of age. Dehydration and protein-losing enteropathies will also affect total protein concentration, so the test should be used only

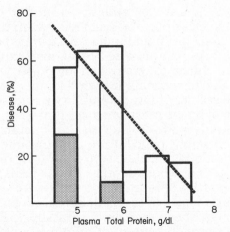

Figure 2–8 Plasma total protein concentration in healthy calves less than eight days of age reflects colostral immunoglobulin status. Calves usually have total proteins between 4.3 and 5.3 gm/dl at birth. Protein concentrations start to rise soon after colostrum feeding but drop in calves fed milk. A plasma total protein concentration of less than 6.0 gm/dl is associated with an increased susceptibility to disease. Total protein estimation by refractometer offers a rapid tool for screening presurgical calves; hypoimmunoglobulinemic animals are particularly prone to develop postsurgical complications. Refractor plasma protein values of less than 6.0 gm/dl often indicate hypoimmunoglobulinemia in foals.

on healthy animals. The technique is thought to be less useful in foals (Rumbaugh et al. 1978), but foals with serum total proteins less than 5.5 gm/dl or plasma proteins less than 6.0 gm/dl have a high incidence of hypoimmunoglobulinemia. Other tests that can be used for assessment of immunoglobulin status in the field are the sodium sulfite precipitation test for calves and the zinc sulfate turbidity test for calves and foals. Interpretation of these tests is also complicated by dehydration and protein-losing enteropathy.

Feeding

Feeding dairy calves usually involves giving milk and milk substitutes for the first 5 to 10 weeks of life at the rate of 8 per cent of body weight a day for the first week, after which it is increased to 10 per cent of body weight a day. Milk is usually fed at room temperature twice a day. When a change in diet is made, for example, following transport to a veterinary hospital, milk intake should be limited to 5 per cent of body weight, with an equal volume of water fed separately to maintain fluid intake. Over the next three days, the amount of milk should be increased and the amount of water decreased until straight milk is fed; this regimen minimizes the risks of diarrhea. Hay, which stimulates rumen development, and grain are generally introduced toward the end of the first week. These should be of good quality to encourage intake and should be fed in amounts that slightly exceed consumption; uneaten feed should be replaced daily to maintain palatability. If diarrhea does develop, milk intake should be temporarily restricted to minimize malabsorption and bacterial overgrowth in the intestine. Milk is gradually reintroduced when the diarrhea ceases. Calves with persistent diarrhea should not be fasted for more than two days. Electrolyte solutions are fed to maintain hydration. Solutions containing electrolytes, glucose, glycine, and citrate provide the best absorption.

Weaning is carried out on the basis of weight and feed consumption rather than age. Holstein calves should consume at least 1 kg of concentrate (calf starter) a day and gain 15 kg by weaning. Milk and milk replacers are expensive, and there are economic advantages to weaning early.

Foals, lambs, and piglets are usually suckled by their dams during early life. If the dam is not available, they can be fostered. Successful fostering is carried out using a combination of restraint of the dam and provision of an appropriate olfactory cue. Piglets can be crossfostered by placing sows with similar farrowing dates in adjacent crates that restrain the sows while allowing the piglet free access. Lambs and calves can be given the smell of the natural offspring by soaking them in water used to clean the natural offspring or by tying the skin of the dead offspring over them. If this is unsuccessful, tying the dam's head and restraining the body so that the lamb or calf can approach and suckle without being sniffed and kicked eventually leads to acceptance. Fostering is most successful when the foster dam has only recently lost her offspring.

When fostering is impracticable or when necessary for other reasons, temporary hand feeding can be accomplished using commercially available milk replacer. There are special formulations for piglets, lambs, and foals. Alternatively, lambs can be fed ewe's milk at 5 per cent of body weight per meal three times daily from an infant's nursing bottle. Neonatal lambs can be fed cow colostrum. Weak lambs should be fed by a tube passed into the stomach to reduce the risk of inhalation pneumonia (Detection 1978). They are also easier to return to their dams (Detection 1978) if fed this way. Foals can be fed mare's milk from a calf feeding bottle or by stomach tube. In an artificial rearing situation, early weaning is usually encouraged to reduce labor costs and the risk of digestive disturbances. The intake of solid feed can be encouraged by feeding fresh, high quality hay and rolled grain mixtures containing molasses, which is often particularly palatable.

FEEDING THE SICK PATIENT

Feed Restriction

Temporary Feed Restriction. This regimen is prescribed for many surgical patients. This practice limits gut fill, reduces the risks of vomition or food reflux during anesthesia, and may decrease the strain on intestinal incisions.

Chronic feed restriction adversely affects immune function and wound healing and can eventually lead to death. For these reasons the clinician may wish to encourage feed intake in animals that are cachectic or that have a history of anorexia. The simplest and safest method of increasing feed intake in sick animals is to offer a variety of palatable feeds.

Except for caesarean section, surgery is usually avoided in heavily pregnant animals. Feed restriction should be practiced with care; several days of poor feed intake may predispose to the development of pregnancy toxemia. Hypocalcemia can develop within 8 to 24 hours when previously well-fed sheep are denied feed.

Improving Feed Intake

Feed Palatibility. The palatability of feed can be improved in a number of ways. Molasses added to grain mixes may increase palatability, especially if the feed is dusty. "Sweet feed," a mixture of rolled grain and molasses, can be particularly palatable to horses and cattle. Salt added to grain can increase feed intake in animals low in sodium. Bran masses are of low palatability for horses, but a moist mash may be preferred by animals with oral ulcers. Sick animals often refuse concentrate but continue to eat roughage, whereas fresh grass is usually eaten when all other feed is refused.

Healthy horses and cows often prefer alfalfa hay over nonlegume hay, although sheep may prefer grass hay. The high protein content of alfalfa hay often makes it a useful feed for the sick patient. Lactating dairy cattle will eat more corn silage than barley silage (Chandler and Walker 1972); corn silage is often more palatable to sick cows. The choice of feed offered to the sick animal should not be restricted to those that the animal prefers when healthy, because some sick animals will eat straw bedding and prefer poor quality hay, particularly grass hay, at this time. It is best to offer a variety of feeds, including grass, and allow the patient to choose. Fresh feed is invariably preferred over stale feed, and feed should be changed regularly and the feed buckets kept clean.

Sudden Dietary Changes. Any sudden dietary change, especially from roughage to concentrates, can cause problems in any animal. Increases in grain intake for mature horses or cows should be limited to 0.5 kg/feeding (1 kg/day). A sudden change from a grass to alfalfa hay can cause diarrhea in horses, and it is best to gradually increase the proportion of alfalfa hay fed over a five-day period.

Antipyretics. These may help increase feed intake in febrile animals. Sheep made febrile with endotoxin have decreased feed intake, and this can be partially alleviated by blocking the fever (Baile et al. 1980).

Analgesics. Feed intake can be improved with analgesics. For example, some horses with chronic skeletal pain eat better when given phenylbutazone.

Centrally Acting Feed Stimulants. These have been used to increase feed intake in sick animals. Diazepam, one of the most readily available benzodiazepines, can increase feed intake in healthy horses (Brown, Houpt, and Schryver

NUTRITION, METABOLISM, AND THE SURGICAL PATIENT / 41

1976), but in sick animals its tranquilizing and sedative actions usually predominate. A related compound, elfazepam, is a potent feeding stimulant. This has been used successfully to increase feed intake in sheep suffering from endotoxemia (Baile et al. 1981) and has been used clinically to treat selected cases of hypophagia in the horse (Della Fera, Naylor, and Baile 1978). In severely ill animals elfazepam is often ineffective in stimulating feeding, and its sedative effects may be observed instead.

Oral Alimentation. Some animals refuse all feed or have physical impairments that make eating impossible. These patients may benefit from tube or intravenous feeding. Tube feeding has several advantages: the solutions are inexpensive and do not need to be sterile. Nutrients are absorbed across the gut wall, and normal homeostatic mechanisms are not bypassed. Oral alimentation for sick animals can take several forms.

SUPPLEMENTS. Protein and vitamin B supplements help spare protein reserves and maintain adequate vitamin B levels; B vitamins are often administered parenterally. Adult animals have large reserves of the fat-soluble vitamins, and energy deficits can be met by mobilizing fat. For example, it has been shown that positive nitrogen balance can be maintained in fasting people by feeding maintenance protein without another energy source (Blackburn et al. 1973). About 600 gm of crude protein or 300 gm of digestible protein is needed to satisfy the maintenance requirements of the adult horse. Dehydrated cottage cheese may be used as a protein supplement for horses; it contains a high proportion of casein, a protein that has a 90 per cent digestibility and high biological value. Horses utilize milk protein more efficiently than linseed oil meal protein (Hintz, Schryner, and Lowe 1971), and the high biological value of dehydrated cottage cheese makes it a particularly useful supplement for sick horses. Protein supplements can be made into a slurry and injected into the mouth using a dose syringe; 50 gm of dehydrated cottage cheese has been given three times daily to horses with poor feed intake.

In ruminants, attempts are made to maintain rumen fermentation and pro-vide nutritional support at the same time. A mixture of 1 kg dehydrated alfalfa meal and 0.5 kg brewer's yeast can be given (the yeast is a source of protein and B vitamins), and up to 0.5 liter of glycerol can be added as a substrate for gluconeogenesis. A total of 30 gm of sodium chloride, 30 gm of sodium bicarbonate, and 30 gm of potassium chloride is added as a source of electrolytes, and the complete mixture is made up with 20 liters of water. Alfalfa meal will expand if allowed to soak in water for a long time, and the mix becomes unmanageable. Dextrose should not be given orally to ruminants because it is rapidly fermented to lactic acid; furthermore, there is no beneficial effect on blood glucose concentrations. The electrolyte and water mix is half isotonic with plasma; adding extra salt or reducing the volume of water can result in salt poisoning. Many dehydrated cattle will drink the electrolyte and water mixture voluntarily. Allowing dehydrated cattle access to a bucket of electrolytes and water (Table 2–3) in addition to plain water can be a very simple and effective way of hydrating them and can be very useful in the support of cattle postsurgically.

COMPLETE NUTRITIONAL SUPPORT. This regimen is indicated for some patients, particularly animals that are cachectic or when poor feed intake for more than five days is anticipated. Such animals can be fed slurries or refined diets by stomach tube.

Slurries can be made either from ground feeds or by soaking pelleted feeds in water. In ruminants, the rumen is large and a large-bore stomach tube can be passed. It is more difficult to meet the maintenance requirements of a horse with slurry; the capacity of the stomach is small and thick slurries clot the tube.

A semiliquid diet that will pass

Table 2–3 ELECTROLYTE MIXTURES FOR VOLUNTARY INTAKE IN DEHYDRATED ANIMALS*

	Sodium Bicarbonate	Sodium Chloride	Potassium Chloride
Acidotic patients	30	30	30
Alkalotic patients		60	30

*All values in grams.
Note: Dissolve electrolytes in 20 liters of water and offer free choice together with plain water.

Table 2–4 MAINTENANCE ELECTROLYTE MIXTURE*

Electrolyte	Amount (gm)
Sodium chloride (NaCl)	10
Sodium bicarbonate (NaHCO₃)	15
Potassium chloride (KCl)	75
Potassium phosphate (dibasic anhydrous) (K₂HPO₄)	60
Calcium chloride (CaCl₂ · 2H₂O)	45
Magnesium oxide (MgO)	25

*One day's requirement for a 450-kg horse.

through a stomach tube has been developed to support sick horses. The diet has been used successfully to support patients that were unable to ingest feed because of esophageal ulceration and spasm secondary to choke, pharyngeal problems, or botulism. Horses refusing feed because of toxemia associated with severe infections or unable to eat because of irreversible nervous derangements caused by protozoal myelitis have not benefited from this semiliquid diet. Ten patients requiring long-term nutritional support were tube fed for an average of 15 days; four recovered (at least two of these owed their survival to nutritional support).

The liquid diet for horses contains electrolytes (Table 2–4), dextrose, dehydrated cottage cheese, and dehydrated alfalfa meal (Naylor 1977). The mixture is low in sodium and rich in potassium, like many natural horse feeds, and the electrolyte proportions are suitable for maintenance but not for replacement purposes. Horses with fluid losses as a result of diarrhea or sweating require additional sodium. Horses have been successfully maintained on this electrolyte mixture for up to four weeks. Routine supplements of additional sodium salts are not recommended, but if hyponatremia develops, 15 gm of sodium chloride can be added daily. The proportions of electrolytes, energy, protein, and fiber are given in Table 2–5. The diet is rich in highly digestible protein and should induce positive nitrogen balance. The values for digestible energy contents in Table 2–5 are estimates, but the diet provides most of the maintenance energy requirements of the normal horse. The diet can be increased to maintenance by addition of .75 liter of glycerol or 1 kg of alfalfa meal per day. Water intake is more than sufficient for maintenance purposes, and the urine is often dilute. Sometimes an improvement in hydration is noted following the use of this regimen even though the horse had previously been receiving intravenous fluids. The diet is introduced gradually and is slowly increased in maintenance amounts (see Table 2–5).

The diet is usually administered by a nasogastric tube but may also be given through a cervical esophagotomy (Fig. 2–9). Difficulties may be encountered because the diet is viscous. The limiting factor is the amount of dehydrated alfalfa meal added. Alfalfa swells in water and should be added immediately before the mix is poured into the stomach tube. A large-diameter tube facilitates passage of the mix, and if persistent difficulties occur, the alfalfa meal can be put back to 600 gm/feeding.

Two problems seen in horses fed this

Table 2–5 RECOMMENDED TUBE FEEDING SCHEDULE*

Feed	Day						
	1	2	3	4	5	6	7
Electrolyte mixture (gm)	230	230	230	230	230	230	230
Water (liter)							
Dextrose (gm)	21	21	21	21	21	21	21
Dehydrated cottage cheese (gm)	300	400	500	600	800	800	900
	300	450	600	750	900	900	900
Dehydrated alfalfa meal (gm)	2,000	2,000	2,000	2,000	2,000	2,000	2,000
Megacalories/day (DE)	7.4	8.4	9.4	10.4	11.8	11.8	12.2

*These recommendations are for a 450-kg horse. The allowances should be divided up and fed three times daily. Maintenance requirements for a 450-kg horse are 15 Mcal of digestible energy (DE) and 580 gm of crude protein.

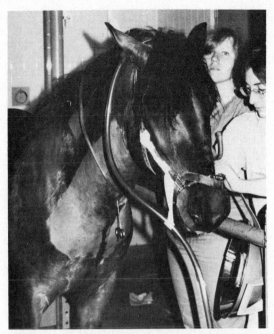

Figure 2–9 Cervical esophagotomy can be used to permanently place a small diameter stomach tube directly into the esophagus. The large-diameter tube hanging from the halter was passed nasally to outline the esophagus during the surgery. The surgery can be performed in the standing horse. It should be performed only when other methods of feeding are not feasible and the possible complications of cellulitis and possible damage to the left recurrent laryngeal nerve can be justified on the basis of an improvement in the horse's well-being (see Freeman and Naylor: JAVMA 172:314, 1978 for details).

Table 2–6 FORMULATION OF INTRAVENOUS FEEDING SOLUTION

Item	Amount
5% amino acid solution	1,000 ml
50% dextrose	500 ml
Potassium chloride	30 mEq
Sodium bicarbonate	30 mEq
Injectable multivitamins	

Note: These items are mixed aseptically to yield a solution with a final volume of 1,500 ml. The solution is hypertonic and is administered at the rate of 3 L/day to a 45-kg foal.

diet are diarrhea and laminitis. The risk of laminitis can be minimized by avoiding the diet in horses that are foundering or those that have chronic laminitis or rotation of the pedal bones. Diarrhea associated with the diet is not accompanied by fever or changes in the hemogram and responds to withdrawal or restriction of the diet and intravenous electrolyte solutions to maintain hydration. Diarrhea is not usually seen in horses on the diet for less than five days, and the incidence can be greatly reduced by making sure that alfalfa meal is not left out of the oral alimentation mix.

Intravenous Alimentation. This feeding method is both costly and time-consuming; solutions and infusion sets must be sterile. Particular care must be taken with catheter placement because solutions are hypertonic. The catheter should be in a large vessel to minimize the risk

of thrombosis. The catheter should be placed using an aseptic technique following thorough scrubbing of the skin (Burrows 1982). The catheter and tubing should be changed regularly to decrease the risk of contamination (Flack et al. 1971). Another problem with intravenous nutrition is that large loads of glucose are given by a route that bypasses the liver and many of the homeostatic mechanisms of the gut (Chandra 1972). Hyperglycemia may develop, particularly in septic patients. Fat would be particularly useful as an alternative energy source, and Intralipid has been used successfully in horses (Greatorex 1975).

Intravenous feeding may be indicated in the treatment of foals and calves with diarrhea. The smaller body size reduces some of the costs of intravenous feeding, and a formulation for calves has been reported (Hoffsis et al. 1977; Hoffsis 1977) (Table 2–6) (Fig. 2–10).

Sick animals are more prone to derangements of glucose metabolism than healthy animals, and blood glucose should not be allowed to rise above 200 to 300 mg/dl. Hyperglycemia will result in urinary loss of glucose and osmotic diuresis; very high glucose concentrations may induce convulsions (Goldberger 1975).

When feeding intravenously, the flow of nutrients should be kept as even as possible. Nutrient intake should be increased from half maintenance to maintenance over the course of two days. Additions to the fluid bottles should be minimized and should be made using a closed technique, preferably under a laminar flow hood, because additions to intravenous solution bottles in a laboratory resulted in a 25 per cent contamination rate (Dionigi et al. 1977; Flack et

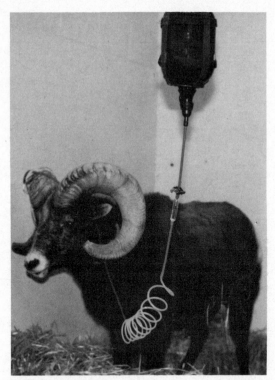

Figure 2–10 Valuable animals can be supported by intravenous feeding with dextrose, amino acids and electrolytes.

al. 1981). The addition of a broad spectrum antibiotic to the intravenous fluid may limit bacterial growth. When mixing before infusing, remember that incompatibilities may not be physically evident, e.g., the addition of vitamin complexes and tetracycline can produce precipitates, and antibiotics are best given through a separate catheter.

REFERENCES

Allden, W. G.: The effect of nutritional deprivation on the subsequent productivity of sheep and cattle. Nutr. Abs. Rev. 40:1167, 1970.

Asirvadham, M.: The bone marrow and its leukocytic response in protein deficiency. J. Infect. Dis. 83:87, 1948.

Baetz, A. L., and Mengeling, W. L.: Blood constituent changes in fasted swine. Am. J. Vet. Res. 32:1491, 1971.

Baetz, A. L., and Pearson, J. E.: Blood constituent changes in fasted ponies. Am. J. Vet. Res. 33:1941, 1972.

Baile, C. A., Naylor, J., McLaughlin, C. L., and Catanzaro, C. A.: Endotoxin elicited fever and anorexia and elfazepam-stimulated feeding in sheep. Physiol. Behav. 27:271, 1981.

Baird, G. D., Heitzman, R. J., and Hibitt, K. G.: Effects of starvation on intermediary metabolism in the lactating cow. Biochem. J. 128:1311, 1972.

Barac-Nieto, M., Spurr, G. B., Lotero, H., and Maksud, M. G.: Body composition in chronic undernutrition. Am. J. Clin. Nutr. 31:23, 1978.

Beisel, W. R.: The effect of nutrition on immunological responses of the host: The key role of scarce amino acids. Proceedings of the Western Hemispheres Nutrition Congress IV:313, 1974.

Blackburn, G. L., Bistrain, B. R., Maini, B. S., Schlamm, H. T., and Smith, M. F.: Nutritional and metabolic assessment of the hospitalized patient. JPEN 1:11, 1977.

Blackburn, G. L., Flatt, J. P., Clowes, G. H. A., O'Donnell, T. F., and Hensle, T. E.: Protein sparing therapy during periods of starvation with sepsis or trauma. Ann. Surg. 177:588, 1973.

Blackburn, G. L., Maini, B. S., and Pierce, E. C.: Nutrition in the critically ill patient. Anesthesiology 47:181, 1977.

Bramley, P. S., Denehy, H. L., and Newton, J. E.: The effect of different planes of nutrition before mating on the reproductive performance of Masham ewes. Vet. Rec. 99:294, 1976.

Brandon, M. R., Husband, A. T., and Lascelles, A. K.: The effect of glucocorticoid on immunoglobulin secretion into colostrum in cows. Aust. J. Exp. Biol. Med. Sci. 53:43, 1975.

Brandon, M. R., Watson, D. L., and Lascelles, A. K.: The mechanism of transfer of immunoglobulins into mammary secretions of cows. Aust. J. Exp. Biol. Med. Sci. 49:613, 1971.

Breukink, H. J.: Oral mono- and disaccharide tolerance tests in ponies. Am. J. Vet. Res. 35:1523, 1974.

Brown, R. F., Houpt, K. A., and Schryver, H. F.: Stimulation of food intake in horses by diazepam and promazine. Pharmacol. Biochem. Behav. 5:495, 1976.

Burrows, C. F.: Inadequate skin preparation as a cause of intravenous catheter-related infection in the dog. JAVMA 180:747, 1982.

Buzby, G. P., Mullen, J. L., Matthews, D. C., Hobbs, C. L., and Rosato, E. F.: Prognostic nutritional index in gastrointestinal surgery. Am. J. Surg. 139:160, 1980.

Cakala, S., and Bieniek, K.: Bromosulpthalein clearance and total bilirubin level in cows deprived of food and water. Zentrabl. Veterinaermed. [A] 22:605, 1975.

Chandler, P. T., Walker, H. W.: Generation of nutrient specifications for dairy cattle for computerized least cost formulation. J. Dairy Sci. 55:1741, 1972.

Chandra, R. K.: Immunocompetence in undernutrition. J. Pediatr. 81:1194, 1972.

Cuthbertson, D. P.: Symposium on surgery and nutrition: Historical approach. Proc. Nutr. Soc. 39:101, 1980.

Della Fera, M. A., Naylor, J. M., and Baile, C. A.: Benzodiazepines stimulate feeding in clinically debilitated animals. Fed. Proc. 37:401, 1978.

Detection and treatment of hypothermia in lambs. In. Prac. 4:20, 1982.

de Torre, G. L., and Rankins, B. J.: Factors affecting growth curve parameters of Hereford and Brangus cattle. J. Anim. Sci. 46:604, 1978.

Dickerson, J. W. T., and McCance, R. A.: Severe undernutrition in growing and adult animals. 8. The dimensions and chemistry of the long bones. Br. J. Nutr. 15:567, 1961.

Dionigi, R., Zonta, A., Dominioni, L., Gnes, F., and Ballalio, A.: The effects of total parenteral nutritional on immunodepression due to malnutrition. Ann. Surg. 185:467, 1977.

Downey, N. E., Connolly, J. F., and O'Shea, J.: Experimental ostertagiasis in lambs fed high and low protein (Nx 6.25) grassmeal. Vet. Rec. 85:201, 1969.

Dudrick, S. J., Copeland, E. M., and MacFadyen, B. V.: Long-term parenteral nutrition: its current status. Hosp. Pract. 10:47, 1975.

Flack, H. L., Gans, J. A., Serlick, S. E., and Dudrick, S. J.: The current status of parenteral hyperalimentation. Am. J. Hosp. Pharm. 28:326, 1971.

Fleck, A.: Protein metabolism after surgery. Proc. Nutr. Soc. 39:125, 1980.

Forbes, J. M.: The effect of pregnancy and fatness on the volume of rumen contents in the ewe. J. Agric. Sci. Camb. 72:119, 1969.

Freeman, D. E., and Naylor, J. M.: Cervical esophagastomy to permit extraoral feeding of the horse. JAVMA 172:314, 1978.

Freminet, A., Poyart, C., Leclerc, L., and Gentil, M.: Effect of fasting on glucose recycling in rats. Febbs Letters 61:294, 1976.

Goldberger, E. (ed.): A Primer of Water, Electrolyte, and Acid-Base Syndromes, 5th ed. Philadelphia: Lea & Febiger, 1975.

Good, R. A., Fernandes, G., Unis, J., Cooper, W. C., Jose, D. C., Kramer, T. R., and Hansen, M. A.: Nutritional deficiency, immunologic function and disease. Am. J. Pathol. 84:599, 1976.

Greatorex, J. C.: Intravenous nutrition in the treatment of tetanus in the horse. Vet. Rec. 97:498, 1975.

Heard, C. R. C., Frangi, S. M., Wright, P. M., and McCartney, P. R.: Biochemical characteristics of different forms of protein energy malnutrition. An experimental model using young rats. Br. J. Nutr. 37:1, 1977.

Hill, J. R., Lamond, D. R., Hennicks, D. M., Kickey, J. F., and Niswender, G. D.: The effects of undernutrition on ovarian function and fertility in beef heifers. Biol. Reprod. 2:78, 1970.

Hillman, D., Armstrong, D. V., Newman, L. E., Ellis, D. J., and Boyd, J. S.: Raising calves to improve the dairy business. Cooperative Extension Service Bulletin 412. East Lansing, MI: Michigan State University, 1982.

Himal, H. S., Allard, J. R., Nadeau, J. E., Freeman, J. B., and MacLean, L. D.: The importance of adequate nutrition in closure of small intestinal fistulas. Br. J. Surg. 61:724, 1974.

Hintz, H. F.: Growth rate of horses. In Proceedings of the American Association of Equine Practitioners 24:455, 1978.

Hintz, H. F., Schryver, H. F., and Lowe, J. E.: Comparison of a blend of milk products and linseed meal as protein supplements for young growing horses. J. Anim. Sci. 33:1274, 1971.

Hoffsis, G. F.: Saving the valuable calf. Proc. Bov. Pract. 10:119, 1977.

Hoffsis, G. F., Gingerich, D. A., Sherman, D. M., and Bruner, R. R.: Total intravenous feeding of calves. JAVMA 171:67, 1977.

Holmes, J. H. G., and Lambourne, L. J.: The relation between plasma free fatty acid concentration and the digestible energy intake of cattle. Res. Vet. Sci. 11:27, 1970.

Irving, T. T.: Effects of malnutrition and hyperalimentation on wound healing. Surg. Gynecol. Obstet. 146:33, 1978.

Keusch, G. T.: Effects of malnutrition on immunological functions. Proceedings of the Western Hemispheres Nutrition Congress IV:319, 1974.

Klain, G. J., Sullivan, F. J., Chinn, K. S. K., Hannon, J. P., and Jones, L. D.: Metabolic responses to fasting and subsequent refeeding in the pig. J. Nutr. 107:426, 1977.

Kronfeld, D. S.: Feeding, nutrition and gastrointestinal disorders. In Veterinary Gastroenterology. Philadelphia: Lea and Febiger, 1980, pp. 239–240.

Kronfeld, D. S.: Ketosis in pregnant sheep and lactating cows, a review. Aust. Vet. J. 48:680, 1972.

Kronfeld, D. S., and Raggi, F.: Irregular plasma glucose concentrations, elevated plasma nonesterified fatty acid concentrations and unchanged glucokinase activities in brain, muscle and liver during pregnancy toxaemia in sheep. Res. Vet. Sci. 7:493, 1966.

Law, D. K., Dudrick, S. J., and Abdou, N. I.: The effect of dietary protein depletion on immunocompetence. Ann. Surg. 179:168, 1974.

Lintern-Moore, S.: A differential effect of protein and calorie deficiency on ovarian follicular growth in the sow. Mech. Aging Dev. 7:199, 1978.

Logan, E. F.: The influence of husbandry on colostrum yield and immunoglobulin concentration in beef cows. Br. Vet. J. 133:120, 1977.

Lymphocyte number and function in protein malnutrition. Nutr. Rev. 34:208, 1976.

Manston, R., Russel, A. M., Dew, S. M., and Payne, J. M.: The influence of dietary protein upon blood composition in dairy cows. Vet. Rec. 96:497, 1975.

McCance, R. A.: Severe undernutrition in growing and adult animals. 1. Production and general effects. Br. J. Nutr. 14:59, 1960.

McCance, R. A., Ford, E. H. R., and Brown, W. A. B.: Severe undernutrition in growing and adult animals 7. Development of the skull, jaws and teeth in pigs. Br. J. Nutr. 15:213, 1961.

McFarlane, H., and Hamid, J.: Cell-mediated immune response in malnutrition. Clin. Exper. Immunol. 13:153, 1973.

McGarry, J. D., Meier, J. M., and Foster, D. W.: The effects of starvation and refeeding on carbohydrate and lipid metabolism in vivo and in the perfused rat liver. J. Biol. Chem. 248:270, 1973.

Morrison, F. B.: In Feeds and Feeding. 20th ed. Ithaca, New York: Morrison Publishing Co., 1944, p. 79.

Morrow, D. A.: Fat cow syndrome. J. Dairy Sci. 59:1625, 1976.

Morrow, D. A., Hillman, D., Dade, A. W., and Kitchen, H.: Clinical investigation of a dairy herd with the fat cow syndrome. JAVMA 174:161, 1979.

Mullen, J. L., Buzby, G. P., Matthews, D. C., Smale, B. F., and Rosato, E. F.: Reduction of operative morbidity and mortality by combined preoperative and postoperative nutritional support. Ann. Surg. 192:604, 1980.

Murray, M. J., and Murray, A. B.: Anorexia of infection as a mechanism of host defense. Am. J. Clin. Nutr. 32:593, 1976.

Naylor, J. M.: Unpublished data, 1982.

Naylor, J. M.: Colostral immunity in the calf and the foal. Vet. Clin. North Am. Large Anim. Prac. 1:331, 1979.

Naylor, J. M.: The nutrition of the sick horse. J. Eq. Med. Surg. 1:64, 1977.

Naylor, J. M.: Studies on an all-liquid, zero-fiber, elemental diet in the horse. Am. J. Dig. Dis. 22:570, 1977.

Naylor, J. M., and Kenyon, S. J.: Effect of total calorific deprivation on host defense in the horse. Res. Vet. Sci. 31:369, 1981.

Naylor, J. M., Kronfeld, D. S., and Acland, H.: Hyperlipemia in horses: Effects of undernutrition and disease. Am. J. Vet. Res. 41:899, 1980.

Naylor, J. M., Kronfeld, D. S., Bech-Neilsen, S., et al.: Plasma total protein measurement for prediction of disease and mortality in calves. JAVMA 171:635, 1977.

Naylor, J. M., Kronfeld, D. S., and Johnson, K.: Fasting hyperbilirubinemia and its relationship to plasma free fatty acids and triglycerides in the horse. Proc. Soc. Exp. Biol. Med. Sci. 165:86, 1980.

Newton, D. J., Clark, R. G., and Woods, H. F.: The nutritional fate of the undernourished surgical patient in convalescence. Proc. Nutr. Soc. 39:141, 1980.

Palmblad, J.: Fasting (acute energy deprivation) in man: Effect on polymorphonuclear granulocyte functions, plasma iron and serum transferrin. Scand. J. Haematol. 17:217, 1976.

Parker, B. N. J., and Blowey, R. W.: Investigations into the relationship of selected blood components to nutrition and fertility of the diary cow under commercial farm conditions. Vet. Rec. 98:394, 1976.

Pomeroy, R. W.: The effect of a submaintenance diet on the composition of the pig. J. Agric. Sci. 31:50, 1941.

Reddy, V., Jagadeesan, V., Ragharumulu, N., Bhaskharam, C., and Srikantia, S. G.: Functional significance of growth retardation in malnutrition. Am. J. Clin. Nutr. 29:3, 1976.

Richard, J. R.: Current concepts in the metabolic responses to injury, infection and starvation. Proc. Nutr. Soc. 39:113, 1980.

Robinson, J. J.: Some aspects of ewe nutrition. Vet. Rec. 92:602, 1973.

Rumbaugh, G. E., Ardans, A. A., Ginno, D., et al.: Measurement of neonatal equine immunoglobulins for assessment of colostral immunoglobulin transfer: Comparison of single radial immunodiffusion with the zinc sulfate turbidity test, serum electrophoresis, refractometry for total serum protein and the sodium sulfite precipitation test. JAVMA 172:321, 1978.

Saudek, C. D., and Felig, P.: The metabolic effects of starvation. Am. J. Med. 60:117, 1976.

Schryver, H. F., and Hintz, H. F.: Feeding horses. Extension Information Bulletin 94. Ithaca, NY: Cornell University, 1975.

Selman, I. E., McEwan, A. D., and Fisher, E. W.: Absorption of immune lactoglobulin by newborn dairy calves. Res. Vet. Sci. 12:205, 1971a.

Selman, I. E., McEwan, A. D., and Fisher, E. W.: Studies on dairy calves allowed to suckle their dams at fixed times post partum. Res. Vet. Sci. 12:1, 1971b.

Selman, I. E., McEwan, A. D., and Fisher, E. W.: Studies on natural suckling in cattle, during the first 8 hours post partum. I. Behavioural studies in dams. Anim. Behav. 18:276, 1970a.

Selman, I. E., McEwan, A. D., and Fisher, E. W.: Studies on natural suckling in cattle during the first 8 hours post partum. II. Behavioural studies in calves. Anim. Behav. 18:284, 1970b.

Seth, V., and Chandra, R. K.: Opsonic activity, phagocytosis, and bactericidal capacity of polymorphs in undernutrition. Arch. Dis. Child. 47:282, 1972.

Sirisinha, S., Suskind, R., Edelman, R., Charupatana, C., and Olsen, R. E.: Complement and C3-proactivator levels in children with protein calorie malnutrition and effect of dietary treatment. Lancet 1:1016, 1973.

Skinsnes, O. F., and Woodridge, R. L.: The relationship of biological defense mechanisms to the antibiotic activity of penicillin. 1. The modifying influence of penicillin on the pattern of pneumococcic infection and the immune response in the protein depleted rat. J. Infect. Dis. 83:78, 1948.

Smythe, P. M., Schonland, M., Bereton Stiles, G. G., Coovadia, H. M., Grace, H. J., Loening, W. E. K., Mafoyane, A., Parent, M. A., and Vos, G. H.: Thymolymphatic deficiency and depression of cell mediated immunity in protein calorie malnutrition. Lancet 2:939, 1971.

Spivey, J., and Johnston, I. D.: The effect of environmental temperature and nutritional intake on the metabolic response to abdominal surgery. Br. J. Surg. 59:93, 1972.

Stephenson, L. S., Pond, W. G., Krook, L. P., and Nesheim, M. C.: The relationship between ascaris infection, dietary protein level and intestinal pathology in growing pigs. Fed. Proc. 36:1181, Abst. 4816, 1977.

Voitk, A. J., Brown, R. A., McArdle, A. H., Hinchey, E. J., and Gurd, F. N.: Clinical uses of an elemental diet—preliminary studies. Can. Med. Assoc. J. 107:123, 1972.

Wensing, T. H., Schotman, A. J. H., and Kronman, J.: Various new clinical chemical data in the blood of normal ponies and ponies affected with hyperlipemia (hyperlipoproteinemia). Tijdschr. Diergeneeskd. 98:673, 1973.

Widdowson, E. M., Dickerson, J. W. T., and McCance, R. A.: Severe undernutrition in growing and adult animals 4. The impact of severe undernutrition on the chemical composition of the soft tissues of the pig. Br. J. Nutr. 14:457, 1960.

Wildman, E. E., et al.: A dairy cow body condition scoring system and its relationship to selected production characteristics. J. Dairy Sci. 65:495, 1982.

Witherspoon, D.: Nutrition and breeding management of problem mares. Mod. Vet. Prac. 58:459, 1977.

CHAPTER 3

THE HEMATOPOIETIC SYSTEM

VICTOR PERMAN, D.V.M., PH.D.

The indications for hematological examination of the surgical patient vary with the nature of the surgical procedure and the species of animal. Preoperative considerations may be the establishment of a data base or a definition of the surgical problem. Monitoring of the patient during surgery is frequently necessary. Postoperative considerations relate to monitoring therapy and defining complications that may arise. At times, preoperative and postoperative laboratory examinations are performed without a time factor constraint. Emergency surgical intervention usually demands readily available laboratory services. These circumstances may determine the usefulness of the various laboratory tests. A determination will have to be made regarding tests to be provided within a practice and those that should be sent to a central laboratory for analysis.

It is the intent, in this chapter, to provide the most important aspects of hematological examination for the veterinary surgeon relevant to surgical problems. It is not intended to provide all the basic information presented in the excellent textbooks of veterinary hematology and clinical pathology.

INDICATIONS FOR HEMATOLOGICAL EXAMINATION

The clinical indications for presurgical hematological examination may be subdivided into those desired for establishment of a data base and those necessary for diagnostic evaluation. For a presurgical data base, a panel of tests may be designed based on ease of monitoring and economic considerations. When hematological examination is necessary for definition of the diagnosis, selection of tests may extend well beyond the minimal data base.

The nature of the surgical problem and the species involved will influence the selection of tests. The horse with colic will require frequent evaluation of certain parameters. Under these circumstances, the tests selected should be simple, should require a minimum period of time, and should be proved to generate useful clinical information.

Postoperative hematological evaluation will vary, depending on many factors. Most frequently, the surgeon is concerned with evaluation for complications. The selection of tests will generally include the minimal data base; it may be expanded to assess certain cellular and biochemical parameters.

MATERIALS AND METHODS FOR HEMATOLOGICAL EXAMINATIONS

The quality specimen is essential for quality laboratory results. Presampling considerations should include the necessary equipment and supplies for the situation. Factors of importance will be emphasized.

Laboratory Report Form. A form to identify and accompany the specimen should include animal identification, date, and time of collection. Appropriate notations should be made regarding previous medication, method of restraint, and status and reaction of the animal at the time of sampling. Such information may seem superfluous at the moment, but it may be difficult to recall or obtain when the generated data is interpreted.

The Specimen. For a hematological examination, the specimen is a carefully drawn and appropriately preserved blood sample. The anatomic sites and approaches to drawing a blood specimen are amply illustrated (Schalm, Jain, and Carroll 1975; Archer and Jeffcott 1977).

Equipment. The equipment usually includes a syringe and needle or the standard needle holder–vacuum tube system. The effect of needle size and blood flow on hemolysis is a matter of frequent controversy (Moss and Staunton 1970). It is commonly thought that one should use a large bore needle to avoid hemolysis. This is, in fact, erroneous. Hemolysis is affected by the velocity of blood flow and the nature of the entrance and exit sites. Small bore needles have a lower potential blood velocity. Aspiration through 20-, 22-, and 25-gauge needles should not be associated with hemolysis under usual sampling conditions. Shorter needle lengths and larger bores increase the velocity of flow, thereby increasing the potential for hemolysis. Well-rounded entrance sites are less hemolytic than are sharp-edged entrance sites. Removing the needle from the syringe to fill the sample tube will minimize hemolysis. Jeffcott found that suction apparatus (e.g., Vacutainer, Becton, Dickinson) contributes to appreciable hemolysis, rendering the system impracticable for diagnostic tests for that species that require hemolysis-free specimens (1977).

Anticoagulant. The anticoagulant of choice for hematological examination is the dipotassium salt of ethylenediaminetetraacetic acid (EDTA). The concentration of EDTA used is 1.0 to 2.0 mg/ml of blood. Excess EDTA (more than 2 mg/ml of blood) should be avoided since it causes shrinkage of the erythrocytes. Changes in erythrocyte volume due to anticoagulant excess may invalidate the packed red cell volume (PCV) and erythrocyte indices (Penny et al. 1970). Properly preserved blood maintained at 4°C will be satisfactory for erythrocyte parameters and leukocyte counts for up to 48 hours (Penny et al. 1970). Deterioration of specimens occurs more rapidly at higher temperatures and with freezing. The effects of the disease state may hasten sample deterioration.

When EDTA-preserved blood is used for the preparation of blood smears, critical observations are not always possible. The blood film should be made as soon as possible and, preferably, from fresh, unanticoagulated blood.

Blood Film. A properly prepared fresh blood film made by the slide or coverslip method is essential for hematological examination (Schalm, Jain, and Carroll 1975). Properly prepared blood smears are achieved when both the preparation and examination are conducted by the same individual, one who has a knowledge of what constitutes an acceptable smear. When glass slide or coverslip smears of blood are made, the cellular elements do not distribute randomly. The cells distribute according to mass and composition, i.e., the heavy, dense cells settle out first and larger, low-density cells tend to be carried toward the feathered end. These light cells include platelet clusters, reticulocytes, and the following leukocytes: neutrophils, eosinophils, basophils, and monocytes with abundant cytoplasm. This distribution phenomenon is accentuated when the viscosity of blood is decreased, as in the anemic patient.

Preparation of the Blood Smear. Schalm, Jain, and Carroll (1975) have described slide and coverslip methods for blood smear preparation. Because of the importance of a quality blood smear, an additional technique for slide preparation is described. Clean slides are placed on a flat, firm surface. A small drop of blood, free of air bubbles, is placed at least 1 cm from the end of the slide. The pusher slide should be clean and free of nicks. The pusher slide is held lightly and placed at a 30 to 45° angle on the slide to be spread. As the pusher slide is drawn back to cover the drop of blood, there is the tendency to allow the blood to flow to the margins before advancing the pusher slide. This is followed by a slow forward motion, which will usually affect the uniform spreading of cells. Variations in this step of the smear process will improve cell distribution. The pusher slide is drawn back to cover the drop of blood and is immediately advanced forward. The motion is that of a pendulum, back through the drop and forward without stopping. When this procedure is continuous, the speed of the pusher slide is faster and more constant, resulting in more uniform distribution of cells. The decreased viscosity of blood in the anemic patient is controlled by reducing the size of the drop of blood and increasing the speed of movement of the pusher slide. The smear shape is rather constant. The edges of the smear are parallel but away from the sides of the slide, and the feathered end remains in the middle portion of the slide so that it may be easily examined under the microscope.

The blood smear should be dried rapidly. Under humid and/or cold conditions it is necessary to provide heat or forced air to hasten the drying. Warming plates, hair dryers, or a fan may be used. Slow drying is objectionable because it results in the crenation of erythrocytes and enhances precipitated stain formation.

Laboratory. Whether the laboratory tests are performed within the veterinary hospital or by an outside laboratory depends on the circumstances peculiar to each veterinary practice. When outside laboratories are used, it is important to know that the methods and instruments used are proper for animal bloods. Knowledge of species differences and a quality control program are necessary. Know your laboratory, whether it is within your hospital or an outside service. This is most important when veterinary practices use the services of a human hospital laboratory. Species differences may require adjustments in methods and instrumentation. Knowledge of quantitative and qualitative species differences are necessary for the proper handling of veterinary specimens.

Tests. The laboratory tests conducted will be influenced by need, availability, and usefulness of data generated. Significant factors concerning each test will be discussed. Appropriate methods are available in standard veterinary textbooks.

ERYTHROCYTES

The packed cell volume (PCV), hemoglobin (Hb), and erythrocyte count (RBC) are commonly performed tests. Erythrocyte morphology may yield useful information.

Packed Cell Volume

The PCV as determined by the microhematocrit method provides the most useful measurement of the erythron. Technical aspects of the method are of sufficient importance to require comment. The suspension stability of erythrocytes in ruminants is good, whereas erythrocytes of the horse and pig settle more rapidly. Complete mixing of blood prior to filling the microhematocrit tubes is essential for accurate results. Centrifuge maintenance is required to ensure high speeds. Blood tubes should be filled to the proper amount. EDTA excess may result in a decrease in PCV of 25 per cent or more (Penny et al. 1970). The hematocrit (Hct) calculated from instrument measurement of the mean red cell volume and the red cell count eliminates the effect of trapped plasma and is, therefore, a lower value than the PCV.

The PCV is influenced by the red cell mass and plasma volume. These determinations are seldom made in veterinary practices.

Splenic contraction associated with excitement and epinephrine release may greatly increase the PCV in some species. The status of the spleen and the degree of contraction at the time of sampling is unknown and a matter of interpretation. Splenic dilation may occur with chemical restraint, anesthesia, or drug therapy, resulting in a lowered PCV.

Alterations of the plasma volume occur in dehydration states, with a resultant increase in the PCV, a state of hemoconcentration. The plasma proteins usually increase concurrently. The plasma volume may increase during persistent hyperproteinemic states, thus lowering the PCV.

Hemoglobin

There are several methods for determining the hemoglobin concentration of blood. The cyanmethemoglobin method determines total hemoglobin and is the accepted standard method. The accuracy of this spectrophotometric method is ±

0.5 gm/dl. Hemoglobin determination should not be performed in lieu of the PCV determination. Its usefulness lies principally in the calculation of the red blood cell indices. Hemoglobin determination provides a more valid assessment of circulating red cells than the PCV when excess EDTA effects are present.

Red Blood Cell Count

The red blood cell count, (RBC), when measured accurately with electronic or photoelectric instrumentation, is used to determine the mean corpuscular volume (MCV) and mean corpuscular hemoglobin (MCH). The usefulness of these determinations in large animal surgical practice is limited. Within species, breed- and age-dependent values from previous data bases should be available. Reference values for breed, age, and sex may be inadequate for meaningful comparison.

Erythrocyte Indices

The red cell indices or mean cell constants, based on the method used for humans (Wintrobe 1974), provide useful clinical information only when the limitations of the method and normal values are understood. The MCV, MCH, and mean corpuscular hemoglobin concentration (MCHC) may be calculated using the following equations:

$$MCV \text{ (femtoliters)} = \frac{PCV \times 10}{RBC \text{ count in millions}}$$

(Example: PCV 35; RBC = 7.0 million

$$MCV = \frac{35 \times 10}{7} = 50 \text{ fl})$$

$$MCH \text{ (picograms)} = \frac{Hb \times 10}{RBC \text{ count in millions}}$$

(Example: Hb = 12.0; RBC = 6.0 million

$$MCH = \frac{12.0}{6.0} \times 10 = 20 \text{ pg})$$

$$MCHC \text{ (g/dl)} = \frac{Hb}{PCV} \times 100$$

(Example: Hb = 12; PCV = 36

$$MCHC = \frac{12}{36} \times 100 = 33 \text{ g/dl})$$

Red cell index values based on the PCV and the Hct are different because of non-equivalence of the methods.

MEAN CORPUSCULAR VOLUME

The MCV is determined by calculation or by direct volume measurement with electronic particle counters. Both methods require attention to specimen management to avoid in vitro changes in erythrocyte volume. In controlled studies, the MCV may be the most sensitive method of detecting increased erythrogenesis. Microcytosis is most accurately determined by MCV measurements. Reference values for the MCV may be unreliable because of age, breed, and within-breed differences. Baseline values for the population in question are required.

MEAN CORPUSCULAR HEMOGLOBIN

The MCH is useful in evaluating iron and copper deficiencies when low values are found. The limitations of the MCH are similar to those associated with the MCV.

MEAN CORPUSCULAR HEMOGLOBIN CONCENTRATION

The MCHC is relatively constant among mammals and ranges from 31 to 36 g/dl. MCHC values above 36 g/dl reflect errors in Hb or PCV determinations, except for members of the family Camelidae, in which higher values occur. Values of 30 g/dl or less indicate decreased hemoglobin content of erythrocytes. The MCHC may be low in two different conditions: 1) in the presence of intense erythrogenesis during which high numbers of reticulocytes are present, and 2) in cases of iron and copper deficiencies, in which virtually no reticulocytes are found; the decrease is due to a lack of hemoglobin. Reticulocytes are low in hemoglobin because of the size of the reticulocytes and incomplete hemoglobin synthesis. As the reticulocyte matures, a full complement of hemoglobin is formed. In species releasing large numbers of reticulocytes, the indices must be interpreted in light of the reticulocyte count. Similarly, a classification of anemias based on red cell indices may be confusing, since marked species variations occur in reticulocyte release.

Reticulocyte Counts

Evaluation of the anemic patient includes determination of the state of erythrogenesis. Increased erythrogenesis is seen following blood loss and blood destruction, in newborns of some species, and in bone marrow repopulation following recovery from hypoplasia of the bone marrow. In the cow, sheep, goat, and pig (but not in the horse), reticulocytes may be released into the peripheral blood when the stimulus for erythropoiesis is great. The horse does not release reticulocytes from the bone marrow; equine evaluation is made based on bone marrow reticulocyte levels.

The reticulocyte may be demonstrated by one of several methods: 1) polychromasia on a Wright's stained blood smear, 2) supravital stains, which aggregate or accentuate reticulocytes, or 3) new methylene blue on an air-dried blood smear (Schalm 1964). In ruminants, the polychromatophilic erythrocyte may appear as basophilic stippling and both are enumerated to determine the reticulocyte count.

Smears made too slowly will result in large, low-density cells (such as reticulocytes) being drawn to the feathered end in greater than normal numbers. The count may be expressed as absolute reticulocyte number, reticulocyte percentage, or a semiquantitative score such as slight, moderate, and marked. The absolute reticulocyte count is based on reticulocyte percentage and the red cell count. This method of expressing results is used when easily obtained and accurate RBC counts are available. The reticulocyte percentage method is recommended for each species. The semiquantitative score requires the technician to make an interpretation based on knowledge of the physiological response of that species. This judgment should only be made by the veterinarian.

LEUKOCYTES

The method of choice for leukocyte counting in veterinary practice is the hemocytometer method. Instrument counting of leukocytes is used in central laboratories and in veterinary practices in which frequent determinations are made. The use of cell counters necessitates well-trained staff. Some instruments require calibration for each animal species. Internal and external quality control programs are advised when cell-counting instruments are used. Gross errors in leukocyte count may be readily apparent from smear examination.

Differential Cell Counts

The quality of the differential cell count is dependent on the technician, the quality of the smear, and the technique employed. The usual procedure is to count at least 100 leukocytes while systemically scanning the smear in an area of good cell distribution. Distribution errors are reduced as more cells are enumerated. Confidence limits, from which one may estimate the probable error of a different cell count, are reported in Table 3–1 (Cartwright 1968).

Leukocyte differential cell counts are usually made under 1000× magnification. Differential cell counts should be made at 400 to 500× magnification. When the standard 40× objective is used, a drop of immersion oil is placed on the smear and a glass coverslip is applied. This allows cells to be viewed with suffi-

Table 3–1 95 PER CENT CONFIDENCE LIMITS FOR DIFFERENTIAL LEUKOCYTE COUNTS*

Percentage of Given Cell Type	100 Cells Counted	200 Cells Counted
0	0.0–3.0	0.0–1.5
1	0.5–4.7	0.2–3.1
2	0.4–6.3	0.7–4.6
4	1.4–9.1	2.0–7.2
5	2.0–10.5	2.7–8.5
10	4.0–16.0	5.8–14.2
20	12.0–28.0	14.3–25.7
30	20.8–39.2	35.5–36.5
40	30.2–49.8	33.1–46.9
50	50.0–60.0	42.9–57.1
60	50.2–69.8	53.1–66.9
70	60.8–79.2	63.5–76.5
80	72.0–88.0	74.3–85.7
90	84.0–96.0	85.8–94.2

*From Cartwright: Diagnostic Laboratory Hematology. New York: Grune & Stratton, 1968. Reprinted courtesy of the author and Grune & Stratton.

Note: For percentages of 5 or less, the limits were derived assuming a Poisson rather than a binomial distribution.

cient clarity for differential cell counts. Furthermore, cell identification is easier when large populations of cells are viewed.

Differential cell counts should be made on smears prepared from fresh blood. Morphological changes occur in leukocytes when anticoagulant blood is used. Blood that has been preserved with anticoagulant should be refrigerated if smears are not made immediately. Although it is possible to differentiate cells on smears made from anticoagulant blood preserved for as long as 24 hours, morphological changes will preclude precise evaluation.

Leukocyte Responses

Species response differences require that variables be recognized for precise interpretation of data. In addition to differences among the species, variables include breed, sex, age, stage of lactation, environment, latent diseases, seasonal changes, and sampling differences.

The total leukocyte count should not be interpreted unless the blood smear is examined for cellular constituents. The differential cell count allows quantification of each leukocyte. Absolute values for each leukocyte type are preferable to percentages or ratios.

NEUTROPHILS

Neutrophils are categorized according to location. The bone marrow is the site for proliferation, maturation, and storage of reserve cells. The reserve or storage pool releases neutrophils in response to stimuli from inflammatory sites. Storage pool release of neutrophils results from high levels of exogenous or endogenous steroids. A similar response is elicited with low-dose endotoxin (Jain and Lasmanis 1978). Animals with subclinical, low-level demands for neutrophils may lack sufficient reserve cells to elicit a significant release response to appropriate stimuli. Species variability in replenishment of the granulocyte reserve and response to neutropenic conditions is important to interpretation (Valli et al. 1969). The degree of response to

release of storage neutrophils through noninflammatory and inflammatory stimuli varies among different species, and young animals tend to be more responsive than adults.

The neutrophils in the blood stream are in transport from sites of production to sites of utilization and natural destruction. Two compartments exist in blood, the circulating and marginated pools. The marginated pool of cells is released with excitement and fright, i.e., the so-called epinephrine effect. Variability in neutrophil counts in part relates to sampling conditions that affect the number of circulating cells. Conversely, drugs that decrease heart rate and blood flow may decrease the white blood cell count, probably by increasing the marginated pool of cells (Usenik and Cronkite 1965).

NEUTROPENIA

The mechanism of neutropenia is varied. Production failure in pancytopenic condition reflects injury to stem cells. Neutropenia is commonly found in association with severe inflammation. Endotoxin produces a neutropenia in animals when administered extravascularly (Jain, Schalm, and Lasmanis 1978; Burrows 1979) or intravascularly (Jain and Lasmanis 1978). The mechanism of endotoxin-induced neutropenia is activation of complement via the alternate pathway (Jacob et al. 1980). The complement appears to cause vascular leukostasis through granulocyte aggregation (Jacob et al. 1980). Toxins of other bacteria that activate complement within the vascular system would have a similar mechanism for inducing neutropenia.

The effect of toxins on cells in the proliferative and maturation compartments is variable. Neutrophil production may be adversely affected. Maturation aberrations occur in that polyribosome aggregates persist in maturing cells, giving rise to basophilia of the cytoplasm in Wright's stained smears (the "toxic neutrophil"). Invariably, a degenerative left shift is present when toxic neutrophils are observed. The clinical interpretation is that of overwhelming bacterial sepsis and/or toxemia.

NEUTROPHILIA

Increased numbers of circulating neutrophils may reflect inflammatory or noninflammatory release of cells from the production area. In inflammation-induced neutrophilia, a left shift may be seen, which is usually absent in steroid or stress neutrophilia. The magnitude of the neutrophilia and the degree of left shift may be more dependent on species response variations than on the inciting disease process.

EOSINOPHILS

Eosinophil leukocytes appear to participate in an array of disease processes including allergic disorders, metazoan parasitic infestations, and some neoplasias (Bass 1979). In some species, the numbers of circulating eosinophils clearly reflect response to disease. In the cow, high numbers of eosinophils were found in a random sample of dairy cattle (Perman et al. 1970). These values differ from those reported for cattle in other geographical areas (Schalm, Jain, and Carroll, 1975). The significance of these differences and the high eosinophil numbers for some species is unknown.

BASOPHILS

The response of basophils in disease is seen in some species. When increased basophils are found, the stimulus for the response is similar to that for eosinophils. Basophils interact with homocytotropic antibodies. Basophils release mediators in anaphylaxis and participate in cell-mediated hypersensitivity reactions.

MONOCYTES

Monocytes are bone marrow-derived cells that are part of the monocyte-macrophage system. The fixed phagocytic cells of the blood stream are located in the spleen and liver. Monocytes are distributed in the blood stream in the circulating and marginated pools.

Administration of corticosteroids may induce significant monocytosis in some species (Schalm, Jain, and Carroll 1975). In general, those species that respond with significant neutrophilia to corticosteroids develop significant monocytosis.

Monocytes function as phagocytic cells (Territo and Cline 1975). Diseases resulting in excessive intravascular debris are associated with monocytosis, such as is seen in severe hemolytic crises. Monocyte levels may increase during the recovery period in inflammatory disease. However, the connotation that monocytosis is equated with chronicity is misleading. In some species, a significant monocytosis may be seen in acute disease processes. The nature of the stimulus and the species response must be considered in interpretation.

LYMPHOCYTES

Lymphocyte numbers are influenced by species and age. Species with short gestation periods, i.e., those giving birth to immature young, tend to have low lymphocyte numbers in the neonatal period. This is followed by increased lymphocyte numbers as immunological experiences are encountered. Thereafter, there tends to be a fall in lymphocyte numbers throughout the life of the animal. Species differences are significant. Conditions of sampling may affect lymphocyte numbers, particularly in young animals (Schalm, Jain, and Carroll 1975).

Lymphocyte responses in disease relate to physiological effects of corticosteroids and immunological cellular functions. The general response of lymphocytes to stress, whether related to functional or organic disease, is a decrease in number. Severe lymphopenia may be either hereditary or acquired. Agents may directly affect lymphocyte number through decreased production. Lymphocyte increases in response to disease are not common, and most increases relate to immunologically mediated mechanisms.

PLATELETS

The blood platelet count may be made on EDTA-preserved samples for up to 24 hours when specimens are properly refrigerated. Instrument counts are possible on most species. Hemocytometer counts by phase contrast or light microscopy are standard methods. Platelet estimates made from stained blood smears have been shown to correlate well with direct counts (Abbey and Belliveau, 1978). In the author's laboratory, each platelet in the red cell area of the blood smear approximates 15,000 platelets (at 1000× magnification). Platelet clumping invalidates this method of platelet estimation. However, large platelet clumps are indicative of adequate numbers of platelets for effective hemostatic mechanisms.

EXAMINATION OF THE BLOOD SMEAR

Examination of erythrocytes, leukocytes, and platelets on stained blood films for morphological changes and inclusions provides information that may not be evident from quantitative studies. The quality of the smear and stain is the principal limiting factor for the technician and veterinarian. After the blood smear has been examined for the differential cell count, it is examined in a systematic manner for other changes. The shape of the smear and the staining density on direct visual observation yield information regarding quality of the smear and stain. The following protocol may be used for the summary of findings.

Platelets	Erythrocytes	Leukocytes
Number	Size	Number
Morphology	Color	Differential
	Shape	Morphology
	Inclusions	

The microscopic examination should begin with the scanning 4.0× objective (40×). A sweep of the feathered end and the deeper portions of the slide is made for unusually large cells and formed structures. The 10× objective (100×) will define cell distribution. Gross impressions may be made of the leukocyte count as to leukopenic, normal, or elevated. At 100×, it is possible to identify most white cells. Changes in erythrocytes and platelets may be apparent at this magnification.

At 400×, most changes in the formed elements are recognizable. Estimates of the differential cell count are made. At this magnification, the red cell area of the smear is localized. The red cell area of a blood smear is that portion of the slide in which erythrocytes are in sufficient amounts of plasma to assume shape changes; there is uniform distribution of erythrocytes with minimal overlapping of cells. When the area is too thin, erythrocytes are stretched, and shape changes will be altered. In the thin area the cells are all round and without central pallor. In areas that are too thick, rouleau formation may be present, and drying artifacts, such as punched-out centers or stomatocyte-like shapes, are more pronounced.

The red cell area is examined under 1000× for platelet number and morphological changes. The erythrocytes are examined for reticulocyte count and changes in size, color, and shape. Inclusions are evaluated at this magnification.

Definitive changes in leukocyte morphology and the presence and absence of inclusions are best seen at this magnification. For the hematologist, the blood smear is the most critical and useful portion of the hematological examination for yielding significant clinical information. It should be likewise for the veterinary surgeon.

TOTAL PLASMA PROTEIN (TPP)

The TPP may be determined with the use of a temperature-compensated refractometer, which measures the refractive index. Through the use of tables or direct reading refractometers, the TPP is measured. Hemolysis and lipemia interfere and yield erroneous results. The TPP of animals is age dependent. Newborn animals have low TPP values, which increase with stimulation of the immune system. Increases in plasma proteins occur with dehydration and disease in which immunoglobulin production is markedly stimulated for long periods of time (the polyclonal gammopathies) (Schalm 1970a). Decreases in TPP reflect protein loss, production failure, and hemodilution phenomena.

FIBRINOGEN

Fibrinogen precipitates at 56° to 58°C, whereas other plasma proteins remain in solution. Kaneko and Smith (1967) applied this principle to animal blood for determination of fibrinogen. Increases in plasma fibrinogen correlate with the degree of inflammation present. Fibrinogen levels are usually increased in acute and chronic inflammatory disease and may be more sensitive than leukocyte elevation in detecting inflammatory and neoplastic diseases (Schalm 1970a; 1970b; Schalm, Smith, and Kaneko 1970). Decreased fibrinogen levels occur with fibrinolysis. Thromboplastin release into the circulation in disseminated intravascular coagulation results in fibrinolysis and a decline in fibrinogen levels. Schalm, Jain, and Carroll (1975) recommend a plasma protein:fibrinogen ratio (PP:F) as useful in interpreting disease in the presence of dehydration. The ratio is determined by subtracting the fibrinogen level from TPP and dividing the remainder by the fibrinogen value. Ratios below 10:1 indicate a marked increase in fibrinogen for most species (Schalm, Jain, and Carroll 1975).

SEDIMENTATION RATE

The sedimentation rate of animal blood is species dependent and is influenced by both the PCV and composition of plasma proteins. The sedimentation rate, when corrected for influence of the PCV, does correlate with the quantity and quality of plasma proteins. However, it is species dependent. The sedimentation rate as a test for latent disease is seldom used in large animal practice since the TPP and fibrinogen determination yield similar information. Harkness (1971) feels that determination of plasma viscosity offers several advantages over sedimentation rate determination. Archer (1977) gives normal plasma viscosity values for the horse, cow, and dog.

BLOOD TYPING

Blood typing of animals is restricted to a limited number of laboratories because of the complexity of animal blood groups and because of economic considerations. Blood group antigens vary in antigenicity. Naturally occurring antibodies to a few red cell antigens are found. Specific antiserums for blood typing are almost all prepared by isoimmunization. Reagents tend to be species specific with some known cross reactivity.

Blood group determination is useful in genetics and breeding studies. Parentage determination and selection of blood donor animals are of importance to the veterinary surgeon. Leukocyte and platelet antigens and antibodies do occur.

CROSSMATCHING OF BLOOD

Although it is a generally accepted principle in veterinary medicine that the first blood transfusion can be given safely without crossmatching for compatibility, crossmatching is advised for the initial transfusion and required for subsequent transfusions with intervals of four or more days. Properly matched blood should be given to females to avoid primary sensitization and subsequent risk of hemolytic disease to offspring.

CLASSIFICATION OF ANEMIA

Classification of anemias based on quantitative and morphological criteria provide useful information in clinical diagnosis. The erythrocyte indices are advocated by Schalm (1974) to classify anemias based on cell volume and hemoglobin content. This approach is based on the premise of accurate erythrocyte counts. Erythrocyte counts should be made by electronic (or the equivalent in accuracy) cell counters. The hemocytometer method of erythrocyte counting is not of sufficient accuracy to give consistently reliable indices. The microhematocrit method for PCV determination is accurate. Current spectrophotometric measurements by the cyanmethemoglobin method are accurate with clear plasma.

Schalm's classification based on indices is as follows (1974): I. macrocytic normochromic anemia; II. macrocytic hypochromic anemia; III. normocytic normochromic anemia; IV. microcytic hypochromic anemia. The major factor to be considered in the application of this classification to all species is differences in response to disease.

Macrocytic normochromic anemia has been related to aberrations in cell proliferation associated with DNA and RNA synthesis alterations. These changes, common with vitamin B_{12} and folate deficiencies in some species, have not been reported in cobalt deficiency of ruminants. The macrocytic normochromic anemia may reflect malnutrition effects rather than those of vitamin B_{12}.

The typical macrocytic hypochromic anemias are those of blood loss, blood destruction, and bone marrow recovery. Macrocytosis appears to be a constant finding and the MCV the most sensitive measurement of intensified erythropoiesis among the various species. Macrocytosis persists after the reticulocytes have fallen to normal levels (Schnappauf et al. 1967). The hypochromasia present relates to the incomplete hemoglobinization of reticulocytes. High reticulocyte levels are necessary for the development of the hypochromic parameter, a phenomenon common to dogs and pigs. The hypochromic effect is not seen in horses (Schalm 1975b) or in ruminants, a factor that may be misleading in the interpretation of erythrocyte indices.

The normocytic normochromic anemias are appropriately classified by this method when age-related reference values are considered in the interpretation of the MCV.

Microcytic hypochromic anemias occur in iron and copper deficiency states. The microcytic nature of the erythrocyte transcends most animal species. In milk-fed iron-deficient veal calves, the hypochromic nature of the cell is not reflected in a significant change in the MCHC, and the cells are normally hemoglobinized (Doxey 1977). The morphological appearance of hypochromasia so apparent in Wright's stained blood smears of the dog and pig is lacking in the horse and ruminants.

When the limitations of the classification of anemias based on the indices are known, the usefulness of the method in clinical diagnosis is apparent. In the absence of accurate erythrocyte counts, erythrocyte responses based on blood smear examination are useful in classification of the anemias as either regenerative or nonregenerative. The method is limited because of variability and duration of reticulocyte responses and visual perception of changes in size and color saturation.

The more common classification of anemias is based on etiology (Schalm, Jain, and Carroll 1975). The logical course of evaluation of the anemic animal is determination of the mechanism for the anemia. The erythrocyte indices and blood smear examination are useful in this determination.

MONITORING THE SURGICAL PATIENT

The indications for monitoring the surgical patient relate to the animal species and the procedure involved. This is of great concern to the equine surgeon in cases in which the nature of the surgical procedure may necessitate monitoring the patient during surgery and, more importantly, in the immediate postoperative period.

The hematologic parameters selected relate to their value and ease of determination. A minimal data base for monitoring the surgical patient is necessary for a reference. Thereafter, PCV, TPP, and blood smear aid in assessing dynamic changes. The blood smear allows evaluation of changes in neutrophil morphology and platelet estimates. This does not preclude counting and differentiating leukocytes when necessary for more critical assessment. The activated clotting time (ACT) and measurement of fibrinfibrinogen split products (FSP) is necessary when disseminated intravascular coagulation (DIC) is considered.

Care must be exercised in interpretation of the PCV and TPP. Sequestration of erythrocytes in animals under chemical restraint or anesthesia may result in a decreased PCV and no change in the TPP. Changes in plasma volume may be endogenous or may be associated with fluid administration. In acute blood loss, the PCV and TPP do not reflect loss of cells and protein until the plasma volume is replenished, which may take several hours after hemorrhage decreases.

Leukocyte counts in the immediate postsurgical period may fluctuate relative to physiological and nonpathogenic mechanisms. The WBC usually decreases in anesthetized animals. Recovery from anesthesia may be associated with a typical stress response and significant neutrophilia when the bone marrow storage pool is adequate and cells are released.

Manifestation of inflammation and DIC may occur in the immediate postrecovery period. A data base is required to assess change or status quo regarding leukocyte responses. Anticipation of DIC will include collection of the appropriate specimens. In general, platelet numbers may be estimated from the blood smear, FSP may be evaluated by the protamine sulfate test, which detects fibrin monomers, and early FSP may be evaluated by gelation or by fibrin strands when plasma is mixed with 1% protamine sulfate at pH 6.5 (Dodds 1980). A latex-agglutination method for measuring FSP* in human blood can be used for

several animal species (Dodds 1980). A special tube for blood collection is provided with the test kit.

THE HORSE

Erythrocytes

REFERENCE VALUES

There is considerable variation in reference values in the hemogram of horses of different breeds, ages, and sexes. The breed difference is considerable between hot-blooded horses (those of considerable Arabian ancestry) and cold-blooded horses. The hot-blooded horses have higher erythrocyte numbers, but the erythrocytes are smaller than those of cold-blooded horses. Normal erythrocyte parameters in hot-blooded horses are compiled in Table 3–2. Data on cold-blooded horses and ponies is limited and mostly collected prior to the use of electronic particle counters and modern, quality-controlled hematological procedures. Normal values for cold-blooded equine are compiled in Table 3–3.

---

*Thrombo-Wellcotest, Burroughs Wellcome Co., Research Triangle Park, NC.

Table 3–2 ERYTHROCYTE VALUES OF HOT-BLOODED HORSES OF DIFFERENT AGES

Reference	Age (Number Examined)	RBC ($\times 10^6/\mu l$)	Hb (g/dl)	PCV (%)	MCV (fl)	MCH (pg)	MCHC (g/dl)
Schalm (1975b)	8–18 mos (8)	8.60 ±0.58	11.8 ±1.6	34.5 ±3.8	40.1 ±2.9	13.7 ±1.3	34.1 ±1.4
	2 yrs (27)	9.88 ±1.34	14.7 ±1.6	41.4 ±4.2	42.7 ±2.8	14.9 ±1.1	34.9 ±1.3
	3–4 yrs (50)	9.10 ±1.16	14.3 ±1.4	40.8 ±4.3	44.8 ±3.4	15.7 ±1.2	35.2 ±1.5
	5 yrs (62)	8.57 ±0.98	14.4 ±1.6	40.8 ±4.1	47.8 ±4.0	16.8 ±1.3	35.4 ±1.4
Allen and Archer (1973)*	21 mos (78)	9.85 ±1.31	13.6 ±1.9	37.8 ±5.0	38.5 ±2.49	13.8 ±1.07	36.1 ±1.62
	1–9 mos (75)	10.33 ±1.24	12.7 ±1.55	35.3 ±4.4	34.3 ±2.93	12.3 ±1.23	36.1 ±2.25
	yearling (100)	9.91 ±1.11	13.7 ±1.44	37.5 ±3.89	37.9 ±1.90	13.8 ±0.68	36.6 ±1.36
	2 yrs (308)	9.86 ±0.98	14.6 ±1.44	39.9 ±3.99	40.6 ±2.53	14.7 ±0.87	36.2 ±1.02
	3 yrs (353)	9.71 ±1.06	15.1 ±1.52	41.4 ±4.18	42.7 ±2.54	15.6 ±0.83	36.5 ±1.07
	4 yrs (138)	9.28 ±0.98	15.0 ±1.65	40.8 ±4.65	44.3 ±2.43	16.7 ±0.86	36.5 ±1.30
	>4 yrs (302)	8.80 ±1.09	14.6 ±1.61	39.8 ±4.70	45.5 ±2.56	16.6 ±9.1	36.5 ±1.36

*English Thoroughbreds.

Table 3–3 ERYTHROCYTE VALUES FOR COLD-BLOODED EQUIDAE

Reference	Type of Animal (No. examined)	RBC (× 10⁶/μl)	Hb (g/dl)	PCV (%)	MCV (fl)	MCH (pg)	MCHC (g/dl)
Jones (1976)	Adult ponies (27)	7.39 ±1.07	12.81 ±1.65	32.0 ±11.0	48.2 ±4.0	17.4 ±1.3	36.2 ±1.1
	Crossbred ponies from one stud (22)	7.65 ±0.75	12.17 ±1.02	30.1 ±10.0	44.8 ±4.3	16.0 ±1.7	34.7 ±1.9
Steward and Holman (1940)	Clydesdales (36)	5.7–8.8 (6.95)	8.1–11.0 (9.55)	24–34 (27)	–	–	–
Trum (1952)	Percherons (11)	5.7–9.65 (7.39)	10.1–14.5 (11.67)	–	–	–	–
Jones (1976)	Adult donkeys (16)	6.4 ±1.04	12.8 ±1.91	36.9 ±6.0	57.8 ±3.0	20.1 ±0.9	34.9 ±1.3
	Donkey foals (6) (6–12 mos)	7.05 ±0.15	11.9 ±0.24	33.9 ±1.3	47.98 ±3.9	16.95 ±1.4	35.3 ±1.3

Erythrocyte parameters of hot-blooded horses are significantly influenced by release of erythrocytes from the splenic circulation during the stress of excitement, restraint, or exercise. Schalm, Jain, and Carroll (1975) showed an increase of 18.3 per cent (range of 14 to 64 per cent) in the PCV of 24 horses restrained on an operating table before anesthesia. Under halothane or halothane plus barbiturate anesthesia, the average PCV was 37.0 per cent, which is close to the preanesthesia resting PCV of 38.2 per cent. Similar drops occur in the PCV of excitable horses tranquilized with promazine hydrochloride (Schalm, Jain, and Carroll 1975).

The effect of age on erythrocyte parameters is most pronounced in hot-blooded foals (Schalm, Jain, and Carroll 1975). There is an early drop in PCV (nadir 8 to 12 days) followed by a gradual increase in PCV and Hgb and insignificant increases in RBC count. These changes are associated with a decrease in RBC size with a change in MCV from 40 to 32 fl. Jeffcott (1977) found erythrocyte parameters in ponies to decrease after birth for the first year. A drop in MCV and MCH with a nadir at three months was followed by a return to normal levels at one year. Thus, a significant change in erythrocyte size occurs during the first year of life in horses. Catling, as reported by Jeffcott (1977), found a significant increase in erythrocyte parameters of Thoroughbreds from the onset of training at 20 months to the end of the third year.

The average PCV of 35 per cent increased to 43 per cent during the first nine months of training.

As horses age, the RBC count decreases while the PCV remains constant (see Table 3–2). This is a result of an increase in the MCV. Aged animals are reported to have high MCV values (Jeffcott 1977).

Sex differences in erythrocyte parameters exist but appear to be of low magnitude (Schalm, Jain, and Carroll 1975).

MORPHOLOGY

The morphology of equine erythrocytes is determined by location on the blood smear. At the feathered end, the erythrocytes are round and without central pallor. In the red cell area, they are round, slightly variable in size, and the central pallor is minimal. In the thicker portion of the red cell area, sufficient depth of plasma allows for rouleau formation, a feature common to all Equidae.

ERYTHROPOIESIS

Horses do not release reticulocytes from the bone marrow in response to increased erythropoiesis, regardless of the magnitude of stimulation. In severe anemia, the regenerative response is associated with a release of macrocytic erythrocytes, and an increase in anisocytosis is found. Schalm, Jain, and Carroll (1975) report an increase of 10 to 15 fl in the MCV after massive hemorrhage. The best approach to evaluation of the intensity of erythropoiesis in the anemic animal appears to be bone marrow examination. Schalm (1975b) states that the number of reticulocytes in the bone marrow combined with a myeloid:erythroid ratio (M:E) is a better indication of erythropoietic activity than the M:E ratio alone. The crest core bone marrow biopsy is a useful adjunct to determine total cellularity.

On rare occasions, reticulocytes, nucleated red blood cells, and Howell-Jolly bodies may be seen in the peripheral blood. This is not necessarily a reflection of increased erythrogenesis.

Sedimentation Rate

The sedimentation rate of erythrocytes of horses increases as the PCV decreases. Diphasic sedimentation is seen in severe anemia.

Icterus Index

The icterus index of the horse ranges in health from 7.5 to 25 units (Schalm, Jain, and Carroll 1975) and varies directly with increasing PCV values.

Leukocytes

REFERENCE VALUES

Total leukocyte and differential cell counts are influenced by age (Kielstein 1959; Jeffcott 1977; Schalm 1975a). Neutrophil numbers are variable but are not significantly age dependent. Lymphocyte counts increase in foals and peak during the first year (Jeffcott 1971). Lymphocyte counts decrease in animals older than one year. Schalm (1975a) found the neutrophil:lymphocyte ratio (N:L) in blood of horses over five years of age to be 1.5:1.0. The N:L of aged horses was 2.0:1.0. Eosinophils are low at birth and increase to normal adult values by two to three months of age (Jeffcott 1977). Basophils and monocytes are not significantly age dependent. Normal leukocyte and different cell counts are compiled in Table 3-4.

MORPHOLOGY

The horse neutrophil has a very coarse chromatin structure to the lobes, giving it the appearance of hyperlobation. The lobes are indistinct, and usually only one short filament is found per cell. The female sex chromatin body is seen in some neutrophils. Persistent hypersegmented neutrophils have been described in one horse by Praase, George, and Whitlock (1981).

The band neutrophil has a more delicate chromatin structure. A left shift is indicated by a count of more than 200 bands/μl (Schalm 1975a). Hence, band neutrophils are rarely found in healthy horses, and their presence is highly significant.

Horse neutrophils may contain Döhle's bodies when responding to bacterial stimuli. Döhle's bodies are viewed as the pending development of toxic neutrophils. The toxic neutrophil contains diffuse light blue cytoplasm, which is related to altered maturation during states of severe bacterial toxemia. The toxic neutrophils are seen accompanying marked shifts in immaturity. The term degenerative left shift with toxic neutrophils implies a serious and usually rapidly deteriorating condition of bacterial origin. The leukocyte count may be low.

Severe disorders of the gastrointestinal tract may result in a degenerative left shift with toxic neutrophils. Moderate thrombocytopenia may occur. Endotoxin from gram-negative bacteria results in similar responses and probably plays a major role in later stages of equine colic (Burrows 1979).

The lymphocytes are mainly of the small type with limited cytoplasm. Occasionally, azurophilic granules are present in the cytoplasm. Large lymphocytes with blastic features are present in small numbers in immunologically responsive states. Eosinophils, basophils, and monocytes are distinctive and easily recognized.

Platelets

The horse platelet stains lightly with most Wright's stains. The cytoplasm is pale blue, and fine azurophilic granules are present. Platelets are usually round

Table 3-4 NORMAL LEUKOCYTE AND DIFFERENTIAL CELL COUNTS OF VARIOUS EQUIDAE

| Reference | Type of Animal (No. examined) | WBC (× 10⁶/μl) | Neutrophils (× 10⁶/μl) | | | | | | Eosinophils | | Basophils | | Lymphocytes | | Monocytes | |
			Juv.	Stabs No.	Stabs %	Segs No.	Segs %		No.	%	No.	%	No.	%	No.	%
Schalm (1975a)	Hot-blooded (8) 8–18 mos	10,812 ±1,874	–	16 ±28	0.1 ±0.2	4,658 ±745	43.8 ±7.0		478 ±403	4.1 ±2.9	43 ±47	0.4 ±0.5	5,210 ±1,250	47.9 ±6.0	398 ±278	3.6 ±2.0
	(27) 2 years	9,678 ±1,883	–	39 ±81	0.4 ±1.1	4,805 ±1,196	50.1 ±10.1		278 ±232	2.8 ±2.1	33 ±58	0.3 ±0.5	4,059 ±1,456	41.4 ±10.5	445 ±255	4.7 ±2.8
	(50) 3–4 years	8,666 ±1,560	–	48 ±153	0.4 ±1.2	4,568 ±1,189	52.5 ±8.0		278 ±218	3.2 ±2.6	34 ±46	0.4 ±0.5	3,376 ±787	39.3 ±7.7	360 ±176	4.2 ±2.0
	(62) 5+ years	8,822 ±8,760	–	22 ±57	0.3 ±0.7	4,877 ±1,316	55.0 ±7.7		316 ±231	3.6 ±2.6	60 ±72	0.7 ±0.8	3,146 ±826	36.0 ±7.4	385 ±240	4.4 ±2.6
Knill et al. (1969)	Thoroughbreds Mares (28) Stallions (11) Geldings (11)	8,900 ±1,700	–	–	–	–	47.0 ±8.2		–	3.7 ±2.4	–	0.1	45.1 ±8.9	–	–	4.0 ±3.0
Jeffcott (1977)	in training (611)	4,540 ±8,830	–	–	–	–	–		–	–	–	–	–	–	–	–
	Adult ponies (27)	8,440 ±1,460	27	25	–	4,370 ±140	–		272 ±206	–	22	–	3,960 ±130	–	13	–
	Crossbred ponies (22)	10,340 ±1,530	2	18	–	4,890 ±142	–		541 ±362	–	26	–	4,950 ±940	–	76	–
	Adult donkeys (16)	10,900 ±1,460	8	81	–	4,970 ±1,180	–		574 ±281	–	6	–	5,150 ±1,800	–	88	–
	Donkey foals (6) 6–12 mos	14,700 ±3,120	36	72	–	4,840 ±1,740	–		310 ±262	–	47	–	10,260 ±240	–	102	–

to oval, although unusual forms may be found. The horse has lower platelet values than other animals. The count may be as low as 100,000/μl, ranging to 400,000/μl. There appear to be no significant breed differences, and age differences have not been reported.

Plasma Components

The normal plasma of the horse is more yellow than that of other species; the color is directly proportional to the PCV (Schalm, Jain, and Carroll 1975). The plasma bilirubin, which contributes to the color, is normally high. The plasma bilirubin increases markedly in fasting states or with diseases of the gastrointestinal system. The presence of a high icterus index and a low PCV should lead to a suspicion of hemolytic anemia. However, a high icterus index with a normal or elevated PCV is not indicative of hemolytic disease.

PLASMA PROTEINS

The total plasma proteins of the horse are low in the newborn foal and increase following nursing owing to absorption of immunoglobulins (Jeffcott 1974). Thereafter, the plasma proteins increase gradually. Normal adult values are found at three months of age. Schalm, Jain, and Carroll (1975) found the plasma proteins to range from 6.0 to 8.5 g/dl in 147 clinically normal horses and the fibrinogen to range from 1.0 to 4.0 g/liter.

LIPEMIA

Lipemia in horses is clinically significant. Schotman and Kroneman (1969) reported lipemia in periparturient mare ponies associated with anorexia. Baetz and Pearson (1972) found the most marked change in fasted ponies to be lipemia. Schalm, Jain, and Carroll (1975) feel that marked lipemia is indicative of severe liver disease. Lipemia caused by a variety of known causes may be found in other species.

Anemia

Clinical evaluation of the anemic horse differs from that of other species in that severe anemia is not associated with a blood reticulocyte response. Morphological changes in blood may be seen as anisocytosis. In mild anemia, anisocytosis is not discernible. Examination of the bone marrow is required to properly assess the status of the erythron as to degree of erythrogenesis (Schalm 1975b). Smith and Agar (1976) studied erythrocyte metabolism during active erythropoiesis following phlebotomy and concluded that erythrocyte adenosine-5-triphosphate may be used to determine intensity of cell production.

Measurement of the TPP is useful in evaluation of acute blood loss (Schalm 1975b). The decrease in TPP occurs in conjunction with the decrease in PCV in acute blood loss as fluid balance is reestablished.

Polycythemia

Splenic contraction induced by excitement at sampling increases the PCV without increasing the TPP. Hemoconcentration due to plasma fluid loss is reflected in an increase of PCV and TPP.

Primary polycythemia has not been reported in the horse.

Leukocyte Responses

Leukocyte values are useful as a data base when elective surgical procedures are considered. Evaluation of the acute surgical patient requires consideration of physiological effects on the hemogram (the steroid response). This is particularly applicable to the colic patient. The neutrophilia and eosinopenia seen reflect endogenous corticosteroid release, i.e., mobilization of the neutrophil reserve from the bone marrow and sequestration of eosinophils. Dynamic changes occur in colic when major segments of the intestinal tract are significantly compromised. Absorption of endotoxin may result in leukopenia and the rapid development of a degenerative left shift. Toxic neutrophils may be found after a day of significant toxemia. Progression of the course in the colic patient is best monitored and interpreted when examination of peritoneal fluid and blood are made simultaneously. The transport system reflects changes in the inflammatory cells of peritoneal fluid. In acute colic, exudation of high numbers of inflammatory cells into peritoneal fluid does not usually occur. When great numbers are present, they tend to reflect antecedent disease of a purulent nature.

Inflammation of several days' duration is accompanied by an increase in fibrinogen levels (Schalm 1975a). Chronic inflammation of a purulent nature may lead to mild anemia, the anemia of infection.

Blood Coagulation

Presurgical screening for platelet numbers may be evaluated by blood smear examination. The functional status of the coagulation cascade may be examined for gross abnormality by the ACT. Rawlings and associates (1975) reported ACT times of 158 seconds for normal ponies. The platelet count and ACT are practical screening approaches to the surgical patient.

When coagulation abnormalities, including DIC, are considered, determination of FSP is indicated (Dodds 1980). Evaluation of the coagulation cascade and factors require the services of a coagulation laboratory. In that event, a properly preserved plasma specimen is necessary. The anticoagulant of choice is 3.8% trisodium citrate (one part to nine parts blood). A control specimen, drawn under similar conditions, is also necessary.

THE OX

Recent advances in the use of hematology in the diagnosis of diseases of cattle stem from the principle that cattle are regarded as a herd rather than individual animals. Selective examination of small groups of cattle within herds provides a profile to aid diagnosis of mismanagement practices (Payne et al. 1970). This approach does not preclude hematological study of individual animals to establish a data base for the surgical plant.

Erythrocytes

Cattle erythrocyte variables are related to age, management practices, stage of location, and season of the year.

REFERENCE VALUES, CALVES

Doxey (1977) compiled data from several authors on normally reared and milk-fed veal calves (Table 3–5). These average values indicate a slight decline in PCV and Hgb with age in normally reared calves. Calves fed wholly milk replacer diets had marked declines in PCV and Hgb associated with reduced serum iron levels. Bremner and colleagues (1976) reviewed data from several authors on the microcytic normochromic anemia in milk-fed veal calves. The practice of feeding calves liquid milk replacer and low-iron diets and confining

Table 3–5 NORMAL ERYTHROCYTE VALUES FOR CALVES (BIRTH TO ONE YEAR)*

Type of Animal	RBC (× 10⁶/μl)	Hb (g/dl)	PCV (%)	MCV (fl)	MCH (μg)	MCHC (g/dl)	Fe (μmol/liter)	Reticulocytes (%)
Normally reared calves								
Birth	8.38	43.0	12.5	51.3	14.9	29.1	–	0.2
1 week	8.04	36.3	11.1	45.1	13.8	30.5	13.2	0.05
1 mo	8.06	33.7	10.4	41.8	12.9	30.8	13.4	–
3 mos	8.36	33.0	10.9	39.4	13.0	33.0	28.1	0.07
6 mos	8.06	36.1	11.7	44.8	14.5	32.4	25.9	0
12 mos	7.57	35.9	9.7	47.4	12.8	27.0	23.2	0
Veal calves								
Birth	7.68	39.3	12.3	51.2	16.0	31.2	12.6	–
3 mos	6.65	23.6	7.4	35.4	11.1	31.3	–	–
4½ mos	6.74	27.0	9.0	40.0	13.3	33.3	5.7	–

*From Doxey *In* Archer and Jeffcott (eds.): Comparative Clinical Hematology. Oxford: Blackwell Scientific Publications, 1977. Reprinted courtesy of Doxey and Blackwell Scientific Publications.

Table 3–6 ERYTHROCYTE, HEMOGLOBIN, PACKED CELL VOLUMES, AND INDICES
ON HOLSTEIN CATTLE IN MINNESOTA, MEAN AND STANDARD DEVIATION

Age (yrs)	Number Examined	RBC ($\times 10^6/\mu l$)	Hb (g/dl)	PCV (%)	MCV (fl)	MCH (μg)	MCHC (g/dl)
2	36	7.26 ±0.69	11.3 ±1.18	33.6 ±2.7	46.3	15.6	33.6
3	136	6.89 ±0.83	11.1 ±1.23	32.8 ±2.9	47.6	16.1	33.8
4	129	6.82 ±0.72	11.2 ±1.12	33.4 ±3.1	48.9	16.4	33.5
5	122	6.76 ±0.74	11.2 ±1.29	33.1 ±3.6	59.0	16.6	33.8
6	141	6.76 ±0.70	11.4 ±1.27	33.8 ±3.3	50.0	16.9	33.7
7	115	6.50 ±0.75	11.3 ±1.21	33.2 ±3.5	51.1	17.4	34.0
8	68	6.57 ±0.92	11.1 ±1.45	32.6 ±4.1	49.6	16.9	34.0
9	36	6.21 ±0.77	10.7 ±1.37	31.5 ±3.5	50.7	17.2	34.0
>10	56	6.26 ±0.83	11.1 ±1.45	32.8 ±3.9	52.4	17.7	33.8
All ages	839	6.70 ±0.80	11.2 ±1.27	33.1 ±3.4	49.4	16.7	33.8

them to restrict movement is used to produce pale colored carcasses, termed high-quality veal. Bremner and coworkers (1976) found that milk-substitute diets containing iron concentrations of 25 to 30 mg/kg dietary dry matter were sufficient for normal appetite and growth and still yielded pale carcasses at slaughter. Iron concentrations above 40 mg/kg dietary dry matter led to significant increases in myoglobin formation in skeletal muscles.

REFERENCE VALUES, ADULT CATTLE

The PCV and Hgb of adult dairy cows are relatively constant regardless of age of animal (Wingfield and Tumbleson 1973). An age-related decrease in erythrocyte numbers and increased erythrocyte volume, however, does occur (Table 3–6). Mean erythrocyte values for adult cattle reported by Schalm, Jain, and Carroll (1975), Stevens and associates (1976), and Doxey (1977) are similar to those found in Table 3–6. Significant differences in erythrocyte parameters relate to season of year, lactation (Rowlands et al. 1979), and level of production (Stevens et al. 1976). Rowlands and colleagues (1979) concluded that differences due to season and herd, in definition of normal ranges, are at the level of one standard range for interpretation of metabolic profiles. However, differences between nonlactating or low-yielding cows and lactating cows at peak production of about 3.0 per cent PCV and 1.0 g/dl Hgb below average values should be considered normal. Bulls have higher PCV (37.8 to 45.9 per cent) and Hb (12.2 to 16.0 g/dl) levels than cows.

MORPHOLOGY

The shape of the bovine erythrocyte is biconcave, with minimal central pallor observed in Wright's-stained blood smears. The erythrocyte size decreases from birth to a nadir at three months and then increases gradually to constant volumes by five years of age (see Table 3–6). Anisocytosis is prominent in cattle, with the greatest variability in calves.

RETICULOCYTES

The normal reticulocyte level of cattle blood is very low (see Table 3–5). In blood loss experiments, removal of 5 to 10 per cent of the calculated erythrocyte mass over 10 days until a total of 60 to 70 per cent had been removed caused only slight or no reticulocytosis (Schnappauf et al. 1967). A sudden loss of 30 to 40 per cent of the erythrocyte mass resulted in slight reticulocytosis. In two calves, phlebotomy and reinfusion of plasma to create a 65 per cent deficit in erythrocyte mass resulted in 9 and 14 per cent peak reticulocyte responses on the sixth day (Schnappauf et al. 1967). Furthermore, these investigators demonstrated that reticulocytes were no longer released after the PCV reached 60 per cent of its original value 11 days after phlebotomy. Macrocytosis was prominent with cells in the 78- to 150-fl range. The reticulocytes observed appeared as polychromatophilic cells or demonstrated basophilic stippling in Wright's stained smears.

Basophilic stippling of some immature bovine erythrocytes on Romanowsky's stained blood smears is considered normal to any regenerative anemia

Table 3–7 NORMAL LEUKOCYTE VALUES* FOR CALVES, BIRTH TO ONE YEAR†

Age	WBC	Neutrophils	Lymphocytes	Monocytes	Eosinophils	Basophils
Birth	9.40	6.20	2.80	0.30	0.09	0
1 week	7.46	3.80	3.40	0.20	0.06	0
3 mos	9.30	2.50	6.00	0.60	0.20	0
1 year	9.9	2.50	6.58	0.65	0.25	0

*All values $10^3/\mu$l
†From Doxey In Archer and Jeffcott (eds.): Comparative Clinical Hematology. Oxford: Blackwell Scientific Publications, 1977. Reprinted courtesy of Doxey and Blackwell Scientific Publications.

(Schalm, Jain, and Carroll 1975). The cells are counted as polychromatophilic erythrocytes in assessing the regenerative response.

SEDIMENTATION RATE

The suspension stability of bovine erythrocytes is great. Wintrobe sedimentation rates of less than a 2-mm fall in eight hours are normal for the author's laboratory. Increased sedimentation rates of greater than a 4-mm fall in eight hours are considered prolonged and are indicative of chronic inflammation of a purulent nature.

Leukocytes

Leukocytes show an age-dependent variation. Leukocytes are quite variable in young calves. The trend is toward higher total leukocyte counts in calves and growing animals (Schalm, Jain, and Carroll 1975). High neutrophil numbers are found at birth with lower lymphocyte values (Tennant et al. 1974). Reversal occurs during the first week of life, with neutrophils at normal adult levels and lymphocytes at high values.

REFERENCE VALUES

The leukocyte values in Table 3–7 for calves are summarized by Doxey (1977). The total leukocyte count decreases with age in apparently healthy cattle (Perman et al. 1970). This age-dependent decrease is most marked in lymphocyte number. Neutrophils decrease slightly, whereas monocytes and eosinophils maintain near constant values. Eosinophils, which are in low numbers in calves (see Table 3–7), attain adult levels by two years of age (Schalm, Jain, and Carroll 1975).

Leukocyte values for healthy adult Minnesota Holstein-Friesian cows are given in Table 3–8 (Perman et al. 1970). The eosinophil values are higher than those reported by Schalm, Jain, and Carroll (1975) and Doxey (1977).

MORPHOLOGY

The mature neutrophil of cattle tends to form discrete lobes separated by fila-

Table 3–8 LEUKOCYTE VALUES OF MINNESOTA HOLSTEIN-FRIESIAN COWS*

Age (yrs)	Number Examined	WBC	Neutrophils	Lymphocytes	Monocytes	Eosinophils	Basophils
2	36	10.3 ±2.1	3.8 ±1.2	5.0 ±1.5	0.3 ±0.2	1.2 ±0.8	0
3	136	9.3 ±1.9	3.0 ±1.1	4.7 ±1.0	0.3 ±0.2	1.3 ±0.7	0
4	129	9.2 ±1.9	3.2 ±1.3	4.5 ±1.0	0.3 ±0.2	1.3 ±0.7	0
5	122	8.5 ±1.7	3.0 ±1.2	4.1 ±1.0	0.3 ±0.2	1.2 ±0.7	0
6	141	8.2 ±1.6	2.7 ±0.9	3.9 ±1.0	0.3 ±0.2	1.3 ±0.7	0
7	115	8.0 ±1.5	2.8 ±1.0	3.7 ±0.8	0.2 ±0.2	1.3 ±0.7	0
8	68	7.8 ±1.7	2.5 ±1.1	3.6 ±0.9	0.3 ±0.2	1.4 ±0.7	0
9	36	7.4 ±1.7	2.5 ±1.1	3.4 ±1.2	0.2 ±0.1	1.2 ±0.5	0
>10	56	7.5 ±1.7	2.6 ±1.3	3.3 ±0.9	0.2 ±0.2	1.4 ±0.6	0
All ages	839	8.5 ±1.9	2.9 ±1.1	4.1 ±1.1	0.3 ±0.2	1.3 ±0.7	0

*All values $10^3/\mu$l

ments. The lobes are smooth with coarse internal chromatin. Granules are dust-like when demonstrated. The lymphocytes are small to large. The typical small lymphocyte nucleus has a dense, coarse chromatin structure. The nucleus is cleaved or round and surrounded by scanty blue cytoplasm. Medium and large lymphocytes are most numerous. The cytoplasm is abundant and light blue in color. Azurophilic granules of varied sizes are seen relatively frequently in bovine lymphocytes but not in all animals.

Platelets

The platelet counts of cattle are age dependent, with mean values of 820,000/μl seen in young calves (Perman et al. 1956). Thereafter, the platelet levels drop slowly with adult levels of 2.0 to 6.0 × 10^6 platelets by two years of age (Pritchard et al. 1956).

Plasma Components

The plasma proteins of caesarean-delivered calves range from 4.0 to 5.3 gm/dl with a mean value of 4.7 gm/dl (Schalm, Smith, and Kaneko 1970). The routine values of total plasma protein in most species are 5.0 to 7.0 gm/dl. The routine fibrinogen values are 1 to 5 gm/liter. Colostrum absorption increases the plasma proteins to 6.5 ± 0.83 gm/dl. A common range for yearlings is 6.8 to 7.5 gm/dl and for mature cattle 7.0 to 8.5 gm/dl (Schalm, Jain, and Carroll 1975).

The fibrinogen level of newborn calves is 1.55 ± 1.32 gm/liter and ranges from 3.0 to 7.0 gm/liter in growing and mature cattle.

Anemia

The clinical signs of anemia in cattle are not usually manifest until the anemia is severe. Anorexia, weight loss, and decreased milk production may be recognized. The systemic effects relate to weakness or downer cows. Lighting conditions are usually inadequate to perceive pallor of mucous membranes.

Mild anemia is diagnosed when blood samples are taken for examination; it is not recognized on physical examination.

Definition of mild anemia in lactating dairy cattle requires knowledge of the effect of high milk production on erythrocyte parameters (Rowlands et al. 1979; Stevens et al. 1976). The mean PCV for Holstein-Friesian cows of 33.1 per cent± 3.4 SD is significantly related to lactation. Stevens and coworkers (1976) report a PCV of 34.4 per cent ± 2.03 SD for cows that are dry or producing less than 20 lbs of fat-corrected milk (FCM), a PCV of 32.8 per cent ± 2.03 SD for cows producing 20 to 40 lbs of FCM, and a PCV of 31.8 per cent ± 1.64 SD for cows producing more than 40 lbs of FCM.

The anemias of importance for presurgical consideration are mainly those of blood loss and nutritional deficiencies and the anemia associated with chronic inflammation. Internal bleeding from abomasal ulcers usually presents as a regenerative anemia with polychromasia and basophilic stippling. A complete coverage of anemia is provided in standard texts (Schalm, Jain, and Carroll, 1975; Archer and Jeffcott 1977).

The application of metabolic profile testing has revealed the importance of nutrition in the development of anemia in dairy cattle (Payne et al. 1970; Stevens et al. 1976). Factors of importance appear to be quality and quantity of protein, iron, copper, and cobalt.

The anemia associated with chronic inflammation is of frequent occurrence and importance to presurgical examination. The mechanism of anemia in inflammatory disease is related to the unavailability of storage iron (Feldman, Kaneko, and Farver 1981). The presence of normocytic normochromic anemia and indication of chronic inflammation by fibrinogen, plasma protein, and leukocyte responses forewarns of the magnitude and long duration of the inflammatory process.

Leukocyte Responses

The leukocyte responses of cattle to the stress of disease and to the nature of the disease process differ from the general patterns of other species in magnitude and time relationships. The corticosteroid response is seen during parturition and stressful conditions whether or not it is disease related. For example, transportation for several hours and displaced abomasum both produce similar changes. Neutrophils are released from the storage pool and may increase two- to fourfold. Lymphocytes decrease by less than half the normal number. Eosinophils are the most stress-sensitive cells and may disappear from the blood. Monocytes increase to levels of less than 1000/μl.

The leukocyte response to inflammatory stimuli is dependent on the nature and duration of the stimulus. The response to gram-negative organisms relates to the endotoxemia produced (Schalm, Jain, and Carrol 1975). The response to endotoxin injected into a lactating mammary gland (Jain, Schalm, and Lasmanis 1978) and into the circulation (Jain and Lasmanis 1978) is similar. High levels of endotoxin in the circulation produce severe leukopenia through leukoaggregation and destruction (Jacob et al. 1980). The bone marrow reserve is depleted (Jain, Schalm, and Lasmanis 1978). Recovery from the leukopenia depends on the persistence of the endotoxemia. The delayed recovery of the bone marrow and the slow re-establishment (seven days) of peripheral blood granulocytes is normal for the cow (Valli et al. 1971). The leukopenia of gram-negative sepsis is associated with a degenerative left shift and "toxic" neutrophils. Examination of the blood smear reveals the reaction. Concurrent with the severe endotoxin-induced neutropenia is platelet destruction, and severe thrombocytopenia may develop. Persistent gram-negative sepsis leads to acute disseminated intravascular coagulation that may be manifest in severe bleeding.

Less virulent microorganisms inciting inflammation cause leukocyte numbers in the blood transport system to reflect the nature and extent of the inflammatory process. The quantitative changes may be within normal limits for neutrophils. The presence of a left shift and elevated fibrinogen levels is a more sensitive indicator of an inflammatory process and distinguishes it from the stress response.

In chronic suppurative disease, the neutrophils tend to be mature. The process must be extensive before elevated counts are found. A neutrophil count of 20,000 to 40,000/μl is seen occasionally with massive suppurative lesions associated with low-virulence microorganisms. The fibrinogen and plasma proteins are markedly elevated in these cases.

Eosinophil numbers may be high in apparently healthy adult cattle. The mean eosinophil count for dairy cattle in Steele County, Minnesota, was 1300/μl with a range to 3000/μl (Perman et al. 1970). The association of high eosinophil numbers with disease was not made. The absence of eosinophils in adult cattle is a reflection of severe stress or stress of disease, even of metazoan etiology.

Lymphocyte values in dairy cattle are age dependent. A persistent lymphocytosis of apparently normal cattle is associated with endemic bovine leukemia infection on a herd basis (Bendixen 1965). Lymphocyte counts of up to 100,000/μl with normal morphology have been observed. The frequency of persistent lymphocytosis is variable (Bendixen 1965).

Lymphocytes decrease in number in stressful situations and reflect the usual response to inflammatory disease. Viral infections in general cause lymphopenia, which may be severe when the virus has a predilection for lymphoid tissue. Lymphocytosis may occur in blood parasitic diseases.

Monocytosis is not commonly found as a response in cattle. When observed, it may be associated with acute and chronic diseases. Schalm, Jain, and Carroll (1975) report a significant monocytosis in normal parturition and with retained placentae. Monocytes may be in low numbers in the acute phases of disease and in higher numbers in chronic inflammatory diseases.

Leukemia

Leukemia in cattle affects the lymphocytes to the exclusion of other cellular elements. A leukemic phase may be observed in about 5 to 10 per cent of animals with bovine leukemia. The leukemic cells are recognized by blastic features and increased numbers. A wide range of morphological forms are seen with no apparent significance to the type found. Diagnosis is best made by tissue biopsy, cytology, and histopathology.

Table 3–9 NORMAL HEMATOLOGICAL VALUES FOR SHEEP*

	Mean	Range
Erythrocytes	12×10^{12}/liter	$9–15 \times 10^{12}$/liter
PCV	0.33 liter/liter	0.26–0.42 liter/liter
Diameter	4.5 μm	3–8 μm
Volume (MCV)	32 fl	28–40 fl
Hb	12 g/dl	8–16 g/dl
MCH	10 pg	8–12 pg
MCHC	33 g/dl	31–138 g/dl
Leukocytes	8×10^9/liter	$4–12 \times 10^9$/liter
Lymphocytes (%)	63	50–75
Neutrophils (%)	30	10–50
Eosinophils (%)	4	2–12
Basophils (%)	< 0.5	0–1
Monocytes (%)	3	2–8
Platelets	450×10^9/liter	$250–750 \times 10^9$/liter

*From Greenwood: *In* Archer and Jeffcott (eds.): Comparative Clinical Hematology. Oxford: Blackwell Scientific Publications, 1977. Reprinted courtesy of Greenwood and Blackwell Scientific Publications.

Blood Coagulation

The activated coagulation test (ACT) as a measure of blood clotting appears less variable than the Lee White tube method. Riley and Lassen (1979) report ACT means of 145 seconds with a range of 120 to 180 seconds. The platelet count ACT and measurement of FSP are useful screening tests for problems of hemostasis.

THE SHEEP

The hematology of sheep resembles that of cattle. A wide range of hematological values has been summarized (Schalm, Jain, and Carroll 1975). The

Table 3–10 ABSOLUTE LEUKOCYTE NUMBERS FOR SHEEP*

	Mean Absolute Numbers ($\times 10^9$/liter)
Total	8.00
Lymphocytes	5.00
Neutrophils	2.40
Eosinophils	0.32
Basophils	0.03
Monocytes	0.25

*From Greenwood: *In* Archer and Jeffcott (eds.): Comparative Clinical Hematology. Oxford: Blackwell Scientific Publications, 1977. Reprinted courtesy of Greenwood and Blackwell Scientific Publications.

variation in erythrocyte parameters may relate to sampling conditions, parasitic disease, and husbandry practices. The data of Greenwood (1977) summarize normal values for adult sheep (Tables 3–9 and 3–10).

Erythrocytes

REFERENCE VALUES

Erythrocyte values of sheep are quite variable owing to excitement and splenic contraction at the time of sampling. The spleen contains one-seventh of the total blood volume and one-fourth of the circulating red cell mass (Turner and Hodgetts 1959). Interpretation of data for erythrocyte values may be misleading unless sampling conditions are referenced.

The erythrocytes of sheep are of small diameter, and central pallor is minimal. Reticulocytes are released when erythropoiesis is intensely stimulated (Mohandas et al. 1980). These investigators demonstrated a macrocytosis on the day following phlebotomy relating to the stimulatory pulse of erythropoietin. Reticulocytosis developed by the fourth day, peaked on the seventh day, and returned to base line values by the eleventh day following a single stimulatory phlebotomy. Macrocytosis was present throughout the entire period.

Sheep have two main types of hemoglobin, HbA and HbB. The genes that control and express each type are codominant; animals may have either one or both types. Animals with HbA or HbAB produce a third hemoglobin, HbC, when erythropoiesis is intensified. HbC is found in lambs up to three months of age and in severely anemic sheep with regenerative responses. The implications of hemoglobin switching are reviewed by Young and Nienhuis (1978). It has been demonstrated that sheep red cells with HbA or HbAB may be induced to sickle in vitro (Greenwood, 1977). Hb switching occurs in goats in which in vivo morphological changes in erythrocytes have been demonstrated (Jain et al. 1980).

RETICULOCYTES

Low numbers of reticulocytes are normal in newborn lambs. Reticulocytes are essentially absent from nonanemic adult sheep. The reticulocyte response to blood loss and blood destruction is modest in comparison to that of the dog and pig (Mohandas et al. 1980).

Leukocytes

Leukocyte morphology, quantitative values, and responses in disease resemble those of cattle. The neutrophil:lymphocyte ratio is high at birth and reaches adult values within a few weeks. Eosinophil levels are low in lambs (similar to those in calves). Eosinophils comprise 18.5 per cent of the nucleated cells of the bone marrow (Grunsell 1951). The blood transport system does not reflect the responsive nature of these cells adequately.

Platelets

Platelet numbers in sheep range from 250,000 to 900,000/μl, with somewhat higher numbers in young animals.

Plasma Proteins

Schalm, Jain, and Carroll (1975) report normal fibrinogen levels of 1.0 to 5.0 g/liter. Elevations of fibrinogen of up to 16.0 g/liter occur in disease processes. Elevations in fibrinogen in general relate to inflammatory disease.

The total plasma protein for adult sheep range from 6.5 to 7.5 g/dl (Schalm, Jain, and Carroll 1975). Elevations in plasma proteins are related to other causes in other species, namely, dehydration and inflammatory disease.

THE GOAT

Erythrocytes

REFERENCE VALUES

The hematology of goats has received scant attention regarding population studies and reference values. The data compiled by Greenwood (1977) serves as a useful basis for clinical study (Tables 3–11 and 3–12).

MORPHOLOGY

The erythrocytes of goats are small in diameter, 3.2 μm, with a range of between 1.5 and 5.0 μm (Holman and Dew 1963). The erythrocytes of the young kid (1 to 13 months) and of the anemic goat in recovery exhibit marked poikilocytosis. Jain and Kono (1977) reported the occurrence of fusiform and spindle-shaped erythrocytes in some normal Angora goats. Subsequently, it was shown that the fusiform cells decreased to low levels when goats were made anemic by bleeding (Jain et al. 1980). The disappearance of the fusiform erythrocyte was associated with the appearance of discoid and odd-shaped (anisocytosis) erythrocytes. Goats switch hemoglobin when subject to intense erythropoietin stimulation. Hemoglobin switching to HbC was demonstrated in these studies.

RETICULOCYTES

The goat responds with a small increase in reticulocytes (Jain et al. 1980). A reticulocyte response of 2.5 to 4.2 per cent was associated with a near 50 per cent deficit in Hb. The magnitude of the response is not unlike that of sheep and cattle.

Young and Nienhuis (1978) stated that

Table 3–11 NORMAL HEMATOLOGICAL VALUES FOR GOATS*

	Mean	Range
Erythrocytes	14×10^{12}/liter	7–21×10^{12}/liter
PCV	0.29 liter/liter	0.19–0.40 liter/liter
Diameter	3.2 μm	1.5–5 μm
Volume (MCV)	21 fl	15–39 fl
Hb	11 g/dl	8–16 g/dl
MCH	6.9 pg	5.3–8.4 pg
MCHC	37 g/dl	32–40 g/dl
Leukocytes	8×10^9/liter	4–15×10^9/liter
Lymphocytes (%)	49	45–60
Neutrophils (%)	42	40–50
Eosinophils (%)	6	2–10
Basophils (%)	<0.5	0–1
Monocytes (%)	3	2–6
Platelets	450×10^9/liter	400–500×10^9/liter

*From Greenwood: *In* Archer and Jeffcott (eds.): Comparative Clinical Hematology. Oxford: Blackwell Scientific Publications, 1977. Reprinted courtesy of Greenwood and Blackwell Scientific Publications.

all goats produce HbC during neonatal life and periods of erythropoietic stress. The association of odd-shaped erythrocytes and HbC formation appears to be a useful clinical indicator of intense erythropoiesis and should be interpreted as for increased reticulocytes.

Leukocytes

Holman and Dew (1965) reported that the leukocyte count increases after birth to a peak level of 18,000/μl at three months, followed by a decrease to 8,000/μl by age two years. Lymphocytes account for the higher leukocyte values in this age group.

Table 3–12 ABSOLUTE LEUKOCYTE NUMBER FOR GOATS*

	Mean Absolute Numbers ($\times 10^9$/liter)
Total	8.00
Lymphocytes	3.90
Neutrophils	3.40
Eosinophils	0.43
Basophils	0.03
Monocytes	0.24

*From Greenwood: *In* Archer and Jeffcott (eds.): Comparative Clinical Hematology. Oxford: Blackwell Scientific Publications, 1977. Reprinted courtesy of Greenwood and Blackwell Scientific Publications.

MORPHOLOGY

The morphology of the various leukocytes of the goat are similar to that of sheep and cattle.

Platelets

The platelet count for goats ranges from 250 to 900 $\times 10^3$/μl (Perman 1980). The morphology is similar to that of sheep and cattle.

THE PIG

Hematological values for pigs are affected by age, nutrition, and management. Imlah and McTaggart (1977) state that "normal" values, which refer to all pigs, are of limited value because of factors known to affect hematological parameters.

Erythrocyte Values

The newborn pig is affected by a dietary lack of iron and rapid growth. Iron stores at birth are lacking based on the Prussian blue reaction. Hypochromic erythrocytes in low numbers may be demonstrated in the blood of newborn pigs. The newborn pig doubles its weight during the first week of life and hence its

Table 3–13 ERYTHROCYTE VALUES OF PIGS

Reference	Age	RBC (× 10⁶/µl)	Hb (g/dl)	PCV (%)	MCV (fl)	MCH (pg)	MCHC (g/dl)	Reticulocytes (%)
Miller et al. (1961)	Birth	6.20	12.6	40.0	64.8	20.5	31.5	0.65
	3 days	4.57	9.3	31.0	—	—	20.1	5.25
	7 days	5.26	9.1	31.0	—	—	—	7.25
	12 mos.	7.52	14.2	44.0	64.3	—	31.2	—
Schalm, Jain, and Carroll (1975)	3½ to 4 mos	7.1	12.0	40.0	57.0	—	30.0	—
	Males, 1 year and older	6.7	14.1	45.0	66.0	—	31.0	—
	Females, 1 year and over; not pregnant	6.0	12.1	38.0	64.0	—	31.0	0
	Females, 1 year and over; pregnant 2½ to 3½ mos	6.4	12.8	42.0	65.0	—	31.0	—
Imlah and McTaggart (1977)	Pigs as a whole	7.2 (6.0–9.0)	14.0 (11.0–17.0)	42.0 (37.0–50.0)	—	—	—	—

Table 3–14 LEUKOCYTE VALUES OF PIGS*

Reference	Age or Weight	WBC	Neutrophils		Eosinophils	Basophils	Lymphocytes	Monocytes
			Stabs	Segs				
Schalm, Jain, and Carroll (1975)	Duroc-Jersey both sexes, 3½–4 mos	26.9	0.54	7.26	0.66	0.13	16.95	1.35
	Duroc-Jersey males, 1 year and older	13.3	0.08	4.26	0.47	0.12	7.32	1.06
	Duroc-Jersey females, 1 year and older, pregnant, 2½ to 3 mos	16.4	0.11	5.90	0.66	0.05	8.86	0.80
McTaggart and Rowntree (1965)	Minimally diseased pigs, 90 kg	15.9	—	3.06	0.58	0.07	11.02	0.95
	Conventional pigs, 90 kg	19.6	—	6.31	0.98	0.13	10.57	1.25
Schalm, Jain, and Carroll (1975)	Pigs as a whole	16.0 (11.0–22.0)	0.16	5.92	0.56	0.08	8.48	0.80

*All values × 10³/µl.

red cell mass. Sow's milk provides approximately one-seventh of the necessary iron for hemoglobin formation of this expanding cell mass. The erythrocyte parameters observed during this period of rapid growth are influenced by iron supplied and may not reflect significant age variations (Miller et al. 1961). Oral iron compounds are effective in supplying the requirement when the chemical form and dosage are correct. Parenterally injected iron dextran given during the first days of life maintains adequate erythrocyte parameters (Kernkamp 1957). Although several chemical forms of iron administered orally will provide adequate iron, the ease of parenteral injection of iron compounds will continue to be the major reason for the popularity of this method of iron administration.

Vitamin E deficiency has been stated to be associated with anemia in pigs (Lynch et al. 1977). In studies on vitamin E and selenium deficiency in young pigs, it was found that vitamin E is not a limiting factor for normal erythropoiesis. Erythropoiesis appeared to be slightly decreased in selenium-deficient pigs (Fontaine, Valli, and Young 1977; Fontaine et al. 1977).

Tumbleson and coworkers (1969) found slightly increased hemoglobin, PCV, MCV, and MCH values on Hormel miniature swine from four to nine months of age. Erythrocyte parameters decreased during pregnancy, probably owing to the dilution effect of increased plasma volume (Tumbleson et al. 1970; Imlah and McTaggart, 1977).

Management may influence erythrocyte parameters in the postweaning period. Pigs kept under minimal disease conditions may have higher PCV, Hb, and RBC counts than conventionally reared pigs (McTaggart and Rowntree 1969). Erythrocyte values are given in Table 3–13.

Leukocyte Values

The leukocytes of the pig have significant age-related changes. The newborn pig invariably has more neutrophils than lymphocytes. At about one week, the lymphocytes become more numerous than the neutrophils. Lymphocyte counts may show distinct peaks during the 9- to 15-week age period (McTaggart 1975), with counts as high as $30.0 \times 10^6/\mu l$. Such peaks are of short duration. Leukocyte values are given in Table 3–14.

Leukocyte responses in disease are similar to those of other animals in general terms. However, specific diagnostic attributes of leukocyte responses are lacking in the literature. A postweaning pig with a total leukocyte count of under 10,000 is considered to be leukopenic. Variable causes are known for leukopenia in pigs, as for other species.

Platelets

The platelet counts of pigs are age variable, with the lowest counts reported for two-day-old pigs (mean $241,000/\mu l$) and a range for older pigs of 250,000 to $700,000/\mu L$ (Imlah and McTaggart, 1977).

Plasma Proteins

The plasma proteins are age variable. Schalm, Jain, and Carroll (1975) report total plasma proteins for pigs under one month of age to be less than 6.0 g/dl; for pigs two to six months of age, 6.0 to 7.0 g/dl; and for pigs over one year of age, 7.0 to 8.0 g/dl.

REFERENCES

Abbey, A. P., and Belliveau, R. R.: Enumeration of platelets. Am. J. Clin. Pathol. 69:55, 1978.

Allen, B. V., and Archer, R. K.: Studies with normal erythrocytes of the English Thoroughbred horse. Equine Vet. J. 5:135, 1973.

Archer, R. K.: Technical methods. In Comparative Clinical Haematology, Archer, R. K., and Jeffcott, L. B. (eds.). Oxford: Blackwell Scientific Publications, 1977, p. 575.

Archer, R. K., and Jeffcott, L. B. (eds.): Comparative Clinical Haematology. Oxford; Blackwell Scientific Publications, 1977.

Baetz, A. L., and Pearson, J. E.: Blood constituent changes in fasted ponies. Am. J. Vet. Res. 33:1941, 1972.

Bass, A. D.: The function of eosinophils. Ann. Intern. Med. 91:120, 1979.

Bendixen, H. J.: Bovine enzootic leukosis. Adv. Vet. Sci. 10:129, 1965.

Bremner, I., Brockway, J. M., Donnelly, H. T., and Webster, A. J. F.: Anemia and veal calf production. Vet. Rec. 99:203, 1976.

Burrows, G. E.: Equine Escherichia coli endotoxemia: Comparison of intravenous and intra-peritoneal endotoxin administration. Am. J. Vet. Res. 40:991, 1979.

Cartwright, G. E.: Diagnostic Laboratory Hematology. New York: Grune & Stratton, 1968.

Dodds, W. J.: Hemostasis and coagulation. In Clinical Biochemistry of Domestic Animals, 3rd ed. Kaneko, J. J. (ed.). New York: Academic Press, 1980.

Doxey, D. L.: Hematology of the fox. In Comparative Clinical Hematology. ed. by Archer, R. K., and Jeffcott, L. B. (eds.) Oxford: Blackwell Scientific Publications, 1977.

Feldman, B. F., Kaneko, J. J., and Farver, T. B.: Anemia of inflammatory disease: Availability of storage iron in inflammatory disease. Am. J. Vet. Res. 42:558, 1981.

Fontaine, M., Valli, V. E. O., and Young, L. G.: Studies on vitamin E and selenium deficiency in young pigs. III. Effect on erythrocyte production and destruction. Can. J. Comp. Med. 41:57, 1977.

Fontaine, M., Valli, V. E. O., Young, L. G., and Lumsden, J. H.: Studies on vitamin E and selenium deficiency in young pigs. I. Hematologic and biochemical changes. Can. J. Comp. Med. 41:41, 1977.

Grunsell, C. S.: Bone marrow biopsy in sheep. 1. Normal. Br. Vet. J. 107:16, 1951.

Harkness, J.: The viscosity of human blood plasma: Its measurement in health and disease. Biorheology 8:171, 1971.

Holman, H. H., and Dew, S. M.: The blood picture of the goat. IV. Changes in coagulation times, platelet counts and leukocyte numbers associated with age. Res. Vet. Sci. 6:510, 1965.

Holman, H. H., and Dew, S. M.: The blood picture of the goat. I. The two-year-old female goat. Res. Vet. Sci. 4:121, 1963.

Imlah, P., and McTaggart, H. S.: Hematology of the pig. In Comparative Clinical Hematology. Archer, R. K., and Jeffcott, L. B., (eds.). Oxford: Blackwell Scientific Publications, 1977.

Jacob, H. S., Craddock, P. R., Hammerschmidt, D. E., and Moldow, C. F.: Complement-induced granulocyte aggregation. N. Engl. J. Med. 302:379, 1980.

Jain, N. C., and Kono, C. S.: Fusiform erythrocytes resembling sickle cells in angora goats: Light and electron microscopic observations. Res. Vet. Sci. 22:169, 1977.

Jain, N. C., Kono, C. S., Myers, A., and Bottomly, K.: Fusiform erythrocytes resembling sickle cells in angora goats: Observations on osmotic and mechanical fragilities and reversal of cell shape during anemia. Res. Vet. Sci. 28:25, 1980.

Jain, N. C., and Lasmanis, J.: Leukocytic changes in cows given intravenous injections of Escherichia coli endotoxin. Res. Vet. Sci. 24:386, 1978.

Jain, N. C., Schalm, O. W., and Lasmanis, J.: Neutrophil kinetics in endotoxin-induced mastitis. Am. J. Vet. Res. 39:1662, 1978.

Jeffcott, L. B.: Clinical haematology of the horse. In Comparative Clinical Haematology. Archer R. K., and Jeffcott, L. B. (eds.). Oxford: Blackwell Scientific Publications, 1977.

Jeffcott, L. B.: Haematology in relation to performance and potential. 2. Some specific aspects. J. S. Afr. Vet. Assoc. 45:278, 1974.

Jones, D. M.: The husbandry and veterinary care of wild horses in captivity. Equine Vet. J. 8:40, 1976.

Kaneko, J. J., and Smith, R.: The estimation of plasma fibrinogen and its clinical significance in the dog. Calif. Vet. 27:21, 1967.

Kernhamp, H. C. H.: A parenteral hematinic for the control of iron-deficiency anemia in baby pigs. North Am. Vet. 38:6, 1957.

Kielstein, P.: Der Einfluss des Alters auf das Differentialblutbild des Pferdes. Vet. Diss. Leipzig, 1959. (Abstr. JAVMA 137:59, 1960).

Knill, L M., McConaughy, C., Camerena, I., and Day, M.: Hemogram of the Arabian horse. Am. J. Vet. Res. 30:295, 1969.

Kociba, G. J.: Disseminated intravascular coagulation. In Current Veterinary Therapy VI. Kirk, R. W. (ed.). Philadelphia: W. B. Saunders, 1977, p. 448.

Lynch, R. E., Hammar, S. P., Lee, G. R., and Cartwright, G. E.: The anemia of vitamin E deficiency: An experimental model of human congenital dyserythropoietic anemia. Am. J. Hematol. 2:145, 1977.

McTaggart, H. S.: Lymphocytosis in normal young pigs. Br. Vet. J. 131:574, 1975.

McTaggart, H. S., and Rowntree, P. G. M.: The haematology of "minimal disease" bacon pigs: A comparison with genetically-related conventionally-reared pigs. Br. Vet. J. 125:240, 1969.

Miller, E. R., Ullrey, D. E., Ackermann, I., Schmidt, D. A., Luecke, R. W., and Hoeffer, J. A.: Swine hematology from birth to maturity. II. Erythrocyte population, size and hemoglobin concentration. J. Anim. Sci. 20:890, 1961.

Mohandas, N., Clark, M. R., Wyatt, J. L., Garcia, J. F., Fisenberg, P. D., and Shohet, S. B.: Erythropoietic stress, macrocytosis and hemoglobin switching in HbAA sheep. Blood 55:757, 1980.

Moss, G., and Stauton, C.: Blood flow, needle size and hemolysis — examining an old wives' tale. N. Engl. J. Med. 282:967, 1970.

Naylor, J. M., Kronfeld, D. S., Bech-Nielsen, S., and Barthalomew, R. C.: Plasma total protein measurement for prediction of disease and mortality in calves. JAVMA 171:635, 1977.

Payne, J. M., Dew, S. M., Manston, R., and Faulks, M.: The use of metabolic profile tests in dairy herds. Vet. Rec. 87:150, 1970.

Penny, R. H. C., Carlisle, C. H., Davidson, H. A., and Gray, E. M.: Some observations on the effect of the concentration of ethylenediamine tetraacetic acid (EDTA) on the packed cell volume of domesticated animals. Br. Vet. J. 126:383, 1970.

Perman, V.: Unpublished data, 1980.

Perman, V., Dirks, V. A., Fangman, G., Snyder, M. M., Sorensen, D. K., Anderson, R. K., Goltz, D. J., Larson, V. L., and Stevens, J. B.: Statistical evaluation of lymphocyte values on Minnesota dairy cattle. Am. J. Vet. Res. 31:1217, 1970.

Perman, V., Rehfeld, C. E., Sautter, J. H., and Schultze, M. O.: Bioassay for toxic factor in trichloroethylene-extracted soy bean oil meal. Agri. Food Chem. 4:959, 1956.

Praase, K. W., George, L. W., and Whitlock, R. H.: Idiopathic hypersegmentation of neutrophils in a horse. JAVMA 178:303, 1981.

Pritchard, W. R., Rehfeld, C. E., Mizuno, N. S., Sautter, J. H., and Schultze, M. O.: Studies on trichloroethylene-extracted feeds. I. Experimental production of acute aplastic anemia in young heifers. Am. J. Vet. Res. 17:425, 1956.

Rawlings, C. A., Byars, T. D., Van Nay, M. K., and Bugard, C. E.: Activated coagulation test in normal and heparinized ponies and horses. Am. J. Vet. Res. 36:711, 1975.

Riley, J. H., and Lassen, E. D.: Activated coagulation times in normal cows. Vet. Clin. Pathol. 8:31, 1979.

Rowlands, G. J., Little, W., Stark, A. J., and Manston, R.: The blood composition of cows in commercial dairy herds and its relationships with season and lactation. Br. Vet. J. 135:64, 1979.

Schalm, O. W.: A simple and rapid method for staining blood films with new methylene blue. JAVMA 145:1184, 1964.

Schalm, O. W.: Equine hematology as an aid to diagnosis. In Proceedings of First International Symposium on Equine Hematology. Kitchen, H., and Krehbiel, J. D. (eds.). American Association of Equine Practitioners, Golden, CA. 1975a.

Schalm, O. W.: Bone marrow erythroid cytology in anemias of the horse. In Proceedings of First International Symposium on Equine Hematology. Kitchen, H., and Krehbiel, J. D. (eds.). American Assocation of Equine Practitioners, Golden, CA, 1975b.

Schalm, O. W.: Morphologic classification of the anemias. Calif. Vet. 28:30, 1974.

Schalm, O. W.: Clinical significance of plasma protein concentration. JAVMA 157:1627, 1970a.

Schalm, O. W.: Plasma protein: Fibrinogen ratios in disease in the dog and horse — Part II. Calif. Vet. 24:19, 1970b.

Schalm, O. W.: Plasma protein: Fibrinogen ratios in routine clinical material from cats, dogs, horses and cattle — Part III. Calif. Vet. 24:6, 1970c.

Schalm, O. W., Jain, N. C., and Carroll, E. J.: Veterinary Hematology, 3rd ed. Philadelphia; Lea & Febiger, 1975.

Schalm, O. W., Smith, R., and Kaneko, J. J.: Plasma protein: fibrinogen ratios in dogs, cattle and horses. Part I. Influence of age on normal values and explanation of use in disease. Calif. Vet. 24:9, 1970.

Schnappauf, H., Stein, H. B., Sipe, C. R., and Cronkite. E. P.: Erythropoietic response in calves following blood loss. Am. J. Vet. Res. 29:1991, 1967.

Schotman, A. J. H., and Kroneman, J.: Hyperlipemia in ponies. JAVMA 155:757, 1969.

Smith, J. E., and Agar, N. S.: Studies on erythrocyte metabolism following acute blood loss in the horse. Equine Vet. J. 8:34, 1976.

Stevens, J. B., Anderson, J. F., Olson, W. G., Perman, V., and Schlotthauer, J. C.: Metabolic profile test design for dairy herd application. Proceedings of Technicon International Conf., NY, Dec. 1976.

Stewart, J., and Holman, H. H.: The "blood picture" of the horse. Vet. Rec. 52:157, 1940.

Tennant, B., Harrold, D., Reina-Guerra, M., Kendrick, J. W., and Loben, R. C.: Hematology of the neonatal calf: Erythrocyte and leukocyte values of normal calves. Cornell Vet. 64:516, 1974.

Territo, M. C., and Cline. M. J.: Mononuclear phagocytic proliferation, maturation and function. Clin. Haematol. 4:685, 1975.

Trum, B. F.: Normal variances in horse blood due to breed, age, lactation, pregnancy and altitude. Am. J. Vet. Res. 13:514, 1952.

Tumbleson, M. E., Burks, M. F., Spote, M. P., Hutcheson, D. P., Middleton, C. C.: Serum biochemical and hematological parameters of Sinclaire (5–1) miniature sows during gestation and lactation. Can. J. Comp. Med. 34:312, 1970.

Tumbleson, M. E., Middleton, C. C., Tinsley, O. W., and Hutcheson, D. P.: Serum biochemic and hematologic parameters of Hormel miniature swine from four to nine months of age. Lab. Anim. Care 19:345, 1969.

Turner, A. W., and Hodgetts, V. E.: The dynamic red cell storage function of the spleen in sheep. 1. Relationship to fluctuations of irregular hematocrit. Aust. J. Exp. Biol. Med. Sci. 37:399, 1959.

Usenik, E. A., and Cronkite, E. P.: Effects of barbiturate anesthetics on leukocytes in normal and splenectomized dogs. Anesth. Anal. 44:167, 1965.

Valli, V. E. O., Holland, T. J., McSherry, B. J., Robinson, G. A., and Gilman, J. P. W.: The kinetics of hematopoiesis in the calf. I. An autoradiographic study of myelopoiesis in normal, anemic and endotoxin treated calves. Res. Vet. Sci. 12:535, 1971.

Valli, V. E. O., McSherry, B. J., Robinson, G. A., and Willoughby, R. A.: Leukophoresis in calves and dogs by extracorporeal circulation of blood through siliconized glass wool. Res. Vet. Sci. 10:267, 1969.

Wingfield, W. E., and Tumbleson, M. E.: Hematologic parameters as a function of age, in female dairy cattle. Corn. Vet. 63:72, 1973.

Wintrobe, M. M.: Clinical Hematology, 7th ed. Philadelphia: Lea & Febiger, 1974, p. 119.

Young, N. S., and Nienhuis, A. W.: Hemoglobin switching in sheep and man. In The Year in Hematology. Silber, R., LoBue, J., and Gordon, A. S. (eds.). New York: Plenum Publishing, 1978.

CHAPTER 4

THE NERVOUS SYSTEM

I. G. MAYHEW, B.V.SC., PH.D.
Ted S. STASHAK, D.V.M., M.S.

INTRODUCTION

The major objectives of a neurological examination are, firstly, to determine whether a neurological deficit exists and, secondly, to determine the site(s) of the lesion(s). At the conclusion of the neurological examination, the clinician should be able to localize the site of the lesion within one or more of the general areas — *cerebrum, brainstem, cerebellum, spinal cord, peripheral nerves,* and *muscles.* The more detailed and precise the examination, the more accurate the localization of the lesion. After the site of the lesion is determined, the clinician may consider the possible etiological mechanisms and the therapy and management of the case.

This chapter is designed firstly as a guide for the clinician in performing a neurological examination in any large animal, in reaching an anatomic and etiologic diagnosis, and in utilizing pertinent ancillary aids. Chapter 17 is designed as an introduction to neurosurgical procedures that have been, or could be, utilized in large animals. Emphasis is given to the more frequently occurring diseases in which neurosurgical intervention must be considered. The methodology for the neurological examination is based on the works of deLahunta (1977), Howard (1968), Mayhew and Ingram (1978), Palmer (1976), and Rooney (1971). The reader is referred to deLahunta (1977), Getty (1975), and Jenkins (1977) for further reading on the neuroanatomical basis of the neurological examination.

DIAGNOSTIC NEUROLOGY FOR LARGE ANIMALS

Approach to the Neurological Case

Evaluation of large animals suspected of having neurological disease can be one of the most fascinating and rewarding challenges in veterinary clinical diagnosis. Establishing, performing, and recording a thorough neurological examination are the essential components that must be mastered to meet this challenge. Added to this, a basic understanding of the nervous system's structure and function and an ability to observe carefully and reason logically will then result in accurate evaluation of a neurological case. Most veterinarians are capable of achieving this, but all too often omission of a thorough neurological examination thwarts all efforts aimed at successful case management.

Experience and logic have shown that a neurological examination informs us of the presence and site of a lesion — not the cause. This information, along with information obtained from the history, physical examination, and ancillary procedures, can then result in a differential diagnosis, a prognosis, and a suitable plan for therapy. Neurological examinations often must be repeated. Subtle changes may alter the prognosis or the required therapy and may even affect the diagnosis. Thus, results of a neurological examination must be recorded — they cannot be left to memory.

The aims of the clinician evaluating a large animal suspected of having a neurological disease should be (1) to determine if a neurological deficit exists; (2) to determine the site of the lesion; (3) to determine what is causing the lesion; and (4) to treat the animal.

Neurological Examination

The nervous system can be regarded as a relatively hidden body system insofar as it is not accessible to the preliminary clinical examination procedures of observation, palpation, percussion, and auscultation. Also, the functions of the nervous system are observed by its effects on other body systems, notably the musculoskeletal system. These effects may be altered by providing the nervous system with information via its sensory pathways. The neurological examination is thus a series of observations of the functions of the many systems that are affected by the nervous system and alterations in these symptoms as a result of specific standardized stimuli to the afferent pathways. To evaluate the nervous system one must *make* these observations and *perform* these standardized tests.

The order in which a neurological examination is carried out is important; omission is the most common mistake in performing the examination. In this text, a precise practical format is given that is logical in sequence and easy to remember with practice and that emphasizes the necessity of an *anatomical* diagnosis (where is the lesion?) before an *etiological* diagnosis (what causes it?).

The rationale for the sequence of the neurological examination is threefold. First, the examination starts at the head and proceeds caudally to the tail. Second, the same procedure is used in all species, whether the patient is ambulatory or recumbent. Third, the anatomical location of a lesion is considered as the examination proceeds.

Evidence of a lesion in the brain is sought initially. If there are no head signs, then the lesion is likely to be in the spinal cord, peripheral nerves, or muscles. If there are signs of a lesion in the brain, then an attempt is made to explain all abnormalities in the rest of the examination as a result of such a lesion. If this cannot be done, then more than one lesion must be present. Examination of the gait follows to give an overall assessment of the limbs. This is followed by specific evaluation of the neck and forelimbs. If neurological signs exist in the forelimbs and they cannot be explained by evidence of a lesion in the brain, then a lesion is present between C_1* and T_2 (including spinal and peripheral nerves). The back and hind limbs are then assessed. Again, if any neurological signs present cannot be explained by evidence of a lesion cranial to T_3, then a lesion is present between T_3 and S_2. Finally, the tail and anus are assessed. If a neurological deficit exists in this area and cannot be explained by evidence of a lesion cranial to S_2, then a lesion exists between S_3 and the last caudal segment. The overall sequence of evaluation for the neurologic examination is as follows:

1. Head
   a. Behavior
   b. Mental status
   c. Head posture and coordination
   d. Cranial nerves
2. Gait and posture
3. Neck and forelimbs
4. Back and hind limbs
5. Tail and anus

HEAD

Behavior. The owner should be questioned about the patient's behavior and normal responses. Age, breed, and sex may influence behavior. An animal that is recumbent owing to cervical spinal cord disease will not usually have altered behavior. Occasionally, some animals (particularly horses and wild cattle) that are recumbent owing to spinal cord disease, fractured long bones, myopathy, aortic thrombosis, and even acute vestibular disease will be delirious and even aggressive in their frantic struggle to get up.

Close observation may be required to observe seizures in an animal in which they have been documented historically. Auditory and tactile stimulation will

---

*C = cervical, T = thoracic, L = lumbar, S = sacral, Ca = caudal (coccygeal) spinal cord regions. Subscript number denotes specific segment within each region.

sometimes elicit seizure activity. It has been observed in mares that recurrent bouts of seizures associated with several different brain lesions occur at the time of estrus. Any seizure activity must be recorded accurately to assist in determining the progression of disease and response to therapy.

Bizarre and inappropriate behavior, such as head pressing, compulsive wandering, circling, changes in voice and appetite, licking objects, and aggressiveness, are easy to recognize and are usually regarded as signs of cerebral disease. Remarkable alterations in behavior in the horse occur with hepatoencephalopathy. Calves with many diffuse encephalopathies, particularly those associated with lead poisoning, will show odontoprisis (teeth grinding). Also, cattle with lead poisoning and rabies may bellow continually, foals with neonatal meningitis and cerebral hemorrhage may bark like dogs, and pigs with salt poisoning often do not squeal, even with noxious stimuli.

Although behavioral abnormalities cannot usually be defined as asymmetrical, an animal with a cerebral lesion, if it circles compulsively, will tend to circle toward the side of the lesion. This may be seen, for example, with a cerebral hematoma in a calf and with a cerebral abscess in a horse.

Mental Status. An assessment is made of the patient's state of awareness or consciousness. This level of responsiveness of an animal to its internal and external environment is affected by the ascending reticular activating system (ARAS) in the brainstem and by the cerebral cortex. These areas can be affected by stimuli received by the sensory nervous system. Thus, in evaluating the mental status of an animal, the response to visual, tactile, auditory, painful, olfactory, and gustatory (nursing) stimuli should be considered.

Coma is a state of complete unresponsiveness to noxious stimuli. The deepest comas in animals are usually related to brainstem, particularly midbrain, lesions. Head trauma, with or without skull fracture, often results in hemorrhages in the brainstem and varying degrees of unconsciousness.

Semicoma is a state of partial responsiveness to stimuli. An animal in semicoma does not respond to the environment or to minor stimuli (e.g., visual) but responds, usually in an altered manner, to noxious stimuli. Voluntary movements occur with stimulation. Other less profound levels of loss of awareness are variously described as stupor, obtundation, somnolence, deliriousness, lethargy, and depression. These states often result from lesions affecting the cerebral cortex, such as severe hydrocephalus and hepatoencephalopathy.

Animals that are recumbent owing to spinal cord disease are usually bright and alert. However, particularly with heavy animals and those that struggle, some depression is often observed because of exhaustion, anorexia, dehydration, decubital sores, and myositis.

Head Posture and Coordination. All normal animals maintain the head in a certain posture and maneuver it quickly and smoothly to perform certain acts (e.g., prehension of food). Abnormal input from the vestibular system often affects the mechanisms maintaining head posture, resulting in a head tilt. Such a vestibular head tilt is characterized by the poll being deviated to one side and the muzzle being deviated to the opposite side. In comparison, an animal with a cerebral lesion that continually turns in circles often has the whole head (and neck) deviated to one side. In this circumstance, the poll is not rotated about the muzzle, and there is a slight scoliosis of the neck to one side.

The cerebellum modulates movements of the head as well as locomotion. With cerebellar disease, the fine control of head positioning is often lost, resulting in awkward, jerky movements. Often, even at rest, the lack of control is seen as bobbing movements of the head. This bob can be exaggerated by increasing the voluntary effort of the head positioning, such as offering the animal some feed or forcing it to watch something intently. The resulting fine jerky movements of the head are called intention tremor. Cerebellar degeneration in Arabian foals, cerebellar abiotrophy in Yorkshire pigs, and in utero infection of calves with bovine virus diarrhea are examples of cerebellar diseases often producing these head signs.

Cranial Nerves. Abnormalities in the cranial nerve (CN) examination are most helpful in localizing a lesion in the brain. The examiner starts with the most rostral nerve and proceeds caudally, assessing the function of each cranial nerve.

I.* OLFACTORY NERVE. Clinical deficit of smell (anosmia) is rarely encountered in large animals. Such a deficit may, however, be significant in localizing a lesion to the frontal lobes or the limbic system resulting in behavioral changes. Normal function is usually equated with the patient's ability to smell the hand of the examiner or its feed. Further assessment should entail the use of pure aromas like citrol rather than substances that are irritants to the nasal mucosa such as ammonia and cigarette smoke.

II. OPTIC NERVE. An owner may indicate that a patient has been acting as if it were blind, but the observations leading to this interpretation must be questioned; a depressed animal or one with vestibular disease may stumble over objects without being blind.

The visual pathway of animals is tested by the menace (blink or eye preservation) response. A threatening gesture of the hand toward the eye will elicit immediate closure of the eyelids, and the head may be jerked away. In the sheep and horse, approximately 90 per cent of fibers in the optic nerve cross over to the opposite (contralateral) side at the optic chiasm (Cummings and deLahunta, 1969). Thus, for practical purposes in large animals, vision in one eye is perceived by the visual cortex of the contralateral cerebral hemisphere. The incoming or afferent pathway for this menace response is the ipsilateral eye and optic nerve, the optic chiasm, and the contralateral optic tract, lateral geniculate nucleus (thalamus), optic radiation, and occipital cortex. The outgoing or efferent pathway of the menace response is from this contralateral visual cortex to the ipsilateral facial nucleus affecting closure of the eyelids. A jerking away of the head would be affected by the accessory

nucleus and probably other lower motor neurons to the somatic musculature of the neck.

When checking the menace response, it is important to avoid touching the face or creating air currents that may be felt, either of which can allow a blind patient to perceive the menace and close the eyelids. On the other hand, some stoic, depressed, or even excited animals may not respond by closing the eyelids or may keep the eyelids closed. In such cases a light tap on the head near the eye with the menacing hand will often attract the patient's attention so that the test can then be performed. Neonatal animals, although sighted, often do not respond and may become refractory to repeated menace testing.

If there is any question whether or not the menace response is present, a true visual deficiency may be detected while the animal moves about its environment, when objects are placed in front of it, or when nonaromatic objects are dropped noiselessly in its visual fields. Nyctalopia or night blindness, such as occurs in Appaloosa horses and in growing or adult cattle with vitamin A deficiency, may best be demonstrated by moving the animal through a maze in dim light. To better assess a unilateral blindness, blindfolding each eye in turn while the animal maneuvers through the maze can be helpful. Unilateral blindness (hemianopia) can be very difficult to assess in some cases, and it may take repeated efforts to determine this abnormality. Often the examiner must resort to sneaking up to the patient's stall and making noiseless gestures, first from one visual field (side) and then the other.

Ophthalmoscopic examination of the fundus should be included in the neurological evaluation. This may show congenital optic nerve hypoplasia, as reported in the horse and in vitamin A–deficient calves. Swelling of the optic disc may be associated with optic neuritis.

Lesions of the eye and optic nerves, such as periorbital masses, cranial trauma with contusion of the optic nerve, and optic nerve hypoplasia, can result in ipsilateral blindness. Lesions of the optic tracts and lateral geniculate nucleus cause contralateral blindness.

Space-occupying cerebral lesions, such

---

*The classic notation of Roman numerals I through XII will be used to identify the cranial nerves.

as hematomas and abscesses caused by *Streptococcus equi* and *Corynebacterium pyogenes*, frequently result in blindness. This can be the result of direct involvement of the central visual pathways. More frequently the blindness arises from the pressure and cerebral edema caused by the mass; the occipital lobes are forced caudally into the tentorium cerebelli and herniate under this rigid part of the calvarium. The resulting blindness will be contralateral to the lesion but is often bilateral because of the associated diffuse brain swelling. Overzealous use of a hot iron or caustic chemicals when dehorning young kid goats can cause necrosis of the thin bones of the skull and extensive malacia of the underlying cerebrum, resulting in blindness. Embolism to the cerebral circulation can give rise to infarction of central visual pathways and blindness. This can be seen with thrombosis of the cerebral vessels as seen in *Hemophilus somnus* infection in cattle and arteritis of the blood vessels supplying the head of the horse in *Strongylus vulgaris* infestation.

With involvement of the central visual pathways, the pupillary light responses will be intact. However, with involvement of the eyeball, optic nerves, or chiasm, the pupillary light responses will be abnormal.

All species of large animals with various diffuse cerebellar diseases have been observed to have bilaterally deficient menace responses, although neither blindness nor facial paralysis has been present to explain this finding. It is assumed that the efferent pathway for the menace response passes from the contralateral occipital cortex, through the ipsilateral cerebellum, to the facial nucleus.

III. OCULOMOTOR NERVE. The diameter of the pupillary aperture is controlled by the constrictor muscles of the pupil innervated by the parasympathetic fibers in the oculomotor nerve and by the dilator muscles of the pupil innervated by the sympathetic fibers from the cranial cervical ganglion. These autonomic innervations have their upper motor neurons in the brainstem and change pupil diameter in response to light (oculomotor nerve), fear, and excitement (sympathetic).

The first observation to be made is the size and symmetry of the pupillary apertures, taking into consideration the amount of ambient light and the emotional status of the patient. The response of the pupils to light directed into each eye — the pupillary light responses — can then be noted after observing the eyeballs for any lesion that may interfere with the response of the pupil such as adhesions or lesions caused by iritis, iris atrophy, or glaucoma. The normal response to light directed into one eye is constriction of both pupils; this is referred to as a direct response in the eye in which the light is shone (ipsilateral) and a consensual response in the other (contralateral) eye. The afferent pathway for this reflex is similar to that for the menace response to the level of the thalamus. The pathway is through the optic nerve, optic chiasm, where some crossing occurs, through both optic tracts lateral and dorsal to the thalamus without synapsing, then ventrally into the midbrain. Crossing occurs at this site, and axons pass to the parasympathetic oculomotor nuclei in the midbrain on both sides. The motor (efferent) pathway is from these nuclei via the oculomotor nerves to the ciliary ganglia behind the eyeballs and to the constrictor muscles of the pupils.

This pupillary light reflex is within the brainstem and is not affected by lesions involving the visual cortex. A widely dilated (mydriatic) pupil in an eye that has normal vision suggests an oculomotor nucleus or nerve lesion. Such a pupil will be unresponsive to light directed into either eye. The pupil in the contralateral eye will respond to light directed into either eye. A retrobulbar lesion involving the optic and oculomotor nerves will also be seen as a mydriatic pupil that is unresponsive to light shone in either eye, but in addition there will be a visual (menace) deficit in the eye.

Cranial injury can result in concussion, contusion, and hemorrhage in the brainstem with effects on the oculomotor nuclei and nerves. Also, because of their position on the ventral aspect of the brainstem, the oculomotor nerves are subject to damage by any swelling (e.g., edema) or space-occupying lesion (e.g., abscess) in the forebrain exerting pressure on the brainstem. With asymmetrical swelling of the cerebral tissue, greater pressure may be applied to one oculomotor nerve, resulting in anisocoria (asymmetrical pupils), which is usually evident as ipsilateral pupillary dilation. Severe brainstem contusion can produce various pupillary abnormalities in association with coma or semicoma, which can change rapidly in the first few hours following injury. Progressive bilateral dilation following cranial injury warrants a grave prognosis.

Horner's syndrome in the horse is an easily recognizable entity, although it can be readily overlooked in the cow and especially so in the sheep and goat (Smith and Mayhew, 1977). The upper motor neuron cell bodies of the sympathetic nervous system are located in the hypothalamus, midbrain, pons, and medulla. These areas, particularly the hypothalamus, receive input of various modalities (e.g., pain, fright, cardiovascular function, and so on) from the rest of the nervous system. Neuronal fibers descend through the midbrain, medulla, and cervical spinal cord in the lateral tectotegmentospinal tract to synapse on preganglionic cell bodies in the lateral intermediate gray column of the thoracolumbar spinal cord. The preganglionic sympathetic cell bodies supplying the head are situated in this position in the cranial thoracic segments (T_1–T_3). Axons leave these segments of the spinal cord, traverse the thorax, and ascend the neck with the vagus nerve in the vagosympathetic trunk to the cranial cervical ganglion. In the horse, the cranial cervical ganglion lies on the caudodorsal wall of the medial compartment of the guttural pouch below the atlanto-occipital articulation. In ruminants, the ganglion is closer to the base of the cranium and lies medial to the tympanic bulla. Postganglionic sympathetic fibers leave the cranial cervical ganglion to innervate the glands, smooth muscles, and blood vessels of the eyeball, head, and cranial cervical area (deLahunta, 1977; Getty, 1975).

Damage to the sympathetic supply of the eyeball results in Horner's syndrome. In the horse this is seen as a slight ptosis of the upper lid, a miosis (constriction of the pupil), and a slight protrusion of the nictitating membrane; vision and the pupillary light response are unaffected. In the cow, sheep, and goat these signs can be very subtle. These components of Horner's syndrome may be seen with a lesion involving the postganglionic fibers to the eyeball after they have left the cranial cervical ganglion. Lesions involving the sympathetic supply to the head give rise to signs of Horner's syndrome and additional signs. In the horse, these additional signs include a dilation of facial blood vessels, hyperemia of nasal and conjunctival mucous membranes, increased temperature, and sweating of the face. This latter sign is most prominent at the base of the ear and is present over the face and neck down to the level of the axis. Sweating may be only a temporary finding, although the other signs may persist. All these signs have been produced experimentally in the horse and have been seen with involvement of the sympathetic pathways in guttural pouch mycosis and surgery following trauma, focal infection, or neoplasia in the area of the cervical vagosympathetic trunk and with a space-occupying lesion (melanoma) at the thoracic inlet (Smith and Mayhew, 1977). In cattle, the additional signs caused by involvement of the entire sympathetic supply to the head are distension of vasculature and cutaneous warming of the pinna and a *reduced* production of beads of sweat over the nostril on the affected side. Only ophthalmic signs of Horner's syndrome have been recorded in goats and sheep. Signs of Horner's syndrome can also present with lesions involving the descending sympathetic pathways in the brainstem and cervical spinal cord. In the horse, such a lesion affects the entire spinal cord sympathetic outflow, resulting in increased cutaneous blood flow (heat) and sweating on the same side of the body as the lesion. This sign would be expected only in horses.

III. OCULOMOTOR NERVE; IV. TROCHLEAR NERVE; VI. ABDUCENT NERVE. In addition to innervation of the pupillary constrictor muscles, the oculomotor nerve also innervates the extraocular muscles along with the trochlear and abducent nerves. The function of these muscles and nerves is tested by observing normal position of the eyes within the orbits and eye movement. An abnormal position (strabismus) results when these nerves or muscles are damaged.

Consideration must be given to the normal response of the eyes to head posture and movement. When the nose of a large animal is elevated (head extended), the eyes tend to maintain a horizontal position and thus move ventrally in the orbits. Rotation of the head about its long axis results in dorsal movement of the eye in the orbit on the side to which the head is rotated and ventral movement of the eye on the other side. This is most pronounced in cattle. While the head is moved to one side, the eyes move in a rhythmical manner instead of remaining fixed in the center of the bony orbit. There is a slow phase of movement in the direction opposite that of head movement followed by a fast phase in the direction of head movement. These rhythmical eye movements continue until the head comes to rest and the eyes return to the center of the orbits. These eye movements are regarded as normal vestibular nystagmus and result from connection between the vestibular nuclei (balance centers) in the medulla and the nuclei of the cranial nerves controlling eye movement (III, IV, VI). Vestibular nystagmus thus requires an intact vestibular system; intact cranial nerves III, IV, and VI; and the direct connection between these structures.

The exact neurological findings with specific paralysis of each of these three cranial nerves are not known in large animals. The oculomotor nerve innervates the dorsal, ventral, and medial recti and the ventral, oblique, and levator palpebral muscles. Paralysis of the oculomotor nerve should thus produce a lateral and ventral strabismus. A ptosis of the upper eyelid should arise from paralysis of the levator palpebral muscle. Mydriasis and absent pupillary light reflex may also be present due to paralysis of the pupillary constrictor muscles as discussed previously. Paralysis of the trochlear nerve, which innervates the dorsal oblique muscles, should result in dorsal rotation of the medial aspect of the pupil. A rotational strabismus such as this (described as dorsomedial) is regularly seen in cattle with polioencephalomalacia. This is possibly due to the peculiar sensitivity of the trochlear nerve neurons to damage from the metabolic defect produced by thiamine deficiency. The abducent nerve innervates the lateral rectus and retractor bulbi muscles. Thus, damage to this nerve might produce a medial strabismus and a lack of the ability to retract the globe in the orbit. This latter response is tested in the corneal reflex. When the eyelids are held open and the cornea is gently touched, the globe is withdrawn in the orbit, resulting in passive protrusion of the third eyelid. The afferent component of this reflex is the ophthalmic branch of the trigeminal nerve. The efferent pathway involves the abducent nerve and the retractor oculi muscle, but probably also the oculomotor and trochlear nerves and involvement of all the extraocular muscles. Spasm of the extraocular muscles resulting in eyeball retraction and protrusion (flicking) of the nictitating membrane is frequently seen in tetanus in all large animal species, particularly the horse. This probably results from a predilection of the tetanus toxin for the internuncial neurons in these three cranial nerve nuclei, particularly those of the abducent nuclei.

The forms of strabismus described for paralysis of each of these nerves should be present in all positions of the head. The eyes should not be able to be moved to the position opposite the direction of strabismus because of muscle paralysis. Such examples of true strabismus are rarely encountered in large animals but may be expected with severe brainstem lesions. A deviation of the eyeballs resulting from a disturbance of the vestibular system that alters the normal tonic mechanism controlling eye position is more frequently seen. This vestibular strabismus is usually seen as a ventral deviation of the eyeballs. The important difference is that the eyeballs can be moved out of this position and will usually respond with vestibular nystagmus when the head is rotated. With unilateral vestibular system disease, such as otitis media, otitis interna, or listeriosis, this vestibular strabismus involves the eyeball on the ipsilateral side.

One further mechanism can result in abnormal eye positions without damage to the innervation of the extraocular muscles. With some asymmetrical cerebral lesions there can be a tendency for the animal to turn and walk in the direction of the lesion. Occasionally in an animal with such a lesion, all responses of the head and body will be directed toward that one side. Thus, movement in response to a visual, tactile, or auditory stimulus on either side will always be toward the side of the lesion. These movements can also involve the extraocular muscles with resulting bilateral strabismus, lateral on the side of the lesion and medial on the contralateral side. The syndrome can be regarded as an aversion phenomenon toward the side of the lesion. Again, the eyeballs are not fixed in the abnormal position owing to muscle paralysis.

V. TRIGEMINAL NERVE. This large cranial nerve contains motor nerve fibers to the muscles of mastication in the mandibular branch and sensory nerve fibers from most of the head in all three branches — mandibular, maxillary, and ophthalmic. As well as these three branches being separate nerves after exiting the cranium, the motor and sensory nuclei of the trigeminal nerve are quite separate within the brainstem. Thus, lesions can quite readily involve only parts of this cranial nerve, necessitating a critical evaluation of each function.

Loss of motor function of the mandibular nerve bilaterally results in a dropped jaw and an inability to close the mouth. The tongue may appear to protrude because it drops forward in the mouth. Saliva dribbles from the mouth because of the lack of jaw movement. Unilateral lesions usually result in weak jaw tone. Atrophy of the temporal and masseter muscles and the distal belly of the digastricus muscle also occurs; asymmetrical lesions will result in asymmetrical muscle atrophy.

Pituitary abscesses in cattle and sheep often spread rostrally and caudally to involve cranial nerves as they exit the cranium. Cranial nerves II through XII can be involved, although the oculomotor and trigeminal nerves are most frequently affected, resulting in mydriasis and a dropped jaw. In listeriosis in ruminants, there can be microabscessation of the motor nucleus of the trigeminal nerve with weak jaw tone or a dropped jaw. Injury to the head and jaws in a squeeze chute can result in a dropped jaw with no evidence of fracture or dislocation of the mandible. This syndrome may result from bilateral injury to the mandibular nerve. A severe myopathy involving these muscles with resulting atrophy can obviously mimic these findings; electromyography may be the best method of differentiation.

Function of the sensory branches of this cranial nerve is tested reflexly and directly by assessing sensation to the head. Gentle pricking of the ear stimulates sensory nerve endings in the maxillary branch and results in reflex flicking of the ear. Gentle palpation of the medial (ophthalmic branch) and lateral (maxillary branch) margins of the eyelids results in closure of the eyelids. Pin pricking of the upper lip and nostrils tests the maxillary nerve; the response is a movement of the lips and nostrils. Similarly, pricking the lower lip and cheek tests the sensory branch of the mandibular nerve and results in movement of the lips. The motor pathway of all these reflexes, resulting in movement of the ears, eyelids, nostrils, and lips, is in the branches of the facial nerve. The corneal reflex, as described previously, is tested by gently touching the cornea with the eyelids held open; withdrawal of the eyeball and passive protrusion of the nictitating membrane indicate a normal reflex. This reflex involves the sensory ophthalmic nerve and the motor nerve fibers supplying the muscles that withdraw the eyeball (III, IV, and VI).

Sensation of the head should be assessed in the distribution of each of the major branches of the trigeminal nerve. This can be achieved by observing a cerebral response (pulling the head, shaking the head, attempts to bite, phonation, and so on) at the time of reflex testing. Sensation from at least the lateral and medial canthi of the eyelids and the cheek should be tested to evaluate the maxillary, ophthalmic, and mandibular nerves, respectively. In stoic or depressed animals, sensation may be assessed by lightly pricking sensitive membranes of the internal nares and nasal septum. Lesions that affect the motor function of the trigeminal nerve can also result in hyporeflexia and hypalgesia of the face from involvement of the sensory components. Lesions of the spinal tract and sensory nucleus of the trigeminal nerve on the side of the medulla can result in facial hypalgesia and hyporeflexia without weakness of the muscles of mastication. In the horse, at least, this may result in feed impacting in the rostral cheek pouch because the horse cannot feel the feed. Horses that acquire the syndrome of continually rubbing one side of their face, even to the point of self-induced injury, are said to have idiopathic hyperesthesia, which is referred to as trigeminal neuralgia. This may be similar to head shyness, which some horses can develop. The etiology of this syndrome is usually unknown; however, several horses with guttural pouch mycosis have been reported to show this, although no association with the trigeminal nerve could be made (Cook 1968). It has been observed that extensive cerebral and thalamic lesions can produce a contralateral facial hypalgesia that is most evident in the nasal septum, without hyporeflexia. This is thought to be due to involvement of the sensory parietal cortex with sparing of the trigeminal nuclei and reflex pathways in the brainstem. Lesions resulting in this sign include thalamic abscesses in cows and cholesterol granulomata of the lateral ventricles, cerebral protozoal myeloencephalitis lesions, and those lesions deriving from intracarotid injections and cerebral contusions in horses.

VII. FACIAL NERVE. This is predominantly a motor nerve innervating the muscles of facial expression and the lacrimal and certain salivary glands. This nerve contains the lower motor neurons of many of the reflexes tested previously. Initial evaluation of the facial nerve involves observation of those reflexes that result in closure of the eyelids (menace, palpebral, and corneal reflexes) and movement of the ears, eyelids, lips, and nostrils. In large animals a facial paralysis is generally seen as a drooping of the ear, ptosis of the upper eyelid, drooping of the lips, and a pulling of the nostrils to the unaffected side. It is worth remembering that a ptosis of the upper eyelids is not what would be expected and is not seen in small animals with facial paralysis. This is because the facial nerve innervates the muscles that close the eyelids (musculus orbicularis oculi). A paralysis of these muscles perhaps would be expected to result in a wider palpebral fissure. It is probable that the bulk of atonic orbicular muscles of the eye weighs down the upper eyelid, partly closing it. General inspection for symmetry of facial expression is a useful way to detect a unilateral facial paresis. An evaluation of the tone in the orbicular muscles that close the eyelids can be helpful. This is achieved by placing a finger lightly on each cornea to detect the force of eyelid closure. Detection of a deviation of the nasal philtrum, especially in the pig, can best be achieved by looking down on the face (i.e., a dorsal view). Some normal horses do appear to have a subtle deviation of the nostrils to one side when viewed from the front. Movement of the nares during respiration must be observed, as a lack of flaring on one side during inspiration may be one of the earliest findings in facial paresis.

Observation of the use of the muzzle, lips, and cheeks during prehension and mastication should be observed. A cow, sheep, goat, or horse with unilateral facial paresis can lose feed out of the side of the mouth; there can be difficulty in moving feed such as hay into the mouth so that it remains in the lips on the affected side longer; and occasionally a small amount of feed may remain in the cheeks on the affected side. This must not be confused with the dysphagia that results from sensory and/or motor trigeminal paralysis. The tone present in the lips can be evaluated by grasping the lips at the commissures and detecting resistance to movement. Because of the lack of muscle tone, saliva may drool from the corners of the lips in facial paralysis. If there is only weakness of the lips and a deviated nasal philtrum without a drooped ear and ptosis, it is most likely due to involvement of only the buccal and nasal branches, indicating the presence of a peripheral lesion involving the facial nerve along the side of the face. This can be seen with direct injury or following prolonged recumbency. The facial nucleus can be involved in lesions of the medulla caused by equine protozoal myeloencephalitis, listeriosis in ruminants, and cerebrospinal nematodiasis (caused by migrating parasites such as *Parelaphostrongylus tenuis*) in goats and sheep. As with other cranial nerves, the diagnosis of a central (versus peripheral) nerve lesion can be made by identifying involvement of adjacent structures in the medulla oblongata. Often, with facial nuclear lesions, there will be depression due to reticular formation involvement and signs of damage to vestibular nuclei and other cranial nerve nuclei (V through XII). Most particularly, there will often be a gait abnormality in the limbs on the same side as the lesion, originating from ascending proprioception tract and descending motor tract involvement. Facial nerve paresis can be seen with meningitis in any large animal. An idiopathic facial paralysis has been seen, at least in horses, that is transient and presumed to be a selective viral or allergic neuritis. The chronic, diffuse, granulomatous neuritis that affects the cauda equina of the horse (cauda equina neuritis, polyneuritis equi) can also involve other spinal and cranial nerves including the facial nerve. In otitis media that extends to produce an otitis interna and resulting vestibular signs, there is often an accompanying facial nerve paralysis. This is because the facial nerve lies in the facial canal of the petrous temporal bone and is separated from the tympanic cavity by only a thin membrane. Lack of involvement of other areas of the brainstem is used to differentiate such signs of peripheral facial and vestibular nerve disease from involvement of these nerves as they leave the medulla together and from involvement of their nuclei within the medulla oblongata. In the horse the facial nerve lies on the dorsolateral aspect of the wall of the lateral compartment of the guttural pouch where it is near the mandibular nerve (V) and the maxillary artery. Guttural pouch mycosis has been associated with facial paralysis (Björklund and Palsson 1970).

VIII. VESTIBULOCOCHLEAR NERVE. The cochlear division of this nerve transmits impulses involved with hearing. Bilateral otitis media–otitis interna would result in deafness, but unilateral hearing loss associated with unilateral otitis media–otitis interna is very difficult to detect.

The vestibular division of the eighth cranial nerve supplies the major input to the vestibular system. Fibers carrying impulses from the receptor end-organs in the semicircular canals, saccule, and utricle pass in this nerve through the internal acoustic meatus with the cochlear division, through the vestibular ganglion in the petrosal bone, penetrating the lateral medulla oblongata and terminating in the vestibular nuclei. A few fibers pass directly to small parts of the cerebellum that are in the vestibular system: the fastigial nuclei and the flocculonodular lobes. The vestibular system receives input from many higher centers and from the cerebellum and functions in controlling orientation of the head, body, limbs, and eyes in space.

Signs of vestibular disease can be seen with lesions involving any part of the vestibular system. Changes in normal head posture have been described, and alterations in body and limb orientation seen with vestibular disease will be examined under gait. The abnormal eye positions that frequently occur with vestibular system disorders have been described.

In evaluating normal vestibular function, the eyeballs are checked for normal position in the bony orbits with the head in normal and extended positions and for normal vestibular nystagmus when the head is moved from side to side. The presence of nystagmus with the head resting in a normal position (spontaneous) or with the head held still in various abnormal positions (positional) is regarded as abnormal and is indicative of a disorder of the vestibular system. The direction of nystagmus can be helpful in determining the site of the vestibular lesion and is always described by referring to the fast phase. In peripheral vestibular system disorders such as trauma to the petrous temporal bone and otitis media–otitis interna, the nystagmus (fast phase) is always directed away from the side of the lesion and the direction of head tilt. It is usually horizontal, although it may be rotary or arc shaped. During the acute phase of a vestibular system disease there is often a spontaneous nystagmus that is seen with the head in a normal position. Later in the course of the disease this nystagmus may be seen only when the head is placed in an abnormal position such as extended or flexed to one side. With peripheral vestibular disease, this induced or positional nystagmus is always in the same direction. With lesions involving the central components of the vestibular system, spontaneous and positional nystagmus may be horizontal, vertical, or rotary and may also change direction with changes in head posture. This is frequently seen in diseases such as listeriosis in ruminants, *Parelaphostrongylus tenuis* infection in goats, and head trauma in the horse with hemorrhage within the medulla oblongata. Lesions involving the vestibular nuclei in the medulla oblongata will frequently affect adjacent structures such as the descending motor tracts effecting voluntary limb movement and the reticular formation, resulting in tetraparesis and depression, respectively.

Some animals, particularly horses, may become frantic at the onset of an acute vestibular disorder. This is probably associated with the profound disorientation that must be experienced. Particularly with peripheral vestibular disease, the changes seen in head posture, eye position, movement, and gait will often improve markedly within several days and may resolve in several weeks with mild nonprogressive diseases. This is assumed to be due to a central accommodation wherein the vestibular system can utilize input of other modalities (vision, touch, proprioception, and so on) to correct the abnormal input being received from the diseased portion of the vestibular system. Consequently, by blindfolding an animal that has accommodated to a vestibular disease, the signs will often exacerbate immediately. Partly because the vestibular portions of the cerebellum are relatively small, there are often no signs of vestibular disease with lesions affecting the cerebellum. This is the case with the majority of congenital cerebellar disorders in all species.

IX. GLOSSOPHARYNGEAL NERVE; X. VAGUS NERVE; XI. ACCESSORY NERVE. The major role of these cranial nerves is innervation of the pharynx and larynx with both sensory and motor fibers. The functions of these nerves are tested by listening for normal laryngeal sounds, observing normal swallowing of food and water, assessing the swallowing reflex by passage of a stomach tube, assessing the gag reflex by placing the fingers in the pharynx, and, finally, inspecting the larynx and pharynx, with an endoscope if necessary. The major nucleus for motor control of the pharynx and larynx via these three cranial nerves is the nucleus ambiguus in the caudal medulla oblongata. The key clinical signs of a deficit in this nucleus or in these three cranial nerves are related to paralysis of the pharynx and larynx. The severity of signs will depend on whether there is uni- or bilateral involvement. In pharyngeal paralysis there is usually feed and water seen at the nostrils. Because physical obstructions between the pharynx and stomach (choke) are the most frequent cause of these signs, an attempt must be made to pass a stomach tube. This is to check the patency of the upper gastrointestinal tract and to assess sensation from the pharynx and the swallowing reflex. The swallowing reflex can also be evaluated in an animal with dysphagia (e.g., a dropped jaw) by elevating the head and observing for swallowing movements; saliva and feed will run caudally from the mouth and nasal passages into the pharynx to stimulate swallowing movements. The pharynx and larynx should be observed clinically when possible and also palpated, both externally and via the mouth utilizing a protective glove in listeriosis and rabies suspects. Use of a rhinolaryngoscope to observe pharyngeal and laryngeal function may then be required. By this stage of the examination, physical causes of dysphagia such as choke, pharyngeal phlegmon, and cleft palate will have been detected.

Many diffuse infectious and noninfectious encephalopathies can result in dysphagia. These include the equine viral encephalitides (WEE, EEE, and VEE), bacterial meningoencephalitis in neonatal animals, salt poisoning in pigs, and hepatoencephalopathy due to liver disease in all species. This form of dysphagia probably results from the generalized depression of voluntary movement (weakness) seen in such disorders but does not affect reflex swallowing of a stomach tube, for example.

For further evaluation, the various sites for neuromuscular dysphagia must be considered. Lesions in the nucleus ambiguus and swallowing center in the medulla oblongata will usually affect adjacent structures, resulting in depression, ataxia, weakness, and signs of other cranial nerve involvement. Listeriosis is the commonest cause of CNS dysphagia in ruminants. The equine protozoal myeloencephalitis agent can affect these areas of the medulla oblongata. Dysphagia is a frequent finding in rabies and presumably arises from lesions in the medulla oblongata. Owing to their close association with the guttural pouch, cranial nerves IX, X, and XI) can become involved with guttural pouch disease. The diffuse granulomatous lesions seen with neuritis of the cauda equina in the horse can involve these cranial nerves to produce difficulty in swallowing. Dysphagia is often present with the diffuse lower motor neuron–neuromuscular paralysis of botulism. In chronic lead poisoning in horses, there is frequently a polyneuropathy involving the pharyngeal (and laryngeal) nerves producing dysphagia. There is a specific polymyopathy that involves the muscles of mastication in the horse, which can also affect the pharyngeal and lingual muscles resulting in dysphagia. This disease may be related to cachexia and vitamin E and selenium status. Affected muscles are swollen, and attempts at swallowing are usually distressful. Affected animals can die from acute cardiac involvement. It should be remembered that inhalation pneumonia is an important sequela of dysphagia.

Paralysis of the larynx with stertorous breathing that is particularly noticeable during inspiration may be detected with most of the diseases that result in pharyngeal paralysis. The abnormal bellowing, often with an altered pitch, that can be heard with rabies and lead poisoning in cattle may result from central and peripheral involvement of these cranial nerves, respectively. Chronic lead poisoning in horses does result in a peripheral neuropathy and inspiratory dyspnea. The more frequent syndrome of laryngeal hemiplegia (roaring) in horses is usually the result of neurogenic atrophy of the muscles innervated by the left recurrent laryngeal nerve and consequent failure to abduct the vocal fold during inspiration. The cause is still obscure, but it has been suggested that the fiber degeneration and segmental demyelination and remyelination observed may result from ischemia of the recurrent laryngeal nerve due to stretching as it passes around the aortic arch within the thorax.

XII. Hypoglossal Nerve. This last cranial nerve has its cell bodies in the hypoglossal nucleus of the caudal medulla oblongata and is the motor nerve to the tongue muscles. The tongue must be inspected for symmetry, normal movement, and evidence of atrophy. Normally there is strong resistance to withdrawing the tongue from the mouth. A unilateral lesion of the nucleus or nerve will result in unilateral atrophy of the tongue with weak retraction, although it will usually not remain protruding from the mouth. Bilateral involvement will interfere with prehension and swallowing, the tongue will usually protrude, and the animal will not be able to draw it back into the mouth.

In animals with severe cerebral lesions resulting in marked depression without focal brainstem involvement, the tongue may remain protruded and may be slow to return to its normal position when pulled out of the mouth. This is similar to the ineffective swallowing efforts made by animals suffering from such lesions previously described. That the animal can pull the tongue back into the mouth and that there is no resulting atrophy indicate that this finding is not the result of a lesion in the hypoglossal nucleus or nerve. The voluntary control pathways from higher centers are interfered with in these instances, resulting in a supranuclear or pseudobulbar palsy without involving the hypoglossal nucleus or nerve (i.e., an upper motor neuron lesion). A profound defect in tongue movement (dystonia) is seen with the upper motor neuron lesion in nigropallidal encephalomalacia (Yellow star thistle poisoning) of horses.

Many focal brainstem diseases, such as listeriosis and equine protozoal myeloencephalitiis, can involve the hypoglossal nuclei and paralyze the tongue. Excessive physical manipulation can result in paralysis of the tongue in cattle and horses. This is usually temporary. Fracture of the hyoid bone in any species can result in tongue paralysis due to the close proximity of this bone to the hypoglossal nerve. A unilateral hypoglossal palsy has been seen in association with a locally malignant parotid adenocarcinoma in an aged thoroughbred mare; there was concurrent unilateral involvement of cranial nerves II, V, VII, IX, X, and XI. Finally, pituitary abscesses in cattle have been seen to result in basilar epidural empyema with partial involvement of cranial nerves II through XII (Espersen 1975). In the latter disease there is frequently an associated star-gazing attitude and bradycardia.

GAIT AND POSTURE

Having completed the examination of the head, the examiner then evaluates the gait and posture of the animal as a general assessment of brainstem, spinal cord, and peripheral nerve and muscle function. If evidence of a lesion has been detected in the examination of the head, then an attempt is made to explain any abnormalities found during the rest of the examination as being caused by such a lesion above the level of the atlantooccipital junction. If this cannot be done, then there must be at least two lesions or a diffuse disease. If no deficits are found in examining the head, then the lesion is assumed to be in the spinal cord or peripheral nerves or muscles.

Unless there is a suspicion of a bone fracture, every effort should be made to assist a tetraplegic animal to stand and walk. This will often require "tailing" the patient, and a lot of information can be gained by observing a few steps taken by such an animal. This is particularly so with a heavy cow, horse, or pig when performed early in the course of recumbency, before secondary problems of decubital sores, decreased blood supply to limbs, and dehydration make evaluation difficult.

The first observation to be made in evaluating the gait is which limbs have an abnormal gait and, second, whether there is evidence of lameness suggesting a musculoskeletal component to any change in gait. The essential components of a neurologic gait abnormality are weakness, ataxia, spasticity, and dysmetria. Each limb must be evaluated for evidence of these. This is done while the animal is walking and trotting in a straight line, walking in circles, turning tightly (pivoting), and backing. To detect subtle asymmetry in the length of stride it helps to walk parallel to the animal, matching step for step. If possible, the gait should also be evaluated while the animal is blindfolded, walking up and down a slope, walking with the head and neck held extended, and running free in a field. Very often subtle alterations will not be evident at normal gaits but will be seen as consistent mistakes while the animal performs these more involved gait maneuvers.

Weakness is often evidenced by an animal dragging the limbs, by worn hooves, and by a low arc to the protraction phase of the stride. When an animal bears weight on a weak limb, the limb will often be seen to tremble, and the animal may even collapse on that limb because of lack of support. Classical weakness is seen as difficulty in rising on the affected limbs from a sternal position even though the feet are positioned correctly. While circling, walking on a slope, and walking with the head elevated, an animal will frequently stumble on a weak limb and knuckle over on the fetlock. With severe weakness in all four limbs but no ataxia and spasticity, one must strongly consider neuromuscular diseases. Profound weakness in only one limb is suggestive of a peripheral nerve or muscle (lower motor neuron) lesion in that limb. Weakness will occur with descending motor pathway (upper motor neuron) lesions in the brainstem and spinal cord and is present in the limbs caudal to, and on the same side as, the lesion.

Ataxia, or proprioceptive deficit, is poor coordination in moving the limbs and body. It is seen as a swaying of the pelvis, trunk, and, sometimes, the whole body from side to side and as a weaving of the limb during the protraction phase. This often results in an abducted or adducted foot placement and crossing of the limbs or stepping on the opposite foot, especially while the animal is circling or turning tightly. Circumduction of the

THE NERVOUS SYSTEM / 87

outside limbs when turning and circling is also regarded as a proprioceptive deficit. Walking an animal on a slope with the head elevated will often exaggerate an ataxia, particularly in the pelvic limbs. When a weak and ataxic animal is turned sharply in circles, it will often leave an affected limb in one place and pivot around it. This may also occur when backing such an animal. Blindfolding does not appear to exacerbate any weakness and ataxia caused by spinal cord disease. However gait abnormalities seen with vestibular and cerebellar diseases will often worsen with blindfolding. Ataxia resulting from vestibular disease is frequently characterized by staggering. An ataxic gait may be most pronounced when an animal in moving freely in a paddock at a trot or canter, especially when attempting to stop, when the limbs may be wildly adducted or abducted. Proprioceptive deficits are caused by lesions affecting the general proprioceptive sensory pathways that relay information on the position of the limbs and body to the cerebellum (cerebellar proprioception) and to the thalamus and cerebral cortex (conscious proprioception). Often it is difficult to differentiate weakness from ataxia, but in most instances this is unimportant. This is because the descending upper motor neuron tracts and the ascending general proprioceptive tracts are closely related in the white matter of the brainstem and spinal cord.

Spasticity, stiffness, or hypometria is seen as very little flexion of the joints, particularly the carpal and tarsal joints, generally indicating a lesion affecting the descending motor pathways (upper motor neuron) to that limb. Spasticity is seen with a few diseases in which there may be involvement of sensory pathways from a limb, e.g., periodic spasticity in cattle and stringhalt in horses. A spastic gait, particularly in the thoracic limbs, may best be seen when the animal is backed or when maneuvering on a slope with the head elevated. The thoracic limbs may move almost without flexing under these circumstances, as in the manner of a marching tin soldier. Spasticity may be the most obvious deficit in thoracic limbs with cervical spinal cord disease.

Dysmetria is the term used to describe an altered limitation and direction of motion. This is usually seen as an overreaching of the limbs with excessive joint movement, called hypermetria. Decreased range of motion of limb joints is essentially spasticity as described previously. Hypermetria and ataxia, without weakness, are characteristic of cerebellar disease. In diffuse cerebellar disease, a head (intention) tremor is usually present and a depressed menace response will often be seen; only rarely are there signs of vestibular disease. A unilateral cerebellar lesion will usually result in a gait alteration on the same side as the lesion. The short-strided, staggery gait seen with acute vestibular disease may also be regarded as hypometria.

Grading the Gait Abnormality. The degree of weakness, ataxia, spasticity, and dysmetria should be graded for each limb. An arbitrary scale of 0 to 4+ has been described for the degree of abnormality (Mayhew et al. 1978). A 1+ gait change indicates that the signs are just detectable in the limb. A 2+ change indicates that the signs are detectable at a normal gait and are exaggerated with backing, turning, neck extension, and so on. A grade of 3+ indicates that the signs are easily detected as soon as the animal moves, and turning, neck extension, maneuvering on a slope, and so on causes the animal to stumble regularly. When an animal stumbles and possibly falls at normal gaits it is said to have a 4+ neurologic gait abnormality.

Generally, with focal cervical spinal cord and brainstem lesions, signs of ataxia, weakness, and spasticity are one grade more severe in the pelvic limbs than in the thoracic limbs. Thus, with a mild focal cervical spinal cord lesion there may be a 1+ change in the pelvic limbs with no signs in the thoracic limbs. In such cases, the clinician can state only that there is a mild brainstem or spinal cord lesion. A 3+ or 4+ abnormality in the pelvic limbs and no neurological signs in the thoracic limbs are consistent with a thoracolumbar spinal cord lesion. With a 1+ and 4+ gait abnormality in the thoracic and pelvic limbs, respectively, one must consider a severe thoracolumbar lesion and a mild cervical lesion or a diffuse spinal cord disease. A 4+

abnormality in the thoracic limbs with a 1+ abnormality in the pelvic limbs is also not consistent with a single focal cervical lesion. Such neurological signs are suggestive of either a lesion of the brachial intumescence (C_6-T_2) with involvement of gray matter supplying the thoracic limbs (lower motor neuron lesion) or a diffuse spinal cord lesion. A severe gait alteration (3+ or 4+) in the thoracic limbs with normal pelvic limbs indicates lower motor neuron involvement of the thoracic limbs — ventral gray columns at C_6 to T_2, peripheral nerves, or muscle. Gait abnormalities can occur in all four limbs, with lesions affecting the white matter in the caudal brainstem. In these cases, head signs such as depression and cranial nerve deficits are used to define the site of the lesion. Lesions affecting just the cerebrum do not usually result in any changes in gait. If a cerebral lesion such as an abscess or hematoma results in increased intracranial pressure, then the brainstem may be compressed, resulting in a neurologic gait abnormality and cranial nerve signs. With an acute cerebral lesion there may be some abnormalities detected in the use of the limbs in complex maneuvers such as hopping and standing up from lateral recumbency. These signs will be seen in the limbs contralateral to the lesion and have been detected only during the acute or progressive phase of a lesion. Caudal to the red nucleus in the midbrain, a lesion will result in an alteration in the gait, usually on the same side as the lesion.

NECK AND FORELIMBS

Following an overall evaluation of gait, attention is focused on the neck and thoracic limbs. If an abnormal gait was detected in the thoracic limbs and there were no head signs, then this part of the examination attempts to confirm involvement of the spinal cord from C_1 to T_2 and localize the lesion within these segments.

Observation and palpation of the neck and forelimbs will detect gross skeletal defects, asymmetry in the neck, and muscle atrophy, all of which may be associated with neurological disease and will, therefore, be localizing findings.

Scoliosis has been reported in foals (Mayhew, Watson, and Heissan, 1978) and calves (White, Pennock, and Seiler, 1978) with various congenital occipito-atlanto-axial malformations (OAAMs). Palpation of the affected area in such animals will often reveal the malformed bones and restricted movement arising from atlanto-occipital fusion. Cervical scoliosis and kyphosis have been seen with trauma to the neck in cattle, horses, and goats. When the cervical distortion is extreme it is termed torticollis or wry neck and may or may not be associated with evidence of spinal cord disease (compression). The transverse processes of the cervical vertebrae can be palpated in most large animals except adult swine and bulls. These processes can be quite prominent at C_4 and particularly at C_5. It is more difficult to palpate the intervertebral articulations.

Sweating can be an extremely helpful localizing sign in the horse and usually indicates a lesion involving the sympathetic nervous system. In Horner's syndrome in the horse, there is sweating of the head and cranial cervical area to the level of C_2. Involvement of the peripheral pre- and postganglionic sympathetic neurons in the horse results in focal patches of sweating. With a profound lesion of the cervical spinal cord there can be involvement of the descending sympathetic tectotegmentospinal tracts with resulting sweating on the whole ipsilateral side of the body as well as Horner's syndrome. This has been seen with an asymmetrical equine protozoal myelitis lesion at C_6.

The neck should be manipulated to assess normal range of movement. Evidence of a stiff neck, such as reluctance to flex the neck or pain on flexing the neck, needs careful appraisal before any conclusions are drawn. Pain can be demonstrated when flexing a horse's neck toward the side of an enlarged intervertebral articular process that compresses the intervertebral spinal nerve.

When the skin of the lateral neck of a horse above the jugular groove is tapped lightly with a blunt pointed object, there is contraction of the cutaneous muscle that results in a flicking of the skin. The brachiocephalic muscle often contracts also, causing the shoulder to be pulled cranially. There is also a flicking of the ear rostrally, and the other facial muscles will contract briefly. These are the cervical and cervico-facial responses. The anatomical pathways are not known, although they must involve several cervical segments and probably the facial nucleus in the medulla. Severe focal cervical lesions that involve gray and white matter, such as compression of C_1 due to an OAAM and extensive equine protozoal myelitis involving cervical segments, can result in depressed or absent cervical responses.

An assessment of sensory perception from the neck and forelimbs must be made. This can be observed by a cerebral response at the time of observing the cervical responses and continuing the skin pricking over the shoulders and down the limbs.

Pushing against the shoulders to force the animal to first resist and then take a step laterally is a test of the sway reaction for the thoracic limb. It is performed on horses and cattle and can be done while the animal is standing still or walking forward. This is a type of postural reaction involving connections to higher motor centers. This is used in adult large animals in place of the thoracic limb hopping reaction. Weakness can be evidenced by a lack of resistance to lateral shoulder pressure. Weakness and ataxia may result in tripping and stumbling on the forelimbs when taking lateral steps. By pulling laterally on both the tail and the halter simultaneously, an assessment of the resistance (strength) on each side of the body can be made. Pinching and pressing down with the fingers on the withers of a normal animal results in some arching (lordosis), but there is resistance to the downward force. An animal that is weak in the thoracic limbs may not be able to resist this force and may arch the back more than normal and even buckle in the thoracic limbs. These tests can be helpful in determining an asymmetrical thoracic limb deficit.

In the smaller and younger large animals, other postural reactions can be elicited. These are most beneficial in detecting signs of subtle proprioceptive and upper motor neuron (higher centers and white matter) lesions when the gait is normal. Wheelbarrowing the patient by making it walk on just the thoracic limbs, hopping it to the left and right on each thoracic limb in turn, and hemistanding/hemiwalking the animal by making it stand and then walk sideways on both left then both right limbs are three useful postural reactions to test. A slow response will usually indicate some motor impairment. This will be present in the limbs on the same side if a lesion is between the red nucleus and T_2. A postural reaction deficit may be present in a thoracic limb on the side opposite the side of a cerebral lesion. Cerebellar diseases usually result in a delayed onset but exaggerated (spastic) response to postural reaction testing. These abnormalities occur in the limbs on the same side as the cerebellar lesion.

If it is feasible to cast the animal, this should be done to assess the spinal reflexes. Otherwise, if an animal is ambulating well it is usual to assume that the spinal reflexes are intact.

Recumbent Patient. A large animal that has recently become recumbent but uses the thoracic limbs well in an attempt to get up most likely has a lesion caudal to T_2. If such an animal cannot attain a dog-sitting posture, the lesion is likely to be in the cervical spinal cord. It is important to assess voluntary effort in the neck in such a tetraplegic animal. If only the head, i.e., not the neck, can be raised off the ground, there is probably a severe cranial cervical lesion. With a severe caudal cervical lesion, e.g., at C_6, the head and neck can usually be raised off the ground although thoracic limb effort will be decreased and the animal usually will not be able to maintain sternal recumbency or a dog-sitting posture. No assessments of limb function in adult cattle and horses should be done while the animal is lying on the limb being tested. The amount of voluntary motor activity present in each thoracic limb is assessed. This can best be done while observing the animal in its attempts to get up. In addition, the muscular tone can be determined by manipulating each limb. A flaccid limb with no motor activity is typical of a lesion in a lower motor neuron to that limb. The examiner should be aware that in heavy animals that are down for a day or so there frequently is poor tone and very little voluntary effort observable in a limb that has been lain upon. A severe upper motor neuron lesion to the thoracic limbs (cranial to C_6) will result in decreased or absent voluntary effort, but there will be normal, or more likely increased, muscle tone in the limbs. This is because there is usually a release of the lower motor neuron from the calming influences of the descending upper motor neuron pathways.

Finally, spinal reflexes are tested in the thoracic limbs. One must remember that a spinal reflex can be intact without the animal perceiving the stimulus and showing a cerebral response. A spinal reflex requires a peripheral sensory nerve, one or a few segments of spinal cord, a peripheral motor nerve, and effector muscles to be intact. Perception (sensation) of the stimulus used for the reflex requires ascending sensory pathways to the forebrain to be intact. This sensation is usually seen as a cerebral response on the part of the patient in the form of changes in facial expression, moving the head, or phonating. The flexor reflex in the thoracic limb involves stimulation of the skin of the distal limb with artery forceps and observing for flexion of the digits, carpus, elbow, and shoulder. This reflex arc involves sensory fibers in the median and ulnar nerves, spinal cord gray matter in segments C_6 to T_2, and motor fibers in the axillary, musculocutaneous, median, and ulnar nerves. Thus, if this reflux is absent in an animal that is recumbent owing to spinal cord disease and this deficit cannot be accounted for by prolonged recumbency with decubital changes, the lesion most likely involves the gray matter at C_6 to T_2. Conscious perception of the stimulus will be intact as long as the afferent fibers in the median and ulnar nerves, the dorsal gray columns at C_6 to T_2, and the ascending sensory pathways in the cervical spinal cord and brainstem are intact. Lesions cranial to C_6 may release this reflex from the calming effect of the upper motor neuron pathways and result in an exaggerated reflex with rapid flexion of the limb, which may remain flexed for some time. Such lesions may also result in a crossed extensor reflex. This is seen as an exaggerated flexion of the limb being tested and a forceful extension of the opposite limb. The crossed extensor reflex usually occurs only with severe upper motor neuron lesions, and thus the animal will usually have very poor voluntary motor activity in the limbs being tested. Normal neonatal animals may have hyperactive, and even crossed extensor, reflexes.

The triceps and particularly the biceps reflexes are not easily detected in normal adult large animals, although these reflexes are readily elicited in the smaller patients. If these reflexes are found to be easily elicited, it is likely that there is an upper motor neuron lesion cranial to the spinal cord segments involved, i.e., cranial to C_7 to T_1. A test of the biceps reflex is performed by placing two or three fingers firmly on the biceps and brachial muscles on the dorsum of the elbow joint, balloting them with a plexor, and feeling for contraction of these muscles and observing for flexion of the elbow. On adult cattle and horses the muscle bellies themselves can be percussed with a neurology hammer or similar plexor. This reflex has its afferent and efferent pathways in the musculocutaneous nerve and involves spinal cord segments C_7 and C_8 lying within the sixth and seventh cervical vertebrae. To test the triceps reflex the relaxed limb is held slightly flexed and the distal portion of the long head of the triceps and its tendon of insertion is ballotted with a plexor while observing and palpating for contraction of the triceps muscle, which causes extension of the elbow. The triceps reflex involves the radial nerve for its afferent and efferent pathways, the lower motor neurons being in spinal cord segments C_7 to T_1, which lie within the sixth and seventh cervical vertebrae.

By this stage of the examination the clinician should have a clear idea of the presence and location of lesions in the brain, the spinal cord cranial to T_2, and the peripheral nerves and muscles of the thoracic limbs. The more peripheral the lesion, the better defined the sensory and motor deficits. Syndromes resulting from lesions involving the peripheral nerves of the thoracic limb involve characteristic gait abnormalities, paralysis of specific muscles with resulting muscle atrophy, specific reflex loss, and sensory deficits that are briefly described below. The reader is referred to specific descriptions of these syndromes (deLahunta, 1977; Hamilton, 1964; Vaughan, 1964) for more details.

Suprascapular paralysis ultimately results in atrophy of the supra- and infraspinatus muscles and in the horse and calf will result in abduction of the shoulder and a subtle circumduction of the limb during the protraction phase of the stride that improves with time.

Musculocutaneous paralysis would possibly not alter the gait although the elbow may be overextended. There would ultimately be atrophy of the biceps and brachial muscles.

Radial paralysis results in a dropped elbow with an inability to extend the digits and support weight. This causes difficulty in advancing the limb, dragging the digits on the ground, and attempts to support weight on the dorsum of the pastern. In the cow there may be decreased sensation from the dorsal and possibly the medial aspect of the pastern and claws. The triceps reflex will be absent (not abnormal in itself) and there will ultimately be atrophy of the triceps muscles and the extensor muscles of the carpus and digits. If the radial nerve is damaged distal to the triceps innervation, then the animal should be able to support weight, but, because of lack of carpal and digital extension, weight will be supported on the dorsum of the pastern while the animal walks.

Median and ulnar paralysis in the calf results in a stiff, goose-stepping gait with hyperextension of the carpal, fetlock, and pastern joints. There is cutaneous analgesia of the plantar and lateral surfaces of the limb from the elbow to the coronet.

TRUNK AND HIND LIMBS

If the examination of the head, gait, or neck and thoracic limbs reveals evidence of a lesion, then an attempt should be made to explain any abnormalities in the trunk and hind limbs as arising from such a lesion. If signs are present only in the trunk or hind limbs, then the lesion must be between T_2 and S_2, and this part of the examination will help to localize the lesion better. The examiner should remember, however, that with a subtle (grade 1+) change in the gait of the pelvic limbs the lesion may be anywhere cranial to the midsacral spinal cord. Mature cattle and horses that are paraplegic and can "dog sit" for several minutes should be regarded as having a lesion between T_2 and S_3.

The trunk and hind limbs must be observed and palpated for malformations, fractures, and asymmetry. Lesions affecting thoracolumbar gray matter can result in muscle atrophy, which is a very helpful localizing finding. With marked asymmetrical myelopathies, there will often be a scoliosis of the vertebral column, the concave side being opposite the lesion (i.e., the curve toward the side of the lesion, which will be the weakest side of the animal). In many normal large animals, particularly calves, there is an apparent palpable groove in the tip of the dorsal spinous processes of the thoracolumbar vertebrae. Thus, caution must be used when diagnosing such malformations as *spina bifida* in these animals. Malformations of the vertebral column may be present with or without malformations of the spinal cord, and clinical signs of spinal cord compression from such bony deformities as congenital thoracolumbar scoliosis associated with a wedge vertebra may not be present at birth and may become evident only as the animal matures. Signs of spinal cord disease resulting from congenital malformations of the spinal cord, such as diplomyelia or syringomyelia, will usually be apparent as soon as the animal is fully ambulatory.

Sweating in the horse, which may occur over the trunk and hind limbs, will usually indicate sympathetic involvement.

Sensation over the trunk and hind limbs should be evaluated at this stage of the examination. Degrees of hypalgesia and analgesia have been detected caudal to the sites of severe thoracolumbar spinal cord lesions. The cerebral response to testing for sensation must be identified separately from the panniculus response, which may also be helpful in identifying the location of a thoracolumbar lesion. Gentle pricking of the skin over the trunk, particularly the lateral aspects of the body wall, results in contraction of the cutaneous trunci muscle seen as a flicking of the skin over the trunk. The sensory stimulus travels to the spinal cord in the dorsal branches of the thoracolumbar spinal nerve level with the site of stimulation. Transmission is then via the spinal cord white matter to the gray matter of the brachial intumescence (probably C_8–T_1), where the lower motor neuron cell bodies of the lateral thoracic nerves are stimulated, causing contraction of the cutaneous trunci muscle. This response is most prominent in horses and easiest to initiate over the midthorax. Lesions anywhere along this pathway may result in a suppression of the response, which is easiest to detect with an asymmetrical lesion.

Pushing against the pelvis or pulling on the tail to feel the resistance given by the animal and observe any resulting movement of the pelvic limbs is a good test of the sway reaction for the pelvic limbs. An animal that shows a spastic ataxia may resist this maneuver strongly (spastically). As with the sway reaction for the thoracic limbs, this test can also be performed while the animal is walking forward. A weak animal will be easily pulled and pushed laterally while walking. Proprioceptive deficits in the pelvic limbs can be observed by marked overabduction and crossing of the limbs when a step is taken to the side. This test can be very helpful to detect asymmetry, weakness, and/or ataxia in the pelvic limbs of adult cattle and horses.

Pinching and pressing down with the fingers on the thoracolumbar paravertebral muscles will cause a normal animal to fix the thoracolumbar vertebral column in slight extension (lordosis) but resist the pressure and not flex the thoracic or pelvic limbs. Similar pressure on the sacral and caudal paravertebral muscles will result in fixation of the thoracolumbar vertebral column in slight flexion (kyphosis), again resisting the pressure and not flexing the pelvic limbs. Obviously the pressure applied, for example, to a foal or calf, can be so great that even a normal animal may collapse. A weak animal will usually not be able to resist the pressure and fix the vertebral column and will overflex or extend the back and begin to buckle in the limbs.

The postural reactions, i.e., wheelbarrowing, hopping, hemistanding, and hemiwalking, have been described previously. With lesions involving one cerebral hemisphere, such as a hematoma or abscess in a calf, there will often be an abnormal hopping response in the contralateral limbs. This is seen as a slow onset of movement with stumbling on the feet, indicating some degree of weakness. With asymmetrical lesions involving the upper motor neuron to the pelvic limbs in the brainstem and spinal cord cranial to L_3, there will be a slow hopping response in the ipsilateral pelvic limb. Lower motor neuron lesions in one pelvic limb will result in poor tone, paresis, and often an extremely slow or absent hopping response in that limb. Also, in smaller patients, the pelvic limb wheelbarrowing and extensor postural thrust reactions can be tested. This is performed by holding the patient around the thorax with the pelvic limbs off the ground and lowering it to the ground, observing the supporting movements of each pelvic limb. The animal is then made to walk forward and backward, supporting weight on just the pelvic limbs. As with other postural reactions, observations are made on the symmetry, strength, and coordination of movement of the limbs.

Recumbent Patient. It is generally assumed that an animal that is ambulating well on the pelvic limbs has intact spinal reflexes in those limbs. The pelvic limb spinal reflexes must be evaluated in all animals with marked gait deficits in the pelvic limbs that can be restrained in lateral recumbency and in all recumbent animals. In addition, the amount of voluntary effort and muscle tone present in the pelvic limbs is assessed by watching the animal in its attempts to get up or in its struggling in response to stimuli while lying in lateral recumbency. It is worth re-emphasizing that the absence of voluntary movement in a limb that is flaccid and areflexic is strongly suggestive of a lower motor neuron lesion. Asymmetry in voluntary efforts to stand and in muscle tone in the pelvic limbs is helpful in lateralizing a spinal cord lesion.

The patellar reflex and the flexor reflex are the two main spinal cord reflexes involving the pelvic limbs, and, as with thoracic limb reflexes, they should not be attempted on a limb on which the animal is lying. A test of the patellar reflex is performed by supporting the limb in a partly flexed position, tapping the intermediate patellar ligament, and observing for a reflex contraction of the quadriceps muscle resulting in extension of the stifle. A small animal (human) neurology hammer is ideal for this test in foals, calves, goats, sheep, and pigs, but a heavier instrument such as a short piece of iron pipe is more suitable for adult horses and cattle. The sensory and motor fibers for this reflex are in the femoral nerve, and the spinal cord segments involved are predominantly L_4 and L_5. The flexor reflex test of the pelvic limbs is performed as in the thoracic limbs by stimulating the skin of the distal limb with artery forceps and observing for flexion of the limb. As with the thoracic limbs, a stronger stimulus, such as an electric prod, may be necessary to elicit this reflex in a large animal that has been recumbent on a limb for some time. The stimulus can slowly be increased until a reflex response is obtained or until the patient shows obvious discomfort from the stimulus. The afferent and efferent pathways to this reflex are in the sciatic nerve, although the site of the stimulus dictates which branch of the sciatic relays the sensory stimulus. Flexion of the hip is mediated via all lumbar spinal nerves. Again, normal neonatal animals have quite hyperactive reflexes.

At this stage of the neurological evaluation, the clinician should have a clear idea of the probable site of any brain lesion and any lesion resulting in an abnormal gait or recumbency. As for the thoracic limbs, lesions of the peripheral nerves to the pelvic limbs result in specific syndromes that can be reviewed in the references. These syndromes are summarized below.

Femoral paralysis is seen as an inability to support weight on the limb owing to lack of stifle extension. At a walk, the limb is advanced with difficulty, the length of stride being considerably reduced. The limb buckles when an attempt is made to bear weight on the limb. In the horse the stifle collapses (flexes) and the hock and fetlock flex automatically. Thus, the horse rests with all the joints flexed in an affected limb. Atrophy of the quadriceps muscle is evident within one to two weeks, and the patellar reflex is absent. The sensory branch (the saphenous nerve) separates from the femoral nerve at the level of the iliopsoas muscle and innervates the medial leg from the midthigh to the hock. Bilateral femoral paralysis has been seen in calves following dystocia in a hip or stifle lock position, resulting in stretching of the femoral nerves.

Obturator paralysis results in a lack of adductor function because the obturator nerve supplies the adductor muscles of the pelvic limb. Experimentally in the calf, there is some abduction of the pelvic limbs evident with bilateral neurectomy. This abduction was unnoticeable at rest and slightly evident at a walk but marked when the calf was running.

In the adult cow, the signs of unilateral obturator paralysis are more evident, with abduction and circumduction of the limb at a walk and difficulty standing up due to a lateral slipping of the affected leg. Bilateral obturator sectioning in the cow results in collapse of the pelvic limbs because of total abduction. The syndrome of paraparesis and paraplegia in postparturient cattle occurs from damage to the ventral spinal nerve roots from the lumbar spinal cord within the pelvic canal as they form the lumbosacral plexus and divide into the peripheral nerves supplying the pelvic limbs. Such postcalving paralyses are the result of damage to more than just the obturator nerves, although pelvic limb abduction is often the most striking sign.

Sciatic paralysis results in very poor limb flexion, with the stifle and hock extended and the fetlock flexed when the animal is not bearing weight on the leg. Weight can be supported on the limb if the digits are extended; otherwise, weight is taken on the dorsal surface of the foot and the hock is overflexed. There may be limb hypalgesia from the stifle down, except for the medial surface between the stifle and hock. Sciatic paralysis undoubtedly adds to the deficit seen with coxofemoral luxations and proximal femoral fractures in cattle. Sciatic paralysis, sometimes bilateral, has been observed with intramuscular injections into the caudal thigh in calves and may be expected in all species under these circumstances.

Tibial paralysis in the horse is reported to result in a hypermetric or stringhalt-like gait and flexion of the hock (dropped hock). In the calf there is hock flexion at rest, and the fetlock is knuckled forward while the hooves remain flat on the ground. There is excessive jerky hock flexion when walking, and there is no dragging of the toes. Sensation is lost from the caudal aspect of the metatarsus in the calf and, probably, the caudal leg distal to the midtibia in the horse. Tibial paralysis appears to be uncommon in large animals.

Peroneal paralysis results in an inability to flex the hock and extend the digits. In the horse and calf there is hyperextension of the hock and hyperflexion of the fetlock and interphalangeal joints so that the animal drags the fetlock along the ground. There is a shorter protraction phase to the stride, and weight is taken with the dorsal surface of the foot on the ground. If the foot is placed in a normal position, weight can be taken until the animal attempts to walk, at which time the fetlock will again knuckle. There is hypalgesia to the cranial portion of the leg from the level of the stifle to the fetlock area. The peroneal nerve is subject to injury as it passes across the lateral surface of the tibia. Peroneal paralysis is thus seen in adult cattle that are recumbent in the postpartum period, in horses recumbent for anesthesia, and in those receiving a kick to the side of the leg.

Cranial gluteal paralysis results in very little alteration in gait. There may be a slight abduction or outward rotation of the stifle at the end of the propulsive phase of stride. Ultimately, there will be atrophy of the gluteal region, predominantly involving the middle gluteal muscle. The cranial gluteal nerve can be damaged with fractures of the pelvis as it traverses the shaft of the ilium. Cranial gluteal nerve damage has also been observed in horses with protozoal myeloencephalitis when the lesion is confined to the ventral gray columns at L_6.

TAIL AND ANUS

This final component of the neurological examination is an evaluation of the function of organs and structures innervated by nerves from the sacral and coccygeal spinal cord segments. Once again, if there is evidence of a lesion in the examination up to this point, then an attempt is made to explain any findings from this part of the examination as arising from such a lesion. If this cannot be done, then there must be a lesion affecting the sacrococcygeal spinal cord segments or nerves or the peripheral nerves or innervated structures.

Tail tone can be assessed just prior to testing the perineal reflex. There is a marked variation in tail tone between and within species. Thus, just because a pig has a straight tail instead of a curled tail, one must not conclude that the flaccid tail is caused by a coccygeal lower motor neuron lesion. However, the completely flaccid tail having no voluntary movement, as if a caudal epidural anesthetic had been given, is easily detected and indicative of a lower motor neuron lesion. Animals with spinal cord lesions cranial to the coccygeal segments may have decreased tail movement because of upper motor neuron paresis, but tail tone will be normal. This can be rather subjective to assess in an individual animal, and usually the spinal cord lesion must be severe for the weakness to be apparent. Some horses are regarded as natural "tail wringers" and will flick their tails up and down and laterally while moving. This feature can also be observed with painful musculoskeletal diseases and has been observed to be acquired by horses that have later been determined to have spinal cord disease; thus, it is not a reliable neurological finding.

The perineal reflex is elicited by lightly pricking the skin of the perineum and observing reflex contraction of the anal sphincter and flexion (clamping down) of the tail. The sensory fibers are contained within the perineal branches of the pudendal nerve (S_1–S_3). Contraction of the anal sphincter is mediated via the caudal rectal branch of the pudendal nerve and tail flexion by the sacral and coccygeal segments and nerves (S_1–C_0). An animal with a flaccid tail and anus due to a lower motor neuron lesion will not have an anal (or tail) reflex. However, it may still have normal sensation from the anus and tail if the sensory nerves and spinal cord and brainstem white matter pathways to the sensory cortex are intact. Thus, as with all other reflex testing, the sensory perception of the stimulus must be evaluated separately from the segmental reflex action.

It should be remembered that the spinal cord ends within the cranial sacrum in large domestic animals (midsacrum in the pig). Thus, focal lesions of the last lumbar, sacral, and coccygeal vertebrae may involve the cauda equina and, thus, the lower motor neurons (spinal nerves) from many sacrococcygeal spinal cord segments. Depending on the level, this will result in varying degrees of hypalgesia, areflexia, and hypotonia of tail, anus, perineum, hips, and caudal thighs. As with peripheral nerve lesions, the fibers in the nerve roots of the cauda equina affected last by compression or injury are those transmitting the modality of pain. Analgesia thus warrants a poorer prognosis than do other deficits.

A rectal examination may detect space-occupying lesions such as lymphomas in cattle and melanomas in horses or abscesses, vertebral fractures, and luxations in any animal. In addition, an assessment should be made of urinary bladder volume and the tone of the bladder wall and rectum. Large animals, particularly adult horses, that are recumbent for any reason will often not urinate and thus usually have a distended bladder that eventually spills over. Manipulating such animals to assist them to stand or violent attempts by such animals to stand up can result in a ruptured bladder.

An animal that is ambulatory and has nonobstructive distention of the bladder and urinary incontinence probably has a lesion affecting the sacral spinal cord segments or the pelvic nerves. In such cases, there will usually be excessive feces in the rectum, but this will usually not result in overt constipation unless there is a dense, diffuse, sacral lower motor neuron lesion (e.g., cauda equina neuritis). A clinical characteristic of horses with equine herpesvirus 1 (rhinopneumonitis) myelopathy is urinary incontinence, even with mild to moderate degrees of pelvic limb ataxia and weakness. This paresis of the urinary bladder has not been related specifically to lower motor neuron (gray matter) lesions in the sacral spinal cord segments. However, the lesions in this disease are usually widespread throughout the spinal cord. Some horses and cattle with rabies have been seen to have a hypotonic and hypalgesic tail and anus, presumably owing to lower motor neuron involvement of the ventral gray matter in the sacrocaudal spinal cord.

Paraplegic cattle, horses, and pigs frequently contuse their perineum and tail while dog sitting and in their attempts to stand. Also, tail ropes and various forms of sling support frequently result in damage to these areas. An assessment of neurological function must be made as soon as possible because perineal and tail contusion results in edema, quickly followed by hypotonia, areflexia, and hypalgesia.

Anatomic Diagnosis

After completing the neurological examination, the clinician first decides on the most probable site of the lesion within one or more of the major areas of the nervous system.

Cerebrum. With cerebral lesions there is frequently a depressed mental status, behavioral abnormalities, seizures, and central blindness. If circling occurs, it is generally toward the side of the lesion. There is no alteration in gait, although there may be postural reaction deficits in the limbs contralateral to the lesion. Upper motor neuron (pseudobulbar) cranial nerve palsies are seen.

Brainstem. The characteristics of brainstem diseases are marked depression or coma and cranial nerve deficits. There may also be behavioral changes and seizures. With caudal brainstem lesions there will be a gait abnormality (paresis, ataxia, spasticity), usually in the limbs on the same side as the lesion. The various cranial nerve deficits are most helpful in localizing a lesion within the brainstem.

Cerebellum. Diffuse cerebellar disease results in a lack of a menace response without blindness, a head tremor, and an abnormal gait characterized by hypermetria and ataxia without paresis. There is sometimes a truncal tremor or swaying at rest but only rarely are there vestibular signs.

Spinal Cord. Typically there is a neurologic gait abnormality and postural reaction deficit in the limbs on the same side as, and caudal to, the lesion. Focal cervical spinal cord lesions produce a slightly more severe gait defect in the pelvic limbs than the thoracic limbs unless the lesion involves the gray matter or nerve roots from C_6 to T_2. Such thoracic limb lower motor neuron lesions may make the gait worse in the thoracic limbs than in the pelvic limbs. Lower motor neuron signs, such as profound paresis, areflexia, and hypotonia, and sensory deficits are helpful in localizing a spinal cord lesion. Horner's syndrome may be present with severe cervical spinal cord lesions or lesions involving gray matter at T_1 to T_3.

Peripheral Nerves and Muscles. Single peripheral nerve lesions produce well-defined motor deficits but less well-defined sensory deficits in large animals. Involvement of peripheral cranial nerves results in typical syndromes without other evidence of brainstem disease.

Myopathies result in focal or diffuse weakness without sensory deficits, and they may be painful. Suppression of spinal reflexes often occurs with diffuse myopathies. This can be quite helpful in a tetraplegic animal when attempting to distinguish between a diffuse myopathy and spinal cord disease.

Etiological Diagnosis

After localizing the lesion, the clinician can then give consideration to the possible cause of the lesion.

Malformation. Signs caused by congenital malformations of the nervous system are usually stable and first occur when the animal ambulates. In comparison, malformations of the calvarium and vertebral column may produce neurological signs later in life, and they may progress during growth. Such malformations usually act by compressing nervous tissue. Some malformations, such as hydrocephalus, may be acquired by almost all other mechanisms of disease discussed hereafter. Radiography is an extremely helpful diagnostic aid.

Infection and Inflammation. This includes viruses, bacteria, fungi, protozoa, helminths, idiopathic inflammation, and immune mechanisms. Signs may be acute or insidious but usually progress. Signs may be diffuse, but asymmetrical and multifocal lesions are more typical in individual animals. Outbreaks may occur. Regression of signs occurs with some infections. Cerebrospinal fluid analysis and specific serological tests are frequently helpful in diagnosing infectious diseases. Slow degenerations can occur, particularly with certain viruses.

Trauma. Neurological signs resulting from trauma are usually sudden at onset and stabilize within 24 hours. Unless the traumatic insult continues, the signs will frequently improve. Secondary effects of edema, further hemorrhage, and swelling of nervous tissue may result in fluctuation and progression of signs. Bony exostoses may occur later and may produce secondary clinical signs.

Toxic, Nutritional, and Metabolic Disease. Signs are frequently acute or subacute in onset, symmetric and often diffuse, and generally progress or fluctuate. Slow degenerations may occur. Quick response to early therapy is often a good diagnostic aid. Outbreaks may occur.

Vascular Disease. This mechanism of disease includes emboli, thrombi, aneurysms, and inflammatory vascular lesions. Signs are usually acute in onset and stabilize rapidly, as with traumatic diseases.

Degenerative Disease. Many degenerative diseases of the nervous system are the result of inborn errors in metabolism, whereas others are associated with viral, immunological, vascular, endocrine, and nutritional diseases. As more is understood about the etiology of such diseases they are relegated to other categories. Signs are generally symmetrical and relentlessly progressive.

Neoplastic Disease. Primary neoplasms of nervous tissue, with the exception of nerve sheath tumors in cattle, are rare in domestic large animals. Disseminated lymphosarcoma masses frequently compress the spinal cord in cattle. However, other forms of secondary involvement of the nervous system by neoplasms are a rare occurrence. Signs can be peracute with spinal cord or peripheral nerve involvement but are generally chronic and progressive.

Ancillary Aids

CLINICOPATHOLOGICAL TESTS

A routine hemogram can be helpful in diagnosing some infectious diseases and lymphosarcoma and in cases of trauma with blood loss.

Routine blood chemistry tests assist in defining many metabolic diseases affecting the nervous system, particularly liver disease, hypocalcemia, hypomagnesemia, and hypoglycemia. Special serum enzyme assays may be run to confirm liver and muscle disease.

Serum titers, particularly acute and convalescent titers, are very helpful for diagnosing some infectious diseases, and blood and tissue toxin levels can assist in diagnosis of intoxications.

CEREBROSPINAL FLUID ANALYSIS

The collection and analysis of cerebrospinal fluid (CSF) from large animals has been described (Mayhew 1975; 1981). Simplified techniques for analysis are also published (Mayhew and Beal 1980). The results of CSF analysis can be considered to reflect diseases in the brain and spinal cord, as does the hemogram for many systemic diseases. Thus, CSF analysis is one of the most helpful aids in determining the cause of lesions.

In most malformations the CSF will be normal. If a malformation of the calvarium or vertebral column results in damage to underlying nervous tissue, the CSF may reflect trauma and possible subtle hemorrhage.

Infectious diseases often result in a CSF pleocytosis and protein elevation. The cell type present varies considerably, although generally there will be neutrophils with bacterial diseases and small mononuclear cells with viral diseases. Fungal and protozoal diseases usually result in mixed cell responses. Protozoal and particularly helminth parasite infestations may result in an eosinophilic response in the CSF as well as hemorrhage. In most chronic inflammatory states and in diseases in which there is much CNS tissue necrosis, the CSF can contain many large mononuclear cells or macrophages.

With traumatic injury to the CNS there will often be some hemorrhage into the CSF with resulting yellow discoloration. This xanthochromia remains after red cells have been centrifuged off. Trauma also results in leakage of red cells and some protein into the CSF, particularly if meningeal vessels are damaged. Neutrophils, followed by macrophages, will usually appear in the CSF as a result of such hemorrhage.

In most toxic, nutritional, and metabolic neurologic diseases, the results of routine CSF analysis are normal. However, in those diseases in which there may be considerable tissue destruction such as lead poisoning, polioencephalomalacia in ruminants, and moldy corn encephalomalacia in horses, there may be some protein leakage and a large mononuclear cell response in the CSF.

There is typically leakage of protein and some evidence of hemorrhage (i.e., xanthochromia) without any significant pleocytosis in many vascular diseases. If the hemorrhage is marked, then neutrophils and macrophages may also be seen.

Degenerative diseases do not result in any typical changes in CSF, and most frequently the CSF analysis is normal.

Neoplasms can act like other space-occupying lesions such as abscesses and hematomas and increase the CSF pressure. The most frequent change in CSF in patients with neoplasia is a slight elevation in protein content. Only rarely will there be atypical lymphocytes in CSF from cattle with CNS lymphosarcoma; more frequently there will be evidence of mild injury, i.e., xanthochromia and a few macrophages.

ELECTRODIAGNOSTIC TESTING

Electroencephalography, electromyography, and nerve stimulation and conduction testing are aids to a complete neurological evaluation of humans and small animals (Klemm 1976; Hoerlein 1978). The techniques used in large animals are the same as those in small animal neurology. Considerable experience with the use of these ancillary aids is required to be able to interpret electroencephalograms and nerve conduction studies in large animals, because the findings in normal animals are not yet well defined. This fact and the expense of the equipment make these procedures somewhat prohibitive to most large animal clinicians.

Needle electromyography to detect abnormal electrical activity seen in muscle that has been denervated and in several myopathies can be just as useful in helping to localize neurological lesions in large animals as it is in small animals. The reader is referred to other literature for description of the methodologies and interpretation of electromyography in animals (Hoerlein 1978; Mayhew et al., 1978).

NEURORADIOLOGY

Radiography of the calvarium and vertebral column is indispensable for identifying bony malformations, fractures, displacement, and osteomyelitis.

The techniques of positive contrast myelography and vertebral venography have been described in the horse (Stowater et al., 1978; Mayhew et al., 1978; Beech, 1979; Rendano, 1978; Nyland et al., 1980). These procedures are useful for defining spinal cord compression and swelling of the spinal cord. Some experience is required to be able to obtain satisfactory studies; complications do occur, and the procedures can be prolonged and distressful to the patient. Consequently, it is suggested that these procedures be done only by an experienced radiologist with the correct equipment and only in clinical cases in which the clinician is prepared to attempt whatever surgical and medical therapy is indicated or to perform euthanasia if necessary at the termination of the procedure.

REFERENCES

Beech, J.: Metrizamide myelography in the horse. J. Am. Vet. Rad. Soc. 20:22, 1979.

Björklund, N. E., and Palsson, G.: Guttural pouch mycosis in the horse. A survey of 7 cases and a case report. Nord. Vet. Med. 22:65, 1970.

Cook, W. R.: Headshaking in horses. Part 4: Special diagnostic procedures. Equine Pract. 2:7, 1980.

Cook, W. R.: The clinical features of guttural pouch mycosis in the horse. Vet. Rec. 83:336, 1968.

Cummings, J. F., and deLahunta, A.: An experimental study of the retinal projections in the horse and sheep. Ann. NY Acad. Sci. 167:293, 1969.

deLahunta, A.: Veterinary Neuroanatomy and Clinical Neurology. Philadelphia: W.B. Saunders, 1977.

Espersen, G.: A hypophysis-abscess-syndrome in cattle. I. Clinical investigations. Nord. Vet. Med. 27:465, 1975.

Getty, R. (ed.): Sisson and Grossman's The Anatomy of Domestic Animals, 5th ed. Philadelphia: W. B. Saunders, 1975, chap. 24.

Hamilton, G. F.: Diseases of peripheral nerves. In Current Veterinary Therapy, Food Animal Practice. Howard, J. L. (ed.). Philadelphia: W. B. Saunders, 1981, pp. 1097–1101.

Hickman, J.: Veterinary Orthopaedics. Edinburgh: Oliver & Boyd, 1964.

Hoerlein, B. F.: Canine Neurology: Diagnosis and Treatment, 3rd ed. Philadelphia: W. B. Saunders, 1978.

Howard, J. R.: Neurologic examination of cattle. Vet. Scope 13:2, 1968.

Jenkins, T. W.: Functional Mammalian Neuroanatomy. Philadelphia, Lea & Febiger, 1977.

Klemm, W. R. (ed.): Applied Electronics in Veterinary Medicine and Animal Physiology. Springfield, IL: Charles C Thomas, 1976.

Mayhew, I. G.: Cerebrospinal fluid. In Current Veterinary Therapy, Food Animal Practice. Howard, J. L., (ed.). Philadelphia: W. B. Saunders, 1981, pp. 1078–1080, 1981.

Mayhew, I. G.: Collection of cerebrospinal fluid from the horse. Cornell Vet. 65:500, 1975.

Mayhew, I. G., et al.: Spinal cord disease in the horse. Cornell Vet. 68(Suppl. 6):1, 1978.

Mayhew, I. G., and Beal, C. R.: Techniques of analysis of cerebrospinal fluid. Vet. Clin. North Am. Small Anim. Pract. 10(1):155, 1980.

Mayhew, I. G., and Ingram, J. T.: Neurologic evaluation of the horse. Proceedings of the American Association of Equine Practitioners:525, 1978.

Mayhew, I. G., Watson, A. G., and Heissan, J. A.: Congenital occipitoatlantoaxial malformations in the horse. Equine Vet. J. 10:103, 1978.

Nyland, T. G., et al: Metrizamide myelography in the horse: Clinical, radiographic and pathologic changes. Am. J. Vet. Res. 41:204, 1980.

Palmer, A. C.: Introduction to Animal Neurology, 2nd ed. Oxford: Blackwell Scientific Publications, 1976.

Rendano, V. T., and Quick, E. B.: Equine radiology — the cervical spine. Mod. Vet. Pract. 53:921, 1978.

Rooney, J. R.: Clinical Neurology of the Horse. Kennett Square, PA: KNA Press, 1971.

Smith, J. S., and Mayhew, I. G.: Horner's syndrome in large animals. Cornell Vet. 67:529, 1977.

Vaughan, L. C.: Peripheral nerve injuries: An experimental study in cattle. Vet Rec. 76:1293, 1964.

White, M. E., Pennock, P. W., and Seiler, R. J.: Atlantoaxial subluxation in five young cattle. Can. Vet. J. 19:79, 1978.

CHAPTER 5

FLUID, ELECTROLYTE, AND ACID-BASE THERAPY IN LARGE ANIMAL SURGERY

WILLIAM J. DONAWICK, D.V.M.

Maintenance of normal water, electrolyte, blood-gas, and acid-base balance in large animals unable to meet their own needs poses the ultimate challenge to the most talented veterinary surgeon. Fortunately, in large animals the incidence of accompanying renal disease is low, thus permitting the surgeon to make estimates of the patient's general and special needs with full realization that minor miscalculations will be compensated for by the kidney and through changes in respiration.

The purpose of supplemental oral and parenteral therapy is to maintain the intake of water, electrolytes, and essential minerals, vitamins, and micronutrients when disease has curtailed normal ingestion. In general, the ability to maintain a large animal patient with parenteral therapy must be thought of as a temporary and inadequate substitute for normal oral intake. Thus, for the large animal surgeon, it is of paramount importance that an accurate diagnosis be arrived at quickly, followed by performance of the right operation with the finest operative technique with the aim of restoring the natural desire and ability of the animal to provide for its own needs.

TOTAL BODY WATER

The largest single component of an animal is water. In the case of cattle, for example, 95 per cent of an embryo shortly after conception is water, whereas at birth the percentage is 75 per cent or more, decreasing sometimes to 40 per cent at maturity.

This water is divided into three functional compartments. The largest of these areas of distribution is intracellular water. Here 60 per cent or more of the total body water can be found. Intracellular water content is in direct proportion to the amount of muscle mass present in the animal, for there is less water in other tissues of the body such as fat and bone.

The second major compartment of body water is extracellular fluid (ECF), which is distributed intravascularly as plasma and between cells as interstitial water. ECF in normal animals accounts for approximately 30 per cent of the total body weight.

The third, much smaller, compartment is made up of transcellular fluid. The total volume of these often specialized fluids under normal conditions is small.

These fluids are found in joints, pleural and peritoneal cavities, and the cerebral spinal space and as secretions in the gastrointestinal tract. With the onset of disease, excessive secretion, sequestration, or continued loss of these transcellular fluids may result in large total body deficits of water, severely taxing the animal's homeostasis if the losses are not promptly replaced.

Water is easily diffusible from one compartment to another in the normal animal, but the percentage of total body water in each of the three compartments stays reasonably constant. For instance, the plasma volume is generally 5 per cent of total body weight even though the molecules of water in the plasma at any given moment may later be found in the ECF or the intracellular compartment.

Osmotic Pressure and Osmolality

Osmotic pressure and osmolality of extracellular fluids, especially as measured or estimated in plasma, are important in the maintenance of a normal distribution and balance of water within the major compartments of the body. Water is freely diffusible across cell membranes, which collectively make up the semipermeable membranes separating the theoretical water compartments. Slight alterations in osmotic pressure (or osmolality) can result in major water shifts.

Approximately four-fifths of the total osmotic activity of plasma and the interstitial fluid is caused by sodium and chloride ions, whereas one-half of the intracellular osmotic pressure is maintained by potassium ions. Sodium is freely diffusible from the intravascular to the interstitial space but under normal circumstances is actively prevented from reaching equilibrium in the intracellular fluid. In contrast, potassium is primarily an intracellular ion with an intracellular concentration nearly 30 times that of ECF. These major ions, combined with the contributions of many other soluble diffusible and non-diffusible ions and molecules found in varying concentrations on either side of the semipermeable cell membranes, create an osmotic pressure of more than 5,400 mm Hg and an osmolality of 285 ± 10 mOsm/liter of water. The osmotic pressure and osmolality of the interstitial and intracellular fluids are identical, but those of plasma are slightly higher owing to the presence of dissolved, negatively charged (anion) proteins, which do not readily diffuse into interstitial fluid.

Albumin and, to a lesser extent, globulin and fibrinogen create what is known as a colloid osmotic pressure or oncotic pressure of approximately 28 mm Hg. This small increase in plasma pressure over that of interstitial fluid plays an exceedingly important role in the maintenance of normal blood and interstitial fluid volumes, which, if altered, have a rapid and often deleterious effect on the health of every cell of the animal. The presence of these plasma proteins diminishes the forces at the arterial end of capillaries, causing fluids to leave the intravascular space for the interstitial fluid, and creates the forces favoring reabsorption of most of the lost water at the venous end of the capillaries. Thus, from a clinical standpoint, two factors, plasma osmolality and plasma protein concentration, stand apart in importance in the maintenance of normal water equilibrium. Both can be accurately and quickly measured, and, where necessary, steps can be taken to correct deficiencies or excesses. Osmolality is most commonly determined by a freezing-point depression method, and plasma proteins are routinely measured with the aid of a refractometer, which provides sufficient accuracy in clinical situations.

We rely on changes in plasma composition to indicate irregularities in body patterns of water, electrolytes, and acid-base balance because plasma is easily obtained and analyzed. Although this does provide a "tunnel vision" view of the derangements of the body as a whole, the picture is far from complete, for disease is primarily a cell-related event and distant sampling may reflect the cell's condition poorly or not at all. Measurement of intracellular osmolality, although desirable, is not yet available, leaving the clinician one step away from the knowledge that all is well at the cellular level.

CLINICAL SIGNIFICANCE OF OSMOLALITY VALUES

A high measured serum osmolality (>300 mOsm/L) can occur in water loss, diabetes, and uremia and rarely with sodium excess. A low measured serum osmolality (< 270 mOsm/L) can occur with water excess or sodium loss (often associated with renal disease) or following large infusions of dextrose and water. The presence of excess protein, lipids, and glucose can significantly change the osmolality when the serum water concentration of sodium is normal.

CLINICAL SIGNIFICANCE OF PLASMA PROTEIN VALUES

High plasma proteins (> 8 gm/dl; 10 gm/dl in swine) can occur with salt depletion and chronic infections and commonly in diseases of the gastrointestinal system, especially when water and electrolytes, but not protein, are selectively lost through or sequestered in the gastrointestinal tract. When high plasma proteins occur in association with an elevated serum sodium level and increased packed cell volume, high plasma proteins help to confirm the presence of dehydration.

Low plasma proteins can occur after severe acute or chronic hemorrhage, renal disease, acute and chronic diarrhea and other protein-losing enteropathies of the intestinal tract, peritonitis, pleuritis, other diseases that have as a feature the loss or sequestration of plasma, such as burns and loss into the intestinal tract following strangulation and devitalization of the intestine, and massive infusion of protein-deficient fluids in the management of dehydration and shock.

Because of the importance of plasma proteins, mainly albumin, in maintaining colloid osmotic pressure to preserve body water equilibrium, low plasma proteins cannot be ignored. The plasma volume of animals is 5 per cent of body weight, and, since plasma proteins can be thought of as restricted to the intravascular space, deficits can be estimated quite accurately. For example, a horse weighing 450 kg has a measured plasma protein concentration of 3.5 gm/dl. Assuming no further loss, how many liters of plasma with a protein concentration of 8 gm/dl would have to be transfused to increase the plasma proteins to 6 gm/dl?

The plasma protein concentration immediately after transfusion would be less than calculated, because plasma is 93 per cent water with a normal complement of electrolytes, which temporarily increase the plasma volume. In addition, a small part of the infused protein will normally be lost to the interstitial fluids. The more rapid the rate of administration of plasma, the greater the expansion and apparent dilution.

If whole blood is needed or is given, more whole blood will be required to provide for the protein deficit. Since generally 40 per cent of whole blood is made up of red blood cells, plasma volume and therefore the amount of plasma proteins administered will be proportionately decreased. In general, the percentage increase of whole blood that would have to

---

Solution: Weight of horse: 450 kg
Desired plasma protein: 6 gm/dl
Actual plasma protein: 3.5 gm/dl
Protein deficit: 2.5 gm/dl

$$\text{liters donor plasma required} = \frac{\text{body weight (kg)} \times 0.05 \text{ (protein deficit in gm/dl)}}{\text{protein concentration donor plasma (gm/dl)}}$$

$$= \frac{450 \times 0.05 \, (2.5)}{8} = 7.03$$

be transfused is equivalent to the per cent packed cell volume of the transfused blood.

Useful Conversion Formulas

It is often necessary to convert units of measure to determine electrolyte deficits and to calculate the amount of salts needed to restore normal concentrations in body fluids. Serum concentrations of many ions, including the cations sodium (Na^+), potassium (K^+), calcium (Ca^{++}), and magnesium (Mg^{++}) and the anions chloride (Cl^-), phosphate (PO_4^{--}), and bicarbonate (HCO_3^-), can now be measured quickly and with a high degree of accuracy. Although serum electrolytes are commonly reported in milliequivalents per liter (mEq/L), some laboratories report part or all results of ion concentrations in plasma and serum in milligrams per deciliter (mg/dl) or milligrams per 100 milliliters (mg/100 ml) or milligrams per cent (mg %). Conversion factors for commonly reported plasma electrolytes are provided in Table 5–1. Armed with this plasma electrolyte information, it is often possible, especially for predominantly extracellular ions, to estimate total body deficits or excesses based on total body weight.

To prepare ion solutions for administration, weight units of salts must be converted to ion concentration in solution before the substance is useful to the clinician. It is common practice to make up solutions containing ion concentrations in mEq/L. An mEq/L of an ion is equal to the molecular weight in milligrams divided by its valence per 1000 ml (1 liter). In the case of commonly used salts the mEq/L of the cation and anion of the salt can be determined by substituting the formula or molecular weight of the substance for the atomic weight of a specific ion.

It is easiest for the clinician to think in terms of equivalent weights (mg/mEq) when calculating the number of milliequivalents in any given weight (mg or gm) of a substance, and vice versa. The equivalent weights of commonly used cations, anions, and salts are given in Tables 5–1 and 5–2. Examples of a few clinical situations follow to illustrate the ease of calculation if the equivalent weight of a substance is known.

Example 1: How many mg of potassium citrate ($K_3C_6H_5O_7 \cdot H_2O$, equivalent weight 108) will be required to have 1 mEq of potassium K^+?

Formula: Equivalent weight (mg/mEq) × mEq desired = mg of salt required

Solution: 108 × 1 = 108 mg of potassium citrate

Example 2: A patient is known to have a deficiency of 200 mEq of magnesium. How many mg (or gm) of magnesium sulfate, USP (Mg_2SO_4; chemical formula $Mg_2SO_4 \cdot 7H_2O$; equivalent weight 123) will be needed to correct the deficiency?

Formula: Total mEq deficit × equivalent weight (mg/mEq) = $\dfrac{mg}{1000}$ = gm of Mg_2SO_4 required.

Solution: 200 × 123 = 24,600 mg or 24.6 gm of Mg_2SO_4

Example 3: Conversion of mg to mEq. 30 gm of potassium bicarbonate ($KHCO_3$; equivalent weight 100) was added to a bucket containing 4 liters of water. How many mEq of K^+ and HCO_3 will the patient receive if all the water is consumed?

Formula: $\dfrac{\text{Weight of salt (mg)}}{\text{Equivalent weight (mg/mEq)}}$ = mEq.

Solution: 30 gm of $KHCO_3$ = 30,000 mg of $KHCO_3$

$\dfrac{30,000}{100} = \dfrac{300\,mEq\ of\ K^+\ and}{300\ mEq\ of\ HCO_3^-}$

Example 4: Formulating solutions. A solution is needed that contains 3 mEq/L of Mg and 27 mEq/L of acetate. How many gm of magnesium chloride, USP ($MgCl_2 \cdot 6H_2O$; equivalent weight 101.5) and sodium acetate, USP ($C_2H_3O_2Na$; equivalent weight 82) will have to be added to each liter?

Formula: $\dfrac{\text{Desired mEq/L} \times \text{equivalent weight (mg/mEq)}}{1000}$

= gm/L of salt required.

Solution: A. To obtain 3 mEq/L of magnesium from magnesium choride:

$\dfrac{3 \times 101.5}{1000} = \dfrac{0.305\ gm}{MgCl_2 \cdot 6H_2O}$

B. To obtain 27 mEq/L of acetate from sodium acetate:

$\dfrac{27 \times 82}{1000} = 2.214\ gm\ C_2H_3O_2Na$

Table 5–1 CONVERSION FACTORS FOR PLASMA OR SERUM ELECTROLYTE CONCENTRATIONS OF mEq/L OR mg/dl (mg %; mg/100 ml)

Substance	Chemical Formula	Atomic Weight or Formula Weight (mg/mMOL)	Equivalent Weight (mg/mEq)	Valence (mEq/mMOL)	Conversion Factors*
Cations					
Sodium	Na^+	23.0	23.0	1.0	2.3
Potassium	K^+	39.0	39.0	1.0	3.9
Hydrogen	$[H^+]$	1.0	1.0	1.0	1.0
Ammonium	NH_4^+	18.0	18.0	1.0	1.8
Calcium	Ca^{++}	40.0	20.0	2.0	2.0
Magnesium	Mg^{++}	24.0	12.0	2.0	1.2
Anions					
Chloride	Cl^-	35.5	35.5	1.0	3.5
Bicarbonate	HCO_3^-	77.0	77.0	1.0	2.2 (as CO_2 content)
Carbonate	CO_3^{--}	60.0	30.0	2.0	3.0
Phosphate	PO_4^{--}	31.0 (as phosphorus)	17.2	1.8†	1.7
Lactate (as lactic acid)	$CH_3CHOHCOOH$	90.0	90.0	1.0	9.0
Protein	—	—	—	—	0.41

*To convert from mg/dl to mEq/L, divide by the number indicated. To convert from mEq/L to mg/dl, multiply by the number indicated.

†The phosphate is calculated as phosphorus, with a valence of 1.8 because at the normal pH of extracellular water, 20 per cent of the phosphate ions are in a form with one sodium equivalent (NaH_2PO_4) and 80 per cent are in the form of sodium equivalents (Na_2HPO_4). The total valence is therefore $(0.2 \times 1) + (0.8 \times 2) = 1.8$.

Table 5–2 EQUIVALENT WEIGHTS OF COMMONLY USED SUBSTANCES FOR REPLACEMENT THERAPY IN LARGE ANIMALS

Substance	Chemical Formula	Atomic Weight or Formula Weight (mg/mMOL)	Equivalent Weight (mg/mEq)	Valence (mEq/mMOL)	Approximate Milliequivalents (mEq/gm)
Dextrose USP (D-glucose monohydrate)	$C_2H_{12}O_6 \cdot H_2O$	198.0	—	—	—
Magnesium chloride USP (hexahydrate)	$MgCl_2 \cdot 6H_2O$	203.0	101.5	2	9.9 (magnesium and chloride)
Sodium acetate USP (anhydrous)	$C_2H_3O_2Na$	82.0	82.0	1	12.2 (sodium and acetate)
Sodium lactate USP (anhydrous)	$C_3H_5NaO_3$	113.0	113.0	1	9.0 (sodium and lactate)
Sodium gluconate	$C_6H_{11}NaO_7$	218.0	218.0	1	4.6 (sodium and gluconate)
Sodium phosphate (dibasic, anhydrous)	Na_2HPO_4	142.0	47.3	3	21.0 (phosphate)
Sodium proprionate	CH_3CH_2COONa	96.0	96.0	1	10.4 (sodium and gluconate)
Ammonium chloride	NH_4Cl	53.5	53.5	1	18.7* (hydrogen and chloride)
Hydrochloric acid 10%, dilute, USP	HCl	36.5	36.5	1	2.7† (hydrogen and chloride)
Sodium bicarbonate	$NaHCO_3$	84.0	84.0	1	12.0 (sodium and bicarbonate)
Calcium borogluconate	$C_{12}H_{20}B_2CaO_{16}$	482.0	241.0	2	4.1 (calcium)
Magnesium sulfate USP	$MgSO_4 \cdot 7H_2O$	246.5	123.0	2	8.1 (magnesium)
Calcium gluconate	$C_{12}H_{22}CaO_{14} \cdot H_2O$	448.0	224.0	2	4.46 (calcium)
Calcium chloride	$CaCl_2$	111.0	55.5	2	18.0 (calcium)
Potassium bicarbonate	$KHCO_3$	100.0	100.0	1	10.0 (potassium and bicarbonate)
Potassium citrate	$K_3C_6H_5O_7 \cdot H_2O$	324.0	108.0	3	9.3 (potassium)
Potassium chloride	KCl	74.5	74.5	1	13.4 (potassium and chloride)
Sodium chloride	$NaCl$	58.5	58.5	1	17.1 (sodium and chloride)

*Given as 0.9% NH_4Cl solution (168 mEq/L).

†Given slowly IV at rate of 100 mEq/L[H^+]; or 37 ml 10% HCl/L 5% dextrose in water.

BASELINE REQUIREMENTS OF WATER, THE FORGOTTEN NUTRIENT

Most of the water that is utilized by the animal body is ingested, and under normal circumstances, animals are able to adjust water intake to meet their needs provided fresh water is readily available. Normal metabolic processes of glucose, protein, and fat also contribute to the animal's total water turnover. Oxidation of fat provides slightly more than 1 ml of water/gm of fat oxidized. Endogenous water derived from each kilogram of skeletal muscle lost is 850 ml. Glucose yields 60 per cent of its weight as water. Many conditions determine the amount of water an animal will consume. Important among these to the large animal surgeon are ambient temperature, humidity, body size, heredity, diet, milk yield, stage of pregnancy, the species involved, and body temperature.

There is an increasing need for water as ambient and body temperature increase, body size and humidity decrease, and dry matter, salt, and the percentage of protein in the diet increase. Of all the farm animals, lactating cows require the greatest amount of water in proportion to their size. Late gestation also increases water needs.

Because the water requirements can be met so easily in normal animals without thought or calculation, the continuing need for water during sickness is easily overlooked until the accumulated deficit has a detrimental effect on the patient. In many instances the deficit may even exceed the capabilities of the surgeon to replenish the loss. Several special problems confront the large animal surgeon with regard to water balance: (a) body size of patients may vary from 1 kilogram for a newborn piglet to 1000 kilograms or more for a mature bull; (b) water and nutrient needs vary with body size, use, and stage in life, with the greatest need seen in the suckling neonate; (c) the daily amount of water required may become tremendous in heavy patients suffering severe extraordinary losses, as in the case of profuse diarrhea associated with salmonellosis or the sequestration of water in the abomasum in volvulus; and (d) the equipment and time necessary to administer the needed water may be unavailable or the expense may prohibit extended treatment.

In general, daily requirements for water are closely related to the metabolic body size. A convenient, although empirical, way to describe metabolism of different species, and in turn the daily water needs, is as an exponential rate of weight in kilograms. The net energy for maintenance of homeotherms is generally agreed to be: $140–160 \ W(kg)^{0.75}$. The coefficient 140–160 represents an average value for the kilocalories of maintenance energy needed or produced per unit of metabolic size. This formula takes into account the fact that heat production and water needs per kilogram body weight are greater in smaller animals than in large animals, reflecting the relatively large surface area and more active body mass of smaller animals.

Macfarlane and Howard (1970) have proposed that a more appropriate formula for the estimation of daily water turnover is $W(kg)^{0.82}$. Using this formula and the water turnover rates per 24 hours as measured in various species, Figure 5–1 was developed to permit estimation of daily baseline water requirement in animals weighing from 1 to 1000 kg. In this figure the daily water requirement is equal to $150 \ W(kg)^{0.82}$. For example, using this figure it can be estimated that an animal weighing 50 kg would need 3.7 liters of water/24 hr, whereas an animal weighing 500 kg would have a baseline requirement of 24 liter/24 hr. In the case of lactating animals, 1 liter of water should be added to the baseline water requirement for each liter of milk produced per day, since milk is approximately 87 per cent water.

With the onset of fever, base line water requirements increase 13 per cent above normal with each degree (centigrade) increase in body temperature. Since there is a relatively constant increase in metabolic rate with each degree rise in temperature, an empirical formula was written to reflect the corresponding increase in water required. This formula is:

$$(0.15 + 0.02 \ \triangle \ T) \ W^{0.82} = L \ of \ water/24 \ hr$$

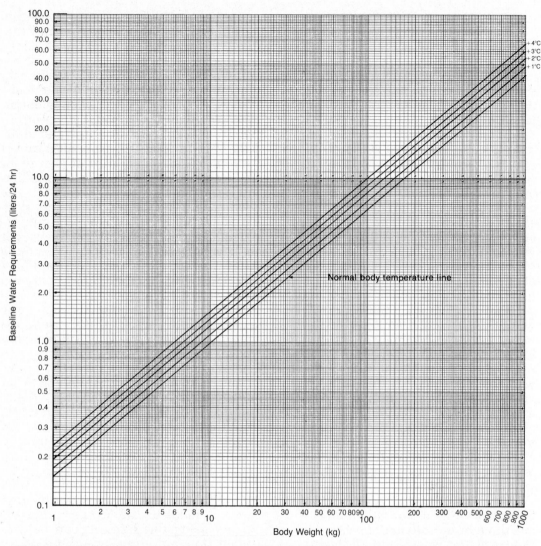

Figure 5–1 Daily baseline water requirements (liters/24 hrs) for normal and febrile animals unwilling or unable to consume water or purposefully denied access to water for per os consumption. To the baseline requirements should be added 1 liter for each liter of milk produced/day, and an estimate (in liters) of all extraordinary water losses.

Where $\triangle$ T is the change in temperature in degrees above normal. For convenience, Figure 5–1 can be used to estimate for each degree increase in body temperature.

All extraordinary losses must be added to the estimated daily baseline water requirements determined by Figure 5–1. Such losses occur with profuse diarrhea, sequestration of water in the gastrointestinal tract associated with ileus or any disease obstructing the normal passage of ingesta, abnormally high urine output with altered kidney function, drainage from the gastrointestinal tract through a nasogastric tube, excessive sweating, peritonitis, pleuritis, edema, ascites, burns, severe trauma, excessive strenuous activity, hemorrhage, shock, diabetes insipidus, and high ambient temperature. In some instances these losses can be measured, but in most the loss can only be estimated. Urine can be collected with relative ease, as can blood lost during surgery. Drainage from a nasogastric tube, pleural and peritoneal cavities, abomasum, and cecum can also be measured with relative ease.

Diarrheic calves develop a rapid disproportionate loss of water, with the blood vascular system sustaining nearly 50 per cent of the total loss. Their water needs may more than double owing to the water loss caused by the diarrhea. Under most clinical circumstances it is nearly impossible to make an accurate assessment of total fecal water loss associated with acute diarrhea. It is known that feces contain approximately 75 per cent water, whereas in acute diarrhea the percentage of water increases to more than 90 per cent. Carlson (1979) has estimated that the fecal water loss in acute diarrhea in an adult horse may vary widely from 15 to 80 liters per day beyond baseline requirements. Such a wide range makes it impossible to estimate the water needed for replacement without consideration of the clinical signs and clinical laboratory studies.

Clinical assessment of the degree of dehydration based on the skin turgor, moistness of the mucous membranes, and character and placement of the eye is very subjective and is not accurately expressed as a percentage of dehydration, although attempts are often made to do so. Single measurements of the packed cell volume (hematocrit), plasma protein (or total solids), and serum Na^+ concentration are not effective diagnostic aids for assessing water needs, as they normally vary over a wide range. However, serial samples are useful in determining the adequacy of initial therapy and in estimating future needs.

Evaluation of Accumulated Deficits

Water deficits begin accumulating soon after the normal ingestion of water ceases. This may vary somewhat depending on the anatomical form of the digestive tract; i.e., a fully developed ruminant stomach may be capable of holding many liters of water "in reserve" as compared with the small simple stomach of the young pig, in whom the reserve volume is very small.

In clinical settings it is convenient to use the onset of illness as the starting point in determining accumulated deficits if the animal has not continued to consume its usual daily water intake.

It is useful to bear in mind that a patient denied water will die within a few days, whereas a patient deprived of food may survive for many weeks. Since the ability of the animal to conserve water is limited, it can be generally stated that the water deficit is equivalent to the daily baseline requirements multiplied by the number of days of water deprivation.

It has become common practice to attempt to express water needs as a percentage of body weight using the following formula; a moderately dehydrated animal might be assumed to be 10 per cent dehydrated and a severely dehydrated patient to be 15 per cent dehydrated (Table 5–3).

Body weight (kg) × % dehydration = replacement water needs (liters)

Since an accurate weight before or during sickness is rarely available, use of this formula is inevitably prone to serious miscalculation. As routinely applied, a 450-kg horse estimated to be 10 per cent

Table 5–3 "RULE OF THUMB" APPROXIMATIONS FOR FLUID AND BICARBONATE THERAPY IN HORSES AND RUMINANTS WITH SEVERE ACUTE DIARRHEA*

Estimated Degree of Dehydration	Total Fluid Loss (liters)	Approximate Base Deficit (mEq/L)	Immediate HCO_3^- Needs (as $NaHCO_3$)	
			(mEq)	(gm)
10% body weight (depressed, sunken eyes; dry skin; ambulatory or sternal)	4.50	15–20	270–360	25–30
15% body weight (Moribund, lateral recumbency, decreased temperature)	6.75	25–30	455–545	40–45

*Example is a 100-lb (45-kg) calf.
Notes: For a 1000-lb cow, multiply the above figures by 10. 50 gm of $NaHCO_3$ yields approximately 600 mEq of HCO_3^-. Do not exceed 50 gm $NaHCO_3$ per liter of IV fluid.

dehydrated would require 45 liters of water to replenish its loss.

450 kg × 0.10 = 45 liters of water deficit

Route and Rate of Water Administration

Water lacking salts or sugars, which makes it isotonic or nearly so, can only be administered safely into the gastrointestinal tract. If a patient cannot or will not consume sufficient water to meet all or part of its estimated water requirements, water can be given per os after passage of a nasogastric tube or placement of an esophagotomy tube. Of course, the prefered oral route of administration can only be used when normal passage through and absorption from the gastrointestinal tract is possible. The amount and frequency of per os administration of water depend on the capacity of the stomach and the amount needed. It is best to give water with sufficient time between treatment intervals so as to be able to determine if normal passage and absorption of the water are taking place. Administration of water into the colon through a tube placed rectally has been advocated periodically, but this route cannot be supported because of the danger of rectal or colon damage including perforation.

When the oral route cannot be used to meet daily water needs, the preferred route of administration is intravenous injection (IV). If fluids must be given rapidly, IV isotonic solutions are preferred. The hypotonic limit for safe IV infusion of fluids is about 180 mOsm/L. Hypertonic fluids in excess of 300 mOsm/L should be given with caution and may be inappropriate for correction of primary water deficits because of their tendency to result in a shift of water from cells to extracellular fluid (ECF).

Calculated deficits and baseline requirements of water are best given by slow continuous IV administration unless life-threatening dehydration dictates rapid replacement of a portion of the needs. In such instances one-third to one-half of the fluid needs are given rapidly through a large central vein. There are many commercially available IV solutions designed for rapid, safe IV use. A partial listing of these is provided in Table 5–4. A practical balanced electrolyte solution can also be prepared from readily available salts (Table 5–5). Balanced solutions approximating the electrolyte concentration of plasma but lacking dextrose are best for rapid IV infusion. If 5% dextrose in water is used for rehydration it is well to remember that the rate of glucose removal following IV administration does not exceed 0.75 gm glucose/kg body weight/hr. Administration at a rate in excess of metabolization will cause hyperosmolality, hyperosmotic diuresis, and renal excretion of water intended for rehydration.

Unless extraordinary losses are present, IV administration at a rate of 2 to 4 ml/kg/hr should be adequate. In extreme circumstances multiple veins can be cannulated, allowing the administration of fluids under pressure at flow rates up to 200 ml/kg/hr.

Percutaneous catheters 12 cm or more in length placed aseptically in a large vein, usually the external jugular or cephalic vein (Brownlow and Hutchins, 1981) provide the safest avenue for IV treatment. If kept under bandage, these catheters can usually be left in place for 72 hours before replacement.

In special circumstances it may be necessary to reduce calculated baseline water requirements or slow the rate of administration because of overriding considerations. An example of this is severe hypoproteinemia, which would result in pulmonary edema if the protein was diluted by expansion of the intravascular plasma volume. Here, plasma, whole blood, or a concentrated source of protein would be required before aggressive correction of dehydration could be undertaken.

Measurement of central venous pressure (CVP) and arterial blood pressure offers a practical means of monitoring patients to determine a safe rate of fluid administration. Expansion of the intravascular volume causes an increase in intrathoracic venous pressure (usually measured in cm H_2O). Dangerous fluid overloads are signaled by elevations of CVP above 15 cm H_2O.

Table 5-4 COMMON COMMERCIAL IV SOLUTIONS*

| Product | Electrolyte Composition (mEq/L) | | | | | Buffer Source (mEq/L) | Toxicity | pH | Caloric Value (per L) | Indications |
	Na+	K+	Ca++	Mg++	Cl-					
Balanced Electrolyte Solutions										
Lactated Ringer's	130	4	3	—	109	Lactate 28	Isotonic	6.5	9	To correct fluid and electrolyte deficits and mild acidosis.
Ringer's injection	147	4	5	—	156	—	Isotonic	5.8	—	To correct fluid and electrolyte deficits in the presence of metabolic *alkalosis.*
Normosol-R†	140	5	—	3	98	Acetate 27 Gluconate 23	Isotonic	6.4	18	All-purpose replacement fluid used to correct fluid and electrolyte deficits and moderate to severe metabolic acidosis.
Normosol-R pH 7.4	140	5	—	3	98	Acetate 27 Gluconate 23	Isotonic	7.4	18	To correct fluid and electrolyte deficits and moderate to severe metabolic acidosis. Particularly indicated in small neonates.
Normosol-R and 5% dextrose	140	5	—	3	98	Acetate 27 Gluconate 23	Hypertonic	5.7	185	To correct fluid and electrolyte deficits and moderate to severe metabolic acidosis when added calories are needed.
Normosol-M and 5% dextrose	40	13	—	3	40	Acetate 16	Hypertonic	5.5	175	To maintain physiologic fluid and electrolyte balance in patients with restricted oral intake.
Saline/Carbohydrate Solutions										
0.9% Normal saline inj., USP	154	—	—	—	154	—	Isotonic	5.4	—	To restore extracellular volume when renal tubules are damaged.
5% Saline inj.	856	—	—	—	856	—	Hypertonic	—	—	To correct severe sodium and chloride deficits.
5% Dextrose in water	—	—	—	—	—	—	Isotonic	5.0	170	To correct hypoglycemia, as additive to other solutions when added calories are needed, and for rehydration.
Dextrose 2.5% in 0.45% saline	77	—	—	—	77	—	Isotonic	4.8	85	For rehydration and to improve renal function.
5% Dextrose and 0.9% sodium chloride inj., USP	154	—	—	—	154	—	Hypertonic	4.7	170	For rehydration and to improve renal function.
Dextrose 50% in water	—	—	—	—	—	—	Hypertonic	4.2	1700	To correct hypoglycemia.

Table continued on following page

Table 5-4 COMMON COMMERCIAL IV SOLUTIONS (*Continued*)*

Product	Electrolyte Composition (mEq/L)					Buffer Source (mEq/L)	Toxicity	pH	Caloric Value (per L)	Indications
	Na$^+$	K$^+$	Ca^{++}	Mg^{++}	Cl$^-$					
Special Solutions										
5% Sodium bicarbonate inj., USP	595	—	—	—	—	Bicarbonate (HCO$_3^-$)595	Hypertonic	7.8	—	Buffering solution to correct metabolic acidosis common in gastrointestinal diseases, shock, and renal impairment.
Sodium bicarbonate 8.4% (50 mEq/50 ml)	1000	—	—	—	—	Bicarbonate (HCO$_3^-$)1000	Hypertonic	—	—	Buffering solution to correct metabolic acidosis common in gastrointestinal diseases, shock, and renal impairment.
Potassium chloride (40 mEq/20 ml)	—	2000	—	—	2000	—	—	4.5	—	To correct acute potassium deficits.
Dextan 6% W/V in 0.9% saline	154	—	—	—	154	—	Hypertonic	—	—	For plasma expansion.
Calcium borogluconate 23% solu.	—	—	943	—	—	—	Hypertonic	—	—	To treat calcium deficiencies.
Aminosyn 5% (crystalline amino acid solu.)	—	5.4	—	—	—	—	Hypertonic	5.3	345	To provide amino acid source for stressed, anorexic, or debilitated patients.

*Adapted from a table distributed by CEVA Laboratories, Inc., 10560 Barkley, Overland Park, KS 66212.
†Normosol, Abbott Laboratories, North Chicago, IL 60064.

Table 5–5 A BALANCED, BUFFERED, MULTIPLE-ELECTROLYTE SOLUTION FOR INTRAVENOUS AND ORAL USE IN REPLACEMENT THERAPY IN LARGE ANIMALS

Total Cations	(mEq/L)		Total Anions	(mEq/L)
Sodium	140		Chloride	98
Potassium	5		Acetate	27
Magnesium	3		Proprionate	23
Total	148		Total	148

Solution	mg/L
Sodium chloride (NaCl; F.W. 58.44)	526
Potassium chloride (KCl; F.W. 74.56)	370
Magnesium chloride (MgCl$_2$·6H$_2$O; F.W. 203.33)	303
Sodium acetate USP (C$_2$H$_3$O$_2$Na; F.W. 82.03) (anhydrous)	222
Sodium proprionate (NaC$_3$H$_5$O$_2$; F.W. 96.06)	221

Note: pH adjusted to approximately 6.4 with hydrochloric acid.

MANAGEMENT OF ELECTROLYTE DISORDERS

Although the sum of cations and anions must be equal, abnormalities in the concentration of various electrolytes are common in surgical patients and, if left unattended, may result in prolonged morbidity or, worse, loss of the patient. Laboratory tests are now commonly available that permit rapid, accurate determination of the concentration of blood, plasma, and urine; sodium, potassium, calcium, magnesium, and hydrogen ion cations; and bicarbonate, chloride, phosphate, lactate, and protein anions (Table 5–6). Additionally, the trace elements zinc and iron are now commonly measured.

Sodium

Sodium (Na$^+$) is the most plentiful cation in the body, with approximately 45 mEq, or 1 gm, of sodium distributed in each kg of body weight. As an extracellular ion, found primarily within the vascular system and the interstitial tissues, it is the main cation responsible for osmolality and maintenance of extracellular volume. The normal concentration of

Table 5–6 NORMAL ELECTROLYTES, PROTEIN, BLOOD-GAS, AND ACID-BASE VALUES FOR SERUM, PLASMA, AND BLOOD OF LARGE ANIMALS*

Test	Bovine	Equine	Caprine	Ovine	Porcine	Useful reference numbers
Cations						
Sodium (Na$^+$) mEq/L	132–152	132–146	142–155	139–152	135–150	140.0
Potassium (K$^+$) mEq/L	3.9–5.8	2.4–4.7	3.5–6.7	3.9–5.4	5.5	4.0
Calcium (Ca^{++}) mg/dl	9.4–12.2	11.2–13.6	10.3	8.2–12.8	8.6–10.6	10–12
Magnesium (Mg^{++}) mg/dl	1.0–2.9	1.6–2.5	2.5	1.7–2.1	1.9–3.2	2.0
Anions						
Chloride (Cl$^-$) mEq/L	97–111	99–109	99–110	95–103	94–106	100.0
Bicarbonate (HCO$_3^-$) mEq/L	21–29	24–34	21	20–25	18–27	24.0
Phosphate (PO$_4^{--}$) mg/dl (as phosphorus)	4–7	3–7	6–8	4–7	4–7	5.0
Total protein (gm/dl)	5.7–8.0	5.3–7.6	6.3	5.2–6.4	7.0–10	7.0
pH (arterial) pH units	7.31–7.53	7.32–7.44	7.35	7.32–7.53	7.38	7.4
pO$_2$ (arterial) torr	70–95	70–95	90	80–95	80–95	90.0
pO$_2$ (venous) torr	34	36–46	45	41	42	40.0
pCO$_2$ (arterial) torr	35–44	35–38	37	38	34	40.0
pCO$_2$ (venous) torr	47	44	47	45	57	45.0

*Adapted in part from Formulary, Colorado State University, Veterinary Teaching Hospital, September, 1976.

plasma sodium is 132 to 155 mEq/L, depending on the species and environmental conditions. Before, during, and after surgery, sodium concentration, if abnormal, may be high (hypernatremia) or low (hyponatremia).

HYPONATREMIA

Hyponatremia is present when the plasma sodium concentration is less than 132 mEq/L. The clinical signs associated with hyponatremia are dependent on the rapidity of sodium loss. With a gradual loss of sodium, there is muscle weakness, inappetence, listlessness, and low blood pressure. If the loss occurs very acutely, the result is shock. The causes of hyponatremia can be found in Table 5–7.

The treatment of hyponatremia is directed toward stopping further Na^+ loss and giving sufficient Na^+ to restore normal extracellular concentrations. When Na^+ is lost as a part of gastrointestinal secretions, potassium as well as sodium is lost and must be replaced. Usually, Na^+ is replaced by the administration of normal saline (154 mEq/L Na^+ and Cl^-), unless this results in volume overload, in which case 3% saline (30 gm sodium chloride per liter; Na^+ concentration 513 mEq/L) or 5% saline (50 gm sodium chloride per liter; sodium concentration 855 mEq/L) is administered.

The volume of solution given is based on the patient's needs and the concentration of sodium in the solution. Patient needs are calculated from the formula below. The Na^+ deficit (in mEq) is divided by the concentration of sodium in normal saline (154 mEq/L), 3% saline (513 mEq/L), or 5% saline (855 mEq/L), to determine the liters of solution required. In many instances, 3 or 5% saline is preferable to normal saline for IV administration because the deficits are so large that if normal saline were given, the volume of fluid needed would cause an overload of the ECF.

It must be remembered that when sa-

Table 5–7 CAUSES OF HYPONATREMIA AND HYPERNATREMIA IN LARGE ANIMALS

Hyponatremia
Fluid sequestration, as occurs in peritoneal cavity with rupture of bladder in newborn foals
Body fluid loss without adequate replacement, as with severe, profuse diarrhea of salmonellosis
Major surgery when patients are given excessive water (usually iatrogenic) or dextrose in water IV
Chronic wasting disease, as seen with chronic infections, liver disease, hypoproteinemia
Intrinsic kidney disease and diuresis following administration of potent diuretics such as furosemide
Gastrointestinal fistulas
Severe hemorrhage
Loss of sodium through skin from extensive sweating
Adrenal crisis (rare in large animals)

Hypernatremia
Dehydration owing to loss of hypotonic fluid (desiccation), prolonged exposure to dry heat, respiratory loss with fever
Deprivation of adequate water
Excessive solute loading associated with feeding of highly concentrated foodstuffs without adequate supplemental water or use of isotonic electrolyte solutions as total source of water intake
Excessive salt intake without adequate water

line is administered in any concentration, the mEq of chloride given will equal that of sodium. Since the concentration of chloride in normal plasma is 100 mEq/L, administration of normal or concentrated saline solutions can cause dramatic changes in serum chloride. Should the patient be acidotic, saline administration is contraindicated because it will enhance acidosis and elevate the already high plasma chloride concentration. In hyponatremic acidosis, 5% sodium bicarbonate (595 mEq/L Na^+ and HCO_3^-), sodium lactate (lactated Ringer's solution, USP; 28 mEq/L), or another bicarbonate precursor should be given.

HYPERNATREMIA

Hypernatremia occurs when the plasma sodium is greater than 155 mEq/

$$\frac{(140 - \text{measured plasma } Na^+[\text{mEq/L}]) \times \text{weight (Kg)}}{3} = \text{mEq } Na^+ \text{ needed for replacement}$$

L. Increases in Na^+ concentration indicate a *relative* water deficit in which more water than sodium has been lost. The causes of hypernatremia are listed in Table 5–7.

Hypernatremia often can be corrected simply by providing free-choice fresh water for ingestion when the cause is excessive salt intake or solute loading, water deprivation, or dehydration due to loss of hypotonic fluid. When the alimentary route cannot be used to correct hypernatremia, IV correction is best accomplished by administration of 5% dextrose in water and 0.45% saline in 2.5% dextrose, a polyionic *maintenance* electrolyte solution (containing approximately 40 mEq/L of sodium). The object is to provide water with little or no sodium in a form acceptable for IV administration. The volume of fluid required cannot be accurately calculated. The volume required will depend on the initiating disease or circumstance, rate of continued water loss, degree of hypernatremia, sodium content of the fluid given, rate of administration, antidiuretic hormone level, aldosterone response, and kidney function. Clinical judgment must be used to determine an approximate dosage, followed by frequent reassessment of osmolality or plasma sodium concentration.

Potassium

Only a small amount of the total body potassium (K^+) is present in the extracellular fluid; the vast majority resides within cells. Large fluctuations in total body potassium can occur without causing corresponding changes in plasma potassium concentration. In fact, often the plasma K^+ concentration changes in an inverse relationship to the loss or gain of total body potassium. Thus, plasma K^+ concentration is not a reliable index of total body potassium, nor is it a reliable indicator for the administration of potassium. Unfortunately, there is still no clinically applicable test to determine intracellular potassium deficits or excesses. The normal plasma potassium is 2.4 to 6.7 mEq/L, depending on the species.

A transient increase in plasma K^+ concentration is common after major surgery or extensive trauma (Table 5–8). The increase in plasma concentration and urine excretion of potassium is associated with the catabolic breakdown of cells, especially skeletal muscle, that follows as a normal sequence of healing.

Respiratory and metabolic acidosis, renal failure, trauma, and major surgery tend to raise the plasma K^+ concentration through the transfer of intracellular potassium to extracellular fluid. In general, modest increases in plasma potassium concentration are well tolerated, but elevations beyond 7.5 mEq/L may be life-threatening and must be dealt with promptly.

Alkalosis causes potassium to enter cells, resulting in a lowered plasma K^+. As a general rule, potassium loss causes metabolic alkalosis; conversely, a metabolic or respiratory alkalosis causes hypopotassemia. When potassium is lost from cells, sodium and hydrogen ions

Table 5–8 COMMON CAUSES OF HYPOKALEMIA OR HYPERKALEMIA IN LARGE ANIMALS

Hypokalemia
Metabolic alkalosis from loss of hydrochloric acid in gastric juice by aspiration of stomach contents in horses
Sequestration of abomasal contents in cattle with volvulus of abomasum, diarrhea, intestinal fistulas
Curtailed ingestion of potassium due to anorexia
Dilution, as when large amounts of potassium-free-fluid are given rapidly by intravenous injection
Renal loss of potassium due to renal tubular dysfunction, use of organomercurial- and thiazide-derived diuretics or adrenal mineralocorticoid steroids, massive doses of sodium penicillin intravenously
Excessive administration of bicarbonate or other alkalizing salts
Surgical treatment or anesthesia with major urinary loss of potassium, usually with reduced potassium intake

Hyperkalemia
Acute or chronic renal failure
Excess potassium ingestion
Tissue trauma liberating intracellular potassium
Severe metabolic or respiratory acidosis
Rapid infusion of penicillin G, potassium in a small patient
Hemolysis of blood specimen or laboratory error
Acute dehydration or adrenal insufficiency
Rupture of bladder in newborn foals
Overly rapid infusion of potassium salts

move from the extracellular water into the cells to replace the potassium. In exchange for every three K^+ ions lost from cells, two Na^+ ions and one $[H^+]$ ion enter. This causes a decreased hydrogen ion concentration in the extracellular water, resulting in metabolic alkalosis. In primary alkalosis, the opposite occurs: $[H^+]$ ions move from the cell to the extracellular water in an attempt to lower the pH in exchange for K^+, resulting in a hypopotassemia.

HYPOKALEMIA

Hypokalemia, a plasma potassium concentration of less than 2.5 mEq/L, may be accompanied by muscle weakness of both skeletal and smooth muscle, resulting in intestinal ileus, peripheral muscle weakness, and flaccid paralysis. Changes in the electrocardiogram, characteristic of hypokalemia in humans, are usually not seen in large animals.

Hypokalemic alkalosis often occurs in cattle with abomasal volvulus and in horses that have lost chloride, hydrogen ions, and potassium from the gastrointestinal tract, usually following the repeated removal by stomach tube of large amounts of gastric reflux.

Whenever an animal is anorexic or known to be losing potassium, treatment with potassium salts should be begun early (within two days) before the total body loss of potassium is so great as to cause serious decreases in the plasma potassium concentration.

Treatment of Hypokalemia

Hypokalemia is usually treated with potassium chloride IV or PO. Potassium bicarbonate or potassium citrate may also be given if there is no chloride deficit.

Since only a small part of the total exchangeable potassium is present in the extracellular fluid and since time is required for the transfer of potassium across cellular membranes to the intracellular compartment, care must be exercised in the IV administration of potassium chloride to prevent unwanted and dangerous hyperkalemia. In adult large animals, limits to the rate of administration will usually prevent the inadvertent

development of hyperkalemia. In neonatal and small species of large animals, more care must be exercised in the administration of potassium, as hyperkalemia may develop.

The length and type of illness can provide valuable information when determining the amount of potassium needed and the rate and route for safe administration. The rate of intravenous administration of potassium probably should not exceed 100 to 150 mEq/hr in large (300 kg and more) animals unless frequent laboratory assessments of potassium can be made to determine the onset of hyperkalemia. It is important to ensure that there is reasonable kidney function before rapid administration of potassium is begun or before large total doses of potassium are given. As a general rule, a safe initial dosage can be calculated using the following formula: calculated extracellular deficit × total body weight.

Example: Weight of animal: 500 kg
Measured plasma potassium: 1.8 mEq/L
Normal plasma potassium: 3.5 mEq/L

$(3.5 - 1.8) \times 500 = 850$ mEq KCl (63.4 gm) initial IV or PO dosage

If frequent laboratory assessments are not possible, it is best to administer potassium chloride, orally, well diluted in water, at the rate of 0.5 to 1.5 mEq KCl/kg body weight/day.

Since hundreds of mEq may be needed to replenish a total body potassium deficit, several days of continuous or periodic treatment may be required to correct the accumulated loss. Treatment should be continued until the plasma potassium concentration returns to and remains within the normal range.

HYPERKALEMIA

Fortunately, hyperkalemia (plasma potassium concentrations above 6.8 mEq/L) is rare in large animals. Before emergency treatment is undertaken to lower an extremely high plasma K^+ concentration, it should be determined that there is no laboratory error and that the sample used for the determination was not hemolyzed.

Electrocardiographic changes in ponies and calves do not occur until the plasma potassium exceeds 7 mEq/L (Fig. 5–2). When the potassium values are greater than 7.5 mEq/L, the QRS duration increases progressively and there is a loss of the P wave and an increase in the amplitude of the T wave. Hyperkalemia cannot be diagnosed with certainty on the basis of T wave changes alone, because the T wave is strongly influenced by the relative tone of the autonomic nerve supply, and, in the equine EKG, the T wave is the most variable wave form.

The chief danger associated with hyperkalemia is ventricular fibrillation or cardiac arrest.

Treatment of Hyperkalemia

The aim of treatment is to find the cause of the hyperkalemia and correct it if possible. Unfortunately, sustained high plasma K$^+$ concentrations in large animals (excluding rupture of the bladder in foals and metabolic acidosis) are often associated with renal failure. If immediate steps are necessary to lower the plasma K$^+$ concentration, they should include the following:

1. IV administration of $NaHCO_3$ to correct acidosis and shift potassium to the intracellular compartment;

2. administration of 0.5 gm/kg of dextrose and 0.1 unit/kg body weight of insulin IV to take up potassium for glycogen synthesis; and

3. IV administration of calcium gluconate to temporarily alleviate the effects of hyperkalemia on the heart.

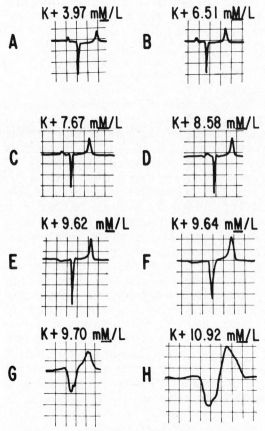

Figure 5–2 Progressive changes in ECG with induced hyperkalemia in ponies (Lead III). *A*, Plasma K$^+$ value of 4.0 mM/L. Control. *B*, Plasma K$^+$ value of 6.5 mM/L. Notice increase in T-wave amplitude. *C*, Plasma K$^+$ value of 7.7 mM/L. Notice increase in P-wave duration. *D*, Plasma K$^+$ value of 8.6 mM/L. Notice decrease in P-wave amplitude. *E*, Plasma K$^+$ value of 9.6 mM/L. Notice PR segment shift. *F*, Plasma K$^+$ value of 9.6 mM/L. Notice inversion of P wave and prolongation of QRS. *G*, Plasma K$^+$ value of 9.7 mM/L. Notice marked intraventricular block. *H*, Plasma K$^+$ value of 10.9 mM/L. Notice sinusoidal-shaped QRS-T complex. Terminal cardiac arrest was noticed at plasma K$^+$ (12.4 mM/L). (Reprinted with permission from Glazier, Littledike and Evans: Am. J. Vet. Res. 43:1935, 1982.)

Calcium

Although there is an enormous reservoir of skeletal calcium, almost all is found in crystalline apatite of bone and is not immediately available in the event of a sudden drain on plasma calcium. The classic example of this in large animals is parturient paresis in the dairy cow, in which the early demands of milk production after parturition decrease plasma calcium faster than the homeostatic mechanisms can mobilize calcium from bone. Although severe hypocalcemia may be present in large animal surgical patients, especially if presented near parturition, it is more common to encounter patients with moderate (7 to 9 mg/dl) hypocalcemia resulting from inappetence or intestinal disease.

HYPERCALCEMIA

Hypercalcemia occurs when the plasma calcium concentration is greater than 14 mg/dl. The incidence of hypercalcemia is rare in large animals with the exceptions of transient iatrogenic hypercalcemia resulting from rapid IV infusion or absorption after subcutaneous injection of large amounts of calcium borogluconate to treat parturient paresis and hyperparathyroidism and hypercalcemia associated with certain cases of chronic renal disease by an unknown mechanism. Hypercalcemia causes a decreased neuromuscular excitation. Signs of hypercalcemia include muscular weakness or incoordination.

HYPOCALCEMIA

Hypocalcemia is present with plasma calcium concentration of less than 9 mg/dl. Although long neglected, moderate hypocalcemia brought on in part by inappetence may play an active role in many diseases of large animals. Indirect evidence for this includes improved arterial blood pressure and slowing of the heart following IV infusion of calcium during anesthesia and improved skeletal muscle tone and an increase in intestinal activity following treatment with calcium. Left untreated, hypocalcemia may result in inability to stand, hyperactive reflexes such as snapping shut of the eyelids, depressed consciousness, intestinal stasis, and, ultimately, circulatory collapse. Hypocalcemia may also be due to magnesium depletion with a low plasma magnesium, which will respond to the administration of magnesium within a few hours. Hypocalcemia may also be seen in hypoparathyroid states, hypoproteinemia, acute and chronic renal failure, and hypoxic acidosis.

Treatment of Hypocalcemia and Hypercalcemia

Iatrogenic hypercalcemia need not be treated; the plasma calcium will return to normal concentration within hours. The hypercalcemia associated with chronic renal disease is as yet difficult to treat specifically. Fortunately, hyperparathyroidism is not frequently encountered in large animals.

With moderate hypocalcemia, cardiac function during anesthesia can often be improved with as little as 0.2 mEq/kg body weight of calcium borogluconate given IV. Persistent moderate hypocal-

cemia during inappetence or restricted oral intake can usually be corrected by the continuous slow IV infusion of 1 to 2 mEq/kg/24 hr of calcium, usually as calcium borogluconate, diluted in daily maintenance fluids.

Hypocalcemia associated with parturient paresis in cattle is treated by the cautious intravenous administration of 1 mEq/kg body weight of calcium borogluconate (500 ml of a 23% solution of calcium borogluconate). If, during infusion, heart irregularities are noted, treatment should be discontinued immediately and the remainder of the calcium given by subcutaneous injection.

Magnesium

Magnesium is the fourth most common cation in the body; most is either within the crystalline structure of bone or, like potassium, intracellular. Magnesium is an essential component of virtually all enzyme systems and is necessary in the activation of enzymes transferring high-energy phosphate radicals to and from adenosine triphosphate (ATP). High plasma concentrations of magnesium (greater than 2.7 mEq/L) behave similarly to calcium by depressing the activity of myoneural junctions. Also as seen with calcium, a deficiency in magnesium (plasma concentration usually less than 0.4 mEq/L) results in neuromuscular irritability. The central nervous system depression caused by magnesium ions is so great that magnesium administered in high concentrations can be used as a general anesthetic.

HYPOMAGNESEMIA

Hypomagnesemia is a condition in which the plasma magnesium concentration is less than 1 mg/dl (0.8 mEq/L) (0.5 mg/dl [0.4 mEq/L] in sheep). Ruminants may be especially vulnerable with regard to magnesium deficiency because there is no readily mobilizable large store of magnesium in the body; therefore, the delicate balance of extracellular magnesium depends largely on the daily intake of magnesium in the diet. Short periods of starvation (24 to 48 hours) in lactating cows and ewes are capable of causing a significant, sudden depression of plasma magnesium (and a decrease in calcium) concentration. Diarrhea is commonly associated with hypomagnesemia of cattle on lush spring pastures. The average lactating dairy cow needs to ingest 20 gm of magnesium and absorb 4 gm of magnesium daily. Other causes of hypomagnesemia can be found in Table 5–9.

The major clinical signs of hypomagnesemia are incoordination, hyperesthesia, tonic and clonic muscular spasms, and convulsions, with death due to respiratory failure. The signs are similar to those resulting from hypocalcemia, and treatment with calcium will have a temporary beneficial effect, even though hypomagnesemia is the primary cause.

Treatment with magnesium should be considered in large animal surgical patients that have been fed on pastures low in magnesium and during seasonal fluctuations when the plasma magnesium is low. If the animal is anorexic or unable to eat, has diarrhea, or has been housed where the environmental conditions favor hypomagnesemia, treatment with magnesium should also be considered.

Empirical treatment with magnesium may be indicated, provided there is normal kidney function, in patients with postoperative ileus, in the absence of obstruction or other cause, in patients receiving long-term parenteral fluid therapy, in patients with diarrhea, in patients with chronic wasting, when hyperparathyroidism is suspected, and in

young surgical patients more than two months of age still receiving primarily whole milk, which is low in magnesium.

Treatment of Hypomagnesemia

Magnesium can be administered orally, intramuscularly, subcutaneously, or intravenously. Parenteral therapy is usually accomplished by the administration of $MgSO_4 \cdot 7H_2O$. The slow IV administration of 1 mEq/kg body weight of magnesium as a 20% solution will maintain normal plasma levels for three to six hours. Plasma levels can be maintained longer if the magnesium is given by subcutaneous injection. Concurrent administration of calcium is usually advisable.

HYPERMAGNESEMIA

Hypermagnesemia with serum plasma concentrations in excess of 3.2 mg/dl (2.7 mEq/L) is not commonly recognized in large animal surgical patients except following iatrogenic administration. Unless clinical signs of weakness leading to paralysis, bradycardia, and coma occur, no treatment is needed. Acute signs may be temporarily alleviated by the slow intravenous administration of calcium chloride.

Chloride

For practical purposes, chloride (Cl^-) can be thought of as an extracellular anion, although some chloride is intracellular. Chloride is the most plentiful extracellular anion, with a normal plasma concentration of 95 to 111 mEq/L, depending on species, age, housing conditions, and availability of fresh water. Plasma chloride is normally held within narrow limits, but when primary Cl^- imbalance occurs, usually there is also a change in bicarbonate to compensate for the increase or decrease in chloride. For instance, with the onset of hypochloremia, the plasma bicarbonate concentration increases, generally in proportion to the decrease in chloride owing to reabsorption of bicarbonate by the kidney. In this way hypochloremia will result in metabolic alkalosis. Persistent hypochloremia will result in bicarbonate reabsorption in spite of the

Table 5–9 COMMON CAUSES OF HYPOMAGNESEMIA AND HYPERMAGNESEMIA

Hypomagnesemia
  Seasonal fluctuations in ruminants
  Inadequate energy intake while grazing lush
    pasture low in magnesium
  Starvation, anorexia, or deliberate withholding
    of feed
  Low dietary content of magnesium
  Exposure to cold, wet, windy conditions
  Diarrhea
  Hyperparathyroidism
Hypermagnesemia
  Administration of magnesium cathartics to
    horses with impaction
  Acute or chronic renal failure
  IV anesthesia or treatment with solutions
    containing magnesium

presence of metabolic alkalosis. Replacement of the plasma chloride deficit will result in excretion of the excess bicarbonate.

HYPOCHLOREMIA

Hypochloremia, a plasma chloride concentration of less than 94 mEq/L, is commonly encountered in cattle with gastrointestinal obstruction, i.e., volvulus of the abomasum and cecum, and intestinal obstruction, and in horses when repeated emptying of the stomach by nasogastric tube is necessary. Other causes of hypochloremia are listed in Table 5–10.

Since chloride is the only quantitatively important reabsorbable anion, its loss becomes critical in maintenance of the extracellular fluid volume during hypochloremia. When both dehydration and hypochloremia are present, the body will choose to maintain volume at the expense of the extracellular pH. Sodium conservation will prevail in spite of developing hypochloremia and progressive metabolic alkalosis. As strict renal sodium conversion continues while plasma chloride falls owing to sequestration without replacement, the reabsorption of

Table 5–10 COMMON CAUSES OF HYPOCHLOREMIA AND HYPERCHLOREMIA IN LARGE ANIMALS

Hypochloremia
  Chloride loss from gastrointestinal tract, especially common in horse following repeated nasogastric drainage of gastric secretions and intestinal reflux
  Sequestration of abomasal secretions with volvulus of abomasum in cattle
  Reflux and sequestration of chloride-rich fluid in rumen in cattle
  Combined with elevated bicarbonate and pH and low plasma potassium concentration in hypokalemic hypochloremic alkalosis
  As a result of administration of diuretics, with a loss of chloride in excess of sodium and loss of potassium in urine
  In chronic renal disease and acute renal failure
Hyperchloremia
  Combined with hypernatremia in desiccation dehydration, with excess solute loading
  Iatrogenic, with excessive administration of ammonium chloride, hydrochloric acid, or sodium chloride

bicarbonate increases, creating a severe metabolic alkalosis.

Hypochloremia does not by itself produce direct recognizable clinical signs. In compensation for the resultant metabolic alkalosis, the rate and depth of respiration may be decreased. Determination of hypochloremia is based on measurement of plasma chloride, usually by a titration method.

Since chloride is freely diffusible throughout the extracellular fluid, replacement must be based on calculation of the entire ECF volume.

HYPERCHLOREMIA

Acute and chronic salt intoxication has been reported in sheep, cattle, and swine that results in hyperchloremia, a plasma chloride concentration in excess of 110 mEq/L. Excess salt intake usually occurs by ingestion. With acute toxicity gastroenteritis occurs because of the irritating effects of high concentrations of salt. In chronic cases, animals are anorexic and weak, lose weight, and occasionally develop diarrhea. When large amounts of sodium chloride are infused or ingested, metabolic acidosis may occur as a direct result of the high plasma Cl^- and as an indirect effect of the increased volume of extracellular water that follows salt overloading. The excess sodium cations can be excreted by the kidney as sodium bicarbonate, but the overabundant chloride ions are retained along with an equal quantity of hydrogen ions, causing acidosis. A dilution acidosis can occur if large quantities of isotonic or hypotonic saline are given because the infused fluid is lacking in normal buffering capacity.

Treatment of Hypochloremia and Hyperchloremia

Moderate to severe hypochloremia is best treated by the IV administration of 0.9% saline or, in severe cases, 3 or 5% saline. Intravenous administration of chloride-rich solutions improves hydration and slows the inappropriate renal reabsorption of bicarbonate.

If the plasma Cl^- is known, the liters of 0.9% saline required to correct the deficiency can be estimated as follows:

$$\frac{\text{body weight (kg)}}{3} \times \text{plasma Cl}^- \text{ deficit} = \text{mEq Cl}^- \text{ required}$$

$$\frac{\text{mEq Cl}^- \text{ required}}{154} = \text{liters of 0.9\% saline required}$$

where one-third of the body weight (kg) is an estimate of extracellular fluid volume; plasma Cl^- deficit is the difference between normal plasma Cl^- (100 mEq/L) and the measured concentration; and 154 is the concentration of Cl^- in 0.9% saline solution (mEq/L).

In cattle with volvulus of the abomasum, when serum Cl^- has not been measured, an estimate of the Cl^- deficit can be made by classifying the severity of the torsion based on clinical signs, the quantity of fluid drained from the abomasum at surgery, and the degree of dehydration (Smith 1978). Based on Table 5–11, an estimate of the chloride deficit can be made.

It is unwise to give the entire calculated amount of Cl^- by rapid IV administration. It is better to give one-half to two-thirds of the calculated dose rapidly, with the remainder given over several hours.

Hyperchloremia is best treated by the cautious IV infusion of an isotonic balanced electrolyte solution or 5% dextrose in water. Since hyperchloremia may result in acidosis, a solution containing bicarbonate is preferable to dextrose in water.

When hyperchloremia is the result of the ingestion of salt, provision of fresh water must be limited to small quantities or the absorption of more salt may intensify the toxicity.

BLOOD GASES AND ACID-BASE BALANCE

The rapid availability of reliable information on the status of blood gases and acid-base balance has made these measurements vital elements in the management of large animal surgical patients. Serious abnormalities in pH, bicarbonate, oxygen, and carbon dioxide tension are often encountered, which, if left unattended, are life-threatening.

Heparinized arterial blood collected anaerobically is submitted for determination of pH, carbon dioxide tension (Pa_{CO_2}), and arterial oxygen tension (Pa_{O_2}), the latter two values reported in torr units (previously mm Hg) usually corrected to the patient's body temperature. The bicarbonate (HCO_3^-) content of blood can be calculated with the aid of the Henderson-Hasselbalch equation or a nomogram if the pH and Pa_{CO_2} are known. Alternatively, HCO_3^- can be measured indirectly by a method that employs liberation of CO_2 from plasma or determines the buffering capacity of plasma by the addition of acid.

Often acid-base reports also include the base excess (deficit) calculated from a nomogram based on the patient's bicarbonate and hemoglobin concentrations. Base excess is of special value to the clinician in determining the amount

Table 5–11 SEVERITY OF AND SERUM CHLORIDE LEVEL IN RIGHT-SIDED TORSION OF THE ABOMASUM (RTA)*

Classification of Severity	Description	Serum Cl⁻ (mEq/L ± SD)
RTA I	Abomasum distended primarily with gas	100 ± 7.5
RTA II	Abomasum distended with gas and fluid; surgical reduction possible without removal of fluid	91 ± 5.4
RTA III	Abomasum distended with gas and fluid; 1 to 29 L	87 ± 8.6
RTA IV	Abomasum distended with gas and fluid; ≥ 30 L fluid removed before reduction of torsion	73 ± 10.7

*Adapted from Smith: JAVMA *173*:108, 1978.

of HCO_3^- necessary for replacement therapy.

Venous blood may be substituted for arterial blood if the primary derangement is known to be metabolic rather than respiratory. Results from venous blood will usually provide worthwhile information on the pH, P_{CO_2}, and HCO_3^- provided a large vein is used for sampling and systemic circulation is normal or near normal. Adequacy of oxygenation cannot be reliably determined with analysis of venous blood.

pH

The normal pH is 7.40 (no units are usually assigned), with a usual range of approximately 7.35 to 7.45, depending on the species, the sensitivity of the measuring electrode, the collection technique, and the extent of laboratory error. A pH of less than 7.35 signifies acidosis (also called acidemia), whereas a pH in excess of 7.45 indicates alkalosis (alkalemia).

Because pH has a logarithmic derivation, if the pH changes by 0.3 unit, the hydrogen ion [H^+] concentration doubles or halves in an inverse relationship. If the pH decreases from 7.4 to 7.1 (0.3 pH unit), the [H^+] concentration will double. Should the pH decrease to 6.8, the [H^+] concentration in blood will be four times normal. Conversely, if the pH should increase to 7.7, the [H^+) concentration will be one-half normal. Thus, it can be seen under normal circumstances that the [H^+] concentration of the blood is held within very narrow limits with usually a pH change of no more than 0.05 before homeostatic readjustment. Close control of pH is accomplished by a series of buffers in the extracellular fluids, primarily the bicarbonate–carbonic acid system, but also protein, hemoglobin, and phosphate as intracellular buffers. Gram for gram, hemoglobin is almost twice as potent a buffer as protein, and because the total mass of hemoglobin in blood is twice that of protein, the buffering action of hemoglobin in blood is four times that of protein. For this reason, hemoglobin is taken into account in the calculation of base deficits.

Hydrogen ion concentration is a mathematical expression of a ratio of base to acid. Written in terms of the Henderson-Hasselbalch equation, the bicarbonate–carbonic acid ratio at pH 7.4 is 20:1:

$$pH = pK + \log\frac{HCO_3^-}{Pa_{CO_2} \times 0.03}$$

$$= 6.1 + \log\frac{24}{40 \times 0.03} = 7.4$$

where
  pK is the pH of carbonic acid in blood when 50 per cent of it is dissociated, also known as the dissociation constant = 6.1;
  HCO_3^- is equal to the bicarbonate, normally 24 mEq/L;
  Pa_{CO_2} is equal to arterial blood–carbon dioxide tension, 40 torr; and
  0.03 is equal to the solubility factor of CO_2 in water, which creates carbonic acid (H_2CO_3) in the presence of carbonic anhydrase (expressed in mEq/L).

Although there is an abundance of CO_2 as an end product of metabolism, the amount of carbonic acid (H_2CO_3) and hydrogen ions [H^+] formed is limited by the dissociation constant (pK) of H_2CO_3 and the amount of dissolved CO_2.

$$H_2O + CO_2 \xleftrightarrow[\text{anhydrase}]{\text{carbonic}} (H_2CO_3)$$

$$H_2CO_3 \xleftrightarrow[6.1]{pK} [H^+] + [HCO_3^-]$$

Each step in the preceding equation is reversible. The volatile weak acid (H_3CO_3) can be quickly converted to CO_2 and water or bicarbonate. The CO_2 formed is eliminated by the lungs.

The basis of the bicarbonate–carbonic acid buffer system is the fact that as strong acids accumulate and contribute [H^+] ion, sodium bicarbonate (the base) will combine with the [H^+] ion of the strong acid to form carbonic acid (weak) and a neutral salt.

$$\frac{[H^+] \text{ acid}}{\text{(strong)}} + NaHCO_3 \rightleftarrows H_2CO_3 + NaSALT$$

Carbon Dioxide Tension (Pa_{CO_2})

The second essential component for the assessment of acid-base balance is arterial blood carbon dioxide tension (Pa_{CO_2}). The normal range of Pa_{CO_2} is 36 to 44 torr, with a mean of 40 torr. Pa_{CO_2} is controlled by ventilation. Hyperventilation causes a decrease in Pa_{CO_2} below 35 torr and an increase in pH, termed respiratory alkalosis. When effective ventilation decreases, there is hypoventilation, an increase in Pa_{CO_2} above 45 torr, a decrease in pH, and the onset of respiratory acidosis.

Increases and decreases in Pa_{CO_2} brought about by changes in ventilation do not change the overall sodium bicarbonate content of the buffer system because an acid cannot react with its own salt. Hence, $NaHCO_3$ is not depleted as CO_2 and carbonic acid increase; only the ratio between carbonic acid and sodium bicarbonate changes, resulting in respiratory acidosis or alkalosis.

There are three "Golden Rules" of acid-base balance, and Golden Rule 1 relates to the change in pH with changes in Pa_{CO_2}. Golden Rule 1 states that a change in Pa_{CO_2}, either up or down, of 10 torr is associated with an increase or decrease in pH of 0.08 units, i.e., an increase or decrease in carbonic acid. Thus, as Pa_{CO_2} increases 10 torr, pH will fall 0.08, and if Pa_{CO_2} falls 10 torr, pH will increase 0.08.

In application, if Pa_{CO_2} is 40 torr, pH will be 7.4, or normal, in the absence of metabolic acidosis. However, if Pa_{CO_2} increases to 50 torr, pH will fall to 7.32, thereby signifying hypoventilation, or respiratory acidosis. Should Pa_{CO_2} fall to 30 torr, pH will rise to 7.48, thereby indicating hyperventilation, or respiratory alkalosis.

Bicarbonate (HCO_3^-)

Rapid indirect measurement of bicarbonate (HCO_3^-) is now commonplace, but usually, when reported as a part of the acid-base balance, bicarbonate is determined from a nomogram based on the Henderson-Hasselbalch equation and direct measurement of pH and Pa_{CO_2}. Increases or decreases in HCO_3^- concentration are mainly regulated by the kidneys. Renal excretion or conservation of bicarbonate is slow, and its effect on pH is delayed in comparison with the rapid changes possible with changes in ventilation. Commonly, HCO_3^- is thought of as the "metabolic" component of acid-base balance. Increases and decreases in HCO_3^- have a direct relationship to pH. When the HCO_3^- concentration increases above 26 mEq/L, the pH will increase, resulting in metabolic alkalosis. A decrease in HCO_3^- concentration below 22 mEq/L will cause a decrease in blood pH and, therefore, metabolic acidosis. An overabundance of strong acids, such as the accumulation of lactic and pyruvic acids in shock, will also result in metabolic acidosis as the bicarbonate–carbonic acid buffer system is depleted in an attempt to neutralize the strong acids and maintain body pH.

The second rule, Golden Rule 2, provides that a pH change of 0.15 is the result of a base change of 10 mEq/L. Thus, if the pH increases by 0.15, there will be an increase in HCO_3^- of 10 mEq/L. If the HCO_3^- decreases by 10 mEq/L, there will be a decrease in pH by 0.15.*

Oxygen Tension (Pa_{O_2})

Although determination of the partial pressure of O_2 (Pa_{O_2}) in arterial blood is not an integral part of acid-base balance, it is one of the two blood gases (the other being Pa_{CO_2}) normally reported. Pa_{O_2} determination is made possible by diffusion of O_2 across the polypropylene membrane to an electrode containing a platinum cathode and a silver anode. The diffused O_2 sets up a current flow in proportion to the O_2 in the test sample. The normal Pa_{O_2} while breathing room air (20.93% O_2) is 90 torr, with a range of 70 to 95 torr depending on the species, rate and depth of respiration, and the animal's position, i.e., standing or re-

---

*If the HCO_3^- increases from a normal of 24 mEq/L to 34 mEq/L (10 mEq/L), the change in pH using the Henderson-Hasselbalch equation will be:

$$pH = 6.1 + \log \frac{34}{40 \times 0.03} = 7.55$$

or a pH change of 0.15.

cumbent. A Pa_{O_2} of 70 torr at pH 7.4 represents an oxygen saturation of the blood of approximately 94 per cent, still a most acceptable level of saturation under normal circumstances. A low oxygen tension regardless of the percentage of inspired O_2 is defined as hypoxemia.

Base Excess/Deficit (BE)

Actual base excess (BE) is an expression used to describe metabolic imbalance. BE represents the approximate amount of strong acid or base that would be required to return the pH of whole blood at 37°C to pH 7.4 if the Pa_{CO_2} were maintained at 40 torr. BE takes into account the buffering capacity of hemoglobin in whole blood but does not compensate for equilibration in the interstitial fluid compartment. When metabolic acidosis exists, BE is reported as a negative value, i.e., -5 mEq/L. Because this often causes confusion, base deficit is often substituted for BE when the reported value is negative, reserving BE for those situations in which there truly is a base excess.

In actual practice, a negative BE (or base deficit) is used to estimate the amount of HCO_3^- needed to return extracellular fluid pH to 7.4. Similarly, a positive BE can be used to determine the amount of a strong acid that might be needed to correct an extracellular metabolic alkalosis.

Interpretation of Blood-Gas/Acid-Base Analyses

Assessment of acid-base and blood-gas reports is best completed by following a standard format to prevent misinterpretation of results. The steps are as follows:

1. Examine the pH. Is the pH within the normal range (7.36 to 7.44)? If not, is it high or low? If low, the patient is acidotic; if high, the patient is by definition alkalotic. Alkalosis (pH > 7.44) can be caused by (a) hyperventilation and a low Pa_{CO_2}, (b) excessive HCO_3^-, (c) $[H^+]$ ion depletion, or (d) overzealous use of $NaHCO_3$. Acidosis (pH < 7.36) may be caused by (a) hypoventilation and a high Pa_{CO_2}, (b) excessive $[H^+]$ ion concentra-

tion, (c) depleted HCO_3^- ion concentration, or (d) hypoxemia.

The pH may be low because a venous sample, either intentionally or unknowingly, was submitted. Check the Pa_{O_2} to confirm that an arterial sample was submitted. While breathing room air and in the absence of severe pulmonary disease, the Pa_{O_2} should be at least 50 torr; that of venous blood will be lower.

2. Examine the Pa_{CO_2}. Is the Pa_{CO_2} within the normal range (34 to 45 torr)? If low, the patient is hyperventilating, perhaps to compensate for a metabolic acidosis or hypoxemia or perhaps in response to pain.

If the Pa_{CO_2} is high, the patient is hypoventilating and is hypocapneic. The most common cause of a high Pa_{CO_2} in large animal surgical patients is hypoventilation associated with general anesthesia. Alternatively, with hypoventilation, the patient may be breathing rapidly but ineffectually as a result of severe pneumonia, pneumothorax, pyothorax, or other pulmonary disease hampering normal ventilation. The conscious patient may also be attempting to compensate for metabolic alkalosis by decreasing the rate and depth of respiration consistent with minimal oxygen needs. Normal carbon dioxide tension of venous blood (Pv_{CO_2}) is higher than that of arterial blood, so again a check should be made to be sure an arterial sample was submitted.

3. Examine the HCO_3^-. If the HCO_3^- is greater than normal (22 to 26 mEq/L) and the pH is elevated, the patient has metabolic alkalosis. If the HCO_3^- is low with a corresponding decrease in the pH, the patient has a metabolic acidosis.

4. Examine the Pa_{O_2}. A low Pa_{O_2}, less than 70 torr, indicates hypoxemia due to limited pulmonary exchange, decreased O_2 content of the inspired air, or measurement of venous rather than arterial blood. On occasion there may be cause to measure fetal blood Pa_{O_2}. In this instance, arterial blood P_{O_2} will be less than ($Pa_{O_2} = 26 \pm 1.6$ torr) venous blood ($Pv_{CO_2} = 38 \pm 1.5$ torr).

A high Pa_{O_2}, greater than 95 torr, is possible if the patient is breathing oxygen-enriched air; a patient breathing 100 per cent O_2 may have a Pa_{O_2} in excess of 600 torr.

5. Determine the presence and extent of compensation and examine the results for evidence of simultaneous disturbances.

In most instances, the body attempts to correct for changes in pH through compensation (Table 5–12). With time, primary metabolic or respiratory imbalances affecting pH are partially compensated for by either changes in ventilation to effect a change in Pa_{CO_2} or excretion or conservation of HCO_3^- by the kidney. Ventilatory compensation for obvious reasons can occur more rapidly than HCO_3^- readjustment by the kidneys. Compensation is usually not complete.

Simultaneous or mixed disturbances may be present. The recognition of the simultaneous occurrence of more than one acid-base problem may be difficult, especially for clinicians who deal infrequently with such disturbances. A useful clinical tool that facilitates recognition of simple and complex acid-base disturbances is depicted in Figure 5–3. If a patient's Pa_{CO_2} and pH lie outside one of the significant bands, there is a high probability that there is a mixed disturbance. If a patient's Pa_{CO_2} and pH fall within one of the significant spans, it does not automatically follow that there is a single disturbance.

An alternative method for determining the presence of simultaneous disturbances is to calculate changes based on Golden Rules 1 and 2. Unexplained differences indicate the presence of simultaneous acid-base imbalances. If, for example, the Pa_{CO_2} was measured at 50 torr and the pH at 7.26, the increase of 10 torr Pa_{CO_2} would indicate respiratory acidosis. The calculated pH for this abnormality would be 7.32. Since the measured pH is 7.26, there is an unexplained pH difference of 0.06. Thus, based on Golden Rule 2, metabolic acidosis with a bicarbonate of 20 mEq/L is present as well as respiratory acidosis.

TREATMENT OF BLOOD-GAS AND ACID-BASE DISORDERS IN LARGE ANIMALS

Metabolic Acidosis

Metabolic acidosis is by far the most common naturally occurring metabolic derangement of large animal surgical patients. Respiratory compensation of slight to moderate metabolic acidosis is quite effective in maintaining pH through hyperventilation and the resulting decrease in Pa_{CO_2}. When respiratory compensation is inadequate to maintain pH, treatment of metabolic acidosis must be begun and should be directed toward the two basic causes of acidosis: (1) excessive accumulation or retention of strong acids, and (2) the abnormal loss of base.

Usually, excess accumulation of acid, in the form of lactic or pyruvic acid from anaerobic glycolosis, is the result of poor circulation, due to dehydration, decreased blood volume, and diminished cardiac output, or hypoxia. Hypoxia is most often encountered in large animal surgical patients during recovery from general anesthesia while breathing room air but may also be encountered in patients with upper airway obstruction and extreme abdominal distention, which causes thoracic compression and compromise of pulmonary function. Allevia-

Table 5–12 CHARACTERISTICS OF THE PRIMARY ACID-BASE DISORDERS*

Disorder	pH	[H+]	Primary Disturbance	Compensatory Response
Metabolic acidosis	↓	↑	↓ [HCO$_3^-$]	↓ P$_{CO_2}$
Metabolic alkalosis	↑	↓	↓ [HCO$_3^-$]	↑ P$_{CO_2}$
Respiratory acidosis	↓	↑	↑ P$_{CO_2}$	↑ [HCO$_3^-$]
Respiratory alkalosis	↑	↓	↓ P$_{CO_2}$	↓ [HCO$_3$]

Note: To return the pH toward normal, the compensatory response always changes in the same direction as the primary disturbance.

*Reprinted with permission from Rose: Clinical Physiology of Acid-Base and Electrolyte Disorders. New York: McGraw-Hill, 1977, p. 299.

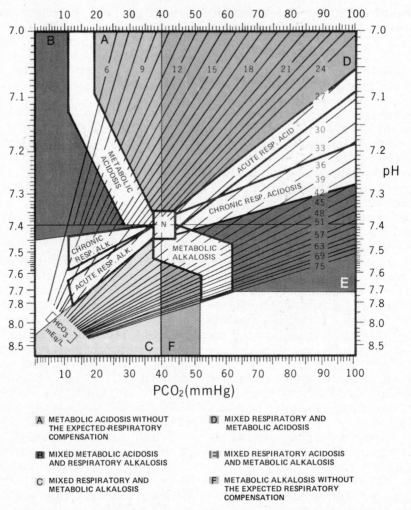

A   METABOLIC ACIDOSIS WITHOUT THE EXPECTED RESPIRATORY COMPENSATION

D   MIXED RESPIRATORY AND METABOLIC ACIDOSIS

B   MIXED METABOLIC ACIDOSIS AND RESPIRATORY ALKALOSIS

E   MIXED RESPIRATORY ACIDOSIS AND METABOLIC ALKALOSIS

C   MIXED RESPIRATORY AND METABOLIC ALKALOSIS

F   METABOLIC ALKALOSIS WITHOUT THE EXPECTED RESPIRATORY COMPENSATION

Figure 5–3 Acid-base map. The significance bands for the various simple disorders are labeled on the map. Probable interpretations for points falling in the tinted areas are suggested below the map. (Reprinted with permission from Myers and Pennock: Res. Staff Phys. May:49, 1979.)

tion of hypoxia is often all that is necessary to correct the progression of metabolic acidosis.

Hypoxia following anesthesia can be treated by intranasal or endotracheal administration of 100 per cent O_2 (at a rate of at least 15 L/min in the adult horse), hyperinflation of the lungs to decrease compressant and positional atelectasis, which develops during surgery, tracheostomy to bypass an upper airway obstruction, and trocarization of gas-distended abdominal organs to relieve impingement on thoracic space.

Metabolic acidosis due to retention of acids normally produced occurs in many acute and chronic renal diseases in which sulfuric and phosphoric acids, in

particular, are retained as well as other metabolic acids. Treatment consists of increased water intake orally by free choice or given by nasogastric tube, IV administration, combined with the administration of $NaHCO_3$ as a buffer, and specific antimicrobial treatment to eliminate renal infection, if present. Diminished oxygen delivery to cells resulting from poor circulation requires prompt expansion of the intravascular and extravascular fluid compartments, preferably by the IV administration of an isotonic balanced electrolyte solution containing bicarbonate or bicarbonate precursors such as acetate or gluconate. The rate and amount of fluid needed will depend on patient size, degree of dehydration, and extent of continuing loss during treatment. Measurement of central venous and arterial blood pressures is the most practical aid for determining a safe rate of administration and the return of normal circulation.

Metabolic acidosis due to loss of base occurs with loss of intestinal secretions, severe diarrhea, or small bowel fistulas. In the intestine, bicarbonate formed by epithelial cells passes into the lumen of the gut. When diarrhea occurs, large amounts of bicarbonate (as well as water) are secreted into the gut and excreted in the feces. With small intestinal fistulas, the bicarbonate of the ingesta is lost before it can be reabsorbed in the colon. When severe diarrhea occurs or an intestinal fistula is left unattended, dehydration, poor circulation, and acid accumulation may be present as well, contributing to the metabolic acidosis. In severe diarrhea, treatment consists of determining the etiology, controlling the diarrhea, correcting the dehydration, and replacing the lost base. Intestinal fistulas must be plugged or surgically eliminated as an important first step in management.

SODIUM BICARBONATE FOR TREATMENT OF METABOLIC ACIDOSIS

Sodium bicarbonate is specifically indicated for acute, severe metabolic acidosis because it has a rapid effect when given IV. The magnitude of arterial blood pH change induced by sodium bicarbonate varies with the dose and rate of administration and severity of the metabolic acidosis, as this influences the rate at which bicarbonate enters intracellular fluid. Although guidelines for estimating a patient's dose requirement are available (see Table 5–3), the most accurate method is calculation after measurement of pH and Pa_{CO_2} with derivation of HCO_3^- or base deficit (or a negative base excess) or measurement of bicarbonate by acid titration.

Replacement bicarbonate therapy can also be determined if only arterial blood pH and Pa_{CO_2} are known based on Golden Rules 1 and 2. For example, a patient with a pH of 7.17, a Pa_{CO_2} of 52 torr, and a weight of 500 kg has respiratory acidosis and is hypoventilating because the Pa_{CO_2} is increased 12 torr. According to Golden Rule 1, an increase in Pa_{CO_2} of 12 torr can be responsible for a pH change to 7.30, leaving an unexplained pH difference of 0.13. Calculating the bicarbonate based on Golden Rule 2 (with each change in pH of 0.15, there is a change in base of 10 mEq/L) reveals a bicarbonate change of 9 mEq/L. For practical purposes the calculated bicarbonate change can be substituted for base deficit (or excess). This patient has respiratory acidosis and metabolic acidosis. The respiratory component should be treated by increasing ventilation. The metabolic component should be treated with bicarbonate administered according to Golden Rule 3 (see below).

If only HCO_3^- is known, an approximation of base deficit can be made by subtracting measured HCO_3^- from the normal of 24 mEq/L. For example, if measured HCO_3^- is 13 mEq/L, the approximate base deficit is 11 mEq/L $(24 - 13 = 11 \text{ mEq/L})$.

When base deficit is known, Golden Rule 3 may be applied to determine the approximate number of millequivalents of base required to correct the deficit. Golden Rule 3 is as follows:

$$\text{Base required (mEq)} = \text{base deficit (mEq/L)} \times \frac{\text{body weight (kg)}}{3}$$

The ECF volume in liters is equal to about one-third of body weight in kilograms.

One-half to two-thirds of the deficit can be corrected over a 30-minute period, with the remainder given over several hours. As a general rule, rapid and complete correction of acidosis is undesirable because of the possibility of causing hyperosmolality, hypokalemia, impairment of oxygen release from hemoglobin, and cerebrospinal fluid acidosis.

Combining sodium bicarbonate with other drugs can affect efficacy. Bicarbonate mixed with calcium-containing fluids will cause formation of insoluble complexes, rendering both drugs ineffective. The action of epinephrine and other catecholamines may be impaired if administered with $NaHCO_3$.

A practical example of the use of Golden Rule 3 can be illustrated as follows. The following data concerning a horse with an acute abdomen are known: weight 450 kg, pH of arterial blood 7.30, Pa_{CO_2} 30 torr, actual bicarbonate 14 mEq/L, BE -10.5 mEq/L. These data indicate a partially compensated metabolic acidosis. Since the base deficit (BE) is 10.5 mEq/L and ECF = 1/3 of body weight $\left(\dfrac{450}{3}\right)$, the amount of sodium bicarbonate required is:

$$10.5 \times \frac{450}{3} = 1{,}575 \text{ mEq NaHCO}_3 \text{ or } 2.6$$

liters of 5% sodium bicarbonate

TREATMENT OF METABOLIC ACIDOSIS WITH BICARBONATE PRECURSORS

The bicarbonate precursors in common use are lactate, acetate, gluconate, and proprionate. In general, bicarbonate precursors are slower to produce maximal changes in pH because they must be metabolized before their buffer action is effective.

Lactate induces alkalinization following hepatic metabolism by the following simplified chemical equation. The first equation summarizes gluconeogenesis and the second, anion oxidation.

$$2CH_3CHOHCOO^- + 2H^+ \rightarrow C_6H_{12}O_6$$
$$CH_3CHOHCOO^- + H^+ + 3O_2 \rightarrow 3CO_2 + 3H_2O$$

The precursor acetate is converted to acetyl-CoA, which enters the tricarboxylic acid cycle and is oxidized to CO_2 and H_2O, resulting in alkalinization. This process does not depend on the liver.

Gluconate is commonly used in combination with acetate as an alkalizer. An advantage of this combination is that gluconate is metabolized more slowly.

Proprionate is also an effective alkalizer that functions in a manner similar to acetate.

Administration of lactate to hypovolemic patients with severe lactic acidosis has been questioned because of the backlog of lactic acid awaiting metabolism in a liver with compromised circulation. In such cases it is best to administer bicarbonate to partially correct pH before commencing administration of lactated fluid.

Metabolic Alkalosis

Respiratory compensation for metabolic alkalosis through hypoventilation and an increase in Pa_{CO_2} is usually not effective because of the overriding homeostatic mechanisms designed to maintain adequate oxygen saturation and prevent hypercapnia. Treatment of metabolic alkalosis is directed, whenever possible, toward prompt correction of the cause. Volvulus of the abomasum in cattle, which causes sequestration of $[H^+]$- and Cl^--rich fluids and prevents normal passage and absorption of feeds high in K^+, requires prompt surgical correction. If possible, the sequestered fluids should not be drained from the abomasum prior to surgical correction of the volvulus, so that later intestinal absorption of the accumulated ions may occur. This will aid in correction of the existing hypochloremic, hypokalemic alkalosis.

It may not be possible to discontinue gastric drainage in horses, to prevent continued loss of hydrochloric acid, for fear of gastric rupture. The resulting dehydration, hypochloremia, and rise in pH usually can be treated with saline IV containing added potassium chloride. In extreme cases, ammonium chloride or dilute hydrochloric acid (1 liter of 0.1N H_4Cl contains 100 mEq of $[H^+]$ and Cl^- ions) may also be required.

Alkalosis caused by excessive bicarbonate therapy and following the administration of diuretics will usually correct itself on cessation of therapy.

Whenever metabolic alkalosis is either suspected, based on clinical signs, or known to be present, bicarbonate and solutions containing bicarbonate precursors should be avoided. In most instances 0.9% saline, USP, is the fluid of choice. It may be supplemented with KCl, HCl, NH_4Cl, and/or calcium borogluconate as required based on clinical laboratory results. Calculation of chloride replacement has been described under treatment of chloride deficits.

Respiratory Acidosis and Hypoxia

Hypoxia is often associated with hypercapnia of respiratory acidosis. Thus, initial treatment of respiratory acidosis should be directed toward ensuring adequate oxygenation as well as improving ventilation. Supplemental O_2 given cautiously by intranasal or transtracheal catheter or through an endotracheal tube, when tolerated, will improve the Pa_{O_2}. A mechanical respirator may be needed to improve ventilation. If upper airway obstruction is present, a tracheostomy or placement of an endotracheal tube may be required to decrease respiratory effort and provide adequate ventilation. Placing a laterally recumbent large animal patient in sternal recumbency, in many instances, is all that is needed to provide adequate oxygenation and ventilation.

Respiratory Alkalosis

Clinically significant respiratory alkalosis is rare in large animal patients, with the exception of large animals overventilated on a mechanical respirator during anesthesia. Severe respiratory alkalosis produces hypocapneic vasoconstriction, which reduces cerebral circulation. Readjustment of the rate and depth of respiration provided by a respirator usually is all that is needed to correct respiratory alkalosis.

TREATMENT OF COMBINED ACID-BASE BALANCE ALTERATIONS

When combinations of metabolic and respiratory changes in acid-base balance occur that are not compensating for the initial derangement, the coexisting abnormalities require treatment. For instance, respiratory acidosis resulting from hypoventilation during anesthesia in a patient with moderate to severe metabolic acidosis should be corrected quickly with a mechanical ventilator.

Nutrition and the Surgical Patient

The stress of disease, pain, fever, septicemia, and surgery increases an animal's protein and energy requirements and causes catabolism of body protein beyond that seen in simple starvation. Malnutrition has been demonstrated to severely compromise an animal's immunocompetency. Until recently, little attention was given to parenteral nutritional supplementation before or after surgery in large animals. Surgical patients are often anorexic, or the clinician is obliged to withhold feed because of dysfunction of the gastrointestinal tract. Such patients, when left unsupplemented, have had to turn to endogenous sources of water, energy, stored minerals, and vitamins for survival and convalescence. Mobilization of body fat stores and the use of endogenous fatty acids provide the greatest sources of energy and water when oral intake ceases. Catabolism of skeletal muscle is the other major source of energy.

The purpose of oral and parenteral nutritional supplementation is to hasten recovery by providing the patient's daily needs of calories, vitamins, and trace minerals as well as the water and electrolytes classically given (see Chapter 2).

CATION-ANION BALANCE AND THE CLINICAL SIGNIFICANCE OF ANION GAP

All of the cations (Na^+, K^+, Ca^{++}, Mg^{++}) in plasma or serum can be and often are measured clinically, and together they total approximately 155 mEq/L. The sum of the anions must always equal the total cation concentration, but, in the case of the anions, routine clinical measurement, until recently, has been limited to chloride. The recent development of a practical means for determining bicarbonate concentration in blood and plasma has made it possible to gain valuable information concerning abnormal accumulations of organic acids usually associated with metabolic acidosis or renal failure.

The sum of the residual unmeasured anions composed of phosphates, sulfates, negatively charged proteins, and organic acids, when added to the known concentration of chloride and bicarbonate, produces cation-anion balance. Under normal circumstances, these residual ions total 25 mEq/L. Thus, the following relationship exists between cations and anions:

$$Na^+ + K^+ + Ca^{++} + Mg^{++} = (HCO_3^- + Cl^-) + 25$$

where 25 is the normal complement of residual ions (R) in mEq/L.

A number of formulas have been advanced for calculation of the anion gap, which is the difference between the routinely measured cations and anions. Normal values or ranges will vary depending on the formula chosen. If all of the cations have been measured along with chloride and bicarbonate the following formula is appropriate:

$$\text{anion gap} = Na^+ + K^+ + Ca^{++} + Mg^{++} - (HCO_3^- + Cl^-)$$

It must be remembered that calcium and magnesium as well as all other cations and anions must be entered in the formula in mEq/L. Here again, the normal anion gap is 25 mEq/L. A simplified formula has been advocated by Feldman and Rosenberg (1981). Their formula omits calcium and magnesium.

$$\text{anion gap} = (Na^+ + K^+) - (Cl^- - HCO_3^-)$$

Here the normal range is 12 to 16 mEq/L for dogs and presumably nearly the same for large animals. The exclusion of calcium and magnesium may be inappropriate in the calculations of anion gap in large animals; marked changes in these ions are encountered and thus their contribution may take on additional importance.

Important among the causes of increased anion gap is the accumulation of organic acids associated with metabolic acidosis. The clinical utility of determining the anion gap is the ability to gather useful information without additional expenditure.

REFERENCES

Blood, D. C., Henderson, J. A., and Radostits, O. M.: Veterinary Medicine, 5th ed. London: Builliere and Tindall, 1979.

Brownlow, M. A., and Hutchins, D. R.: A technique for the continuous administration of intravenous fluid therapy in the horse. Aust. Vet. Pract. 11:258, 1981.

Carlson, G. P.: Fluid therapy in horses with acute diarrhea. Vet. Clin. North Am. 1:313, 1979.

Feldman, B. F., and Rosenberg, D. P.: Clinical use of anion and osmolal gaps in veterinary medicine. JAVMA 178:396, 1981.

Gingerich, D. A., and Murdick, P. W.: Paradoxic aciduria in bovine metabolic alkalosis. JAVMA 166:227, 1975.

Glazier, D. B., Littledike, E. T., and Evans, R. D.: Electrocardiographic changes in induced hyperkalemia in ponies. Am. J. Vet. Res. 43:1934, 1982.

Gulick, B. A., and Meagher, D. M.: Evaluation of an intravenous catheter for use in the horse. JAVMA 178:272, 1981.

Hartsfield, S. M., Thurmon, J. C., and Benson, G. J.: Sodium bicarbonate and bicarbonate precursors for treatment of metabolic acidosis. JAVMA 179:914, 1981.

MacFarlane, W. V., and Howard, B.: Water in the physiological ecology of ruminants. In Physiology of Digestion and Metabolism in the Ruminant. Phillipson, A. T. (ed.). Newcastle-upon-Tyne, England: Oriel Press Ltd., pp. 362–374.

Moon, H. W.: Mechanisms in the pathogenesis of diarrhea: a review. JAVMA 172:443, 1978.

National Research Council, Committee on Animal Nutrition: Nutrient Requirements of Horses, 4th ed. Washington, D.C.: National Academy of Science, 1978.

Rose, B. D.: Clinical Physiology of Acid-Base and Electrolyte Disorders. New York: McGraw-Hill Book Co., 1977.

Rumbaugh, G. E., Carlson, G. P., and Harrold, D.: Clinicopathologic effects of rapid infusion of 5% sodium bicarbonate in 5% dextrose in the horse. JAVMA 178:267, 1981.

Sladen, A.: Acid-base balance. In Textbook of Advanced Cardiac Life Support. McIntyre, K. M., and Lewis, A. J., (eds.). Dallas: American Heart Association, 1981, Chap. 10.

Smith, D. F.: Right-side torsion of the abomasum in dairy cows: classification of severity and evaluation of outcome. JAVMA 173:108, 1978.

CHAPTER 6

SURGICAL MICROBIOLOGY

JOHN P. HEGGERS, PH.D.
PAUL B. JENNINGS, JR., V.M.D., M.S.

MANAGEMENT OF WOUND INFECTIONS IN LARGE ANIMALS

Most traumatic wounds in large domestic animals are already colonized with bacteria by the time the wound is presented for treatment. Therefore, the veterinary surgeon should have a knowledge of the potential microflora involved in large domestic animal wounds and an understanding of the basic principles of wound microbiology and treatment.

Unfortunately, the veterinary literature does not provide us with statistics of the incidence of large animal wound infections and response to treatment. The authors have surveyed several veterinary clinical laboratories for their impressions (Table 6–1).

ACKNOWLEDGMENTS

The authors wish to thank Ann Wilkinson, Elaine K. Longstreth, and Mary Beth Schario for their assistance in preparation of this manuscript.

Table 6–1 INCIDENCE OF ORGANISMS IN LARGE ANIMAL WOUND INFECTIONS (IN ORDER OF FREQUENCY)

Equine*
   Streptococcus zooepidemicus (accounts for 90 per cent of infections)
   Streptococcus equisimilis
   α-hemolytic streptococcus species
   Staphylococcus aureus
   Escherichia coli
   Proteus species
   Pseudomonas aeruginosa
   Gram-negative anaerobes
   Actinobacillus equuli

Bovine*
   Corynebacterium pyogenes (most common)
   α-hemolytic streptococci
   E. coli
   Proteus species
   Gram-negative anaerobes
   Clostridium perfringens

Porcine*
   Corynebacterium pyogenes (most common)
   Streptococcus equisimilis
   Streptococcus suis
   Other β-hemolytic streptococci
   Gram-negative anaerobes
   Pasteurella multocida

Porcine (*Continued*)
   E. coli
   Proteus species
   α-hemolytic streptococci
   Clostridium perfringens
   Clostridium septicum

Sheep and Goats*
   Corynebacterium pyogenes
   Corynebacterium pseudotuberculosis
   α-hemolytic streptococci
   E. coli
   Proteus species

Equine†
   β-hemolytic streptococci, rarely *Staphylococcus* (joint surgery)
   Proteus and *Pseudomonas* species (granulating wounds)
   Streptococcus, Proteus, etc. (osteomyelitis)
   Streptococcus (abscesses)
   Coliforms (peritonitis)

Bovine†
   Corynebacterium (osteomyelitis)
   Corynebacterium (abscesses)
   Rumen flora (peritonitis)

*Hogle, R. M.: Personal communications, 1977.
†Fessler, J. F.: Personal communication, 1977.

MICROBIAL RESIDENTS WITH PATHOGENIC POTENTIAL

Most resident organisms giving rise to infections fall into two distinct categories as distinguished by their gram staining reaction. Gram-positive organisms include those of the families Micrococcaceae, Streptococcaceae, and Bacillaceae; the order Actinomycetales; and the genus *Corynebacterium* (Buchanan and Gibbons, 1974).

GRAM-POSITIVE PATHOGENS

MICROCOCCACEAE

Among the genera recognized in the Micrococcaceae are *Micrococcus, Staphylococcus,* and *Planococcus*. Both *Micrococcus* and *Planococcus* are ubiquitous and exist as amphibionts (Rosebury 1968) but should not be ruled out as potential pathogens. The important pathogens for animals are the staphylococci, and only these organisms will be discussed.

There are three species of importance in this group of organisms, which frequently elicit suppurative processes. The most virulent is *Staphylococcus aureus,* followed by *Staphylococcus epidermidis,* a less virulent but frequently opportunistic pathogen. The third organism, *Staphylococcus saprophyticus,* often regarded as nonpathogenic, has been implicated in urinary tract infections. Like its sister organisms, it is found in urine, air, soil, dust, and dairy products and on animal carcasses.

Staphylococcus aureus and Staphylococcus epidermiditis. These organisms are not uncommon in animal infections. When encountered in a suppurative process in animals, their specific role is not entirely clear, primarily because of their association in a suppurative material with other species of bacteria. Those strains eliciting a disease process in animals are similar to those found in man.

Morphologically, staphylococci appear as gram-positive spheres of uniform size (0.5 to 1.5 mm in diameter) grouped in irregular clusters. This type of arrangement is often encountered in pyogenic exudates as well as in tissue samples. When isolates are inoculated to sheep blood agar (SBA), colonies of staphylococci appear as porcelain-white to yellowish-orange with or without zones of hemolysis.

The staphylococci are catalase positive. *S. aureus* produces coagulase, which is a soluble, enzyme-like product that converts the fibrinogen in human or rabbit plasma into fibrin. This test can be performed by either a slide technique or tube assay. Negative slide tests should be confirmed by the tube assay before being classified as coagulase negative. This is the primary diagnostic test for *S. aureus* (Buchanan and Gibbons 1974; Ellner 1978; Gibbs 1966).

Other virulence factors, besides coagulase, that aid the organism in overcoming the bodies' host defense mechanisms and allow survival and colonization of tissue include the various toxins. There are four exotoxins

1. Alpha-toxin is characterized by its ability to hemolyze sheep and rabbit erythrocytes and to kill macrophages (leukocidal); it is cytotoxic and dermonecrotic.

2. The Panton-Valentine (P-V) leukocidin is a nonhemolytic toxin that kills segmented neutrophils and macrophages without lysis.

3. Beta-toxin is a weakly hemolytic toxin found in strains of animal origin.

4. Delta-toxin, is hemolytic for human, rabbit, sheep, guinea pig, and horse erythrocytes. It is dermonecrotic, leukocidal, leukolytic, and cytotoxic.

The enterotoxin, an intestinal toxin, is peculiar to those *S. aureus* strains in phage group III.

Primary isolation of staphylococci from biological specimens can best be accomplished by inoculating the specimen to a SBA plate. After 18 to 24 hours incubation at 37° C, isolated colonies may produce a golden-yellow to porcelain-white pigment. The staphylococci may elaborate soluble hemolysins, which produce a clear zone of hemolysis. The lack of golden-yellow pigment or hemolysis is not a valid means of separating the two staphylococci species.

The two major tests for speciation are coagulase and mannitol fermentation. By definition, all strains of *S. aureus* are coagulase positive; however, this may not be manifest on primary isolation.* The mannitol fermentation test should be employed when primary isolates render a negative coagulase test. *S. aureus* will usually ferment mannitol within 24 to 48 hours, whereas *S. epidermidis* will not ferment mannitol (fermentation is an anaerobic process). Alternatively, a mannitol-salt-agar plate can be streaked with the isolate. *S. aureus* colonies will be surrounded by a yellow zone indicating fermentation of mannitol (Table 6–2) (Raymond and Traub 1970; Ellner 1978).

Staphylococcal infections in large domestic animals are of no less importance than are those caused by streptococci. Botryomycosis may occur after castra-

*False positive tests may occur with mixed cultures or with pure cultures of some gram-negative rods, e.g., *Pseudomonas*.

tion of the stallion. Once thought to be a fungus infection, it is now attributed to *S. aureus*. This organism is isolated in pure culture, often found encased in small granules resembling those of actinomycosis. The bovine udder is also susceptible to staphylococcal botryomycosis.

Staphylococcal bovine mastitis is becoming more prevalent with the emergence of penicillin-resistant *S. aureus* (McDonald 1977). It has been found that 41 per cent of swine udder infections are caused by *S. aureus*. This organism also has been incriminated in causing swine abortion (Bruner and Gillespie 1973).

STREPTOCOCCACEAE

The family Streptococcaceae consists of five distinct genera. All are homofermentative and catalase negative. Only three of the genera are of importance: *Streptococcus*, *Aerococcus*, *(Gaffkya)*, and *Gemella*.

The genus *Streptococcus* contains 21 distinct species plus 11 subspecies. Of these, over 50 per cent either live as commensalistic parasites or are capable of producing an infectious disease process. Morphologically, the streptococci are not unlike the staphylococci in that they are gram-positive spheres, averaging about 0.8 mm in diameter; they occur in pairs and are seen as short to moderate chains on slides made from clinical material and as long chains in liquid media. On SBA, the streptococci demonstrate varying degrees of hemolysis due to the

Table 6–2 CHARACTERISTICS DIFFERENTIATING SPECIES OF THE GENUS *Staphylococcus*

Test	*S. aureus*	*S. epidermidis*	*S. saprophyticus*
Catalase	+	+	+
Coagulase	+	−	−
Mannitol	+		
Acid aerobically	+	V[a]	V
Acid anaerobically	+	−	−
15% NaCl	+	V	V[b]
40% bile	+	V	−
Novobiocin sensitivity[c]	+	+	−

V = Variable
a = some strains positive; some negative
b = grown in at least 5% NaCl
c = + is sensitive = MIC (minimum inhibitory concentration) 0.6 mg/ml
   − is resistant = MIC 2.0 mg/ml

presence or absence of soluble hemolysins (streptolysins).

The degrees of hemolysis are as follows: (1) Alpha (α) hemolysis: manifested by a green or brown discoloration of the area immediately surrounding the streptococcal colony. Organisms producing this type of hemolysis are usually from the viridans or enterococcus group; (2) Beta (β) hemolysis: manifested by a clear, colorless area immediately surrounding the streptococcal colony. A number of different streptococcal groups possess this hemolytic capability; (3) Gamma (γ) hemolysis: no apparent discoloration or hemolytic area in the immediate proximity of the streptococcal colony.

The streptococci do not produce catalase, whereas the staphylococci do. Therefore, this can be used as a presumptive differentiation. The streptococci can be further differentiated based on specific soluble substances (SSS), which are group-specific polysaccharide antigens present as structural components of the cell wall. Based on Lancefield's identification schema, there are 17 serological groups, sequentially identified by the letters A through S (I and J have been omitted). Those streptococci of importance as obligate parasites giving rise to infections will be discussed individually.

Streptococcus pyogenes. The group A, beta-hemolytic streptococci are those organisms that give rise to malignant suppurative infections, predominantly in man. Although group A streptococcal diseases are only of importance in human infections, some knowledge of *S. pyogenes* as to its cultural, morphological, and biological characteristics is necessary to differentiate it from those streptococcal diseases peculiar to large animals. As Lancefield's schema denotes, group A is beta-hemolytic, one of the many groups that produce this type of hemolysis. The major means of differentiating group A from the other beta-hemolytic groups is with the use of the differential bacitracin disc, which contains 0.04 unit of bacitracin. Only the group A streptococci will show susceptibility to the minimal concentration of bacitracin (Gunn 1976).

Streptococcus agalactiae. This organism is a highly contagious obligate parasite of the bovine mammary gland. This microbial agent belongs to Lancefield's group B, beta-hemolytic streptococci. It is implicated as one of the etiological agents not only in bovine intramammary infection (IMI) but also in neonatal meningitis and genitourinary infections in humans (McDonald and McDonald 1976; Bailey and Scott 1974). However, McDonald and coworkers demonstrated that human strains of *S. agalactiae* are more pathogenic for bovine mammary glands than are the *S. agalactiae* strains of bovine origin (McDonald, McDonald, and Anderson 1976).

The three microbiological tests used for presumptively identifying *S. agalactiae* are the CAMP test, esculin hydrolysis, and hippurate hydrolysis (Table 6–3) (McDonald, McDonald, and Anderson

Table 6–3 DIFFERENTIATION OF STREPTOCOCCI

Group	Representative Species	Hemolytic Reaction	Bacitracin Sens.	SXT	CAMP	Bile Esculin	Na Hippurate	Tol. 6.5% NaCl
A	S. pyogenes	β (rarely γ)	S	V	−	−	−	−
B	S. agalactiae	β γ α	R	R	+	−	+	V
C	S. equi	β α γ	R	S	−	−	−	−
D	Enterococci S. faecalis S. faecium	γ β α	R	S	−	−	V	+
	Nonenterococci S. bovis S. equinus	γ β α	R	S	−	+	−	−
G	S. canis	β α γ	R	S	−			
Nongroupable								
	Viridans	α β γ	V	S	−	−	−	−
	S. uberis	γ α	R	S	V	+	+	−

1976; Gunn 1976; Christie, Atkins, and Munch-Peterson 1944).

Group C Streptococci. Of the four species included in this group, *S. zooepidemicus* (sometimes called animal pyogenes type A), *S. equi,* and *S. dysgalactiae* are most important. *S. zooepidemicus* causes septicemia in cows and swine and is frequently isolated from wound infections in horses. It has been found in the equine and bovine fetus and has been isolated in cases of metritis in both horses and cows. *S. equi,* a distinct species, is peculiar only to horses. It causes equine strangles and has been isolated from mucopurulent discharges of the equine upper respiratory tract including abscesses in submaxillary glands. *S. dysgalactiae* is another streptococcus encountered in IMI. McDonald and associates reported a 9.0 per cent incidence of *S. dysgalactiae* in IMI (McDonald, McDonald, and Anderson 1976). The members of group C do not give a positive CAMP reaction; however, *S. zooepidemicus* and *S. equi* produce a beta-hemolytic reaction on SBA, whereas *S. dysgalactiae* produces a strong alpha reaction. (For specific reactions to differentiate these species, refer to Table 6–3.)

Group D streptococci. These organisms fall into two distinct categories, dependent upon locality of isolation. Those of the viridans group, a normal commensal of the oropharynx, are frequently isolated from the feces of man and animals. *S. bovis* and *S. equinus* belong to this group. Organisms of the viridans group grow well at 45° C. Those organisms of the enterococci group (*S. faecalis* and *S. faecelis,* subsp. *liquefaciens* and *zymogenes*) are also frequently isolated from the feces of man and animals. These organisms not only grow at 45° C but grow at 10° C, differentiating them from organisms the viridans group. *S. faecium (S. durans)* is another of the group D enterococci found in the feces of man and animals (Buchanan and Gibbons 1974).

The remaining two organisms of group D., *S. uberis* and *S. suis,* are known pathogens for cattle and swine, respectively. A high incidence of mastitis in cattle has been reported owing to *S. uberis* (56.5 per cent), whereas *S. suis* has been seen in septicemia in swine. *S. uberis* has SSS antigenic properties comparable to groups E, D, and G and biochemical characteristics of *S. agalactiae* in that some organisms (27.2 per cent) are CAMP positive and hippurate positive. Group D streptococci can be differentiated from group B streptococci (see Table 6–3) by esculin hydrolysis when CAMP positive strains are encountered. *S. suis* is biochemically similar to the Streptococcus family but falls into Lancefield's group E (McDonald, McDonald, and Anderson 1976).

Streptococcus pneumoniae (Diplococcus). This organism has been implicated in sudden death of sheep and goats and has been involved in mastitis in cattle. *S. pneumonaie* type III is most frequently encountered. *S. pneumoniae* can be differentiated from the alpha-hemolytic streptococci by either a bile solubility test or an optochin disc test. Pneumococci are sensitive to the reagent impregnated in the disc (ethylhydrocupreine hydrochloride), whereas other alpha-hemolytic streptococci are not.

BACILLACEAE

The next family of importance is the Bacillaceae. This group is divided into two classifications: aerobic spore formers, *Bacillus* sp., and anaerobic spore formers, *Clostridium* sp. The most devastating organism of the former group is obviously *Bacillus anthracis,* the causative agent of anthrax. All *Bacillus* species are gram-positive rods and form spores within the matrix of the cell. Herbivorous animals, i.e., cattle, sheep, deer, horses, and buffalo, are most susceptible to anthrax. Specimens from suspect animals should be handled with care, as the human form can be fatal. Cultural aspects are distinctive for *B. anthracis.* It grows readily on solid media with a ground-glass appearance and "Medusa-head" colony formation. The gram stain shows a bacillus with square ends, about 1×5 mm in size. Kingsley utilized a phenyl ethyl alcohol and chloral hydrate selective media to differentiate *B. anthracis* from *B. cereus* (Kingsley 1966) (Table 6–4). *Bacillus* species other than *B. anthracis* have been reported as etiological agents of

Table 6–4 DIFFERENTIATION OF THE GENUS *Bacillus*

	(SBAP) Hemolysis	Motile	PEA*	CH†	Pen Agar	Nitrate Red
B. anthracis	−	−	−	−	−	+
B. cereus	+	V	+	+	+	+
B. subtilis	+	+	+	V	+	+
B. megaterium	+	+	−	+	+	−

*PEA = phenyl ethyl alcohol
†CH = chloral hydrate

diseases; these include bacteremia, bronchopneumonia septicemia, and meningitis (Coonrod, Leadley, and Eickhoff 1971; Pennington et al. 1976). Turnbull and coworkers reported a severe necrotic enterotoxin produced by *Bacillus cereus* (Turnbull, French, and Dowsett 1977; Turnbull, Nottingham, and Ghosh 1977). Routinely, when *Bacillus* species are encountered in a surgical wound or body fluid, these organisms are considered innocuous and are ignored, even if they are the only organism isolated. The authors feel that closer attention should be paid to this particular group of organisms.

The anaerobic member of the family Bacillaceae is the genus *Clostridium*. Those clostridia frequently encountered in large animal practice will be discussed. All clostridia are gram-positive spore formers and require an anaerobic environment for growth. Those species of importance are *C. botulinum*, *C. chauvoei*, *C. haemolyticum*, *C. novyi*, *C. perfringens*, *C. septicum*, *C. sordellii*, and *C. tetani*.

Six types of *C. botulinum* (A–F) are now recognized, based on antigenic specificity of the neurotoxins produced by the organisms. *C. botulinum* type A is the predominant type in the Pacific Coast states and the Rocky Mountain states, as well as in Maine, New York, and Pennsylvania.

Those strains found in the Mississippi River Valley and the Great Lakes region are of the type B variety. *C. botulinum* type C has been isolated from soil samples throughout the United States, whereas type D organisms seem to inhabit only the southwestern area. Type E *C. botulinum* appears to be aquatic in nature. It is frequently isolated from lake sediment and coastal areas of the United States. Type F is widely distributed throughout the United States.

Specimens suspected of containing clostridia should be inoculated directly to pre-reduced enrichment medium, i.e., sheep blood agar or egg yolk agar, and placed in an anaerobic environment. The Brewer jar with gas pack is adequate for small laboratories. All plates should be examined for anaerobes after 48 hours of incubation. Spore selection methods are often advantageous. The alcohol method is an easy method and might be useful in treating some types of clinical material. Equal portions (V/V and W/V) of the specimen and absolute alcohol are mixed and remain at room temperature for one hour, with mixing or shaking every 10 to 15 minutes. The suspension is then inoculated to an enrichment medium containing 0.2% starch.

The heat method takes less time but requires a burner and a beaker of boiling water. The specimen is inoculated into pre-reduced chopped meat medium with 0.2% starch, placed in boiling water for 10 minutes, and then incubated in an anaerobic atmosphere for 48 hours. Serum can be substituted for starch, and the boiling water level should be 1 inch above the inoculated medium. A control tube inoculated with the specimen but not heated should be prepared as a viability test. All the clostridia being discussed produce hemolysis on blood agar (sheep or rabbit), including all types of *C. botulinum* (Table 6–5). Indeed, primary enrichment cultures may also be tested for *C. botulinum* toxin prior to plating. Although identification of *C. botulinum* may be made from the culture, producing a toxin that is neutralized by specific *C. botulinum* antitoxin, the cultural properties of the organism must be examined as well. All types of *C. botuli-*

num digest gelatin and are lecithinase negative and lipase positive. Types A, B, and F produce a black color and digest milk with the same reaction in meat; they also digest serum. Types B, C, D, and E, on the other hand, produce acid in milk and no reaction in either meat or serum (see Table 6–5). Types C and D primarily affect ruminants, possibly by the animals' ingesting toxic hay or silage. Immunofluorescence can be used to identify *C. botulinum* types A, B, C, and E.

C. chauvoei, the etiological agent of blackleg in cattle, sometimes affects sheep and goats. Frequently isolated from the soil, *C. chauvoei* is thought to inhabit the intestines of the ruminant as an obligate parasite. Gram staining characteristics are often a key to the identification of this organism. The cells are quite pleomorphic, swollen, citron-like, and unevenly stained. The spores are oval and frequently appear to deform the bacilli. *C. chauvoei* produces hemolysis on blood agar, gelatin is liquified after a few days of incubation, a small amount of gas may be produced, and the milk is made acid. A soft clot often forms after a week of incubation (see Table 6–5).

C. haemolyticum is a pathogen of animals that is closely related to *C. novyi*. This organism is the etiological agent of bacillary hemoglobinuria or redwater disease of cattle. The organ frequently involved is the liver. Petechiae are often noted in clinical evaluation. The small intestine is hemorrhagic, and the urine has a color compatible with port wine. Specimens containing this organism, when inoculated with blood agar, will produce hemolytic colonies. Indole is formed in large quantities and may be a key test for a tentative identification of *C. haemolyticum*. Gelatin is liquified, and milk is usually coagulated.

C. novyi exists as three immunological types, A, B, and C. Type C has slight or no virulence. *C. novyi* inhabits the soil, sea sediments, and parts of the animal body. When examining the organism under the microscope, there is a perceptible difference in size when comparing type A with type B. Type A is approximately 4 to 8 mm long × 1 mm wide. Type B is frequently twice this size. The spores of both types are extremely resistant to heat and can withstand boiling for 30 minutes. This organism is found as the cause of malignant edema in cattle and sheep; however, horses, goats, and pigs are also susceptible. Black disease, sometimes known as infectious necrotic hepatitis, is the disease most frequently associated with this organism in sheep.

Suspect specimens inoculated to blood agar yield hemolytic colonies 3 to 8 mm in diameter. The zones of hemolysis around type B colonies may be wider

Table 6–5   ABBREVIATED LIST OF CHARACTERISTICS OF THE ANIMAL CLOSTRIDIA

Species	Hemolysis	Lecithinase	Lipase	Urease	Gelatin	Milk	Meat	Serum	Nitrate	Indole	Motility
C. botulinum A, B, F	+	−	+	−	L	B , L	B, L	L	−	−	+
C. botulinum B, C, D, E	+	−	+	−	L	A	−	−	−	−	+
C. chauvoei	+	−	−	−	L	A	G	−	+	−	+
C. haemolyticum	+	+	−	−	L	A	−	−	−	+	+
C. novyi A	+	+	−	−	L	A	G	−	−	−	+
C. novyi B	+	+	+	−	L	A	G	−	−	−	+
C. perfringens	+	+	−	V	L	−	B	−	−	−	−
C. septicum	+	−	−	−	L	A	G	−	V	−	+
C. sordelli	+	+	−	+	L	B, L	B, L	L	−	+	+
C. tetani	+	−	−	−	L	−	V	−	−	+	+

L = liquified
B = black
A = acid
G = gas
V = variable

than those around type A colonies. Gelatin is liquified, nitrates usually are reduced, and H$_2$S is formed. Indole and urease are not produced, and milk is slowly clotted. Type B strains digest milk, whereas type A strains do not (see Table 6–5). Blood agar for isolation of type B must be fresh, using plates that have been just prepared or that have been placed in a pre-reduced environment and refrigerated.

The organism referred to as the gas bacillus or, more commonly, *C. perfringens*, is more widely spread than is any other pathogenic bacterium. Its domicile includes the soil and the intestinal tracts of both animals and man. This member of the genus *Clostridium* contains five types, A through E.

The hemolytic pattern on blood agar is distinctive for this clostridial organism, often termed target zone hemolysis. The colony is generally surrounded by a complete hemolytic zone owing to the theta toxin, which is subsequently surrounded by a wider zone of incomplete hemolysis, attributed to the alpha toxin. These zones are usually perceptible after an overnight incubation.

A tentative identification of *C. perfringens* can be made when an anaerobic gram-positive rod is encountered that is nonmotile, hydrolyzes gelatin, forms lecithinase, and ferments lactose and sucrose (see Table 6–5). H$_2$S is produced in most media, indole is not formed, and nitrates are reduced by most strains. The type B and E strains of *C. perfringens* produce urease.

In sheep, *C. perfringens* type B, also known as the LD bacillus, has been implicated as the etiological agent in the disease known as lamb dysentery. Type C has been isolated from enterotoxemia

of lambs, calves, and piglets. Type D is commonly found in a destructive disease of sheep, known as pulpy kidney disease, enterotoxemia, and overeating disease. Type E causes dysentery and enterotoxemia in lambs and calves. Identification of these types is primarily accomplished by neutralization studies. The specificity of the clostridial antitoxins to the toxigenic type of *C. perfringens* is presented in Table 6–6.

Generally called the malignant edema bacillus, *C. septicum* is relatively widespread in nature; it exists in fertile soil and in the intestinal tracts of herbivorous animals. Infections in cattle caused by this bacillus sometimes resemble blackleg. Wound infections with this etiological agent are generally fatal, with the demise of the animal lasting from a few hours to one to two days after onset of intoxication. *C. septicum* causes infection in cattle and sheep and also has been seen in horses and swine.

The ubiquitousness of this organism frequently presents problems in identifying the true etiological agent of disease. Its nutritional requirements are less fastidious than are those of most other members of the clostridial group; and it frequently overgrows the others in both in vivo and in vitro environments. Batty and Walker, using fluorescent-labeled antisera to the somatic agents of *C. septicum*, differentiated between *C. septicum* and *C. chauvoei* in tissue sections as well as in smears from cultures (Smith and Holdeman 1968).

The cultural characteristics of *C. septicum* are unremarkable when compared with the other members of the clostridial group. It is hemolytic on blood agar, is extremely motile, and literally swarms over the agar surface. Nitrate reduction is

Table 6–6 TOXINS NEUTRALIZED BY *C. perfringens* ANTITOXIN

Antitoxins	Toxins According to Type					
	A	B	C	D	E	F
A	+	–	–	–	–	–
B	+	+	+	+	–	+
C	+	–	+	–	–	+
D	+	–	–	+	–	–
E	+	–	–	–	+	–

variable, and serum is coagulated. H_2S and indole are not formed, nor is lipase or urease produced (see Table 6–5).

C. sordellii and C. bifermentans are similar both in cultural and morphological characteristics. Both species grow well in most media. They are both moderately proteolytic and they liquify gelatin, digest coagulated serum, and produce indole. The key biochemical test that helps distinguish between these two species is the urease reaction test. C. sordellii is urease positive, whereas C. bifermentans is urease negative (see Table 6–5). Wound infections caused by C. sordellii resemble those produced by C. novyi; however, the edema that occurs with C. sordellii infections is rose colored or blood tinged, whereas C. novyi infections are colorless. Evidence implicating this organism as the causative agent of infection is, as yet, somewhat inconclusive. C. sordellii infections may mimic liver infections characteristic of those of C. novyi type B.

The last important member of the clostridial group is C. tetani. This member can be found in soil and in the intestinal contents of both man and animal. Although hemolysis is produced, this reaction may only be observed on the underside of the blood agar plate, since many strains are motile and swarm over the entire plate. The outstanding morphological feature of C. tetani is the classic spherical terminal spore. Owing to its appearance, this terminal spore has often been termed the "drum stick" or "tennis racket." Carbohydrates are not fermented, gelatin is usually liquified, and coagulated serum is softened and digested.

All clostridial species grow well on prereduced sheep blood agar and on CDC-supplemented thioglycolate broth (Smith and Holderman 1968; Buchanan and Gibbons 1974; Dowell et al., 1977).

ACTINOMYCETALES

This order includes two families of importance: Actinomycetaceae and Nocardiaceae. The genus Actinomyces in the family Actinomycetaceae contains one species important to animals, A. bovis.

This organism is the cause of the disease of cattle known as actinomycosis or lumpy jaw. In lesions, A. bovis is usually seen as a tangled mass of filaments in the classic "sulfur granule," with a periphery of acidophilic capsular material. The filaments stain gram-positive. However, when the granule is crushed, a wide variety of forms are observed; cocci, rods of varying size, filaments, branching forms, and club-shaped elements may be seen. This organism is not positive for the acid-fast stain. This organism is a facultative anaerobe and grows best in an atmosphere of 10 to 15 per cent CO_2 (Buchanan and Gibbons 1974). A. bovis is serophilic, requiring the presence of animal fluids in the medium for optimum growth.

Loeffler's serum agar slants are recommended for isolation of A. bovis. No growth occurs on Sabouraud's glucose agar. The organism takes five to six days at 37° C to achieve maximum size on Loeffler's agar.

Actinomycotic lesions are characterized by the initial formation of soft, granulomatous tissue. Afterward this tissue exhibits necrotic areas that break down to abscesses, forming sinuses or fistulous tracts. At the same time, the connective tissue hardens into dense, tumor-like masses. The pus exuding from these lesions often contains cheese-like granules.

The Nocardiaceae family contains several species; however, N. farcinica is apparently the animal variety of N. asteroides. Lesions of N. farcinica may resemble those of A. bovis, yet, when gram-stained, the filaments may break into fragments resembling bacilli. If they are stained with acid-fast stain, they may be confused with Mycobacterium species. N. farcinica grows well on SAB agar or blood agar plate (BAP) under aerobic conditions at 37° C. Colonies usually appear in four to six days, producing a whitish aerial mycelium. N. farcinica hydrolyzes esculin, Tween 20, and urea. Like A. bovis, N. farcinica is sensitive to antibiotic-treated media, particularly those containing sulfonamides. Some characteristics peculiar to the Actinomycetaceae family are described in Table 6–7 (Blair et al. 1974).

Table 6–7 CHARACTERISTICS OF *Actinomyces* AND *Nocardia*

	Aerobic Growth	Anaerobic Growth (10–15% CO_2)	Acid Fast	Penicillin Sensitivity
A. bovis	−	+	−	S
N. farcinica	+	−	+	R*

*5 I.U. discs

CORYNEBACTERIUM

The coryneform bacteria present a number of unresolved problems in taxonomy and classification. The animal and human parasites in the genus *Corynebacterium* show a number of features that indicate a rather close relationship to mycobacteria and nocardia. Recent work on lipids of mycobacteria, corynebacteria, and nocardia has re-emphasized this relationship, particularly the similarity in content of mycolic acids (Etamadi and Lederer 1965; Senn et al. 1967). With the widespread use of the terms coryneform and diphtheroid, considerable confusion exists as to which organism should properly constitute the genus *Corynebacterium*.

Of the many species of *Corynebacterium*, only four are of primary concern in large animal microbiology. *C. pyogenes* is a pus-forming organism frequently found in cattle, swine, and sheep. It is a gram-positive rod, and it frequently forms chains, giving the appearance of streptococcal chains. This organism has been implicated in such disease states as abscesses, cardiac valvular vegetations, granulomatous tumors, necrotic and suppurative pneumonia, destructive arthritis, and purulent metritis. Growth is definitely enhanced by the addition of animal body fluids to the isolation media and incubation in an environment of 5 to 10 per cent CO_2 (Buchanan and Gibbons 1974; Blair et al. 1974).

C. renale is a rather large, irregularly staining bacillus, often with pointed ends. This organism is the etiological agent of infections of the urinary bladder and kidney in cattle. It grows on ordinary laboratory media; however, growth is favored by the addition of animal body fluids. Colonies are generally dry and granular and may have a pale yellow pigment. Metachromatic granules or bars are easily demonstrated with the methylene blue stain.

Another *Corynebacterium* causing infections in animals is *C. equi*. It gives rise to a suppurative pneumonia in young foals and has been found in uterine discharges in a number of aborting mares (Bruner and Gillespie 1973). Infection with the organism produces a cervical lymphadenitis in swine. Pleomorphic forms are characteristic of this species. Rods may vary in length from coccoid to long, curved, clubbed forms. It grows well on all ordinary media, forming mucoid and pink colonies. Optimal growth is observed at 37° C; however, it will grow equally well at 20° C.

Ulcerative lymphangitis in horses may be confused with cutaneous glanders. The etiological agent of this disorder is *C. pseudotuberculosis*. The green pus exuding from the fetlock area may give an appearance similar to that of a *Pseudomonas* infection. In sheep it gives rise to a disease called caseous lymphadenitis. These gram-positive rods stain irregularly, are small, and vary in shape, with many club forms. Their appearance on agar is similar to the gravis type of *C. diphtheriae*.

Colonies on BAP are small with a narrow zone of hemolysis, generally producing a yellowish-white pigment (Buchanan and Gibbons 1974; Blair et al. 1974). Table 6–8 describes some of the characteristics of these *Corynebacterium* species.

GRAM-NEGATIVE PATHOGENS

These organisms render a red color when gram stained. Although many gram-negative organisms are involved in disease processes of animals, those important in surgical wound infections are limited to representatives of the families Enterobacteriaceae and Bacteroidaceae

Table 6–8 CHARACTERISTICS OF THE *Corynebacterium* SPECIES

Species	Hemolysis BAP	Urea	Catalase	Nitrate	Maltose
C. pyogenes	β	−	−	−	+
C. renale	−	+	+	−	−
C. equi	−	V	+	V	−
C. pseudotuberculosis	β	+	+	+	+

V = variable

and the genera *Pseudomonas* and *Alcaligenes*.

The Enterobacteriaceae family comprises the largest group of septic invaders. All organisms within this group grow readily on most ordinary laboratory media. Frequently, specimens suspected of containing this group of organisms are inoculated to MacConkey's agar (MAC) or eosin–methylene blue agar (EMB) and BAP with phenethyl alcohol (PEA).

Both MAC and EMB contain dye and are classified as differential media. Colonies absorbing the dye incorporated within the media are considered lactose fermentors. Those that remain clear and/or colorless are nonlactose fermentors. The incorporation of PEA in BAP inhibits the swarming organisms such as those of the *Proteus* species. Another medium employed in the presumptive identification of organisms of the Enterobacteriaceae family is triple sugar iron agar (TSI). This medium contains three sugars: lactose, sucrose, and glucose, with ferrous sulfate (*Diagnostic Procedures* 1963). Table 6–9 describes the reactions peculiar to the genera frequently encountered.

The first species of concern is *Escherichia coli*. This organism is a normal inhabitant of the gastrointestinal tract of warm-blooded animals. Along with *S. aureus*, it has been the major violator in surgical wound sepsis (Robson and Heggers 1969; Robson, Krizek, and Heggers 1973), accounting for over 50 per cent of all infections. Endotoxic shock is a major sequela found concomitant with *E. coli* sepsis (Osborne and Meredith 1970; Hinshaw, Reine, and Hill 1966; Beadle and Huber 1977). Hemolytic strains are often found in swine (Buchanan and Gibbons 1974). Usually *E. coli* is observed as a short, plump, gram-negative rod. It may or may not be motile, produce gas as an end product of glucose fermentation, or ferment lactose. All strains are indole and methyl red (MR) positive and Voges-Proskauer (VP) negative (Blair et al. 1974).

Although *Salmonella* and *Shigella* species are of economic importance as disease producers, their frequency in surgical wound sepsis is virtually nil.

The *Klebsiella* and *Enterobacter* genera contain five major species and share common capsular antigens (Ewing and Edwards 1972; Buchanan and Gibbons 1974).

The *Klebsiella-Enterobacter* group (K-E) are gram-negative rods and are either motile or nonmotile. *Klebsiella pneumoniae* (*Aerobacter aerogenes*)

Table 6–9 BIOCHEMICAL REACTIONS ON KLIGERS IRON AGAR (KIA)

Bacterial Species	KIA Reactions			
	Slant	Butt	Gas	H$_2$S
Escherichia coli	A (K)*	A	+ (−)	−
Klebsiella-Enterobacter group	A	A	+	−
Serratia marcescens	K or A	A	−	−
Proteus vulgaris	A(K)	A	+	+
Proteus mirabilis	K(A)	A	+	+
Morganella morganii	K	A	− (+)	−
Providencia sp.	K	A	t or −	−

*A = acid; K = alkaline; ( ) designates variation of reaction

Table 6–10 BIOCHEMICAL DIFFERENTIATION OF SOME MAJOR ORGANISMS IN THE ENTERIC GROUP

Bacterial Species	Test or Substrate							
	Indole	MR	VP	Urease	Citrate	KCN	Motility	H₂S
Escherichia coli	+	+	−	−	−	−	V	−
Klebsiella sp.	−	−	+	V	+	+	−	−
Enterobacter sp.	−	V	V	V	+	V	+	−
Serratia marcescens	−	V	+	−	+	+	+	−
Proteus sp.	V	+	−	+	V	+	+	+
Providencia sp.	+	+	−	V	+	+	+	−
Morganella morganii	+	+	−	+	−	+	+	−

Notes: MR = methyl red
VP = Voges-Proskauer
KCN = potassium cyanide
V = variable reaction

has been implicated in urogenital infections in mares (Greenwood and Ellis 1976; Bruner and Gillespie 1973; Buchanan and Gibbons 1974). Biochemical differences of *Klebsiella* and *Enterobacter* species are included in Table 6–10.

The family Pseudomonadaceae contains several genera that one may encounter in surgical wound sepsis. Of this group, organisms of the *Pseudomonas* genus are most frequently encountered in a wide variety of wounds. Earlier encounters with this genus were ignored, as the organisms were considered saprophytes. These organisms are also gram-negative and motile and utilize carbohydrates through an oxidative process rather than through fermentation.

Pseudomonas aeruginosa has been isolated from abscesses of the spleen and liver of both cattle and swine; it has also been seen in traumatic pericarditis of cattle (see Table 6–11).

Alcaligenes faecalis, another gram-negative motile rod, is also considered a

Table 6–11 CHARACTERISTICS OF *Pseudomonas* AND *Alcaligenes*

Test	*Pseudomonas*	*Alcaligenes*
Hemolysis BAP	β	α
Citrate	+	−/+
Urea	V	−
Nitrate	+	−
Oxidative utilization glucose	+	−

V = variable

saprophyte. It too, however, must be considered as a potential pathogen.

The Neisseriaceae family consists of a diverse group of organisms that vary from the diplococcal kidney-bean shape of *Neisseria* to the short, plump rods of *Acinetobacter*, formerly called the tribe *Mimeae*. The pathogenicity of *Neisseria* organisms found in wound infections is minimal, if at all. *Moraxella* is a known pathogen in animal disease, but there are no available reports implicating it in surgical wound sepsis. The *Acinetobacter* organisms, on the other hand, are known etiological agents of septicemia, wound infections, and endocarditis (Goldberg 1971; Graber 1970). Formerly of the tribe *Mimeae*, they are frequently found in clinical specimens from various animals. Table 6–12 describes some of the characteristics of the family Neisseriaceae.

The gram-negative anaerobic bacilli are found as inhabitants of both man and animals. The most frequently encountered organisms are those of the family Bacteroidaceae, of which two genera, *Bacteroides* and *Fusobacterium*, play a formidable role in surgical infections in man (Felner and Dowell 1971). Members of this family inhabit the intestinal tract of man, the reticulorumen of cattle, and the cecum and respiratory tract of swine (Buchanan and Gibbons 1974). Quantitatively, anaerobes outnumber the facultative species (e.g., *E. coli*) by a ratio of 1000:1 in the intestinal tract of man (Nichols and Smith 1975). Ruminants, on the other hand, live in a symbiotic

Table 6–12 CHARACTERISTICS OF NEISSERIACEAE

Tests/Characteristics	Genus		
	Neisseria	Moraxella	Acinetobacter
Shape	Cocci	Rod	Rod[a]
Hemolysis	V	−	−
Catalase	+	V	+
Oxidase	+	+	−
H_2S	+[b]	−	−

a = may appear as diplococci
b = four or six are positive; N. gonorrhea and N. meningitis are negative

relationship with a wide variety of anaerobes. If one were to quantitate anaerobes in the rumen fluid, the counts per volume of fluid would be 1×10^{11}/ml. Bacteroides amylophilus constitutes 10 per cent of the bacterial population (Bryant and Robinson 1961), whereas B. succinogenes is presumed to be the predominant species in the ruminant (Buchanan and Gibbons 1974). B. putredinis and B. nodosus are both found in foot rot in sheep, with B. nodosus considered the true etiological agent.

On the other hand, Fusobacterium necrophorum, normally found in the cecum of swine and in the alimentary tract of other species of animals, causes a wide variety of lesions in horses, cattle, sheep, and swine. In horses, the disease takes the form of gangrenous dermatitis of the feet, not unlike foot rot in cattle. However, the exact role of the primary pathogen is still in question, since F. necrophorum is frequently isolated with other major pathogens.

Both Bacteroides and Fusobacterium are obligate anaerobic nonsporogenous rods and, when stained with the gram stain, appear as gram-negative bacilli.

At 37° C on nutrient media (e.g., prereduced SBA) in an anaerobic environment, colonies generally appear after 48 hours of incubation (Buchanan and Gibbons 1974; Dowell and Lombard 1976). Table 6–13 lists characteristics of the Bacteroidaceae family.

REFERENCES

Bailey, R. W., and Scott, E. G.: Diagnostic Microbiology, 4th ed. St. Louis: C. V. Mosby, 1974.

Beadle, R. E., and Huber, T. L.: Blood chemistry changes associated with rapid intravenous administration of Eschericha coli in anesthetized ponies. Equine Med. Surg. 1:137, 1977.

Blair, J. E., et al.: Manual of Clinical Microbiology. Baltimore: Williams & Wilkins, 1974.

Bruner, D. W., and Gillespie, J. H. (eds.): Hagans Infectious Diseases of Domestic Animals, 6th ed. Ithaca, NY: Cornell University Press, 1973.

Bryant, M. P., and Robinson, I. M.: Studies on the nitrogen requirements of genus Ruminococcus. Appl. Microbiol. 9:96, 1961.

Buchanan, R. E., and Gibbons, N. E. (eds.): Bergey's Manual of Determinative Bacteriology, 8th ed. Baltimore: Williams & Wilkins, 1974.

Christie, R., Atkins, N. E., and Munch-Peterson, E.: A note of a lytic phenomenon shown by group B. Streptococci. Aust. J. Exp. Biol. 22:197, 1944.

Table 6–13 BIOCHEMICAL CHARACTERISTICS FOR BACTEROIDACEAE

Species	Indole	Esculin	Nitrate	Hemolysis	Motility
B. ruminicola	−	V	−	−	−
B. amylophilus	−	−	−	−	−
B. clostridiiformis	−	W	+	−	+
B. putredinis	+	−	−	−	−
B. nodosus	−	−	−	−	−
B. succinogenes	−	−	−	−	−
Fusobacterium necrophorum (Fusiformis necrophorus)	+	−	−	B	−

V = variable
W = weak
B = beta hemolysis

Coonrad, J. D., Leadley, P. J., and Eickhoff, T. C.: *Bacillus cereus* pneumonia and bacteremia. Am. Rev. Resp. Dis. *103*:711, 1971.

Diagnostic Procedures — Culture Media, Chapter 4 (4th ed.) New York: American Public Health Assoc., 1963.

Dowell, V. R., Jr., Lombard, G. L., Thompson, F. S. M., and Armfield, A. Y.: Media for Isolation; Characterization and Identification of Obligately Anaerobic Bacteria. U.S. Department of Health, Education, and Welfare. NCDC, November, 1977, pp. 1–46.

Dowell, V. R., Jr., and Lombard, G. L.: Presumptive Identification of Anaerobic Non-spore Forming Gram-Negative Bacilli. U.S. Department of Health, Education, and Welfare. NCDC, 1976, pp. 1–13.

Ellner, P. D.: Current Procedures in Clinical Bacteriology, 2nd ed. Springfield, IL: Charles C Thomas, 1978.

Etemadi, A. H., and Lederer: Sur la structure des acides—mycoliquies de la souche lurmaine test. Bull. Soc. Chim. Fr. *9*:2640, 1965.

Ewing, W. H., and Edwards, P. R.: Identification of Enterobacteriaceae, 3rd ed. Minneapolis: Burgess Publishing, 1972.

Felner, J. M., and Dowell, V. R., Jr.: Bacteroides bacteremia. Am. J. Med. *50*:787, 1971.

Gibbs, B. M., and Skinner, F. A. (eds.): Identification Methods for Microbiologists, Part A. New York: Academic Press, 1966.

Goldberg, M. H.: Mimeae: Opportunistic oral organisms. J. Oral Surg. *29*:715, 1971.

Graber, C. D.: Miscellaneous Bacterial Pathogens and Nosocominants, in Rapid Diagnostic Methods in Medical Microbiology. Baltimore: Williams & Wilkins, 1970.

Greenwood, R. E. S., and Ellis, D. R.: Horses. *Klebsiella aerogenes* in mares. Vet. Rec. *99*:439, 1976.

Gunn, B. A.: SXT and Taxo A disks for presumptive identification of group A and B streptococci in throat cultures. J. Clin. Microbiol. *4*:192, 1976.

Hinshaw, L. B., Reine, D. A., and Hill, R. J.: Response of isolated liver to endotoxin. Can. J. Physiol. Pharmacol. *44*:529, 1966.

Kingsley, R. F.: Selective medium for *Bacillus anthracis*. J. Bacteriol. *92*:784, 1966.

McDonald, J. S.: Streptococcal and staphylcoccal mastitis. JAVMA *170*:1157, 1977.

McDonald, J. S., McDonald, T. J., and Anderson, A. J.: Characterization of and bovine intramammary infection by group B *Streptococci agalactiae* of human origin. *In* Proceedings of the U.S. Animal Health Assoc., Portland, OR, 1975 (1976).

McDonald, T. J., and McDonald, J. S.: Streptococci isolated from bovine intramammary infections. Am. J. Vet. Res. *37*:377, 1976.

Nichols, R. E., and Smith, J.: Clinical aspects of anaerobic infections in the surgical patient. Am. J. Med. Technol. *41*:87, 1975.

Osborne, J. C., and Meredith, J. H.: The influence of environmental and surgical stressors on susceptibility to bacterial endotoxin. Exper. Med. Surg. *28*:39, 1970.

Pennington, J. E., Gibbons, N. D., Strobeck, J. E., Simpson, G. L., and Myerowitz, R. L.: *Bacillus* species infection in patients with hematologic neoplasia. JAMA *235*:1473, 1976.

Raymond, E. A., and Traub, W. H.: Identification of staphylococci isolated from clinical material. Appl. Microbiol. *19*:919, 1970.

Robson, M. C., and Heggers, J. P.: Surgical infection. I. Single bacterial species or polymicrobic in origin? Surgery *65*:608, 1969.

Robson, M. C., Krizek, T. J., and Heggers, J. P.: Biology of surgical infection. Curr. Probl. Surg. 1–62, Mar. 1973.

Rosebury, T.: Microorganisms Indigenous to Man, Chapter 1. New York: McGraw-Hill, 1968.

Senn, M. T., Ioneda, I., Pudles, J., and Cederer, E.: Spectrometrie des masse de glycolipides. I. Structure du "cord-factor," de *Corynebacterium diphtheriae*. Eur. J. Biochem. *1*:353, 1967.

Smith, L. D. S., and Holderman, L. V.: The Pathogenic Anaerobic Bacteria, 2nd ed. Springfield, IL: Charles C Thomas, 1968.

Turnbull, P. C. B., French, T. A., and Dowsett, E. G.: Severe systemic and pyogenic infections with *Bacillus cereus*. Br. Med. J. *1*:1628, 1977.

Turnbull, P. C. B., Nottingham, J. F., and Ghosh, A. C.: A severe necrotic enterotoxin produced by certain food, food poisoning and other clinical isolates of *Bacillus cereus*. Br. J. Exp. Pathol. *58*:273, 1977.

SURGICAL METHODS IN THE MANAGEMENT OF WOUND INFECTIONS

Certain techniques are essential in the surgical treatment of infections and are not made obsolete by the new availability of antimicrobial agents. In this section we will discuss basic principles that are applicable to all species. Later in this text, various authors will cover the specifics of wound treatment in their areas of expertise.

The results of interaction between the bacteria and the host, although under some systemic influence, are ultimately determined by local wound factors. Necrotic tissue, poor blood supply, foreign bodies, hematomas, and dead space all seem to alter the host's resistance and allow infection to occur. Tissue damage, whether chemical, mechanical, or thermal, may result in a lowering of resistance and a greater propensity for a minor contamination to initiate an infection. Using guinea pigs, Silvola and associates (1968) showed that simple compression of incision edges with a hemostat for 30 seconds significantly increased the intensity of infection, even though there was no measurable deterioration of tissue viability.

Another factor is the increased susceptibility to infection due to decreased local wound perfusion. Conolly, Hunt, and Dunphy (1969) found that a wound needs oxygen for collagen synthesis and healing; this calls for local circulation. Hunt and coworkers (1967) have shown that all wounds are hypoxic and, therefore, have only borderline circulation. Consequently, if the local circulation becomes impaired, healing will be affected and the chance of infection will increase. The enhancement of bacterial growth by decreased local perfusion caused by adrenalin was demonstrated by Evans, Miles, and Niven (1948). Miles also showed, using guinea pigs, that the size of the infected lesion could be altered by local injection of epinephrine, provided the injection was made within four hours of the bacterial inoculation (Miles 1956).

Foreign bodies have been associated with decreased host resistance, and the presence of a single 6-0 suture was shown by Elek (1957) to decrease the number of staphylococci necessary to form pus in human volunteers from 1,000,000 to 100, a 10,000-fold decrease. Carpendale and Sereda (1965) demonstrated a greatly increased infection rate in experimentally contaminated skin wounds closed with sutures as compared with those closed with tape. In a thorough study of contaminated wounds, Edlich and associates unequivocally documented the role of percutaneous sutures in causing wound infections (Edlich et al. 1973).

Not only does the presence of sutures increase the susceptibility to infection, but the properties of various suture materials are quite important. Catgut has been shown to cause more infection than silk because of the prolonged inflammatory reaction caused by catgut. Alexander, Kaplan, and Altemeier (1967) and Everett (1970) have reviewed the evidence of suture material causing decreased resistance. They have shown that for each type of suture studied, the monofilament variety results in fewer infections than does the braided variety. Recent studies by Getzen and Jansen (1966) suggest that the sutures act as allergens. These authors correlated the incidence of wound complications with skin reactions to suture material and have observed increases in blood eosinophil counts. Experiments with various biocidal sutures have been intriguing. LeVeen and collaborators (1968), using sutures impregnated with a quaternary ammonion compound, were able to prevent infection in mice that had sutures placed in an area containing 3.9×10^6 staphylococci. Ludewig, Rudolf, and Wangensteen (1968) produced comparable results with iodized gut sutures in mice.

May and associates (1966) and Conolly and Golovsky (1967) reported that up to 30 per cent of clinical wound infections were associated with hematomas. Krizek and Davis (1965) demonstrated quantitatively that a hematoma had a pronounced effect on injected bacteria. When 5×10^7 E. coli organisms were injected subcutaneously, the E. coli were effectively contained at the injection site by natural host defenses. Blood stream cultures or tissue cultures from lung, liver, spleen, and kidney remained at 10^5 or fewer organisms per gram. However, when the same number of bacteria was injected into a hematoma, bacterial counts in the blood and tissues began to rise precipitously within six hours. The counts reached levels of greater than 10^5 organisms per gram, and 80 per cent of the animals died. Thus, the hematomas seemed to prevent the natural defense mechanisms from localizing the bacteria at the injection site.

Hunt and coworkers (1967) developed an experimental rabbit model using wire mesh cylinders to make a reproducible dead space. Employing this model, they showed that dead space alone can increase the susceptibility of tissue to infection. These local wound factors upset the equilibrium. The quantitative increase in bacterial growth reflects these changes.

The contamination/infection risk is definitely related to the type of operative wound involved. The following is a classification of operative wounds in relation to contamination and increasing risk of infections. A *clean wound* is nontraumatic, with no inflammation and no break in surgical technique; it does not involve the respiratory, alimentary, or urogenital system. A *clean contaminated wound* is a wound in which the gastrointestinal and/or respiratory tract is entered without significant spillage. *Contaminated wounds* are those with a major break in technique, including gross spillage from the gastrointestinal tract, or a fresh trau-

matic wound in which the genitourinary and/or biliary tract has been entered in the presence of infected urine or bile. The *dirty infected wound* is one in which an acute bacterial inflammation is present without pus. Such a wound may be present during transsection of clean tissue for the purpose of surgical access to a collection of pus, with a perforation of a hollow viscus, in a traumatic wound with delayed treatment, or with a dirty source (Altemeier et al. 1976).

TREATMENT SEQUENCE FOR WOUND INFECTIONS

1. Remove Devitalized Tissue (Pulaski 1964).

The animal should be situated to allow confinement or restraint during treatment. Physical restraint (halter, stocks, small pen) or chemical restraint may be needed to avoid additional trauma during treatment.

The hair or wool should be removed from around the wound. Hair is a foreign body (and, therefore, a breeding ground for bacteria) and must be removed prior to definitive treatment. Clotted blood and debris may mat hair or wool and clog electric clippers. The hair may have to be washed and combed to remove debris. Shave enough hair away from the wound edges to prevent future irritation, to facilitate cleaning, and to check for additional wounds hidden by the hair coat.

Wash around the wound with mild soap and warm water, using a brush if necessary. Do not use the brush *in* the wound, however, for this will increase the possibility of the wound becoming infected (Custer et al. 1971). When skin abrasions are present around the affected areas, use care and gentle cleansing so as not to produce more trauma than already exists.

Where possible, use protective sterile drapes around the affected area to wall it off. This may be impossible or impractical in a field situation but should be possible whenever definitive surgery is planned under more controlled conditions.

2. Cleanse the Wound

Many methods of applying warm physiological saline to wounds have been suggested. (1) Use gravity flow (to increase the head of pressure of saline entering the wound) by means of an intravenous infusion bottle and set. This helps to flush deeply into the wound. (2) A bulb syringe (also using a pressure effect) may be used to flush the warm saline. To enhance the pressure and effectiveness, use a large bore needle (18 to 19 gauge) and a 35- to 50-ml plastic or glass syringe to deliver the saline at 8 psi (Madden 1971). (3) Pulsating water-jet lavage may be used.

The dental Water Pik (Teledyne Aquatec, Fort Collins, CO) has been modified for use as an instrument to provide pulsating water-jet lavage in the treatment of contaminated wounds (SurgiLav, Stryker Corp., Kalamazoo, MI) (Bhaskar et al. 1971; Grower et al. 1972). Water-jet lavage has been shown to be three times more effective than a bulb syringe in removing tissue fragments and seven times more effective in removing bacteria from contaminated wounds. When used in conjunction with surgical debridement, pulsating jet lavage produces a very clean wound. The optimum pressure at the nozzle is 60 psi; higher pressures cause undue trauma and may, in fact, push bacteria and other materials deeper into the wound. Some workers have recommended adding antibiotics to the lavage solution to enhance the antimicrobial effect, whereas others feel warm saline alone is adequate (Gross et al. 1972).

When debris has blown into a wound or when an animal has been injured and dragged, imbedding debris in the wound, the pulsating water-jet lavage is extremely helpful in removing this material without causing undue trauma to surrounding tissue.

3. Debride the Wound

The most important mode of wound therapy to prevent dead and damaged tissue from serving as a bacterial media is surgical debridement. This means surgical excision of the wound tract, all devitalized tissue, foreign material, clotted blood, and tissue debris. Hemorrhage must be controlled meticulously during the debridement process.

Use a scalpel blade plus noncrushing forceps to remove the shredded muscle, torn fascia, and black discolored skin.

Devitalized muscle is grey in color and crumbles readily. Incise back to where fresh bleeding muscle is present. Remove debris and foreign bodies and probe to the recesses of the wound with gloved fingers to ensure complete exposure. Arteries, veins, nerves, tendons, and ligaments should not be destroyed but should be salvaged to the greatest extent possible. In some cases, the wound will have to be cleaned and made free of bacterial contamination before definitive surgery can be performed to repair these structures. Skeletal bone splinters may be removed surgically or by lavage, but large bone fragments may be left in situ to bridge bone defects. Debride and clean these fragments and they will act as a bone graft.

4. Close the Wound.

Clean wounds less than six to eight hours old can generally be closed primarily. The following types of wounds should be left open for delayed primary closure (closure at four to seven days) or longer, if needed: wounds in which extensive destruction occurs; gunshot wounds; bites; cases of extensive soilage by intestinal contents or external sources; cases in which the clinician is still not convinced his treatment has completely removed contamination (Committee on Trauma 1976). If you are not convinced the wound is clean, leave it open.

Equine leg wounds below the knee and hock may heal with production of exuberant granulation tissue. Meticulous care is needed in this species in approximating tissue and providing strict hemostasis and postoperative immobilization of the limb to prevent irritation to the wound site. For details on treatment of equine wounds, the reader is referred to Chapters 11 and 12.

REFERENCES

Alexander, J. W., Kaplan, J. Z., and Altemeier, W.A.: Role of suture materials in the development of wound infection. Ann. Surg. *165*:192, 1967.

Altemeier, W. A., Burke, J. F., Pruitt, B. A., and Sandusky, W. R. (eds.): Manual of Control of Infection in Surgical Patients, A. C. S. Philadelphia: J.B. Lippincott, 1976.

Bhaskar, S. I. Y., Cutright, D. D., et al.: Pulsating water jet device in debridement of combat wounds. Mil. Med. *136*:264, 1971.

Carpendale, M. T. F., and Sereda, W.: The role of percutaneous sutures in surgical wound infection. Surgery 58:672, 1965.

Committee on Trauma, American College of Surgeons: Early Care of the Injured Patient. Philadelphia: W. B. Saunders, 1976, pp. 11–12.

Conolly, W. B., and Golovsky, D.: Postoperative wound sepsis. Med. J. Aust. 1:643, 1967.

Conolly, W. B., Hunt, T. K., and Dunphy, J. E.: Management of contaminated surgical wounds. Surg. Gynecol. Obstet. 129:593, 1969.

Custer, J., Edlich, R. F., et al.: Studies on the management of the contaminated wound. V. An assessment of the effectiveness of pHisoHex and Betadine surgical scrub solution. Am. J. Surg. 121:572, 1971.

Edlich, R. F., et al.: Physical and chemical configuration of sutures in the development of surgical infection. Ann. Surg. 177:679, 1973.

Elek, S. D.: Experimental staphylococcal infections in the skin of man. Ann. Acad. Sci. 65:85, 1956.

Elek, S. D., and Conen, P. E.: The virulence of Staphylococcus pyogenes for man. A study of the problems of wounds. Br. J. Exper. Pathol. 38:573m, 1957.

Evans, D. G., Miles, A. A., and Niven, J. S. F.: The enhancement of bacterial infections by adrenalin. Br. J. Exper. Pathol. 29:20, 1948.

Everett, W. G.: Suture materials in general surgery. Prog. Surg. 8:14, 1970.

Getzen, L. C., and Jansen, G. A.: Correlation between allergy to suture material and postoperative wound infections. Surgery 60:825, 1966.

Gross, A., Cutright, D. W., et al.: The effect of antiseptic agents and pulsating jet lavage on contaminated wounds. Mil. Med. 137:145, 1972.

Grower, M. F., Bhaskar, S. N., et al.: Effects of water lavage on removal of tissue fragments from crush wounds. Oral Surg. 33:1031, 1972.

Hunt, T. K., Jawetz, E., Hutchinson, J. G. P., and Dunphy, J. E.: Repiratory gas tension and pH in healing wounds. Am. J. Surg. 114:302, 1967.

Krizek, T. J., and Davis, J.H.: The role of the red cell in subcutaneous infection. J. Trauma 5:85, 1965.

LeVeen, H. H., Falk, G., Mazzapica, F. A., and Dennis, C.: The suppression of experimental wound infections by biocidal sutures. Surgery 64:610, 1968.

Localio, S. A., Casale, W., and Hinton, J. W.: Wound healing: Experimental and statistical study. V. Bacteriology and pathology in relation to suture material. Surg. Gynecol. Obstet. 77:481, 1943.

Ludewig, R. M., Rudolph, L. E., and Wangensteen, S. L.: Reduction of experimental wound infections with iodized gut sutures. Surg. Gynecol. Obstet. 133:946, 1971.

Madden, J. D.: Application of principles of fluid dynamics to surgical wound infection. Current topics. Surg. Res. 3:85, 1971.

May, J., Chalmers, J. P., Loewenthal, J., and Rountree, P. M.: Factors in the patient contributing to surgical sepsis. Surg. Gynecol. Obstet. 122:28, 1966.

Miles, A. A.: Nonspecific defense reactions in bacterial infections. Ann. NY Acad. Sci. 66:356, 1956.

Pulaski, E. J.: Common Bacterial Infections. Philadelphia: W. B. Saunders, 1964.

Silvola, H., Laustela, E., Kosunen, T., and Sillanpaa, V.: Tissue trauma in surgical wound infection. Ann. Chir. Gynaec. Fenn. 57:548, 1968.

BACTERIOLOGICAL ASSESSMENT IN THE TREATMENT OF WOUND INFECTIONS

The environment that surrounds both man and animals is not germ-free; it is a balance between a host, its systemic and local protective mechanisms, and a variety of microbial agents, which have the potential to cause infection (Robson, Krizek, and Heggers 1973). Initially, the local defense mechanisms are breached by the disruption of the protective integument. Often, a large inoculum of bacteria is added, coupled with those bacteria that already exist as normal flora on the skin and deep in hair follicles. Normally, bacteria in the recesses of the hair follicles achieve numbers as high as 10^3 organisms per gram of tissue (Pillsbury, Shelley, and Kligman 1956).

All open wounds contain bacteria and remain contaminated with varying quantities of bacteria until successful closure has been accomplished. Regardless of the mode of trauma (acute or chronic), wound closure can only be accomplished if both the local environment and the bacterial flora are in balance (Robson, Krizek; and Heggers 1973).

As mentioned previously, the sine qua non for treatment of such potentially heavily contaminated wounds is adequate surgical debridement. Sir James Learmoth's couplets are most appropriate to this procedure (Whelan, Burkhalter, and Gomez 1968).

Of the edge of skin
take a piece very thin
The tighter the fascia
the more you should slash 'er
Of the muscle much more
'til you see fresh gore
And bundles contract
at least impact
Leave intact the bone
except bits quite alone.

Once adequate debridement is accomplished, the successful closure of either an acute or chronic wound is dependent on the microbial population. If quantitative wound biopsy counts exceed 10^5 organisms per gram of tissue, the wound is not ready for closure. If, however, counts are less than 10^5 organisms per gram of tissue, the wound can be successfully closed (Heggers, Robson, and Ristroph 1969; Robson and Heggers 1969; Krizek and Robson 1975; Levine et al. 1976; Raahave 1976). Exceptions to this general rule are noted below.

Many methods of quantification have been developed. In 1969, Robson and Heggers reported a biopsy technique by which an aliquot of tissue was excised, weighed, homogenized, and subsequently diluted tenfold to achieve a quantitative count. Then, in 1974, Raahave devised a velvet pad technique, employing a 9 cm² × 8 cm² velvet pad affixed to aluminum foil. An impression of the wound was made and transferred to a blood agar plate, yielding information pertinent to wound surface contamination. It is known that normal skin surface contamination generally produces counts of less than 10^3 organisms per gram of tissue (Artz and Moncrief 1969; Pillsbury, Shelley, and Kligman 1956). However, to our knowledge, normal surface contamination figures have not been established for large animals.

The major surface organs of the body responsible for harboring potentially infectious organisms are the hair follicles. The quantitative distribution of bacteria is related to the distribution of hair and has been reported at levels ranging from 5 to 865,000 per sq cm for aerobic varieties and as many as 200,000 per sq cm for the anaerobic types. Combined, this endogenous microbial population achieves numbers sufficient to cause infection.

Levine and coworkers (1976) improved

on the preceding studies with their development of a swab culture technique. Like all standard culture techniques, this, too, suffered from a lack of rapid results, since all biological functions require 18 to 24 hours for growth.

Subsequent to the Robson-Heggers biopsy technique in 1969, Heggers, Robson, and Ristroph in the same year developed a rapid slide procedure. The time interval from obtaining the specimen to examining the gram stain was reduced to 30 minutes.

Today the procedure takes only 10 minutes. The procedural outline follows and only differs from the biopsy procedure in that a *gram stain is performed on the initial 1:10 dilution*. To date, over 9,000 specimens have been examined. When compared with the back plate method, a 98.2 per cent accuracy rate has been achieved.

1. The surface of the open wound (including burn eschar) is cleansed with alcohol (70% isopropyl).

2. A biopsy specimen is obtained with either a 3- or 4-mm dermal punch or a scalpel. In most cases, no anesthesia is required to biopsy an open wound, for the amount of tissue needed is less than 0.5 g and can be cut from the wound site readily.

3. After transport to the laboratory in a sterile tube, the specimen is aseptically weighed.

4. The specimen is then dipped in alcohol, air dried, and flamed to remove surface contamination.

5. After the tissue is diluted 1:10 with supplemented thioglycolate or supplemented brain-heart infusion broth (BHI) (1 ml/g), it is homogenized.

6. Exactly 0.02 ml of the suspension is spread on a glass slide from a 20-lambda Sahli pipette. The inoculum is confined to an area 15 mm in diameter.

7. The slide is oven dried for 15 minutes at 75°C.

8. The slide is stained, using either a gram-stain or the Brown and Brenn modification for tissue staining, to accentuate the gram-negative organisms.

9. The smear is read under a 1.9-mm objective (magnification × 97), and all fields are examined for the presence of bacteria.

10. The presence of even a single organism is evidence that the tissue contains a level of bacterial growth greater than 10^5 bacteria per gram of tissue.

11. The remaining specimen is serial diluted (1:10, 1:100, 1:1,000, and so on) in supplemented thioglycolate or BHI.

This technique, like the quantitative approach, enables the surgeon to know with considerable diagnostic precision in a relatively short period of time not only the relative number of bacteria present in the wound but the organism's specific gram reaction, an indicator that can be used for initiating specific antimicrobial therapy. As stated previously, this technique uses an all-or-none response and simply relies on the mere presence of one organism to be considered positive (Figs. 6–1 and 6–2).

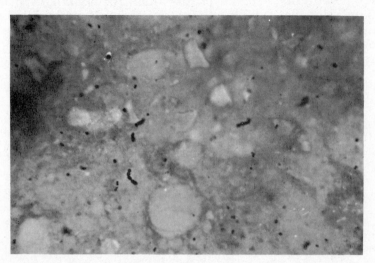

Figure 6–1 Gram stain of a 1:10 dilution of tissue. Rapid slide count greater than 10^5 per gram of tissue. (Streptococci 1000×)

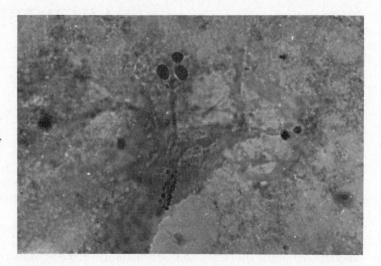

Figure 6–2 Gram stain of a 1:10 dilution of tissue. Rapid slide count greater than 10^5 per gram of tissue. (*Candida* species $1000\times$)

Other rapid techniques have been designed (Levine et al. 1969; Raahave 1976; Bornside and Bornside 1979); however, surface contamination is not as good an indicator of the extent of tissue involvement as is the presence of pyogenic exudates. Bacteriological counts on biopsies, exceeding 10^5 organisms per gram of tissue, yielded 82 per cent pure single species when compared with pyogenic exudates and surface contamination (Robson and Heggers 1969; Krizek, Robson, and Wray 1973).

Despite the number of techniques available to determine the quantity of bacteria in wound tissue, there is surprisingly little difference in the volume of bacteria considered to be critical, ranging in all studies from 10^5 to 10^6 bacteria per gram of tissue (Krizek and Robson 1975).

Before leaving quantitative bacteriology, it should be mentioned that not every species of bacteria appears to adhere to the generalization that a count of greater than 10^5 organisms will produce complications. In particular, the *β-hemolytic streptococci have been demonstrated repeatedly to be clinically significant at a much lower count level*. To date, no other species has proven to be troublesome at a lower level, but this may be a chance phenomenon. It has been the practice of the authors in all operative procedures not to perform a skin graft or close a wound in the presence of β-hemolytic streptococci, regardless of its quantitative level (Krizek, Robson, and Wray 1973; Robson, Krizek, and Heggers 1973; Krizek and Robson 1975; Robson and Heggers 1969).

REFERENCES

Artz, C. P., and Moncrief, J. A.: The Treatment of Burns. Philadelphia: W. B. Saunders, 1969.

Bornside, G. H., and Bornside, B. B.: Comparison between moist swab and tissue biopsy methods for quantitation of bacteria in experimental incisional wounds. J. Trauma *19*:193, 1979.

Heggers, J. P., Robson, M. C., and Ristroph, J. D.: A rapid method of performing quantitative wound cultures. Mil. Med. *134*:666, 1969.

Krizek, T. J., and Robson, M. C.: Evolution of quantitative bacteriology in wound management. Am. J. Surg. *130*:579, 1975.

Krizek, T. J., Robson, M. C., and Wray, R. C.: Care of the burned patient. *In* Management of Trauma. Ballinger W. F., et al. (eds.) Philadelphia: W.B. Saunders, 1973.

Levine, N. S., Lindberg, R. B., Mason, A. D., Jr., et al.: The quantitative swab culture and smear: A quick, simple method for determining the number of viable aerobic bacteria on open wounds. J. Trauma *16*:89, 1976.

Pillsbury, D. M., Shelley, W. B., and Kligman, A. M.: Dermatology. Philadelphia: W. B. Saunders, 1956.

Raahave, D.: Bacterial density in laparotomy wounds during gastrointestinal operations. Scand. J. Gastroenterol. 37:135, 1976.

Robson, M. C., and Heggers, J. P. Bacterial quantification of open wounds. Mil. Med. *134*:19, 1969.

Robson, M. C., and Heggers, J. P.: Surgical infection. I. Single bacterial species or polymicrobic in origin. Surgery 65:608, 1969.

Robson, M. C., Krizek, T. J., and Heggers, J. P.: Biology of surgical infection. Curr. Probl. Surg. 1–62, Mar. 1973.

Whelan, T. J., Jr., Burkhalter, W. E., and Gomez, A.: Management of war wounds. *In* Advances in Surgery, Vol. 3. Welch, C. E. (ed.) Chicago: Yearbook Medical Publishers, 1968.

THE USE OF ANTIMICROBIAL AGENTS

The most important factor introduced in recent years to alter the biological balance between host resistance and microorganisms has been the use of antimicrobial agents. The administration of an antimicrobial agent at the proper time and in sufficient quantity to be therapeutically active should, theoretically, be uniformly effective in preventing or treating infection from susceptible organisms. Furthermore, the expansion of coverage achieved by broad spectrum antibacterial agents should provide the patient with a "blanket of protection" against infection. However, it is clear that the ready availability and wide usage of antibiotics have neither eliminated surgical infection as a threat to the patient nor even reduced the incidence of such infections in most cases (Ellis 1969). In addition, there is evidence that the widespread and often indiscriminate use of antimicrobial agents may be responsible for the changing patterns of bacteria implicated in nosocomial infections and for the emergence of bacterial species – amphibionts – heretofore considered to be nonpathogenic (Adler, Burke, and Findland, 1971; Johnson, 1971; Seneca and Grant 1976). Finally, toxicity and sensitization produced by these agents have introduced a new hazard to the patient (Martin 1966; McGowan and Finland 1974).

As with any potent therapeutic modality, antibacterial agents should be introduced into the host-bacteria equation only with proper and sufficient indications. The potential benefits must be sufficient to warrant whatever potential hazards may be present. When such indications exist, the agent should be chosen on the basis of its known mechanisms of action and with a specificity, wherever possible, determined by the precision of culture and susceptibility testing. It should be given in time, in sufficient dosage, by an appropriate route, and for a duration sufficient to accomplish the goals outlined by the treatment. There must be a clear understanding at all times of the status of systemic and local host-resistant factors, which will ultimately determine the success or failure of the therapy (Kunin 1977).

Surgical infection differs from a medical type of infection in that it lends itself in some form to intervention by some surgical means. Examples of microbial infections that do not require surgery and for which systemic antimicrobial therapy is indicated are uncomplicated pneumonia, pharyngitis, and meningitis. However, complications of these infections, such as development of empyema, parapharyngeal abscess, or subdural collection of pus, may require surgical intervention. Antibiotics alone will not quell the infectious process. The basic treatment principles that cannot be ignored are abscess drainage, debridement, use of biologic wound dressings, and well-timed secondary wound closure. The persistent and, perhaps, illogical use of antimicrobials is no substitute for basic wound management (Dillon, Bowling, and Postelthwait 1972).

There are four major points to be assessed before initiating antimicrobial therapy. (1) The decision to use antimicrobials must be based on the specificity of the antimicrobial and its potential effects on the microorganisms present. (2) This decision cannot be a guess but should be based on culture and susceptibility testing. (3) The time, dosage, and route of administration and duration of therapy necessary to render the microbial invader impotent should be considered. (4) The systemic and local host-resistant factors must be weighed (Kunin 1977). Neu's review of the effects of antimicrobials is recommended as an in-depth publication (1973). Those antimi-

Table 6–14 ANTIMICROBIAL MODE OF ACTION*

Alter Cell Wall Synthesis
 Bacitracin
 Cephalosporins
 Penicillins
 Vancomycin
Alter Cell Membrane Permeability
 Amphotericin B
 Colistin
 Nystatin
 Polymyxin B
Inhibit Protein Synthesis
 Chloramphenicol
 Erythromycin
 Kanamycin
 Lincomycin
 Neomycin
 Streptomycin
 Tetracyclines
Inhibit DNA Synthesis
 Griseofulvin
 Nalidixic acid
Intermediary Metabolism
 Sulfonamides
 Trimethoprim

*Modified after Heggers: Clin. Plast. Surg. 6: 545, 1979.

crobial agents that render the invading microorganisms ineffectual are presented in Table 6–14.

To be effective, antimicrobials, such as penicillins, require an actively metabolizing organism that is in the process of developing a cell wall. They have little or no effect on microbes whose cell walls are completely developed. Those antimicrobials that affect the cell membrane, such as polymyxin B, contain both lipophilic and lipophobic groups, enabling them to invade the lipid protein union that is the foundation of the cell membrane. This distortion destroys the capacity of the membrane to freely diffuse the nutrients required for cell survival. This permanent binding of the antimicrobial to the cytoplasmic membrane is bactericidal.

Inhibition of protein synthesis occurs at two major biosynthetic pathways, the first at transcription, where the coded message is transferred to the M-RNA, and the second at the point at which the RNA prepares to process protein. Rifampin inhibits the initial stage of protein synthesis by binding to RNA polymerase, thus preventing the conformational change needed for the initiation of RNA

production. The other antibiotics render their inhibitory effects at different phases of protein synthesis. The aminoglycosides, such as gentamicin, bind the 30 S ribosomal subunit, inhibiting peptide bond formation, thus forming an inactive 70 S ribosome. Chloramphenicol, on the other hand, binds the 50 S ribosome, inhibiting the attachment of the functional aminoacyl end of aminoacyl plus RNA. Currently, only three antimicrobials have been linked to DNA interference. Nalidixic acid interacts between the stacked bases of DNA, thus interfering with transcription. Novobiocin affects DNA polymermerase, whereas griseofulvin interacts as a purine analogue. The intermediary drugs, such as sulfonamides, act as analogues of paraminobenzoic acid (PABA), thus inhibiting folic acid synthesis (Neu 1973; 1977).

Each organism isolated from a surgical wound should be grown in pure culture and tested by the Kirby-Bauer susceptibility method. This diffusion technique is recommended by the Food and Drug Administration. The agar employed is a Mueller-Hinton agar dispensed in a 150-mm plastic Petri dish. Plates are inoculated with an actively growing pure culture of the organism to be tested. After each culture's turbidity is adjusted to match a 0.5 MacFarland turbidity standard, the antimicrobial-impregnated discs are applied to the agar surface 15 minutes after inoculation. Each disc should be at least 15 mm from the edge of the plate and far enough from the others so that zones of inhibition do not overlap. Generally, 12 to 13 discs can be applied to a 150-mm plate. The plates are then incubated, inverted at 35°C for 16 to 18 hours, and the zones of inhibition are measured (Barry 1976). Table 6–15 gives a suggested battery of antimicrobials for routine susceptibility testing.

Time, dosage, and route of administration of antibiotics are important considerations when treating surgical wounds. Robson, Duke, and Krizek (1973) showed that in 80 per cent of human traumatic wounds presenting in emergency departments, although contamination was evident, the initial bacterial count prior to wound cleansing and debridement was less than 10^5 bacteria per gram of tissue.

Table 6–15 SUGGESTED BATTERY OF ANTIMICROBIALS FOR
ROUTINE SUSCEPTIBILITY TESTING*

Antimicrobial	Gram-Positive Cocci		Gram-Negative Bacteria	
	S. aureus	Enterococci	Enterobacteriaceae	Other
Ampicillin	−	+	+	−
Penicillin G	+	+	−	−
Cephalothin	+	+	+	
Erythromycin	+	+	−	−
Clindamycin	+	−	−	−
Chloramphenicol	+	+	+	+[b]
Tetracycline	+	+	+	+[b]
Gentamycin	+	−	+	+
Cefamandole	+	−	+	+[b]
Tobramycin	+	−	+	+
Kanamycin	−	−	+	+[b]
Oxacillin	+	−	−	−
Polymyxin B	−	−	+	+
Nitrofurantoin	−	−	+[a]	−
Nalidixic acid	−	−	+[a]	−
Sulfonamide	−	−	+[a]	+[b]
Carbenicillin	−	−	−	+
Ticarcillin	+[c]	+	+	+

*Modified after Heggers: Clin. Plast. Surg. 6:545, 1979.
a = urinary tract infections
b = non fermentative bacteria and pseudomonads other than P. aeruginosa
c = non penicillinase producing

The mean time from injury for wounds containing less than 10^5 bacteria per gram was less than three hours. Those wounds with counts greater than 10^5 per gram of tissue had a mean time from injury of 5.17 hours. Interestingly, after wound cleansing these investigators found that bacterial counts were reduced in 57 per cent of the cases, unchanged in 25 per cent of the cases, and increased in 18 per cent of the cases. It was apparent that it made little difference which agent caused the wound, since successful closure correlated directly with the bacterial count rather than with any other single factor. Thus, it appears that as the wound becomes altered, it serves to enhance the metabolic functions of the microbes so that the organisms can achieve tissue levels of greater than 10^5 per gram of tissue, creating a pathogenic and potentially septic situation.

We must recognize that we cannot create a germ-free patient by using antimicrobial agents and that their use is indicated only when the *potential incidence* of infection is real. The timing is particularly important. Within hours after accidental wounding or even planned surgical intervention, it is evi-

dent that bacterial lodgement has occurred (Burke 1961). There is an abundance of experimental and clinical data to indicate that if antimicrobial agents are initiated more than three to four hours after wounding, the desired or anticipated effects of the antimicrobial do not occur in vivo (Ad Hoc Committee on Trauma 1964; Krizek, Koss, and Robson 1975; Neu 1973; 1975; 1977).

Open granulating wounds do not lend themselves to systemic antimicrobial manipulation. A 20 per cent full thickness scald burn was created in a rat as a model of a granulating wound. The wound was then seeded topically with *Escherichia coli, Pseudomonas aeruginosa,* or *Staphylococcus aureus.* The animal was left with a monocontaminated granulating wound that failed to heal after the eschar was removed on the fifth day. Quantitatively, all tissue biopsied yielded counts greater than 10^7 bacteria per gram of tissue. An antimicrobial, specific for each etiological agent, was given systemically to achieve adequate blood and tissue levels. However, the microbial level remained unchanged from the initial count. The wound tissue demonstrated no antimicrobial effects against the particular agent involved, yet blood levels theoretically were adequate to produce the desired antimicrobial effects (Robson et al. 1974). From these studies it appears that, in granulating wounds, successful reduction of bacterial counts to acceptable levels required for wound closure must be achieved by means other than systemic antimicrobial therapy.

In surgical wounds, the controversy over whether or not to use prophylactic antimicrobials still exists. Before using prophylactic antimicrobials, try to place each of these wounds into categories based on a clinical estimate of the degree of contamination; these categories are clean, clean-contaminated, contaminated, dirty, and infected wounds (Altemeier et al. 1976).

As a result of two wound infection studies in man (Howard et al. 1964; Cruse and Foord 1973), it was shown that the incidence of wound infections was approximately 1 in 20. Therefore, if antimicrobials were used prophylactically, the number of individuals who would potentially be exposed to unnecessary risks, such as adverse drug reactions, would be large, encompassing over 75 per cent of the total population of both studies. Consequently, antimicrobial prophylaxis cannot be recommended. Only in cases in which consequences of an infection are considered grave or in which implants are to be used should prophylactic antimicrobials be considered.

The clean-contaminated category includes a number of surgical manipulations in which the degree of contamination is minimal and in which the probability of infection is not significant enough to warrant the risk of antimicrobial prophylaxis. Yet there are some procedures in this category in which it is advisable to initiate prophylactic antimicrobials; these are (1) any surgical procedure involving the abdomen in which vascularity may be compromised, (2) amputation of a poorly vascularized extremity, and (3) those procedures that enter the oropharyngeal cavity.

Prophylactic antimicrobials are obviously recommended in the remaining categories provided they do not meet the criteria described earlier in traumatic (acute) wounds or granulating wounds

(Altemeier et al. 1975; Krizek, Koss, and Robson 1975).

The role of prophylactic antimicrobials in abdominal and extra-abdominal surgery still remains a controversial issue. In a report by Michel and colleagues (1977), their evaluation of prophylaxis in a variety of surgical manipulations revealed that of all the human patients undergoing large bowel surgery, 80 per cent received prophylactic antibiotics and 30 per cent developed postoperative wound infections. The infection rate in gastric surgery in those who received prophylaxis was identical to that in those who received no antimicrobials. In gallbladder surgery, prophylaxis was associated with a high infection rate in both high-risk and low-risk patients.

Stone (1977) feels that the available data unequivocally support the thesis that prophylactic antimicrobial therapy is an effective means of reducing incisional infection in gastric surgery. Yet the effectiveness is solely dependent upon achieving antibacterial levels in the tissue prior to surgical intervention and microbial contamination.

Current trends toward anaerobic infections have opened new vistas in the development of antimicrobials. The cephalosporins apparently have a broad spectrum and are efficacious in anaerobic as well as aerobic infections.

The reduction of anaerobic infections in colonic surgery with the aid of prophylactic therapy is impressive. Yet if one studies the environment of the gut during a surgical procedure, one finds that, immediately upon penetration of the abdominal wall, 95 per cent of all cultures yield anaerobes; this is reduced to 5 per cent in two hours owing to the drastic environmental changes (Polk 1977).

Predisposing or modifying factors notwithstanding, most surgeons tend not to employ prophylactic antimicrobials in plastic and reconstructive surgery (Krizek, Koss, and Robson 1975). In orthopedic surgery, Patzakis and Ivler (1977) reported that prophylactic use of cephalothin reduced the incidence of infection in open fractures when compared with penicillin-streptomycin prophylaxis. Boyd (1977) felt that, in clean orthopedic cases, the routine use of preventive antibiotics was not indicated, that the sur-

Table 6–16 ROUTES OF ADMINISTRATION AND WOUND/TISSUE FLUID LEVELS OF ANTIBIOTICS*

Antibiotic	Dosage	Route	— Concentration (μg/ml) in wound fluid per time (hrs)									
			1/2	1	3	4	5	8	12	16	20	24
Ampicillin	25 mg/kg	IM q6h	2.0			3.5		4.0	6.0	9.0	8.0	8.5
		IV Push q6h	4.0			3.0		4.0	2.0	6.0	6.0	5.0
		IV Cont	1.0			≤2.5		2.5	5.0	6.0	5.0	6.5
	500 mg[b]	IV q6h		3.0	5.0		1.0					
	1.0 g[b]			16.0	8.0		1.5					
Gentamycin	2 mg/kg[a]	IM q6h	0.5			0.75		≥1.0	0.5	1.0	0.75	0.75
		IV Push q6h	0.5			0.75		≤1.0	0.5	1.0	0.75	<0.75
		IV Cont	0.5			0.75		≤0.5	0.5	0.5	0.75	0.5
	1.7 mg/kg[c]	IM		1.36 ± 1.03		0.62 ± 0.33						
Clindamycin	4 mg/kg[a]	IV q6h	<1.0			1.0		<2.0	3.0	4.0	4.0	4.0
		IV Push q6h	<1.0			2.0		2.0	3.0	<2.0	4.0	3.0
		IV Cont	<1.0			<1.0		1.0	<1.0	2.0	<2.0	2.5
Tetracycline	300 mg[b]	IV q6h		5.5	5.5		4.0					
	7 mg/kg	IM q6h	<1.0			<1.0		1.0	1.5	2.0	<2.0	—
		IV Push q6h	<1.0			1.5		3.0	3.0	>3.0	—	—
		IV Cont	<1.0			<1.0		1.5	2.0	8.0	3.0	—
Cephalothin	25 mg/kg[a]	IM q6h	<3.0			6.0		5.5	7.0	8.0	8.0	6.5
		IV Push q6h	<3.0			5.0		7.0	5.0	8.0	4.0	4.5
		IV Cont	<3.0					5.0	7.0	8.0	8.5	6.0
Carbenicillin	1.0 g[b]	IV q6h		7.0	5.0		3.0					
	3.0 g	IV Push		13.67 ± 6.60		2.60 ± 1.84						
Ticarcillin[c]	3.0 g	IV Push		11.71 ± 5.90		2.10 ± 0.71						
Cefazolin	1.0 g[c]	IV Push		2.61 ± 2.80		1.23 ± 0.86						
Tobramicin[c]	500 mg[b]	IV q6h		20.0	16.0		14.0					
	1.0 g[b]			20.0	42.0		35.0					
	1.7 mg/kg	IM		0.84 ± 0.61		0.53 ± 0.38						
Amikacin[c]	7.5 mg/kg	IM		2.16 ± 1.53		2.11 ± 1.23						
Penicillin[a]	5 megaunits	IV Push		3.8 IU/mg		7.2 IU/mg†						
	2 megaunits			1.9 IU/mg		—						
Cephapirin[b]	1.0 g	IV q6h		8.0	4.0		2.0					
Oxacillin[b]	1.0 g	IV q6h		13.0	11.5		4.5					

*Modified after Heggers: Clin. Plast. Surg. 6:545, 1979.
†Three hours
a = Alexander and Alexander: J. Trauma 16:488, 1976.
b = Bagley et al.: Ann. Surg. 188:202, 1978.
c = Tan and Salstrom: Antimicrob. Agents Chemother. 11:698, 1977.
d = Raahave: Scand. J. Gastroenterol. 37 (Suppl.):129, 1976.

geon must evaluate each case on its own merit, and that prophylactic antimicrobials have no place in surgical procedures in which there is only minimal risk involved.

Obviously, the decision to use prophylactic antimicrobials is dependent on the surgeon's past experience and his examination of predisposing factors. Krizek, Koss, and Robson (1975) have presented the following principles for usage of prophylactic antimicrobials in surgery:

1. The potential incidence of and danger from infection must be sufficient to warrant the use of such agents.

2. The agent chosen must be appropriate for the potential infection.

3. The agent must be administered at a time and in a dosage and route most likely to be effective.

Dosage of antimicrobials is of major importance in that the dose administered must deliver a level of drug to the potentially infected area in a minimum inhibitory concentration adequate to prevent that infection. Most manufacturers recommend a therapeutic regimen that delivers to the tissues and blood stream microgram quantities high enough to abrogate or prevent an infection.

It is equally important to know what microbial agents would most likely be encountered in a surgical procedure. Based on bacteriological statistics, i.e., an infection experience factor plus the frequent use of the simple gram stain, the most probable etiological agent responsible for postsurgical infection can be determined and an appropriate antimicrobial can be selected. Robson and Heggers (1969) have shown that 80 per cent of the isolates from biopsied soft tissue wounds in man yielded staphylococci 46 per cent of the time, enterobacteria 22 per cent of the time, and pseudomonads 12 per cent of the time.

After selecting the appropriate antimicrobial, the route of administration is the next most important consideration. Although serum levels achieve bactericidal concentrations within a short period of time (one hour), the antimicrobial concentration delivered to the traumatized or incised tissues is often not sufficient to be effective and depends on two factors: (1) the effectiveness against the etiological agent, and (2) the rapidity of penetra-

tion and ultimate concentration at the site of insult or infection. When administered properly, each antimicrobial arrives at the tissue site in sufficient levels.

Experimental studies have shown that, at 30 minutes, ampicillin concentrations were four times greater with intravenous (IV) push than with a continuous IV. However, after six hours, wound fluid levels were higher when the drug was given by the intramuscular route (Alexander and Alexander 1976). In wound fluid, gentamycin levels were equal with either IM or IV push, whereas tetracycline sustained better levels with continuous IV as opposed to IM or IV push. IV bolus of penicillin achieved antibacterial levels for up to three hours postinjection (Raahave 1976). Bagley and associates recently demonstrated higher wound fluid levels in patients receiving higher doses of cephalosporins, and penicillin derivatives (1975). Wound fluid levels surpassed serum levels after 2.5 hours. Table 6–16 presents some routes of administration and wound/tissue fluid levels at varying time intervals. The recommended antimicrobials for both gram-positive and gram-negative bacteria are compiled for easy reference in Tables 6–17 and 6–18.

FACTORS THAT RENDER ANTIMICROBIALS INEFFECTIVE

The binding of antimicrobials to tissue proteins has been a major topic of discussion. This binding may account for the low tissue levels observed with the aminoglycosides. Insoluble intracellular proteins, such as nucleic acids and acid proteins, are the sites for binding. Polymyxins have been shown to bind on the phospholipids of the tissue membranes, whereas antimicrobials such as penicillin and cephalosporin bind to soluble intracellular protein such as the hemoglobin metabolites found in liver and kidney. Purulent material has been shown to inactivate the action of aminoglycosides. High magnesium and calcium concentrations will reduce the activity of tobramicin and gentamycin. Other factors decreasing the activity of antimicrobials are pH, intracellular location of bacteria, and decreased blood flow. An-

Table 6–17 PRIMARY AND SECONDARY ANTIMICROBIALS
FOR GRAM-POSITIVE BACTERIA

Organism	Antimicrobial	
	Primary	Secondary
Staphylococcus aureus		
Nonpenicillinase	Penicillin G or V	Cephalosporin
Penicillinase	Oxacillin	Cephalosporin
Streptococcus pyogenes	Penicillin G or V	Erythromycin
Streptococcus agalactiae	Penicillin G	Chloramphenicol
Streptococcus viridans group	Penicillin G	Cephalosporin
Streptococcus, enterococcus group	Ampicillin with streptomycin or kanamycin	Vancomycin
Streptococcus pneumoniae	Penicillin G or V	Cephalosporin
Streptococcus, anaerobic	Penicillin G	Clindamycin
Clostridium sp.	Penicillin	Chloramphenicol (*C. perfringens*) Tetracycline (*C. tetani*)
Corynebacterium sp.	Erythromycin	Penicillin G
Listeria monocytogenes	Ampicillin	Erythromycin

aerobic and hypercapnic conditions have been shown to render antimicrobials such as gentamycin, tobramicin, and amikacin inactive or less active against facultative bacteria.

Although nonprotein-bound agents diffuse well into areas containing blood clots, such a condition significantly decreases the antimicrobial effect on enteric or staphylococcal organisms present during surgery. Additionally, inert materials such as fecal contamination can alter the effects or inactivate aminoglycosides (Neu 1975; 1977).

TOPICAL ANTIMICROBIALS

Penicillin, bacitracin, and most sulfa creams are extremely antigenic or ineffective topically. Polymyxin B in combination with other drugs has been used with some success.

Topical antimicrobials have been found to be most efficacious in burn wound sepsis. Sulfamylon (mafenide acetate) is a water-soluble cream. This sulfa cream effectively penetrates the eschar and clinically reduces the microbial flora to less than 10^4 bacteria per

Table 6–18 PRIMARY AND SECONDARY ANTIMICROBIALS FOR
GRAM-NEGATIVE BACTERIA*

Organism	Antimicrobial	
	Primary	Secondary
Enterobacter sp.	Aminoglycosides (gentamycin)	Carbenicillin or ticarcillin
Escherichia coli	Gentamycin	Ampicillin
Klebsiella pneumoniae	Gentamycin	Cephalosporin
Proteus sp. (other than *P. mirabilis*)	Gentamycin	Carbenicillin or ticarcillin
Proteus mirabilis	Ampicillin	Gentamycin or ticarcillin
Pseudomonas aeruginosa	Gentamycin	Polymyxin B carbenicillin
Pseudomonas fluorescens	Gentamycin	Polymyxin B kanamycin
Pseudomonas maltophilia	Polymyxin B	Chloramphenicol
Bacteroides sp. (gastrointestinal)	Clindamycin	Chloramphenicol
Fusobacterium fusiforme	Penicillin G	Tetracycline

*Modified after Heggers: Clin. Plast. Surg. 6:545, 1979.

gram of tissue, a level compatible with the survival of epithelial islands and skin grafts. Its antibacterial spectrum encompasses the major burn pathogens, particularly *Pseudomonas aeruginosa*. It does, however, share the antigenic potential that other sulfa creams elicit. It does absorb well but may produce metabolic acidosis in a debilitated patient.

Silver sulfadiazine, a cream with a compounded silver ion, is also a very effective antimicrobial agent. Its antibacterial spectrum includes *Pseudomonas aeruginosa*, *E. coli*, *Enterobacter*, *Proteus*, and *Staphylococcus aureus*. Recently, the authors have completed a study employing silver sulfadiazine as a topical agent in the management of pressure sores. With the wide variety of microbial agents available and the ineffectiveness of systemic antimicrobial penetration, this drug was found to be most efficacious when applied topically (Robson, Krizek, and Wray 1979).

Gentamycin sulfate (Garamycin) is a broad spectrum antimicrobial with a structure similar to that of neomycin and kanamycin. It has an unusual bactericidal effect on *Pseudomonas aeruginosa*. Toxicity and side effects remain at a minimum. A major disadvantage that accompanies and limits its use is the rapid emergence of resistant strains of pseudomonads.

Compounds such as bacitracin and neomycin are not hampered by clot or fibrin formation. Although incorporated in the clot, they apparently are released in adequate concentrations to inhibit the entrapped bacteria.

Although topical antimicrobials have reduced the incidence of burn wound sepsis and are considered most efficacious, there are a few studies to date to recommend their overall use in other types of wounds. More research is needed in this area. Recently the authors have become aware of a new topical antimicrobial in both liquid and cream base form (Dermaide Aloe*). It has successfully resuscitated three animal species destined for euthanasia.

The first of these were two canines presenting with 35 to 50 per cent dorsal

*Dermaide Aloe, Dermaide Research Corp., Chicago, Ill.

trunk burns. The wounds healed within 25 to 65 days with no apparent scarring of the tissue. The second animal (Rhesus monkey) received a 100 per cent body surface scald burn and was returned to the monkey colony in 30 days with no apparent complications.

The third animal was an equine that received IV Butazolidine for an unrelated lameness problem. Extensive (6 in. deep × 6 in. across) suppurative necrosis of the neck and main muscle mass along the jugular vein was noted two weeks postinjection. A drain was inserted and Dermaide liquid was flushed through the would b.i.d.; Dermaide cream was applied to the surface area. The wound healed within five weeks with a 1 1/2 in. superficial area lacking hair. There was no impairment of front limb movement (Cera 1979; 1980).

DRUG RESISTANCE

The appearance of drug-resistant bacteria has been assumed to be the result of a predictable process: (1) the development of a spontaneous mutation of a bacterium, and (2) the selective multiplication of the resistant strain in the presence of the drug. A more insidious problem is the phenomenon called infectious drug resistance, a process whereby the genetic markers carrying the resistance factors are transferred from the resistant organism to a nonresistant organism of the same species or a different species (Watanabe 1965).

Lacey (1975), describing the ecological relationship of *S. aureus* in man, presents some ominous thoughts. Since *S. aureus* and *S. epidermidis* cohabit man's body surface and nasal and buccal cavities, it is possible that the reservoir for these resistant plasmids originated in *S. epidermidis* and subsequently was transferred to *S. aureus*. The most probable site for transference is the body surface. If this is the case, the use of topical antimicrobials may be contraindicated.

In a study conducted by Siegel, Huber, and Enbe (1974) on the continuous nontherapeutic use of antimicrobials in food-producing animals, the occurrence of drug resistance was staggering. Organisms isolated from fecal material of both swine and cattle showed a minimum of 50 per cent resistance to oxytetracycline and dihydrostreptomycin and as high as 90 per cent in some cases.

Burton and coworkers (1973) found that the administration of tetracycline enhanced the colonization of the intestinal tract of man by an E. coli of animal origin. Subsequently, the use of this antimicrobial influenced the transfer of the resistant factors of man's resident E. coli.

Pasteurellosis as a disease in cattle and swine has been treated with penicillin, tetracycline, and sulfonamides. Chang and Carter (1976) recently reported on the multiple drug resistance to these agents by Pasteurella multocida and P. haemolytica. They proposed that the cause could be attributed to the frequent use of antimicrobial feeds and the transfer of plasmids from other bacteria.

Therapeutic drug combinations are warranted in only a few instances in certain infections. These may be used possibly to prevent the emergence of resistant organisms and to lessen adverse reactions by administering small drug dosages in combination. The use of such combinations should not substitute for determining what single drug is best. The fact is, in most clinical situations, a single drug most frequently produces better results (Jawetz 1967).

REFERENCES

Ad Hoc Committee of the Committee on Trauma, Division of Medical Sciences, National Research Council Report: Postoperative wound infections: The influence of ultraviolet irradiation of the operating room and the influence of various other factors. Ann. Surg. 160 (Suppl.):1, 1964.

Adler, J. L., Burke, J. P., and Findland, M.: Infection and antibiotic usage at Boston City Hospital, January 1970. Arch. Intern. Med. 127:460, 1971.

Alexander, J. W., and Alexander, N. S.: The influence of route of administration on wound fluid concentration of prophylactic antibiotics. J. Trauma 16:488, 1976.

Altemeier, W. A., Burke, J. F., Pruitt, B. A., and Sandusky, W. R.: Manual on Control of Infection in Surgical Patients. Philadelphia: J. B. Lippincott, 1976.

Bagley, D. H., MacLowry, J., Beazley, R. M., et al.: Antibiotic concentration in human wound fluid after intravenous administration. Ann. Surg. 188:202, 1978.

Barry, A. L.: The Antimicrobic Susceptibility Test: Principles of Practices, 1st ed. Philadelphia: Lea & Febiger, 1976.

Boyd, R. J.: Orthopedic surgery. South. Med. J. 70 (Suppl. 1):48, 1977.

Bryant, R. E., and Hammond, D.: Interaction of purulent material with antibiotics used to treat Pseudomonas aeruginosa infections. Antimicrob. Agents Chemother. 6:702, 1974.

Burke, J. F.: The effective period of preventive antibiotic action in experimental incisions and dermal lesions. Surgery 50:161, 1961.

Burton, G. C., Hirsh, D. C., Blendin, D. C., and Zeigler, J. L.: The effects of tetracycline on the establishment of Escherichia coli of animal origin and the in vivo transfer of antibiotic resistance in the intestinal tract of man. In The Normal Microbial Flora of Man, symposium No. 3. Skinner, F. A., and Carr, J. E., eds. New York: Academic Press, 1973.

Cera, L. M.: Personal communication. 1979 and 1980.

Chang, W. H., and Carter, G. R.: Multiple drug resistance in Pasteurella multocida and Pasteurella haemolytica from cattle and swine. JAVMA 169710, 1976.

Condon, R. E., and Nichols, R. L.: Surgical gastrointestinal disease. In Antimicrobial Therapy, 2nd ed. Kagan, B. H., ed. Philadelphia: W. B. Saunders, 1974.

Cruse, P. J. E., and Foord, R.: A five-year prospective study of 23,649 wounds. Arch. Surg. 107:206, 1973.

Dillon, M. L., Bowling, K. A., and Postlethwait, R. W.: Cephaloridine therapy in patients with surgical infections. Surg. Gynecol. Obstet. 134:83, 1972.

Elliot, D. W.: Biliary tract surgery. South. Med. J. 70 (Suppl. 1):31, 1977.

Ellis, H.: The place of antibiotics in surgical practice today. Ann. Royal Coll. Surg. 45:162, 1969.

Galask, R. P., and Ohm, M. J.: Abdominal hysterectomy. South. Med. J. 70 (Suppl. 1):37, 1977.

Heggers, J. P.: The use of antimicrobial agents. Clin. Plast. Surg. 6:545, 1979.

Howard, J. M., Barker, W. F., Culbertson, W. R., Grotzinger, P. J., et al.: Postoperative wound infections: The influence of ultraviolet irradiation of the operating room and of various other factors. Ann. Surg. 160 (Suppl.):1, 1964.

Hummel, R. P., Miskell, P. W., and Altemeier, W. A.: Antibiotic resistant transfer from nonpathogenic to pathogenic bacteria. Surgery 82:382, 1977.

Jawetz, E.: Combined antibiotic action: Some definitions and correlations between laboratory and clinical results. Antimicrob. Agents Chemother. 7:203, 1967.

Johnson, J. E. III: Wound infections. Postgrad. Med. 50:126, 1971.

Krizek, T. J., Koss, N., and Robson, M. C.: The current use of prophylactic antibiotics in plastic and reconstructive surgery. Plast. Reconstr. Surg. 55:21, 1975.

Krizek, T. J., and Robson, M. C.: Evolution of quantitative bacteriology in wound management. Am. J. Surg. 130:579, 1975.

Kunin, C. M.: Antimicrobial prophylaxis in surgery. Isr. J. Med. Sci. 13:547, 1977.

Lacey, R. W.: Antibiotic resistance plasmids of Staphylococcus aureus and their clinical importance. Bacteriol. Rev. 39:1, 1975.

Ledger, W. J., Boice, C., Yonekura, L., and Di Zerega, G.: Vaginal hysterectomy. South. Med. J. 70 (Suppl. 1):40, 1977.

Martin, W. J.: Complications of antibiotic therapy in the management of bacterial infections. Lancet 86:159, 1966.

McGowan, J. E., Jr., and Finland, M.: Usage of antibiotics in a general hospital: effect of requiring justification. J. Infect. Dis. 130:165, 1974.

Michel, J., Sacks, T., and Simchen, E.: Pattern of prophylactic use of antibiotics in six surgical departments of a teaching hospital in Jerusalem. Isr. J. Med. Sci. 13:549, 1977.

Neu, H. C.: Clinical pharmacokinetics in preventive antimicrobial therapy. South. Med. J. 70 (Suppl. 1):14, 1977.

Neu, H. C.: Newer antimicrobial agents. Postgrad. Med. 58:55, 1975.

Neu, H. C.: Antimicrobial agents. Mechanisms and action and clinical usage. Curr. Probl. Surg. 1–64, June, 1973.

Patzakis, M. J., and Ivler, D.: Antibiotic and bacteriologic considerations in open fractures. South. Med. J. 70 (Suppl. 1):46, 1977.

Polk, H. C., Jr.: Antibiotic prophylaxis in surgery of the colon. South. Med. J. 70 (Suppl. 1):27, 1977.

Raahave, D.: Penetration of penicillin into laparotomy wounds to reduce bacterial contamination during intestinal operations. Scand. J. Gastroenterol. 37 (Suppl.):129, 1976.

Robinson, G. N., and Sutherland, R.: The binding of antibiotics to serum proteins. Br. J. Pharmacol. 25:638, 1965.

Robson, M. C., and Heggers, J. P.: Surgical infection. I: Single bacterial species or polymicrobic in origin. Surgery 65:608, 1969.

Robson, M. C., Krizek, T. J., and Heggers, J. P.: Biology of surgical infection. Curr. Probl. Surg. 1–62, Mar., 1973.

Robson, M. C., Duke, W. F., and Krizek, T. J.: Rapid bacterial screening in the treatment of civilian wounds. J. Surg. Res. 14:426, 1973.

Robson, M. C., Edstrom, L. E., Krizek, T. J., and Groskin, M. G.: The efficacy of systemic antibiotics in the treatment of granulating wounds. J. Surg. Res. 16:299, 1974.

Robson, M. C., Krizek, T. T., and Wray, R. C.: Care of the thermally injured patients. In The Management of Trauma. Zuidema, G. D., Rutherford, R. B., and Ballinger, II, W. F. (eds.). Philadelphia: W. B. Saunders, 1979.

Seneca, H., and Grant, J. P.: The changing pattern of bacterial sepsis since the introduction of antibiotic therapy. J. Am. Geriatr. Soc. 24:155, 1976.

Siegel, D., Huber, W. G., and Enloe, F.: Continuous non-therapeutic use of antibacterial drugs in feed and drug resistance of gram-negative enteric flora of food-producing animals. Antimicrob. Agents Chemother. 6:697, 1974.

Stone, H. H., Hooper, C. A., Kolb, L. D., et al.: Antibiotic prophylaxis in gastric, biliary and colonic surgery. Ann. Surg. 184:443, 1976.

Stone, H.: Gastric surgery. South. Med. J. 70 (Suppl. 1):35, 1977.

Tan, J. S., and Salstrom, S. J.: Levels of carbenicillin, ticarcillin, cephalothin, cefazolin, cefamandole, gentamicin, tobramycin and amikacin in human serum and interstitial fluid. Antimicrob. Agents Chemother. 11:698, 1977.

Taylor, W., and Salath, L. D.: Adverse effects of antimicrobial agents. In Antimicrobial Therapy, 2nd ed. Kagan, B. M., ed. Philadelphia, W. B. Saunders, 1974.

Turner, J. R., Preston, D. A., and Wold, J. S.: Delineation of the relative antibacterial activity of cefamandole and cefamandole nafate. Antimicrob. Agents. Chemother. 12:67, 1977.

Wagman, G. H., Bailey, J. V., and Weinstein, M. J.: Binding of aminoglycosides to feces. Antimicrob. Agents Chemother. 6:415, 1974.

Watanabe, T.: Infectious drug resistance. Sci. Am. 217:19, 1965.

SELECTED REFERENCES

Alexander, R. H., Reichenbach, D. D., and Merendino, K. A.: Serratia marcescens endocarditis. Arch. Surg. 98:287, 1969.

Bassett, D. C. J., Stokes, K. J., and Thomas, W. R. G.: Wound infection with Pseudomonas multivarons. Lancet 1:1188, 1970.

Cruse, P. J. E., and Foord, R.: A five-year prospective study of 23,649 wounds. Arch. Surg. 107:206, 1973.

Howe, C. W.: Experimental studies on determinants of wound infection, II. Surgery 60:1072, 1966.

Middleton, J. E.: The sensitivity in vitro of the providencia group of enteric bacteria to 14 antibiotics and nitrofurantoin. J. Clin. Pathol. 11:270, 1958.

Seldon, R., Lee, S., Wang, W. L. L., Bennett, J. V., and Eickhoff, T. C.: Nosocomial klebsiella infections: Intestinal colonization as a reservoir. Ann. Intern. Med. 74:657, 1971.

Solberg, C. O., and Matsen, J. M.: Infection with providence bacilli. A clinical and bacteriologic study. Am. J. Med. 50:241, 1971.

Speller, D. C. E., Stephens, M. E., and Biant, A. C.: Hospital infection by Pseudomonas cepaci. Lancet 1:798, 1971.

Von Graevenitz, A.: Ewinia species isolates. Ann. NY Acad. Sci. 174:436, 1970.

Von Graevenitz, A., and Strouse, A.: Isolation of Ewinia species from human sources. Antonie van Leeuwenhoek 32:429, 1966.

GENERAL REFERENCE

Lennette, E. H., Spauldung, E. H., and Traunt, J. P. (eds.): Manual of Clinical Microbiology, 2nd ed. Washington, D.C.: American Society for Microbiology, 1974.

CHAPTER 7

MANAGEMENT OF SHOCK IN LARGE ANIMALS

WILLIAM J. DONAWICK, D.V.M.

One of the most fundamental biological principles is that the survival of an organism depends on the continuous production and expenditure of energy. The predominant energy source in biological systems is the end-product of hydrolysis of the high-energy phosphate bonds of adenosine triphosphate (ATP) and adenosine diphosphate (ADP). Consequently, depletion of the energy source is detrimental to the health of the organism; if prolonged or severe, it can lead to irreversible changes in cellular function and structural integrity that may cause the death of the cell and, ultimately, the entire organism (Schuler, Erve, and Schumer 1976). Shock in its many forms deprives cells of the building blocks of energy and threatens survival through vasoconstriction, decreased perfusion, and anoxia.

Circulatory collapse and shock are far from uncommon in large animals. Both states carry a continuing high mortality through the combined effects of delayed recognition; inadequate clinical assessment and monitoring; and failure to rapidly restore tissue perfusion, combat acidosis, and locate and eliminate hidden sites of infection.

DEFINITION OF SHOCK

Shock results when the cells of tissues and organs receive blood flow inadequate to sustain normal activities. Thus, shock is an acute circulatory insufficiency characterized by cardiac output inade-quate to provide normal perfusion for the major organs. Whether shock is associated with a generalized increased resistance to blood flow, widespread pooling or loss of blood, marked hypotension, or inability of the heart to pump enough blood peripherally is immaterial. The end result is the same: circulatory blood volume insufficient to ensure adequate cellular perfusion.

Shock is a molecular disease. Metabolic derangements of shock revolve around anaerobic glucose metabolism, which produces increased amounts of lactic acid, amino acids, fatty acids, and phosphoric acids. Metabolic acidemia produces lysosome membrane disruption with the outpouring of the lytic enzymes, causing cellular death. Associated with this anaerobic metabolism is a decreased production of the energy component ATP. This causes a derangement in protein synthesis and cell membrane pump function. Derangement of protein synthesis reduces the ability of the organism to combat shock, especially bacteremic shock, and the cell membrane pump function derangements produce cellular and mitochondrial edema.

CLASSIFICATION OF SHOCK IN LARGE ANIMALS

Shock is usually classified according to its origin: hemorrhagic, traumatic, gram-negative bacterial (also called endotoxin or septic shock), hypovolemic, or cardiogenic. Large animals rarely devel-

160

op cardiogenic, traumatic, or hemorrhagic forms of shock. There are dramatic exceptions, especially hemorrhagic shock when it occurs following laceration of the subcutaneous mammary vein in cattle or massive hemorrhage from the lungs or guttural pouch in horses. Fortunately, the incidence of these forms of severe hemorrhage is infrequent, and the loss of blood is obvious to even the most casual observer.

Unfortunately, shock in large animals usually presents as a complex systemic disease with an admixture of gram-negative bacterial disease (or at least the potential for its development), loss or sequestration of intravascular fluids causing a hypovolemia most commonly associated with the gastrointestinal tract, peritoneal soiling, infection, and acute vascular strangulation with bowel necrosis.

Clinical shock is most commonly seen with (1) severe diarrhea in the neonate, (2) colic in the horse, (3) salmonellosis, (4) gastrointestinal obstruction with or without strangulation in cattle, (5) septic mastitis, (6) peritonitis, and (7) deep wounds and abscesses.

Pathophysiology

Much of the current knowledge of the pathophysiology of shock in large animals has been gained through the study of ponies and horses given intravenous, intraperitoneal, or subcutaneous injections of endotoxin derived from the gram-negative bacterium *Escherichia coli*. These endotoxins are primarily lipopolysaccharides from the cell wall with a mixture of other components such as proteins and amino acids (Burrows 1981). Only minute quantities of endotoxin are required to produce profound effects.

Large animals (calves, horses, ponies, and pigs) appear to have an exquisite natural sensitivity to endotoxin. This sensitivity, combined with the high incidence of gastrointestinal tract disease, providing an opportunity for the uncontrolled growth of gram-negative bacteria, may predispose large animals to the ravages of shock. Compounding the problem of shock in large animals is the insidious

clinical onset often associated with ill-defined signs of disease. Often the seriousness of the disease state is not apparent until shock is well established. Traumatic, hemorrhagic, and cardiogenic shock, common in companion animals and human beings, may be more difficult to recognize and diagnose in large animals, in which these forms of shock are uncommon.

Gram-Negative Bacterial (Endotoxin) Shock in Horses and Ponies

Endotoxins have long been suspected of exerting profound pathophysiological effects in many diseases of large animals, including colic and laminitis in horses and diarrhea, strangulating obstruction of the gastrointestinal tract, trauma, septicemia, and liver disease in all large animal species. The advent of a modified Limulus amebocyte lysate assay for the detection of endotoxin in blood has made possible the laboratory verification of clinical signs indicative of endotoxemia (Meyers et al. 1982). Meyers and colleagues recently demonstrated endotoxin-like substances in horses with spontaneous gastrointestinal disease. The findings of endotoxin in cecal fluid of horses at a concentration of 80 μg/ml by Moore and associates (1981) adds a further dimension to the potential hazards should the mucosal barrier preventing absorption of these endotoxins be altered by disease. These findings have added credibility to the experimental induction of endotoxemia as a method of studying ways to avert the lethal effects of endotoxin in large animals. It is a well-recognized fact that serious errors occur when the results of endotoxin studies are extrapolated from one species to another.

EXPERIMENTAL OBSERVATIONS IN PONIES AND HORSES

When endotoxin or live *Escherichia coli* organisms are injected intravenously or intraperitoneally in ponies and horses, there is an almost immediate dose-related clinical response as well as the onset of widespread derangement of the cardiovascular system. In addition, during the first few hours of experimentally induced lethal shock, a multitude of alterations occur in blood chemical values, regional blood flow, plasma enzymes, blood gases, and available energy supplies. The duration and intensity of these changes often vary with time. The known responses of ponies to endotoxin can be conveniently summarized as follows: clinical signs, cardiovascular effects, hematological alterations, respiratory and blood-gas abnormalities, changes in blood and plasma chemical values, and pathological changes.

Clinical Signs

Within five minutes after the injection of endotoxin the first signs of shock can be seen clinically. There is an increased respiratory rate leading to acute dyspnea, restlessness, depression, and ataxia. The heart rate may decrease briefly during the injection of endotoxin, but this is soon followed by tachycardia. The color of the mucous membranes changes from pink to bluish, and there is an increase in capillary refill time. A characteristic persistent rise in temperature occurs, which is believed to be mediated by prostaglandin. Intermittent abdominal pain is followed by the simultaneous passage of formed and watery feces. If a lethal dose of endotoxin has been given, collapse and death intervene within a few minutes to a few hours.

Cardiovascular Effects

Within the first few minutes after injection of endotoxin, the mean arterial blood pressure decreases, followed quickly by compensation with return of the pressure to near pre-injection levels. After 30 minutes, hypotension returns and systemic arterial pressure remains at a low level until death. The cardiac output decreases, and pulmonary artery pressure increases sharply within minutes after injection of endotoxin, resulting in severe pulmonary hypertension. A decreased blood flow to the lungs and acute respiratory failure are the end results. The pathogenesis of the increase in pulmonary arterial pressure is believed to occur as follows:

1. Platelet and/or leukocyte aggregates form in the peripheral circulation. They filter out in the pulmonary microvasculature and mechanically restrict pulmonary blood flow.

2. Platelets and leukocytes are trapped during passage through the pulmonary vessels by primary endotoxin-induced damage to the vascular endothelium.

3. Platelet aggregates mediate the hypertensive response (the pulmonary pressor response is significantly attenuated in thrombocytopenic animals), and leukocytic aggregates play a less substantial role.

4. Vasoactive substances released by endotoxin-damaged endothelial cells, endotoxin-activated platelets, or leukocytic enzyme–damaged endothelial cells mediate the response (Moore 1982).

Pulmonary hypertension subsides as mean arterial pressure takes its second severe fall. The central venous pressure increases initially, followed by a fall to very low levels with no recovery. Capillary refill time is increased, sometimes exceeding many seconds.

Following exposure to endotoxin, there is an intense vasoconstrictive or vascular occlusion that results in an acute increase in total vascular resistance. There are exceptions to this general increase in vascular resistance: blood flow increases to the gastrointestinal tract, including the stomach and small and large intestines. Here there is a very dramatic vasodilatation of blood vessels with a redistribution of blood flow to the abdominal organs.

Blood flow to skeletal muscle is generally unchanged, as is coronary blood flow. Flow to the lungs and brain is decreased, both of which are significant events in the pathogenesis of shock.

Injection of endotoxin causes pulmonary vascular damage in the form of loss of endothelial surfaces over as much as 70 per cent of the pulmonary arteries studied (Schaub et al. 1982).

Hematological Alterations

Less than five minutes elapse before the onset of a severe leukopenia characterized by a fall in total white blood cell count. If death does not intervene, the leukopenia will be followed by a leukocytosis. Early leukopenia is believed to be due to an increased margination of leukocytes along a vascular endothelium. In some species (Hammerschmidt et al. 1978), leukopenia is complement dependent. The interaction of the toxic lipid A complement of endotoxin with circulating plasma complement activates the complement cascade, producing the margination.

Soon after the injection of endotoxin there is an increase in the packed cell volume owing to splenic contraction and the release of pooled red blood cells into the circulation. The total protein does not increase until late in the shock syndrome.

A thrombocytopenia develops and persists following injection of endotoxin. The greatest number of platelets appear to be trapped within the pulmonary microvasculature. There is evidence that endotoxin binds to the platelets, causing them to adhere to the other platelets or to the vascular endothelium (Spillvogel 1967). There is a prolongation of the activated partial thromboplastin time and an increase in fibrin degradative products indicative of coagulation factor consumption, both of which are suggestive of the presence of diffuse intravascular coagulation.

Respiratory and Blood-Gas Abnormalities

The hyperventilation following endotoxin injection causes a decrease in arterial blood carbon dioxide tension (Pa_{CO_2}) and a respiratory alkalosis. This hypocapnia is maintained because of the continued high respiratory rate.

The arterial blood oxygen tension (Pa_{O_2}) falls dramatically soon after the injection of endotoxin and is partially responsible for the increased respiratory rate. Although Pa_{O_2} decreases and cardiac depression is severe, oxygen delivery is maintained owing to an increased arterial hemoglobin concentration (Sembrat et al. 1981).

Oxygen consumption decreases because oxygen diffusion capacity is decreased. This apparently occurs because of increased peripheral resistance closing the capillaries and arteriovenous shunts, which reduces the available area for oxygen to diffuse. Oxygen diffusion is also slowed by increased capillary-to-mitochondria distance because of increasing amounts of interstitial fluid.

Changes in Blood and Plasma Chemical Values

Early in endotoxic shock there is a hyperglycemia followed by a severe, sustained hypoglycemia. Insulin levels tend to follow glucose concentrations. Endotoxin may induce hypoglycemia by increasing insulin secretion, increasing peripheral utilization of glucose, decreasing gluconeogenesis, or any combination thereof. Since it has been shown that levels of insulin decrease with the onset of hypoglycemia, it appears unlikely that the hypoglycemia is due to an increase in insulin. Since peripheral utilization of glucose decreases but uptake is near normal in shock, it is probable that decreased gluconeogenesis is responsible for the hypoglycemia. Certainly the stress of endotoxin results in the rapid depletion of hepatic glycogen stores.

Blood lactic acid increases significantly and in a linear fashion within the first hour and can reach a maximum of 400 per cent of baseline values at four to six hours. This may be due, in part, to a direct depressive effect of endotoxin on the ability of the liver to metabolize lactate. It seems fairly clear that anaerobic metabolism accounts for the major increase in lactic acid. The accumulation of lactic acid results in a decrease in available bicarbonate, a fall in pH, an increase in base deficit, and metabolic acidosis, which is only partially compensated for by the respiratory alkalosis resulting from tachypnea.

Pyruvate concentration increases, but not in direct proportion to that of lactic acid, and the result is an increasing lactate/pyruvate ratio.

In response to the stress imposed by endotoxin, plasma cortisol concentrations increase greatly. There is also an increase in testosterone and serum muscle enzyme concentrations (Moore, et al. 1983).

Concurrent with the initial pulmonary hypertension, drop in systemic arterial blood pressure, and resultant high central venous pressure is an increased thromboxane A_2 concentration. There is an increase in prostaglandins at the time of the second drop in blood pressure. The discovery of the involvement of these arachidonic acid metabolites in endotoxin shock has sparked great interest in the early use of flunixin meglumine, a drug that effectively blocks prostaglandin release from cells, to counteract many of the effects observed in early shock.

There is an increase in the cellular lysosomal enzyme β glucuronidase level, perhaps originating from the lysosomes of neutrophils. Serum β glucuronidase levels can reach 200 per cent of baseline values by two hours, with a subsequent maximal increase of approximately 350 per cent at eight hours (Burrows 1981).

Finally, β endorphin concentration increases following injection of endotoxin. There is no evidence that β endorphins released during shock are responsible for the changes in hemodynamics, blood flow, or plasma enzymes, because naloxone, an antagonist to β endorphins, was unable to prevent these endotoxin-induced changes.

Pathological Changes

Endotoxin causes widespread hemorrhage throughout the body. Changes in the lungs, some of which may be agonal, consist of pulmonary edema, atelectasis, and emphysema. The adrenal cortex may be darkened, congested, and discolored. Renal cortical necrosis may occur with severe congestion in the renal medulla with accumulation of a proteinaceous type of material in the lumen of distal tubules. There is often prominent submucosal edema, which is most common in the large colon. Occasionally there is vascular congestion and a marked infiltration of eosinophils in the lamina propria or the submucosa. In addition, there is often a variable amount of peritoneal or pericardial fluid.

RESPONSE OF OTHER LARGE ANIMAL SPECIES TO ENDOTOXIN

Endotoxin has been given experimentally to swine (Kurtz and Quast 1982) and calves (Anderson et al. 1975) as well as to ponies and horses. Pigs given continuous IV endotoxin developed early clinical signs, including salivation, retching, vomiting, tachypnea, depression, cyanosis, increased volume and frequency of defecation, urination, pyrexia, weakness, and incoordination. They also had an increased packed cell volume, leukopenia, decreased platelet counts, hypoglycemia, increased blood fibrinogen, and severe pulmonary edema and hemorrhage due to vascular thrombosis at necropsy.

Endotoxin given IV to calves caused an increase in pulmonary artery pressure after a delay of approximately 8 minutes (Anderson et al. 1975), attaining an average value of 74 mm Hg at 15 minutes. There was a fall in systemic arterial pressure and cardiac output. Corresponding to the increase in pulmonary artery pressure was an increase in the concentration of prostaglandin F from the lungs, and it appears that prostaglandin was a mediator of the endotoxin-induced pulmonary hypertension.

MONITORING IN THE MANAGEMENT OF CLINICAL SHOCK IN LARGE ANIMALS

The technology is now available to bring many of the techniques previously reserved for use in the research laboratory stall-side to improve the management of large animals in shock. Both conscious standing and anesthetized recumbent large animal patients can benefit from improved monitoring to pinpoint derangements early, while the opportunity to manage them successfully still exists.

Important, and sometimes crucial, monitoring techniques beyond the usual recording of temperature, pulse, respiration, and capillary refill time include determination of the plasma electrolytes sodium, potassium, calcium, magnesium, chloride, and bicarbonate; periodic measurement of packed cell volume and differential and total white blood cell counts; measurement of blood gases (oxygen and carbon dioxide tension) and acid-base status; determination of arterial blood pressure, central venous pressure, and pulmonary artery and pulmonary capillary wedge pressures; measurement of cardiac output; determination of plasma creatinine and urine output; measurement of plasma lactate; calculation of anion gap; electrocardiographic monitoring; and culture and antimicrobial sensitivity testing of fluid from abscesses, wounds, and cavities.

Since determination of many of these parameters has already become "routine," the discussion will be restricted to techniques not commonly employed.

Mean Arterial Blood Pressure (MABP)

Direct catheterization of an artery provides the best means of measuring arterial blood pressure in large animals in shock. Arteries commonly employed are the lateral tarsal, facial, middle auricular, median, and common carotid. Percutaneous catheterization with an 18-gauge, 5- to 8-cm indwelling plastic catheter permits direct measurement of MABP by connecting the catheter with tubing filled with saline containing 10 units/ml of sodium heparin to either a simple mercury manometer or a transducer and datascope such as the Datascope #865C, Type 2 transducer pressure module.*

A MABP of 80 ± 10 mm Hg has been recorded in normal conscious ponies and should be sought during management of the animal in shock.

Central Venous Pressure (CVP)

Central venous pressure can be measured easily with a water manometer (in cm H_2O pressure) through a 24-inch catheter introduced percutaneously into a jugular vein, passing toward the heart and stopping with the tip well within the thoracic cavity (Klein and Sherman 1977). The catheter is attached by means of tubing containing heparinized saline and a three-way stopcock to a vertical tube backed by a centimeter scale. The third arm of the three-way stopcock leads to a bottle of saline containing heparin sodium (10 units/ml), which can be used to flush the catheter and fill the centimeter tube. The scale is set at 0 by adjusting the height to the sternal midline for horses in lateral recumbency and to the notch on the lateral tuberosity of the humerus for standing horses and those in dorsal recumbency.

Normal CVP in the standing horse is 7.5 ± 1.5 cm H_2O. Administration of acetylpromazine or xylazine causes a decrease in CVP to approximately 1.0 cm H_2O. The normal CVP in horses in lateral recumbency is 21 ± 1.5 cm H_2O. The normal CVP in horses in dorsal recumbency is approximately 6.5 ± 1.5 cm H_2O.

There are several factors that cause changes in CVP. The major determinants are pumping effectiveness of the right heart (CVP is elevated with right ventricular failure) and changes in venous return caused by (1) increased or decreased resistance to blood flow from the arteries and veins, or (2) an increased or decreased ratio of blood volume to vascular-bed holding capacity. It must be remembered that positive pressure ventilation, pneumothorax, obstructive pulmonary disease, and cardiac tamponade will cause an increase in CVP.

In hypovolemic and septic shock of noncardiogenic origin, CVP has been used as a guide to intravascular fluid therapy to maintain optimal cardiac output. Since there are many potential pitfalls to the use of CVP in the management of the patient in shock, treatment would be more precise if it were on pulmonary-capillary wedge pressure, which provides a better assessment of cardiac and pulmonary function and response to therapy.

Cardiac Output (CO)

The practical measurement of cardiac output in large animals during shock must be accurate without the need for complex electronic equipment, must provide immediate results, and must have the capability of frequent and inexpensive measurements. Thermodilution measurement of CO in large animals offers many advantages over the Fick indicator-dilution and Harvey techniques. Thermodilution measurement of CO has been shown to be simple, reliable, and safe with good reproducibility (Muir, Skarda, and Milne 1976). The technique has been used effectively to determine CO in conscious ponies given endotoxin (Sembrat et al. 1981).

To perform the thermodilution measurement of CO, a No. 8 French balloon-tipped flow-directed pulmonary artery catheter is placed in the pulmonary artery and its position verified by pressure values and contour on an oscilloscope. Thirty to forty ml of 5% dextrose at 0° C are injected into the right atrium and the

*Datascope Corp., Paramus, NJ.

effect on probe temperature determined as a measure of CO. Determination of CO by thermodilution in conscious, normal horses (approximately 450 kg) has resulted in a CO of 72.2 ml/kg/min. This figure compares favorably with the results of dye-dilution techniques.

Halothane anesthesia in ponies caused a time-dependent decrease in CO, greatest within 20 minutes of onset of anesthesia and at one hour averaging 30 per cent less, or 61 ± 8.3 ml/kg/min (Hillidge and Lees 1975).

Pulmonary Artery Pressure (PAP) and Pulmonary Capillary Wedge Pressure (PCW)

Placing a balloon-tipped flow-directed thermodilution catheter into the pulmonary artery and allowing it to "wedge" in a small pulmonary end artery will permit measurement of PAP when the balloon is deflated and PCW when the balloon is inflated (Swan et al. 1970). The same catheter can be used to sample pulmonary arterial (mixed venous) blood for oxygen tension. With this information, one can evaluate left and right cardiac ventricular function and pulmonary response during shock, determine safe fluid replacement therapy, and monitor the response to therapeutic interventions with serial measurements (Kaye 1981).

Pulmonary congestion and alveolar edema will cause PCW to rise and can be expected to occur as wedge pressure rises above 20 to 25 mm Hg. Pulmonary hypertension, so characteristic of shock, even in hypovolemic states, upsets pulmonary hemodynamics and can quickly lead to pulmonary congestion and edema.

In contrast, when PCW is low during the advanced stages of shock owing to peripheral vasodilatation, especially of the gastrointestinal tract, and hypovolemia, it can signal the need for additional fluid therapy. PCW has proved to be a reliable guide to fluid therapy, allowing very rapid infusion of crystalloid solutions because repeated measurements will detect the early onset of congestive heart failure or fluid overload. In addition, optimal left heart filling pressure can be determined and maintained by repeated measurements of PCW pressure.

CLINICAL MANAGEMENT OF SHOCK IN LARGE ANIMALS

Provision for Adequate Ventilation and Oxygenation

Inadequate ventilation and oxygenation are often overlooked by the clinician preoccupied with the more obvious and seemingly pressing clinical signs of shock. Adequate ventilation and oxygenation cannot be taken for granted simply because the patient is breathing rapidly and is still able to stand. The common denominator in the shock syndrome is diminished tissue delivery of oxygen, which favors the anaerobic formation of lactic acid from pyruvate. Thus, one of the truly essential drugs in the management of shock is oxygen (O_2) (McIntyre and Lewis 1981).

Maximum oxygen saturation of hemoglobulin is achieved with an arterial blood oxygen tension (Pa_{O_2}) of 100 torr. Room air, which contains 20.93 per cent O_2, rarely has a high enough oxygen content to supply maximum oxygen saturation, even under normal conditions. During shock the large animal patient may be unable to maintain even a normal room air Pa_{O_2} because of abdominal distention, positional atelectasis, or shock-induced intrapulmonary shunting (the shock lung syndrome).

To ensure maximum oxygen hemoglobin saturation, supplemental oxygen should be provided and the flow rate later adjusted based on measurement of the Pa_{O_2} to maintain 100 torr. Supplemental O_2 can be given as humidified 100 per cent O_2 by intranasal or transtracheal catheter, endotracheal tube, or a tube inserted in a tracheostomy. Initially, an O_2 flow rate of at least 15 L/min should be given in the adult (450 kg) large animal. If this is inadequate even when given through a tracheostomy and if other possible steps have been taken to improve ventilation, consideration must be given to mechanical ventilation.

The endotracheal tube, trachea, and major bronchi should be suctioned every one to two hours. If pulmonary edema is present, it may be necessary to suction more frequently.

INCREASED Pa$_{CO_2}$

An increased Pa$_{CO_2}$ indicates hypoventilation. The consequent increased alveolar retention of CO_2 will contribute unwanted hydrogen ions to the acidosis of shock. An increased Pa$_{CO_2}$ is uncommon in large animals until the terminal stages of shock. This is fortunate, because the only treatment beyond percutaneous relief of accumulated gas, causing abdominal distention, relief of airway obstruction, and reduction of pulmonary dead space by tracheostomy, is the use of a mechanical ventilator to lower alveolar CO_2. Such ventilators are most helpful and applicable during general anesthesia but are difficult to incorporate into the management of the standing, mobile, and sometimes fractious large animal.

DECREASED Pa$_{CO_2}$

It is common to encounter a moderately decreased Pa$_{CO_2}$ following hyperventilation in large animals in shock. This is, in part, a compensatory response to an increasing metabolic acidosis and a decreasing pH, but other contributing factors are pain, anxiety, and increased respiratory rate in response to fever and exertion.

A moderate hypocapnia (Pa$_{CO_2}$ 25 to 35 torr) may improve pH until adequate tissue perfusion is restored, and bicarbonate therapy has been given to buffer the accumulated organic acids.

Continued rapid, deep, labored respirations are undesirable because of the accompanying increased exertion and expenditure of precious cellular energy stores.

MECHANICAL VENTILATION

When assisted ventilation is undertaken, it should be given with a volume-limited ventilator. An adequate tidal volume in millimeters can be estimated by multiplying the patient's weight in kilograms by 10. The inspiratory-expiratory ratio, i.e., the ratio of duration of inspiration to expiration, should be 1:2. The initial respiratory rate should be 12 times a minute. The pressure limit should be set at 10 cm H_2O higher than the pressure needed to deliver the tidal volume. The inspired air should contain 90 per cent O_2, because there is evidence that a lack of nitrogen results in complete absorption of O_2 from the alveoli, increased intrapulmonary shunting, and hypoxemia (West 1974).

In summary, the goal of ventilatory therapy is to maintain maximal O_2 hemoglobin saturation with minimal expenditure of energy for respiration. The hypercapnia of hypoventilation should be aggressively treated.

Restoration and Maintenance of Optimal Intravascular Fluid Volume

It is obvious that without restoration and maintenance of an effective circulatory volume to provide adequate tissue perfusion, the shock syndrome, once well entrenched in a large animal patient, cannot be managed successfully. Even with the aggressive use of fluids to expand the intravascular volume and replenish lost extra- and intracellular fluids the results have been discouraging. There are many reasons for this. The volume of fluid needed to resuscitate a full grown, large animal may be monumental. Monitoring of ventilation, perfusion, and cardiac function is often minimal or lacking in the clinical setting.

Yet encouraging progress is being made, especially in our understanding of the derangements caused by hypovolemia and the adaptation of principles and techniques of shock treatment in humans for the assessment of optimal levels of fluid replacement in large animals.

CHOICE OF IV SOLUTION

With the exception of the need for whole blood during massive hemorrhage, isotonic polyionic solutions containing physiologic concentrations of sodium, chloride, and potassium have received the widest acceptance for use in the restoration of intravascular and interstitial fluid deficits in shock. Lactated Ringer's solution probably should not be used in lactic acidosis; other solutions containing bicarbonate precursors are more acceptable. Initially, when large volumes of IV fluids must be administered rapidly, solutions containing dextrose should be avoided. Whenever possible, plasma should also be given, as it will increase oncotic pressure, expand the depleted intravascular volume, and reverse the hemoconcentration and stasis in the capillary circulation.

It is usually difficult to estimate the volume deficit in a hypovolemic patient. As a result, the adequacy of volume replacement must be evaluated from physical examination, clinical monitoring, and laboratory results. Restoration of mean arterial blood pressure to 80 mm Hg and CVP to 10 to 15 cm H_2O, determination of peripheral capillary refill time and heart rate, and auscultation of the lungs are the clinical yardsticks most commonly employed to assess optimal treatment while averting pulmonary edema. In small neonatal large animals, less than one liter of fluid may prove adequate, whereas a 500-kg animal may require large quantities of fluid, often in excess of 75 liters.

RATE OF VOLUME REPLACEMENT

The immediate aim of therapy is to get the patient out of danger. To accomplish this it may be necessary to administer the fluids rapidly through multiple large-bore indwelling venous catheters. Multiple catheters offer the advantage of increased rate of administration with reduced incidence of phlebitis (often caused by the turbulent flow of the fluids given rapidly through a narrow-bore catheter).

If the CVP and mean arterial blood pressure are low, rapid IV administration is safe. With successful treatment both MABP and CVP will increase. An increase in CVP without a corresponding rise in MABP indicates poor cardiac function, which may require specific treatment. Rapid administration of fluids can be continued until the CVP approaches 25 cm H_2O in laterally recumbent patients, after which the rate of fluid administration must be slowed to maintain optimal cardiac and pulmonary function.

Selection and Use of Antibiotics

At the onset of shock in large animals it is often impossible to know whether or not endotoxin produced by bacteria is a contributing factor. Certainly a multitude of microorganisms may be trapped within the strangulated intestine of the horse with an acute abdomen, many of which are capable of proliferating and producing endotoxin. Bacterial infection with production of endotoxin is more obvious in acute septic coliform mastitis in ruminants. In this situation it is sometimes possible to obtain a preliminary identification of a single type of bacteria from the mammary secretion on gram stain. Such is usually not the case in peritonitis, septic metritis, pneumonia, wounds, and abscesses, where often more than one species of bacteria is present and it is not possible to determine their relative contribution to the disease process. Even if a single species is found on culture and identified, the time needed to determine antimicrobial sensitivity will delay selection of the most appropriate antibiotic. With the possible exception of true hemorrhagic or cardiogenic shock, large animals must be treated with antibiotics capable of killing endotoxin-producing bacteria commonly encountered in the species being treated. If a single organism can be found in secretions or aspirates on gram stain and identified, and if the usual antibiotic sensitivity patterns have been established (Table 7–1), the antibiotic choice can be more specific.

When early identification of the bacteria is not possible, shock in large animals should be initially treated with high levels of penicillin G potassium combined with a potent aminoglycoside for the following reasons: (1) high systemic levels of these antibiotics can be achieved quickly; (2) they are highly effective against most strains of gram-positive and gram-negative endotoxin-producing microorganisms; (3) they are bacteriocidal; and (4) they are highly effective against most other bacteria that may be contributing to the disease.

Penicillin G potassium inhibits bacterial cell wall synthesis, resulting in destruction of susceptible bacteria. Penicillin G is particularly effective against gram-positive streptococcal bacteria, the non-penicillinase–producing strains of *Staphylococcus aureus,* and most anaerobic bacteria. Penicillin G is metabolized only to a minor degree but rapidly becomes bound to serum proteins; only unbound drug exerts antibacterial activity. Penicillin G is excreted rapidly and unchanged via renal tubules, so that its half-life is very short. Initially, penicillin G potassium is given at a dosage of 40,000 units/kg body weight IV every four hours. Penicillin G is the treatment of choice for all anaerobic bacterial infections except those caused by *Bacteroides fragilis.* Only clindamycin, chloramphenicol, and metronidazole are consistently effective against *B. fragilis* (Kagan 1980).

Neomycin, kanamycin, gentamicin, tobramycin, and amikacin, all aminoglycosides, are active against most strains of aerobic gram-negative microorganisms including most Enterobacteriaceae, such as *Escherichia coli, Klebsiella* species, *Enterobacter* species, and *Proteus* species. Tobramycin is the most active aminoglycoside against *Pseudomonas aeruginosa,* whereas kanamycin is not active against this bacteria. Gram-positive microorganisms vary in their susceptibility to the aminoglycosides. *Staphylococcus aureus* strains, including β-lactamase producers, are susceptible to aminoglycosides. Aminoglycosides are relatively inactive against anaerobic bacilli and cocci.

Aminoglycosides alter the protein synthesis of susceptible bacteria, causing death, but the exact mechanism remains unclear. They bind to the 30 S ribosomal protein. The aminoglycosides are not metabolized and are excreted primarily by glomerular filtration.

Of the available aminoglycosides, streptomycin, neomycin, kanamycin, and gentamicin have enjoyed widespread use in veterinary medicine. In serious life-threatening shock in which the threat of gram-negative infection is present, the aminoglycosides of choice are kanamycin and gentamicin. Although streptomycin and neomycin are less expensive, their narrow spectrum of activity and toxicity renders them inadequate. Tobramycin and amikacin should be reserved for use with bacteria resistant to other aminoglycosides.

Initially, gentamicin is given at the rate of 2.2 mg/kg body weight every six hours IM or buffered in an equal volume of 8.4% $NaHCO_3$ by slow IV injection. Kanamycin is usually given IM at the rate of 5 mg/kg body weight every six hours.

Some clinicians may choose to substitute ampicillin for penicillin G potassium, but at present there is little indication to do so. If less potent antibiotics are selected because of financial constraints or personal preference, it must be done so with the realization that the effectiveness of the chosen antibiotic is also probably reduced. Frequent re-evaluation of antimicrobial susceptibility patterns is mandatory because of the rapid development of bacterial resistance to commonly used antibiotics. Failure to administer an effective antibiotic may cause complications in addition to those associated with the release of endotoxin. For example, the unbridled growth of bacteria in the blood stream could conceivably cause multiple microemboli.

Penicillin G potassium is generally safe even at high intravenous levels. The use of aminoglycosides is not without risk. Renal dysfunction characterized by an elevated creatinine level is not an uncommon sequela to the systemic use of aminoglycosides.

Antibiotic treatment is not a substitute for correction of the initiating cause of shock. Prompt removal of strangulated intestine with good surgical technique, drainage of abscesses, excision of necrotic tissue, irrigation of the uterus with metritis, drainage of thoracic and peritoneal effusions, and repeated milking of infected mammary glands cannot be overlooked.

Correction of Metabolic Acidosis with Sodium Bicarbonate

Metabolic acidosis is a consistent feature of the shock syndrome regardless of its cause. It is caused by the enhanced production and accumulation of lactate from pyruvate in excess of the liver's

Table 7-1. SUSCEPTIBILITY PATTERNS OF GRAM-NEGATIVE AND GRAM-POSITIVE ORGANISMS IN LARGE ANIMALS*

Organism	No. Isolates	Antibiotic (Percent Susceptible)															
		Amikacin	Ampicillin	Cephalothin	Chloramphenicol	Clindamycin	Erythromycin	Gentamicin	Kanamycin	Methicillin	Neomycin	Nitrofurantoin	Penicillin†	Streptomycin	Tetracycline	Trimethoprim Sulfa	Triple Sulfa
Gram-Positive																	
Staphylococcus aureus	29		28	93	97	97	97	93		97		93	28		93	97	93
Group D streptococci																	
enterococcus	28		79	11	14	18	36	61		0		68	4		32	—	—
not enterococcus	4		100	50	75	100	100	75		25		75	50		25	—	—
Beta streptococcus	19		100	100	89	68	84	100		95		100	100		11	—	—
Alpha streptococcus	3		100	100	100	67	67	100		100		67	100		33	—	—
Gamma streptococcus	2		100	89	100	100	100	100		100		100	100		50	—	—
Streptococcus zooepidemicus	9		100	100	100	78	100	100		89		100	100		0	—	—
S. equi	3		100	100	100	100	100	100		100		100	100		100	100	—
Corynebacterium equi	4		50	0	75	0	100	100		0		50	0		100	100	100
Gram-Negative‡																	
Escherichia coli	106	98	52	12	61			76	38		38	91	—	15	41	59	41
Pasteurella—Actinobacillus spp.	38	89	82	89	92			92	47		39	95	37	21	87	84	71
Pasteurella spp.	15	100	93	100	100			100	87		80	93	67	67	100	93	73
P. multocida	4	100	100	100	100			100	50		50	100	100	25	100	100	75
Pseudomonas aeruginosa	35	94	0	0	0			91	3		0	0		0	0	0	9
P. fluorescens	4	100	0	0	25			100	100		100	0		25	50	25	75
P. maltophilia	2	100	0	0	50			100	50		50	0		0	0	100	100
P. putida	1	100	0	0	0			100	100		100	0		0	0	100	0
Enterobacter cloacae	16	88	0	0	38			50	50		63	63		13	31	50	44

Organism	No.													
E. agglomerans	9	100	67	78	100	89	89	89	89	—	89	89	89	89
E. aerogenes	7	100	14	29	43	71	43	43	43	—	0	29	43	43
E. sakazakii	2	100	0	0	0	0	50	50	50	—	50	50	50	0
Proteus mirabilis	13	92	77	77	23	62	62	92	8	—	31	0	77	54
P. vulgaris	13	100	8	8	23	54	38	54	0	—	38	0	46	46
Morganella morganii	2	100	0	0	50	100	100	50	58	—	50	50	50	50
Klebsiella pneumoniae	12	100	8	67	42	83	75	83	83	—	33	50	58	50
K. oxytoca	6	100	0	67	67	100	67	100	0	—	33	83	67	67
Bordetella bronchiseptica	10	100	0	60	100	100	100	100	0	0	0	100	100	100
Acinetobacter calcoaceticus														
var. anitratus	8	88	0	0	38	63	50	63	0	—	38	63	63	63
var. lwoffi	4	100	100	0	50	100	75	100	25	—	25	50	50	50
Aeromonas hydrophila	6	100	0	0	83	100	83	100	100	—	50	83	83	83
Serratia spp.	2	80	0	0	0	80	100	80	0	—	50	0	100	100
S. marcescens	5	100	0	0	80	100	100	100	25	—	100	33	100	80
S. rubidaea	3	100	0	0	100	100	100	100	100	—	100	100	100	67
S. fonticola	1	50	50	50	25	25	50	50	50	—	100	100	100	100
Alcaligenes spp.	4	100	0	0	0	0	0	25	50	—	0	0	75	75
Citrobacter diversus—Levinea	2	100	0	0	0	0	0	0	100	—	0	0	0	0
C. freundii	2	100	0	0	0	0	0	0	100	—	0	0	0	0
C. amalonaticus	1	100	0	0	100	100	100	100	100	—	100	100	100	100
Providencia stuartii	2	100	0	0	0	0	0	0	0	—	0	0	0	0
P. rettgeri	1	100	0	0	0	0	0	0	0	50	0	0	0	0
Moraxella spp.	2	100	100	100	100	0	0	100	100	—	100	100	100	0
Achromobacter xylosoxidans	2	50	0	0	0	0	100	0	0	—	0	0	100	100

*Data provided by Charles E. Benson, University of Pennsylvania; collected 7/1/82 to 12/31/82.
†Penicillin testing for non-enterobacteriaceae gram-negative organisms only.
‡As identified by analytical profile index, Analytab Products, Plainview, NY.

ability to metabolize these products of anaerobic glycolysis. Lactic acid can be temporarily buffered with sodium bicarbonate, but it will continue to accumulate until adequate circulation is restored, permitting normal tissue delivery of oxygen.

The administration of $NaHCO_3$ results in a simple acid-base reaction in which the HCO_3^- ion combines with $[H^+]$ of the lactic and pyruvic acids in the blood and thereby elevates the blood pH, as in the following equation:

$$HCO_3^- + [H^+] \rightleftarrows H_2CO_3 \rightleftarrows CO_2 + H_2O$$

The carbonic acid, H_2CO_3, formed is a weak acid and is therefore converted to CO_2 and water. The increase in pH that occurs after HCO_3^- administration is dependent on ventilatory elimination of the carbon dioxide produced.

The deleterious effects of metabolic acidosis are well established. Acidosis, particularly if the arterial pH is less than 7.10 to 7.15, can predispose the animal to potentially fatal ventricular arrhythmias and can reduce both cardiac contractility and the inotropic response to catecholamines. This decrease in ventricular function may play an important role in the perpetuation of shock-induced lactic acidosis, and the acidosis may have to be corrected before tissue perfusion can be restored (Rose 1977).

Empirically, a patient in shock should be given 1 mEq/kg body weight of sodium bicarbonate by slow IV injection. The arterial blood bicarbonate concentration should be determined as soon as possible. Subsequently, the bicarbonate or base deficit should be used to calculate bicarbonate needs according to the Golden Rule 3, as follows:

$$HCO_3^- \text{ required (mEq)} = \text{base deficit (mEq/L)} \times \frac{\text{body weight (kg)}}{3}$$

Correction of metabolic acidosis with solutions containing bicarbonate precursors such as lactate, acetate, and gluconate is inappropriate in the treatment of shock because these substances must be metabolized before HCO_3^- can become available as an antacid. Clinical experience indicates that the "bicarbonate equivalents" in solutions containing bicarbonate precursors should be ignored when calculating HCO_3^- replacement therapy, even though such solutions are most appropriate for restoring intravascular fluid volume.

Excessive sodium bicarbonate administration may result in metabolic alkalosis, with displacement of the oxyhemoglobin dissociation curve and consequent impairment of oxygen release to tissues. Hypernatremia and hyperosmolality also may develop. Excess sodium bicarbonate may produce cerebrospinal fluid acidosis because of the rapid diffusion of CO_2 across the blood-brain barrier.

Persistent metabolic acidosis also affects capillary hydrostatic pressure and intravascular fluid volume. Early capillary sphincter adjustments due to the sympathoadrenal responses of shock result in decreased capillary hydrostatic forces with intravascular volume augmentation from the extravascular tissues. Acidosis causes relaxation of the vasoconstriction at the arterial end of the capillary but not at the venous end. The net effect is the pooling of blood in the capillary circulation; hydrostatic pressure increases and fluid is pushed out of the capillaries into the interstitium.

Neither catecholamines nor calcium salts should be mixed with bicarbonate solutions, since catecholamines may be inactivated and calcium salts precipitated.

It must be remembered that the beneficial antacid effects of $NaHCO_3$ can only be achieved by providing for adequate ventilation to eliminate CO_2.

Corticosteroids

Corticosteroids, specifically the glucocorticoids, have been shown to be effective in protecting a variety of animals against shock induced by purified endotoxic lipopolysaccharides. The precise manner in which glucocorticoids protect against endotoxin challenge remains to be clarified. Glucocorticoids are believed to exert their positive effects in shock via a number of mechanisms, including stabilization of lysosomal membranes, promotion of adequate tissue perfusion during endotoxemia through vasodilatation, stimulation of hepatic gluconeogenesis, prevention of excess lactate accumulation, reduction of pulmonary inflammation and edema, prevention of increases in vascular permeability, and reduction of the release of histamine and bradykinin.

Most experimental studies to determine the efficacy of glucocorticoids have involved its use in animals given endotoxin or live *E. coli* organisms capable of producing endotoxin. In these studies the glucocorticoids have their best protective effects if given at the time of introduction of bacteria or toxin to combat the early derangements specific to endotoxin. Dramatic improvements in survival have occurred during the first few hours after treatment with glucocorticoids (Pitcairn et al. 1972). However, if viable bacteria were introduced and continued to multiply, providing a continuing source of endotoxin, a point was reached beyond which the remaining level of glucocorticoids was insufficient to counteract the ever-increasing level of endotoxin. At this point only a combination of a glucocorticoid and an effective antibiotic impeded bacterial multiplication and reduced the degree of endotoxemia (Schuler, Erve, and Schumer 1976). Based on these experimental findings, it is not surprising that dramatic and consistent improvements have not resulted from the administration of glucocorticoids to large animals in shock. Still, the potential benefits of their use far outweigh any theoretical hazards.

Corticosteroid therapy is not a substitute for maintenance of optimal intravascular fluid volume, correction of the initiating cause of shock, continued antimicrobial therapy aimed at controlling gram-negative bacteria, and correction of acidosis with bicarbonate.

Concern remains that any beneficial clinical effects derived from glucocorticoid therapy may be outweighed by its interference with the host's ability to control the infectious process. Glucocorticoids have multiple effects on the host's defense mechanisms against infection including decreased reticuloendothelial phagocytic capacity, inhibition of intracellular destruction of bacteria, retardation of macrophage replication, and

changes in the type of host cellular responses at the site of infection. Certainly, repeated treatments with glucocorticoids can and do manifest these effects, but, as currently recommended, single, large "pharmacologic" boluses have not led to detrimental effects. The use of glucocorticoids has now been established to be highly beneficial in human beings suffering septic shock in both prospective and retrospective studies with minimal complications except when prolonged, multiple-dose administration was given (Schumer 1976).

DOSAGE OF GLUCOCORTICOIDS

To achieve the most beneficial effects from glucocorticoids in the treatment of shock, the cause of the shock, dosage, route of administration, timing of administration with respect to the onset of shock, and commercial form of the glucocorticoid all appear important. Large, single, bolus doses of methylprednisolone sodium succinate, dexamethasone sodium phosphate, or hydrocortisone given IV early after recognition of shock are most beneficial.

For shock, methylprednisolone sodium succinate (30 mg/kg), dexamethasone sodium phosphate (5 mg/kg), and hydrocortisone (50 to 150 mg/kg) are given by slow (15 to 20 min) direct IV bolus. The equivalent doses in a 450-kg horse are 13.5 gm of methylprednisolone, 2.25 gm of dexamethasone, and 22.5 to 67.5 gm of hydrocortisone. There is no documented evidence that increasing body weight reduces the dosage requirement of glucocorticoid. Rather, experimental evidence substantiates the need to maintain the mg/kg dosage when extrapolating from the rat to the dog, humans, and large animals. It must be remembered that the primary effects of glucocorticoids are at the cellular level and that all cells can benefit from treatment.

Nonsteroidal Anti-Inflammatory Drugs (Phenylbutazone and Flunixin Meglumine)

The two drugs that have received the most attention with regard to their ability to abolish some of the deleterious effects of endotoxin in the horse and pony are phenylbutazone and flunixin meglumine.

Phenylbutazone is a classic anti-inflammatory drug now recognized as a prostaglandin synthesis inhibitor. When 15 mg/kg body weight, approximately three times the routine clinical dose, of phenylbutazone was given 30 minutes after an intraperitoneal injection of endotoxin followed by 10 mg/kg at 6 and 12 hours, it had a salutary effect on many of the characteristic changes associated with endotoxic shock. Phenylbutazone treatment blocked hemoconcentration, suppressed hyperglycemia and pyrexia, decreased blood lactate, decreased bicarbonate and blood pH, and prolonged capillary refill time. Treatment with phenylbutazone was not successful in preventing leukopenia, thrombocytopenia, late severe hypoglycemia, or death. The abolition of pyrexia is believed to be related directly to prostaglandin synthesis inhibition. Effects of phenylbutazone on blood lactate, blood pH, and bicarbonate are probably secondary to general improvement in peripheral vascular perfusion.

Flunixin meglumine, an analgesic with anti-inflammatory and antiprostaglandin actions, has been reported to have beneficial effects in ponies and horses when given before or soon after injection with endotoxin. At a dosage of 1.1 mg/kg body weight, flunixin meglumine administered to ponies given endotoxin prevented the development of early hyperglycemia, pulmonary hypertension, the second fall in systemic arterial blood pressure, extensive vasodilatation, increased blood flow to the gastrointestinal organs, decreased blood flow to the brain, lactic acidosis, and hypoxia. Flunixin meglumine appears to prevent increases in thromboxane A_2 (TxA_2) and prostaglandin I_2 (PGI$_2$), both of which are potent vasoactive substances (Bottoms et al. 1982). Thromboxane and prostaglandin are part of the cellular arachidonic acid metabolism. Thromboxane A_2 is produced by blood platelets and induces vasoconstriction and platelet aggregation. Prostaglandin I_2 is synthesized in vascular endothelial cells and is known to be a potent inhibitor of platelet aggregation and to cause vasodilatation. Both thromboxane A_2 and prostaglandin I_2 are unstable, with half-lives of less than three minutes.

The mechanisms of action of endotoxins appear to be complex, and inhibition of specific body responses by prostaglandin-synthesis inhibition does not by itself protect animals from the lethal effects of endotoxin. This should not be interpreted to mean that these mechanisms are not important but should indicate that there are additional mechanisms in operation during the development of the disease. Nonsteroidal anti-inflammatory drugs may provide beneficial effects in the therapy of endotoxemia; however, other therapeutic approaches, perhaps more specifically directed toward the metabolic derangements, must be utilized as well (Burrows 1981).

Heparin

The use of heparin in the treatment of endotoxemia is controversial. The rationale for heparinization evolves from (1) demonstration of endotoxin-induced intravascular thrombi, (2) reports of alterations in coagulation parameters in both clinical cases of sepsis and experimental studies, and (3) increased recognition of the pathological condition of disseminated intravascular coagulation association with endotoxemia (Proceedings 1982).

Studies of the effects of heparin in endotoxin shock have produced conflicting results. When given clinically, the recommended dosage is 150 units of sodium heparin per kg body weight given subcutaneously at multiple sites every 12 hours. This dosage has caused a gradual unexplained decrease in packed cell volume, which returns to normal when treatment is terminated.

Supplemental Treatments

ATROPINE

Atropine sulfate is a parasympatholytic drug. Its cardiac vagolytic action reduces vagal tone and thereby accelerates the rate of discharge of the sinus node of the heart. It may also improve atrioventricular (AV) conduction by the same vagolytic action.

Atropine is useful in treating severe sinus bradycardia accompanied by hemodynamically significant hypotension and when there are frequent ventricular ectopic beats. It may also be used in the presence of high-degree AV block at the nodal level. The customary dosage is 0.5 to 2.0 mg IV, repeated at five-minute intervals until the desired heart rate is achieved.

LIDOCAINE

Clinically, lidocaine may be useful in the suppression of heart dysrhythmias of ventricular origin. Discharge from ectopic foci may be suppressed because lidocaine decreases automaticity by slowing the rate of spontaneous depolarization.

Lidocaine is indicated if there is electrocardiographic evidence of premature ventricular contractions. Treatment consists of a bolus injection of 1 to 2 mg/kg body weight followed immediately by an infusion of 20 to 50 μg/kg/min (Knight 1983). It must be remembered that lidocaine has a half-life of only about eight minutes and that the intention of treatment is to initiate and sustain a therapeutic concentration of lidocaine.

Vasodilator Therapy

ISOPROTERENOL

Isoproterenol hydrochloride is a synthetic sympathomimetic amine. It is nearly a pure beta-adrenergic receptor stimulator. The potent inotropic and chronotropic properties of isoproterenol generally result in an increase in cardiac output. Isoproterenol causes a decrease in peripheral vascular resistance, but systolic pressure is usually maintained or increased after therapeutic doses of the drug owing to a proportionally greater increase in cardiac output. Mean arterial blood pressure and mean perfusion pressure may be reduced.

The recommended infusion rate for isoproterenol is 2 to 20 μg/min titrated according to the heart rate. An IV solution can be prepared by adding two 1-mg vials to 500 ml of 5% dextrose in water, producing a concentration of 4 μg/ml.

SODIUM NITROPRUSSIDE

Sodium nitroprusside is a potent, rapidly acting, direct peripheral vasodilator, affecting both arterial and venous systems. Its effect is immediate and ceases when the infusion is ended. It is useful in reducing peripheral arterial resistance. Direct venodilation decreases left ventricular filling pressure, thereby tending to relieve pulmonary congestion and decrease left ventricular volume.

The recommended average initial dose of nitroprusside ranges from 0.5 to 8.0 μg/kg/min, but much lower dosages may provide adequate vasodilation. Because of its potency and rapid action it should be administered by a microdrip regulating system. To prepare solutions for infusion, the contents of a 50-mg vial of nitroprusside should be dissolved in 2 to 3 ml of dextrose and water and then mixed with 1000 ml of dextrose and water. No diluent other than dextrose and water should be used. The solution must be wrapped promptly in aluminum foil for protection from light, since it deteriorates quickly. Solutions should be used within four to six hours.

PHENOXYBENZAMINE

Phenoxybenzamine (Regitine) is a long-acting vasodilator that acts as an alpha-adrenergic blocking agent. It is capable of releasing arterioles and venules from vasoconstriction owing to sympathoadrenal response. Its use in the experimental management of laminitis in the horse has been reported by Hood, Stephens, and Amoss (1982). The treatment has shown promise when given to horses at a dosage of 1.5 mg/kg body weight diluted in 500 ml of saline IV. One-half the dosage was repeated at 12 hours. This dosage was reported to produce alpha-adrenergic blockade that lasted approximately 72 hours.

REFERENCES

Anderson, F. L., Tsagaris, T. J., Jubiz, W., and Kuida, H.: Prostaglandin F and E levels during endotoxin-induced pulmonary hypertension in calves. Am. J. Physiol. 228:1479, 1975.

Bottoms, G. D., Templeton, C. B., Fessler, J. F., Johnson, M. A., Ewert, K. M., and Adams, S. B.: Thromboxane prostaglandin I_2 (epoprostenol) and the hemodynamic changes in equine endotoxin shock. Am. J. Vet. Res. 43:999, 1982.

Burrows, G. E.: Therapeutic effect of phenylbutazone on experimental acute Escherichia coli endotoxemia in ponies. Am. J. Vet. Res. 42:94, 1981.

Hammerschmidt, D. E., Harris, P., Wayland, J. H., and Jacob, H. S.: Intravascular granulocyte aggregation in live animals: a complement-mediated mechanism in ischemia. Blood 52:125, 1978.

Hillidge, C. J., and Lees, P.: Cardiac output in the conscious and anesthetized horse. Equine Vet. J. 7:16, 1975.

Hood, D. M., Stephens, K. A., and Amoss, M. S.: The use of alpha- and beta-adrenergic blockade as a preventative in the carbohydrate model of laminitis: a preliminary report. Newsletter of the American Association of Equine Practitioners:142, 1982.

Kagan, B. M.: Antimicrobial therapy, 3rd ed. Philadelphia: W. B. Saunders, 1980.

Kaye, W.: Invasive monitoring techniques. In Textbook of Advanced Cardiac Life Support. McIntyre, K. M., and Lewis, A. J. (eds.). Dallas: American Heart Association, 1981.

Klein, L., and Sherman, J.: Effects of preanesthetic medication, anesthesia, and position of recumbency on central venous pressure in horses. JAVMA 170:216, 1977.

Knight, A. P.: ECG of the month. JAVMA 182:126, 1983.

Kurtz, H. J., and Quast, J.: Effects of continuous intravenous infusion of Escherichia coli endotoxin into swine. Am. J. Vet. Res. 43:262, 1982.

McIntyre, K. M., and Lewis, A. J. (eds.): Textbook of Advanced Cardiac Life Support. Dallas: American Heart Association, 1981.

Meyers, K., Reed, S., Kech, M., Clem, M., and Bayly, W.: Circulating endotoxin-like substance(s) and altered hemostasis in horses with gastrointestinal disorders: an interim report. Am. J. Vet. Res. 43:2233, 1982.

Moore, A. B., Roseel, O. F., Fessler, J. F., and Bottoms, G. D.: Effects of naloxone on endotoxin-induced changes in ponies. Am. J. Vet. Res. 44:103, 1983.

Moore, J. N.: Association of endotoxin-induced hematologic alterations and pulmonary hypertension in conscious ponies. Proceedings of the First Equine Endotoxemia-Laminitis Symposium 2:67, 1982.

Moore, J. N., Garner, H. E., Shapland, J. E., and Schaub, R. G.: Equine endotoxemia: an insight into cause and treatment. JAVMA 179:473, 1981.

Muir, W. W., Skarda, R. T., and Milne, D. W.: Estimation of cardiac output in the horse by thermodilution techniques. Am. J. Vet. Res., 36:697, 1976.

Pitcairn, M., Schuler, J., Erve, P. R., Holtzman, S., and Schumer, W.: Glucocorticoid and antibiotic effect on experimental gram-negative bacteremic shock. Arch. Surg. 110:1012, 1975.

Proceedings of the First Equine Endotoxemia-Laminitis Symposium 2:1, 1982.

Rose, D. B.: Clinical physiology of acid-base and electrolyte disorders. New York: McGraw Hill, 1977, p. 341.

Schaub, R. G., Moore, J. N., Garner, H. E., and Shapland, J. E.: Pulmonary vascular damage in a pony induced by endotoxin: effect of lidocaine. Proceedings of the First Equine Endotoxemia-Laminitis Symposium, 2:87, 1982.

Schuler, J. J., Erve, P. R., and Schumer, W.: Glucocorticoid effect on carbohydrate metabolism in the endotoxin-shocked monkey. Ann. Surg. 183:345, 1976.

Schumer, W.: Steroids in the treatment of clinical septic shock. Ann. Surg. 184:333, 1976.

Schumer, W., and Sperling, R.: Shock and its effect on the cell. JAMA 205:215, 1968.

Sembrat, R., DiStazio, J., Maley, W., and Stremple, J.: Oxygen consumption changes in septic pony. Am. J. Vet. Res. 42:1944, 1981.

Spillvogel, A. R.: An ultrastructural study of the mechanisms of platelet endotoxin interaction. J. Exp. Med. 126:235, 1967.

Swan, H. J. C., Ganz, W., Forrester, J., Marcus, H., Diamond, G., and Chonette, D.: Catheterization of the heart in man with use of a flow-directed balloon-tipped catheter. N. Engl. J. Med. 283:447, 1970.

West, J. B.: First annual SCCM lecture: Pulmonary gas exchange in the critically ill patient. Crit. Care Med. 2:171, 1974.

CHAPTER 8

ANESTHESIOLOGY FOR THE LARGE ANIMAL SURGEON

INTRODUCTION

All anesthetic dosages are ordered according to the particular species and the physiological condition of the individual animal. Experience in the "state of the art" technology is important for the anesthesiologist. If you rarely administer anesthetics, you are safest using techniques with which you are familiar rather than adopting new fads with each anesthetic. Once experience with anesthesia is gained, inhalation techniques are the most universal and the most freely extrapolated from case to case. Injectable agents and recipes are the most variable and should not be extrapolated freely from species to species or case to case. In this section, the authors will deal with the safest, most practical technique applicable to each species for the common surgical and anesthetic needs today. Usually, the horse, by its "fight or flight" nature, is given general anesthesia for convenience and safety to the operator and patient. The ruminant accepts mechanical restraint well for local and regional anesthesia but can be given general anesthesia, with more risk owing to respiratory and gastrointestinal functions. Swine are also more at risk and are anesthetized less frequently in practice.

EQUINE INHALATION ANESTHESIA

E. P. STEFFEY, V.M.D., Ph.D.

Inhalation anesthesia is defined as general anesthesia produced by the controlled administration of gaseous or volatile agents via the respiratory system. Its increasing usage in equine medicine and surgery is generally acknowledged as a major factor in reducing patient morbidity and mortality and has supported many important advances in surgical and diagnostic techniques.

The popularity of inhalation anesthesia is primarily dependent upon its ease of control, because the uptake and elimination of inhaled anesthetic agents is largely affected by the respiratory and circulatory systems. Hence, if the level of general anesthesia is insufficient, the inspired concentration of the agent may be elevated. Conversely, if the depth of anesthesia has become excessive, the inspired concentration may be decreased and surplus agent will be eliminated by ventilation.*

Although the relative ease of control of anesthetic depth is of major concern, inhalation anesthesia affords other decided advantages over general anesthesia maintained via intravenous or intramuscular injection. An anesthetic delivery apparatus or machine is usually used to administer the inhaled anesthetic agent. This equipment includes a source of oxygen (O_2), a reservoir rebreathing bag or bellows, and an endotracheal tube or catheter. This equipment contributes significantly to the physiological support of the anesthetized equine patient. For example, supplemental O_2 aids the achievement and maintenance of a suitable alveolar/arterial oxygen concentration. Monitoring rebreathing bag excursions permits an assessment of the anesthetized horse's respiration and, if desirable, permits manual or mechanical compression of the reservoir to improve ventilation. The endotracheal tube permits the maintenance of a patent airway and isolates the respiratory tract from potential contaminants.

Unfortunately, the relative cost of anesthetic vapors, gases, and delivery equipment and the size and seeming complexity of anesthetic delivery equipment and its proper use sometimes limit its clinical availability.

INHALATION ANESTHETIC AGENTS

THE IDEAL AGENT

Unfortunately, the ideal inhalation anesthetic for the horse is not yet available. Presumably this agent should be chemically stable, nonflammable, nonexplo-

sive, economical, compatible with existing anesthetic apparatus and ancillary drugs, and readily accepted by the horse. Such an agent could be either a volatile liquid or a gas. If a liquid, the vapor pressure should be sufficiently high at ambient temperatures to ensure attaining anesthetic concentrations. The solubility of the anesthetic in blood (as evidenced by the blood/gas solubility or partition coefficient) should be low enough so that the agent's partial pressure within the lung may be rapidly changed. This also facilitates a rapid anesthetic induction and recovery. The agent's oil and rubber solubility should be low enough so that little agent is stored in fat and in the anesthetic delivery apparatus. Low solubility in rubber and fat would minimize prolonged anesthetic recoveries.

The agent should be sufficiently potent to produce reversible sleep, profound analgesia, immobility, and skeletal muscle relaxation at concentrations that permit adequate patient oxygenation and tissue perfusion.

The compound should be inert, rapidly and completely eliminated unchanged via the lungs, and nontoxic to all organs of the body.

CURRENT AGENTS

Virtually all inhalation anesthetics available for clinical administration in man have been investigated for use in the horse. Some of these agents have been discarded as others, more promising, have become known.

Currently, halothane is most popular for use in the horse. Methoxyflurane and nitrous oxide (N_2O) are of limited current interest, and their general physical, chemical, and pharmacological properties will be summarized. Discussion of diethyl ether (commonly referred to as ether) and two new isomeric halogenated ethers, isoflurane and enflurane, will also be briefly included. Because this is not intended as an exhaustive compendium, agents such as chloroform and cyclopropane, which in recent times have come to be regarded as unfavorable in the horse owing to their explosiveness, flammability, and toxicity, will not be reviewed.

---

*Although inhalation anesthetic agents are metabolized in the body to varying degrees, metabolism does not represent a major mode of anesthetic agent elimination.

Chemical and Physical Characteristics

The chemical and physical properties of inhalation anesthetic agents of clinical importance to the equine anesthetist are indicated in Table 8–1. For an in-depth review of these properties the reader is referred to a textbook of anesthesia (Adriana 1962; Collins 1976; Gray and Nunn 1981; Hall 1971; Lumb and Jones 1973; Soma 1971; Miller 1981).

Pharmacological Characteristics

POTENCY

The potency of an anesthetic drug is described by the position on a dose response curve of an effective dose within the brain. Because the alveolar concentration of an inhaled anesthetic is the most readily measured index of brain anesthetic tension, potency has come to be defined in terms of this concentration (Eger, 1974). The *minimal alveolar concentration* (MAC) of an inhaled anesthetic is that concentration that just prevents purposeful movement of an unpremedicated animal in response to a painful stimulus. Since potency varies inversely with the magnitude of the dose required to produce a given effect (i.e., purposeful movement), potency may be defined as the reciprocal of MAC (i.e., 1/MAC). MAC is also useful for comparing the pharmacological effects of inhaled anesthetics on an equipotent basis.

MAC values for a variety of inhaled agents have been determined in the horse and are given, along with useful inspired concentration data, in Table 8–2. It must be stressed that MAC implies *alveolar* concentration, which is usually less than the *delivered* (from the vaporizer) or the *inspired* anesthetic concentration. The difference between the alveolar and inspired anesthetic concentrations is related to such variables as agent solubility, carrier gas flows, anesthetic delivery system volume, and efficiency of ventilation (Steffey and Howland 1977). Anesthetic potency and, therefore, MAC are significantly influenced by a variety of clinical variables. For example, hypothermia and concomitant drugs such as barbiturates, narcotics, and ataractics increase anesthetic potency and therefore reduce MAC and the delivered anesthetic concentration required for clinical purposes. Conversely, hyperthermia and youth may increase MAC (Egér 1974). Alveolàr anesthetic concentrations necessary for surgical intervention are generally 20 to 30 per cent greater than MAC.

CIRCULATORY EFFECTS

Inhaled anesthetics without exception depress circulatory function. They diminish myocardial contractility in a dose-related fashion. Only diethyl ether and N_2O in low doses counteract this depression through stimulation of the sympathetic nervous system.

In the horse, dose-related circulatory depression produced by halothane, methoxyflurane, enflurane, or isoflurane is usually manifested by a decrease in arterial pressure, cardiac output, and stroke volume (Hall 1971; Lumb and Jones 1973; Soma 1971; Eberly et al. 1968; Steffey et al. 1977a; Steffey 1978; Steffey and Howland 1978a; 1980). The addition of N_2O to light halothane anesthesia may cause less depression of cardiac output than would an equipotent anesthetic level of halothane-O_2 (Steffey and Howland 1978b). Whereas the horse's heart rate usually decreases from the awake to the anesthetized state, changes in heart rate accompanying alteration in anesthetic depth are more variable and depend on the anesthetic agent and mode of ventilation.

Reductions in circulatory function accompany increasing concentrations of the halogenated compounds. Depressant effects are most profound during controlled mechanical ventilation and, at least during halothane anesthesia, in the absence of surgical stimulation (Steffey 1978; Steffey and Howland 1978a; Hall, Gillespie, and Tyler 1968). Evidence suggests that isoflurane depresses cardiac output and stroke volume significantly less at moderate and deep levels of anesthesia than does halothane (Steffey and Howland 1980).

Inhaled halogenated anesthetics sensitize the myocardium to catecholamines

Table 8–1 SOME PHYSICAL AND CHEMICAL PROPERTIES OF INHALATION ANESTHETIC AGENTS

	Diethyl Ether	Enflurane	Halothane	Isoflurane	Methoxyflurane	Nitrous Oxide
Common name	Ether	Ethrane	Fluothane	Forane	Metofane, Penthrane	Nitrous Oxide
Structure	$CH_3CH_2OCH_2CH_3$	$CHFClCF_2OCF_2H$	$CF_3CHClBr$	$CF_3CHClOCF_2H$	$CHCl_2CF_2OCH_3$	N_2O
Molecular weight	74	184	197	184	164	44
Appearance	Colorless, clear volatile liquid	Colorless volatile liquid	Colorless, clear, volatile liquid	Clear volatile liquid	Colorless, clear volatile liquid	Stored as a gas
Odor	Pungent	Pleasant, ethereal	Sweet, pleasant	Pleasant	Pleasant, fruity	Pleasant
Flammability (in anesthetic range)	Yes	No	No	No	No	No
Vapor pressure (mm Hg at 20°C)	442	180	243	250	23	Gas at room temperature
Vapor concentration (% saturated at 20°C)	58	24	32	33	3	100
Boiling point (C at 760 mm Hg)	36.2	56.5	50.2	48.5	104.7	−88.4
Partition coefficient Blood/Gas (at 37°C)	12.1	1.9	2.3	1.4	13.0	0.47
Oil/Gas (at 37°C)	65	98	224	98	970	1.4
Rubber/Gas (at 23°C)	58	74	120	62	630	1.2

Table 8–2 USEFUL ANESTHETIC CONCENTRATIONS FOR THE HORSE*

	Induction†	Maintenance†	MAC‡
Methoxyflurane	3	0.25–1.5	0.3
Halothane	3–5	1–3	0.9
Isoflurane	3–5	1.2–3.5	1.3
Enflurane	4–7	2–5	2.1
Diethyl Ether	10–30	4–10	(3.0, dog)‡
Nitrous Oxide	50–60	<60	205

*Agents are listed in order of decreasing potency (i.e., increasing MAC)
†Volume per cent
‡MAC values not determined in the horse

and increase the risk of ventricular fibrillation. Subjects anesthetized with halothane appear most sensitive (and with methoxyflurane least sensitive) to the arrhythmic effects of epinephrine (Hunson and Tucker 1975; Johnson, Eger, and Wilson 1976; Zahed et al. 1977; Lees and Tavernor 1970).

RESPIRATORY EFFECTS

Respiratory depression generally accompanies inhalation anesthesia. This concept is based on studies of ventilation and the partial pressure of carbon dioxide in arterial blood ($Paco_2$) during general anesthesia. As alveolar ventilation decreases, $Paco_2$ increases. Hypoventilation exists when $Paco_2$ is above normal resting values (i.e., above 40 mm Hg). Conversely, as alveolar ventilation increases, $Paco_2$ decreases (presuming an unchanging metabolic rate).

Halothane, enflurane, and isoflurane induce hypoventilation in the horse (Steffey et al. 1977a; Steffey 1978; Steffey and Howland 1978a; 1980). The magnitude of hypoventilation is in direct proportion to the alveolar anesthetic dose. Hence, the deeper the plane of anesthesia the greater the reduction in ventilation and the greater the rise in $Paco_2$. Except for the greater absolute $Paco_2$ values for a comparable anesthetic dose in the horse, these trends are similar to findings in other species (Munson et al. 1966; Nunn 1977; Steffey et al. 1975). Comparable studies in the horse involving methoxyflurane are not available. However, little difference is noted in other species in the respiratory depressant properties of approximately equipotent doses of halothane and methoxyflurane

(Larson et al. 1969). Personal clinical and limited laboratory experience suggests that methoxyflurane is no less depressing to ventilation in the horse than is halothane. Similar studies defining the effects of diethyl ether have not been reported for the horse. However, in dogs and humans, ether causes the least depression to ventilation of commonly available agents (Hall 1971; Lumb and Jones 1973; Soma 1971; Larson et al. 1969). At light-to-moderate surgical levels of ether anesthesia of humans, average $Paco_2$ values remain at or below the person's conscious value. This indicates that ventilation is either spared or stimulated at light planes of ether anesthesia.

The respiratory pattern of the unpremedicated, surgically unstimulated anesthetized horse varies with the anesthetic agent and concentration. For example, in a recent study the respiratory frequency (f) of horses anesthetized with halothane remained relatively constant over a wide range of anesthetizing doses (Steffey et al. 1977a; Steffey 1978). On the other hand, if studies in man apply to the horse, an increasing f would be expected as the concentration of methoxyflurane or ether increased. Conversely, horses anesthetized with isoflurane usually breathe at a lower f/min, and increasing alveolar anesthetic concentration may cause a progressive reduction in f (Steffey et al 1977a; Steffey and Howland 1980).

At very deep levels of anesthesia f decreases for all anesthetics. The average alveolar concentration at which the horse's spontaneous respiratory effort ceases for at least one minute (i.e., the apneic concentration) is 2.3 per cent, 3.23 per cent, and 4.91 per cent for halothane, isoflurane, and enflurane, respectively (Steffey et al. 1977a). Although not reported for the horse, alveolar concentrations of about 7.5 per cent for ether and 0.58 per cent for methoxyflurane. (i.e., 2.3 to 2.5 times MAC) would presumably also result in apnea. With the possible exception of diethyl ether, all studied anesthetics induce a decrease in the breath volume (i.e., tidal volume) as anesthetic dose increases (Munson et al. 1966; Nunn 1977; Larson et al. 1969).

Normally, the arterial oxygen concentration (Pao_2) is about 80 to 100 mm Hg in the awake, standing, healthy horse breathing air at sea level. The Pao_2 may be above 100 mm Hg in the horse when the inspired oxygen concentration is high. Values of 450 mm Hg or greater are not uncommon in anesthetized humans and dogs breathing 95 per cent or greater oxygen (Nunn 1977). Studies have shown that adequacy of oxygenation in the horse is particularly sensitive to the effects of general anesthesia and recumbency. Arterial Po_2 is usually less than predicted in the spontaneously breathing, anesthetized horse (Steffey et al. 1977a; Hall, Gillespie, and Tyler 1968; Steffey et al. 1977b; Gillespie, Tyler, and Hall 1969). This observation appears primarily related to the depth of general anesthesia, the body position, and the mode of ventilation rather than to specific inhaled agents. Presumably these findings are a result of hypoventilation, mismatching of ventilation to perfusion, and vascular shunts (Hall, Gillespie, and Tyler 1968; Nunn 1977; Gillespie, Tyler, and Hall 1969). When N_2O is used to supplement general anesthesia in the spontaneously breathing healthy horse, maximal inspired concentrations of 50 per cent or less are usually necessary to ensure an adequate Pao_2 (Steffey and Howland 1978b). Mechanical positive pressure ventilation should accompany the use of N_2O to minimize the influence of hypoventilation on the adequacy of Pao_2. Devices to determine the inspired O_2 concentration or the Pao_2 or both are most helpful if the use of N_2O is frequent.

With the exception of diethyl ether, the inhaled anesthetics currently in use for the horse are not particularly irritating to the upper or lower respiratory tract. Because of the significant increase in respiratory tract secretions, atropine is usually administered prior to ether anesthesia.

OTHER CLINICALLY IMPORTANT EFFECTS

When N_2O is used during induction, a large gradient exists between the inspired gases and the arterial blood. Accordingly, a large volume of N_2O is taken up by the blood during the early moments of anesthesia. This uptake of large volumes of the first or primary gas (i.e., N_2O) accelerates the uptake of a second, concurrently administered gas (e.g., halothane) and is known as the second gas effect. The clinical implication of this effect is a hastened anesthetic induction. It is important to note that this phenomenon is of significance only during the first 5 to 15 minutes of induction, since uptake of large volumes of N_2O is limited to this period (Eger 1974; Epstein et al. 1964).

At the termination of N_2O administration, a large N_2O partial pressure gradient exists between the arterial blood and the alveoli, and a correspondingly large volume of N_2O diffuses into the alveoli. If the patient is allowed to breathe air (i.e., inspired O_2 concentration of about 20 per cent), alveolar O_2 is diluted, decreasing the alveolar partial pressure of O_2 and thus the alveolar-arterial O_2 diffusion gradient. Hypoxemia ensues ($Pao_2 < 80$ mm Hg) (Fink 1955). This may be prevented by allowing the horse to breathe 100 per cent O_2 at high delivery flow rates for at least 10 to 15 minutes prior to termination of anesthesia and air breathing.

The partial pressure of N_2O in blood causes it to diffuse into air-containing cavities until equilibrium is approached. Because N_2 is significantly less soluble in blood than N_2O, air-containing cavities in the body expand as a result of the rapid diffusion of N_2O into the cavity from the blood. This can cause considerable distension of the bowel during prolonged anesthesia (Steffey et al. 1979; Moens and DeMoor 1981). This may be of particular concern in horses prone to aerophagia (cribbing).

Abnormal muscle movements and

EEG evidence of cerebral irritability are common findings during enflurane anesthesia in a variety of species including the horse (Steffey et al. 1977a; Steffey 1978; Klide 1978; Joas, Stevens and Eger 1971; Neigh, Garman, and Harp 1971). Abnormal muscle twitching, especially about the head and forelimbs, is intensified by increasing alveolar doses of enflurane. In some horses, loud noise, vibrations, and painful stimuli intensify the abnormal activity, Similar abnormal activities have not been reported accompanying other inhaled anesthetics in the horse.

The first reported clinical suspect of malignant hyperpyrexia in the horse was reported in 1975 by Klein. A subsequent report verified the anesthetic sensitivity of muscle of some horses (Rosenberg and Waldron-Maese 1977). This syndrome, first noted in the medical literature in 1922, is characterized in humans by an abrupt rise in body temperature (greater than 40° C or 104° F) during the administration of inhalation anesthesia (usually halothane). The rise in core temperature usually begins early in the course of anesthesia and, if not controlled, continues to rise rapidly. Hypercapnia, hypoxemia, metabolic acidosis, cardiovascular collapse, and death ensue (Collins 1976).

The effect of inhaled anesthetics and general anesthesia on hepatic and renal function in the horse has not been extensively evaluated. However, work to date suggests that most general anesthetics do not usually produce marked hepatocellular damage in normal healthy animals (Gopinath, Jones, and Ford 1970; Lees, Mullen, and Tavernor 1973; Steffey et al. 1980; Steffey, Zinkl, and Howland 1979; Wolff, Lumb, and Ramsay 1967). The incidence of liver dysfunction may increase in the presence of certain predisposing factors such as nutritional deficiency, hypoxia, hypercapnia, and hepatic hypoperfusion (Gray and Nunn 1971).

Alterations in renal functions have been observed in a variety of animals with many of the inhalation anesthetic agents in common use. It is probable that most of the observed changes accompanying general anesthesia resulted from variations in renal blood flow and are transient in nature (Gray and Nunn 1971). A toxic nephropathy has been reported in man and some laboratory animals following methoxyflurane anesthesia (Crandell, Pappas, and MacDonald 1966; Mazze, Shui, and Jackson 1971; Mazze, Cousins, and Kosek 1972; Cousins and Mazze 1973). It is characterized by a high output renal failure and is related to the dose and duration of exposure to methoxyflurane and the production of a metabolite, fluoride ion. However, similar observations have not been reported for the horse.

This risk of anesthesia with inhaled anesthetics may not be limited to the patient. Studies with man and animals have called attention to the presence of trace concentrations of anesthetic gases in the operating room atmosphere and suggest a potential health hazard to personnel chronically exposed (Best and McGrath 1977; Cohen, Bellville, and Brown 1971; Cohen et al. 1974; Dreesen, et al. 1981; Mazze 1980; Ward and Byland 1982; Wingfield et al. 1981). Possible hazards include reproductive defects, altered behavior or performance, hepatic and renal disease, and cancer. The data to date remain equivocal and suggest that if a hazard is present the magnitude is very small. The most convincing, though much debated, evidence is an exposure-related increase in the risk of spontaneous abortion among exposed females. In view of the suggestive evidence of human health problems associated with chronic trace anesthetic exposure, methods for reduction and control of anesthetic exposure levels are warranted (Manley and McDonell 1980).

ANESTHETIC DELIVERY APPARATUS

The function of an inhalation anesthetic delivery apparatus is to supply adequate and known quantities of anesthetic and O_2 to the horse's lungs. In so doing, it must *not* significantly compromise the horse's breathing efforts or efficiency by either increasing respiratory dead space and permitting the rebreathing of metabolically produced CO_2 or increasing the resistance to gas flow and ventilation. It is desirable that the apparatus be relatively simple in construction and repair and economical to purchase and maintain. The ability to mechanically assist or control the horse's ventilation is also most helpful.

In general, an anesthetic delivery apparatus includes: 1) gas delivery equipment, 2) volatile liquid anesthetic vaporizer(s), 3) breathing circuit, and 4) endotracheal equipment. The apparatus may also include a mechanical lung ventilator. Space limitations do not permit an extensive review of the individual components, and the reader is referred to appropriate texts and articles for further evaluation of their functions and use.

Gas Delivery Equipment

The function of the gas delivery equipment is the preparation of gas mixtures of pure and precisely known yet variable composition. The gases must be delivered to the vaporizer and/or the breathing system in volumes appropriate for the horse and the individual anesthetic agent or technique. Major components of the equipment include: 1) the gas source; 2) the pressure gauge, which indicates the pressure of the gas at the source (generally a compressed gas cylinder) 3) the gas-reducing valve or regulator, which converts a high, variable gas pressure from the source to a lower, constant pressure suitable for use with flow meters; 4) the flow-control valve and meter, with which the flow rate of the gas is adjusted and measured; and 5) the O_2 flush valve, which directs O_2 at high flows directly to the breathing system. Depending on the manufacturer and the wishes of the anesthetist, the apparatus may also include: 1) a gas cylinder yoke; 2) a gas pipeline connection, which connects a hospital's centralized gas pipeline system to the anesthetic apparatus; 3) an oxygen failure safety valve, which stops the flow of anesthetic gases when O_2 pressure falls below a preset value; 4) an alarm device that warns when O_2 pressure is low; and 5) a back pressure safety device, which prevents the transmission of excessive pressures from the breathing system backing up into the gas delivery equipment (Dorsch and Dorsch 1975).

Vaporizers

The function of the vaporizer is to convert volatile liquid anesthetic to a gas phase of known composition. The vaporizer may be positioned within the circuitry of the gas delivery system (out of circuit) or within the breathing system (in circuit).* The positioning of the vaporizer, in part, determines the requirement for a simple, inexpensive (in circuit) vaporizer or a complex, relatively expensive, precision vaporizer (out of circuit). Each vaporizer position has both advantages and disadvantages, which have been reviewed (Dorsch and Dorsch 1975; Mapleson 1960; Galloon 1960; Mushin and Galloon 1960; Eger and Epstein 1964; Thurmon and Benson 1981). Today, most anesthetic apparatuses commercially available in the United States for equine use are equipped with out of circuit vaporizers.

Breathing Circuit

The function of the breathing circuit (system) is to deliver the intended gaseous mixture to the horse's lungs. A variety of systems are currently available for the horse, with no single system enjoying universal application.

In general, systems for delivering inhalation anesthetics can be divided into four categories. The following simplified classification is adapted from Moyers (1953) and is based on the presence or absence of: 1) a reservoir bag, and 2) the rebreathing of expired gases. The rational selection and clinical use of a technique requires an understanding of its function and method of operation.

OPEN TECHNIQUE

Open circuits are devoid of reservoir bags, and no rebreathing of exhaled gases occurs. They are the simplest of the anesthetic systems and include the anesthetic techniques of open drop and insufflation.

---

*The designations "in circuit" and "out of circuit" have traditionally been related to the breathing circuit or system.

Open drop techniques have been described and used on the horse (Hall 1971). However, they have little importance to contemporary equine inhalation anesthesia.

Insufflation is a technique whereby anesthetic gases and/or O_2 is administered by allowing the gases to flow in the vicinity of the horse's airway. During inspiration, the inhaled mixture is composed of gas coming from the gas delivery equipment and vaporizer via the delivery tube plus room air breathed through the nose. Dead space is minimal. The technique is sometimes employed for brief periods during anesthetic induction of foals (Langley 1972) or severely physiologically stressed horses or during brief periods of inhalation anesthesia in which tracheal intubation is not convenient or possible (Steffey 1979). Oxygen is also frequently administered to the postanesthetic recumbent horse via insufflation.

The principal disadvantages of the technique are the high flows of gas required, the inability to confine anesthetic gas to the breathing system, and the difficulty in maintaining a stable state of anesthesia owing to the dilution of the anesthetic mixture with room air. Dilution is greatest when the patient's respiratory volume and flow rate are greatest and the flow from the delivery machine is lowest.

SEMIOPEN TECHNIQUE

The semiopen technique, if used properly, also does not permit rebreathing of expired gases. A reservoir bag is incorporated within the system. This system is most familiar to the small animal practitioner who commonly anesthetizes patients less than 10 to 15 kg. Systems such as the modified Ayre's T piece and the Magill apparatus are rarely applicable to clinical equine anesthesia and therefore will not be further discussed.

SEMICLOSED AND CLOSED TECHNIQUES

The semiclosed and closed anesthetic delivery techniques are rebreathing techniques and are most commonly employed for equine inhalation anesthesia. The semiclosed circuit includes a reservoir bag. Part of the patient's exhaled gases pass into the atmosphere and part mixes with fresh gases and is rebreathed. Rebreathing of exhaled gases can take place because a chemical absorbent is placed within the breathing circuit, which prevents inhalation of gases rich in CO_2. The closed technique differs from the semiclosed technique only in that complete rebreathing of expired gas occurs and all CO_2 is chemically absorbed. In a completely closed circuit fresh gas inflow is equal to the patient's oxygen requirements (consumption) plus his uptake of anesthetic gases.

Because CO_2 is chemically absorbed, lower total gas flows are possible, providing the advantages over open and semiopen techniques of economy of life support and anesthetic gases and minimal anesthetic pollution of the immediate environment. At the same time, however, circuit denitrogenation is accomplished more slowly and induction of anesthesia and alteration of anesthetic depth is noticeably delayed (Tevik et al. 1969; Steffey and Howland 1977).

The circle and to-and-fro absorber systems are used for the semiclosed and closed anesthetic techniques. Although either system may be used for the inhalation anesthetic management of the horse, the circle system is the most widely used anesthetic delivery circuit in this country (Fisher and Jennings 1957; 1958; Weaver 1960; Tavernor 1961; Fowler et al. 1963; Thurmon 1972; Rex 1972). It is also the most complex and expensive system in use. The components of this system include a CO_2 absorber, a reservoir bag, inspiratory and expiratory valves (which route inspired-expired gases in a one-way circular pattern through the absorber and hence the system's name), a pop-off (gas overflow) valve, two corrugated breathing tubes, a Y piece, and an anesthetic/fresh gas delivery port.

Two system sizes are available for equine use. The adult human circle absorber system, available on most standard (human or small animal) anesthetic delivery apparatuses, is most suitable for foals and small ponies up to about 100 to 150 kg (220 to 231 lbs). The large animal circle absorber system is commercially available for horses. Descriptions and evaluations of available systems appear elsewhere (Hall 1971; Soma 1971; Weaver 1960; Fowler et al. 1963; Thurmon 1972; Rex 1972; Purchase 1965; Short 1970; Thurmon and Benson 1981).

The to-and-fro system is the simpler of the two rebreathing techniques. It consists only of a CO_2 absorber and a reservoir bag positioned in series, a pop-off valve, and an anesthetic/fresh gas delivery port. The expired gases pass to and from the reservoir bag (i.e., to and fro) through the CO_2 absorber. The decided advantage of this system is that it may be easily disassembled and transported. Consequently, it has been favored by some for providing inhalation anesthesia in the field. However, there are hazards of the patient accumulating CO_2 as a small amount of absorbent is exhausted, respiratory gas heat accumulates, and the greater possibility of inhaling dust from the absorbent. Despite its value in certain circumstances, the system enjoys only limited use in this country (Tavernor 1961; Thurmon 1972; Thurmon and Benson 1981).

Face Mask and Endotracheal Equipment

FACE MASK

The use of a face mask enables the anesthetist to administer anesthetic or life-support gases from the anesthetic delivery apparatus without having to intubate the horse's trachea. The face mask is most useful when attempting to induce inhalation anesthesia in awake foals or small ponies and for pre- or postanesthetic supplemental O_2 therapy.

Suitable equine face masks are intermittently commercially available or can be easily fabricated from disposable plastic or rubber bottles.

TRACHEAL TUBES

Intubation of the trachea is advantageous for a host of reasons. A partial list includes the following: 1) the patency of the airway is reasonably assured, 2) anatomical respiratory dead space is reduced, and 3) mechanical control of ventilation is facilitated.

Tracheal tubes are usually made of natural or synthetic rubber or a polymer (e.g., polyvinyl chloride, nylon, and so on) and are available in a variety of sizes (Hodges 1977; Heath 1974; 1976; Lodge 1969). An inflatable balloon or cuff is present on some tracheal tubes, which allows a leak-resistant fit between the tube and the trachea. To prevent tracheal damage, care must be taken not to overinflate the cuff after proper placement. Recently, a "Cole-type" cuffless tube was introduced for use in the horse (Heath 1974; 1976).

In selecting the proper tracheal tube for the horse, due consideration must be accorded anatomical features of the upper airway, possible tramatic airway damage, anatomical dead space, and resistance to respiratory gas flow (Lodge 1969). In general, the largest size endotracheal tube that can be easily passed into the trachea should be used.

Mechanical Ventilator

Various devices have been developed to augment or replace the anesthetized horse's own respiratory efforts when satisfactory spontaneous ventilation is diminished or absent (Hansson and Johannisson 1958; Weaver 1967; Smith 1971; Thurmon, Menhusen, and Hartofield 1975; Beerwinkle and Witzel, 1976). All units in current use for ventilating anesthetized horses operate by raising upper airway pressure to a preset level, thereby producing the necessary pressure gradient needed to move a volume of air into the animal's lungs.

Although a variety of descriptions of positive pressure breathing devices suitable for use on large animal patients have appeared worldwide in the past decade, most devices used in this country incorporate a large animal anesthetic reservoir "bag in a bottle" arrangement. In this system, a bag is suspended within a bottle or sealed drum. The bag is compressed by gas delivered from a ventilator during its inspiratory phase. Most recently, a concertina-type bellows replacement for the bag has become available commercially. Although the reservoir bag offers greater convenience for replacement and economy, the movement of the bellows with inspiration is easier to quantify. The ventilator used to drive the bag in bottle system is usually a modified version of one designed specifically to produce intermittent positive pressure ventilation in humans (Soma 1971; Thurman; Menhusen, and Hartofield 1975; Skarda, Boehes, and Fackelman 1974; Steffey and Berry 1977; Steffey 1981).

Currently, at least two complete intermittent positive pressure anesthesia ventilators are commerically available in this country for use with horses* (Thurmon, Menhusen, and Hartofield, 1975; Beerwinkle and Witzel 1976; Latshaw and Fessler 1976; Steffey 1981). Designs for homemade units have also recently appeared. No attempt will be made to further discuss specific points of design. Interested readers should consult the references for further information.

ANESTHETIC DELIVERY (UPTAKE AND DISTRIBUTION)

General anesthesia results from the interaction of anesthetic molecules with the central nervous system. It is assumed that this interaction is achieved by developing a sufficient partial pressure (concentration) of anesthetic in the brain. Since it is not appropriate to inject inhaled anesthetics directly into the brain, the respiratory and circulatory systems must be relied upon to augment their delivery and removal. In achieving general anesthesia, the selected agent passes down a partial pressure gradient, the greatest tension of the agent being at its source and the least in the brain and other tissues. The development of these gradients determines the course of inhalation anesthesia. The characterization and study of this process is frequently referred to as the uptake and distribution of inhaled anesthetics and has been most actively investigated in recent times by Eger (1974). It is not the purpose of this chapter to thoroughly review principles of uptake and distribution of inhalation anesthetics. This is more adequately presented elsewhere

---

*North American Drager, 148B Quarry Road, Telford, PA 18969; and J.D. Medical Distributing Co., Inc., Phoenix, AZ 85001.

(Eger 1974). However, a number of clinically important points are worthy of emphasis. They relate to the influence of the anesthetic delivery apparatus and pulmonary ventilation on the speed with which inspired and alveolar concentrations of anesthetic and thus the level of central nervous system depression may be altered in the horse.

Vaporizers

The anesthetist relies on the vaporizer to deliver a selected anesthetic concentration to the anesthetic delivery system. Some vaporizers are more efficient than others (Dorsch and Dorsch 1975; Steffey and Howland 1977; Hill 1963; Paterson, Hulands, and Nunn 1969). The glass "ether" jar delivers varying concentrations depending on such considerations as vapor pressure and volume and temperature of the anesthetic liquid. The currently more popular precision vaporizers are far more accurate because they can *partially* compensate for changes in temperature and carrier gas flow rate. However, even the precision vaporizers lose some of their efficiency at relatively high carrier gas flow rates and maximum vaporizer settings (Steffey and Howland 1977, Steffey, Woliner, and Howland 1982; Paterson, Hulands, and Nunn 1969). This limits the delivery of anesthetic vapors to the anesthetic delivery apparatus.

Circle System

One of the greatest decreases in anesthetic partial pressure (concentration) from the anesthetic source to the brain occurs in the circle absorber system. Insertion of a circle system between the anesthetic source and the patient markedly influences the inhaled (inspired) concentration (Eger 1974; Steffey and Howland 1977). The degree of influence relates to the size of the apparatus, the affinity of the anesthetic agent for the components of the system (e.g., rubber), and the fresh gas inflow. Because the gas within the anesthetic delivery system dilutes fresh gases flowing into it, changes in anesthetic partial pressure are buffered. An equine circle absorber system may contain an internal gas volume of 30 to 50 liters depending on the components in use, whereas a circle system commonly used to anesthetize foals or small animals may contain only 5 to 10 liters. For a given fresh gas inflow rate and vaporizer setting, the larger the equine anesthetic delivery system the more slowly changes in inspired anesthetic concentration occur (Steffey and Howland 1977).

Rubber parts of the anesthetic system also limit a rapid change in inspired anesthetic concentration by taking up or giving off anesthetic (Eger 1974; Eger and Brandstater 1963; Titel and Lowe 1968). The amount of anesthetic contained by the rubber is proportional to the rubber/anesthetic gas partition coefficient (Eger and Brandstater 1963; Titel and Lowe 1968) (see Table 8–1).

Finally, the rate of change of anesthetic within the circle absorber system is dependent upon the rate of inflow of fresh gas into the system (Eger 1974; Steffey and Howland, 1977). All things being equal, the greater the fresh gas inflow the more rapid the change in the system's anesthetic concentration. It is of importance to recognize that the system's volume and fresh gas inflow rates do not function independently in their influence on anesthetic concentration.

A delay in the rate of increase of inspired anesthetic concentration is also produced by the equine patient and is in direct relation to its voluminous respiratory system and body size (i.e., tissue uptake of anesthetic). Because of dilution in the lungs of the inspired anesthetic and the uptake of anesthetic by pulmonary blood, expired gas contains less anesthetic than that presented to the system. This further dilutes the anesthetic concentration of inspired gas. This process is particularly of importance during the early phases of anesthetic induction (period of rapid anesthetic uptake).

Ventilation

Development of an adequate alveolar anesthetic concentration sufficient to promote anesthetizing doses of the agent in the arterial blood and hence the brain is of obvious importance. The alveolar concentration is controlled, in part, by the development of an adequate concentration of anesthetic in the delivery apparatus (supra-vida) and, therefore, in the inspired gas and by the ventilation of the lungs. The rate at which anesthetic leaves the lungs via the circulatory system is also a factor but will not be further discussed here. It is probably patently clear that ventilation has a major influence on the rate of change of anesthetic depth. Presuming constant pulmonary blood flow, if ventilation is 0 (i.e., apnea), the alveolar concentration cannot rise (in fact it may fall) regardless of the concentration within the delivery system. Conversely, hyperventilation (via spontaneous or mechanical efforts) will enable the alveolar concentration to more rapidly approach the inspired concentration.

The practical significance to the practicing equine anesthetist of this brief discussion on anesthetic delivery is that, using contemporary methods of inhalation anesthesia, a significantly *longer* period of time is necessary to alter (either increase or decrease) anesthetic depth in the horse than is usually experienced when anesthetizing smaller species. This is in large part owing to the large size of the equine patient and the equipment necessary for inhalation anesthesia and the common clinical use of relatively low fresh gas inflow rates.

GENERAL PRINCIPLES OF CLINICAL INHALATION ANESTHESIA

Preanesthetic Period

The preanesthetic period is a time for evaluating the patient, determining the anesthetic protocol to be used, and anticipating and preparing for anesthetic and postanesthetic needs and complications.

PATIENT EVALUATION

The clinican must adequately assess the patient's physical condition prior to induction of anesthesia. This is the keystone of any anesthetic regimen. A thorough medical history is of undeniable value in alerting the clinician to previous anesthetic complications and/or possible adverse drug reactions. A thorough physical examination should be performed with special emphasis on the life support (i.e., cardiopulmonary, hepatic, and renal) systems and on areas or organ systems directly related to the surgical complaint. Supporting laboratory and radiographic examinations should be performed as indicated. Minimal recommendations should include a direct or indirect evaluation of red blood cell hemoglobin concentration. Special operative, monitoring, or physiological support requirements should be identified and arrangements made for their successful handling. Finally, the owners of the surgical patient should be appraised of any anticipated anesthetic or surgical complications prior to anesthetic induction.

CHOICE OF ANESTHETIC TECHNIQUE

No anesthetic technique is unequivocally the best for all horses, surgical procedures, or veterinarians. The rationale that underlies the selection of an appropriate anesthetic agent and anesthetic protocol includes the anesthetist's capabilities and confidence, the patient's needs, and the surgical requirements. The expressed wishes of the client and the facilities available may also play a role in deciding the most favorable course.

PREANESTHETIC THERAPY AND PREPARATION

Immediately prior to induction of general anesthesia, ataractics (e.g., promazine, acetylpromazine, xylazine), hypnotic-sedatives (e.g., pentobarbital, chloral hydrate), opiates (e.g., meperidine, oxymorphone), and/or anticholinergics (e.g., atropine) may be administered to the horse. The purpose of these premedicant drugs is to facilitate handling of the horse, smooth anesthetic induction, reduce the animal's anesthetic requirement, and minimize certain undesirable effects or reflex responses (Soma 1971). The choice of drug, dosage, and route of administration depends on a multitude of factors including the patient's age and physical status, anesthetic agent, surgical and anesthetic facilities, personal preferences, and so on. Specific guidelines for the use of preanesthetic medicants are provided elsewhere (Collins 1976; Hall 1971; Lumb and Jones 1973; Soma 1971).

Anesthetic equipment and drugs must be thoroughly prechecked and conveniently positioned prior to the induction of general anesthesia. A typical setup for the inhalation anesthetic management of an adult horse would include intravenous anesthetic induction agent(s), suitable size endotracheal tube(s), endotracheal tube lubricant jelly, air syringe to inflate the tracheal tube cuff, clamp for tracheal tube cuff, mouth speculum, anesthetic delivery apparatus, mechanical ventilator, monitoring equipment, intravenous fluids, and miscellaneous drugs. Depending on the patient, anticipated induction technique, and facilities, a special halter, ropes, shipping boots, supplemental body padding, and so on, may also be desirable. All equipment should be clean and working properly.

Immediately prior to anesthetic induction, the horse's oral cavity is flushed clean with a dose syringe and clean water. This is done to reduce the risk of food or foreign matter being introduced into the trachea during intubation. Except for brief periods in which an intravenous anesthetic is not used or intravenous fluid therapy is not anticipated, an appropriate intravenous needle or commercially available catheter is aseptically preplaced in the intended upside (in the recumbent horse) peripheral vein (i.e., external jugular vein) and secured. A 14- to 16-gauge, 5- to 6-in or longer catheter is used to minimize the risk of perivascular infusions, especially during anesthetic induction, and allows rapid infusions of intraoperative support fluids.

Anesthetic Period

ANESTHETIC INDUCTION

Induction of general anesthesia may be accomplished in a variety of ways. The actual drug selected is probably secondary to its proper administration. Most popular present-day practices are to administer a "sleep" dose of an ultrashort-acting thiobarbiturate (e.g., thiamylal or thiopental). Actual barbiturate dosage depends on the size, physical status, and temperament of the horse and its clinical response to any preanesthetic medication. About 4 to 6 mg/kg (2 to 3 g/1000 lbs) is usually sufficient.

Intravenously administered glyceryl guaiacolate (GG), by itself or in combination with an ultrashort-acting thiobarbiturate, chloral hydrate, or xylazine and ketamine may also be used to induce general anesthesia prior to inhalation anesthesia (Hall 1971; Lumb and Jones 1973; Soma 1971; Wolff, Lumb, and Ramsay 1967).

It should be remembered that major emphasis will be placed on the inhalation agent for producing immobility and anesthesia. The purpose of the induction agent is merely to produce transient patient recumbency and restraint with minimal circulatory and respiratory insult.

Foals of less than 90 to 115 kg (200 to 250 lbs) may be safely and conveniently induced with an inhalation agent (e.g., halothane with or without N_2O) via a face mask connected to a standard small animal or human-type semiclosed anesthetic circle system.

TRACHEAL INTUBATION

Immediately following induction of anesthesia, orotracheal intubation of the horse is accomplished without the benefit of an endoscope or direct visualization of the larynx. The tip of the endotracheal tube should be coated with a sterile lubricant. Intubation is performed after opening the horse's mouth and inserting a mouth speculum or bite block. This is to keep the oral cavity open during intubation and throughout anesthesia. The actual method of intubation will depend on the type of tracheal tube in use and the preference and experience of the anesthetist. Various methods have been described (Hall 1971; Soma 1971). In general, the largest size tracheal tube that will easily pass into the trachea should be used. The tongue may be immobilized but should not be pulled forward. The tracheal tube is passed on the midline over the base of the tongue to the level of the larynx. With the horse's head held in extension, the tube is passed into the

larynx during the inspiratory phase of the horse's respiratory cycle. The tube should only be long enough for the tip to be in the mid to lower cervical region. If a cuffed tube is in use, the cuff should not be in the larynx. To ensure minimal mechanical dead space, the distal end of the tracheal tube should be connected to the anesthetic delivery apparatus in the region of the rostralmost portion of the oral cavity. The cuff of the tracheal tube should only be inflated enough to prevent gas from escaping between the tracheal and endotracheal tube walls. Care must be taken to prevent overinflation. Occasionally, it may be undesirable or impossible to position a tracheal tube within the oral cavity. Depending on clinical circumstances, the trachea may also be intubated via the nose (nasotracheal intubation) or a tracheostomy. These techniques are described elsewhere (Steffey 1979).

ANESTHETIC MAINTENANCE

After successfully intubating the horse, the anesthetist connects the tracheal tube to the anesthetic machine and adjusts the anesthetic concentrations and O_2 flows. Considering both patient oxygenation and anesthetic delivery and using a semiclosed anesthetic delivery technique in the absence of N_2O, initial flows for an adult horse of 8 to 10 liters per minute are beneficial. After 10 to 15 minutes, the O_2 flow rate may be reduced to a maintenance level of 3.5 to 5 liters per minute. When anesthetic concentrations need to be altered rapidly, higher O_2 flows may again be required (supra-vida) (Tevik et al. 1969; Steffey and Howland 1977; Gabel et al. 1966).

An in-depth review of the signs and stages of anesthesia is beyond the scope of this chapter and appears elsewhere (Hall 1971; Lumb and Jones 1973; Soma 1971; Manley 1981). In monitoring the anesthetized horse it is important to recall that all signs of anesthesia are influenced by the complex interaction of the physical status of the horse, the inhalation anesthetic and adjuvant drugs in use, adequacy of ventilation and oxygenation, presence or absence of painful stimuli, and so on. Consequently, *no single* sign is a universal reliable indication of the depth of anesthesia. Accordingly, at the very least the horse's heart rate and rhythm, arterial blood pressure, breathing volume and frequency, eye and miscellaneous signs of anesthesia should be assessed and recorded at least every five minutes. Maintenance of the lightest plane of general anesthesia consistent with the surgical procedure is usually warranted. A light plane of anesthesia is usually indicated in the horse by at least some of the following: 1) the presence of a "wandering" eye or frank nystagmus, 2) tearing, 3) brisk corneal and palpebral reflex, 4) tear formation and a moist cornea, 5) increased resistance by the horse to mechanical lung inflation, 6) sweating, 7) breath holding or a rise in respiratory frequency and tidal volume following a painful stimulus, and 8) a rise in arterial blood pressure and heart rate associated with pain.

Alveolar hypoventilation usually accompanies inhalation anesthesia in the spontaneously breathing horse and results in an elevation in $PaCO_2$ and respiratory acidosis (Hall 1971; Lumb and Jones 1973; Soma 1971; Steffey et al. 1977a; Steffey 1978; Hall, Gillespie, and Tyler 1968; Nunn 1977; Steffey et al. 1977b; Gillespie, Tyler, and Hall 1969; Mitchell and Littlejohn 1971). An impairment in oxygenation is also frequently demonstrable and is influenced by body position and time of anesthesia (Munson and Tucker 1975; Nunn 1977; Steffey et al. 1977b; Gillespie, Tyler, and Hall 1969; Mitchell and Littlejohn 1971).

Mechanical ventilators may be used to assist or control the horse's ventilation. Assisted ventilation implies that the horse initiates inspiration by reducing airway pressure, which triggers the ventilator to deliver the desired tidal volume. Since respiratory frequency and, therefore, respiratory minute ventilation are determined by the horse, alveolar hypoventilation may accompany mechanically assisted ventilation during anesthesia. On the other hand, during controlled intermittent positive pressure ventilation all of the work of breathing is accomplished by the ventilator. Both tidal volume and respiratory frequency (and therefore respiratory minute ventilation) are determined by the anesthetist.

Hence, if proper ventilator adjustments are made, $PaCO_2$ will remain normal in the anesthetized horse (Hall 1971; Lumb and Jones 1973; Soma 1971; Hall, Gillespie, and Tyler 1968; Steffey et al. 1977b; Steffey 1981).

Mechanical intermittent positive pressure ventilation may interfere with venous return, lower cardiac output, and cause arterial hypotension. The accompanying reduction in $PaCO_2$, drugs administered during the preanesthetic and anesthetic periods, and hypovolemia may also contribute to a fall in blood pressure. Accordingly, the arterial blood pressure should be closely monitored in horses maintained on mechanical ventilation.

Intravenous fluids are commonly administered intraoperatively to horses undergoing elective operations in an effort to maintain a patent access to the cardiovascular system and to maintain an adequate intravascular fluid volume. Lactated Ringer's solution in a dosage of 5 to 8 ml/kg/hour is commonly administered to the healthy, elective surgical patient. Horses presented for surgical exploration of severe acute abdominal discomfort (e.g., colic surgery) usually require a much greater fluid volume administration. The rate, volume, and type of fluid administered are ultimately dictated by the patient's physical status and intraoperative requirements.

Postanesthetic Period

Because airway patency and adequacy of oxygenation are of major concern even in the young, healthy, postanesthetic, recumbent horse, maintenance of tracheal intubation and supplemental oxygen therapy well into the recovery period is desirable (Steffey et al. 1977b; Steffey 1979; Mitchell and Littlejohn 1971). Tracheal extubation is indicated by adequate ventilation as determined by appropriate clinical signs. Extubation should not be performed before the horse is able to effectively swallow and cough. Oxygen may be administered to the horse via a mask or with an insufflation tube positioned down the tracheal tube or after extubation in one of the nostrils to the level of the pharynx. Oxygen flows of at least 10 to 15 liters per minute are usually necessary to prevent hypoxemia in healthy elective surgical patients. To improve ventilation, animals should be encouraged to assume a sternal recumbent position when clinical conditions warrant.

REFERENCES

Adriani, J.: The Chemistry and Physics of Anesthesia. Springfield, IL; Charles C Thomas, 1962.

Beerwinkle, K. R., and Witzel, D. A.: A pneumatically driven, electronically-controlled respirator for use with large animal inhalation anaesthesia systems. Vet. Anesth. 3:110, 1976.

Best, J. L., and McGrath, C. J.: Trace anesthetic gases: an overview. JAVMA 171:1268, 1977.

Cohen, E. N., Bellville, J. W., and Brown, B. W.: Anesthesia, pregnancy and miscarriage: A study of operating room nurses and anesthetists. Anesthesiology 35:343, 1971.

Cohen, E. N., Brown, B. W., Bruce, D. C., et al.: Occupational disease among operating room personnel: A rational study. Anesthesiology 41:321, 1974.

Collins, V. J.: Principles of Anesthesiology. Philadelphia: Lea & Febiger, 1976.

Cousins, M. J., and Mazze, R. I.: Methoxyflurane nephrotoxicity: A study of dose-response in man. JAMA 225:1611, 1973.

Crandell, W. B., Pappas, S. G., and MacDonald, A.: Nephrotoxicity associated with methoxyflurane anesthesia. Anesthesiology 27:591, 1966.

Dorsch, J. A., and Dorsch, S. E.: Understanding Anesthetic Equipment: Construction, Care and Complications. Baltimore: Williams & Wilkins, 1975.

Dreesen, D. W., Jones, G. L., Brown, J., et al.: Monitoring for trace anesthetic gases in a veterinary teaching hospital. JAVMA 179:797, 1981.

Eberly, V. E., Gillespie, J. R., Tyler, W. S., et al.: Cardiovascular values in the horse during halothane anesthesia. Am. J. Vet. Res. 29:305, 1968.

Eger, E. I. II: Anesthetic Uptake and Action. Baltimore: Wlliams & Wilkins, 1974.

Eger, E. I., and Brandstater, B.: Solubility of methoxyflurane in rubber. Anesthesiology 24:679, 1963.

Eger, E. I. II, and Epstein, R. M.: Hazards of anesthetic equipment. Anesthesiology 25:490, 1964.

Eger, E. I. II, and Saidman, L. J.: Hazards of nitrous oxide anesthesia in bowel obstruction and pneumothorax. Anesthesiology 26:61, 1965.

Epstein, R. M., Rackow, H., Salanitre, E., et al.: Influence of the concentration effect on the uptake of anesthetic mixtures: The second gas effect. Anesthesiology 25:364, 1964.

Fink, B. R.: Diffusion anoxia. Anesthesiology 16:511, 1955.

Fisher, E. W., and Jennings, S.: The use of fluothane in horses and cattle. Vet. Rec. 70:567, 1958.

Fisher, E. W., and Jennings, S.: A closed circuit anaesthetic apparatus for adult cattle and horses. Vet. Rec. 69:769, 1957.

Fowler, M. E., Parker, E. E., McLaughlin, R. F., Jr., et al.: An inhalation anesthetic apparatus for large animals. JAVMA 143:272, 1963.

Gabel, A. A., Heath, R. B., Ross, N., et al.: Hypoxia — its prevention in inhalation anesthesia in horses. In Proceedings of the American Association of Equine Practitioners:179, 1966.

Galloon, S.: The concentration of anesthetics in closed circuits, with special reference to halothane: II. Laboratory and theatre investigations. Br. J. Anaesth. 32:310, 1960.

Gillespie, J. R., Tyler, W. S., and Hall, L. W.: Cardiopulmonary dysfunction in anesthetized, laterally recumbent horses. Am. J. Vet. Res. 30:61, 1969.

Gopinath, C., Jones, R. S., and Ford, E. J. H.: The effect of the repeated administration of halothane on the liver of the horse. J. Pathol. 102:107, 1970.

Gray, T. C., and Nunn, J. F. (eds.): General Anesthesia, 4th ed. London: Butterworths, 1981.

Hall, L. W.: Wrights' Veterinary Anesthesia and Analgesia. London: Bailliere Tindall, 1971.

Hall, L. W., Gillespie, J. R., and Tyler, S. W.: Alveolar-arterial oxygen tension differences in anaesthetized horses. Br. J. Anaesth. 40:560, 1968.

Hansson, C. H., and Johannisson, D.: Inhalation anaesthesia with automatic artificial respiration during succinylcholine relaxation in large animals. Nord. Vet. Med. 10:469, 1958.

Heath, R. B.: Inhalation anesthesia. In Proceedings of the American Association of Equine Practitioners: 335, 1976.

Heath, R. B.: Cole equine endotracheal tube. Vet. Anesth. 1:15, 1974.

Hill, D. W.: Halothane concentrations obtained with a dräger "vapor" vaporizer. Br. J. Anaesth. 35:285, 1963.

Hodges, W. S.: Tracheal tubes for veterinary use. Vet. Rec. 100:201, 1977.

Joas, T. A., Stevens, W. C., and Eger, E. I. II: Electroencephalographic seizure activity in dogs during anaesthesia. Br. J. Anaesth. 43:739, 1971.

Johnson, R. R., Eger, E. I. II, and Wilson, C.: A comparative interaction of epinephrine with enflurane, isoflurane and halothane in man. Anesth. Analg. 55:709, 1976.

Klein, L. V.: Case report: A hot horse. Vet. Anesthesiol. 2:41, 1975.

Klide, A. M.: Cardiopulmonary effects of enflurane and isoflurane in the dog. Am. J. Vet. Res. 37:127, 1976.

Langley, J. A.: Nasal intubation as a method of halothane anaesthesia. In Proceedings of the Association of Veterinary Anaesthesiologists of Great Britain and Ireland:10, 1972.

Larson, C. P., Jr., Eger, E. I. II, Muallem, M., et al.: The effects of diethyl ether and methoxyflurane on ventilation: II. A comparative study in man. Anesthesiology 30:174, 1969.

Latshaw, H. S., Jr., and Fessler, J. F.: Incorporation of a deliberate leak in an equine ventilator-bellows system. Vet. Anesthesiol. 3:96, 1976.

Lees, P., Mullen, P. A., and Tavernor, W. D.: Influence of anaesthesia with volatile agents on the equine liver. Br. J. Anaesth. 45:570, 1973.

Lees, P., and Tavernor, W. D.: Influence of halothane and catecholamines on heart rate and rhythm in the horse. Br. J. Pharmacol. 39:149, 1970.

Lodge, D.: A survey of tracheal dimensions in horses and cattle in relation to endotracheal tube size. Vet. Rec. 85:300, 1969.

Lumb, W. V., and Jones, E. W.: Veterinary Anesthesia. Philadelphia: Lea & Febiger, 1973.

Manley, S. V.: Monitoring the anesthetized horse. Vet. Clin. North Am. 3:111, 1981.

Manley, S. V., and McDonell, W. N.: Recommendations for reduction of anesthetic gas pollution. JAVMA 176:519, 1980.

Mapleson, W. W.: The concentration of anesthetics in closed circuits, with special reference to halothane: I. Theoretical study. Br. J. Anaesth. 32:298, 1960.

Mazze, R. I.: Waste anesthetic gases and the regulatory agencies. Anesthesiology 52:248, 1980.

Mazze, R. I., Cousins, M. J., and Kosek, J.: Dose-related methoxyflurane nephrotoxicity in rats: A biochemical and pathologic correlation. Anesthesiology 36:571, 1972.

Mazze, R. I., Shui, G. L., and Jackson, S. H.: Renal dysfunction associated with methoxyflurane anesthesia: A randomized prospective clinical evaluation. JAMA 216:278, 1971.

Miller, R. D. (ed.): Anesthesia. New York: Churchill Livingstone, 1981.

Mitchell, B., and Littlejohn, A.: Influence of anesthesia and posture on arterial oxygen and carbon dioxide tension, alveolar dead space and pulse rate in the horse. In Proceedings of the Association of Veterinary Anaesthesiologists of Great Britain and Ireland:61, 1971.

Moens, Y., and DeMoor, A.: Diffusion of nitrous oxide into the intestinal lumen of ponies during halothane-nitrous oxide anesthesia. Am. J. Vet. Res. 42:1750, 1981.

Moyers, J.: A nomenclature for methods of inhalation anesthesia. Anesthesiology 14:609, 1953.

Muir, W. W., Skarda, R. T., and Milne, D. W.: Evaluation of xylazine and ketamine hydrochloride for anesthesia in horses. Am. J. Vet. Res. 38:195, 1977.

Munson, E. S., Larson, C. P., Jr., Babad, A. A., et al.: The effects of halothane, fluroxene and cyclopropane on ventilation: A comparative study in man. Anesthesiology 27:716, 1966.

Munson, E. S., and Tucker, W. K.: Doses of epinephrine causing arrhythmia during enflurane, methoxyflurane and halothane anesthesia in dogs. Can. Anaesth. Soc. J. 22:495, 1975.

Mushin, W. W., and Galloon, S.: The concentration of anesthetics with special reference to halothane: III. Clinical aspects. Br. J. Anaesth. 32:324, 1960.

Neigh, J. L., Garman, J. K., and Harp, J. R.: The electroencephalographic pattern during anesthesia with ethrane: Effects of depth of anesthesia, PaCO$_2$ and nitrous oxide. Anesthesiology 35:482, 1971.

Nunn, J. F.: Applied Respiratory Physiology. New York: Appleton-Century-Crofts, 1977.

Paterson, G. M., Hulands, G. H., and Nunn, J. F.: Evolution of a new halothane vaporizer: The Cyprane Fluotec Mark 3. Br. J. Anaesth. 41:109, 1969.

Purchase, I. F. H.: Function tests on four large-animal anaesthetic circuits. Vet. Rec. 77:913, 1965.

Rex, M. A. E.: Apparatus available for equine anaesthesia. Aust. Vet. J. 48:283, 1972.

Rosenberg, H., and Waldron-Maese, E.: Malignant hyperpyrexia in horses: Anesthetic sensitivity proven by muscle biopsy. In Proceedings of the American Society of Anesthesiologists' annual meeting:333, 1977.

Short, C. E.: Evaluation of closed, semiclosed and nonrebreathing inhalation anesthesia systems in the horse. JAVMA 157:1500, 1970.

Skarda, R., Baches, G., and Fackelman, G. E.: Improving pulmonary ventilation in anesthetized horses with the Bird Mark 9 respirator. VM/SAC 69:754, 1974.

Smith, M.: A respirator for large animals. Nord. Vet. Med. 23:537, 1971.

Soma, L. R. (ed.): Textbook of Veterinary Anesthesia. Baltimore: Williams & Wilkins, 1971.

Steffey, E. P.: Mechanical ventilation of the anesthetized horse. Vet. Clin. North Am. 3:97, 1981.

Steffey, E,P.: Anesthetic management of the horse with respiratory disease. Vet. Clin. North Am. Large Anim. Pract. 1:113, 1979.

Steffey, E. P.: Enflurane and isoflurane anesthesia: A summary of laboratory and clinical investigations in horses. JAVMA 172:367, 1978.

Steffey, E. P., and Berry, J. D.: Flow rates from an intermittent positive pressure breathing-anesthetic delivery apparatus for horses. Am. J. Vet. Res. 38:685, 1977.

Steffey, E. P., Farver, T., Zinkl, J., et al.: Alterations in horse blood cell count and biochemical values after halothane anesthesia. Am. J. Vet. Res. 41:934, 1980.

Steffey, E. P., Gillespie, J. R., Berry, J. D., et al.: Circulatory effects of halothane and halothane-N$_2$O anesthesia in the dog: Spontaneous ventilation. Am. J. Vet. Res. 36:197, 1975.

Steffey, E. P., and Howland, D., Jr.: Comparison of circulatory and respiratory effects isoflurane and halothane anesthesia in horses. Am. J. Vet. Res. 40:821, 1980.

Steffey, E. P., and Howland, D., Jr.: Cardiovascular effects of halothane in horses. Am. J. Vet. Res. 39:611, 1978a.

Steffey, E. P., and Howland, D., Jr.: Potency of halothane-N$_2$O in the horse. Am. J. Vet. Res. 39:1141, 1978b.

Steffey, E. P., and Howland, D., Jr.: The rate of change of halothane concentration in a large animal circle anesthetic system. Am. J. Vet. Res. 38:1993, 1977.

Steffey, E. P., Howland, D., Jr., Giri, S., et al.: Enflurane, halothane and isoflurane potency in horses. Am. J. Vet. Res. 38:1037, 1977a.

Steffey, E. P., Johnson, B. H., Eger, E. I. II, et al.: Nitrous oxide: effect on accumulation rate and uptake of bowel gases. Anesth. Analg. 58:405, 1979.

Steffey, E. P., Wheat, J. D., Meagher, D. M., et al.: Body position and mode of ventilation influences arterial pH, oxygen and carbon dioxide tensions in halothane anesthetized horses. Am. J. Vet. Res. 38:379, 1977b.

Steffey, E. P., Woliner, M., and Howland, D., Jr.: Evaluation of an Isoflurane vaporizer: The cyprane fortec. Anesth. Analg. 61:457, 1982.

Steffey, E. P., Zinkl, J., and Howland, D., Jr.: Minimal changes in blood cell counts and biochemical values associated with prolonged isoflurane anesthesia of horses. Am. J. Vet. Res. 40:1646, 1979.

Tavernor, W. D.: A simple apparatus for inhalation anaesthesia in adult cattle and horses. Vet. Rec. 73:545, 1961.

Tevik, A., Sharpe, J., Nelson, A. W., et al.: Effect of nitrogen in a closed-circle system with low oxygen flows for equine anesthesia. JAVMA 154:166, 1969.

Thurmon, J. C.: Some aspects of large animal inhalation anesthetic equipment. In Proceedings of the American Association of Equine Practitioners:465, 1972.

Thurmon, J. C., and Benson, G. J.: Inhalation anesthetic delivery equipment and its maintenance. Vet. Clin. North Am. 3:73, 1981.

Thurmon, J. C., Menhusen, M. J., and Hartofield, S. M.: A multivolume ventilator–bellows and air compressor for use with a Bird Mark IX respirator in large animal inhalation anesthesia. Vet. Anesth. 2:34, 1975.

Titel, J. H., and Lowe, H. J.: Rubber-gas partition coefficients. Anesthesiology 29:1215, 1968.

Ward, G. S., and Byland, R. R.: Concentration of halothane in veterinary operating and treatment rooms. JAVMA 180:174, 1982.

Weaver, B. M. Q.: Mechanical control of ventilation in horses. Vet. Rec. 80:249, 1967.

Weaver, B. M. Q.: An apparatus for inhalation anaesthesia in large animals. Vet. Rec. 72:1121, 1960.

Wingfield, W. E., Ruby, D. L., Buchan, R. M., et al.: Waste anesthetic gas exposure to veterinarians and animal technicians. JAVMA 178:399, 1981.

Wolff, W. A., Lumb, W. V., and Ramsay, M. K.: Effects of halothane and chloroform anesthesia on the equine liver. Am. J. Vet. Res. 28:1363, 1967.

Zahed, B., Miletich, D. J., Ivankovich, A. D., et al.: Arrhythmic doses of epinephrine and dopamine during halothane, enflurane, methoxyflurane and fluroxene anesthesia in goats. Anesth. Analg. 56:207, 1977.

EQUINE INTRAVENOUS ANESTHESIA

R. B. HEATH, D.V.M., M.S.

PHILOSOPHY, GENERAL COMMENTS, AND DEFINITIONS

Intravenous anesthesia is objectively distinct from sedation hypnosis (used for standing procedures) and inhalation anesthesia, even though some of the same drugs may be used. Stated differently, do not stereoscope all drugs and their labels by dosing to the maximum. Rather, dose to the minimum and use judicious objectives in designing combinations. Agents used alone tend to result in short to moderate periods of anesthesia. Only by various recipes and combinations can you *safely* lengthen anesthesia time with intravenous anesthesia. Create specific anesthesia situations for specific patients, surgeons, purposes, and length of procedures. Anesthesia must be planned, especially with respect to time, *in advance*. If possible, when complications occur, switch to inhalation rather than lengthen anesthesia time with injectables. Many IV methods are used only for intubation and volatile vapor induction.

The first objective of intravenous anesthesia is to have a smooth, crisp recovery. The second objective is to use an IV anesthesia that provides enough control and time to complete the procedure. To accomplish these objectives, follow these rules:

1. No horse gets more than 5 grams of any barbiturate, including draft horses.

2. No intravenous program should be longer than one hour total time.

3. Seriously consider inhalation anesthesia if rules 1 or 2 are exceeded. In addition, obey all the standard rules on padding, position, and trauma to the patient and keep excitement out of the situation.

Candidates for intravenous anesthesia are healthy, normal elective Class I or II patients. Those with clinical, laboratory, or physical signs of disease would greatly benefit from oxygen and would be better candidates for inhalation techniques. Patients with blood loss and a packed cell volume below 22 *should not be anesthetized*. They need transfusion and/or rest before proceeding with the surgery. Patients with evidence of respiratory infection and serous nasal discharge develop an alveolar diffusion barrier to oxygen absorption, which will greatly increase risk during anesthesia.

EQUINE INTRAVENOUS ANESTHETIC DRUGS

SEDATIVE/HYPNOTICS

All sedative-hypnotics appear to act as CNS depressants, with dose-dependent respiratory and cardiovascular depression. All are alkaline and caustic and cause intimal irritation as well as severe subcutis irritation if inadvertently injected extravascularly.

Chloral hydrate is currently available in two forms: USP crystals to make your own solutions, and the proprietory chloral, magnesium sulfate, pentobarbital mixture (Chloropent, Fort Dodge Laboratory). When given IV, chloral hydrate is quickly converted to trichlorethanol, which is the active form. It induces a dose-related sedation and can lead to hypnosis and coma. Sedative standing doses are very useful as substitutes for tranquilizers. Chloral hydrate is analgesic and more predictable than phenothiazine tranquilizers. Anesthetic doses give light surgical restraint and result in drunk, barbiturate-like recoveries, which usually last longer than the anesthetic period, hour for hour.

Pentobarbital, an oxybarbiturate, is short in action and has been used as a standing sedative (approximately 10 ml in adults). It is currently available as a 6 per cent solution (Pentobarbital Na, Fort Dodge Laboratory). Used alone, it may occasionally be used in foals in a dose of 15 to 30 mg/kg given slowly and carefully. Since other forms of anesthesia (i.e., inhalation) have so many more advantages, pentobarbital is rarely used today.

Two *thiobarbiturates* are available, thiamylal (Surital, Parke-Davis; Biotal, Burns Lab) and thiopental (Pentothal, Abbott). These agents are highly soluble, sulfur substituted, and ultrashort in action. Thiamylal appears in clinical use to be slightly stronger than thiopental. This is advantageous in equine surgery, giving the operator a bit more control, but gives the patient more toxicity in the form of respiratory and cardiovascular depression. Both thiobarbiturates benefit from use of a preanesthetic, such as a tranquilizer, to potentiate and smooth induction and lessen the dose needed. Alone intravenously for short knockdown, thiamylal at 6.6 mg/kg usually results in 7 to 12 minutes of anesthesia. Thiopental at 6.6 mg/kg usually results in 4 to 9 minutes of anesthesia. With the proper light preanesthetics, you can reasonably expect to double the down times at the same doses.

With these agents, a guideline of *no more than 5 grams of barbiturate* given to any horse will result in optimum recovery characteristics.

Methohexital (Brevane, Lilly) has been used in the horse. Single injections are usually safe but yield only three to four minutes of light restraint. Multiple injections result in life-threatening convulsions and death. Methohexital is an oxybarbiturate with molecular chemistry characteristics barely defining it as a barbiturate, resulting in its undesirable side effect of convulsion.

MUSCLE RELAXANTS

Guaifenesin (also called glyceryl quaiacolate [GG]), used extensively as a base for anesthesia drug combinations, is an internuncial neuron spinal level muscle relaxant. It is in the family of mephenesin and enjoys less hemolysis than its cousin given intravenously. The drug is also used as the main antitussive in cough syrup. It is useful given intravenously to the pig, cow, and horse in 5 per cent concentrations. Ten per cent and higher concentrations appear from time to time, but minimal hemolysis is experienced with 5 per cent, so this concentration is preferred. There is minimal effect on the cardiovascular system and a dose-related depression of ventilation. Used alone, doses of 110 mg/kg result in light unconsciousness, euphoria, and relaxed lateral recumbency for 6 to 10 minutes. Animals will respond slightly to deep pain. A triple dose (330 mg/kg) is usually needed to effect respiratory arrest. The drug is metabolized to catechol and other conjugates with the possibility of high doses resulting in carbonate crystalluria and renal colic. If this complication occurs, it is readily reversed with fluids and a diuretic such as furosemide. Occasionally in smaller patients or in large, fast administrations, a transient muscular rigidity is observed before relaxation. This is rarely seen when guaifenesin is used in anesthetic drug combinations (Garner, Rosborough, and Amend 1972).

Succinylcholine USP is a myoneural junction muscle relaxant of the depolarizing class. Used alone in the horse, it is a pure restraint agent with no analgesia or unconsciousness attached to its pharmacology. Use of this drug must be with direct veterinary supervision, using the guidelines established by the American Association of Equine Practitioners (1971). Much clinical data and compilation of case histories appear in the veterinary literature related to succinylcholine. The summation and essence of these are as follows: 1) extreme physiologic blood pressures are reached (Heath and Gabel 1970); 2) physical performance is risked owing to hypoxic, ecchymotic heart damage (Larsen, Loomis, and Steel 1959); 3) death is seen on occasion. With the advent of newer anesthetic drug combinations, there are better drugs available for chemical restraint.

DISSOCIATIVE AGENTS

Ketamine HCl appears to offer no depression to the central nervous system. Rather, a pharmacological dissociation of the limbic and cortical systems occurs. Available commercially and label approved for cats and primates are Vetalar (Parke-Davis) and Ketaset (Bristol Labs). There are a tremendous number of administrations in common use in all species, with an excellent therapeutic safety record regarding losses related to anesthesia. The drug produces an elevated heart rate and pressure, due partly to increased peripheral resistance, thus increasing heart work. Ketamine used alone is useful in foals for short induction and intubation in dosages of 2.2 to 6.6 mg/kg. In adult horses, it is better used in combination anesthesia.

Drug Combination Anesthesia

Also known colloquially as balanced anesthesia, "recipes," and "garbage anesthesia," there are several useful drug combination programs for intravenous maintenance of the horse. The guidelines mentioned previously should be carefully adhered to, especially rules 1 and 2. To reasonably construct an objective drug program, the clinician must have a close estimate of the time needed to complete the surgery. These "balanced" programs are tuned to time, with an eye to good recovery in each instance.

SHORT TIME PERIOD:
XYLAZINE-KETAMINE

Xylazine (Rompun, Chem-Agro), in doses of 1.1 mg/kg IV, will take effect in two to three minutes. It is a large dose and the effect may be profound, so it is handy to have the animal close to the surgery site. Xylazine used at this dose is usable tranquilization, with tremendous potentiation of other drugs. After effects are noted, administer 1.66 to 2.2 mg/kg Ketamine HCl intravenously. It is best to allow the horse to fall by himself; if you try to hold the animal it will usually feel the restraint during the slow induction and will resist by pulling or trying to compensate sideways and will fall in a more violent fashion. Let the horse assume a sawhorse stance and "melt down" all by itself. The lower dose almost always results in 7 to 12 minutes of down time, whereas 1 mg/lb usually allows 15 minutes of restraint. Occasionally, individuals will be anesthetized for as long as 30 minutes. Each individual will repeat the time and character pattern in subsequent anesthesias.

The advantages of this regimen are smooth induction and very smooth recovery (especially if the patient is allowed to stay quiet). Practitioners like the management of patients with this regimen because it can be accomplished with little or no extra labor handlers. The patient is trustworthy during recovery, even in the hands of inexperienced owners (the patient is almost always up before the instruments are cleaned and put away). There is little depression of respiratory function, with a slight overall increase in blood pressure and cardiovascular function. Disadvantages include total cost per minute realized (although this is often compensated by the time- and labor-saving nature of the combination) and the fact that, occasionally, when xylazine fails in a particular patient, the ketamine will also have little effect. The authors feel it is best to give the agents in separate syringes, waiting for each drug effect to potentiate the situation. Xylazine and ketamine can be mixed in the same syringe, but you get less time and lighter surgical effect for your money and the patient exhibits more muscular rigidity and slight tetany.

LONG TIME PERIOD: GUAIFENESIN-BASED RECIPES

Guaifenesin (GG) at 110 mg/kg in 5 per cent solution, given alone, allows six to eight minutes of anesthetic effect. It must be given in bolus (fast IV administration by large bore needles or pressure apparatus) because the rate of metabolism is high and the effects will wear off in six to eight minutes. Given slowly by cautious drip, there have been instances in which the patient did not go down at all. In fact, used in this way, it is an excellent treatment to relieve the tetany of tetanus, in repeated maintenance doses, leaving the animal relaxed but standing.

Several factors need to be considered when designing the proper regimen with GG. The most important factor is the amount of time needed. To have a reasonable recovery, you must minimize the amount of barbiturate administered. If more than one hour of surgery time is routinely needed, you should consider the advantages of inhalation equipment in your practice. The following individualized anesthetic programs each allow a slightly longer surgical time.

1. 2.2 ml/kg GG given rapidly IV results in the patient going down in about two minutes for about six minutes of light, not quite surgical-level, restraint.

2. Preanesthetizing with phenothiazine tranquilizer and then administering GG at 2.2 ml/kg will take the patient down easier and a bit sooner and will keep him down for about 12 to 14 minutes of light, almost surgical-level, restraint.

3. Preanesthetizing with phenothiazine tranquilizer and adding 3 grams of an ultrashort-acting barbiturate (thiamylal, thiopental) to 1 liter of GG will provide a solution to use as follows: Start the administration fast IV and give approximately 1.1 mg/kg (half the bottle to the average horse). When the horse goes down, stop the administration; you will usually have 12 to 20 minutes of adequate surgical restraint time. The rest of the liter can be used to add time to this patient or can be used to do a second patient. Usually, in a slow-drip maintenance, you can extend useful surgical time to 30 to 40 minutes.

4. For the longest practical IV period using GG-based programs, use xylazine as the preanesthetic to take advantage of its potentiation. Add 3 grams of an ultrashort-acting barbiturate and 1 gram of pentobarbital Na, 6 per cent, to 1 liter of GG. This mixture then gives a little more authority plus has the xylazine to give a more profound starting point to tranquilization. Start the IV rapidly until the patient goes down (this usually requires one-third of the bottle as com-

pared with one-half in recipe 3), then stop the administration. You can expect 15 to 20 minutes of good surgical-level anesthesia. The rest of the liter can be used to extend the time, usually to 40 to 50 minutes and occasionally to 60 to 80 minutes. Remember that those patients that are under longer will have less desirable recoveries.

If more time is needed after xylazine-ketamine procedures, *small amounts* of GG-barbiturate solution can be used to carefully prolong anesthesiá. For GG regimens, some operators like to use a second bottle of GG as a drip to keep the patient under longer. This is acceptable from a management standpoint if it can be done within the guidelines of less than 5 grams of barbiturate and one hour of total intravenous time. If the guidelines cannot be followed, the consequences will be a long, drawn out, drunk barbiturate recovery (Muir 1979)

Occasionally, practitioners object to GG anesthesia as not being fast enough in onset and needing more help in induction stages when the patient is wobbly going down.

Ketamine HCl will give a small crisp takedown to GG programs with xylazine as a preanesthetic, administering approximately 1.1 ml/kg (1/2 liter GG) or until the patient is unsteady on its feet. Then administer 1.65 mg/kg ketamine. The horse will undergo a more predictable anesthetic experience than with either xylazine-ketamine alone or GG alone with plenty of time for a short surgical procedure or intubation and volatile vapor induction.

LONG TIME PERIOD: CHLORAL HYDRATE-BARBITURATE RECIPES

It is possible to establish a reasonable regimen for anesthesia using promazine HCl (.55 mg/kg) or acepromazine (.055 mg/kg) IV as a preanesthetic (Gabel 1962). Give the patient a period of privacy and rest to allow the phenothiazine tranquilizer to have its full effect. This should be at least 30 to 40 minutes. Then intravenously inject a bolus of 120 to 150 ml per average 1000-lb horse of the "Army mixture" (chloral hydrate,

$MgSO_4$, pentobarbital; Chloropent, Fort Dodge Laboratory). This bolus will induce a light stage of restraint, the patient will be down and in approximately stage 2, not quite surgical anesthesia, which will last for about 20 to 25 minutes. Quite a bit of surgery has been accomplished at this stage of restraint, such as simple castration, biopsy, wound debridement, and trauma repair. It is advisable to use some form of mechanical restraint such as a casting harness or sideline. To obtain deeper planes of anesthesia at this point, use dilute 4 per cent solutions of thiobarbiturate in 5-ml doses (it is most convenient to work with a preplaced catheter). Repeat 5-ml doses at 30- to 40-second intervals until the horse is in a *light* plane of anesthesia (this is usually after about three or four 5-ml doses). Be extremely careful not to take the patient too deeply into barbiturate maintenance depth. Here again, a casting harness is recommended. There should be a *strong* palpebral response at all times, occasional deep respiratory sighs up to and including raising the head, and slight to vigorous movement on the part of the patient. This is *light* anesthesia — anything deeper will produce the same consequences as those mentioned for barbiturate recovery. If more surgical control is needed, consider the advantages of inhalation anesthesia.

ADMINISTRATION EQUIPMENT

Disposable intravenous catheters are well worth the money spent if only to avoid inadvertent extravascular injection. A trustworthy catheter can be used if you have an inexperienced helper giving injections under your direction while you are busy with surgery. Many commercial versions are available, both catheter-inside-cannula, which leaves a slightly larger entrance wound, and catheter-outside-stylet, which requires slightly more practice to place correctly. For adult animals, 6-in sizes in 16 or 14 gauge are most useful. For foals, small animal 2- to 3-in sizes in 16 to 20 gauge are adequate. Disposable IV administration sets, compatible with your fluid sources, are readily available from hospital supply houses. Their sterility, convenience, and patient safety are obvious advantages.

IV sets and catheters usually have multiple injection sites (rubber diaphragms) incorporated. Through these injection dams you can repeatedly inject and flush heparinized saline to keep the IV access open to the patient. A simple pressure system can be devised for rapid administration of large volumes (fluid or GG) by replacing the air port of any commercial IV administration set with a bulb syringe attached to a short piece of IV hose with a standard B-P IV tip. The bulb syringes are available at most drug stores as inflation bulbs for orthopedic or decubitis cushions. Caution must be observed with a pressurized IV system; it will deliver *air just as quickly* as fluids when empty or tipped over on an angle.

REFERENCES

American Association of Equine Practitioners: Suggestions for use of succinylcholine chloride. JAVMA *158*:290, 1971.

Catcott, E. J., and Smithcors, F. J. (eds.): Equine Medicine and Surgery, 2nd ed. Santa Barbara: American Veterinary Publications, 1972.

Gabel, A. A.: Promazine chloral hydrate and ultrashort barbiturate anesthesia. JAVMA *140*(6):564, 1962.

Garner, H. E., Rosborough, J. P., and Amend, J. F.: Effects of GG on serum, plasma and cellular parameters in ponies. VM/SAC 67:408, 1972.

Heath, R. B., and Gabel, A. A.: Evaluation of thiamylal, succinylcholine and glyceral guaiacolate in horses. JAVMA *157*(11):1486, 1970.

Larsen, L. H., Loomis, L. N., and Steel, J. D.: Muscle relaxants and cardiovascular damage. Aust. Vet. J. 35:269, 1959.

Muir, W.: Presentation to the Anesthesia Society. Annual convention of American Veterinary Medical Association, Seattle, July, 1979.

Roberts, D.: The role of glyceryl guaiacolate in balanced equine anesthesia. *In* Proceedings of the American Association of Equine Practitioners: 171, 1967.

LOCAL AND REGIONAL ANESTHESIA IN RUMINANTS

R. B. HEATH, D.V.M., M.S.

Mechanical restraint and local anesthesia are the safest procedures when performing surgery on ruminants. For convenience, general anesthesia can be used in food animals, for example, in the surgery of large bulls. General anesthesia may actually save surgery time (by not having to dodge kicks and fight movement). However, the savings in time is offset by the risks of general anesthesia. Another factor, of course, is the level of anatomical expertise of the operator in performing local blocks.

In all procedures, a surgical prep with clipping, detergent, and disinfectant is used to ensure cleanliness. Gloves may or may not be used, depending on the operator's preference and the particular case. The anesthetic agent may also be of the operator's choice. In general, lidocaine has replaced procaine. Procaine works well in food animals, and if it is more economical, it is entirely satisfactory. Experience and anatomical knowledge will serve the operator better than huge doses injected into the general area. A technique called the shaky hand can be used to compensate for anatomical variations by spreading out the injections over the area.

REGIONAL BLOCKS OF THE HEAD

For anesthesia of the horn, block the cornual nerve, which is a branch of the lacrimal portion of the ophthalmic division of the trigeminal nerve. Anatomically, the block is placed under the lateral edge of the supraorbital process of the frontal bone, anterior to the horn and posterior to the medial canthus (Fig. 8–1). Often, blood will be seen emanating from a small vessel near the nerve. Two to five ml of the agent is deposited, using a 22-gauge, 1-in needle. Adult cattle (older than 3 to 4 years) may, in addition, need a local line of infiltration posterior to the horn to block branches of the first cervical nerve innervating the nuchal crest. If it is necessary to perform a local block for a fractured horn involving the frontal bone and sinuses, a complete orbito rotundum foramen block (Peterson 1951) will be necessary.

For ophthalmic anesthesia, the orbit is anesthetized according to the classic description of Peterson (1951). This block anesthetizes all structures of the side of the head except the tongue and mandible. The foramen orbito rotundum and the sensory nerves, including the maxillary and ophthalmic branches of the trigeminal nerve, are blocked using Peterson's method. Motor innervation is provided by the abducent, trochlear, and oculomotor nerves. The foramen is approached by using an 18-gauge, 4- to 5-in needle passed through a 14-gauge, ½-in cannula placed at the junction of the supraorbital process of the frontal bone and the zygomatic arch of the malar bone, ventral and posterior to the medial canthus of the eye (see Fig. 8–1).

The cannula is especially important in this block because it minimizes transport of squamous carcinoma cells to a deep site when dealing with cancer of the eye in cattle. In addition to keeping the deep needle more sterile, the cannula reduces the friction of the skin and allows the operator to feel more acutely with the needle. A slight curve to the needle is described but is not always necessary. Keep the needle in relationship to the planes of the head and insert it straight in, perpendicularly. As the second landmark, walk off the anterior edge of the ramus of the mandible, proceeding to the deepest site. If bone is encountered only two or three inches deep, retract and redirect ventrally to avoid the pterygoid crest. Correct placement of the needle usually results in visible signs from the patient including reaction to pain and a blinking eye reflex. With excessive force, it is possible to penetrate the turbinates and deposit the block in the nasopharynx. Fifteen to 25 ml of agent is deposited in varying locations at the deep site.

The second step of the ocular block is to redirect the 4-in needle posteriorly along the zygomatic arch to block the auriculopalpebral branch of the facial nerve. This is a motor nerve to the upper eyelid and is blocked to aid success of the surgery, especially in large bulls, which are able to close their eye mechanically, stopping surgery. The nerve is palpable in a notch on the arch just anterior to the base of the ear.

REGIONAL BLOCKS OF THE PARALUMBAR FOSSA

Simple infiltration of the incision line or slightly in front of it will suffice for

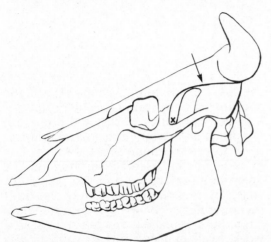

Figure 8–1 Bovine skull. Arrow shows site of cornual block. "X" is landmark for Peterson block.

anesthesia without seriously interfering with healing. Use 22-gauge, 1-in needles with 3/4 to 1 ml of the agent at each site, 3/4 inches apart. Repeat, using a 2-in needle in fat cattle to reach the peritoneum. Use approximately 40 ml total dose.

Two regional techniques are common for paralumbar block. They are widely used, with local or individual operator modifications seen. Farquharson (1940) described a dorsal approach to the intervertebral foramen of T_{13}, L_1, L_2, L_3, and L_4 (also called the Hall or Cambridge method) (Fig. 8–2). First, identify the dorsal vertebral processes and the midline. Palpate the anterior edge of the transverse lumbar processes of L_2 or L_3 (usually the most prominent). The transverse processes of L_1 and L_2 may be obscure in fat cattle. Project an imaginary line to the corresponding process of the opposite side and on a point *no more* than 1¾ inches from the midline place the first subcutaneous wheal for insertion of a cannula. If using the transverse process of L_2, you will actually be in line with the posterior edge of L_1 and its foramen. Insert a 14-gauge short cannula and introduce a 4- to 5-inch, 18-gauge needle. It is advantageous to hit the posterior edge of the transverse process with the needle point as a landmark and then walk the needle off to the ventral surface of the transverse process for the injection. Repeat the imaginary line and cannula placement for L_2 and then use that spacing to judge forward for T_{13}. These three sites are enough for most para-

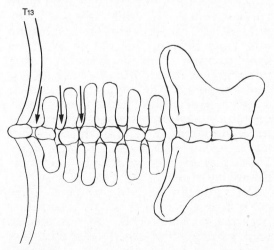

Figure 8–2 Bovine dorsal view. Farquharson paravertebral block.

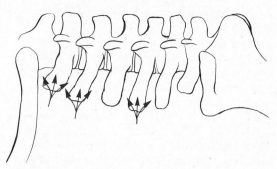

Figure 8–3 Bovine lateral view. Cakala paravertebral block.

lumbar incisions. If teat surgery is contemplated, block L_3 and L_4, which contribute nerves to the inguinal nerve. L_5 may also be blocked to aid in surgery of the tuber coxae.

The volume of local anesthetic used for the Farquharson block is 10 to 12 ml at each site except for 5 to 6 ml at L_3 and L_4. Lumbar nerves 3 and 4 contribute significant branches to the rear limbs, and strength for standing may be affected by anesthesia.

Cakala (1961) described an alternative block, patterned after Magda for approaching the lumbar nerves 1, 2, and 4. Use 3-in needles on the ventral side of the respective lumbar process and inject in a fan-shaped infiltration pattern parallel to the transverse process (Fig. 8–3). Because of the distribution angle, the blocks of L_1, L_2, and L_4 are sufficient to desensitize the whole paralumbar fossa. This block is relatively simple to perform and meets with more success in the hands of operators doing it for the first time, whereas the Farquharson technique is more frustrating to learn and fails occasionally.

EPIDURAL INJECTIONS

There are three different methods of epidural block in cattle. The two most common place a 1½-in, 18-gauge needle at the sacral-coccygeal or coccygeal 1-2 junction. One technique calls for infusion of 3 to 7 ml of anesthetic agent for induction of caudal analgesia. Anesthesia of the tail, perineum, escutcheon, and vaginal vault develops in 8 to 10 minutes.

The second technique is properly called a massive epidural. Using the same anatomical site, increase the volume to 1 ml/4 kg (1 ml/10 lbs). This bathes the nerve roots with the anesthetic agent as far craniad as the thoracic nerves 11 or 12 and gives complete anesthesia and block of parasympathetic innervation below this level. The animal will go down and will experience vasodilation, for which fluids must be given. This technique is useful for all types of surgery and has built-in restraint advantages. In the postoperative management, it is important to leave the animal *unstimulated* until the block is worn off and to ensure good footing during attempts to rise. Tie the rear (hobble) legs together and avoid slippery surfaces to prevent acetabular fracture in splayed out falls.

A third epidural technique was reviewed by Skarda and Muir (1979) and involves a more difficult anatomical placement at the first interlumbar space. Readers are referred to the excellent paper for more details.

General anesthesia should be considered if proper restraint and good anatomical local anesthesia will not suffice or if total immobility is desired.

REFERENCES

References can be found at the end of the chapter.

GENERAL ANESTHESIA IN RUMINANTS

R. B. HEATH, D.V.M., M.S.

LARGE RUMINANTS

Ruminants respond to anesthesia as do brachycephalic species, with the added complication of having a massive GI tract. They are not good respiratory reserve athletes, as are horses. Ruminants have much smaller lung fields than horses and a greater propensity for emphysema problems. The mass of the GI tract weighs on the diaphragm and inhibits its movement. In addition, rumen contents are readily regurgitated, risking aspiration pneumonia.

Prior to surgery, the clinician should institute complete fasting for 24 hours and water deprivation for 12 hours. During hot weather, water does not have to be withheld. Restrain the patient to permit catheterization of a jugular vein with a 6-in indwelling commercially available catheter. Preanesthetic use of tranquilizers is usually not indicated and may only serve to prolong recovery. Occasionally, animals need slight sedation with xylazine (.02 to .05 mg/kg IV) to aid mechanical restraint. Give .132 mg/kg IV atropine SO_4. This prevents regurgitation and lasts through induction. With respect to other authors' opinions on atropinization of ruminants, the author feels that atropine is quite helpful in ruminant surgery. He has not experienced postoperative gastrointestinal problems in the approximately 4000 bovine anesthesia cases on record at Colorado State University coupled with our short fasting management.

For induction, it is desirable to seize control of the airway as in respiratory high-risk patients. This is accomplished well with guaifenesin 1 liter with 3 g thiobarbiturate, administering 1.5 to 2 ml/kg (.6 to .75 ml/lb) of the solution. It is also possible to bolus inject the ultra-short thiobarbiturate of your choice in a dose of 10 mg/kg. Guiafenesin mixtures give more time for intubation and use of volatile vapor for induction, avoiding the crash induction. Large (45 to 50 mm) endotracheal tubes are needed in animals over 350 kg, and a good sealing cuff is desirable to prevent aspiration. Manual placement of the endotracheal tube is the fastest and easiest method. A long speculum may be needed to identify and intubate the arytenoid opening. Any commercial anesthesia machine for large animals may be used with halothane or methoxyflurane maintenance. You will note that ruminants seem to produce more CO_2 than other species, and soda lime may need to be changed more often. During maintenance, choose the lightest anesthesia possible to do the surgery. Monitoring for the palpebral reflex and "reverse bell" eye position will be useful in cattle. Light planes of anesthesia with some swallowing may be deep enough for some surgery, but at this depth the patient often begins to gag on the endotracheal tube and regurgitation may soon follow. Vaporizer settings, usually in the area of 4 per cent for induction and 1¼ to 2 per cent for maintenance will suffice. Doppler pulse detection of blood pressure is useful on the palmar and volar digital arteries of cattle. Nitrous oxide has *not* been a useful adjunct to anesthesia owing to the potential of increasing gas diffusion to the rumen and the risk of bloat intraoperatively. Fluids are recommended at the rate of 6 to 8 ml/kg/hour.

For recovery, lighten the anesthesia consistent with the needs of surgery as it is ending. Return the patient to a sternal position before he awakens and leave the endotracheal tube in place until the patient coughs vigorously and can hold his head up. Cattle have good recoveries, unlike other species, but it is necessary to protect limbs and horns from damage. Provide some support and massage of "sleepy" limbs postoperatively until proprioception returns. Return patients to their own stalls to recover and avoid unnecessary walking postoperatively.

SMALL RUMINANTS

All baby animals can be safely anesthetized with halothane by gentle restraint and face mask. Adult goats and sheep need an induction similar to that of cattle. Usually, thiobarbiturate in a dose of 10 to 12 mg/kg IV is suitable. Goats, sheep, and calves have a prominent anticubital vein similar to dogs except that it runs at a bit more of an angle. Often this is a handier IV injection site than the jugular vein in small ruminants. Dog-size endotracheal tubes and small animal anesthesia machines are used in sheep, calves, and goats under 125 kg (300 lbs). Goats in general are more delicate about pain, and general anesthesia is needed more in this species. Pygmy goats seem to be highly sensitive to injectable agents and must be very carefully weighed for titration of dose. Inhalation mask techniques are safer and more reversible in very small subjects.

Adult goats anesthetize fairly well with a regimen of xylazine in a dose of .22 mg/kg (.1 mg/lb). If deeper anesthesia is needed, 4.4 to 8.8 mg/kg (2 to 4 mg/lb) of ketamine HCl may be added.

Sheep seem to respond less well to xylazine but, with ketamine added to xylazine as in goats, a reasonably good anesthetic is developed.

Guaiafenesin-thiamylal mixtures similar to those used in cattle or horses will also give gentle anesthesia in goats and sheep. Titrate the dose carefully and maintain light reflexes.

PORCINE ANESTHESIA

Management of swine anesthesia presents some difficulties. Hogs resist mechanical restraint more and are physically more difficult to hold than other species. Strong assistance is needed. IV routes are difficult until practiced. The ear vein is the safest and most assessible vein. Good restraint may be instituted with the animal in lateral recumbency or by use of a hog snare. Hold the major vein at the base of the ear by the hand or forceps and create distension/visibility with massage of the ear. Occasionally a skin irritant, such as xylene, will help.

Small animal indwelling 20-gauge catheters, if available, will help maintain the patency of the vein.

The alternate intravenous route commonly mentioned in the literature is the anterior vena cava. This technique is acceptable for drawing blood but is too risky for anesthetic injections because one-fourth to one-third of the anterior vena cava punctures are actually into the brachial artery. This results in a high incidence of dissecting hematomas and cardiac tamponades. Arterial administration of anything but isotonic physiologic fluids is not indicated. Intraperitoneal, intramuscular, and other routes have been used in frustration, but it is still best for anesthetic purposes to attempt intravenous administration. For tranquilization, phenothiazines work well in a wide range of doses, depending on objective. Acetylpromazine may be used in a dose of .05 to .40 mg/kg; promazine is useful in a dose of .5 to 2.0 mg/kg. Cannibalistic or hysterical sows react well to IM doses in the upper limits of the dosage range. For sedation or for light preanesthetic purposes, use the low end of the dosage range and administer intravenously.

Short intravenous anesthesia can be obtained by thiobarbiturates in a dosage of 6.6 mg/kg (3 to 4 mg/lb). Used properly intravenously, thiobarbiturates will produce 7 to 9 minutes of crisp anesthesia sufficient for castration or electrical ejaculation. The speedy recovery and low cost far outweigh the difficulty of hitting the ear vein when compared with the method of intratesticular injection of overdoses, which the author does not favor.

Longer IV programs can be obtained by injectable Valium in a dose of .25 mg/kg, followed by 6.6 to 17.6 mg/kg ketamine IV. Smooth induction and complete anesthetic control, lasting for 20 to 30 minutes, are produced. This regimen is useful for surgery alone or for induction of inhalation anesthesia in swine. Intubation is usually difficult but presents little problem with Valium-ketamine owing to the lack of laryngospasm.

Guaifenesin-thiobarbiturate mixes (2.2 ml/kg) are useful in pigs if a trustworthy and patent intravenous route can be established for the large volumes needed. Xylazine is not effective in swine.

Innovar Vet (Pitman-Moore), in doses useful in dogs, works well in pigs intravenously or intramuscularly for similar short sedation and chemical restraint.

Inhalation anesthesia in the pig is induced by masking with small animal equipment. If intubation is necessary, it is better to use induction with Valium-ketamine. If a fairly short procedure is anticipated and a mask does not interfere, easy induction and fast recovery are produced with simple masking and restraint. Halothane is preferred, but methoxyflurane works well also. With halothane procedures in swine it is possible to encounter malignant hyperthermia, especially in Landrace, large white, or Poland China breeds.

REFERENCES

Bowen, J. M., and Seidel, S.: Anesthesia in the cow. Vet. Anesth. 3(2):100, 1976.

Cakala, S.: Paravertebral lumbar block in cattle. Cornell Vet. 57:64, 1961.

Elmore, R. G.: Food animal regional anesthesia. VM/SAC 75:1174, 1980.

Farquharson, J.: Paravertebral lumbar anesthesia in the bovine species. JAVMA 97:54, 1940.

Gabel, A. A.: Practical technique for bovine anesthesia. Mod. Vet. Prac. Aug.:39, 1964.

Garner, H. E., et al.: Anesthesia in bulls. Can. J. Comp. Med. 39:250, 1975.

Hall, L. W.: Wrights Veterinary Anesthesia and Analgesia, 6th ed. Baltimore: Williams & Wilkins, 1966.

Heath, R. B.: Chemical restraint and anesthesia. In Bovine Medicine and Surgery, 2nd ed. Santa Barbara: American Veterinary Publications, 1980, p. 1125.

Knight, A.: Pig anesthesia. Unpublished data, 1980.

Peterson, D. R.: Nerve block of the eye. JAVMA 118:145, 1951.

Skarda, R. T., and Muir, W. W.: Segmental epidural in cattle. Am. J. Vet. Res. 40(1):52, 1979.

CHAPTER 9

POSTOPERATIVE CARE OF THE PATIENT

JAMES G. FERGUSON, B.SC., D.V.M., M.SC.

GENERAL OBJECTIVES

The purpose of postoperative care is to maintain the patient in an optimal state so that healing of the surgical correction as well as metabolic stabilization can occur in the shortest time possible. The many factors that affect rapid return to function will be considered from various perspectives in this chapter, and it should be understood from the beginning that postoperative care begins before the operation is initiated and may continue for months or years after the actual operation has been completed. It is almost as much an attitude or philosophy as a set of procedures. The characteristics of recovery from a general anesthetic reflect the quality of the induction procedure as well as the agents used; the tendency toward stormy recovery following difficult induction is an obvious example. The selection of immunization programs, such as tetanus prophylaxis, or antibiotic regimens that may begin before, during, or immediately following the surgical procedure may or may not be considered as postoperative management. However, it is imperative that the course of postoperative care be carefully considered and specifically determined before surgery is begun. But even in emergency situations, when time does not allow for extended discussion in the early stages of treatment, management principles and protocols should be adhered to. Although treatment procedures may be revised during the healing proc-ess, basic treatment principles will not change.

The importance of physical control during recovery from general anesthetic varies between large animal species. Cattle, small ruminants, and swine may be allowed to recover in standard housing facilities provided that adequate bedding and nonslip footing are available. For cattle, a thick (10 to 30 cm) manure pack covered with fresh, clean straw is ideal. Alternatively, layers of wet hay and straw can be spread in a clean stall and packed down.

RECOVERY FACILITIES

Equine surgery requires well-designed facilities and an informed team of surgeons and technical support staff to provide for a safe, uneventful recovery from the anesthetic.

The recovery room itself should be located adjacent to or readily accessible to the operative area. Depending on the average patient size, the room may vary as to internal dimensions. An area 350 × 440 cm is considered a moderate-sized room for a 450- to 500-kg horse (Fig. 9–1). Several features may be incorporated into the recovery room, such as a squeeze gate, rings at 2.5 meters (8 ft) on the wall, an escape door, emergency anesthetic gases, suction, reinforced one-way observation ports, and moveable floor units for transportation purposes. The floors and walls must be covered to a

205

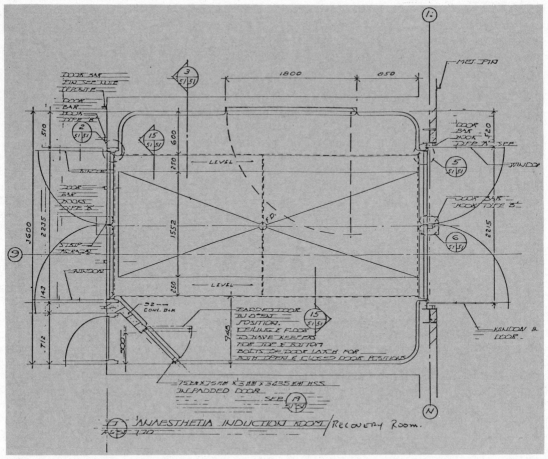

Figure 9–1 Drawing of an induction-recovery room that indicates removable floor sections, recessed squeeze gate, escape/safety door, and dimensions suitable for handling horses of approximately 500 kg.

level of at least 2 meters with durable, thick, energy-absorbing padding material, which significantly reduces the self-inflicted injury that can occur during recovery from anesthetic. It is not necessary to pad the floor to the same degree as the walls. The padding material may be permanently attached to the room or may be hung from the walls as heavy mats, depending on personal preference and financial constraints. The overall design of the room must be very strong, with particular emphasis on hinging and locking devices on exit and entry doors.

The recovery room area must contain ancillary equipment, which may become necessary if unanticipated complications arise. A full complement of emergency anesthetic and monitoring equipment, including tracheostomy and endotracheal tubes, must be readily available. A

surgical pack and sufficient draping material as well as bandaging material, suction hoses, and physical and chemical restraint materials should be accessible in close proximity to the recovery room.

Occasionally it will be necessary to lift or control a horse in the recovery room by means of a sling (Fig. 9–2) for brief or prolonged periods. Regardless of the duration of its use, the sling requires careful and knowledgeable application to ensure effective support. Although many models are commercially available, not all are suitable. The device must be regularly inspected for proper position and adequate support, since the animal will not remain in the same place for any extended time. Initial precautions must be taken to prevent undue excitement or self-inflicted trauma of the horse while it becomes accustomed to the sling.

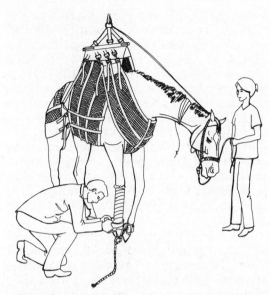

Figure 9–2 Schematic drawing of a horse being supported in a sling that is connected to a ceiling hook by a remote-controlled chain winch. The winch should have a minimum 1000-kg capacity, and the hook should be incorporated into the building design so as to readily support even greater weights without undue stress to the superstructure.

These may include chemical restraint, physical control, and constant attendance by the handler or technical staff. The tendency to turn in circles about the support center is prevented by haltering to a fixed ring.

The design of the recovery room should provide adequate structural strength to safely support a strong ceiling hook, an electrical or mechanical hoist system, and the weight of a large horse without risk of failure. Modifications to existing buildings should involve consultation with appropriate professionals to ensure that design specifications are adequate.

The personnel within the recovery room frequently determine postoperative success or failure. All people working in this area must function as a team, and experience and foresight are required in situations that may become hazardous to the patient and staff alike.

The horse should be removed from the recovery room only when it has fully regained its ability to ambulate. Footing in aisles and in the stall must be dry and secure.

As with many other species, the nature of the recovery process in the horse is in large part related to the quality of the induction procedure. The incidence of stormy recovery increases in proportion to the excitement level of the horse as it is being anesthetized. Hence the need for premedication, reduction of noise, and concentration by all personnel on keeping the horse calm during induction.

PHYSICAL CONTROL DURING RECOVERY

The stormy recovery, or emergence delirium, poses a serious problem for the anesthesiologist-surgeon and strongly tests the physical facilities and the competence of all personnel involved. This condition occurs in a variable percentage of anesthetized horses, depending on anesthetic used, breed, and temperament. The prevention or minimalization of the condition begins preoperatively during the induction process and involves keeping the animal calm and quiet. This is facilitated by the use of adequate premedication such as xylazine.

It may become evident during close recovery monitoring that the horse is becoming increasingly excited, even before strenuous physical actions occur. At this point it is recommended that sedatives or narcotics be given. If there is an increased chance of excitement due to breed, previous incidents, or other reasons, the drugs may be given before the end of the surgical procedure. Although the cause of delirious actions is not always known, any condition causing pain, anxiety, or excitement should be corrected to reduce the consequences of uncontrolled activity in the recovery room. If such movements remain violent and uncontrolled for any length of time, there is a high risk of dehiscence of the surgical wound, fracture of the treated or normal limbs, exertional myositis, generalized trauma to the animal's body, and hazard to recovery room personnel as well as the facility itself.

Violent anesthetic recoveries in cattle, sheep, goats, and pigs are rare and readily controlled. In general following the surgical procedure, these species may be returned directly to their stall and observed until they can maintain themselves in sternal recumbency. They should be encouraged to stand only when total consciousness and coordination have been achieved, i.e., from several minutes to a few hours following the operation. A sow that has received general anesthesia or heavy sedation for a cesarean section should be carefully watched before returning piglets to her to prevent savaging and inadvertent crushing when she lies down.

Bloat is a complication that can arise where there is insufficient time between feeding and the beginning of the anesthetic procedure. Fermentation of gases by ruminal bacteria occurs more rapidly in the engorged condition. In such instances the duration of surgery becomes a factor as well as the early return to the sternal position in the operating room or stall. Lateral recumbency prevents the escape of gas from the esophagus because the opening is usually below the fluid line; in the upright position this positional relationship is corrected. If intraruminal pressure builds to a significant degree, there is severe interference with respiratory excursions and cardiovascular function and the possibility of regurgitation, which may result in aspiration of ruminal contents into the lungs unless a cuffed endotracheal tube is in place.

Whenever cattle struggle on slippery flooring or try to stand before they have recovered their full coordination, damage to the musculoskeletal system may occur. This is best prevented by providing adequate footing, such as a deep, firm manure pack, and encouraging the animal to remain recumbent until fully conscious. It is not uncommon for cows to luxate hips, traumatize skin and teats, and rupture musculotendinous units while attempting to stand under adverse conditions. On the other hand, if larger ruminants remain recumbent for an extended period of time, there is a strong possibility that irreversible damage to muscle groups may occur owing to pressure-related ischemic necrosis, compartment syndrome, or nerve paralysis. These conditions usually develop whenever a heavy adult animal is unable to stand for 36 to 48 hours, regardless of cause. Serum levels of glutamic oxaloacetic transaminase remain markedly elevated, whereas serum creatine phosphokinase levels fall after an initial peak

associated with the early phases of the disease. The muscles primarily affected are the semitendinosus, biceps femoris, and adductors and extensors of the hind limb on the down side (Cox 1981). It is thought that external pressure causes anoxia, which affects the sciatic nerve and the muscle tissues, resulting in vascular leakage into the extracellular compartment. With increased accumulation into the nondistensible compartment, pressure develops, causing further embarrassment of vascular function and leading to ischemia and a self-potentiating cycle.

The contact surface between the stall and the animal must remain dry at all times. In addition to keeping the animal dry and comfortable, it is imperative that undue pressure not be placed for any prolonged period of time on the muscles bearing the weight of the animal in recumbency. For this reason, any recumbent animal should be shifted from side to side at intervals varying between one and three hours on an around-the-clock basis. Whenever the animal is turned over to its new side, the previously "down" muscles should be vigorously massaged, dried if necessary, and handled in a manner that will ensure the maintenance of their function over a prolonged time period. Whenever possible, the animal should be maintained in sternal recumbency rather than lateral recumbency to minimize pressure on muscles and nerves, which will later affect its ability to rise, stand, and walk with minimal damage to the total animal. Although it is difficult to scientifically evaluate the benefits of an animal's attitude on its recovery, many workers feel that, by maximizing all positive reinforcement and encouraging the animal to "want" to get well, the period of immediate postoperative management and the prolonged phase of postoperative care can be effectively reduced.

Rolling small ruminants or swine from side to side is usually a simple matter of one or two people physically rolling the animal over onto a clean, dry, freshly bedded part of the stall; however, the physical limitations of the same procedure become much more complicated as the size of the animal increases to 500 kg or more. When such is the case, short soft ropes should be attached to the down leg either just above or just below the carpus on the foreleg. Then, with one or two people on each rope and an assistant ensuring that the head and neck do not become abnormally twisted, the animal is rolled over onto its back and comes to lie on the previously "up" side of the body. The area where the animal was originally lying is then bedded with fresh straw and the animal made as comfortable as possible.

Occasionally cattle are unable to rise after surgery for a variety of reasons. If the situation continues for more than several hours, efforts should be made to encourage and stimulate the animal to rise with the aid of mechanical devices.

The use of various sling designs has been advocated in the past by many workers; however, it is the author's experience that in large ruminants a body sling is both difficult to apply and frustrating to maintain over any significant period of time postoperatively. The use of slings is not advocated; instead, the hind quarters may be supported and the animal encouraged to rise by the use of hip lifters. It should be mentioned, however, that hip lifters can be significantly damaging to the animal if not carefully and properly applied, primarily because of failure to appreciate the significant mechanical forces involved. Properly placed with firm compression over the wings of the ileum, most hip lifters, when used in conjunction with an electrical or mechanical winch system, enable the surgeon to guide the animal into the standing position in a short period of time. Once this has been accomplished and the animal is seen to be able to support its weight, the hip-lifting device should be loosened to prevent pressure necrosis over the wings of the ileum. The lifting and jack mechanisms are subsequently used only to provide stability to the animal. Once the animal is able to support its weight for 5 to 10 minutes, the hip lifters can be removed as soon as the animal stands. The surgeon or assistant can then help the animal to maintain its balance by controlling the tail and halter. It is usually possible to increase the period of time during which the animal can maintain itself in the standing position over the first few days

after the hip lifter has been applied. If continued, excessive forces are necessary to encourage the animal to stand for even short periods, prognosis for the long term is reduced, and the hip lifters may then become detrimental to the overall welfare of the animal.

Care must be exercised by the operators of the hip lifters for the safety of themselves and their assistants. Placed on an unsteady animal in a confined space such as a box stall, the mechanical device can become hazardous to all personnel in the area if the animal begins to stagger and lose control.

PATIENT MONITORING

The consistent evaluation and re-evaluation of a patient following its recovery from anesthesia are critical parts of good postoperative care. The monitoring process takes into account the preoperative health status, the nature of the surgery, and the parameters measured by the anesthetic and surgical teams and applies them to a protocol of observation and data accumulation, resulting in an accurate assessment of the progress of the animal. Monitoring regimens vary from operation to operation and from patient to patient; however, the principles remain constant and the plan allows for continued reappraisal, changing treatment and tests when appropriate.

A thorough and accurate record is best achieved by using a form that can contain special instructions and considerations as well as provide for the documentation of results that most clearly reveal trends in the criteria being observed. In most instances several team members are responsible for evaluating different parameters. The recording of data from several sources allows the formation of an accurate overall picture by the surgeon in charge of the case and reduces the loss or bias of information being utilized. Since not all tests are performed at the same regular intervals, a written record also reduces the potential confusion over the number of tests being run and allows for the more accurate documentation of costs incurred. Figure 9–3 contains the basics of a simple monitoring protocol worksheet.

INTENSIVE CARE WORKSHEET

CASE NUMBER: NAME: HISTORY:

DATE/TIME	TEMP/RR	PULSE/ QUALITY	MUCOUS MEMBRANE CAP. REFILL TIME (sec)	GUT MOTILITY	CBC	CHEMISTRY, BLOOD GAS, PARACENTESIS	CLINICAL REMARKS, GASTRIC CONTENTS (liters), THERAPY, MEDICATION

Figure 9–3 Simple monitoring worksheet that provides the basis for assessment of patient progress in the immediate postoperative period. Worksheet pages should be numbered to provide a chronological data base in prolonged or more detailed cases.

Regardless of the species being considered, the period during which the animal is removed from the anesthetic machine and its oxygen supply to room air without the benefit of a mechanical airway remains a critical phase in the postoperative interval. It is during this time that the animal undergoes a number of physiological changes and the potential risk of complications is greatest.

In the horse, there is a danger of partial or complete airway obstruction occurring when the endotracheal tube is removed. This possibility must be anticipated in every case and the amount of air moving through the upper airway carefully evaluated. Whenever the tidal volume is considered to be inadequate, an endotracheal tube should be reinserted. If this cannot be accomplished an emergency tracheostomy should be performed through a 10-cm incision directly over the midline approximately one-third of the distance down the neck. After dissecting in blunt fashion down to the trachea, an incision is made in the soft tissue between the cartilaginous rings and a tracheostomy tube inserted to provide the free passage of air into the lungs. Supplemental oxygen may be fed into the airway by means of a small-bore tube connected to a suitable oxygen supply.

When rate and volume of respiration are inadequate, respiratory stimulants, such as doxapram hydrochloride at 0.2 to 0.5 mg/kg, may be given by the intravenous route, particularly if depression is related to xylazine and ultrashort-acting barbiturates. Bronchodilators, such as atropine given intravenously at 0.01 to 0.02 mg/kg, may also be considered (Muir and Bednarski 1983). By encouraging the horse to maintain sternal recumbency as soon as possible, it is thought that pulmonary efficiency is optimized (Boles 1975).

As the horse continues to recover from the procedure and is returned to its stall, hemoglobin and packed cell volumes (PCV) must be regularly evaluated. It is not uncommon for these levels to increase owing to splenic contraction for a few hours after recovery. If, however, there is a progressive elevation not only of PCV (over 45 per cent) but of other parameters, such as total protein levels, fluid administration should be considered to maintain body fluids within normal ranges. Maintaining the operating and recovery rooms at appropriate temperatures helps control body heat or fluid losses and minimizes electrolyte changes, such as those resulting from excessive sweating.

Although the horse should not be forced to stand before it is ready, occasionally a tail rope may be used to balance and support the animal. Such a device may be utilized to provide considerable support, up to the total weight of the animal if necessary. Once full coordination has been achieved, minimal walking on good footing a few hours after recovery will help promote peristalsis, reduce the possibility of laminitis developing, and may improve the horse's attitude.

When intraruminal pressure in ruminants has increased during the surgical procedure, there is a danger that ingesta may be regurgitated into the pharyngeal area. If the endotracheal tube has been removed before effective swallowing reflex has returned, aspiration of digestive fluids and materials may occur. To prevent this, pressure within the rumen should be relieved by inserting a tube through the esophagus into the rumen to release excess gas while the endotracheal tube is in place. The proper dietary management of the animal preoperatively and the reduction of anesthesia and surgery time also minimize the chances of food material entering the respiratory tract. Following removal of the endotracheal tube, the head and neck should be positioned so that any material in the posterior pharyngeal region will drain out the oral cavity rather than back into the trachea and lungs. This is achieved by tilting the chest and posterior body regions above the level of the pharynx, and either placing an elevating object such as a sandbag under the neck near the thoracic inlet or assisting the animal in maintaining sternal recumbency. All of these maneuvers utilize gravitational forces to ensure that aspiration does not occur.

If intraruminal pressure continues to increase and cannot be controlled by esophageal intubation, a rumen trochar may be inserted into the rumen through the upper left paralumbar fossa. This procedure should only be undertaken when its benefits outweigh the consistent development of peritonitis around the insertion site, which may become more generalized in nature.

The most appropriate intervals over which all parameters must be monitored vary with the species, the nature of the surgical problem, and the extent to which complications are expected. Catheters should be left in place whenever possible to facilitate sampling procedures in the immediate postoperative period.

Blood gases may be quantitated after the first hour and thereafter as required based on several clinical parameters. In problem cases PCV and total protein may be tabulated every four hours, as are other values such as temperature, pulse, and respiration. Complete hematological and electrolyte values must be recorded and trends identified on a daily basis. Function of the gastrointestinal tract requires appraisal of vital systems using palpation, auscultation, and visualization of not only the length of the system but also the quality and quantity of the feces.

These suggested intervals should be adjusted so that specific problem areas receive the extra attention required in each case. Some disease processes are predisposed to rapid parameter changes, which must be taken into account for each individual animal.

PAIN CONTROL

The control of pain postoperatively is of major importance in most situations, particularly following gastrointestinal and orthopedic surgery in the horse. In the selection of the most suitable drug, several factors must be taken into consideration. All drugs vary in their effect on different horses and on different body systems; e.g., one that controls low-grade, orthopedic-related pain may be totally inadequate for abdominal pain. Many drugs relieve pain but act over a time period that makes frequent assessment difficult. If pain is to be controlled immediately after anesthesia, hypotensive effects may be critical to the survival of the animal.

Most drugs used to control pain in the postoperative period are categorized as antiprostaglandins, sedatives, or tranquilizers (Table 9–1).

Following abdominal surgery in horses, the control of pain and anxiety will speed recovery, reduce complications, and shorten the convalescent period. The choice of drug must take into account the surgical problem, its expected postoperative sequelae, and the effectiveness of the drug, its side effects, and duration of action.

Gastrointestinal pain is controlled with flunixin meglumine, 2.0 mg/kg IM or IV. It is probably the most effective antiprostaglandin on the digestive tract, with a duration of action ranging from 10 minutes to 6 hours, depending on the amount of pain present. Xylazine HCl is also effective for visceral pain and may be given via the IV route (0.4 to 0.6 mg/kg) or intramuscularly (1.0 to 1.6 mg/kg). This drug has a relatively short duration of action, although it is very effective over that time period. Xylazine has the advantage of minimal side effects on the digestive or cardiovascular system and, owing to its brief duration of action, allows for frequent, accurate re-evaluation of the patient with minimal masking of clinical signs.

Pentazocine, while having few side effects, is not always an effective analgesic for other than mild abdominal pain. The tranquilizers acepromazine and promazine are also relatively ineffective in controlling gastrointestinal pain and, although they do relieve anxiety without affecting intestinal motility, they have a hypotensive effect due to their alpha-adrenergic blocking properties.

Narcotic agents such as meperidine (4.0 mg/kg) or oxymorphone (0.03 mg/kg) are very effective in controlling gastrointestinal pain and do not produce unfavorable side effects in the cardiovascular area but do interfere with peristalsis. This significant side effect, plus the cumbersome nature of handling controlled narcotics, makes their routine use impractical. Methampyrone may be used not only for its analgesic properties but also for its antispasmotic effects. The dose is 10.0 mg/kg IM or IV.

Cattle, small ruminants, and swine rarely require postoperative pain control following gastrointestinal surgery.

Table 9-1. PAIN-RELIEVING DRUGS COMMONLY USED POSTOPERATIVELY

	Generic Name	Trade Name
Antiprostaglandins		
	Acetylsalicylic acid	Aspirin
	Flunixin meglumine	Banamine
	Methampyrone	Dipyrone
	Phenylbutazone	Butazolidin
Sedatives and Tranquilizers		
	Chloral hydrate	
	Pentazocine lactate	Talwin
	Meperidine	Demerol
	Oxymorphone	Numorphan
	Xylazine HCl	Rompun
	Promazine HCl	Promazine
	Acepromazine maleate	Acepromazine

In orthopedic cases, analgesia effects a more quiet, controlled recovery and convalescence, resulting in less stress on the injured and contralateral limbs. With more normal weight-bearing, internal and external fixation devices are allowed to function as designed and are not overchallenged. The other limbs and joints tend not to be unduly stressed, with the net result being rapid healing without complications in the other limbs. The most commonly used pain reliever in orthopedic conditions in the horse is phenylbutazone. Its relative safety, effectiveness, duration of action (12 to 14 hours), and availability in several forms make it universally accepted. Acetylsalicylic acid, another antiprostaglandin, is also indicated in cattle at a dose rate of 100 mg/kg twice daily per os for relief of arthritic pain.

Although not thoroughly documented in animals, the proper use of pressure bandages in humans provides for some pain relief. This is of particular interest to the veterinarian when using pressure bandages over a fractured limb and support bandages on the contralateral limb, which may soon become fatigued and sore owing to increased weight-bearing following injury to the opposite leg.

PHYSICAL MEDICINE

Postoperative care using concepts of physical medicine is not thoroughly considered by most veterinarians, except in equine cases. With increasing technical developments in other fields, the treatment modes of physical therapy in animals will continue to expand.

Considerations for postoperative housing facilities usually take into account the amount of exercise a patient will need. Therapeutic exercise has several benefits regardless of whether the movements are active or passive in nature. If active, direct control over the animal by means of halter or lead shank is recommended to prevent overexuberance and self-trauma. Passive action must be initiated early in the convalescent period and particular care taken to ensure that all tissues and joints are properly manipulated. In evaluating each patient, the affected part, the contralateral part, and the patient's general condition must be accurately assessed. In addition to preventing adhesions and maximizing the range of joint motion, therapeutic exercise restores muscle tone and improves circulation to the part. With better vascular supply, the healing rate is increased owing to such factors as more rapid resorption of waste products, bone response to mechanical stimulation, and a reduction in bone atrophy, which results from decreased limb use. Although the possible "psychological" benefits of exercise are difficult to measure, they may promote the overall well-being of the animal.

Caution must be expressed when considering the benefits of exercise resulting from "turning out" an animal into a medium- or large-sized pasture. Frequently only minimal exercise results, with the affected part not being effectively manipulated and other structures receiving too much stress. "Out of sight, out of mind" is not good therapeutic care.

Physical activity, whether active or passive, has much to offer provided it is performed under controlled situations. Ligaments, ligament-bone junctions, and bone mass are all adversely affected when physical activity is reduced or prevented (Laros, Tipton, and Cooper 1971). It is also believed that passive activity significantly benefits joints, which contain blood as a result of bleeding disorders, trauma, or surgery and, in addition, may reduce the risk of secondary degenerative arthritis (O'Driscoll, Kumar, and Salter 1983).

Faradism

Faradism is the therapeutic use of an interrupted current to stimulate nerves and muscles and is an active, selected form of exercise under the operator's control. The structures exercised are the motor nerve, neuromuscular junction of the muscle, and the muscle group. The current utilized may vary as to pulse, wave form, current, and direction. The manufacturer's guidelines should be followed carefully. One significant advantage of this technique is that one area of the body can be exercised without stressing other areas.

Diathermy

The use of energy in various wavelengths, such as short wave (30 to 33 meters), ultrashort wave (less than 10 meters), and ultrasound, has many medical benefits. It has the advantage of supplying heat directly to deeper structures, whereas other methods heat only the superficial tissues. By heating joints and related articular areas, a significant beneficial result is achieved. The heat is produced in the tissues by conversion of high-frequency vibrations into thermal energy.

Diathermy is indicated for muscle spasm, acute joint and muscle injuries, and old articular and periarticular scars. It can be used near metal implants, where electromagnetic forces should not be used. This therapy mode should not be used around the eye or in patients with infections, malignancies, or bleeding problems. Its use in pregnant animals is in question, and in laminectomy patients its dosage should be reduced. Proper dosage should be utilized in all instances. The patient will indicate pain or discomfort if the dosage is too high. For this reason, denervated areas and twitch restraint should be avoided when using this form of treatment.

Hydrotherapy

Water has a great number of uses in physical therapy in the postoperative period. In the hydrothermal mode, it may be applied as a spray, as hot or cold packs, as baths, or as a wash. Water functions to relieve pain, relax tissues, and stimulate circulation.

The hydrokinetic form of hydrotherapy can be used to provide buoyancy, such as in swimming exercises, which provide shock-free use of limbs, or agitation. Agitation provides mechanical stimulation or massage as well as a cleaning and debriding function by such devices as the whirlpool bath or turbolator boot (Fig. 9–4).

Therapeutic Cold

The application of cold to an area is indicated in conditions of acute trauma, laminitis, and ligament, joint, or muscle injuries referred to as "sprains." Cold reduces the extravasation of blood and

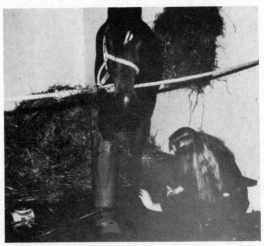

Figure 9–4 Hydrotherapy or turbulator boot in use to encourage healing following implant removal, osteomyelitis, and malunion.

fluids into the tissues and increases their resorption. In addition, the metabolic demands of injured tissues for oxygen and nutrients are reduced and the danger of thrombosis is minimized. The effect of cold on sensory organs reduces pain and decreases muscle spasm associated with pain, thus reducing further spasm, which can result in further ischemic damage. Contraindications to application of cold to an area relate primarily to septic conditions.

Cold is more penetrating than heat owing to natural heat exchange physiology in the body. Methods used to apply this cold are immersion, ice packs, cold compresses, cold water spray, and cold whirlpool baths. The cold is most effective in application periods that extend up to a maximum of 30 or 40 minutes at a time. The treatments may be performed several times a day if necessary. Whenever extensive cold water treatment is undertaken, the skin and feet must be carefully evaluated for potential infections resulting from prolonged exposure to a wet environment.

Therapeutic Heat

When applied to the body, energy in the form of heat has several beneficial results. The local temperature is increased, as are blood and lymph flow, metabolic rate, and phagocytic activity. In addition, pain sensation in some patients is reduced, as healing in the area is maximized. Heat can be applied in many ways, such as heat sources placed directly on the skin (conductive), infared lamps (radiant), warm whirlpool baths (convective), and ultrasound (conversive).

POSTOPERATIVE COMPLICATIONS

Wound Infection

Since wound infection may result from inappropriate postoperative care, prevention begins with concern for tissue handling and good surgical technique during the operation. All maneuvers that unnecessarily traumatize the tissues surrounding the incision interfere with the body's ability to cope with infection. It is

well to recall also that "time is trauma" and that the infection rate increases with the duration of the surgical procedure; hence, expediency reduces complication rate.

With many operations, absolute sterility is not possible and the surgeon must be particularly concerned with facilitating the normal defense mechanisms during and after surgery. Antibacterial therapy should be carefully considered, with culture and sensitivity or previous experience judiciously used to select an appropriate regimen. Occasionally, the accumulation of serum in the immediate vicinity of the wound can result in poor healing, dehiscence, or infection. The surgical placement of drains is indicated in this situation. The proper care of these devices is critical to good wound healing. Drains that are utilized to reduce infection, edema, or fluid accumulation can become pathways of ascending infection if not properly cared for. The most common management problems result from allowing the device to remain in place for too long (four days is the maximum) and inability to keep the drain clean and protected from the environment where it exits from the body. The drain itself should be examined, cleaned, and checked for function several times daily and covered by a sterile dressing to prevent contamination from the outside. An antibacterial ointment may be applied to the drain and the skin at the point of exit to reduce scalding and the chance of retrograde infection.

Infected wounds should be swabbed to identify and monitor bacterial involvement and aid in the selection of the appropriate antibiotic, keeping in mind that microbial populations and sensitivities can change over a short period of time. Cleaning the wound area not only reduces the amount of necrotic debris but also reduces the tendency for scalding of the nearby surfaces. Scalding may also be prevented by liberal application on a regular basis of petrolatum to the area ventral to the draining wound.

The application of bandages over the site restricts further contamination, prevents access by flies, and may aid in controlling pain. It is important that the bandage allow for drainage of the area while still performing its required functions.

Whenever drainage occurs from an incision site, particularly when its location is ventral or at least somewhat dependent, the specter of wound dehiscence and evisceration is present. The decision to surgically re-enter the wound and effect repair or treat more conservatively with supportive body bandaging must be carefully considered, regarding safety, economics, and prognosis.

The postoperative control of wound infection is intimately related to the nature and quality of the surgery that has been performed as well as the age and condition of the animal.

Management is primarily related to maintenance of conditions that reduce the incidence of wound sepsis. Wound or incision sites should be protected from environmental contamination by bandages whenever possible. Not only do such dressings protect the wound from the environment, they can serve as an absorbent that keeps infected material from moving out of the wound. The added padding and pressure prevent further trauma to the wound by preventing either contact with other surfaces or self-trauma. When bandages cannot be applied to specific areas, self-trauma may be limited by muzzles, cross-tying, cradles, narrowed stalls, poles, or other devices.

Although topical wound dressings in spray or powder form have been advocated for many years, their acceptance is far from universal. This also applies to plastic-type aerosol dressings designed to provide a protective impermeable film over the wound. Infected wounds should be cleansed with a mild detergent and debrided to remove necrotic debris and facilitate drainage.

Special care should be given to the provision of suitable bedding that will keep the animal and the wound dry and reduce contamination from feces, urine, or food supplies. The bedding should also be of sufficient thickness to provide protection from pressure and abrasion from the floor.

Wound Dehiscence

Failure of an incision to heal or breakdown of the site resulting in wound de-

hiscence is always a concern of the surgeon regardless of his experience and skill. Wound dehiscence can result in bacterial invasion through the defect and evisceration when the abdominal wall is involved. Causes of wound breakdown may be categorized into those related to healing qualities of the animal such as systemic, vascular, or mechanical factors, including devitalization or inadequate tissue in the suture line; ischemia related to tissue handling or suture placement; and the production of undue forces across the incision line caused by distention of gut, persistent coughing, straining, and violent activity during the recovery or postoperative phase. Specific attention should be directed toward relieving distention with a nasogastric tube when appropriate. Early return of gastrointestinal function will also reduce generalized abdominal pressure. Protective and support bandages will reduce tension across suture lines, particularly in the early postsurgical phase.

The selection and placement of suture materials is a major factor in preventing wound dehiscence. Material should be selected that will maintain its strength for extended time periods, particularly when opposing fascia, which may take months to regain maximum strength. The introduction of suture materials such as polydioxanone suture continues to assist in this regard. Suture patterns that provide maximum strength should be used; however, buried continuous suture patterns are finding favor with many surgeons owing to their ability to reduce operative time.

Early signs of wound breakdown include the continued and progressive seepage of serum from a wound, failure of a serum clot to bridge the edges of the incision, and gaping in the area between skin sutures. When these conditions are observed, supportive bandages should be applied when suitable and a thorough evaluation of the animal performed to establish etiology and prognosis.

Disseminated Intravascular Coagulation and Consumptive Coagulopathy

Disseminated intravascular coagulation (DIC) is a disturbance of the clotting mechanism occurring within the vascular system that results in the uncontrolled consumption of platelets and other clotting factors. The disease is initiated by a number of varied stimuli that can involve the actual surgical procedure performed or the condition responsible for the need for surgical intervention. Whatever the cause, the normal inhibitory feedback mechanism, which is responsible for controlling the coagulation process, fails and allows clotting factors to be used up, resulting in a bleeding tendency. This is demonstrated by intravascular coagulation in the microcirculation, impairment of organ function, platelet consumption, and an inability of the blood to clot. The enzymatic breakdown of the fibrin clots produces fibrinogen and fibrin degradation products (FDP), which in turn tend to inhibit normal coagulation processes.

The surgeon is not usually able to diagnose the disease in the early stages. In its consumptive stage the clinical signs include thrombocytopenia (platelets below 20,000/mm), abnormal partial thromboplastin time, prolonged prothrombin time, markedly depressed fibrinogen values, FDPs detectable in the plasma, and occasionally fragmented erythrocytes. In general, epistaxis and frank hemorrhage are rarely seen, but petechiae and ecchymotic hemorrhages are usually signs leading to laboratory confirmation of the problem.

The surgeon should be acutely aware that this complication can and does arise following surgery for colic, cesarean section, and orthopedic procedures. The prognosis, if the diagnosis is made ante mortem, is guarded at best.

Enteritis

Postoperative enteritis is a complication with minimal clinical significance except in the horse, where it is a constant concern, particularly when repeated operations are performed. The major factor appears to be the stress incurred from the disease process, the surgical manipulations, the anesthetic procedure, or a combination of these factors that allows the development of a Salmonella typhimurium-related diarrhea. Concurrent

antimicrobial therapy with tetracyclines tends to worsen the condition (Ap and Owen 1975).

Transient loosening of the feces frequently occurs as a result of preoperative dietary management or unknown factors affecting the digestive tract. The major concern is when the condition becomes severe and is accompanied by significant fluid and electrolyte imbalances plus the multiplication of the Salmonella organisms, with their inherent adverse effect on the hemogram. Diagnosis is difficult in the early stages owing to inability to isolate the organisms involved. However, isolation procedures should be initiated and treatment begun immediately based on clinical signs and clinical pathology results.

A negative fecal culture from a horse with diarrhea does not rule out Salmonella as a cause of the problem. One of the first signs indicating this organism as a possible cause, other than the diarrhea and fever, is the presence of neutropenia, which may exist for several days before loose feces are seen (Ap et al., 1979).

Affected horses may show rapid alterations in fluid and electrolyte concentrations as well as acid-base abnormalities; hence, careful frequent monitoring of these parameters is imperative. Treatment is aimed primarily at correcting systemic imbalances and secondarily at controlling the causative organism. The surgeon should aggressively seek to correct abnormal values after consulting detailed texts on treatment regimens for the disease.

Paralytic Ileus

Following any surgical procedure involving repair or manipulation of the abdominal viscera, sequelae adversely affecting gut function are of major concern. Ileus, the inhibition of gut motility, is common and an expected finding in many cases; however, the continued lack of function over an extended period of time can become life-threatening. As a result of paralysis of the gut, fluids and electrolytes sequester in the lumen, creating systemic imbalances and interfering with normal return to function in a self-potentiating manner. Causes of ileus include distention of bowel, physical obstruction, peritonitis, excessive handling of gut tissues, and vascular compromise. The presence of serum electrolyte imbalance may also contribute to the syndrome.

Failure to detect normal gut sounds, the lack of fecal production, distention of the abdomen and bowel, or a capricious appetite may be seen. Whenever the stomach of the horse is involved, pain and distress may be observed. In such cases, periodic nasogastric drainage is indicated once the option of maintaining the tube in place for prolonged periods of time is considered. The fluid lost to sequestration should be replaced intravenously so that normal hydration and electrolyte levels are preserved.

Monitoring of fluid volume removed, fluctuations in hemogram, and serum ion levels is mandatory for provision of optimal supportive therapy.

Laminitis

The development of laminitis following surgery should be a major concern for those involved in the postoperative care of horses. It remains a constant threat whenever abdominal surgery is performed, and the incidence increases with concurrent infection, shock, and toxemia. In anticipation of this complication, the animal should be carefully examined several times each day for signs of abnormal stance, reluctance to walk, shifting of body weight, increased periods of recumbency, increased temperature of the feet, and an increase in digital artery pulse.

Flooring of rubber or other substances is thought to reduce the incidence and support the treatment of the condition, pointing strongly to designs of postoperative housing facilities that take these factors into account.

Postoperative Myopathy

One of the most difficult complications to handle is postoperative myopathy, which in its generalized form is related to muscle damage in the fore- and hind quarters. Clinical signs are related to pain and are manifest as colic, sweating, apprehension, and weakness of the affected limbs, which produces struggling due to inability to rise or remain standing. If the horse is able to stand, there is frequently trembling of the affected muscle groups, reflecting pain. Palpation of the affected muscle groups may reveal a flaccid or firm muscle mass, which can become edematous.

Any exertion, whether during the anesthetic recovery phase or during attempts to stand or walk, can potentiate the disease process. The major laboratory findings are related to enzyme release from damaged muscles, primarily elevated serum creatinine phosphokinase (SCPK) and serum asparate aminotransferase levels. With extensive necrosis, myoglobinuria is usually present. The basis for muscle damage appears to be related to pressure of the animal's own weight, which interferes with vascular function to certain muscle groups. This poor tissue perfusion may affect upper or lower limbs if positioning and padding are inadequate and becomes significant during prolonged procedures, if the depth of anesthesia is increased, or when there is a precipitous drop in blood pressure during the operation (Mansmann, McAllister, and Pratt 1982). Many surgeons feel that horses on a high grain ration are more disposed to the condition. Prevention involves dietary management of high risk patients during elective procedures, expedient surgical conduct, proper positioning, and the use of foam, air, or water mattresses during the operation.

Treatment is primarily concerned with alleviating the signs of pain, controlling inflammation, correcting fluid and electrolyte imbalances, and preventing myoglobin deposition in the kidneys. Owing to rapid and varied changes in these parameters, a careful monitoring program should be initiated for the first two or three postoperative days in all animals affected by the myopathy. Exercise should be minimal and at most should consist of hand walking for short distances until signs are greatly reduced. Injectables, such as meperidine or flunixin meglumine, as well as fluid and electrolyte therapy should be administered as clinical signs dictate, and good nursing care should be provided.

Hemorrhage

Whenever bleeding occurs in the postoperative phase the origin and cause should be rapidly established. Many times the problem is minor and can be controlled with minimal effort, e.g., digital pressure or a firm bandage. Often, however, a more radical approach must be used to isolate and ligate the offending vessels or vascular bed to prevent serious blood loss. Whenever this occurs the possibility of systemic clotting problems must be thoroughly investigated and the existence of disseminated intravascular coagulation or other coagulation problems ruled out by evaluating specific laboratory tests for clotting ability.

Airway obstruction may follow removal of the endotracheal tube during the recovery process owing to edema of the larynx, collapse of the soft tissues in that area, or the presence of substances such as blood or a blood clot in the airway. Initial steps should be taken to determine the cause of the obstruction; however, the basis of treatment is reestablishment of patency by use of an endotracheal tube. If bleeding is the source of the problem, a cuffed tube should be applied and ligation, cautery, or pressure used to control the hemorrhage.

Peritonitis

Peritonitis is not an uncommon postoperative complication following abdominal surgery; it is a normal response to physical manipulation as well as chemical or infectious agents. The concern over peritonitis revolves around problems that arise owing to bacterial contamination and free toxins within the abdominal cavity. There are considerable species differences in ability to resist infection within the peritoneal cavity; the bovine is relatively competent and the horse has less capacity to control the disease process. Added to the difficulties in treating peritonitis is the problem of clinical diagnosis in the early stages, when signs can be vague, variable, or almost nonexistent. Diagnosis and treatment of this condition have been discussed in this text previously.

MINIMIZING PHYSICIAN INSULTS

Whenever orthopedic procedures are performed, whether for application or removal of internal fixation devices, the recovery from anesthesia and the first few hours of ambulation are critical for maintaining limb integrity. During these times it is often advisable to apply temporary casts or splints to provide additional support to the limb.

If a cast had been present initially, time and money may be saved by removing the cast using an oscillating saw, making medial and lateral cuts (bivalving). For recovery, one or both halves of the cast may then be reapplied and fixed together with more casting material or other binding devices. Padded bandages that incorporate strong splinting material or various types of casting material may also be used to provide additional support for the first few hours or days.

Total control of exercise must be maintained to ensure that the limb remains protected, particularly after an animal has been closely confined for some time. Improper footing, exercise, or excitement can result in serious complications of refracture, tendon problems, or damage to other body systems. Because of the increased activity, it is important to remove the bivalved cast, bandages, or splints as soon as appropriate to reduce the incidence of abrasions or ulcers from these devices.

IMPLANT REMOVAL

The question of removal of implants has many considerations, indications, and implications, particularly since there is no consensus regarding whether implants need to be removed in any particular situation. The continued presence of metal plates over a healing fracture site is believed to delay remodeling of bone and reduce bone mass, particularly in the case of less flexible bone plates (Uhthoff and Finnegan 1983). However, clinical experience has revealed that animals can function well for prolonged periods despite the continued presence of internal fixation devices.

The most common reason for implant removal is that healing has occurred and the need for the implant no longer exists. The time for healing completion depends on several factors, including the age of the animal, the type and location of the fracture, and the viability of the affected bone. Usually, judgment regarding union is based on a somewhat empirical clinical evaluation and a more objective radiographic analysis of the bone, both of which leave considerable room for personal bias based on past experiences. Other factors that should be considered are the temperament and function of the animal involved as well as the type of implants present. The amount of callus present indicates the type and degree of healing that has occurred and suggests the amount of effort that will be necessary to remove the device. Whenever more than one plate has been applied, the most physiological procedure would be to remove the plates at different stages of healing to allow for a more gradual transition from the rigidly supported to the totally unsupported state. This is considered to best allow for bone remodeling and reduce stress protection within the affected bone. This "staged" removal of plates must be weighed against the benefits of removing all implants at one time including safety, function, and economics.

Occasionally in young animals with fractures in the immediate area of the metaphyseal growth plate it may be necessary to have the plate extend across the physis. In selected cases the end screw may be allowed to remain in the epiphysis for a short time to provide some additional support. It is important, however, that the screw be removed as soon as possible to prevent angulation of the limb due to uneven growth along the physis resulting from the restrictive forces of the plate.

Draining tracts are sometimes seen in association with implants within a few days to weeks following internal fixation. Whenever this condition is related to soft tissue only (implied by lack of bony involvement radiographically), the cause is generally considered to be related to infection or reaction of tissues to the physical or chemical nature of the implant itself. In either case, the treatment of choice is removal of the offending implant provided that stability of the fracture site is maintained until bony union occurs. The same procedure is advocated if the infective process involves bone but only when the osteomyelitis involves bone after fracture healing has occurred or when the area of bony involvement does not involve the healing area.

Whenever an implant fails to provide stability and in fact creates problems around the fracture, such as in the case of a broken or loose implant, the offending device should be removed. In the case of an imbedded and broken screw, the mertis of removal are usually offset by extraction problems and that portion of the screw is usually left permanently in the bone.

Wound care following plate removal is frequently restricted to suction drains applied in the dead space previously occupied by the plate and support and pressure bandages applied to the contralateral and affected limbs for the first few days after surgery.

REFERENCES

Ap, R., and Owen, R.: Post-stress diarrhea in the horse. Vet. Rec. 96:267, 1975.

Ap, R., Owen, R., Fullerton, J. N., Tizard, I. R., Lumsden, J. H., and Barnum, B. A.: Studies on experimental enteric salmonellosis in ponies. Can. J. Comp. Med. 43:247, 1979.

Boles, C.: Post-operative management of equine abdominal patients. Proceedings of the 1st Internal Equine Veterinary Conference 46:123, 1975.

Cox, V. S.: Understanding the downer cow syndrome. Comp. Cont. Ed. Vet. Pract. 3:472, 1981.

Laros, G. S., Tipton, C. M., and Cooper, R. R.: Influences of physical activity on ligament insertions in the knees of dogs. J. Bone Joint Surg. 53A:275, 1971.

Mansmann, R. A., McAllister, E. S., and Pratt, P. W.: Equine Medicine and Surgery, Vols. I and II, 3rd ed. Santa Barbara, CA: American Veterinary Publications, 1982.

Muir, W. W., and Bednarski, R. M.: Equine cardiopulmonary resuscitation—Part II. Comp. Cont. Ed. Vet. Pract. 5:287, 1983.

O'Driscoll, S. W., Kumar, A. L., and Salter, R. B.: The effect of continuous passive motion on the clearance of a hemarthrosis from a synovial joint. Clin. Orthop. Rel. Res. 176:305, 1983.

Uhthoff, J. K., and Finnegan, M.: The effects of metal plates on post-traumatic remodeling and bone mass. J. Bone Joint Surg. 65B:66, 1983.

CHAPTER 10

NEOPLASTIC DISEASE

MICHAEL A. STEDHAM, D.V.M., M.S.

Neoplasms of many varieties present in large animals. Some, such as squamous cell carcinoma of the eye in cattle, occur with relatively great frequency; are rather breed specific; are associated with an inducing factor (sunlight), which is further related to geographical area; are potentially life threatening; occur at specific anatomical sites; and are of economic importance. At the other end of the spectrum there are some tumors, such as myxomas, that occur infrequently; appear in all species and breeds; have no known inducers; are benign; occur in any site that normally contains connective tissue; and are economically insignificant. Between these two extreme examples lie most of the neoplasms to be discussed in this chapter.

The term tumor means, in its broadest sense, a swelling. In common usage, however, tumor is often used interchangeably with neoplasm, which more specifically denotes a new growth of cells that are not under normal control mechanisms.

The neoplasms presented in this chapter have been selected because of their accessibility for surgical intervention, their comparative interest, their high incidence rate, or their economic importance. The last two criteria are, of course, closely related. For a more complete coverage of a greater spectrum of neoplasms in domestic animals, the recent work edited by Moulton (1978) as well as other texts is suggested (Jubb and Kennedy 1970; Smith, Jones, and Hunt 1972).

Neoplasms generally occur in older animals. This is particularly true of carcinomas. Food animals, which are sent to slaughter at a young age, are therefore much less likely to have neoplasms than are animals that are allowed to live out more of their normal life span.

Neoplasms that are easily detected clinically, e.g., those of the skin and subcutis, would be expected to be reported more frequently than occult neoplasms. Likewise, neoplasms that are widely metastatic or that interfere with the normal function of the animal would more likely be detected than would solitary neoplasms or neoplasms that have no effect on the animal. Furthermore, spectacular and unusual neoplasms are most likely reported in the literature more frequently in relation to their true occurrence than are the more mundane neoplasms. The point to be made here is that reported occurrence figures, especially if drawn from clinical material or case reports, do not necessarily reflect the true occurrence in all instances. True figures would be more closely approximated by careful examination of large numbers of necropsy cases in addition to clinical material from a known population.

HORSES

In addition to the general references cited previously, there are several recent reports concerning neoplasms solely in horses (Cotchin 1977; Baker and Leyland 1975; Cotchin and Baker-Smith 1975; Sundberg et al. 1977). Some of these reports, as well as an earlier text (Smith and Jones 1957), contain figures from large surveys. In these surveys and in previous reports referenced in these, neoplasms were found in from 1.75 to 3.1 per cent of clinical or necropsy cases and were seen in 11 per cent of the horses in one abattoir survey (Cotchin and Baker-Smith 1975). This last report had, in addition to a tumor occurrence figure greatly in excess of the other reports, an unusually large percentage of thyroid (47 per cent), adrenal (15.9 per cent), and mesenteric (lipoma) (13.2 per cent) neoplasms. In most reports, however, the greatest number of neoplasms was in the skin, the equine sarcoid being the most common.

Skin and Soft Tissues

Neoplasms of these structures are the most commonly diagnosed neoplasms in the horse and, for the most part, are quite amenable to surgical removal.

Equine Sarcoid (Fig. 10–1). This lesion, although probably not a neoplasm in the strict sense, does form a tumor that has the potential for growth, local invasion, and recurrence after surgical removal. It should not be confused with an entirely different condition in man known as sarcoid or sarcoidosis.

Equine sarcoid is seen in horses, donkeys, and mules and has a worldwide distribution. It is the most common skin tumor in horses. It may be multiple, and it may occur in epizootic form (Ragland, Keown, and Spencer 1970). In addition,

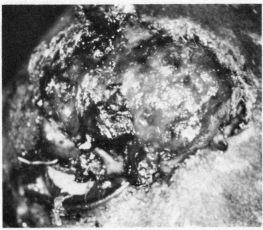

Figure 10–1 Equine sarcoid in the horse. This is a recurrent, fibroblastic-type sarcoid that originated on the eyelid and eventually responded to a combination of immunotherapy and surgery. The eye is at the lower left of this photograph. (Reprinted with permission from Wyman et al. JAVMA 171:449, 1977.)

recurrence within three years has been reported to be nearly 50 per cent (Ragland, Keown, and Spencer 1970).

Although an infectious and probably viral etiology is indicated by the existing evidence, final proof is lacking. Earlier attempts at producing equine sarcoid with bovine papilloma virus (BPV) resulted in fibroblastic tumors with similarities to but also distinct differences from sarcoid (Olson and Cook 1951). The BPV-induced lesions had a short induction period (12 to 27 days), uniform spontaneous regression, and a lack of epidermal proliferation, all of which are not characteristic of sarcoid. In another study, neutralizing antibodies to BPV were not detected in horses with equine sarcoid (Ragland and Spencer 1968). These and other studies militate against BPV as the specific virus that causes equine sarcoid. The electron microscopic finding of intracytoplasmic virus-like particles in cell lines derived from equine sarcoids (England, Watson, and Larson 1973), as well as in the tumors themselves, supports the hypothesis of a viral etiology, as does the tendency for multiple tumors and the report of an epizootic form (Ragland, Keown, and Gorham 1966).

Sarcoids occur most frequently on the head, legs, and ventral trunk, especially the prepuce, and are multiple in about one-third of the cases. There is no apparent age, sex, or breed predilection.

Grossly, sarcoids may present a variety of appearances. These have been categorized as verrucous (warty) type, fibroblastic (proud flesh) type, and mixed type, each of which may be further divided into sessile or pedunculated (Ragland, Keown, and Spencer 1970). Progression from verrucous to fibroblastic type is thought to occur. The tumors vary in size from barely visible to 20 cm or more, with most in the lower end of this range when first detected. The tumors are firm and basically grayish-white with some variations depending on their type and the degree of secondary inflammation, which is commonly seen owing to ulceration of the epidermis. The surface of sarcoids is frequently friable and bleeds easily.

Microscopically, there are two hallmarks of this tumor. One is the acanthotic epithelium with rather extensive epithelial pegs extending deeply into the underlying dermal component. The epithelial component is much more prominent in verrucous sarcoids. The other feature is the proliferation of dermal fibroblasts. Most reports indicate a considerable variation in degree of maturity of the fibroblasts, their patterns, and the amount of collagen, depending on the type of sarcoid. Contrasted with this is the view that sarcoids have more uniform maturity and arrangement of fibroblasts than fibromas, which have more variability both in maturity and arrangement of the fibroblasts (Baker and Leyland 1975).

As the name of the tumor indicates, the tumor may have some sarcoma-like features. Modest anaplasia and mitotic activity may be seen, particularly in more rapidly growing tumors. The cells, which may be plump to spindled, and the accompanying collagen fibers may be primarily parallel to each other, may occasionally be in a herring-bone pattern, or may be very irregularly and randomly arranged. One feature, however, is more constant and is considered by some as an important diagnostic feature of the sarcoid. This is the perpendicular arrangement of the fibroblasts to the epithelium at the dermal-epidermal junction. Another feature of sarcoids is their lack of deep invasion. Underlying muscle or bone is spared.

Although sarcoids may occur in multiple sites, they do not metastasize. Involvement of deep tissues does not occur by either metastasis or extension. Recurrence, however, is common. In addition to routine surgical removal, cryosurgical techniques and immunotherapy have been suggested (Lane 1977; Murphy et al. 1979; Wyman et al. 1977).

Squamous Cell Carcinoma. This malignant neoplasm of squamous epithelial cells may arise in any cutaneous area and at mucocutaneous junctions. Squamous cell carcinomas also occur in the eye and associated structures, in the epithelium lining internal organs, and in the epithelium of some glands, but these will not be discussed in this section. A recent report states that horses with squamous cell carcinomas comprise 20.2 per cent (58 of 287) of the horses with neoplasms in the neoplasm registry of a veterinary school (Strafuss 1976). A further breakdown by anatomical site lists the following frequencies: eye and adnexa (32.6 per cent); anus, vulva, and clitorus (mares) (12.0 per cent); prepuce (27.3 per cent); glans penis (17.0 per cent); and head (10.3 per cent). Another report lists 19 horses with squamous cell carcinomas in a series of 124 horses with neoplasms (Baker and Leyland 1975). Of these, eight arose from the epithelium of the penis and prepuce, eight from the eye, two from the clitoris, and one from the hard palate. As can be seen from these and other reports, squamous cell carcinomas are not uncommon in the horse, but sites other than the skin and mucocutaneous junctions are usually involved.

There is a distinct predilection for involvement of exposed areas in light-haired individuals in some species (cats, cattle). This is related to solar radiation as an inducer of the neoplasms. Whether this occurs in horses is subject to speculation.

The gross appearance of this neoplasm varies somewhat, depending on whether it is productive or destructive. The former type is probably more frequent and has a papillary or cauliflower-like to multinodular appearance and varying degrees of surface ulceration and secondary inflammation. The destructive and invasive type is slightly elevated to mildly depressed or crateriform.

Microscopically, all squamous cell carcinomas are characterized by squamous epithelial cells, which may appear in varying sized nests or cords or may appear individually. The more differentiated neoplasms have larger aggregates of cells and often show some degree of maturation from the periphery to the center of the aggregates. Intercellular bridges are often prominent, and keratinization, sometimes to the point of keratin pearl formation, is seen. In more anaplastic squamous cell carcinomas, the cells usually appear in smaller groups in which the characteristic features of intercellular bridges and keratinization are scant or absent. Occasionally, individual squamous cells are seen in the dermis and subcutis. Mitotic figures may be seen in modest to abundant numbers, the latter situation indicating a more rapidly growing and oftentimes more invasive neoplasm.

Microscopically, the squamous cell carcinoma is not easily confused with other lesions, particularly if the carcinoma is reasonably well differentiated.

As a general rule, squamous cell carcinomas invade locally but are slow to metastasize. Metastasis is to the regional lymph nodes first and then to the lung and other sites.

Cutaneous Papillomatosis. This virally induced condition is relatively common in one- and two-year-old horses. The virus is host specific. Congenital papillomatosis has also been reported in newborn foals, but viral causation remains to be proved (Schueler 1973). The lesions are usually multiple and are most common on the nose and lips.

Grossly, the papillomas are typical in that they grow outward from the surface in a cauliflower-like form. Their size and number vary considerably. In one case of congenital papillomatosis the weight of the lesion caused the lower lip to droop and interfere with suckling (Schueler 1973).

Microscopically, the lesions consist of a central branching dermis-like core of connective tissue and vessels covered by acanthotic and hyperkeratotic epidermis. Varying degrees of cytoplasmic de-

generation may be seen in the stratum spinosum and the stratum granulosum.

The condition is self-limiting and regression occurs in one to three months. Solid immunity follows.

Melanoma (Fig. 10–2). Melanotic neoplasms are of particular biological interest as well as of life-threatening importance in both man and animals. Greatly detailed nomenclature systems have been devised for the various forms of melanotic lesions in man. Of basic importance in man, however, is the primary distinction between nevus, a benign neoplasm, and melanoma, a malignant neoplasm. In animals the term melanoma has been used most often in a nonspecific fashion. Ordinarily, the term malignant is inserted to add specific designation to a malignant neoplasm, whereas benign is used for the benign counterpart. Recent nomenclature, as outlined in recent works (Stannard and Pulley 1978; Weiss and Frese 1974), has somewhat different designations for the benign lesions; however, these seem to be more appropriate for melanotic neoplasms in the dog. In the horse, benign and malignant designations are perhaps less meaningful inasmuch as, although most do not metastasize, cutaneous melanotic neoplasms are considered by some to have a progressive and potentially malignant course, albeit over an extended

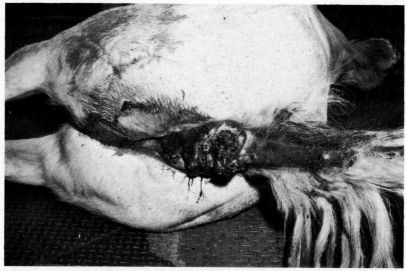

Figure 10–2 Melanoma in the horse. The malignant behavior of this melanoma in the base of the tail was manifested by distant metastasis. (AFIP Photo # 59-1726-3.)

period of time, usually many years (Levene 1971). In contrast to these "less malignant" melanomas, there are a few frankly malignant melanomas that metastasize much more quickly and thus are more equatable with malignant melanomas in some other animals and with melanomas in man. Inasmuch as most, if not all, melanomas in horses are considered to have metastatic potential if given sufficient time, they will be considered as malignant melanomas in this discussion.

Melanomas are among the most common neoplasms of horses. They occur almost exclusively in gray and white horses and increase greatly in numbers with advancing age, particularly over 10 years of age. This increased incidence in aging gray horses is also associated with progressive fading of the hair color. Some breeds or stocks of horses, such as Arabian and Lippizaner horses, both of which are dark at birth and most of which undergo rather dramatic fading, are at an increased risk for melanoma (Levene 1971; Lerner and Cage 1973).

Melanomas are most common in the perineum, tail head, and anus. They also occur in the external genitalia, less frequently in skin in other areas, and, oddly, in the parotid salivary gland (Levene 1971).

Grossly, the earliest detectable lesions are single or multiple dermal swellings. As the swellings increase in size and become more nodular, they become more protuberant and the overlying skin is stretched, sometimes leading to traumatization and ulceration. Inasmuch as the neoplasms are usually in dark-skinned areas, it is difficult to appreciate the deeply pigmented nature of most of them until ulceration occurs or until they are incised. Usually there is a slow progression, often over a span of many years, and the malignant melanoma invades and becomes much more extensive deep to the original dermal lesion. Eventually, metastasis may occur, involving regional lymph nodes and then the peritoneum, spleen, liver, lungs, and other organs.

Microscopically, there are two primary types of pigmented cells in equine melanomas and these appear in various proportions. One cell type is spindled to dendritic in outline and has a medium to large nucleus, usually with a prominent nucleolus. This cell type is clearly melanocytic and contains moderate to abundant amounts of melanin. Occasionally sparsely pigmented neoplasms or neoplasms with areas of sparsely pigmented cells occur. The other cell type is epithelioid in appearance and in most instances is a melanophagic histiocyte. These cells are large, rounded, and typically stuffed with melanin. They have a smaller nucleus, which may be pushed to one side of the cell. Although epithelioid melanomas are described in other species, including man, the occurrence of epithelioid melanocytes as the primary melanocytic cell in horses is probably less frequent. Mitotic activity varies from very slight to moderate. In metastatic lesions in lymph nodes the epithelioid cells, most likely melanophages rather than melanocytes, may be seen by themselves early and probably represent normal lymphatic drainage from the primary lesion. The presence of true melanocytes, however, represents actual metastasis.

As mentioned earlier, the pigmented cutaneous neoplasms of horses have the potential for metastasis, although very long periods of time may be required for metastasis to occur. A few are more frankly malignant. According to one author, excision does not affect the outcome (Levene 1971).

Lipoma. The lipoma is occasionally seen in the dermis or subcutis. It is more common on the trunk but may be seen anywhere. There is no breed or sex predisposition, but older animals are more commonly affected.

Grossly, a firm elevation of the skin is seen. Upon surgical exposure, a white to slightly yellow, rounded or discoid mass that is not attached to the skin or underlying structures is characteristic. Some lobulation may be present. The tumor is greasy to the touch.

Microscopically, lipomas are composed of mature fat cells and cannot be differentiated from normal fat without knowing that the tissue came from a mass.

Lipomas show no tendency for local invasion or recurrence and are easily

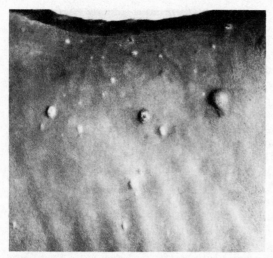

Figure 10–3 Mastocytoma (mastocytosis) in the foal. Multiple cutaneous nodules were located in the skin. In this case, individual lesions grew progressively larger, ulcerated, and regressed. (Photograph courtesy of Dr. Norman Cheville.)

excised. The malignant counterpart, the liposarcoma, is rare.

Mastocytoma (Fig. 10–3). The mastocytoma is less frequent and occurs in the dermis and subcutis of horses. Two forms are seen, the more common one being a single nodule (Altera and Clark 1970) and the other multiple (Cheville et al. 1972; Prasse, Lundvall, and Cheville 1975). The true neoplastic nature of both forms is in some doubt, especially the latter, and the lesions are referred to as mastocytosis. In 12 single lesions and 1 double lesion in which the location was noted, 8 were on the head and neck, 4 were on the body, and 1 was on the legs (Altera and Clark 1970). The age ranged from 1 1/2 to 15 years, and eight horses were eight years old or less. Grossly, the lesions were discrete cutaneous swellings from 2 to 20 cm in diameter, and some were ulcerated.

Microscopically, the major components are variably sized aggregates of mast cells with usually abundant scattered and aggregated eosinophils. Few mitoses are evident. Also seen are macrophages and giant cells, which may be oriented around focal areas of necrosis. Degenerating collagen fibers are often intermingled with the other components.

Metastasis has not been reported, although aggregates of mast cells were found in bone marrow of a case of generalized cutaneous mastocytosis in a foal (Cheville et al. 1972).

Musculoskeletal System

Neoplasms of the locomotor organs in the horse are quite rare. They present problems for surgical removal. Therefore, they will be discussed only briefly. Tumors of striated muscles are so infrequent as to warrant no further mention.

Osteoma. This benign, well-demarcated, slow-growing neoplasm is composed of trabecular bone of varying compactness. It is most common in the bones of the head.

Osteochondroma. This benign neoplasm protrudes from the surface of a bone. It is composed of a base of cancellous bone with marrow and has a cartilaginous cap. It may inhibit locomotion by interfering with muscle attachments or movement and is amenable to removal.

Osteosarcoma. The osteosarcoma is very rare in horses. It arises more commonly in the metaphyseal area of long bones in most species but in the horse is primarily located in the head (Jacobson 1971).

Lymphoid and Hematopoietic Organs

Neoplasms of the lymphoid and myeloid cells are very uncommon in horses, lymphosarcoma being the least uncommon.

Lymphosarcoma. This is the term usually applied to neoplasms of lymphoid cells in animals inasmuch as they almost always form solid masses. Also, the cells do not often appear in the peripheral blood and may not be located primarily or solely in hematopoietic organs; both of these criteria should be met for the designation of leukemia. However, according to one report, 58 per cent of the cases reviewed were leukemic and 15 per cent were leukopenic (Neufeld 1973). Another source states that lymphatic leukemia secondary to lymphosarcoma is not uncommon in the horse, despite the fact that lymphosarcoma may be localized

(Squire 1964). Contrary to findings in several other animal species, no virus has been convincingly incriminated in equine lymphosarcoma. Also, the incidence of lymphosarcoma is less in horses than in many other domestic species (Squire 1964).

The most common sites of involvement are the lymph nodes, liver, spleen, gastrointestinal tract, kidney, lung, heart, skeletal muscle, brain, and meninges, in that order (Neufeld 1973). Other organs are also occasionally involved. The multicentric form of lymphosarcoma is most frequent, followed by the alimentary form. The thymic and skin forms are seldom reported (Moulton and Dungworth 1978).

Grossly, the lesions are usually expansile, nodular to irregular, white to off-white masses that compress and replace tissue of the involved organ. Diffuse infiltration with enlargement of the entire organ is also seen in some parenchymal organs such as the liver and spleen.

Microscopically, a gamut of cell types from undifferentiated (stem) cells to mature lymphocytes may be seen. In a single animal, however, the cell type is rather consistent from one site to another. The neoplastic cells may occur either in broad sheets or as small nests and cords infiltrating pre-existing tissue.

Although neoplastic involvement of the skin and superficial lymph nodes would be particularly accessible to surgery, it is doubtful if removal would alter the course of the disease. The major value of surgery would be to obtain tissue specimens by which to render a definitive diagnosis.

Respiratory Tract

Neoplasms of this system are also rather uncommon, comprising 2.4 per cent of the tumor cases in one report (Baker and Leyland 1975).

Involvement of the nasal cavity and paranasal sinuses is more common than that of the lungs. The pulmonary epithelial and mesenchymal neoplasms of the horse are so uncommon as to warrant no further mention.

Nasal Polyps. These pedunculated inflammatory growths, which mimic neoplasms, arise from the mucous membrane of the nasal passages and are the most common "tumor" of the nasal passages. They are usually relatively small but may become large enough to mechanically interfere with respiration. Polyps may be solitary or multiple but are uncommon bilaterally.

Grossly, the pedunculated mass has a white to pink, smooth, glistening surface, although ulcerations may alter this appearance.

Microscopically, the tissue is covered by a mucous membrane and is composed of loose connective tissue with varying amounts of collagen and myxomatous areas, inflammatory cell infiltrates, and small vessels. In total, it is most like inflammatory granulation tissue. Evidence of secondary bacterial infection may be seen but the inciting cause is ordinarily obscure.

These growths present some problem for surgical removal because they are rather inaccessible and vascular. They do, however, present little potential for recurrence if adequately excised, and they have no potential for metastasis or local invasion. In a few instances, however, recurrence or a new polyp may occur (Stickle 1978).

Carcinomas of Nasal Cavity and Sinuses. A recent compilation of histologically confirmed neoplasms of the nasal passages and paranasal sinuses in horses lists 13 neoplasms from the nasal cavity and 9 from the paranasal sinuses (Madewell et al. 1976). Of the 13 neoplasms in the nasal cavity, 7 were carcinomas including 5 squamous cell carcinomas. Of the nine neoplasms in the sinuses, four were carcinomas including one squamous cell carcinoma. The remainder of the neoplasms were various benign and malignant mesenchymal neoplasms.

Grossly, the carcinomas form masses that are often quite large by the time they are clinically apparent. They protrude into and may obliterate the nasal or sinus spaces, and, in some instances, they may also be quite invasive. Bone may be eroded, and the neoplasm may even extend into the cranial cavity.

Microscopically, the squamous cell carcinomas have typical features for that neoplasm elsewhere including formation of keratin pearls. Squamous cell carcinomas are more common in the maxillary sinus, and the possibility of origin from tooth germ residues or other sources has been reviewed (Moulton 1978). Carcinomas also have somewhat indefinite parentage in that they may arise from the surface epithelium or from the associated serous and mucous glands. They may be solid or they may form glandular structures; both patterns may be seen (Reynolds et al. 1979).

Although these tumors may appear quite malignant histologically, most do not metastasize. If they do it is usually only to the draining lymph node.

Granular Cell Tumor. One interesting neoplasm, the granular cell tumor or granular cell myoblastoma, is also uncommon but three recent reports document eight cases and refer to two additional cases (Misdorp and Nauta-van Gelder 1968; Parker et al. 1979; Parodi, Tassin, and Rigoulet 1974). Most recent evidence indicates that these neoplasms have the same cell of origin as Schwann cells rather than arising from muscle cells, as was once thought and as the name myoblastoma indicates. These tumors may occupy large areas of the lung, are rather solid, and are composed of large, rounded cells with abundant cytoplasmic granules, which are positive when stained by the periodic acid–Schiff procedure.

Digestive Tract

All neoplasms of the equine digestive tract are rare. A few of the more frequently seen entities are briefly discussed here.

Odontogenic Tumors. Adamantinomas, odontomas, and dentigerous cysts are occasionally seen in horses.

Adamantinomas (ameloblastomas) arise from residue of the enamel organ and distend and sometimes cause ulceration of the overlying gingival mucous membrane. They may be multinodular, are usually quite firm, and may invade the underlying bone as well as stimulating new bone formation in their connective tissue stroma. Microscopically, these neoplasms are characteristically composed of nests or cords of epithelial cells that have a peripheral columnar layer of cells. The cells in the center of the nests are less dense, more randomly arranged, and often stellate. These neoplasms do not metastasize but are considered malignant because of their local invasiveness, destruction of tissue, and tendency to recur.

Odontomas are less distinctly neoplastic and are considered by some to be tumor-like malformations (Moulton 1978). They contain epithelial components from the enamel organ as well as mesenchymal components. These components appear in varying proportions and have a variable degree of organization into nearly normal tooth structure in some lesions. They arise in the mandible and maxilla and may connect with existing dental alveoli. Further classification into compound, complex, and ameloblastic odontomata depends on the degree of differentiation and the amount of epithelial derivatives. These tumors are benign but may replace parts of the jaw as well as extend considerably into the soft tissue.

Dentigerous cysts, although uncommon, are more common in the horse than in other species (Moulton 1978). These also are not true neoplasms but are congenital malformations. They occur in younger horses, most commonly in the temporal region near the base of the ear Moulton 1978), but may occur elsewhere as well. The cyst is lined by stratified squamous epithelium and usually contains a single partly or well-formed tooth with the crown of the tooth most commonly projecting into the lumen.

Squamous Cell Carcinoma of the Stomach. Although considered relatively uncommon by some (Moulton 1978), one recent report presents four new cases and gives literature citations of about 50 other cases in horses (Meagher et al. 1974). Adenocarcinomas of the glandular part of the equine stomach are also seen but are much less frequent than squamous cell carcinomas of the nonglandular stomach. There is some speculation as to the relationship of the larvae of *Gasterophilus* spp. and *Habronema megastoma* to gastric squamous cell carcinomas, but a direct causal effect remains unproved (Jubb and Kennedy 1970).

These tumors are considered to be slow growing, often producing large cauliflower-like masses projecting into the lumen and infiltrative cords projecting into the gastric wall before they are detected. The surface of the usually whitish tumor is often ulcerated, infected, and partly covered with dark necrotic debris.

Microscopically, the lesion is rather similar to the squamous cell carcinoma in the skin. Sometimes, extension through and rarely perforation of the gastric wall may lead to implantation on peritoneal surfaces. Metastases to the liver, lymph nodes, spleen, adrenal glands, kidneys, and lungs may also be seen (Moulton 1978).

Lipoma. Lipomas of the serosal surfaces are relatively common in horses (Cotchin 1977). They are discussed with the digestive tract because the only symptoms they produce are associated with intestinal strangulation. This occurs when the peduncle of a mesenteric lipoma winds around the intestine. Nonpedunculate tumors are usually clinically silent. The gross and microscopic appearances of these lipomas are essentially the same as for those in the subcutis.

Liver and Urinary Tract

Neoplasms of these systems do occur in horses but are so uncommon that they are not included.

Reproductive Tract

This organ system, or rather systems in considering the male and female separately, gives rise to some neoplasms with sufficient frequency to be deserving of discussion. Neoplasms of the testicle are very rare in the horse. Although the testicular teratoma is much more common in the horse than in other domestic species, it is nevertheless rare (Moulton 1978). Stromal tumors of the ovary are more frequently reported; however, the external genitalia of both sexes are by far the most frequently involved members of the equine reproductive tract.

Stromal Tumors of the Ovary (Fig. 10–4). These are almost all granulosa cell tumors and are more frequently reported than ovarian teratomas, adenocarcinomas, and other ovarian neoplasms (Norris, Taylor, and Garner). Although they are called granulosa cell tumors, many also contain theca cells or Sertoli-like cells or both. These neoplasms are located in normally positioned ovaries, but, owing to the large size of some, they may extend far beyond the normal bounds of the ovaries.

Most reports in which dimensions or weights are listed give a weight range of from 1 to 8 kg (Fessler and Brobst 1972; Norris, Taylor, and Garner 1968; Stickle et al. 1975) and a size range of from 10 to 27 cm in diameter (Cordes 1969; Fessler and Brobst 1972; Stickle et al. 1975). They may also attain tremendous proportions, however, as indicated by one re-

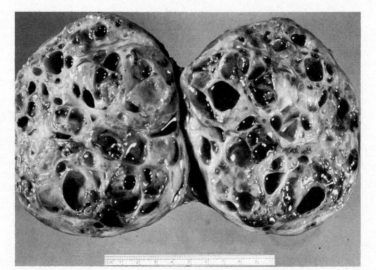

Figure 10–4 Granulosa cell tumor in the horse. This neoplasm exhibits multiple cysts, which are a frequent occurrence. (Reprinted with permission from Stickle et al. JAVMA *167*:148, 1975.)

port of a 23.6-kg tumor with dimensions of 36 by 46 cm (Schmidt, Cowles, and Flynn 1976). Almost all of the tumors are roughly spherical in shape with a few nodular protuberances caused by cysts under the tough capsule. Characteristically, the cysts are multiple and range from barely visible to 5 cm in size. In the few solid tumors, microcysts may be noted histopathologically. The cyst contents vary from clear to red-brown in color, and the tumor parenchyma varies from off-white to gray to yellow.

Microscopically, these tumors feature numerous sheets of cells and solid or microcystic follicular structures in which the granulosa cells toward the center of the follicles have a moderate to abundant amount of clear to lightly eosinophilic cytoplasm and an indistinct rounded to polyhedral outline. At the periphery of the follicles, one or two, and occasionally more, layers of the cells are elongated and radially arranged. Exterior to this basal layer are the theca cells, which are ovoid to spindle shaped and may resemble fibroblasts. True fibroblasts and collagen are also seen in the stroma exterior to the follicles. Hyalinized collagen or poorly formed osteoid has been reported in a few tumors (Cordes 1969; Fessler and Brobst 1972).

Although one source states that more metastasis is seen with the equine ovarian stromal tumors (Moulton 1978), none of the other references cited in this section report on metastasis. Surgical removal is usually curative and, in addition to removing the neoplasms, corrects the abnormalities of the estrous cycle and behavior, which are often present owing to the variable sex steroid secretion by the neoplasms.

Squamous Cell Carcinoma of the Penis, Prepuce, and Vulva (Fig. 10–5). The most significant neoplasm of the external genitalia in both sexes is the squamous cell carcinoma. One report of primarily biopsy specimens lists eight squamous cell carcinomas of the penis and prepuce and two of the clitoris out of a total of 124 horses with neoplasms (Baker and Leyland 1975). Other frequency figures have been listed under squamous cell carcinomas of the skin.

In the male, the squamous cell carcinoma occurs most commonly on the glans penis (Moulton 1978). It also occurs on the inner surface of the prepuce and on the vulvar mucosa in the mare. The neoplasms vary greatly in size, are sessile, and have a cauliflower-like configuration. Microscopically, they are similar to their cutaneous counterparts.

These neoplasms have a tendency to recur after surgical removal and, less frequently, may metastasize to regional lymph nodes and the lungs.

Nervous System

One source indicates no species differences, with a few exceptions, for neoplasms of the central nervous system (Cordy 1978). Another recent work, however, which included compiled data from

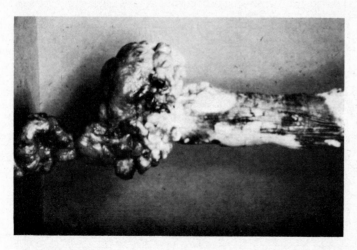

Figure 10–5 Squamous cell carcinoma in the horse. A papillary to multilobulated mass of neoplastic tissue extensively involves the end of the penis. (AFIP Photo # 56-20547.)

11 veterinary school clinics and hospitals, reports that all of the 28 neoplasms seen in horses were of peripheral nerve origin (Hayes, Priester, and Pendergrass 1975). This is in contrast to neoplasms of the nervous systems of dogs and cats, in which the glial and meningeal neoplasms outnumbered those of the peripheral nerves. Another lesion seen with some frequency in horses is the cholesterol granuloma of the choroid plexus.

Cholesterol Granuloma. These lesions, also known as cholesteatoma or cholesteatosis, are non-neoplastic masses in the choroid plexus of older horses. They are formed from breakdown products and the reaction thereto of congestive hemorrhage into the choroid plexus. They may be located in the fourth ventricle or in the lateral ventricles. In the latter location they may attain a large size and may cause an obstructive hydrocephalus with clinical signs (Jubb and Kennedy 1970). Otherwise, they are incidental findings at necropsy.

Grossly, the granulomas vary from smaller multinodular lesions to, more frequently, larger, single masses. They may be gray, white, yellowish, or a combination of these colors, and they may also have some areas of brown coloration.

Microscopically, a granulomatous inflammatory reaction of varying chronicity, usually including foamy and hemosiderin-laden macrophages, and, in particular, cholesterol clefts, characterizes the lesions.

Nerve Sheath Tumors. The nomenclature of these neoplasms is still a subject of controversy. Most sources designate two separate entities, the Schwannoma (neurilemmoma) derived from the Schwann cell and the neurofibroma derived from the perineurial connective tissue. Problems arise in attempting to microscopically distinguish the neoplasms because of overlapping features; some sources consider them as one with the possible participation of perineurial cells in the Schwannomas (Cordy 1978). Inasmuch as they are often very similar and sometimes indistinguishable and the biological behavior is similar, they will be discussed here as one entity, the neurofibroma.

Although these tumors are relatively uncommon, one study lists them as comprising 4.2 per cent (10 of 217) of equine neoplasms (Sundberg et al. 1977). Neurofibromas may arise from any peripheral nerve, and there is no apparent site of predilection in the horse.

Grossly, the neoplasms are firm to gelatinous, white to gray, glistening nodules that are rather well circumscribed (Cordy 1978). They are ideally seen arising from a nerve, but finding the nerve may be difficult.

Microscopically, the neoplasms are characterized by spindle cells with elongated, often wire-like processes. These cells may be in a variety of configurations from interweaving bundles to the more diagnostic palisading rows and tactile corpuscle-like arrangements that mimic Meissner's tactile corpuscles or Verocay bodies. Separating the denser cellular areas are variably sized areas and trabeculae with fewer cells and more intercellular space containing a mixture of collagen fibers, reticulin fibers, and ground substance. The former, denser areas are known as Antoni type A pattern, the latter, looser areas as Antoni type B pattern.

Neurofibromas are considered benign neoplasms although they do have rare histologically malignant counterparts, which may metastasize (Cordy 1978).

Endocrine System

Although most of the compilations of equine neoplasms mentioned in the first part of this section list few to no neoplasms of the endocrine system, one abattoir survey had strikingly different results (Cotchin and Baker-Smith 1975). In this report of 244 tumorous growths from 155 horses, 71 were in the thyroid gland and 24 were in the adrenal gland. The thyroid neoplasms were adenomas of imprecise (follicular or parafollicular) origin. The exact nature of the adrenal neoplasms was also not known, but the majority were thought to be pheochromocytomas (Cotchin and Baker-Smith 1975). Inasmuch as description of these neoplasms was not presented and pictures were not included, it is not possible to comment further on the interpretation of these lesions as neoplasms in contrast to hyperplasia. Additionally, they were all incidental findings at necropsy and no clinical signs were reported.

Adenoma of the Pars Intermedia. Although they are uncommon in the overall incidence of equine neoplasms, adenomas of the pars intermedia are the most common neoplasms of the pituitary, affecting older horses and with a higher frequency in females (Capen 1978).

Grossly, these neoplasms cause enlargement of the pituitary gland and extend out of the sella turcica, resulting in compression of the overlying hypothalamus. They are yellowish-gray to white.

Microscopically, adenomas of the pars intermedia are usually sharply demarcated from the pars distalis, which may be compressed (Capen 1978). The tumor cells are similar to normal cells of this origin. Large cuboidal to columnar to somewhat spindled basophilic cells appear in nests and in rows, sometimes in palisades along the fine fibrovascular stroma.

Although these neoplasms are histologically benign and no metastasis has been reported, they may exert functional malignancy by destroying hypothalamic tissue. This causes a variety of signs including diabetes insipidus, somnolence, hyperpyrexia, hirsutism, and others (Capen 1978; Gribble 1972).

Special Senses

Neoplasia of the ear in horses is very uncommon, with the exception of the previously discussed equine sarcoid. Primary neoplasia of the eye, with the exception of squamous cell carcinoma of the limbus, is also uncommon. The ocular adnexa, however, are more frequently affected, and the eye itself can be involved by extension or invasion.

Squamous Cell Carcinoma of the Eye and Adnexa (Fig. 10–6). This neoplasm is by far the most common in the eye and adnexa. In one report of 68 cases of neoplasms in the eye, adnexa, and orbit, 49 were squamous cell carcinomas (Lavach and Severin 1977). Most of these involved the membrana nictitans and eyelids, but the limbus was the primary site

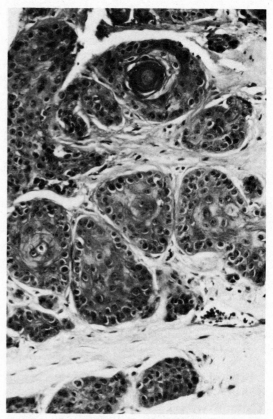

Figure 10–6 Squamous cell carcinoma of the eye in the horse. This neoplasm arose at the limbus and had variably sized nests of cells penetrating downward from the surface epithelium. A keratin pearl is seen near the top of the photograph. (AFIP Photo # 80-582.)

in some cases. The ages ranged from 3 to 19 years with a mean of 9.4 years. Other surveys that included squamous cell carcinomas of all sites in horses listed eye and adnexa as the site in 35 of 54 cases and 19 of 58 cases, respectively (Runnells and Benbrook 1942; Strafuss 1976).

Another report lists 26 cases of conjunctival squamous cell carcinoma, with the nictitating membrane being more frequently affected than the bulbar and palpebral conjunctiva (Gelatt et al. 1974). Metastasis occurred in 4 of the 26 cases. In another report, 10 per cent of the squamous cell carcinomas of the eye and adnexa exhibited metastasis (Lavach and Severin 1977). This reference lists only 3 papillomas as compared with 49 squamous cell carcinomas.

The gross appearance is varied, with some small neoplasms being detected only by careful examination, whereas others are reported up to 10 cm in diameter (Runnells and Benbrook 1942). They may be relatively well-defined, plaque-like, whitish lesions or they may be irregular and more invasive with some discolored areas indicating necrosis or hemorrhage.

Microscopically, these neoplasms are similar to the squamous cell carcinomas described in the skin. The faster-growing and more invasive tumors reflect their greater malignant potential by having less cellular differentiation and more mitotic activity.

CATTLE

Owing to the nature of commercial cattle operations, greatly reduced numbers of males are in the population at risk in comparison with the number of females. It is to be expected that the number of neoplasms associated with older cattle, e.g., ocular squamous cell carcinomas, would be larger in females. In contradistinction, neoplasms of younger animals, e.g., virus-induced papillomas, should have more nearly equal sex distribution.

In attempting to cite meaningful occurrence figures, a note of caution must be injected inasmuch as the figures are gleaned from a variety of sources including clinical biopsy and necropsy material, abattoir surveys, and literature compilations. This variation in sources leads to variation in figures, in addition to the geographical variation that might be seen and the expected variation due to sampling. In any event, several sources were found to be useful in comparing frequencies of neoplasms from large surveys in cattle (Anderson, Sandison, and Jarrett 1969; Cotchin 1960; Misdorp 1967; Monlux, Anderson, and Davis 1956; Monlux and Monlux 1972; Smith and Jones 1957).

Skin and Soft Tissues

A smaller percentage of the total number of neoplasms is reported in these structures in cattle as compared with horses. This is particularly true after exclusion of carcinomas of ocular andexa, which will be discussed later. Another fact that keeps the reported incidence relatively low is that papillomatosis, the most common cutaneous neoplasm, ordinarily undergoes spontaneous regression and does not show up in abattoir surveys. Also, it is not usually a life-threatening or debilitating condition; thus, it does not command a great deal of attention.

Cutaneous Papillomatosis. This is the name most frequently used to specify the virus-induced papillomas of younger cattle. They may also be referred to as infectious fibropapillomas, warts, and infectious verrucae. Some investigators use fibropapilloma to denote a similar lesion, often of the external genitalia. Cutaneous papillomatosis is common in cattle less than two years old and is caused by a DNA virus of the papovavirus group. The papillomas are usually multiple, occasionally become quite massive, and most frequently are found on the head, neck, shoulders or brisket or a combination of these locations. Occasionally they also involve the esophagus, rumen, or teats.

Grossly, the papillomas extend outward from the skin surface in cauliflower- or frond-like projections but may also have plaque or fungoid configurations.

Microscopically, there is a central single or ramifying dermal connective tissue core, which is mildly hyperplastic. The epidermis is much more severely affected, showing extreme degrees of acanthosis and hyperkeratosis. In the acanthotic prickle-cell layer, swelling and degeneration of individual cells and small groups of cells may be seen.

Although these lesions may become extensive and may persist for several months, regression occurs and some degree of immunity is present. Occasionally vaccination is indicated in severe outbreaks. Surgery is rarely indicated in individual animals.

Squamous Cell Carcinoma. This neoplasm occurs much less frequently in the skin than in the eye and ocular adnexa of cattle. It is amenable to surgical removal inasmuch as the metastatic potential of this neoplasm is usually realized only after the prolonged presence of the primary lesion.

The gross and microscopic appearances are similar to those in the horse.

Lipoma. This benign neoplasm comprises a small percentage of reported bovine neoplasms (0.1 to 1.0 per cent) in the works cited in the introduction to neoplasms in cattle. Inasmuch as they are easily recognized grossly because of their lack of local attachment and their fatty appearance and texture, it is probable that most are not submitted for histopathological examination and thus would be underrepresented in reports dealing with clinical biopsy material. Remarks as to morphology of lipomas in horses are also pertinent to lipomas in cattle.

Melanoma. Although melanomas in horses and pigs are better known, one previously cited report lists melanomas as comprising 5.8 per cent of bovine neoplasms (Cotchin 1960), and an additional report lists melanomas at 5.7 per cent (Priester 1973). The other previously cited references in cattle, however, list melanomas at 0.2 to 1.6 per cent of bovine neoplasms. In cattle, melanomas are usually located in the subcutis, but no particular anatomical distribution is known. They may occur in young cattle (Crowell, Chandler, and Williams 1973).

In cattle, as in other species, most melanomas are recognizable as variably pigmented, bulging subcutaneous masses. The amount of pigment is usually great when examined microscopically, and the sections must be bleached to evaluate cellular details to assess malignancy. The features of the recently devised classification system (Stannard and Pulley 1978; Weiss and Frese 1974) are less applicable to bovine melanomas than to canine melanomas. Standard indicators of malignancy need to be assessed, such as high mitotic rate, large nuclei, prominent or multiple nucleoli, and, a conclusive factor, metastatic lesions. Most of the bovine melanomas are benign (Crowell, Chandler, and Williams 1973).

Other. Several other soft tissue neoplasms occur with somewhat less frequency than those already discussed. Among these are hemangioma and fibroma as well as their malignant counterparts.

Musculoskeletal System

Neoplasms of these tissues are very uncommon and will not be discussed.

Lymphoid and Hematopoietic Organs

Neoplasms of these organs are among the most important in cattle because of their grave prognosis and high incidence.

Lymphosarcoma (Fig. 10–7A and B). This neoplasm is also known as malignant lymphoma, leukosis, lymphoma-

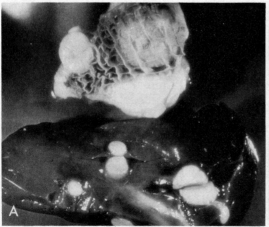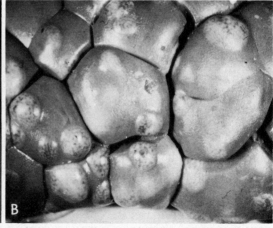

Figure 10–7 Lymphosarcoma in cattle. Variably sized pale nodules may be seen in a variety of organs in addition to enlarged lymphoid organs. *A,* The reticulum and liver are involved. *B,* The kidney is affected. (AFIP Photo # 56-20050-62 and # 53-7646.)

tosis, and, if peripheral blood is involved, lymphoid leukemia. In most reports, it is the most frequently seen neoplasm in cattle.

Lymphosarcoma probably has no breed or sex predisposition, the greater number of affected females being explained by the greater number of females at risk and the greater prevalence in dairy breeds possibly owing to closer contact with other animals. Some familial predisposition has been suspected, though.

Although all ages may be affected, there are distinct age ranges for lymphosarcomas, and these are related to the type of involvement. The most frequently affected age range is from five to eight years (Moulton and Dungworth 1978). These cattle usually have a multicentric form of the disease, whereas the thymic form is most frequently seen in cattle from 6 to 30 months old. Younger animals may also have lymphosarcoma, and there are even reports of the neoplasm in fetuses (Macklin and Miller 1971; Sheriff and Newlands 1976).

Bovine lymphosarcoma had long been suspected to be of viral origin, but it was not until 1969 that a method was devised for culture and demonstration of bovine leukemia virus (Miller et al. 1969). Evidence of this virus as the cause of bovine lymphosarcoma is now rather conclusive. It has also been shown experimentally that the bovine leukemia virus will infect and induce lymphosarcoma in sheep (Olson et al. 1972).

The distribution of lesions in the individual animal usually falls into one of several categories. In addition to the multicentric and thymic forms mentioned previously, the less frequently seen skin form and rare solitary form also occur in cattle. An excellent review of the forms and their age distribution is available (Olson 1974).

The lymph nodes are most frequently affected, usually being greatly enlarged. The color is similar to a normal node, although the amount of grayish-white to pinkish-tan or cream, cortical-appearing tissue predominates. Other organs more commonly involved are the heart, peritoneal cavity (serosa, omentum and so on), spleen, kidneys, skeletal muscle, uterus, and liver, in descending order of frequency (Smith 1965). These organs may have either discrete nodular enlargements or a more diffuse infiltrative involvement, which imparts a paleness.

Microscopically, the cell types may be lymphocytic, prolymphocytic, lymphoblastic, and histiocytic, in order of decreasing frequency (Moulton and Dungworth 1978). In addition, mixed cell types occur fairly frequently, and some variations may be seen in different sites in the same animal.

Although regression is reported (Miller and Olson 1971), the outcome is almost universally fatal.

Thymoma. Although this is a rare neoplasm in cattle, it is mentioned here to emphasize its distinction from thymic lymphosarcoma. The true thymoma is composed of cells that resemble the epithelial cells of the thymus. There are two survey reports in the current literature that describe 20 thymomas in cattle and refer to previous reports (Parker and Casey 1976, Sandison and Anderson 1969).

These neoplasms are, of course, located in the thymic area and may be visible in the thoracic inlet. They may compress vital structures in the neck and anterior mediastinum. Thymomas are usually encapsulated and nodular.

Although some variations and special features may be seen, such as cystic spaces and mineralized bodies, the cells are primarily ovoid and spindle shaped (Parker and Casey 1976). The accompanying population of lymphocytes varies.

Respiratory Tract

Although ethmoidal carcinomas have, in the past, been seen in Sweden and are currently reported in other areas of the world in endemic form (Cotchin 1967; Pospischil, Haenichen, and Schaeffer 1979), neoplasms of the respiratory tract of cattle are generally considered to be rare and are not of economic importance in the United States (Migaki, Helmboldt, and Robinson 1974).

Digestive Tract

Papilloma and Squamous Cell Carcinoma of the Esophagus and Forestomachs (Fig.

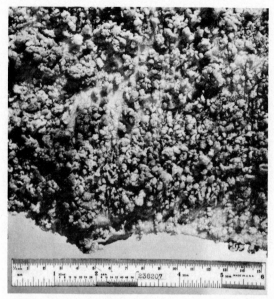

Figure 10–8 Papillomas of the esophagus in cattle. In some instances papillomas cover the entire mucosa (papillomatosis). (AFIP Photo # 53-7639.)

10–8). These are the most common primary neoplasms of the digestive tract, yet they comprise only 0.3 to 1.2 per cent of bovine neoplasms in the large surveys previously referenced. The papillomas are often associated with cutaneous papillomatosis and have a similar appearance. The squamous cell carcinoma of these organs is not related to cutaneous involvement or viral causation but has similar gross and histological morphology. One report lists a seemingly high number (six) of squamous cell carcinomas of the upper alimentary tract in the West of Scotland and draws attention to a possible causative role for bracken fern, which is prevalent in that area (Pirie 1973).

Liver

Although most of the previously referenced surveys list hepatocellular neoplasms as being more frequent than bile duct neoplasms in cattle, the converse is true in two reports (Anderson, Sandison, and Jarrett 1969; Plummer 1956). In an additional survey, hepatocellular carcinomas were not only more frequent than bile duct neoplasms, they were more frequent than any other carcinoma (Vitovec

1976). In general, although hepatic neoplasms are not overly common, they are by no means rare.

Hepatocellular Adenoma and Carcinoma. Use of the term hepatoma is purposely avoided because its use in the past has variously referred to a malignant hepatocellular neoplasm, any neoplasm of hepatocytes, or hepatocellular adenoma.

Both the benign and malignant versions are usually large when detected, often 10 to 20 cm in diameter (Monlux and Monlux 1972), but even larger neoplasms occur. Adenomas are well circumscribed, and carcinomas may be circumscribed or only partly so. Intrahepatic satellites (metastases) are often seen late in the course of hepatocellular carcinoma. These neoplasms are slow growing; thus, they expand slowly and compress adjacent liver tissue. The neoplasms are of a consistency similar to that of the normal liver but are usually lighter in color.

Microscopically, adenomas are composed of rather well-differentiated hepatocytes in cord-like arrangement, mimicking normal structure. There are, however, no portal areas or distinct central veins, thus differentiating this lesion from nodular hyperplasia. Bile production is often seen in either adenoma or carcinoma, and, inasmuch as there is no effective bile ductular system, small amounts of bile may accumulate. It is difficult and probably arbitrary to differentiate adenoma from carcinoma in borderline cases. In obviously malignant tumors, i.e., those with intrahepatic or distant metastases, the use of microscopic criteria to ascribe malignancy is unnecessary. In the absence of metastasis, however, some of the general criteria indicating malignancy apply, e.g., vascular invasion, aggressive invasion into adjacent tissues, loss of trabecular structure, and large hyperchromatic nuclei. Mitotic activity is usually not prominent, even in malignant neoplasms of hepatocytes. In some neoplasms cytoplasmic vacuolation is a feature.

Metastases from adenocarcinomas are most frequent within the liver and then to the adjacent lymph nodes and the lungs.

Cholangiocellular Carcinoma (Bile Duct Carcinoma). These neoplasms often have a rather distinct gross appearance of multiple, irregularly rounded to fungiform whitish nodules in the parenchyma of the liver. Single neoplasms may also be seen. It is often difficult to differentiate multiple cholangiocellular carcinoma from metastatic carcinoma, but it is easier to distinguish it from hepatocellular carcinoma because of the whiter color and the greater connective tissue component of the former.

Microscopically, the cells are cuboidal to columnar or polyhedral, are usually smaller than neoplastic hepatocytes, and ordinarily have a ductular arrangement in at least some part of the neoplasm. In well-differentiated carcinomas, distinct ductular structures may be seen, although this is more common in adenomas. Mucins are ordinarily produced by these neoplasms and are detectable by these neoplasms and are detectable by special staining techniques.

Metastasis is common in cholangiocellular carcinoma, both within the liver and to lymph nodes and lung. Intraabdominal spread by extension may also be seen.

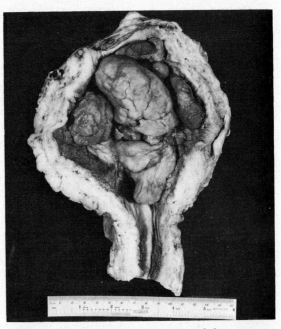

Figure 10–9 Papillary carcinoma of the urinary bladder in cattle. In this case the carcinoma has encroached extensively into the lumen. (AFIP Accession # 201628.)

Urinary Tract

Neoplasms of the kidney are rare in cattle and offer difficulties both in diagnosis and surgical removal. More frequently seen are neoplasms of the urinary bladder (Fig. 10–9). These neoplasms may occur spontaneously but also are experimentally inducible by feeding bracken fern (Pamukcu, Price, and Bryan 1976). In the latter instance they are often accompanied by easily detectable hemorrhage (enzootic hematuria) and have a distinct geographical pattern accompanying areas where bracken fern is plentiful (the Pacific Northwest of the US). A recent review of this syndrome is available (Pamukcu, Price, and Bryan 1976). In this report, naturally occurring and fern-induced bladder tumors were 35 per cent epithelial, 55 per cent mixed epithelial and stromal, and 10 per cent nonepithelial. The neoplasms were usually polypoid, papillary, or fungoid, and in 83 per cent of the animals they were multiple. Both benign and malignant neoplasms occur. Some growths may be both luminal and invasive but are usually easily seen from the luminal surface of the bladder.

Microscopically, most lesions contain discernible transitional epithelium but may have areas of squamous or glandular differentiation; rarely there may be areas of undifferentiated carcinoma cells. These other epithelial types also may occur in the absence of a transitional component, although this is less frequent. Any of these types may be mixed with mesenchymal neoplasms, usually hemangioma or hemangiosarcoma (malignant hemangioendothelioma). Of the purely nonepithelial tumors, smooth muscle–derived tumors are more frequent in sporadic cases and endothelium-derived tumors are more frequent in fern-associated neoplasms.

There probably is not enough evidence to strongly correlate the histomorphology of the epithelial neoplasms with their clinical behavior, yet it would be expected that the more anaplastic and more invasive neoplasms would have a greater potential for metastasis. Pamukcu, Price, and Bryan (1976) reported metastasis to the iliac lymph nodes in 10 per cent of their carcinomas. In a few animals other organs, especially the lungs, may also be involved.

Reproductive Tract

Many parts of the reproductive tract (ovary, uterus, external genitalia of both sexes) are reported to have neoplasms ranging roughly from less than 1 per cent to about 8 per cent of the total of all neoplasms in cattle. There are differences in the surveys as to both the organs most frequently involved and the most commonly found neoplasm in each organ. In considering the high frequency of neoplasms in the testicles in the dog, it is surprising to note the paucity of testicular neoplasia in bulls even after taking into account the relatively small population of bulls as compared with cows.

Granulosa Cell Tumor. Other ovarian stromal tumors (Sertoli cell tumor and arrhenoblastoma) are less frequently reported. Inasmuch as both the morphology of the neoplasms and the behavior of the animals are similar and often overlapping, it has been suggested that these neoplasms all be considered as merely stromal tumors (Norris, Taylor, and Garner 1969). However, in keeping with the vast majority of reports, granulosa cell tumor is used here. Of the previously cited surveys all but one (Anderson, Sandison, and Jarrett 1969) list it as the most common of the ovarian neoplasms in cattle. The previous Anderson paper and one dealing only with neoplasms of the female genitalia (Anderson and Sandison 1969) list adenocarcinomas as being more frequently found in the bovine ovary, but, inasmuch as essentially the same population of animals was used in both papers, they should be considered as one.

Bovine granulosa cell tumors usually involve only one ovary and are irregularly round, with a size range of about 10 to 20 cm. It may be difficult to find normal ovarian tissues, especially in the larger neoplasms. A fibrous capsule is usually seen, as well as irregular fibrous septa. Oftentimes numerous cysts are present. The color is basically a whitish- or grayish-yellow, usually with variable foci and areas of reddening. Frank hemorrhage and necrosis are frequently seen.

Microscopically, the cells resemble the granulosa cells or theca cells of the normal ovary; however, they are in great abundance and are not related to other structures in the normal ovary. The cells are fairly large and polyhedral to spindled with a relatively large amount of cytoplasm and a small nucleus. The cells are mostly arranged in trabeculae and solid sheets, usually with at least some attempt at follicle or gland formation. In some follicles the peripheral cells will have their long axis in a radial orientation.

Granulosa cell tumors may be large and locally destructive and sometimes secrete estrogens or androgens. They are not considered highly malignant, although some do metastasize.

Adenoma and Adenocarcinoma of the Ovary. These neoplasms, reported as being either less frequent or slightly more frequent than granulosa cell tumors, are usually smaller than the granulosa cell tumors. They do, however, share the common trait of having cysts. In fact, they are often referred to as cystadenomas and cystadenocarcinomas. They expand the mass of the ovary and, especially the adenocarcinomas, break through the capsule of the ovary.

Both the benign and the malignant neoplasms are composed of epithelial cells supposedly derived from the ovarian germinal epithelium. The cells are often in a papillary arrangement, which sometimes is visible grossly and which often partly fills cystic spaces, which are usually present. The cuboidal to columnar nature of the epithelial cells is more easily detected when they line papillae in a single layer with their long axes perpendicular to the connective tissue stalk. The cells may also be multilayered or in solid areas. Serous or mucous secretions may be abundant.

Adenocarcinomas of the ovary have a propensity for transcoelomic spread, often extensively seeding the peritoneal cavity. In this form they may easily be mistaken grossly for a mesothelioma. In some cases the similarity to mesothelioma is also striking at the microscopic level. True metastasis may also occur but is less frequent than extension and seeding.

Adenocarcinoma of the Uterus. This neoplasm also is variably reported as comprising 0 to 3 per cent of the total neoplasms in cattle (Anderson, Sandison, and Jarrett 1969; Monlux and Monlux 1972). Even though it may have a relatively low prevalence, it is of some interest because of its often striking appearance and its possible confusion with other neoplasms.

Grossly, the uterus may be enlarged with a thickened wall, but often the primary lesion is small and sclerotic (Migaki et al. 1970). Sometimes an annular constriction is formed. The neoplasm is often paler than the uterine tissue because of its great fibrous content.

Microscopically, the neoplasms are composed of large epithelial cells, which are rather pleomorphic and which usually exhibit at least a modest number of mitotic figures. The cells, even though they may be irregular, often form rather distinct glands. Solid nests and trabeculae of tumor cells are common, and often very small accumulations of cells and individual neoplastic cells are detected. Mucous secretion is prominent in some neoplasms. In any of the epithelial configurations, an abundant proliferation of collagenous stroma is usual.

Transplantation to adjacent organs occurs, and metastasis appears to be frequent. In one report of 192 cases of uterine adenocarcinoma in cows, metastatic neoplasm was found in the internal iliac lymph nodes in 164 cases, the sublumbar lymph nodes in 92 cases, the lungs in 169 cases, the mediastinal lymph nodes in 131 cases, and the bronchial lymph nodes in 101 cases (Migaki et al. 1970).

Fibropapilloma of the Penis, Vulva, and Vagina. These lesions are similar to cutaneous papillomatosis in cattle in that they are caused by the same virus and they occur primarily in younger cattle. The virus is transmitted during coitus.

The fibropapilloma is usually a single lesion but is often extensive, sometimes interfering with function, particularly in breeding bulls. The term fibropapilloma is somewhat misleading in this case because the gross morphology of the neoplasm is rarely papillary. Most often it is sessile and fungiform. The color ranges from pink to gray or white, and areas of necrosis or hemorrhage may be seen.

Microscopically, there is a distinct difference between the fibropapilloma and cutaneous papillomatosis in that the former has a very prominent fibrous component with relatively mild hyperplasia of the epithelium, whereas the converse is true of the latter. The fibrous component of a fibropapilloma is essentially the same as a fibroma in another location, although young tumors may mimic fibrosarcomas because of the less differentiated fibroblasts and mitotic figures (Monlux and Monlux 1972).

These neoplasms are benign, but surgical removal is indicated when they obstruct urinary outflow or when they interfere with breeding functions or parturition. Fibropapillomas may recur after removal, but the total course of the neoplasm is usually a matter of several months (Moulton 1978).

Nervous System

Neurofibroma (Fig. 10–10A and B). This is the only neoplasm of the nervous system occurring with sufficient frequency to warrant discussion here. The highest percentage in a large survey was one in which 29 cases of neurofibromas (Schwannomas) were found in a total of 208 cattle with neoplasms (13.9 per cent) from an abattoir in Holland (Misdorp 1967). Primarily involved were the nerves of the heart, mediastinum, brachial plexus, intercostal spaces, and esophagus. Other surveys report lesser percentages and additional involved organs.

The discussion of neurofibroma versus Schwannoma in the section on equine neural tumors applies here also.

Grossly, enlargement of the peripheral nerves is seen. This may be segmental to diffuse or nodular or both. Often, multiple nerves are involved. The neoplasms are white to off-white or gray and are glistening.

Microscopically, these neoplasms are rather polymorphic but the predominant cell is spindled, having an ovoid to frankly spindled nucleus and an elongated, sometimes wire-like cytoplasmic outline, often with a modest amount of accompanying collagen. Other areas may have cells that are much more plump. Often densely packed cellular areas will be interspersed in looser areas (Antoni type A and type B patterns). Many neoplasms contain numerous parallel spindled cells

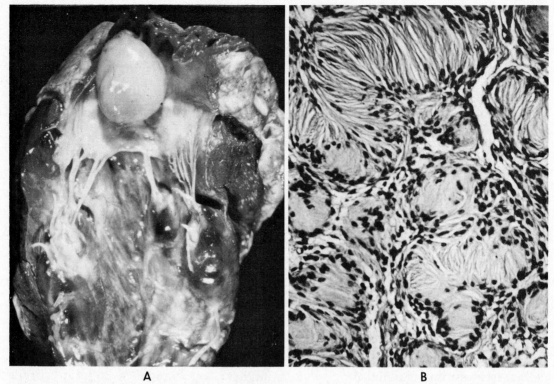

Figure 10–10 Neurofibroma in cattle. *A*, This neoplasm in the atrium demonstrates the typical pale, glistening appearance. (AFIP Photo # 80-584). *B*, This photomicrograph shows the palisading of cells and Verocay bodies that are best exemplified in neurofibromas of cattle. (AFIP Photo # 75-10898.)

with nuclei adjacent to one another (palisading) or whorled, onion skin configurations of spindled cells.

By definition, the neurofibroma is a benign tumor and, as such, does not metastasize, although local infiltration may be seen. Rarely, neurofibrosarcomas are seen.

Endocrine System

Neoplasms of the endocrine organs in cattle are found primarily in the adrenal (both cortex and medulla) and the thyroid, being more frequently reported in the former. The frequency of neoplasms of all the endocrine organs ranges from roughly 2.5 to 11.6 per cent of the total tumors, the average being closer to the lower end of the range. Only the adrenal neoplasms will be discussed here. The reader is guided to the references in the introduction to this chapter for additional information.

Adrenal Cortex. Adenomas are far more frequent than carcinomas and will be the primary focus of this discussion. Because adrenal cortical adenomas are ordinarily nonfunctional in cattle and they usually are not large enough to compress adjacent structures, they are clinically silent and are found as incidental lesions at necropsy.

Grossly, adenomas are single, well-demarcated lesions and, if large, distort the rest of the adrenal gland. They are at least partly encapsulated; this may be detectable grossly. The color is similar to that of the normal cortex, for the most part, but it is ordinarily slightly different, and, especially in larger adenomas, areas of necrosis or hemorrhage may be seen. Hyperplasia is differentiated from adenoma by the presence of multiple nonencapsulated or poorly encapsulated foci. Carcinomas are usually larger, lack encapsulation, and often have more discolored areas due to hemorrhage and necrosis.

Microscopically, the cells of adrenal cortical adenomas are easily recognized as cortical cells. They usually differ from the adjacent cortical cells by being larger, often more highly vacuolated, and frequently arranged in trabeculae several cells wide. Cells of the carcinoma are less like normal cortical cells and may be difficult to identify positively, especially in metastatic sites. These cells often have hyperchromatic nuclei and may have many mitotic figures. Although less well organized than adenomas, carcinomas have some trabecular or cord formation. In addition to the hemorrhage and necrosis mentioned in the gross description, carcinomas are usually characterized by variably thick fibrous stroma.

Adrenocortical carcinomas may grow through the wall of the posterior vena cava, and metastasis to multiple organs is frequently seen.

Pheochromocytoma. This is the most common neoplasm arising in the adrenal medulla. Although they may attain a large size, up to 12 cm in greatest dimension, no clinical signs of functional activity are noted (Monlux and Monlux 1972). Pheochromocytomas are solid neoplasms that compress the adjacent tissue but do not ordinarily invade it and are various shades of white, yellow, or gray. Areas of necrosis and hemorrhage may impart reddish and dirty-brown colors to parts of the neoplasm. Although it is generally held that application of some chromates or iodates to the fresh specimen results in a brown color (Capen 1978), one source indicates that application of chromates to animal pheochromcytomas does not result in a brown color as it does in human pheochromocytomas (Monlux and Monlux 1972).

Microscopically, the cells of the pheochromocytoma may be quite varied from one to the next and even within the same neoplasm. Basically, the cells are polyhedral to cuboidal and are organized into packets by a delicate fibrovascular stroma. Careful examination at high magnification usually reveals at least some fine brownish dust-like granularity in the cytoplasm of the cells similar to that seen, albeit with less difficulty, in the normal cells of the adrenal medulla.

Pheochromocytomas rarely metastasize in cattle.

Special Senses

The only neoplasm of consequence, and it is of great consequence, in these organs is the squamous cell carcinoma in and around the eye.

Squamous Cell Carcinoma (and Associated Neoplasms) of the Eye and Associated Epithelium (Fig. 10–11A and B). These neoplasms comprise from 4.6 to 79.5 per cent of the total bovine neoplasms in the previously cited survey reports. The median is much closer to the lesser figure. The greater figure reflects an accumulation of neoplasms from abattoirs serviced by a laboratory in Denver, Colorado, and

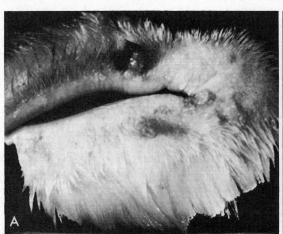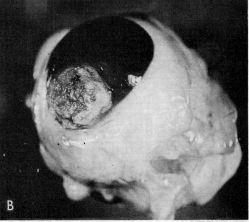

Figure 10–11 Squamous cell carcinoma of the eye and associated epithelium in cattle. *A,* This small papillary lesion of the eyelid is an early carcinoma. (AFIP Photo # 56-20050-112.) *B,* This carcinoma involves much of the cornea but most likely arose at the limbus, the site of origin of almost all squamous cell carcinomas involving the globe itself. (AFIP Photo # 53-7650.)

drew from a population composed of 82 per cent Herefords (Monlux, Anderson, and Davis 1956), a breed with known predisposition to "cancer eye" presumably because of a lack of pigmentation around the eye. Furthermore, the high altitude and high percentage of sunny days in that area intensify the actinic radiation and additional contributing factors to the development of these neoplasms. Other breeds of cattle are much less frequently afflicted. Older cattle are primarily involved. Most are over five years old, and involvement of animals less than one year old is rare (Russell, Wynne, and Loquvam 1956).

The neoplasms of the eye, conjunctiva, and adjacent skin are generally classified as papillomas, epidermal plaques, and squamous cell carcinomas (Monlux and Monlux 1972; Cordy 1978). The squamous cell carcinomas, a small percentage of which are considered noninvasive, greatly outnumber the epidermal plaques and papillomas. As implied by its name, the papilloma is a sharply protruding lesion, whereas the plaque is a superficial broad elevation. Both are white to off-white. The papilloma is more often multiple, and individual lesions may be complex, consisting of multiple finger-like or fungoid projections. Squamous cell carcinomas are usually larger proliferative masses, invade deeper tissues, and more often contain necrotic and hemorrhagic areas. All of these lesions may arise from the cornea, conjunctiva, and adjacent skin, but if the cornea is the primary site it is at the limbus in the vast majority of the cases. Squamous cell carcinomas of the eye are found at the corneal-bulbar conjunctival junction in over 50 per cent of the cases (Monlux and Monlux 1972).

Microscopically, these lesions are all composed of squamous epithelium, but the epithelium is arranged differently and has different degrees of maturity. In the epidermal plaque the epithelium is uniformly thickened with a relatively smooth, nonhyperkeratotic outer surface and a sharp line of demarcation from the underlying stroma. The papilloma, as in papillomas of the skin, has single or multiple, often ramifying, stromal cores with proliferating but essentially normal squamous epithelium, which is covered with an excessive keratin layer. The squamous cell carcinomas have varying appearances, but the epithelial cells are less well differentiated and may even be difficult to recognize as squamous cells. Many are frankly invasive with small fingers and nests of neoplastic cells extending into the underlying tissues. Atypia and mitotic figures are seen more frequently in the aggressive neoplasms.

Although squamous cell carcinomas are malignant, they tend to metastasize only after a considerable length of time, first to the draining lymph nodes. They do, however, invade locally and, in most instances, cause considerable destruction of tissues. Surgical intervention is indicated as early in the course of the condition as is possible. This is true for the papillomas and epidermal plaques as well, because they are considered to be preneoplastic lesions that will eventually become carcinomatous.

SHEEP

The literature states that tumors occur less frequently in sheep than in the other domestic animals and that sheep are probably less susceptible to neoplastic growths (Marsh 1958). Although exact incidence figures may be impossible to obtain because of an unknown population at risk in most reports, at least the relative frequencies of neoplasms in slaughter animals should be roughly comparable.

In one large, year-long survey in Britain, the total number of neoplasms in slaughtered animals at 100 abattoirs was recorded and compared with the total number of animals slaughtered (Anderson, Sandison, and Jarrett 1969). A rate of 2.4 neoplasms per 100,000 slaughtered sheep was obtained, in comparison with 3.6 for pigs and 23.0 for cattle.

In another large survey in New Zealand, the number of neoplasms per 100,000 slaughtered sheep was 252, which was further broken down by age to reveal a rate of 2.2 for lambs (six to nine months) and 1,396 for aged ewes (five to seven years) (Webster 1967). An inordinate number of intestinal neoplasms were seen in this survey. These and other geographical peculiarities will be further addressed.

Other reports from various sources, i.e. biopsy, necropsy, slaughter, or a combination, and from various countries are of interest in comparing the number of different types of neoplasms (Cordes and Shortridge 1971; Cotchin 1960; McCrea and Head 1978; Monlux, Anderson, and Davis 1956; Smith and Jones, 1957).

Skin and Soft Tissues

Neoplasms of these tissues occur much less frequently in sheep than in horses and cows.

Papillomas. These are not reported in most of the surveys of ovine neoplasms previously referenced and the greatest number was four, which accounted for 1.6 per cent of the neoplasms in one survey (Cordes and Shortridge 1971). Viral causation has not been proved in papillomas in sheep.

Although a predilection for the skin of the head and neck is mentioned (Stannard and Pulley 1978), another source states that there is no particularly favored location (Monlux and Monlux 1972). Extensive or multiple involvement is not mentioned in any of the referenced surveys. It is assumed, therefore, that the lesions are primarily solitary. Although the papillomas are quite accessible to surgical removal, there is no need for removal except perhaps for cosmetic purposes in a show animal.

Microscopically, the features of the ovine papilloma are similar to those of the papillomas previously described in horses and cattle.

Squamous Cell Carcinoma. These cutaneous neoplasms also are generally reported less frequently and in lesser numbers in sheep than in cattle and horses. One exception to this, however, lists squamous cell tumors as comprising 6 per cent of ovine tumors (Monlux and Monlux 1972). It is further suggested that sunlight is a contributing factor inasmuch as these lesions are common in the skin of the frontal-parietal area in sheep from the Southwestern United States where sunlight is intense (Monlux and Monlux 1972). Squamous cell carcinomas of the ear and other poorly covered areas were more common in sheep in the hot, dry environment of northwestern Queensland as contrasted with sheep at greater latitudes in Australia (Ladds and Entwistle 1977).

Gross and microscopic features are not sufficiently different from those of bovine or equine squamous cell carcinomas to warrant additional description.

Surgical removal would be beneficial inasmuch as these neoplasms have the potential for metastasis. In one report, metastasis had occurred in 4 of 33 affected sheep that had been thoroughly necropsied (Ladds and Entwistle 1977).

Connective Tissue Tumors. A variety of neoplasms, such as those of fat, collagenous connective tissue, and blood vessels, occur in the connective tissue underlying the skin and in other locations; however, they are infrequent for the most part. There is one recent report of 45 fibrosarcomas in a total of 86 neoplasms from a restricted area of England (McCrea and Head 1978). Most (41) of these fibrosarcomas were of the jaws and appeared to develop deep in the gums. These neoplasms were fast growing and eventually interfered with mastication. No mention was made of surgical attempts.

Musculoskeletal System

Primary neoplasms of these structures are uncommon in sheep. The least uncommon is the chondrosarcoma, probably being more common than the osteosarcoma (Pool 1978). In one abattoir survey, chondrosarcomas comprised 4.5 per cent of all ovine neoplasms (Monlux and Monlux 1972).

Chondrosarcoma. These neoplasms, and the less frequently seen chondroma (Fig. 10–12), occur primarily where cartilage is normally located, i.e., at the epiphyses and articulations of bones and in cartilage of the respiratory passages. In sheep, the ribs and scapula are at greatest risk.

Grossly, these neoplasms are usually rather large when first detected, attaining a weight of up to 10 pounds (Monlux and Monlux 1972). Chondrosarcomas

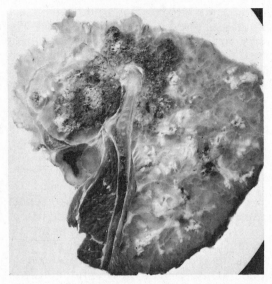

Figure 10–12 Chondroma in the sheep. The large expanding neoplasm arose from the scapula. It has a somewhat lobulated pattern and many small chalky areas of mineralization or ossification. The dark irregular areas are hemorrhages or necroses. Differentiation from chondrosarcoma is often difficult. (AFIP Accession # 218883-15.)

are usually quite firm, are partly or completely encapsulated, have a somewhat knobby surface, and are white to off-white. These characteristics vary, depending on how much mature hyaline-like cartilage is present. Areas of ossification, mineralization, or myxomatous change will alter this appearance. The cut surface usually reveals sublobulations and a glistening appearance. In any event, the neoplastic mass is attached to, and at least partly replaces, the tissue from which it arose.

Microscopically, identification of the tissue as being of cartilaginous origin is usually not difficult, although adequate sampling must be performed to avoid selecting only areas of myxomatous degeneration or reactive proliferation. Chondromas are less cellular, chondrosarcomas being more cellular and having less cartilaginous matrix. Differentiation between benign and malignant lesions often presents a diagnostic problem because of the inherent difficulty in borderline cases and the often limited samples in comparison with the size of the lesion. In general terms, dense cellularity, plump nuclei, hyperchromatic nuclei, and prominent nucleoli are sugges-

tive of malignancy, whereas mitotic activity is somewhat more conclusive.

Chondrosarcomas in sheep tend to grow more slowly and metastasize at a later time than osteosarcomas (Pool 1979).

Lymphoid and Hematopoietic Organs

Thymomas and granulocytic sarcomas have been reported in sheep, but by far the most important neoplasm of the lymphoid and hematopoietic organs is the lymphosarcoma.

Lymphosarcoma. Although the rate of occurrence of lymphosarcoma per 100,000 slaughtered animals over a 10-year period in the United States revealed the rate in sheep to be considerably less than the rate in cattle, calves, goats, pigs, horses, and mules (Migaki 1969), lymphosarcoma in the previously referenced surveys is one of the most commonly occurring neoplasms in sheep. In one report, a remarkable 58 per cent (533) of neoplasms in slaughtered sheep in New Zealand were primary lymphosarcomas of the spleen (Webster 1967). Using the figures in this report, equally remarkable rates of occurrence per 100,000 slaughtered sheep were obtained for sheep of all ages (146/100,000) and for aged ewes (816/100,000). These extremely high figures raise some doubts as to the true neoplastic nature of the condition. In this same population seven other nonsplenic lymphosarcomas were reported. In other countries considerably smaller figures are given (Bostock and Owen 1973). Lymphosarcomas are found primarily in older sheep. No sex or breed predisposition is known.

Grossly, lymphosarcomas are characterized by nodular or diffuse, glistening, gray-white enlargement of the involved organs, most frequently the lymphoid organs. More complete descriptions are available (Johnstone and Manktelow 1978; Migaki 1969). In one of these reports in which adequate information was available for 22 affected sheep, the most common location of the neoplasm was the lymph nodes (19 sheep), spleen (14), liver (13), kidney (10), small intestine (9), and heart (9) (Johnstone and Manktelow 1978). The distribution was considered to be multicentric in 14, alimentary in 6, skin in 1, and thymic in 1. A compilation of information from other papers in the same reference yields the following distribution: 97 multicentric, 25 alimentary, 14 thymic, 20 skin, and 1 other.

Microscopically, the neoplasms are characterized by infiltrations of lymphoid cells with occasional phagocytic histiocytes imparting a "starry-sky" appearance to many of them. In one report of 17 lymphomas, 10 were lymphocytic and 7 were histiocytic (Migaki 1969), whereas another report of 37 lymphosarcomas listed them all as lymphocytic or some variation thereof (Johnstone and Manktelow 1978).

As with lymphosarcoma in other species, surgery is useful only as a biopsy procedure for making or confirming the diagnosis.

Respiratory Tract

Although there are reports of secondary neoplastic involvement of the respiratory organs and a very few other primary neoplasms, the most frequently reported are the ethmoid tumors and pulmonary adenomatosis.

Ethmoturbinate Tumors. These neoplasms are also known as nasal adeno-papillomas (Njoku et al. 1978) and adenocarcinoma of the olfactory mucosa (McConnell, van Rensburg, and van Wyk 1970). They are reported in many countries including the United States (Young et al. 1961; Duncan et al. 1967) where the incidence is endemic within particular flocks. Epidemiological circumstances and transmission experiments incriminated an infectious agent (Cohrs 1953), and virus particles similar to a visna-maedi virus have been seen in electron microscopic studies (Yonemichi et al. 1978).

These neoplasms arise from the mucosa of the nasal cavity and may grow to occupy a large part of the cavity, especially the area of the turbinates, as well as invading the sinuses and even penetrating the skull. They are white or pinkish fleshy masses and have irregular surfaces.

Microscopically, they are more or less well-differentiated epithelial growths showing varying degrees of maturation into ducts and acini with columnar to cuboidal epithelium or remaining as more solid epithelial growths. The amount of stroma is variable, and papillomatous projections are frequently seen. Depending on the degree of differentiation, the neoplasms are referred to as adenomas and papillomas or carcinomas. The histological separation seems to be strictly academic inasmuch as metastasis is not reported.

Pulmonary Adenomatosis. This condition, also known as jaagsiekte in South Africa where it was first reported, has an almost worldwide distribution and an incidence rate of 0.2 to 0.9 per cent (Moulton 1978). Its primary occurrence in older sheep is at least partly related to the long incubation period of the inducing virus, most commonly thought to be a herpes virus. In the past, this condition has been confused with and has sometimes been seen simultaneously with maedi or progressive pneumonia, a virally caused chronic infectious disease.

Gross lesions vary depending on the stage of the disease. Early, small off-white foci are seen primarily in anteroventral parts of the lung. Later in the course of the disease, large areas become off-white to gray, are enlarged and firm, and fail to collapse upon opening the thoracic cavity.

The microscopic hallmarks of this disease are the proliferation of columnar epithelial cells lining the alveoli and the formation of intra-alveolar papillary projections covered by these epithelial cells. This is more readily seen in the advanced stages. Varying amounts of inflammatory cells and fibrosis are seen both within the adenomatous lesions and in adjacent lung tissue. It is sometimes difficult to differentiate this condition from progressive pneumonia.

Whether pulmonary adenomatosis of sheep is truly a neoplastic disease has been a point of discussion, but the presence of metastases in some cases would seem to heavily support the neoplastic concept (Moulton 1978).

Inasmuch as thoracic surgery in sheep is not a practical procedure and diagnosis of this condition in its early, more limited stages is very difficult, surgery is of no real consideration. Nevertheless, the condition has been discussed because of its widespread and common occurrence.

Digestive Tract

An occasional papilloma or squamous cell carcinoma of the upper tract is seen (Anderson, Sandison, and Jarrett 1969; Cordes and Shortridge 1971; McCrea and Head 1978) as well as a few other epithelial and connective tissue neoplasms, but the most interesting neoplasm of the digestive tract is the carcinoma of the small intestine.

Carcinoma of the Small Intestine. This neoplasm is discussed because of its common occurrence in several countries, although it has not been reported in the United States. The greatest numbers have been reported in New Zealand (Dodd 1960; Cordes and Shortridge 1971; Simpson and Jolly 1974; Webster 1967), although an incidence of 0.97 per cent was reported in Icelandic sheep (Georgsson and Vigfusson 1973) and an outbreak on an individual farm was reported in Australia (McDonald and Leaver 1965). Also, 11 cases were reported in a limited geographical area in England (McCrea and Head 1978).

The cause of these neoplasms is not known but the high incidence in certain areas may indicate an environmental carcinogen.

Intestinal carcinomas are most frequently seen in older sheep and near the middle of the small intestine.

Grossly, these neoplasms are first seen as a cord-like mass of white to off-white tissue encircling the intestine. Later, lymphatic invasion and peritoneal seeding lead to much more extensive involvement of lymph nodes and serosal surfaces. Extension to the thoracic cavity via lymphatic drainage may even be seen, but hematogenous spread is very rare.

Microscopically, the early neoplasms may be seen to arise from the mucosa with later extension to involve other layers of the intestine as well as the serosal surfaces. In the intestinal wall the neoplasm consists of sheets, glands, or small nests of cuboidal to columnar epithelial cells, many of which have mucus-containing vacuoles. In contrast to the intestinal lesions, serosal extensions and lymph node metastases may contain extensive fibrous reactions to the neoplastic cells.

Liver

As in cattle, the hepatocellular carcinoma in sheep (Fig. 10–13) is more frequent than cholangiocellular carcinoma (Moulton 1978). In one abattoir survey, a combination of benign and malignant neoplasms of hepatocytes comprised 11 per cent of all neoplasms in sheep (Monlux and Monlux 1972). Other surveys

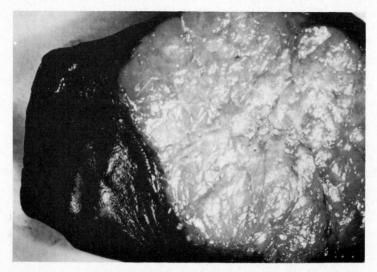

Figure 10–13 Hepatocellular carcinoma in the sheep. This large hepatic neoplasm has a relatively regular outline but has compressed adjacent liver parenchyma. This neoplasm is typically lighter in color than normal liver. (AFIP Photo # 56-20050-34.)

ranged from 3.5 to over 20 per cent. The features of these neoplasms in sheep are essentially the same as those in cattle and the reader is therefore referred to their discussion in cattle.

Urinary and Reproductive Tracts and Nervous System

Neoplasms of these systems are infrequent and do not warrant detailed discussion.

Endocrine System

Adrenal Cortical Neoplasms. Although one source states that adenomas are seen sporadically and carcinomas rarely (Capen 1978), another lists these neoplasms as comprising 8 per cent of the total in an abattoir survey (Monlux and Monlux 1972). Other sources list a smaller figure or none at all. Carcinomas of the sheep adrenal are more likely to metastasize than are those in cattle (Monlux and Monlux 1972).

The gross and microscopic morphologies are essentially the same as those in cattle and will not be reiterated.

Pheochromocytoma. Again, this neoplasm is similar to its bovine counterpart except that in some reports a higher frequency is noted, e.g., 14 per cent in one survey (Monlux and Monlux 1972).

Special Senses

Squamous Cell Carcinoma of the Eye. This is a relatively uncommon neoplasm in sheep and no specific anatomical site is favored; i.e., conjunctiva, limbus, cornea, and eyelid are all sites of this carcinoma (Cordy 1978).

The accessibility to surgical procedures and the characteristic of late metastasis of squamous cell carcinomas should make this neoplasm one of the few in sheep that would be amenable to surgery on a practical basis.

GOAT

The goat is raised in rather small numbers in comparison with the other large domestic animals in the United States and, according to one large abattoir survey, has a relatively low tumor frequency when compared with cattle or horses but a higher frequency when compared with swine and sheep (Brandly and Migaki 1963). Another source states that neoplasms in the goat are rare in relation to tumors of other farm or zoo animals (Zubaidy 1976). Few reports of large series of caprine neoplasms were found, the previously cited work by Brandly and Migaki being the largest with 40 neoplasms (1963). How much of this apparent paucity of neoplasms is dependent upon the young age of most goats at slaughter or is owing to the lack of reporting is conjectural.

Inasmuch as only a few neoplasms are to be discussed, the organization by organ system used in previous parts of this chapter will not be used here.

Cutaneous Papillomatosis. Although this neoplasm is reported to be infrequent in goats (Stannard and Pulley 1978), it is mentioned here because of its ease of diagnosis and accessibility to surgical procedures. The condition is more frequent in adults and in females. Papillomas of the udders of Saanen milking goats and their cancerous potential have been reported (Moulton 1954). Other sites of reported predilection are the head and neck (Sastry 1959).

The papillomas are most often multiple, and the gross and microscopic appearances are not sufficiently different from those in cattle or horses to warrant separate description.

Because some cancerous potential has been reported (Moulton 1954) and because curative surgery is easily performed, removal seems warranted.

Squamous Cell Carcinoma. This neoplasm may be anywhere in the skin of goats but is reportedly found more frequently on the udder of Saanen goats (Moulton 1954) and in the perineal region of White Angora goats (Zubaidy 1976). In Iraq, squamous cell carcinoma is the most important malignant epithelial neoplasm (Zubaidy 1976). The overall frequency of the squamous cell carcinoma, however, may be relatively low in the United States and England as reflected by its absence in two large surveys (Brandly and Migaki 1963; Cotchin

1960). In addition to the previously mentioned sites of predisposition, there is a tendency for the squamous cell carcinoma to develop in nonpigmented and sparsely haired areas that are exposed to excessive sunlight.

No information was found to indicate that the gross and microscopic appearances of this neoplasm in goats differ significantly from the appearance in the previously described species. It is also assumed that the characteristic of metastasis occurring only after prolonged presence also exists in goats. If this be true, surgery would be a practical procedure.

Melanoma. Melanotic tumors are not of great importance in goats. They do, however, occur with a similar frequency as compared with cattle, occur with a greater frequency than in sheep, and occur with a lesser frequency than in horses and pigs (Stannard and Pulley 1978). In one abattoir survey, though, malignant melanomas comprised a large portion of all malignant tumors reported (5 of 26) and equaled lymphosarcomas in occurrence (Brandly and Migaki 1963). One report indicates the perineal region as the most common site in goats (Mustafa, Cerna, and Cerny 1966). Another lists two melanomas of the coronet and one of the udder (Damodaran and Parthasarathy 1972). The perineal melanomas were considered to be malignant by histopathological criteria, and metastasis was noted in one of four.

Carcinoma of the Lung. Adenomatosis, previously described in sheep, also occurs in goats but is less frequent. In fact, primary pulmonary tumors in goats must be considered quite rare inasmuch as only 1 was found in 900,000 slaughtered sheep (Brandly and Migaki 1963). There is, however, a report of 15 pulmonary mucoepidermoid neoplasms in a necropsy survey of 2,500 goats that were five years of age or older (Altman et al. 1970). Although none metastasized, these neoplasms were locally invasive. They contained both squamous and mucus-producing areas.

Thymoma. The correct definition of this neoplasm includes the neoplastic growth of the epithelial component of the thymus, although there may be an admixture of lymphocytes. At some time in the past, thymic lymphosarcomas may have been reported as thymomas. Two reports include substantial numbers of thymomas. One was from a large abattoir survey in which 12 out of a total of 40 neoplasms were thymomas (Brandly and Migaki 1963). The other report documents 17 thymomas found in 67 dairy goats mainly of Saanen breeding and over two years of age (Hadlow 1978). In the latter report, small lymphocytes predominated in 16 goats but all contained epithelial cells, Hassall's corpuscles, and myoid cells. Also, in 16 of the cases, the neoplasm was located in the cranial mediastinal cavity; the other was in the thoracic inlet. The thymomas were nodular to multinodular, encapsulated, and sometimes cystic.

Lymphosarcoma. In two abattoir surveys in the United States, five and two lymphosarcomas were reported, respectively, but the survey periods overlap and some duplication may exist (Brandly and Migaki 1963; Migaki 1969). Three of the four caprine neoplasms in a survey in England were lymphosarcomas (Cotchin 1960). Of these three, two had lesions in the cranial mediastinum, which raises some question about thymic origin. In the two cases described in some detail, both had multiple lymph node involvement and one also had involvement of the heart, liver, and lungs (Migaki 1969). Microscopically, one of these was of the lymphocytic type and one was of the histiocytic type. Further details of gross and microscopic appearances are omitted because they are similar to those of lymphosarcomas in the previously described species.

Miscellaneous. Many other types of neoplasms are reported but their numbers are so small as to be considered of even less significance than those discussed.

PIG

The previous format of listing the neoplasms by organ systems will be discarded for the porcine neoplasms as for the caprine inasmuch as the neoplasms to be discussed are so few. Reports indicate that they are fewer than the bovine or equine in variety of neoplasms and in percentage of animals affected. The latter comparison, however, is probably deceptive because large surveys have drawn largely upon abattoir figures, and, of course, pigs are routinely slaughtered at an earlier stage of life than are cattle or horses. The former comparison regarding variety of neoplasms also requires comment. Although a wide variety of neoplasms may be seen, they are seen in very small numbers in comparison with lymphosarcoma, embryonal nephroma, and melanoma. In several surveys the composite percentage of total porcine neoplasms, which these three neoplasms comprised, ranged from 54.8 to 89.3 per cent (Anderson, Sandison, and Jarrett, 1969; Cotchin 1960; Fisher and Olander 1978; Misdorp 1967; Monlux, Anderson, and Davis 1956; Plummer 1956; Smith and Jones 1957). Therefore these neoplasms will be stressed even though surgery is impractical or would have little curative effect except perhaps in some melanomas.

Melanoma. There are some similarities between equine and porcine melanomas. One is their relatively common occurrence. Another is their predilection — in horses for gray-coated animals and in pigs for members of the Duroc breed and for Hormel and Sinclair miniature pigs (Stannard and Pulley 1978). Two striking differences exist, however. In pigs the neoplasms are common in young animals. A recent report lists the ages of seven swine with melanomas as two, three, four, and nine weeks; six months (two pigs); and six years (Fisher and Olander 1978). Congenital melanomas are not uncommon (Case 1964; Hjerpe and Theilen 1964; Manning et al. 1974). Another difference is that the location of melanomas in the pig is more random than in the horse, in which a perineal preponderance is seen.

Terminology of melanomas is a problem, and much of the discussion of equine melanomas applies for the porcine. In pigs, however, spontaneous regression is seen more frequently than in horses. Although the cutaneous melanomas may metastasize, they are reported by some to do so only after prolonged presence in the pig (Ramsey and Migaki 1975).

The cutaneous lesions may be single or multiple, are usually highly pigmented, and can be exophytic or invasive or both. Cutaneous ulceration is not uncommon. Involvement of noncutaneous sites is more commonly seen accompanying cutaneous involvement; however, it may rarely occur without skin lesions. The regional lymph nodes are commonly involved, and widespread visceral invasion is seen in frankly malignant neoplasms.

A confusing lesion is melanosis, in which pigmented foci are seen in the skin as well as in visceral sites. The differentiation between this lesion and melanoma is often quite difficult and perhaps arbitrary. Grossly, both the neoplastic (melanoma) and the non-neoplastic (melanosis) lesions are pigmented and may be multiple. Melanosis, however, disturbs the architecture of the involved site to a much lesser extent or not at all. So, a small or early melanoma would be difficult to differentiate from melanosis. In larger lesions and in ones in which ulceration has occurred, the cells are more likely to be neoplastic.

Microscopically, the same dilemma can occur because it may be quite difficult to differentiate a melanophage (melanin-laden macrophage) from an epithelioid melanocyte. This may be done with more assurance by use of special stains or electron microscopy. If the melanin-bearing cells are spindled, they are more assuredly identified as melanocytes, thus indicating a neoplasm rather than melanosis. Furthermore, assessing malignancy by histological criteria is fraught with some hazard because melanomas are usually accompanied by some degree of melanophagia by macrophages. Accumulations of pigmented cells in draining lymph nodes must be assessed as to whether they are melanophages or melanocytes. The latter would indicate a malignant melanoma. In addition to identification of metastatic tumor cells, malignancy may also be considered when mitotic activity is prominent, when nuclei are large and hyperchromatic, and when prominent multiple nucleoli are a feature.

Papilloma. This neoplasm is infrequently reported, although a recent reference cites three cases in diverse locations (oral, penile, and cutaneous) (Fisher and Olander 1978). Although

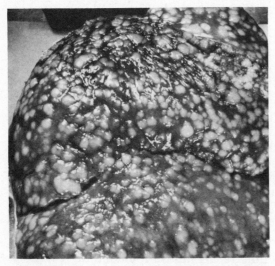

Figure 10–14 Lymphosarcoma in the pig. This liver has disseminated foci of lymphosarcoma. Enlargement of lymph nodes is more commonly seen. (AFIP Photo # 68-6492-12.)

there is no confirmatory evidence for a viral cause of these lesions, there is a previous report of transmissible genital papillomas in pigs (Parish 1961). In the latter referenced cases the lesions regressed spontaneously. In the former cases, the penile papilloma apparently interfered with breeding function and would therefore have benefited from surgery. There is no evidence of any of the porcine papillomas having malignant potential.

Gross and microscopic structures are similar to those previously described in the other species.

Lymphosarcoma (Fig. 10–14). This neoplasm is the most common neoplasm of pigs and commonly affects pigs less than one year old, although the age range is wide (Moulton and Dungworth 1978). Lymphosarcoma accounts for 23 to 51 per cent of all condemnations for neoplasms in swine in abattoirs in the United States (Bostock and Owen 1973). The occurrence is generally sporadic but in one report 53 cases of lymphosarcoma in a large herd were apparently associated with an autosomal recessive gene (Head et al. 1974). Transmissibility and C-type viral causation have been suspected but conclusive proof is lacking (Moulton and Dungworth 1978).

Although any of the anatomical forms of lymphosarcoma may occur in swine, the multicentric form is most commonly seen (Moulton and Dungworth 1978). The visceral lymph nodes are usually more severely involved than are the peripheral nodes.

Microscopically, there is nothing about the porcine lymphosarcoma that is markedly different from lymphosarcoma in the previously described species. Again, the primary value of surgery is to obtain material from which to render a definitive diagnosis.

Embryonal Nephroma (Nephroblastoma) (Fig. 10–15). This neoplasm is considered by some to be the most common neoplasm of pigs (Migaki, Nelson, and Todd, 1971; Monlux, Anderson, and Davis 1956), whereas others rank it behind lymphosarcoma (Anderson, Sandison, and Jarrett 1969; Cotchin 1960; Fisher and Olander 1978; Misdorp 1967; Plummer 1956). Some of the apparent

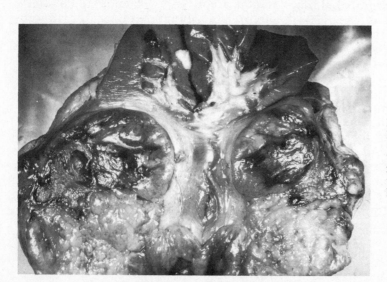

Figure 10–15 Embryonal nephroma in the pig. This neoplasm, which has an irregular shape and color, is quite large when compared with the small remnant of normal kidney at the top of the photograph. (AFIP Photo # 68-7200.)

discrepancies in these reports may merely reflect geographical variations or different populations. Embryonal nephromas are primarily seen in younger pigs.

Embryonal nephromas are usually unilateral and most often are connected to or replace much of the parenchyma of the kidney. They are lobulated or multinodular, are usually covered with a fibrous capsule, which may also extend into and subdivide the neoplasm, and are usually firm, although some areas of necrosis may be seen. The neoplasms are whitish-gray to pink and quite variable in size (1 to 40 cm in diameter and up to 34.1 kg [75 lb] (Migaki, Nelson, and Todd 1971).

Microscopically, the embryonal nephroma is a treat for the microscopist because it contains a variety of components in a variety of configurations. Epithelial and mesenchymal components may be relatively undifferentiated, but, ideally, the epithelial cells will be formed into tubular structures with some configurations of epithelial cells resembling embryonic glomeruli. The mesenchymal tissue usually consists of variably plump spindled cells representing embryonic "blastema." Not infrequently, more mature fibrous tissue is seen and occasionally smooth muscle or even skeletal muscle development is noted.

Although rapid growth is attested to by the large size of these neoplasms often seen in young pigs, metastasis is an infrequent occurrence. Most of the embryonal nephromas are incidental findings at necropsy or postmortem examination.

REFERENCES

Altera, K., and Clark, L.: Equine cutaneous mastocytosis. Vet. Pathol. 7:43, 1970.

Altman, N. H., Streett, C. S., Whitmire, R. E., Terner, J. Y., and Squire, R.: Primary pulmonary mucoepidermoid tumors in the goat. Cancer 26:726, 1970.

Anderson, L. J., and Sandison, A. T.: Tumours of the female genitalia in cattle, sheep and pigs found in a British abattoir survey. J. Comp. Pathol. 79:53, 1969.

Anderson, L. J., Sandison, A. T., and Jarrett, W. F. H.: A British abattoir survey of tumours in cattle, sheep and pigs. Vet. Rec. 84:547, 1969.

Baker, J. R., and Leyland, A.: Histological survey of tumours of the horse, with particular reference to those of the skin. Vet. Rec. 96:419, 1975.

Bostock, D. W., and Owen, L. N.: Porcine and ovine lymphosarcoma: A review. J. Natl. Cancer Inst. 50:933, 1973.

Brandly, P. J., and Migaki, G.: Types of tumors found by federal meat inspectors in an eight-year survey. Ann. NY Acad. Sci. 108:872, 1963.

Capen, C. C.: Tumors of the endocrine glands. In Tumors in Domestic Animals, 2nd ed. Moulton, J. E. (ed.). Berkeley; University of California Press, 1978, pp. 372–429.

Case, M. T.: Malignant melanoma in a pig. JAVMA 144:254, 1964.

Cheville, N. F., Prasse, K. W., van der Maaten, M., and Booth, A. D.: Generalized equine cutaneous mastocytosis. Vet. Pathol. 9:394, 1972.

Cohrs, P.: Infektiose Adenopapillome der Riechschleimhaut beim Schaf. Berl. Muench. Tieraerztl. Wochenschr. 66:225, 1953.

Cordes, D. O.: Equine granulosa tumours. Vet. Rec. 85:186, 1969.

Cordes, D. O., and Shortridge, E. H.: Neoplasms of sheep: A survey of 256 cases recorded at Ruakura Animal Health Laboratory. NZ Vet. J. 19:55, 1971.

Cordy, D. R.: Tumors of the nervous system and eye. In Tumors in Domestic Animals, 2nd ed. Moulton, J. E. (ed.). Berkeley; University of California Press, 1978, pp. 430–455.

Cotchin, E.: A general survey of tumours in the horse. Equine Vet. J. 9:16, 1977.

Cotchin, E.: Spontaneous neoplasms of the upper respiratory tract in animals. In Cancer of the Nasopharynx. Muir, E. S., and Shanmugaratnam, K. (eds.). Union Against Cancer Monograph Series. No. 1. Flushing, NY: Medical Examiners Publishing Co., 1967, pp. 203–259.

Cotchin, E.: Tumours of farm animals: A survey of tumours examined at the Royal Veterinary College, London, during 1950–1960. Vet. Rec. 72:816, 1960.

Cotchin, E., Baker-Smith, J.: Tumours in horses encountered in an abattoir survey. Vet. Rec. 97:339, 1975.

Crowell, W. A., Chandler, F. W., and Williams, D. J.: Melanoma in cattle: Fine structure and a report of two cases. Am. J. Vet. Res. 34:1591, 1973.

Damodaran, S., and Parthasarathy, K. R.: Neoplasms of goats and sheep. Indian Vet. J. 49:649, 1972.

Dodd, D. C.: Adenocarcinoma of the small intestine of sheep. NZ Vet. J. 8:109, 1960.

Duncan, J. R., Tyler, D. E., van der Maaten, M. V., and Anderson, J. R.: Enzootic nasal adenocarcinoma in sheep. JAVMA 151:732, 1967.

Empringham, R. E., and Wilkins, J. N.: Cutaneous melanoma in Hampshire swine. Can. Vet. J. 20:112, 1979.

England, J. J., Watson, R. E., and Larson, K. A.: Virus-like particles in an equine sarcoid cell line. Am. J. Vet. Res. 34:1601, 1973.

Fessler, J. F., and Brobst, D. F.: Granulosa cell tumor. Cornell Vet. 62:110, 1972.

Fisher, L. F., and Olander, H. J.: Spontaneous neoplasms of pigs: A study of 31 cases. J. Comp. Pathol. 88:505, 1978.

Gelatt, K. N., Myers, V. S., Perman, V., and Jessen, C.: Conjunctival squamous cell carcinoma in the horse. JAVMA 165:617, 1974.

Georgsson, G., and Vigfusson, H.: Carcinoma of the small intestine of sheep in Iceland: A pathological and epizootiological study. Acta Vet. Scand. 14:392, 1973.

Gribble, D. H.: The endocrine system. In Equine Medicine and Surgery. Catcott, E. J., and Smithcors, J. R. (eds.). Wheaton, Ill: American Veterinary Publications, 1972, pp. 433–457.

Hadlow, W. J.: High prevalence of thymoma in the dairy goat: Report of seventeen cases. Vet. Pathol. 15:153, 1978.

Hayes, H. M., Jr., Priester, W. A., and Pendergrass, T. W.: Occurrence of nervous-tissue tumors in cattle, horses, cats and dogs. Int. J. Cancer 15:39, 1975.

Head, K. W., Campbell, J. G., Imlah, P., Laing, A. H., Linklater, K. A., and McTaggart, H. S.: Hereditary lymphosarcoma in a herd of pigs. Vet. Rec. 95:523, 1974.

Hjerpe, C. A., and Theilen, G. H.: Malignant melanomas in porcine littermates. JAVMA 144:1129, 1964.

Jacobson, S. A.: The Comparative Pathology of the Tumors of Bone. Springfield, IL: Charles C Thomas, 1971.

Johnstone, A. C., and Manktelow, B. W.: The pathology of spontaneously occurring malignant lymphoma in sheep. Vet. Pathol. 15:301, 1978.

Jubb, K. V. F., and Kennedy, P. C.: Pathology of Domestic Animals, 2nd ed. New York; Academic Press, 1970.

Ladds, P. W., and Entwistle, K. W.: Observations on squamous cell carcinomas of sheep in Queensland, Australia. Br. J. Cancer 35:110, 1977.

Lane, J. G.: The treatment of equine sarcoids by cryosurgery. Equine Vet. J. 9:127, 1977.

Lavach, J. D., and Severin, G. A.: Neoplasia of the equine eye, adnexa, and orbit: A review of 68 cases. JAVMA 170:202, 1977.

Lerner, A. B., and Cage, G. W.: Melanomas in horses. Yale J. Biol. Med. 46:646, 1973.

Levene, A.: Equine melanotic disease. Tumori 57:133, 1971.

Macklin, A. W., and Miller, L. D.: Disseminated malignant lymphoma in a bovine fetus. Cornell Vet. 61:310, 1971.

Madewell, B. R., Priester, W. A., Gillette, E. L., and Snyder, S. P.: Neoplasms of the nasal passages and paranasal sinuses in domesticated animals as reported by 13 veterinary colleges. Am. J. Vet. Res. 37:851, 1976.

Manning, P. J., Millikan, L. E., Cox, V. S., Carey, K. D., and Hook, R. R., Jr.: Congenital cutaneous and visceral melanomas of Sinclair miniature swine: Three case reports. J. Natl. Cancer Inst. 52:1559, 1974.

Marsh, H.: Newsom's Sheep Diseases. Baltimore: Williams & Wilkins, 1958, pp. 260–261.

McConnell, E. E., van Rensburg, I. B. J., and van Wyk, J. A.: A case of adenocarcinoma of the olfactory mucosa in a sheep of possible infectious origin. J. S. Afr. Vet. Med. Assoc. 41:9, 1970.

McCrea, C. T., and Head, K. W.: Sheep tumours in North East Yorkshire. I. Prevalence on seven Moorland farms. Br. Vet. J. 134:454, 1978.

McDonald, J. W., and Leaver, D. D.: Adenocarcinoma of the small intestine of Merino sheep. Aust. Vet. J. 41:269, 1965.

McFadyean, J.: Equine melanomatosis. J. Comp. Pathol. 46:186, 1933.

Meagher, D. M., Wheat, J. D., Tennant, B., and Osburn, B. J.: Squamous cell carcinoma of the equine stomach. JAVMA 164:81, 1974.

Migaki, G. M.: Hematopoietic neoplasms of slaughter animals. In Symposium on Comparative Morphology of Hematopoietic Neoplasms. Lingeman, C. H., and Garner, F. M. (eds.). Bethesda, MD: National Cancer Institute Monograph 32. August, 1969, pp. 121–151.

Migaki, G., Carey, A. M., Turnquest, R. U., and Garner, F. M.: Pathology of bovine uterine adenocarcinoma. JAVMA 157:1577, 1970.

Migaki, G., Helmboldt, C. F., and Robinson, F. R.: Primary pulmonary tumors of epithelial origin in cattle. Am. J. Vet. Res. 35:1397, 1974.

Migaki, G., Nelson, L. W., and Todd, G. C.: Prevalence of embryonal nephroma in slaughtered swine. JAVMA 159:441, 1971.

Miller, J. M., Miller, L. D., Olson, C., and Gillette, K. G.: Virus-like particles in phytohemagglutinin stimulated lymphocyte cultures with reference to bovine lymphosarcoma. J. Natl. Cancer Inst. 43:1297, 1969.

Miller, L. D., and Olson, C.: Regression of bovine lymphosarcoma. JAVMA 158:1536, 1971.

Misdorp, W.: Tumours in large domestic animals in the Netherlands. J. Comp. Pathol. 77:211, 1967.

Misdorp, W., and Nauta-van Gelder, H. L.: "Granular cell myoblastoma" in the horse: A report of 4 cases. Vet. Pathol. 5:385, 1968.

Monlux, A. W., Anderson, W. A., and Davis, C. L.: A survey of tumors occurring in cattle, sheep, and swine. Am. J. Vet. Res. 17:646, 1956.

Monlux, W. S., and Monlux, A. W.: Atlas of Meat Inspection Pathology. Agriculture Handbook No. 367. Washington, DC: U.S. Dept. of Agriculture, 1972.

Moulton, J. E. (ed.): Tumors in Domestic Animals, 2nd ed. Berkeley: University of California Press, 1978, Chaps. 6, 7, 8, and 10.

Moulton, J. E.: Cutaneous papillomas on the udders of milk goats. N. Am. Vet. 35:29, 1954.

Moulton, J. E., and Dungworth, D. L.: Tumors of the lymphoid and hemopoietic tissues. In Tumors in Domestic Animals, 2nd ed. Berkeley: University of California Press, 1978, pp. 150–204.

Murphy, J. M., Severin, G. A., Lavach, J. D., Hepler, D. I., and Lueker, D. C.: Immunotherapy in ocular equine sarcoid. JAVMA 174:269, 1979.

Mustafa, I. E., Cerna, J., and Cerny, L.: Melanoma in goats. Sudan Med. J. 4:113, 1966.

Neufeld, J. L.: Lymphosarcoma in the horse: A review. Can. Vet. J. 14:129, 1973.

Njoku, C. O., Shannon, D., Chineme, C. N., and Bida, S. A.: Ovine nasal adenopapilloma: Incidence and clinicopathologic studies. Am. J. Vet. Res. 39:1850, 1978.

Norris, H. J., Taylor, H. B., and Garner, F. M.: Comparative pathology of ovarian neoplasms. II. Gonadal stromal tumors of bovine species. Vet. Pathol. 6:45, 1969.

Norris, H. J., Taylor, H. B., and Garner, F. M.: Equine ovarian granulosa tumours. Vet. Rec. 82:419, 1968.

Olson, C.: Bovine lymphosarcoma (leukemia) — a synopsis. JAVMA 165:630, 1974.

Olson, C., and Cook, R. H.: Cutaneous sarcoma-like

lesions of the horse caused by the agent of bovine papilloma. Proc. Soc. Exp. Biol. Med. 77:281, 1951.

Olson, C., Miller, L. D., Miller, J. M., and Hoss, H. E.: Transmission of lymphosarcoma from cattle to sheep. J. Natl. Cancer Inst. 49:1463, 1972.

Pamukcu, A. M., Price, J. M., and Bryan, G. T.: Naturally occurring and bracken-fern-induced bovine urinary tract tumors. Clinical and morphological characteristics. Vet. Pathol. 13:110, 1976.

Parish, W. E.: A transmissible genital papilloma of the pig resembling condyloma acuminatum of man. J. Pathol. Bacteriol. 81:331, 1961.

Parker, G. A., and Casey, H. W.: Thymomas in domestic animals. Vet. Pathol. 13:353, 1976.

Parker, G. A., Novilla, M. N., Brown, A. C., Flor, W. J., and Stedham, M. A.: Granular cell tumour (myoblastoma) in the lung of a horse. J. Comp. Pathol. 89:421, 1979.

Parodi, A. L., Tassin, P., and Rigoulet, J.: Myoblastome a Cellules Granuleuses. Trois Nouvelle Observations a Localisation Pulmonaire Chez le Cheval. Rec. Med. Vet. 150:489, 1974.

Pirie, H. M.: Unusual occurrence of squamous carcinoma of the upper alimentary tract in cattle in Britain. Res. Vet. Sci. 15:135, 1973.

Plummer, P. J. G.: A survey of six hundred and thirty six tumours from domesticated animals. Can. J. Comp. Med. 20:239, 1956.

Pool, R. R.: Tumors of bone and cartilage. In Tumors in Domestic Animals, 2nd ed. Moulton, J. E. (ed.). Berkeley: University of California Press, 1978, pp. 89–149.

Pospischil, A., Haenichen, T., and Schaeffer, H.: Histological and electron microscopic studies of endemic ethmoidal carcinomas of cattle. Vet. Pathol. 16:180, 1979.

Prasse, K. W., Lundvall, R. L., and Cheville, N. F.: Generalized mastocytosis in a foal, resembling urticaria pigmentosa of man. JAVMA 166:68, 1975.

Priester, W. A.: Skin tumors in domestic animals. Data from 12 United States and Canadian colleges of veterinary medicine. J. Natl. Cancer Inst. 50:457, 1973.

Ragland, W. L., Keown, G. H., and Gorham, J. R.: An epizootic of equine sarcoid. Nature 210:1399, 1966.

Ragland, W. L., Keown, G. H., and Spencer, G. R.: Equine sarcoid. Equine Vet. J. 2:2, 1970.

Ragland, W. L., and Spencer, G. R.: Attempts to relate bovine papilloma virus to the cause of equine sarcoid: Immunity to bovine papilloma virus. Am. J. Vet. Res. 29:1363, 1968.

Ramsey, F. K., and Migaki, G.: Tumors, intestinal emphysema, and fat necrosis. In Diseases of Swine, 4th ed. Dunne, H. W., and Leman, A. D. (eds.). Ames, IA: Iowa State University Press, 1975, pp. 1032–1045.

Reynolds, B. L., Stedham, M. A., Lawrence, J. M., III, and Heltsley, J. R.: Adenocarcinoma of the frontal sinus with extension to the brain in a horse. JAVMA 174:734, 1979.

Runnells, R. A., and Benbrook, E. A.: Epithelial tumors of horses. Am. J. Vet. Res. 3:176, 1942.

Russell, W. O., Wynne, E. S., and Loquvan, G. S.: Studies on bovine ocular squamous carcinoma ("cancer eye"). I. Pathological anatomy and historical review. Cancer 9:1, 1956.

Sandison, A. T., and Anderson, L. J.: Tumours of the thymus in cattle, sheep, and pigs. Cancer Res. 29:1146, 1969.

Sastry, G. A.: Neoplasms of animals in India. An account of neoplasms collected in 12 years. Vet. Med. 54:428, 1959.

Schmidt, G. R., Cowles, R. R., Jr., and Flynn, D. V.: Granulosa cell tumor in a broodmare. JAVMA 169:635, 1976.

Schueler, R. L.: Congenital equine papillomatosis. JAVMA 162:640, 1973.

Sheriff, D., and Newlands, R. W.: A case of foetal leukemia in a calf. Vet. Res. 98:174, 1976.

Simpson, B. H., and Jolly, R. D.: Carcinoma of the small intestine in sheep. J. Pathol. 112:83, 1974.

Smith, H. A.: The pathology of malignant lymphoma in cattle. A study of 1113 cases. Vet. Pathol. 2:68, 1965.

Smith, H. A., and Jones, T. C.: Veterinary Pathology. Philadelphia: Lea & Febiger, 1957.

Smith, H. A., Jones, T. C., and Hunt, R.: Veterinary Pathology, 4th ed. Philadelphia: Lea & Febiger, 1972.

Squire, R. A.: Hematopoietic tumors of domestic animals. Cornell Vet. 54:97, 1964.

Stannard, A. A., and Pulley, L. T.: Tumors of the skin and soft tissues. In Tumors in Domestic Animals, 2nd ed. Moulton, J. E. (ed.). Berkeley: University of California Press, 1978, pp. 16–74.

Stickle, R. L.: Nasal polyp in a horse. Follow-up of a previously reported case. VM/SAC 73:911, 1978.

Stickle, R. L., Erb, R. E., Fessler, J. F., and Runnels, L. J.: Equine granulosa cell tumors. JAVMA 167:148, 1975.

Strafuss, A. C.: Squamous cell carcinoma in horses. JAVMA 168:61, 1976.

Sundberg, J. P., Burnstein, T., Page, E. H., Kirkham, W. W., and Robinson, F. R.: Neoplasms of equidae. JAVMA 170:150, 1977.

Thirloway, L., Rudloph, R., and Leipold, H. W.: Malignant melanomas in a Duroc boar. JAVMA 170:345, 1977.

Vitovec, J.: Statistical data on 370 cattle tumors collected over the years 1964–1973 in South Bohemia. Zentralbl. Veterinaermed [A] 23:445, 1976.

Webster, W. M.: A further survey of neoplasms in abattoir sheep. NZ Vet. J. 15:51, 1967.

Weiss, E., and Frese, K.: Tumors of the skin. Bull. WHO 50:79, 1974.

Wyman, M., Rings, M. D., Tarr, M. E., and Alden, C. L.: Immunotherapy in equine sarcoid: A report of two cases. JAVMA 171:449, 1977.

Yonemichi, H., Ohgi, T., Fujimoto, Y., Okada, K., Onuma, M., and Mikami, T.: Intranasal tumor of the ethmoid olfactory mucosa in sheep. Am. J. Vet. Res. 39:1599, 1978.

Young, S., Lovelace, S. A., Hawkins, W. S., and Catlin, J. E.: Neoplasms of the olfactory mucous membrane of sheep. Cornell Vet. 51:96, 1961.

Zubaidy, A. J.: Caprine neoplasms in Iraq: Case reports and review of the literature. Vet. Pathol. 13:460, 1976.

CHAPTER 11

THE SKIN AND SUBCUTANEOUS TISSUE

THE ANATOMY OF THE SKIN

TED S. STASHAK, D.V.M., M.S.

The skin is the largest and, certainly, one of the most important organs that the surgeon encounters. It is derived from two embryonic germ layers, the epidermis from ectoderm and the dermis (corium) from mesoderm. Skin thickness varies from area to area within and between species. In the horse, skin thickness varies from 1.0 to 5.0 mm (Boyd 1967). The skin's primary function is to protect the underlying structures from environmental temperature changes, dehydration, and penetration by bacteria, chemicals, and other noxious substances (Muller and Kirk 1976; Swaim 1980).

EPIDERMIS

The epidermis is made up of a basal lamina and five stratified squamous cell layers, which are divided into the stratum basale, stratum spinosum, stratum granulosum, stratum lucidum, and stratum corneum (Fig. 11–1). The epidermis derives its nourishment by diffusion of fluids from the capillary beds in the reticular layer of the dermis (Doering and Jenson 1973).

The stratum basale (base layer) constitutes the deepest layer of the epidermis and is responsible for the production of the cells that overlay it (Muller and Kirk 1976; Swaim 1980). Most of the cells of this layer are keratinocytes, which are constantly reproducing themselves and pushing upward toward the surface to replace cells that have been sloughed off (Muller and Kirk 1976). The other cell types present in this layer are the melanocytes. These cells are responsible for producing the melanin that gives hair and skin its color (Muller and Kirk 1976; Swaim 1980).

The stratum spinosum (prickle-cell layer) is two to three cell layers thick and is composed of cells from the basal layer. These cells appear to be joined together by fine spines referred to as tonofibrils (Muller and Kirk 1976). It is hypothesized that these fibrils interconnect the cells to provide reinforcement to the epidermal layers (Muller and Kirk 1976; Swaim 1980; Troutmann and Fiebiger 1957). Cells in this layer are nucleated and become activated to reproduce when the outer layers of skin are stripped off. The stratum spinosum plus the stratum basale are considered the two layers that make up the stratum germinativum (Swaim 1980; Troutmann and Fiebiger 1957).

The stratum granulosum (granular cell layer) is reported to be from 1 to 15 cell layers thick (Muller and Kirk 1976; Troutmann and Fiebiger 1957). It is composed of cells that are in the process of dying with nuclei that are shrinking and

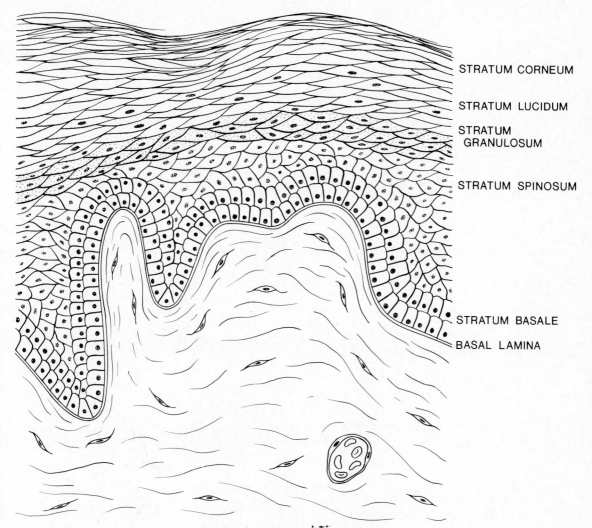

STRATUM CORNEUM

STRATUM LUCIDUM

STRATUM GRANULOSUM

STRATUM SPINOSUM

STRATUM BASALE

BASAL LAMINA

Figure 11–1 Layers of the epidermis.

undergoing chromatolysis (Troutmann and Fiebiger 1957). This layer derives its name from the shiny keratohyalin granules that are present (Swaim 1980).

The stratum lucidum (clear cell layer) is a thin compact layer made up of nonnucleated keratinized cells (Muller and Kirk 1976). This layer is only present in hairless areas of the body (Muller and Kirk 1976; Swaim 1980).

The stratum corneum (horny cell layer) is composed of fully keratinized dead cells that run parallel to the body surface and are constantly being shed from the surface as scales (Muller and Kirk 1976; Swaim 1980). This layer is of varied thickness and forms a barrier zone that protects the underlying skin from irritation, invasion of bacteria and

noxious substances, and fluid and electrolyte losses (Muller and Kirk 1976; Swaim 1980).

DERMIS

The dermis (corium) can be divided into the papillary layer, which lies below the epidermis, and the reticular layer, which extends from the papillary layer down to the subcutaneous tissue (Sisson 1975; Swaim 1980). The dermis contains a rich supply of blood vessels, lymphatics, and sensory nerve endings. The dermal papillae of the reticular layer contain the vascular supply that provides nutrients via diffusion to the overlaying epidermal cells (Muller and Kirk 1976;

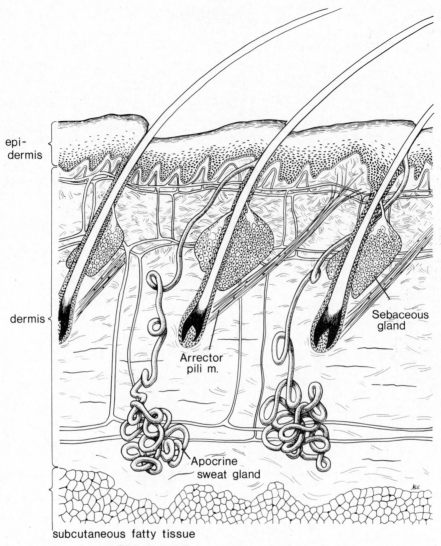

epi-
dermis

dermis

Sebaceous
gland

Arrector
pili m.

Apocrine
sweat gland

subcutaneous fatty tissue

Figure 11–2 Basic anatomy of the skin.

Swaim 1980) (Fig. 11–2). Collagenous, reticular, and elastic fibers present in this layer are suspended in a mucopolysaccharide ground substance made up of hyaluronic acid and chondroitin sulfate (Swaim 1980). The three major cell types present in this layer are the fibroblasts, histiocytes, and mast cells (Muller and Kirk 1976; Swaim 1980). Fibroblasts, of course, are responsible for the production of topocollagen fibrils (immature collagen fibers) and elastic and reticular fibers. The histiocytes possess a phagocytic capability, and the mast cells are responsible for the production of heparin and histamine, which are released during injury to dermal tissues (Muller and Kirk 1976; Swaim 1980).

REFERENCES

Boyd, C. L.: Equine skin autotransplants for wound healing. JAVMA *151*:1618, 1967.

Doering, G. G., and Jenson, H. E.: Clinical Dermatology of Small Animals: A Stereoscopic Presentation. St. Louis: C. V. Mosby, 1973.

Muller, G. H., and Kirk, R. W.: Small Animal Dermatology, 2nd ed. Philadelphia: W. B. Saunders, 1976, pp. 3–20.

Sisson, S.: Common integument. *In* Sisson and Grossman's The Anatomy of the Domestic Animals, Vol. 1, 5th ed. Getty, R. (ed.). Philadelphia: W. B. Saunders, 1975, pp. 247–249.

Swaim, S. F.: Anatomy and physiology of the skin. *In* Surgery of Traumatized Skin. Philadelphia: W. B. Saunders, 1980, pp. 3–39.

Troutmann, A., and Fiebiger, J. F.: The Fundamentals of the Histology of Domestic Animals. Ithaca, NY: Comstock Publishing Associates, 1957.

BOVINE SKIN AND MAMMARY GLAND

F. D. HORNEY, D.V.M.

BOVINE SKIN

Anatomy

The environment of most domestic animals is such that their skin is subjected to a constant barrage of physical and chemical forces. These forces occasionally break down the very effective barrier that the skin provides, resulting in lesions or disease. Numerous infectious, neoplastic, and metabolic diseases also are characterized by skin changes. One therefore wonders why veterinarians are not constantly treating skin problems.

The skin provides a complete covering for the animal except at the mucocutaneous junctions of the body orifices. The subcutaneous tissue attaches the skin to the underlying tissues. Fat deposits may be quite extensive in areas that require additional protection. A considerable area of subcutis is occupied by cutaneous muscle. This muscle provides additional protection and, because of its mobility, a unique twitching property in areas where these muscle fibers enter the skin. There are very few areas of attachment of the skin to the skeleton; therefore, there is not much of a problem with disfiguring scar contracture following trauma.

Cattle have the thickest skin of the large domestic animals. The epidermis consists of a keratinized layer and a germinal underlayer. The germinal underlayer is further subdivided into four layers. The dermis is the fibrous connective tissue of the skin, made up almost entirely of collagen. The hypodermis consists of loose connective tissue joining the skin to the underlying structures. Specialized epithelium, such as hair, horns, and hoofs, provides additional protection to the body and also provides a means of defense.

Physiology

The skin responds to insult as does any other tissue, and its inflammatory response is considered a normal part of any operation regardless of how aseptic the surgery. This inflammatory response is basically the formation of an inflammatory exudate, which is designed to neutralize and remove the irritant. The amount of exudate produced depends on the nature of the irritant. The extent of repair of defects and injuries to an area is species dependent. Lower life forms show a more complete repair process; they are able to replace organs and appendages. In domestic animals, as in humans, all that one can hope for is regeneration of lost tissue. Unfortunately, the more highly developed the tissue, the less power it has to regenerate. Only connective tissue, periosteum, and epidermis can regenerate.

Repair, as it concerns the surgeon in veterinary medicine, is divided into healing of an incised wound and healing of a wound with loss of substance. The end result is either resolution, suppuration with tissue death, or repair by fibrosis.

Lacerations

Cattle either on pasture or permanently housed seldom are involved in situations that result in high-energy wounds such as are encountered in horses. On pasture, attempts to reach pasture on the other side of a fence will cause lacerations if the fence is in poor repair (Fig. 11–3). Any sudden, unusual noise may cause a fright-and-flight response in cattle. In such situations, they are prone to attempt escape through inadequate openings, even doors with glass windows, and in the process are injured.

257

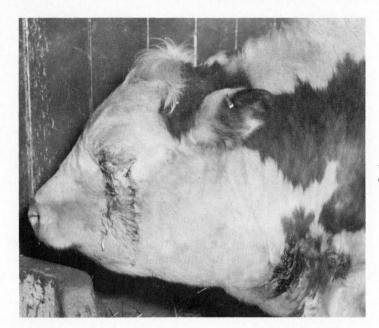

Figure 11–3 Nonspecific cellulitis following laceration (inframandibular phlegmon).

Most wounds so inflicted are usually not observed at the time of occurrence and, as a result, become grossly contaminated and are seldom suitable for complete surgical closure. After adequate debridement, they may be partially closed to minimize scarring. However, adequate drainage is essential if such an approach is used.

On rare occasions, nose rings, a necessary control measure in bulls, accidentally catch on some object or are pulled forcefully, tearing the nasal septum. Debridement and suture will re-establish continuity, but the healing process is unlikely to provide suitable strength for future ring insertion.

Occasionally, grotesque disturbances can arise as the skin accommodates lesions such as subcutaneous and intramuscular swellings (Fig. 11–4A and B). The elastic nature of the skin helps it return to its previous state once the injury is corrected (Fig. 11–4C). It is, however, frequently necessary in such instances to remove some of the excess skin. Failure to obliterate dead space in tissues will result in a collection of serum, providing a favorable medium for possible nourishment of bacterial opportunists that are ever present in the environment.

Neoplasms affecting the skin are not an important part of cattle practice. Fibropapillomata are annoying and appear and disappear without cause, frequently in regions such as the head and neck. Whereas individual lesions may be removed surgically, multiple lesions are usually encountered in areas in which surgical excision of all lesions would be impossible (Fig. 11–5). Varied results are obtained with commercial and autogenous bacterins. When results following vaccination are unsatisfactory, the surgical removal or even crude avulsion of an individual lesion will frequently result in regression of the remaining lesions.

The cutaneous form of lymphosarcoma, although rare, is occasionally encountered (Fig. 11–6). Squamous cell carcinoma is considered a problem in breeds lacking pigment, especially in the region of the eyes. Breeding to eliminate this factor decreases the incidence of carcinoma or cancer. The conjunctiva and lids are usually affected and, when involvement is minimal, excision of the lesion or excision followed by beta radiation is effective. Other forms of treatment that have been used successfully include radon implant therapy, cryosurgery, autogenous bacterins, and BCG treatment (Spradbrow et al., 1977). The economics of veterinary practice necessitate minimal expense. Therefore, ablation or enucleation is frequently advocated rather than expensive plastic surgery or expensive forms of radiation therapy.

Regional anesthesia of the eye (Fig.

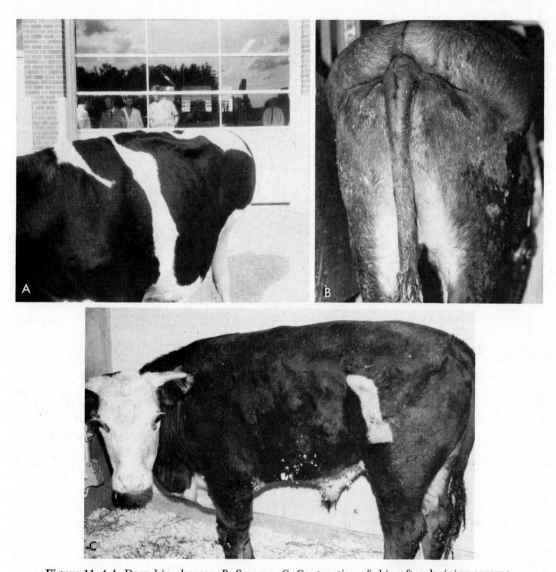

Figure 11–4 *A*, Deep hip abscess. *B*, Seroma. *C*, Contraction of skin after draining seroma.

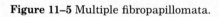

Figure 11–5 Multiple fibropapillomata.

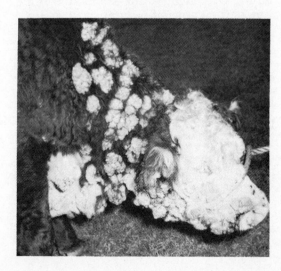

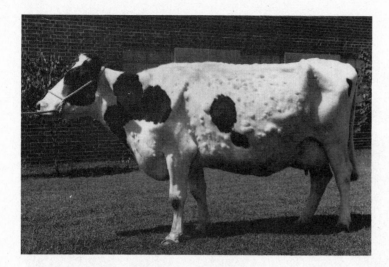

Figure 11–6 Cutaneous lymphosarcoma.

11–7), while reasonably successful, is too often insufficient for major surgery such as eye ablation or enucleation (Peterson, 1951). This technique, if not exercised with care, also carries the risk of introducing infection in the postorbital region. Supplemental sedation or light anesthesia helps provide a more suitable surgical situation regardless of the type of anesthesia used.

Interdigital Fibromata

This growth is classified as a blemish that is tolerated in cattle as long as there is no lameness associated with the fibroma. As the size increases, the pinching that occurs during locomotion causes gait disturbances, and the abrasive contact with the ground results in ulceration. This ulcer or an associated infection is the cause of lameness.

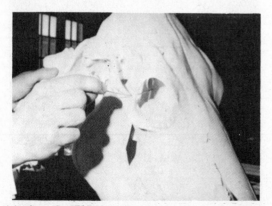

Figure 11–7 The Peterson eye-block approach to the orbitorotundum foramen.

Various treatments have been used, including electrocautery, cryosurgery, and the topical application of caustics, with varying degrees of success. Restraint for surgical excision presents a problem, since squeeze chutes are generally unsatisfactory. In recent years, neurolepto-analgesics, in conjunction with local or regional blocks, have provided better restraint for this surgical procedure. A satisfactory method is sedation with xylazine and regional intravenous anesthesia. Excision is best carried out by an inverted-V incision and careful dissection of the fibroma from the fat pad (Fig. 11–8). The fat pad should not be invaded if it can be avoided, and, should the capsule be accidentally opened, all of the fat should be removed. Postoperative bandaging or wiring of the toes will protect the surgical site and will limit movement until the wound heals.

Iatrogenic Lesions

Skin trauma is frequently the result of surgical intervention, since the skin is opened and closed in most operations. Very little consideration is given to this aspect of surgical intervention except in plastic surgery. Ironically, the need for plastic surgery may be caused by poor healing following a poorly performed routine incision. The nature of many surgical procedures, whether a stab wound for life-threatening bloat or a cesarean section on an immature heifer with dystocia, carries with it the risk of gross con-

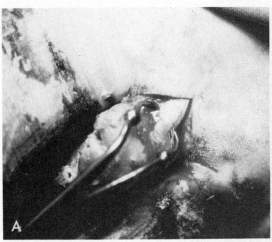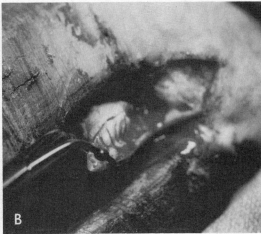

Figure 11–8 Excision of interdigital fibroma. *A,* Inverted-V incision. *B,* Preserving capsule of fat pad.

tamination from the rumen ingesta. Contamination is frequent in the emergency trocarization of the rumen or when the environment for a cesarean section on an exhausted and moribund heifer is a straw-filled stall. Such surgeries, although not relished by today's veterinary surgeon, are occasionally unavoidable and are attended by only minor complications if done judiciously, Wound dehiscence, when it occurs, usually involves the skin and cutaneous muscle (Fig. 11–9). Even if deeper muscle involvement and peritonitis develop, the ruminant has the unique ability to wall off infection in the peritoneal cavity.

Routine elective surgery, which in practice is confined to celiotomy through the paralumbar fossa or ventral abdominal wall, is commonplace in bovine practice, and first intention healing of the celiotomy wound is usually achieved. This is expected in an institution, since an aseptic approach is more easily carried out here than when dealing with emergency procedures under field conditions.

Avoiding contamination in procedures that are likely to result in spillage of ingesta (rumenotomy) can be done by numerous means, the least complicated of which is the simple suturing of the rumen to the skin. Most celiotomy incisions are high in the paralumbar fossa (laparotomy) in the standing animal because there is less difficulty with escape or prolapse of viscera through a high flank incision. Better exposure of viscera can be obtained with a routine vertical paralumbar fossa incision in the standing animal. Incisions made in animals restrained or positioned in lateral recumbency permit variation in the location and configuration of the incision. Those incisions encroaching on the fold of the flank (Fig. 11–10) are, in the author's experience, more prone to wound dehiscence, because of tension on the suture line during locomotion and the inability to eliminate dead space in the region of the flank fold.

In all but sublumbar fossa incisions, some form of local nerve block must be used to give adequate analgesia, because a regional paravertebral block densensitizes only the paralumbar fossa. In practice, this is usually achieved by linear infiltration or field block. The use of lidocaine with epinephrine is helpful in pro-

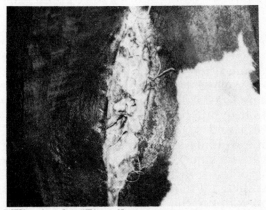

Figure 11–9 Wound dehiscence of the flank.

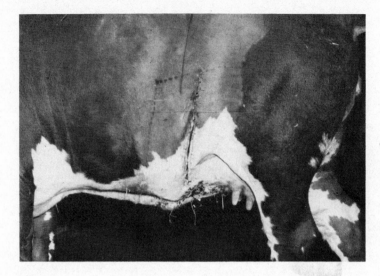

Figure 11–10. Low flank incision encroaching on the flank fold.

viding a longer duration of anesthesia but may be attended by superficial skin sloughing due to ischemia of the skin vessels if too much anesthetic agent is injected in the subcutaneous tissue. Paravertebral block may result in subcutaneous emphysema if the needle is withdrawn without depressing the skin. Tenting of the skin as the needle is withdrawn causes air to enter the subcutaneous tissue. A more serious complication, although fortunately rare, is that the lumbodorsal fascia, if tensed suddenly, is capable of shearing the shaft of the paravertebral needle, imbedding the broken end deeply in the lumbar muscle.

Burdizzo castration, if one improperly, may result in necrosis of the scrotal skin (Fig. 11–11). Occasionally, lay people, in their attempt to correct umbilical her-

nias by ligation, may complicate the condition (Fig. 11–12).

Cosmetic Surgery

Congenital and acquired blemishes may detract from the value of an animal. Owners are therefore anxious to eliminate such problems to improve the esthetic quality and value of the animal. In past years, tie cutting was a practice resorted to on occasion in beef animals, particularly breeding and show stock of the Hereford breed. In the author's region (Eastern Canada), this has not been a common practice in recent years.

Fibrotic thickening of the umbilical vessels is more commonly regarded as an undesirable trait even though there is no evidence of herniation. The excess skin and fibrosed umbilical vessel remnants are removed to improve the animal's appearance.

Rarely, supernumerary appendages may be encountered and, while economically not feasible, may be removed by amputation (Fig. 11–13).

Crushed tails are frequently encountered in feeder animals on slatted floors and should be amputated before bacteremia and systemic complications occur. Short stalls are considered contributing factors since many wounds of the udder and teats in stabled animals are self-inflicted. Frequently in rising, the animal may injure the teats with the dew claw or the edge of the hoof. Amputation of the

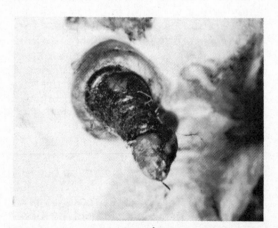

Figure 11–11 Scrotal granulation tissue mass due to improper Burdizzo castration.

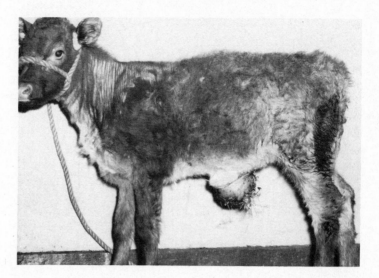

Figure 11–12 Prolapse of hernial sac after attempted repair by ligation.

medial dew claws of the hind legs is carried out as a preventive measure on replacement heifers. This is done when the calves are checked for supernumerary teats, which, if present, are also removed (Anderson, Arnold, and Farnsworth 1976).

MAMMARY GLAND

The importance of this specialized skin gland in the food-producing animal should not be underestimated. Although clinicians are prone to forget anatomical nomenclature, a good working knowledge of the udder is necessary for a veterinarian in a dairy practice. A gland of such size requires a firm suspension, which is provided by the suspensory ligaments. Inadequate support will result in a pendulous udder. The greater elasticity of the median ligament permits an outward protrusion of the teats. Depending on which suspensory ligament is deficient or injured, the gland will be pulled in the direction of the intact ligamentous attachment. The subpubic and prepubic tendons provide attachment for the lateral suspensory ligament, and, while rupture of the prepubic ligament is not a common cause of pendulous udder, it must be considered (Fig. 11–14).

The udder of a cow is completely divided into equal halves. Each half is less well defined into quarters but there is no communication between the quarters. The surgeon needs to have a detailed knowledge of the anatomical features of the teats to do justice to any surgical intervention. The common problem areas are depicted in Figure 11–15. The

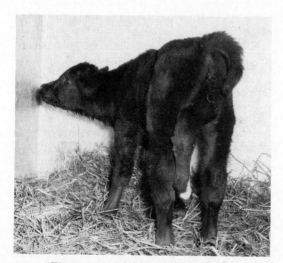

Figure 11–13 Supernumerary limb.

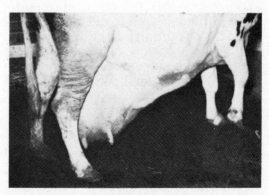

Figure 11–14 Prepubic tendon tear.

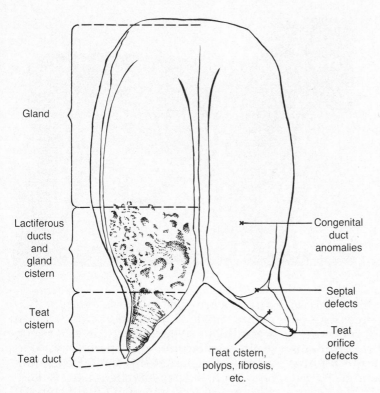

Gland

Lactiferous
ducts
and
gland
cistern

Teat
cistern

Teat duct

Congenital
duct
anomalies

Septal
defects

Teat cistern,
polyps, fibrosis,
etc.

Teat
orifice
defects

Figure 11–15 Structure of the teat. (After Getty: The Anatomy of the Domestic Animals, 5th ed. Philadelphia: W. B. Saunders, 1975, p. 952.)

secretory system is composed of glandular tissue, milk-collecting ducts, gland cistern, teat cistern, and teat orifice. The hind quarters are larger than the front quarters. The milk-collecting ducts are composed of a progressively enlarging collecting system of approximately 12 ducts meeting at the bottom of the quarter. The gland cistern is a multilocular vault with a capacity of approximately 200 to 300 milliliters. Mucous membrane folds form thin partitions between the gland cistern and the teat. The teat cistern is the dilated portion, and the streak canal is the constricted portion of the teat.

The main arterial supply to the udder is through the external pudic and perineal arteries. The branches of the external pudic usually occupy a lateral position in the teat. This may be taken into consideration by surgeon. Venous drainage is through the external pudendal vein, the subcutaneous abdominal vein (milk vein), and the less important perineal veins. The nerve supply is primarily through the inguinal nerves. Ventral deep branches of the first and second lumbar nerves may supply the extreme anterior part of the gland,

Physiology

The mammary gland, while developed to nourish the newborn, now has a more formidable task of feeding humans. Dairy cows are kept primarily to produce milk. Since most milk given at any one milking is already present in the udder at the time of milking, anything that delays, interferes with, or stops the removal of milk will increase intramammary pressure. Rapid removal and atraumatic milking will reduce wear and tear on the teat and udder.

Milk production is less important in beef animals. Of more importance is the reproductive capability of the animal. The quantity of milk produced in beef animals must only be adequate for the calf to remain well nourished. Colostrum, of course, is required by calves as a source of antibodies and vitamin A.

Mammary development usually commences with puberty and develops rapidly through the first pregnancy. Various problems associated with mammary development occur in late gestation and after parturition but are not surgical in nature. Examples include congestion, prepartum edema, and hemorrhage.

Examination

A thorough inspection of the udder and teat is necessary. Radiographical examination for in vivo determination of the anatomy of the bovine teat canal has provided much valuable information. Contrast radiography can be used in situations in which internal lesions may be obscure and not easily identified by palpation (McDonald 1968; Kubicek 1972).

Surgical Conditions

The following prerequisites for successful teat surgery have been suggested by Amstutz (1978).

1. An occluded teat should be opened only when the affected gland is lactating.
2. An interested and cooperative caretaker must be available if surgery on an occluded teat is to be successful.
3. Closure of a teat fistula is best accomplished when the affected gland is not lactating.
4. When a teat sphincter has been completely removed, a true sphincter will not re-form.
5. A severely damaged teat sphincter will rarely, if ever, completely regain its normal function.
6. Strict asepsis should always be maintained when performing teat surgery.
7. Some degree of mastitis will almost always occur when the teat sphincter or teat cistern is severely injured.
8. Antibiotics should be routinely infused into the teat whenever the teat cistern or sphincter is damaged.
9. The use of an indwelling teat dilator or bougie should be avoided if at all possible.

Anesthesia

With the introduction of xylazine to clinically sedate and render cattle more amenable to handling, minor surgical procedures are more easily accomplished as long as there is adequate anesthesia of the surgical site. Adequate anesthesia is also necessary to maintain strict asepsis. When anything more than a simple incision is required, and certainly when su-

turing is necessary, adequate restraint is also required. This can best be achieved by the use of a surgical table. A mobile, hand-operated table, such as is popular in Germany, is very useful, especially in practices involved in a great deal of dairy cattle work. The instillation of 10 to 20 ml of lidocaine provides adequate anesthesia for minor procedures involving the streak canal or lining of the teat cistern. For minor lacerations and contusions, infiltrating the base of the teat with a ring block will provide adequate anesthesia for the surface of the teat. For more involved surgical procedures, the paravertebral block is preferred for more uniform anesthesia (Fig. 11–16).

Congenital Anomalies

Poor udder and/or teat conformation is usually self-limiting and therefore of little concern to the surgeon, primarily because replacement stock is selected on the basis of good conformation. Various anomalies have been described in the literature. Even absence of a portion of the gland (amastia of the rear quarters) has been reported (Alikutty 1978).

Occasionally, the mucous membrane folds between the gland cistern and teat cistern are complete. Most veterinarians prefer to leave these folds intact if they cannot be opened with a simple operation using instruments such as the Hudson probe or teat bistoury. One such congenital anomaly has been reported by Irwin (1957). It was slightly unusual in that two septae were present, one separating the teat from the gland and one obstructing the anterior portion of the gland. The obstruction was relieved by mastotomy.

SUPERNUMERARY TEATS

These are common in both beef and dairy cattle and, when present, usually number from one to three and are situated posterior to the normal teats (Fig. 11–17). Supernumerary teats are best removed when the calf is young and certainly before breeding the animal. If for any reason there has been an oversight and supernumerary teats are present in heifers approaching the last month of

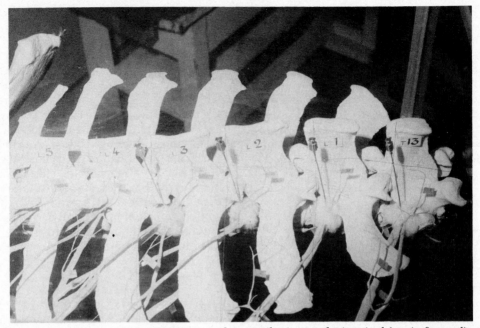

Figure 11–16 Lumbar nerves showing L2, 3, and 4 contributions to the inguinal (genitofemoral) nerve.

gestation, amputation should be avoided because there is likely to be interference with healing should udder edema develop (Fig. 11–18). If a lactating cow has a supernumerary teat and the owner wants it removed, removal should be done during the dry period.

There may be difficulty in differentiating supernumerary teats from normal teats in very young animals. However, with care, proper identification is possible. A curved, sharp scissor is the best instrument to remove small supernumerary teats. In older animals, the use of a Burdizzo emasculator to crush the tissue at the base of the supernumerary teat will provide better hemostasis. Placement of the Burdizzo emasculator on a line with the tension that will occur as the udder develops will avoid problems with healing. A sharp scissor or scalpel is used to sever the teat along the inner aspect of the jaws of the Burdizzo emasculator.

In mature cattle, particularly cows that have previously lactated, surgical excision of supernumerary teats is preferred, using an elliptical incision followed by meticulous suturing of the defect.

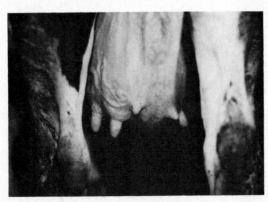

Figure 11–17 Supernumerary teats.

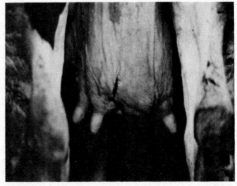

Figure 11–18 Postsurgical draining sinuses in a mature cow following excision of supernumerary teats.

Acquired Anomalies

IMPERFORATE TEATS

The absence of an opening at the end of a teat is seen as a congenital anomaly on occasion and may range from a simple atresia of a teat orifice to a completely fibrosed streak canal and teat cistern. Generally, however, obstruction to milk outflow is acquired as a result of trauma inflicted by milking procedures during lactation. The membranous occlusion of the teat at its base, as described under congenital anomalies, may also be acquired and would be handled as indicated earlier.

Midteat cistern inflammatory or neoplastic lesions may lead to an acquired obstruction to outflow and may be handled by curettage. Abnormal cases with very thick partitions may not be identified until the first calving, when irregular filling of the teat cistern occurs. This may suggest that the occlusion is above some of the lactiferous ducts, preventing the main milk supply from getting to the teat cistern. Conversely, there may be a small hole that permits only a small amount of milk to enter the teat cistern. The Hudson teat probe and bistoury or teat knife slitter is adequate for minor membranous folds, but there is no solution short of radical surgery for heavy fibrous partitions blocking the outflow of milk. Economically, the risk of mastitis or other complications outweighs the loss that might be occasioned by drying off the affected quarter.

CONTRACTED SPHINCTERS—HARD MILKERS

The contracted sphincter is by far the most common teat condition requiring surgery. The most successful method of overcoming this problem is to divide the sphincter muscle in one or more places using a Case teat bistoury, a Stoles teat bistoury, a Lichty teat knife, or similar instrument with a small, narrow blade and a probe point. For this operation, a nose lead and tail hold will suffice for restraint. The instrument is passed into the teat orifice and inserted as far as the sphincter extends. The knife is then drawn downward or the teat is rolled over the blade in one or more places, cutting the sphincter only from within. The cuts are made deep enough to allow dripping of the milk from the teat orifice. Should hemorrhage follow the operation, a stream of milk should be forced from the teat at 10-minute intervals until blood is no longer seen. There may be some postoperative tenderness, and the end of the teat may tend to seal. This can be handled by soaking the teat in warm water for a few minutes and then forcing a few streams of milk out vigorously. A teat dilator may be used but some surgeons feel that, in the farmer's hands, lack of cleanliness may lead to mastitis.

LEAKING TEAT

The risk of infection due to the increased patency of a teat orifice necessitates correcting a leaking teat as soon after calving as possible. Injections of sclerosing substances such as iodine will close down the orifice by stimulating fibroplasia and narrowing of the teat opening. The injections are made into the tissues around the teat orifice.

Traumatic Lesions

Injuries to the end of the teat are aggravated by milking unless the milking is done by hand and the milker uses extreme care and applies pressure only at the base of the teat. The more damage that is inflicted and the more the lesion is aggravated, the more extensive the fibrous tissue proliferation and resulting obstruction to the milk flow. When damage during milking cannot be prevented, this quarter should be dried off or a teat cannula (unscrew the cap of a cannula such as the Ohio teat tube) should be used to remove the milk. Polyethylene tubing taped in place may also be used (Fig. 11–19A). The exposed end of the tubing may be heat fused and opened only at milking times by snipping off the fused portion. The risk of mastitis from teat cannulae or dilators is always present.

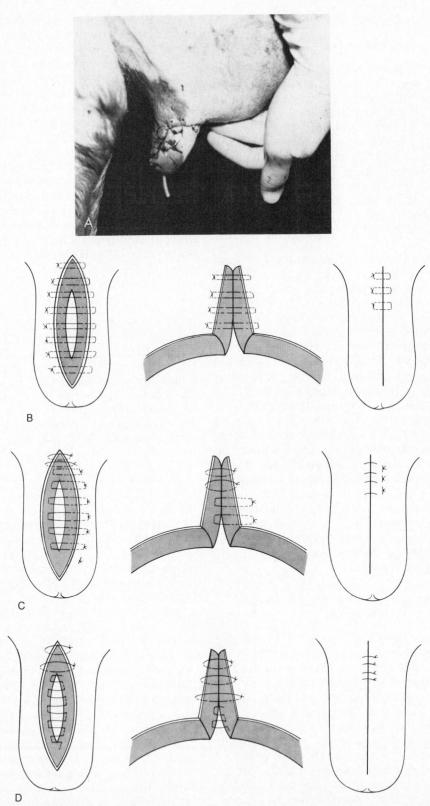

Figure 11–19 *A*, Polyethylene tubing in place of a ridid teat cannula. *B, C,* and *D*, Various suture patterns. *B*, Vertical mattress, nonabsorbable suture. *C*, Deep horizontal mattress, superficial simple interrupted nonabsorbable suture. *D*, Deep continuous mattress, absorbable suture, oversewn simple interrupted nonabsorbable suture.

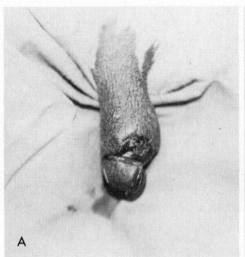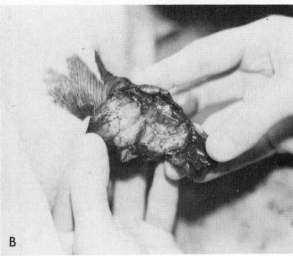

Figure 11–20 *A*, Teat laceration. *B*, Extent of damage on closer observation.

Lacerations

Accidental wounds to the teat and udder present a real problem to dairy cattle practitioners. The prognosis in such cases is always guarded when lacerations extend into the teat cistern or streak canal. Rarely are teat lacerations clean, straight, incised wounds. Many are flap wounds with irregular shapes and depths of penetration. They may be divided conveniently into those not penetrating the milk cistern and those penetrating the milk cistern.

Those not penetrating the milk cistern are usually skin flap wounds with V- or L-shaped configurations. Most will heal as long as they are properly debrided even though they may be unsuitable for suturing. Cleaner wounds may be sutured successfully, and favorable recoveries usually occur in those cases in which there is minimal delay between injury and surgical treatment. In all cases, avoid burying suture material (Fig. 11–19B, C, and D) if possible.

Penetrating lacerations that extend into the teat cistern should be sutured regardless of the irregularity of the laceration or the amount of contamination. When the defect is linear, suturing, while not easy, can be achieved, When the defect is irregular, there is much greater difficulty in apposing tissue and there may be considerable tension on the suture line. Since there is always a delay in having these wounds attended to, adequate debridement is necessary. All too frequently, what appears to be an innocuous wound, on closer inspection, is found to be extensive and irregular (Fig. 11–20).

Teat Fistula

Milk fistulae are usually acquired as a result of injury. In lactating cows, laceration or incisions into the teat or gland cisterns or into one of the lactiferous ducts, even if produced by suturing, may develop into draining fistulae later.

Surgical debridement and meticulous suturing are required following injury (Fig. 11–21A). Should a fistula develop later, an elliptical incision to appose healthy tissue is required (Fig. 11–21B). The use of a Vogelin teat-holding forcep helps identify the teat cistern during repair (Fig. 11–21C).

Suture patterns for teat surgery vary depending on the preference of the operator. The suture pattern should appose, insofar as possible, the tissues between the teat cistern and the teat surface with a noncapillary, inert suture material. A combination technique employing deep mattress tension sutures that do not enter the teat cavity and a simple interrupted skin suture pattern is preferred by many surgeons.

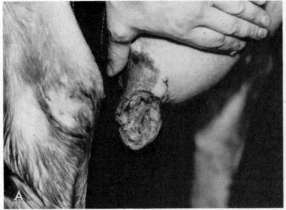

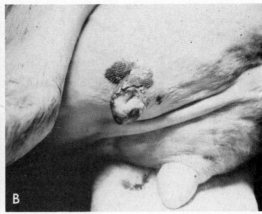

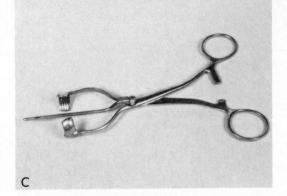

Figure 11–21 A, Teat laceration postcalving. B, Fistula resulting from the laceration in B as it appeared during the dry period. C, Vogelin forcep.

Septic Mastitis

Both coliform and gangrenous mastitis produce a severe toxic state in most cattle. Affected animals are far from suitable candidates for a radical mastectomy or amputation of the udder. Even in those cows that appear able to withstand radical surgery, the operation presents difficulties in handling the bulk of a mature bovine udder and in attempting to quilt the skin to obliterate dead space

after amputation. The surgery can be made easier by elevating the udder once the patient is in dorsal recumbency (Kerr and Wallace 1978).

An alternative to radical amputation has been described (Little and Plastridge 1947). However, the success rate appears to be much lower in cattle than in sheep, perhaps owing to the prominence of the perineal artery and its anastomosis to the caudal mammary artery in some cattle.

The procedure calls for ligation of the

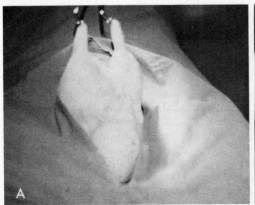

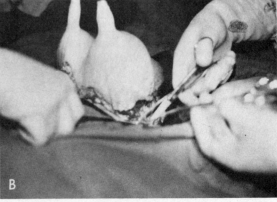

Figure 11–22. Ligation of the external pudic artery.

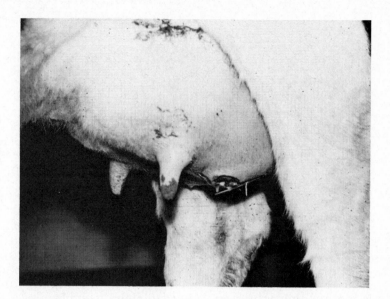

Figure 11–23 Teat amputation after ligation of the external pudic artery.

external pudic artery on the affected side in cases of septic or gangrenous mastitis (Fig. 11–22). Both quarters on the affected side have the same blood supply, so essentially half of the udder will be deprived of blood following this operation. There is no difficulty with hemorrhage after ligating the artery when drainage is established by amputating the teats (Fig. 11–23). Separation of the necrotic area of the affected gland occurs much more quickly after ligation, ahd the animal appears much less toxic (Fig. 11–24). Improvement following surgery is rapid. The ease with which the procedure can be performed and the savings in time and expense (by minimizing the rigorous regimen of drug therapy) make this procedure more attractive than amputation.

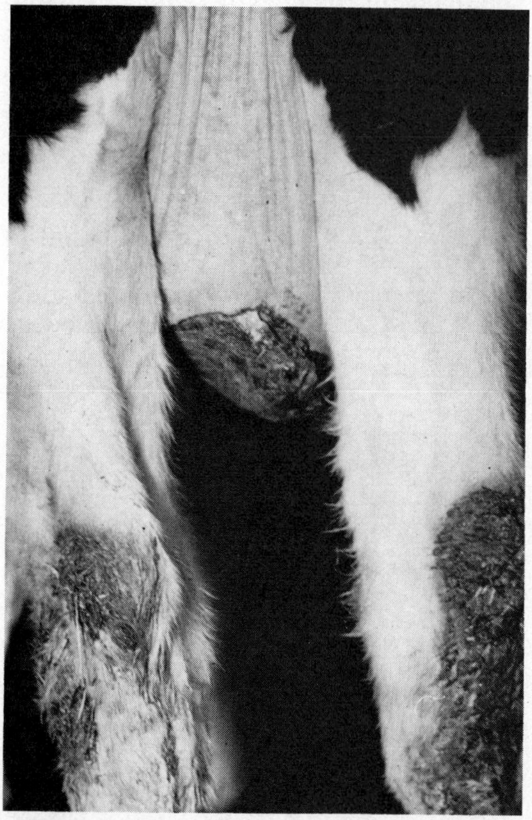

Figure 11–24 Separation of necrotic tissue several days after ligation.

REFERENCES

Alikutty, K. M.: Amastia of rear quarters in a cow. Mod. Vet. Pract. 59:623, 1978.

Amstutz, H. E.: Teat surgery. Mod. Vet. Pract. 59(9):674, 1978.

Anderson, J. F., Arnold, J. P., and Farnsworth, R. J.: VM/SAC 71:73, 1976.

Irwin, D. H. G.: Surgical correction of a congenital mammary abnormality in a heifer. JAVMA 131(4):186, 1957.

Kerr, H. J., and Wallace, C. E.: Mastectomy in a goat. VM/SAC 73(9):1177, 1978.

Kubicek, J.: Radiographic diagnosis of teat abnormalities. Tierärztl. Umsch. 27(3):119, 1972.

Little, R. B., and Plastridge, W. N.: Bovine Mastitis. New York: McGraw-Hill, 1946, pp. 30–31.

McDonald, J. S.: Radiographic method for anatomic study of the teat canal: Observations on twenty-two lactating dairy cows. Am. J. Vet. Res. 29(6):1315, 1968.

Peterson, D. R.: Nerve block of the eye and associated structures. JAVMA 118(888):145, 1951.

Spradbrow, P. B., Wilson, B. E., Hoffman, D., Kelly, W. R., and Francis, J.: Immunotherapy of bovine ocular squamous cell carcinomas. Vet. Rec. 100:376, 1977.

SHEEP AND GOATS

Don E. Bailey, D.V.M.

DEHORNING

Dehorning is an important aspect of goat veterinary practice. Adult goats with horns are dangerous to each other, for they are in constant battle to establish social structure. Owners are soon aware of the danger to themselves, both by accident and intentionally. Many goats are kept and cared for by children, increasing the danger of injury to them. Many fairs and goat shows bar animals with horns.

Scars and regrowth are often common sequelae when horn surgeries are not radical enough. Especially in the Alpine breed, dehorning is most successful if performed before the kids are 7 to 10 days of age. After that age, surgery is more difficult and regrowth is more common.

Polled genes do exist within goat breeds, and ideally selecting for polled genetic strains would be desirable. Unfortunately, polled genes are usually accompanied by intersex recessive genes.

The nerve supply to the horn of the goat consists of the cornual branch of the lacrimal nerve and the infratrochlear nerve. To block the cornual branch of the lacrimal nerve, the needle should be inserted to a depth of 1.0 to 1.5 cm, as close to the caudal ridge of the root of the supraorbital process as possible. The site for local anesthesia of the infratrochlear nerve is the dorsal medial margin of the orbit (this nerve may be palpated in some goats). The needle should be inserted as close as possible to the margin of the orbit to a depth of about 0.5 cm. Approximately 2 to 3 ml of 2% lidocaine should be deposited at each site. Recent publications have advocated the use of xylazine or ketamine for neurolepto-analgesia prior to placement of the local nerve blocks.

Dehorning Baby Goats

Dehorning in the baby goat (under 10 days of age) is termed disbudding by the goat raiser. It is done with an electric dehorner with a ½-in copper pipe burner. The inside of the burning end is tooled to a sharp edge with the outside of the straight burning point (Fig. 11–25). The baby goat is anesthetized with 1 to 3 mg xylazine IM, allowing five minutes for the anesthesia to take effect. This drug is not approved for use in ruminants at this time but is frequently used by veterinary surgeons. Another method of inducing anesthesia is to locally block the infraorbital and lacrimal nerves, as for adult goats. The author has not had success with this method because of the fearful

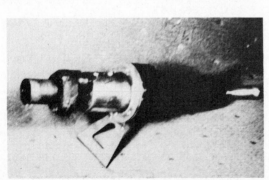

Figure 11–25 Dehorner.

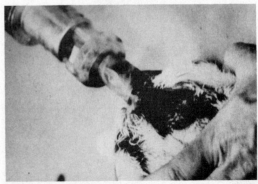

Figure 11–26 Removing the horn button. (Courtesy of Dr. Christine Williams.)

272

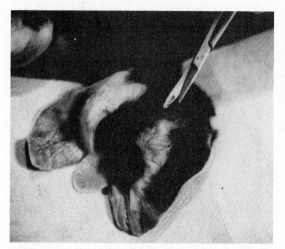

Figure 11–27 Using scissors to remove the horn bud.

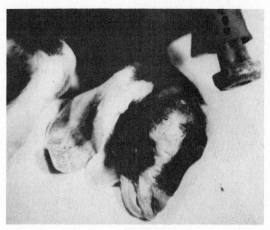

Figure 11–28 Cauterizing the horn bud.

nature of kids; they react to restraint by wiggling, kicking, and screaming. If a tranquilizer, such as acepromazine, is used preceding a nerve or infiltration block, the nerve block is more acceptable. The author has used xylazine, followed by local infiltration of procaine or lidocaine (2%), for disbudding of baby goats.

When anesthesia is not satisfactory, complete infiltration anesthesia, working each horn separately, should be successful in blocking the horn. The tip of the dehorning iron should be cherry red and should never be held on the head for more than 10 seconds. Repeat applications can be done if a cooling off time between applications is observed. A quick turn of the dehorning tip after the horn area is penetrated scoops out the

horn button (Fig. 11–26). Sometimes pushing with the operator's thumb and using scissors will finish removing the horn bud (Fig. 11–27). Reapplication of the *hot* iron to the skin and subcutaneous area (Fig. 11–28) until it is a leather brown color is desirable (Fig. 11–29). Two hundred units tetanus antitoxin or a herd program of tetanus toxoid at dehorning time, with a follow-up booster in two weeks, is indicated.

Dehorning Young Goats

Anesthesia is accomplished by using a combination of xylazine and a ring block of each horn with 2% xylocaine or procaine (Fig. 11–30). After clipping and scrubbing the surgical site, a suitable disinfectant is applied. An amputation or dehorning saw or gigli wire is used to re-

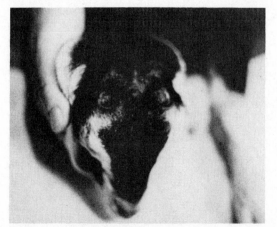

Figure 11–29 "Leather brown" color of horn area, indicating complete cauterization.

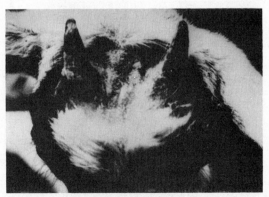

Figure 11–30 Dehorning of young adult goat. (Courtesy of Dr. Christine Williams.)

move the horn. It is important to stay close to the skull and to include a ring of hair when removing the horn. In goats of this age, the top of the cornual sinus will be removed with the horn. This exposes the cornual sinus. The cranial cavity is in close proximity at the posterior medial edge of this sinus. Care must be taken not to invade the cranial cavity. When using a gigli wire, starting at the top of the horn and extending ventrally poses less of a danger of invading the sinus cavity. If a saw is used, it is important to always start at the top and saw down and out to avoid the cranial cavity. Blood vessels that are located are pulled or ligated.

Postoperative care consists of bandaging the area after an application of a disinfectant powder such as nitrofurazone or sulfa powder. The area is rebandaged every three to four days until the skin grows over the cornual sinus and healing occurs (average of two to six weeks). Five hundred units tetanus antitoxin or a two-injection method of tetanus toxoid treatment should precede the dehorning.

Dehorning Adult Goats

Dehorning adult goats is not for softhearted veterinarians. Bleeding is extensive and the amount of horn and cornual sinus removed gives the appearance of complete decapitation. An analgesic dose of xylazine, 1 mg per 10 lb of body weight, is administered. Inhalation anesthesia

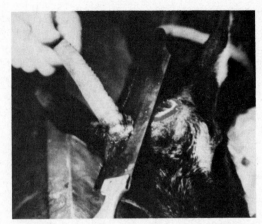

Figure 11–32 Using a dehorning saw.

using halothane or methoxyfluorane works well also. The hair is clipped around the head, and the skin in the area is scrubbed and a suitable disinfectant applied. An infiltration or ring block of 2% lidocaine or procaine is used (Fig. 11–31). A gigli wire or dehorning saw is used (Fig. 11–32), beginning at the top of the horn base and including a generous ring of skin and hair (Fig. 11–33). It has been reported by some veterinary surgeons that complete decapitation is performed, removing both horns with the same cut. Once again, it is important not to cut too close to the posterior medial area so as not to invade the cranial cavity. If regrowth occurs, it will generally occur in the same area, so experience is needed to get just the right amount of horn and cornual sinus. Using a cadaver might be a good way to learn.

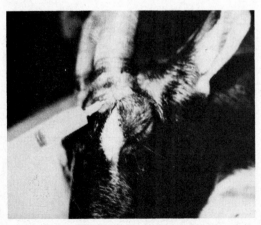

Figure 11–31 Anesthetizing the horn area.

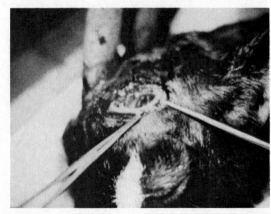

Figure 11–33 Dehorning also includes a ring of skin.

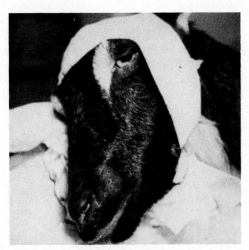

Figure 11–34 Bandaging following dehorning.

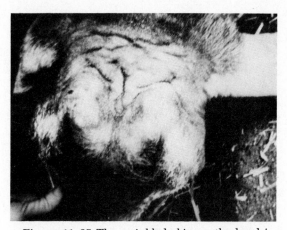

Figure 11–35 The wrinkled skin on the head is also removed when deodorizing the male goat. (Courtesy of Dr. Christine Williams.)

Aftercare for this surgery can extend for months, up to a year. The skin is slow to grow over the large area, and redressing the wound with antibiotic powders and fly repellant is important. Tetanus protection through the use of antitoxins is sufficient, but two injections of tetanus toxoid would protect longer. Owners should be informed of postoperative complications and the possible incidence of regrowth.

Bandaging (Fig. 11–34) is continued until the opening left by the dehorning is closed. In large bucks, this might be six months or more. Antibiotic powders or ointments are applied at each rebandaging. If regrowth starts to appear, the area should be cauterized as soon as possible after it is noticed. Very often anesthesia is not needed.

DEODORIZING THE MALE GOAT

Adult male goats derive most of their pungent odor from the sebaceous cell manes in the skin located on the top of the head (Fig. 11–35). This area is wrinkled, folded, and hairless and is located posteriorly and medially from the horn area. In the case of polled or dehorned bucks, the entire posterior half of the head will be wrinkled and will contain the specialized sebaceous cells. During breeding, bucks have a habit of urinating on their beards, ears, and front legs, resulting in another strong odor.

When dehorning or debudding the young male goat, deodorizing can be accomplished simultaneously by cauterizing a slim area posterior to the horns. A crescent-shaped area of skin is burned, the electric dehorner held vertically to the area and turned sideways as it burns. The burn measures less than 2.5 cm long by 1 cm wide. Removing this tissue will eliminate much of the buck odor and will help eliminate the "goaty" flavor sometimes present in the milk of females.

To remove this tissue surgically, it is necessary to anesthetize the animal. The hair is clipped around the head and the skin is scrubbed. A local anesthetic block of 2% lidocaine is administered around the tissue to be removed. An incision is made about ½ in from the edge of the wrinkled skin down to the bone. This incision is continued across the back of the head to the other side (Fig. 11–36). Be

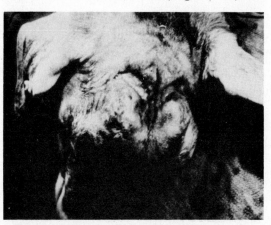

Figure 11–36 Surgically descenting the goat. (Courtesy of Dr. Christine Williams.)

sure to include all of the wrinkled, shiny skin. After this skin is removed, the edge of the incisions are brought together using synthetic suture. Suitable antibiotics are administered for three to five days. A bandage over the head and under the throat for three to five days will reduce swelling.

Owners report that deodorized bucks are less appealing to the does after surgery. Sometimes it is necessary to obtain an intact buck to stimulate estrus in females. An alternative method for stimulating estrus is to rub a sack across the head of an intact buck and hang the sack on a fence where the does are penned.

CHAPTER 12

PLASTIC AND RECONSTRUCTIVE SURGERY

WOUND HEALING

TED S. STASHAK, D.V.M., M.S.

Wound healing is classically divided into four separate stages: the inflammatory stage, the debridement or destructive stage, the proliferative or repair stage, and the maturation stage (Peacock and Van Winkle 1976; Swaim 1980). Each author who has studied this phenomenon describes a sequence of events that usually follows this basic design. However, it is important to remember that these stages are described to facilitate discussion. In reality, wound healing is a continuous process with much overlapping of stages within a given wound (Peacock and Van Winkle 1976). The purpose of this section is to review the basics of wound healing and cover some of the factors that influence it.

INFLAMMATORY STAGE

It is self-evident that all tissue entry, whether as a result of surgical intervention or traumatic injury, is associated with inflammation. Within limits, the inflammatory response observed follows a dose-response curve, which is usually dictated by the severity of the injury (Peacock and Van Winkle 1976). Inflammation is characterized by a vascular and cellular response that protects the wound against excessive blood loss and invasion of foreign substances. It also serves to dispose of dead and dying tissues in preparation for the repair process that follows (Milne 1978; Peacock and Van Winkle 1976; Swaim 1980). The inflammatory stage can be subdivided, but not separated, into vascular and cellular reactions and is thought to last from about zero to six hours after wounding (Peacock and Van Winkle 1976; Swaim 1980). Of course, this stage can be prolonged depending on the degree of wound trauma.

Vascular and Cellular Reactions

Initially after wounding, small vessels adjacent to and within the wound become constricted and occluded (Peacock and Van Winkle 1976; Swaim 1980). This serves to limit the amount of hemorrhage into the wound and subsequent blood loss. After approximately 5 to 10 minutes, vasoconstriction ceases and active vasodilatation occurs (Milne 1978; Peacock and Van Winkle 1976; Swaim 1980). Concurrent with these initial vascular reactions, leukocytes in adjacent vessels become sticky and adhere to the endothelium of the venules, Simultaneous with vasodilatation, a plasma-like fluid fills the wound area and plugs the damaged lymphatics with fibrin (Peacock and Van Winkle 1976; Swaim 1980). Since the lymphatics can no longer drain the injured area, a localized inflammatory response is observed. During this localizing response, leukocytes are observed passing through the vessel walls by a process called diapedesis. Initially, the most prominent white blood cells present are the polymorphonuclear leukocytes. These cells are very short-lived, and, when lysed after their death, their enzymes also contribute to the inflammatory reaction. The fibrocellular clot that fills the wound serves to bind the wound together initially. However, after the clot matures and dehydrates to form a scab, it acts like a bandage by protecting the wound from external contamination (Fig. 12–1). This fibrocellular clot is also responsible for maintaining internal hemostasis as well as providing a scaffold for future repair (Milne 1978; Peacock and Van Winkle 1976; Swaim 1980). Although a scab performs an important function, it is not required for

Wound healing. In fact, it has been shown that wounds heal more rapidly when kept moist under a bandage without scab formation (Peacock and Van Winkle 1976; Swaim 1980). This fact may be important when considering second intention healing of large surface wounds on the cannon bone in the horse.

When suturing the wound, the blood clot that forms should just fill the wound deficit (Fig. 12–2). Excess hemorrhage can lead to pressure necrosis, increased pain, excessive scar tissue formation, and delayed healing and can provide an excellent nutrient medium for bacterial growth (Swaim 1980).

DEBRIDEMENT STAGE

The debridement stage begins approximately six hours after wounding and is classically described as lasting up to about 12 hours. During this stage, the white blood cells (polymorphonuclear cells and monocytes) that were chemotactically stimulated to migrate into the

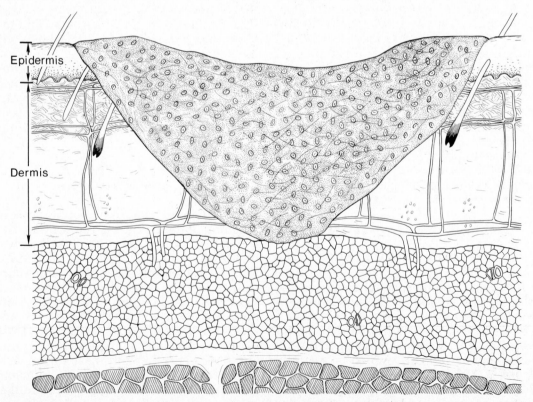

Figure 12–1 Inflammatory stage. Blood and cellular elements fill the wound gap to form a fibrocellular clot. It binds the wound together initially and becomes a scab after it dehydrates.

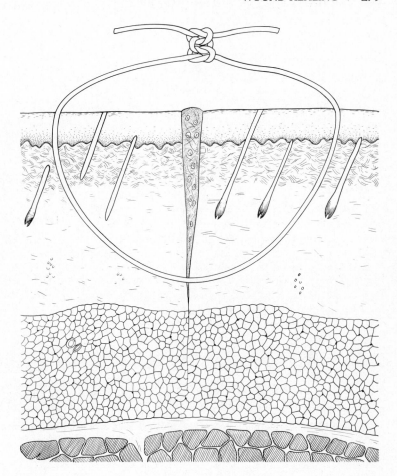

Figure 12–2 Inflammatory stage. A fibrocellular clot is formed in the sutured wound.

wound now begin the clean-up process (Fig. 12–3). Initially, it was thought that polymorphonuclear cells (neutrophils) arrived first, followed by monocytes. However, it has been shown that both of these white blood cell types arrive at the same time and in the same proportions as in the circulating blood, but the neutrophils die early, leaving an apparent increase in the number of monocytes left behind (Peacock and Van Winkle 1976).

The primary function of the neutrophil is the ingestion of microorganisms by phagocytosis. After its death, the lysosomal enzymes of the neutrophil aid the mononuclear cells in further breakdown of necrotic debris. In the absence of infection, healing could progress without the polymorphonuclear cell (Peacock and Van Winkle 1976; Swaim 1980).

Monocytes, on the other hand, are necessary for wound healing. They become macrophages when they enter the wound and phagocytize dead and necrotic tissue plus extraneous debris. In addition to forming macrophages, monocytes also have the capability to coalesce and form multinucleate giant cells or to become histiocytes or epithelioid cells (Swaim 1980). One of the monocyte's important functions is to attract fibroblasts into the wound and, perhaps, stimulate these cells to undergo maturation for collagen synthesis (Peacock and Van Winkle 1976; Swaim 1980).

The duration of the debridement is obviously dependent upon the amount of debris and degree of contamination present. The importance of thorough surgical debridement, good hemostasis, and adequate drainage of the infected wound becomes clear when this stage is understood.

PROLIFERATIVE OR REPAIR STAGE

The repair process involves re-epithelialization of the surface of the wound, migration of fibroblasts necessa-

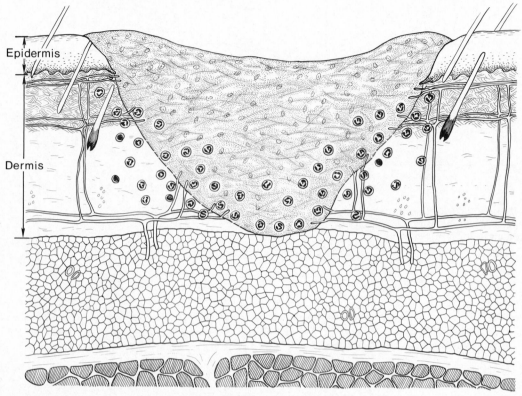

Figure 12–3 Debridement stage. White blood cells migrate into the fibrocellular clot to remove bacteria and extraneous debris. Epithelial cells are beginning to migrate.

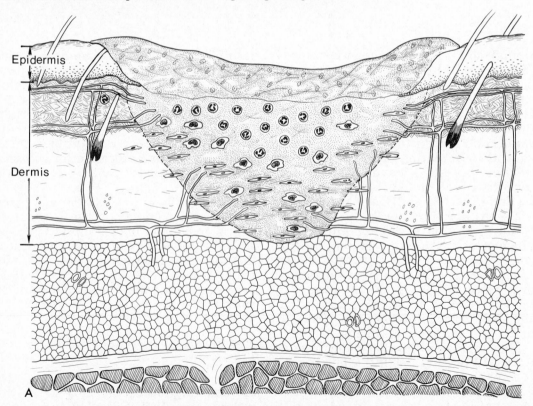

Figure 12–4 Legend on following page.

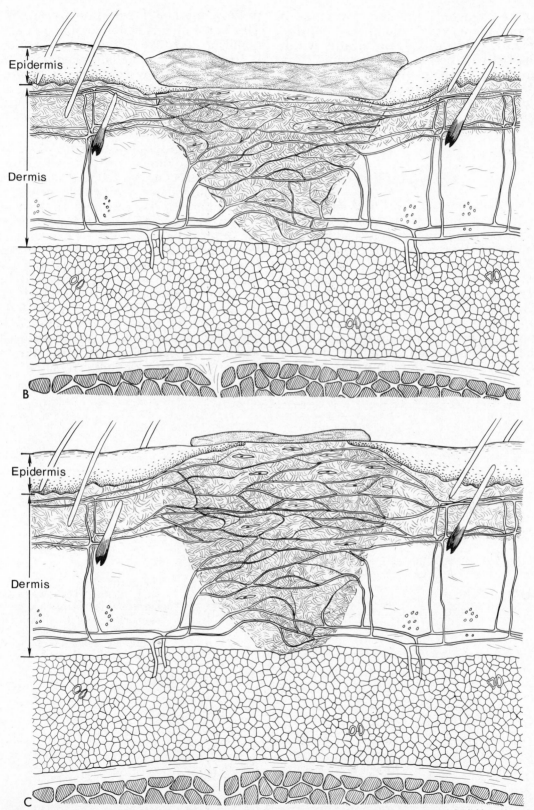

Figure 12–4 A-C Proliferative stage. Epithelial cells migrate under the scab until like cells are contacted. Fibroblasts migrate into the fibrin clot to produce ground substance and early collagen. Budding capillaries revascularize the clot, and granulation tissue is formed. Wound contraction takes place.

ry for collagen formation, formation of granulation tissue, and wound contraction. This stage typically begins within the first 12 hours after wounding and proceeds when barriers, such as blood clots, necrotic tissue, debris, and infection, have been removed (Peacock and Van Winkle 1976; Swaim 1980).

Epithelialization

Epithelialization, the first sign of repair, is recognized at about 12 hours postwounding and is evidenced by a flattening of the rete pegs of the epidermis (Peacock and Van Winkle 1976) (Fig. 12–4). This flattening has a tendency to force adjacent cells toward the wound edges. Simultaneously, the basal cells of the epidermis begin to separate, duplicate, and migrate toward the area of cell deficit. As described by Peacock and Van Winkle, Chalone is responsible for con-

trolling epithelial cell mitosis (1976). This substance is water soluble and epinephrine sensitive. Its primary function is to limit the epithelial cell mitosis in intact skin. After wounding, a diminished concentration of this substance is noticed at the wound edges; this frees the epithelial cell for duplication (Peacock and Van Winkle 1976).

Epithelial migration appears to occur by contact guidance with like cells. However, it has been reported that some cells do migrate independently to the center of the wound. It is presumed that these cells have some directional influence on the other cells that follow (Peacock and Van Winkle 1976; Swaim 1980). If a scab is present, the epithelial cells migrate underneath the scab and detach it by secreting a proteolytic enzyme called collagenase (Peacock and Van Winkle 1976; Swaim 1980). Once epithelialization is complete, the scab falls off. In sutured wounds, the epithelial cells also migrate down suture tracts and, in some in-

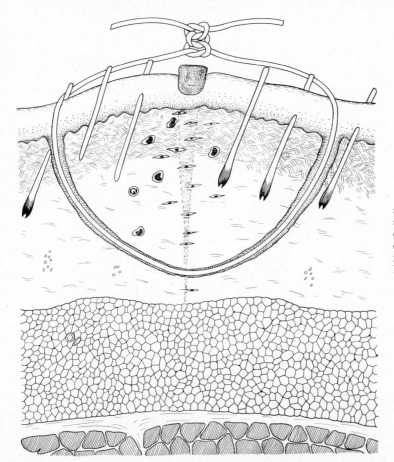

Figure 12–5 Proliferative stage. Epithelial cells cover the surface of the wound and have completed their migration down suture tracts. Scar tissue is present under the epithelial layer.

stances, become keratinized, which may cause local inflammation (Peacock and Van Winkle 1976). The most severe cases may lead to stitch abscess formation (Fig. 12–6) (Peacock and Van Winkle 1976). Generally, epithelial cells continue to migrate until like cells are contacted. Factors that may arrest epithelialization prematurely include infection, excessive production of granulation tissue, repeated dressing changes, extreme hypothermia, and reduced oxygen tension (Swaim 1980). In the incised suture wound, epithelialization completely covers the wound in 12 to 24 hours (see Fig. 12–5) (Peacock and Van Winkle 1976; Swaim 1980). However, in the full thickness open wound, a granulating bed must be formed before epithelialization can occur (Fig. 12–7). In this situation, there is usually a lag period of four to five days before the epithelial tissue begins to migrate (Peacock and Van Winkle 1976). It may take several weeks to months for a large defect to become com-

pletely covered. The rate of epithelialization varies with the region of the body (Milne 1978). In the horse, 400-mm^2 defects on the flank epithelialize at a rate of 0.2 mm/day, whereas similar defects on the lower limb epithelialize at a rate of 0.09 mm/day (Wolton and Neal 1972).

When several layers of epithelial cells cover the wound, cell differentiation and keratinization begin (see Fig. 12–7D). Eventually, these cells come to lay on the smooth undersurface of connective tissue that forms a loose bond, making it easy to disrupt or strip off epithelial cells, This surface lacks the adnexal structures of normal skin and is referred to as scar tissue epithelium (Peacock and Van Winkle 1976) (see Fig. 12–9).

Fibroplasia

Fibroblasts originating from undifferentiated mesenchymal cells in nearby connective tissue move into the wound

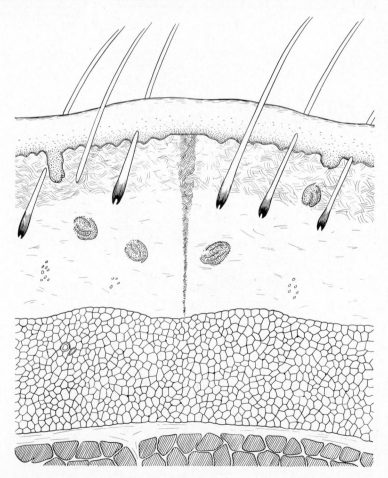

Figure 12–6 Sutures are removed. Keratinized epithelial pearls remain in the dermis associated with suture tracts. They can produce a foreign body reaction and a sterile abscess.

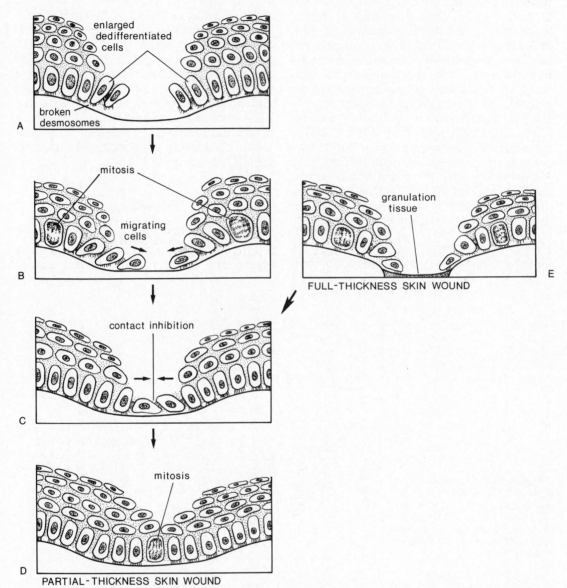

Figure 12–7 Basic process of epithelialization in a partial thickness and a full thickness skin wound. (After Swaim: Surgery of Traumatized Skin. Philadelphia: W. B. Saunders, 1980, p. 84.)

by advancing along the previously formed fibrin clot (see Fig. 12–4). They move by forming cytoplasmic extensions, which extend out from the cells and attach to the solid substrate. The cells then move in the direction of the cytoplasmic extension. Cell movement is directed by contact guidance and ceases when like cells are contacted (Swaim 1980). Fibroblasts usually appear by about the third or fourth day after wounding and remain very active to the fourteenth to twenty-first day (Peacock and Van Winkle 1976; Swaim 1980).

Immediately after entering the wound, fibroblasts begin secreting a protein polysaccharide and glycoprotein, which are necessary components of the ground substance. This ground substance reaches its greatest development at about three to five days and is felt to be necessary for the collagen deposition that follows. Collagen is synthesized by the fibroblasts from hydroxyproline and hydroxylysine. Its formation begins by about the fourth to fifth day and is initiated by the extrusion of the tropocollagen molecule into the extracellular spaces. As these immature fibrils are produced, they begin to bind together to form a mature collagen fiber. As collagen content increases, ground substance content decreases (Peacock and Van Winkle 1976; Swaim 1980).

It is generally believed that the early rise and gain in tensile strength of wounds is a result of collagen formation, whereas later gains in strength result from maturation of the scar (Peacock and Van Winkle 1976; Swaim 1980). The major gain in tensile strength is observed from 5 to 15 days, after which much slower increases are observed. Only 80 per cent of the original tensile strength is reached at one year (Swaim 1980).

The cessation of collagen production may be noted when reduced populations of fibroblasts are seen, which indicate the beginning of the maturation phase of healing. There also appears to be an equilibrium established between collagen production and collagen lysis (Peacock and Van Winkle 1976; Swaim 1980).

Initially, the fibrin lattice, fibroblasts, and early collagen are oriented in a vertical position. However, as the wound matures, collagen fibers become aligned parallel to the skin surface. This realignment of collagen is thought, in part, to be owing to tensional forces produced at wound edges (Peacock and Van Winkle 1976; Swaim 1980).

Granulation Tissue

Granulation tissue begins to appear in the open wound about three to six days after injury (Peacock and Van Winkle 1976; Swaim 1980). The granular appearance of this tissue is a result of proliferating capillaries that form vascular loops. These loops grow behind the fibroblasts and form multiple anastomoses (Swaim 1980) (see Fig. 12–4). Vascular endothelial cells that migrate into the wound contain plasminogen activators responsible for fibrinolysis of the fibrin network (Peacock and Van Winkle 1976; Swaim 1980). As the capillaries develop, so do the lymphatics. However, they do so at a slower rate (Swaim 1980). Granulation tissue formation in an open wound is beneficial for several reasons. (1) It provides a surface for epithelial cells to migrate over. (2) It is resistant to infection. (3) The process of wound contraction is centered around its development. (4) It carries the fibroblasts responsible for collagen formation.

Studies on the dynamics of skin wound healing have shown that the horse is capable of collagen formation as early as one day after wounding (Chvapil et al. 1979). More typically, this capability is reached at about the third or fourth day postwounding. These investigators also found an increased formation of collagen and collagenase in horses' wounds when compared with similar wounds in the rat. They concluded that the healing in the horse is prompt and excessive and tends toward abnormal repair (Chvapil et al. 1979).

Wound Contraction

Wound contraction is a process whereby an open skin defect is reduced in size by the centripetal movement of full thickness skin (Johnston 1979; Milne 1978; Peacock and Van Winkle 1976;

Swaim 1980) (see Fig. 12–4). This movement occurs between the third and fourth days postwounding and appears to be independent of the epithelialization process occurring at the same time. Skin movement is thought to result from the contractile properties of a modified fibroblast, called a myofibroblast, that is found in granulation tissue adjacent to the wound. This cell has good cell-to-cell and cell-to-stroma contact, and it has many properties of smooth muscle including its ability to contract (Peacock and Van Winkle 1976; Swaim 1980). As these cells contract, they draw the surrounding full thickness skin toward the center of the wound. In so doing, the surrounding skin becomes temporarily stretched and thinned. Gradually, new collagen is added to the dermis as new cells are added to the epithelium. This process restores skin thickness and reduces tension and is referred to as intussusceptive growth (Peacock and Van Winkle 1976; Swaim 1980).

Wound contraction works best in loose-skinned areas and is usually sufficient to bring about a closure of the entire wound with minimal scar formation (Peacock and Van Winkle 1976; Swaim 1980). In tight-skinned areas, contraction may not reach an ideal conclusion, and, as a re-sult, a wider scar is formed (Peacock and Van Winkle 1976; Swaim 1980). This occurs in situations in which contraction forces equilibrate with skin tension forces before wound edges are apposed. The rate of wound contraction also varies with lesion location (Milne 1978). In the horse, 400-mm^2 defects on a flank contract at a rate of 0.8 to 1.0 mm/day, whereas similar wounds on the lower limb contract at a rate of 0.2 mm/day (Chvapil et al. 1979).

The shape of the wound also has an effect on the wound's ability to contract. In general, angular defects that are square, rectangular, or triangular contract more rapidly and heal more cosmetically than do circular wounds (Peacock and Van Winkle 1976; Swaim 1980). These angular wounds tend to contract until a stellate scar is formed (Fig. 12–8A, B, and C), whereas circular wounds contract in a crumpled, unpredictable manner at a 30 per cent slower rate (Fig. 12–8D) (Swaim 1980). The clinical implication of this pattern of contraction has yet to be thoroughly defined in the horse.

Wound contraction ceases when (1) contact inhibition of like cells occurs; (2) tension of the surrounding skin equilibrates with the pulling forces of contrac-

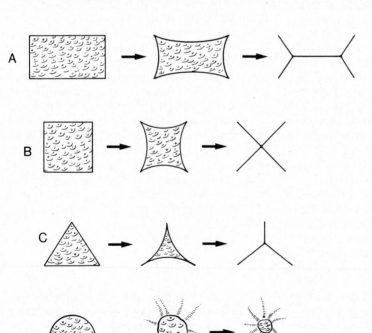

Figure 12–8 Contraction patterns of various wound shapes. (After Swaim: Surgery of Traumatized Skin. Philadelphia: W. B. Saunders, 1980, p. 95.)

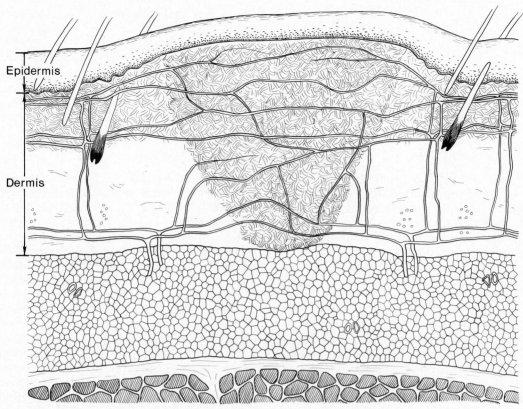

Figure 12–9 Maturation stage. The wound is covered by an epithelial layer with scar tissue replacement of the dermis. A decreased number of fibroblasts and blood vessels are present.

tion; or (3) exuberant granulation tissue inhibits the wound's ability to contract.

MATURATION STAGE

The start of the maturity stage is a reduction in fibroblast numbers with an equilibration between collagen production and lysis (Fig. 12–9). At this point, functionally oriented collagen fibers begin to predominate as nonfunctional ones are dissoved. Despite the reduction in fibroblasts, blood vessels, and dissolving collagen fibrils, the tensile strength of the wound increases. This increase results from collagen molecular orientation along lines of tension, intramolecular crosslinking of collagen, and the formation of more contact bundles. The junction between adjacent collagen bundles becomes less distinct as the fibers interlock. Although the scar formation increases in tensile strength over a prolonged period of time, it still remains 15 to 20 per cent weaker than the surround tissue (Peacock and Van Winkle 1976; Swaim 1980).

REFERENCES

Chvapil, M., Pfister, T., Escalada, S., Ludwig, J., and Peacock, E. E.: Dynamics of the healing of skin wounds in the horse as compared with the rat. Exp. Mol. Pathol. 30:349, 1979.

Ehrlich, P. H., Grislis, G., and Hunt, T. K.: Evidence for the involvement of microtubules in wound contraction. Am. J. Surg. 133:706, 1977.

Johnston, D. E.: The healing processes in open skin wounds. Cont. Ed. 1:789, 1979.

Milne, D. W.: Wound healing and management. In Proceedings of the American Association of Equine Practitioners:349, 1978.

Peacock, E. E., and Van Winkle, W.: Wound Repair, 2nd ed. Philadelphia: W. B. Saunders, 1976.

Swaim, S. F.: Wound healing. In Surgery of Traumatized Skin. Philadelphia: W. B. Saunders, 1980, pp. 70–115.

Wolton, G. S., and Neal, P. A.: Observations on wound healing in the horse. The role of wound contraction. Equine Vet. J. 4:93, 1972.

FACTORS THAT AFFECT
WOUND HEALING

Since the beginning of time, man has been confronted with the problems of wound healing. Only recently, with the aid of extensive research and a better understanding of normal wound healing, have we come to realize a role in providing optimal conditions for wound healing to occur. The major contributions in providing these conditions include (1) the understanding of a contaminated versus an infected wound; (2) the development of aseptic surgical technique; (3) the use of debridement; (4) the development of suturing techniques; and (5) the identification of factors that influence healing. This section will focus on the local and systemic factors that influence wound healing.

PATIENT'S CONDITION

In general, young patients of normal weight on an adequate plane of nutrition and in good general health heal most rapidly. Older patients heal more slowly because of a decreased ability to form granulation tissue; they also have an increased susceptibility to infection (Peacock and Van Winkle 1976; Swaim 1980). Patients with nutritional deficiencies, endocrine imbalances, and hepatic, renal, and cardiac disease also tend to exhibit a delay in wound healing (Swaim 1980). In situations in which elective surgery is contemplated, an attempt should be made to correct any deficiency before proceeding with surgery.

HYPOPROTEINEMIA

Protein deficiencies delay wound healing by reducing the number and activity of the fibroblasts in the granulation tissue (Peacock and Van Winkle 1976; Swaim 1980; Viljanto 1980). This results in a reduction in collagen production, a reduction in wound tensile strength, and an increased tendency for wound disruption (Madden 1977; Peacock and Van Winkle 1976). It appears that the effect of protein on wound healing can be correlated with the degree of deficiency. In situations in which serum protein levels fall to 6.0 g/dl, wound healing is slowed. When serum protein levels fall to 2.0 g/dl, wound healing is markedly inhibited (Swaim 1980; Turner 1978). Experimentally, it has been shown that animals placed on high-protein diets have a more rapid gain in wound tensile strength with less edema formation when compared with animals on protein-deficient diets (Swaim 1980).

ANEMIA PLUS BLOOD LOSS

Normovolemic anemia does not appear to affect wound healing (Swaim 1980). However, it has been well documented that hypovolemic anemia does impair healing. It is thought that the reduced blood volume, with its alteration in vascular dynamics, leads to local hypoperfusion and hypoxia (Swaim 1980). Within limits, the reduced number of red blood cells present does not appear to be a factor in the reduced rate of wound healing (Peacock and Van Winkle 1976; Swaim 1980; Turner 1978).

BLOOD SUPPLY PLUS OXYGEN TENSION

It is well recognized that wound healing depends on adequate local microcirculation to supply nutrients and oxygen. Injury to the microcirculation can occur from (1) bandages or cast applied too tightly; (2) seroma formation; (3) sutures tied too tightly; (4) local trauma; or (5) use of local anesthetics with vasoconstrictors (Swaim 1980; Turner 1978). Adequate oxygen tension is required for cell migration and multiplication and protein collagen synthesis in the healing wound.

Since maintenance of the appropriate oxygen tension is the responsibility of the microvasculature, anything that impairs the blood flow and subsequent delivery of this oxygen will retard wound healing. Although there is some experimental evidence that shows that increased oxygen tension will accelerate wound healing, its clinical application has yet to be defined (Peacock and Van Winkle 1976; Swaim 1980).

TEMPERATURE

Wounds have been shown to heal faster at ambient temperatures of 30°C than at more normal room temperatures of 18 to 20°C (Swaim 1980). Lower temperatures ranging from 12 to 20°C decrease tensile strength in the wound by about 20 per cent. Alternating warm and cold also appears to delay wound healing (Peacock and Van Winkle 1976; Swaim 1980). The inhibitory effect that lower temperatures have on wound healing appears to be a direct result of reflexive vasoconstriction, with subsequent reduction of local blood supply (Peacock and Van Winkle 1976; Swaim 1980). Elevation of local wound temperatures by application of moist heat above 60°C results in thermal injury to the cells. On the other hand, moist heat at 49°C applied to the recently incised wound appears to be optimum for the acceleration of hemostasis (Niemezura and DePalma 1979).

Li and associates compared the effect of full thickness skin burn and freeze-induced injuries on wound healing (1980). They found that the freeze-induced wounds did not contract, whereas the burn-created wound contracted to one-third its original diameter in 21 days. Evidently, slow removal and tissue replacement of the residual frozen tissue matrix prevented contraction. Histologically, the burn wound contained three times the amount of collagen found in normal skin and the freeze-injured skin contained only one and three-fourths times the amount found in normal skin. They concluded that freeze-induced wounds healed more cosmetically than burn-injured skin.

INFECTION

Wound infection results when the number of microorganisms reaches a concentration of 10^6 organisms per gram of tissue. At this point, the organisms have exceeded the capabilities of local tissue defenses (Peacock and Van Winkle 1976; Swaim 1980). Contaminated wounds with lesser concentrations of microorganisms may become infected when (1) foreign bodies are present; (2) excessive necrotic tissue is left in the wound; or (3) local tissue defenses are interfered with, such as in burn patients or patients with immunosuppressive drug therapy. High doses of local irradiation, particularly within the first 4 to 48 hours after wounding, make the contaminated wound more susceptible to infection (Ariyan et al. 1979; Madden 1977). Foreign bodies, including organic material commonly found in the grossly contaminated wound, bone sequestra, suture material, glove powder, and bone plates and screws, promote infection by providing a protective surface area for bacteria to grow on (Turner 1978). An important point to remember is that the lower the inoculum of microorganisms, the longer it will take for the organisms to reach the point of clinical infection and the greater the chances that host defenses will curtail the formation of active infection (Swaim 1980).

Infection delays healing by mechanically separating the wound edges, reducing the vascular supply, and increasing the cellular response, which in turn results in prolongation of the debridement phase of healing (Peacock and Van Winkle 1976; Swaim 1980). Bacteria also produce toxic necrotizing enzymes with specific actions that retard healing (Swaim 1980).

As stated by Peacock and Van Winkle, the best way to deal with infection is to prevent it (1976). The best way to prevent infection is to follow aseptic technique. In the traumatized patient, this means thorough debridement, wide excision, meticulous hemostasis, thorough lavage, elimination of dead space, and the use of proper suturing techniques.

DEHYDRATION AND EDEMA

Dehydration has been shown to reduce the rate of epithelialization and, in general, delays wound healing (Swaim 1980). Edema, on the other hand, has a temporary inhibiting effect on wound healing. However, this delay appears to be more mechanical than biochemical in nature (Peacock and Van Winkle 1976).

BANDAGING AND BIOLOGICAL DRESSINGS

Although bandaging a wound with nonadherent dressings has no effect on the epithelial cell mitotic rate, it does appear to enhance the epithelial migration across the wound. In studies involving human subjects, it was noted that sutured wounds covered with nonadherent dressings had epithelial coverings in 24 hours, whereas subjects with similar wounds without bandages did not have epithelial coverings for 72 hours (Rovee et al. 1972). It is thought that slower epithelial migrations in open wounds result from desiccation of the peripheral epithelial cell and the formation of a thick scab, requiring the migrating epithelial cells to cleave deeper planes underneath the scab (Swaim 1980). The bandaged wound maintains a moist microenvironment, which allows for freer epithelial movement. Whereas nonadherent dressings are beneficial, adherent dressings are detrimental because fluid and cells accumulate and become entrapped in the interstices of the dressing and are removed at each dressing change. However, some like to use this principle for early debridement of wounds that are to heal by second intention or delayed primary closure (Bojrab 1981).

Porcine xenographs, referred to as biological dressings, have low antigenic properties and have proved to be beneficial in the treatment of large surface defects in animals and man (Diehl and Ersek 1980; Madden and Smith 1970; Morris and Tracey 1977). These grafts can be sutured or simply applied topically to the wound like a nonadherent dressing of the wound. Bandages are usually changed every four to five days, and the graft is removed and replaced at this time. This is repeated until the desired result is obtained. The benefits of biological dressings include (1) immediate reduction in wound pain; (2) prevention of dehydration; (3) reduction in protein and electrolyte losses; (4) stimulation of granulation tissue; (5) enhanced epithelialization; (6) decreased scar tissue formation; and (7) a reduced incidence of infection (Diehl and Ersek 1980; Madden and Smith 1970).

SUTURING TECHNIQUES

Suturing techniques as well as the materials selected have an influence on wound healing (Stashak 1978). When simple interrupted sutures were compared with the simple continuous sutures in animal models, the simple interrupted apposed wounds had less edema, an increased microcirculation (assessed by fluorescein dye), and a 30 to 50 per cent greater tensile strength at 10 days postsuturing (Speer 1979). These results support the use of interrupted sutures rather than continuous sutures in situations in which impaired healing is anticipated and excessive tension is present.

POVIDONE IODINE

Povidone iodine is a potent, relatively nonirritating antiseptic agent when applied to intact skin. It is also very popular for use in surgically clean and contaminated skin wounds. Clinical and laboratory studies have shown that contaminated wounds irrigated with povidone iodine have a decreased infection rate (Mulliken, Healey, and Glowaoki 1980). It also appears that povidone iodine does not affect epithelialization, wound contraction, or tensile strength gain in healing wounds (Mulliken, Healey, and Glowaoki 1980). One investigator noted an increased inflammation and stagnation of the microcirculation in povidone iodine–irrigated wounds. However, these adverse effects could be reversed with subsequent irrigation with sterile physiologic saline (Branemark and Ekholm 1967; Mulliken, Healey, and Glowaoki 1980).

Recently, a human prospective study has shown an increased incidence of infection in wounds sprayed with 5 per cent povidone iodine as compared with controls sprayed with saline. When 1 per cent povidone iodine was used and compared with controls, the opposite was true. It was shown that 5 per cent povidone iodine inhibits leukocyte migration ability to ward off infection (Viljanto 1980).

Another human clinical study on burn patients found that 8 out of 58 patients treated with polyvinylpyrolidone-iodine suffered local wound irritations; the treatment was quite painful in children (Schneider et al. 1976). Clinical symptoms of hyperthyroidism were present in three patients, and this was verified by elevated T_3 levels (Schneider et al. 1976).

Amber and associates (1983) reporting on the antimicrobial efficacy and tissue reactions of four antiseptic agents, found that chlorhexidine 0.5 or 1.0 per cent was more effective than benzalkonium chloride, povidone iodine, or pluronic polyol applied to experimentally created wounds on dogs.

CARTILAGE

Cartilage or cartilage extracts, applied directly or implanted adjacent to the wound, have proved to be beneficial in wound healing (Madden 1977; Madden and Smith 1970; Pruddin, Wolarsky, and Balassa 1969). This cartilage can be applied topically, such as pieces of ear cartilage sutured over a wound, it can be made in a powder, or it can be solubilized into a fluid extract and injected adjacent to the wound or produced in pellet form (Swaim 1980). Histological studies suggest that cartilage increases the number of fibroblasts and subsequent formation of collagen during the early phases of wound repair (Madden 1977). However, the exact mechanism for stimulation of healing by implantation of cartilage is unknown at this time.

BETA-AMINOPROPIONITRILE (BAPN) AND PENICILLAMINE

The lathyritic agents BAPN and penicillamine appear in certain situations to be able to control the amount of fibrosis in a healing wound. BAPN's mode of action is to block the covalent crosslinking bond of collagen by irreversibly inhibiting the enzyme lysyl oxidase. This action alters the physical properties of fibrous tissue without altering the rate of collagen synthesis (Jackson 1979). Penicillamine, on the other hand, blocks the next step after lysyl oxidase in collagen crosslinking. Clinically, penicillamine appears to be effective in the treatment of the active phase of scleroderma when collagen biosynthesis is taking place (Jackson 1979). Neither of the agents appears to be effective in modifying scar tissue formation after fibrosis has occurred (Arem, Misiorowski, and Chvapil 1979; Jackson 1979). The effect of these agents has not been adequately evaluated in the horse.

NEOPLASIA

Neoplasia, whether directly associated with the wound or present at some remote site, has a tendency to delay wound healing. The local or adjacent factors responsible for delayed wound healing are a result of tumor cells seeding the remaining incision, whereas the often debilitating systemic effect of neoplasms is thought to be responsible for poor healing in wounds in other sites (Peacock and Van Winkle 1976; Swaim 1980; Turner 1978).

MOVEMENT

Movement of one portion of the wound with respect to the other can disrupt neovascularization, cell migration, and the formation of early stromal elements of the wound (Swaim 1980). This results in prolonged wound healing and promotes excessive scar tissue formation (Swaim 1980). Good suturing techniques, plus the use of appropriate bandaging and splinting techniques, can reduce the detrimental effects of movement.

LOCAL IRRADIATION

High doses of local irradiation, particularly within the first 4 to 48 hours after wounding, not only retard normal wound healing but make the contaminated wound more susceptible to infection (Ariyan et al. 1979; Madden 1977). It is reported that radiation alters wound healing by depressing the formation of normal fibroblasts. It also decreases capillary proliferation, collagen formation, and wound contraction (Russell and Billingham 1962). Because of this deleterious effect, it is recommended that wounds requiring radiation after surgery not be irradiated sooner than five to seven days after the procedure is completed (Schilling 1976). In situations in which the wound is irradiated prior to surgery, it is recommended that surgery be delayed for 30 to 45 days, at which time total excision of the lesion is advised (Schilling 1976).

SEROMA AND HEMATOMA

Collection of blood or serum within the tissue can delay healing by mechanically separating the wound. If the expanding pressure is sufficient, it can also alter the local vascular dynamics enough to reduce the blood supply. In addition, this accumulation of fluid provides an excellent nutrient environment for bacterial growth and also lengthens the debridement phase of wound healing (Swaim 1980). Meticulous hemostasis, elimination of dead space, proper drainage procedures, and appropriate bandaging techniques will reduce the incidence of this problem.

LOCAL ANESTHETICS

Local anesthetics with or without adrenalin have been shown to adversely affect wound healing (Chvapil et al. 1979; Morris and Tracey 1977; Turner 1978). When lidocaine and bupivacaine effects were tested on tissue cultures of newborn rat skin and granulation tissue of rats, a reduction in major structural macromolecules, collagen formation, and glycosaminoglycans was noted (Chvapil et al. 1979). Lignocaine administered intradermally and subcutaneously will also reduce the number of leukocytes sticking to endothelium, which reduces their migration to ward off infection (Morris and Tracey 1977). The incorporation of adrenalin appears to potentiate the detrimental effect of local anesthetics on wound healing because of its vasoconstrictive effect, reducing blood supply to wound edges (Morris and Tracey 1977). It has been recommended that local anesthetics be administered at sites far removed from the wound (Turner 1978). However, from a practical standpoint, the author finds this difficult to recommend unless local regional selective nerve blocks can be easily performed.

NONSTEROIDAL ANTI-INFLAMMATORY DRUGS

Since inflammation plays an important role in wound healing, it is logcal that anti-inflammatory drugs, such as phenylbutazone, aspirin, and indomethacin, have an effect on wound healing. In a study performed on horses, oxyphenbutazone, administered in a loading dose of 12 mg/kg (two days) and a maintenance dose of 6 mg/kg (five days), significantly reduced granulation tissue formation and inflammation in artificially created incisions (Gorman et al. 1968). It is theorized that phenylbutazone acts by decreasing capillary permeability, which, in turn, alters early fluid and cellular responses in the wound healing process. Aspirin and indomethacin appear to act by reducing the effect of prostaglandins (Peacock and Van Winkle 1976; Swaim 1980). However, it should be noted that excessive amounts of these drugs are required to alter wound healing; when they are used in therapeutic doses, no alteration in the quality of wound healing is observed (Swaim 1980). Most clinicians find these drugs useful because they diminish pain from inflammation, improve overall well being, and encourage ambulation, resulting in increased circulation, especially to the distal limbs (Arem, Misiorowski, and Chvapil 1979; Turner 1978).

STEROIDS

Steroids, when given in moderate and large amounts within the first five days after injury, significantly retard the wound healing process (Peacock and Van Winkle 1976; Swaim 1980). However, it is important to note that although wound healing is retarded, it eventually occurs at a much slower rate. It appears that steroids retard healing by stabilizing the lysosomal membranes, which in turn prevent the release of enzymes responsible for initiating the inflammatory response. They are also reported to suppress fibroplasia, ground substance formation, collagen formation, capillary proliferation, and granulation tissue formation. In addition, they retard wound contraction and delay the gain in tensile strength within the wound. Steroids may also retard epithelialization, but not all experimenters agree on this point (Swaim 1980). Steroids are most effective in delaying healing when they are administered before inflammation starts.

TOPICAL INSULIN

Insulin, applied topically to wounds, is reported to increase protein synthesis, cellular multiplication, and fat deposition (Swaim 1980; Turner 1978). It also enhances phagocytosis, increases wound contraction, and reduces tissue edema (Edmonds 1976; Swaim 1980). In a limited study on a lower leg wound in a horse, insulin promoted wound integrity and reduced the inflammatory response (Edmonds 1976). Insulin's positive effect on wound healing was thought to result from its ability to increase the rate of cell multiplication (Edmonds 1976).

VITAMINS

Vitamin A. The anti-inflammatory effects of steroids that occur at the lysosomal level can be counteracted by the topical application or systemic administration of vitamin A (Peacock and Van Winkle 1976; Ehrlich 1968). Vitamin A acts as a lysosomal labilizer, antagonizing the lysosomal stabilizing effect of steroids and vitamin E so that wound healing can progress at a normal rate (Swaim 1980). This antagonism also counteracts the steroid's effect on tensile strength (Swaim 1980). Experimentally induced vitamin A deficiencies cause retardation in epithelialization, wound closure, collagen synthesis, and collagen crosslinking (Peacock and Van Winkle 1976; Swaim 1980). Some recent studies on wounds produced in rats indicate that vitamin A has an accelerating effect on healing skin incisions by enhancing epithelialization and the formation of reparative granulation tissue (Peacock and Van Winkle 1976).

Vitamin K. Vitamin K, being essential for blood clot formation, is an important part of wound healing. A deficiency in vitamin K may result in excessive bleeding, impairment of healing, and increased susceptibility to infection (Peacock and Van Winkle 1976; Swaim 1980).

Vitamin E. Vitamin E, like steroids, has a tendency to stabilize cellular membranes and, in doing so, alters the normal inflammatory process. In high doses, vitamin E may inhibit wound repair (Peacock and Van Winkle 1976; Swaim 1980).

Vitamin C. The observations during the 1600s that scurvy (vitamin C deficiency) caused delayed wound healing set the stage for studies that have defined the clinical and biochemical role of ascorbic acid in wound repair. Vitamin C appears to be necessary for normal epithelialization, blood vessel formation, and the synthesis of collagen.

In reality, vitamin deficiencies are probably not a problem in large animal patients. However, in those situations in which animals are chronically debilitated and undernourished, vitamin supplementation may be considered.

REFERENCES

Amber, E. I., Henderson, R. A., Swaim, S. F., and Gray, B. W.: A comparison of antimicrobiol efficacy and tissue reaction of four antiseptics on canine wounds. J. Vet. Surg., 12:63, 1983.

Arem, A. J., Misiorowski, R., and Chvapil, M.: Effects of low dose BAPN on wound healing. J. Surg. Res. 27:228, 1979.

Ariyan, S., Marfuggi, R. A., Harder, G., and Goodie, M. M.: An experimental model to determine the effects of adjuvant therapy on the incidence of postoperative wound infection: Evaluating preoperative radiation therapy. Plast. Reconstr. Surg. 65:328, 1979.

Beeman, G. M.: A surgical approach to the repair of equine wounds. In Proceedings of the American Association of Equine Practitioners:163, 1972.

Bojrab, M. J.: A Handbook of Veterinary Wound Management. Boston: Kendall Co., 1981.

Branemark, P. I., and Ekholm, R.: Tissue injury caused by wound disinfection. J. Bone Joint Surg. 49A:48, 1967.

Chvapil, M., Hameroff, S. R., O'Dea, K., and Peacock, E. E.: Local anesthetics and wound healing. J. Surg. Res. 27:367, 1979.

Diehl, M., and Ersek, R. A.: Porcine xenografts for treatment of skin defects in horses. JAVMA 177:625, 1980.

Edmonds, T.: Evaluation of topical insulin on wound healing in the distal limb of the horse. Vm/SAC 71:451, 1976.

Ehrlich, H. P., Tarver, H., and Hunt, T. K.: Effects of cortisone and vitamin A on wound healing. Ann. Surg. 167:324, 1968.

Gorman, H.A., Wolff, W. A., Frost, W. W., Lumb, W. V., and Nelson, A. W.: The effect of oxyphenyl butazone on surgical wounds of the horse. JAVMA 152:487, 1968.

Jackson, D. S.: Possible modification of scar tissue by biochemical methods. Equine Vet. J. 11:102, 1979.

Li, A. K. C., Chir, B., Erlich, H. P., Trelstad, R. L., Koroly, M. J., Schattenkerk, M. E., and Malt, R. A.: Differences in healing of skin wounds caused by burn and freeze injuries. Ann. Surg. 191:241, 1980.

Madden, J. W.: Wound healing: Biologic and clinical features. In Davis-Christopher Textbook of Surgery, 11th ed. Sabiston, D. C. (ed.). Philadelphia: W. B. Saunders, 1977.

Madden, J. W., and Smith, H. C.: The rate of collagen synthesis and deposition in dehisced and resutured wounds. Surg. Gynecol. Obstet. 130:417, 1970.

Morris, T., and Tracey, J.: Lignocaine: Its effects on wound healing. Br. J. Surg. 64:902, 1977.

Mulliken, J. B., Healey, N. A., and Glowaoki, J.: Povidone-iodine and tensile strength of wounds in rats. J. Trauma 20:323, 1980.

Niemezura, R. T., and DePalma, R. G.: Optimum compress temperature for wound hemostasis. J. Surg. Res. 26:570, 1979.

Peacock, E. E., and Van Winkle, W.: Wound Repair, 2nd ed. Philadelphia: W. B. Saunders, 1976.

Pruddin, J. F., Wolarsky, E. R., and Balassa, L.: The acceleration of healing. Surg. Gynecol. Obstet. 128:1321, 1969.

Rovee, D. T., Kurowsky, C. A., Labun, J. et al.: Effects of local wound environment on epidermal healing. In Epidermal Wound Healing. Maibach, H. I., and Rovee, D. T. (eds.). Chicago: Year Book Medical Publishers, 1972, p. 159.

Russel, P. S., and Billingham, R. E.: Some aspects of the repair process in mammals. Prog. Surg. 2:1, 1962.

Schilling, J. A.: Wound healing. Surg. Clin. North Am. 56:859, 1976.

Schneider, W., Ahuja, S., and Klebe: Clinical and bacteriological studies of the polyvinyl-pyrrolidone-iodine complex. In Proceedings of the World Congress on Antisepsis: 100, 1976.

Speer, D. P.: The influence of suture techniques on early wound healing. J. Surg. Res. 27:385, 1979.

Stashak, T. S., and Yturraspe, D. J.: Consideration for selection of suture materials. J. Vet. Surg. 7:48, 1978.

Swaim, S. F.: Surgery of Traumatized Skin. Philadelphia: W. B. Saunders, 1980, pp. 100–115.

Turner, A. S.: Local and systemic factors affecting wound healing. In Proceedings of the American Association of Equine Practitioners: 355, 1978.

Viljanto, J.: Disinfection of surgical wounds without inhibition of normal wound healing. Arch. Surg. 115:253, 1980.

SUTURE PATTERNS USED FOR WOUND CLOSURE IN VETERINARY SURGERY

CLASSIFICATION OF SUTURE PATTERNS

Suture patterns can be divided into simple, mattress, tension, and pull-out sutures. A simple suture directly apposes tissue by a single passage through the tissue on each side of the incision, after which it is tied. Mattress sutures appose tissue by two passages of the needle on each side of the incision. Tension sutures are usually mattress sutures that are preplaced well back from the skin edges and tied so that tension is reduced on the primary suture line (Stashak 1977). Pull-out sutures are used in situations in which it is undesirable to bury sutures in deeper tissues. They are placed so that they can be removed after healing. These suture patterns are classified as apposing, everting, or inverting, depending on the position of the wound edges following suture placement (Knecht et al. 1975).

The surgeon may choose to place the sutures in either an interrupted or a continuous pattern. Interrupted sutures are tied and cut after one or two passages in tissue. Continuous sutures, on the other hand, are placed in an uninterrupted manner from their point of origin to some relatively distant end point (Knecht et al. 1975).

SUTURE PLACEMENT

Most surgeons tend to place sutures ritualistically. Few realize that after wound closure the edges become weakened by collagenolysis and suture holding power is impaired (Forrester 1975). Sutures placed more than 0.5 cm from the wound edge apparently are not affected by collagenolysis (Forrester 1975; Pullen 1975). Because inflammation also reduces holding power, it may be wise to place sutures further than 0.5 cm from the edge in severely traumatized wounds (Forrester 1975). Recommendations have also been made concerning the number of sutures required to close a wound (Forrester 1975; Menendez 1968; Price 1948; Swaim 1980). The more sutures used, the less strain on any one individual suture, up to a point (Forrester 1975). It appears that maximal wound-holding strength is obtained with sutures placed 0.5 cm apart (Forrester 1975). When sutures are placed closer than this, they delay healing by causing excessive tissue reaction and by compromising the blood supply to the wound edges (Swaim 1980). A good rule to follow is to place a sufficient number of sutures to provide good coaptation of wound edges. In general, spacing between sutures can be increased in thick-skinned areas and areas in which incisions or lacerations

are parallel to skin tension lines (Swaim 1980).

SELECTION OF SUTURE PATTERNS

The choice of suture pattern is most important. A continuous suture may be the simplest to apply and may provide the most uniform support, but a single break can be disastrous (Forrester 1975; Stashak 1977). Also, because of their helical design, simple continuous sutures have a tendency to reduce the microcirculation to the wound edges. This prolongs the destructive phase of wound healing and increases edema formation (Speer 1979). A more rapid gain in tissue tensile strength is obtained with simple interrupted sutures when compared with simple continuous sutures (Speer 1979). Statistically, simple interrupted sutures are stronger than simple continuous sutures (Larsen and Ulin 1970; Speer 1979). In general, interrupted suture placement is preferred when strength, tissue mobility, and distensibility are required (Forrester 1975; Speer 1979; Stashak 1977).

Interrupted Sutures

SIMPLE INTERRUPTED SUTURE

The simple interrupted suture is the most widely used and perhaps the most versatile of the suture patterns (Stashak 1977). When placed properly, it maintains good wound apposition, acts independently of other sutures in the suture line, and allows tissue mobility between sutures.

Tension on each interrupted suture is inversely proportional to the number of sutures utilized (Stashak 1977). As previously mentioned, there is no tensile strength advantage to placing sutures closer than 0.5 cm apart (Forrester 1975). The technique for placement is easy and rapid (Fig. 12–10A). Sutures are placed by directing the needle through the tissue greater than 0.5 cm lateral to the cut edge (Stashak 1977). The suture is inserted perpendicularly through the tissue on one side, passed through an equal amount of tissue on the opposite side, and tied (Knecht et al. 1975; Swaim

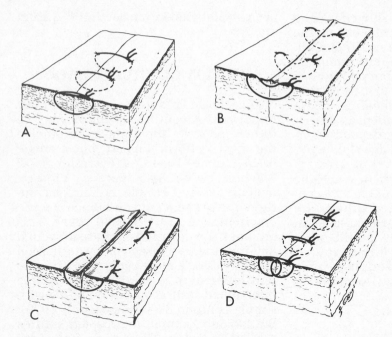

Figure 12–10 *A*, Placement of simple interrupted sutures. *B*, Placement of vertical mattress sutures. *C*, Placement of horizontal mattress sutures. *D*, Placement of far near–near far sutures. (Reprinted with permission from Stashak: JAVMA *170*:144, 1977.)

1980). Knots should be offset so that they do not rest upon the incision (Knecht et al. 1975). Suture ends (ears) are cut short if the suture is to be buried but are left 0.5 to 1.0 cm long when used in the skin. The next simple interrupted suture is placed close enough to prevent gaping of the wound edges (Stashak 1977). Surgeons should take advantage of the field of incision and their own dexterity by placing sutures from right to left in a horizontal incision if right-handed and from left to right if left-handed (Knecht et al. 1975). When suturing a vertical incision, the surgeon usually starts from the most distant end and sutures toward the closest end (Knecht et al. 1975). The simple interrupted suture is an apposing suture, but if excessive tension is applied, it will generally cause undesirable inversion and a dimple-like scar formation after healing. Proper placement of sutures and tying of knots with moderate tension will provide consistently satisfactory results (Knecht et al. 1975).

The advantages of the simple interrupted suture include ability to adjust the tension of each suture independently, a more rapid gain in tissue tensile strength, and decreased tissue edema of the healing wound with simple interrupted sutures when compared with simple continuous patterns (Speer 1979). Interrupted sutures can also be used to de-

crease a small amount of dead space by placing the deep component of the suture into fascia underlying the skin (Speer 1979; Swaim 1980). The disadvantages of interrupted sutures are that more suture materials is used and the overall time involved in tying and cutting is increased when compared with continuous sutures. Also, if buried, the presence of additional amounts of suture material in the tissues in the form of knots causes increased tissue reaction, and the knots may be palpable for some time after surgery (Knecht et al. 1975).

VERTICAL MATTRESS SUTURES

The vertical mattress suture pattern provides precise edge-to-edge apposition with slight eversion of the skin edges when the suture is tied. To achieve this apposition, the first bite is placed more than 0.5 cm from the cut edge and the second bite splits the thickness of the skin (1 mm into the dermis) (Stashak 1977) (Fig. 12–10B). The advantage of a vertical mattress suture is twofold: there is minimal alteration of blood supply, and, if placed well back from the wound edge, the vertical mattress suture can be used as a tension suture in support of the primary suture line (Stashak 1977). Disadvantages include increased time for suture placement and increased inflammation owing to four penetrations with the needle. These sutures should be placed according to tension (Stashak 1977).

HORIZONTAL MATTRESS SUTURE

The horizontal mattress suture, if placed properly, forms a perfect square, with both ends of the suture exiting on the same side of the wound's edge (Swaim 1980) (Fig. 12–10C). Skin penetration is well back from the wound edges, resulting in slight eversion of the edges after the sutures are tied (Stashak 1977). This suture pattern is particularly useful when suturing wounds under moderate tension. The advantages of the horizontal mattress suture are (1) less suture material is used; (2) it can be rapidly applied; (3) it can be used as a tension suture when placed well back from the skin edges; and (4) it can be used to close dead space (Stashak 1977; Swaim 1980). The primary disadvantages of the horizontal mattress suture are the relative difficulty of applying it in skin, excessive scar formation because of skin eversion, and its tendency to reduce the blood supply to skin edges when placed under tension (function of geometric design) (Stashak 1977). If the mattress suture is applied so that it angles through the skin and passes just below the dermis and if the knots are tied just tightly enough for the skin edges to meet, eversion is less likely to occur (Fig. 12–11) (Knecht et al. 1975).

A modified placement of the horizontal mattress suture has proved to be effective in closing the point (apex) of a V-shaped wound (Swaim 1980). To achieve this, the suture that passes through the V point is placed in the dermis instead of exiting through the skin (Fig. 12–

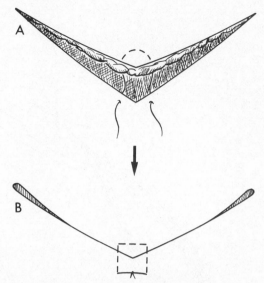

Figure 12–12 *A*, A modified horizontal mattress suture passes through the dermis of the V point and does not exit through the skin. *B*, The suture is tied. (After Swaim: Surgery of Traumatized Skin. Philadelphia, W. B. Saunders, 1980, p. 281.)

12A). The suture is tied on the skin surface opposite the V point (Fig. 12–12B). This pattern has the advantage of providing good apposition of the V point with a reduced incidence of V-tip necrosis seen with other suture patterns (Swaim 1980). This suture pattern has also been referred to as a three-point suture closure (Swaim 1980).

CRUCIATE MATTRESS AND FIGURE-EIGHT MATTRESS SUTURES

In this modification of the mattress suture, the needle is introduced on one side of the incision and is passed perpendicularly across the incision line, after which a second passage is made through the tissues parallel to and 5 to 10 mm from the first passage (Fig. 12–13A). The suture origin on one side is tied to the contralateral end on the other side, forming an X (Knecht et al. 1975; Swaim 1980). The cruciate mattress has an advantage over a horizontal mattress in that it does not reduce the blood supply to the wound edge when tied under tension. Cross mattress sutures also prevent eversion. An alternate method is the figure-eight mattress suture (Fig. 12–13B).

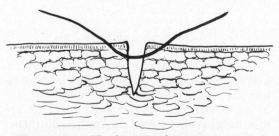

Figure 12–11 The horizontal mattress suture is angled through the skin for better apposition.

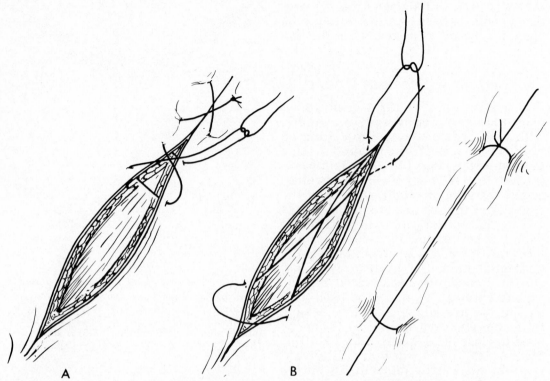

Figure 12–13 *A*, Cruciate mattress suture. *B*, Figure-eight mattress suture.

FAR NEAR–NEAR FAR SUTURE

This suture pattern, referred to as a pulley suture, has been described as a combination tension and apposition suture (Swain 1980). It is advantageous to use this suture pattern when skin margins require mild tension for reapposition (Stashak 1977). The far component takes up the tension while the near component holds skin margins in apposition (see Fig. 12–10D) (Stashak 1977; Swaim 1980). Excessive tightening should be avoided to prevent inversion at the incision line (Speer 1979). The mean tensile strength of this pattern is greater than that achieved with simple interrupted and mattress patterns (Stashak 1977).

BURYING THE KNOT

In certain situations, it is desirable to bury the knot beneath the tissue surface to prevent excessive irritation. Catgut sutures placed in subcutaneous and intradermal tissues are frequently buried; if they are not and if a large knot is formed immediately below or within the skin surface, it may cause excessive pressure and local necrosis of the skin (Knecht et al. 1975). For subcutaneous closure, the knot is buried by introducing the needle deep in the subcutaneous tissues and passing the suture toward the dermis. The exit point of the suture is the incision line beneath the dermis. The suture is then passed across the incision line, introduced in the subcutaneous tissue close to the dermis, incorporating subcutaneous tissues, and recovered deep in the subcutaneous tissue (Fig. 12–14 (Knecht et al. 1975). Burying the knot for intradermal closure is the same, except the sutures pass through the dermis.

Continuous Sutures

Continuous sutures are neither knotted nor cut after each introduction or pair of introductions through the tissue (Knecht et al. 1975). The advantages of continuous sutures are speed of application, the minimal number of knots and suture material required, ease of removal, and

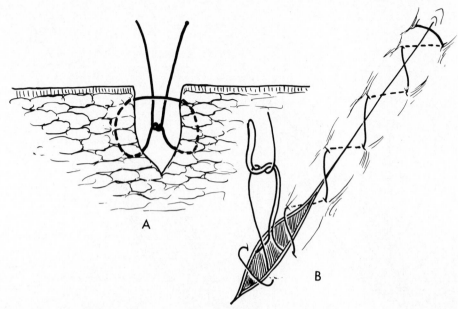

Figure 12–14 *A,* To bury the knot, the suture begins deep in the subcutaneous tissues, exits and re-enters just below the dermis, and exits deep to be tied. *B,* The knot is buried after a running suture placement in the subcutaneous tissue.

more complete tissue apposition. In situations in which simple interrupted sutures may cause a curtaining effect between sutures, a continuous pattern will firmly appose the adjacent tissues and prevent fluid or tissue leakage through the incision line (Knecht et al. 1975). The primary disadvantage of the continuous suture pattern is that knot slippage or suture breakage is likely to cause failure of the entire suture line. Needless to say, particular attention must be paid to the integrity of the suture material used and the knots tied when continuous sutures are used (Knecht et al. 1975). One investigator reported increased wound edema, decreased blood supply, and reduced tensile strength in wounds sutured with continuous sutures compared with those sutured with interrupted sutures (Speer 1979). Continuous suture patterns are felt to be undesirable for wounds that are under tension and that are subjected to increased mobility and distension pressures (Speer 1979; Stashak 1977).

SIMPLE CONTINUOUS SUTURE

The simple continuous suture consists of a series of simple uninterrupted sutures that are only tied at the beginning and end of the pattern (Knecht et al.

1975). The end with the needle is advanced and introduced through the tissue perpendicular to the incision line (Fig. 12–15A). The suture is advanced and reintroduced in the same direction as the previous sutures (Knecht et al. 1975). At the end of the incision line or at a distance not usually exceeding 13 cm, the suture is tied with four single throws (Knecht et al. 1975). A modification of the simple continuous suture is the running suture (Fig. 12–15B). The running suture is a simple continuous suture in which both the deep and superficial portions advance, rather than the deep portion passing perpendicular to the incision line (Knecht et al. 1975). Because of its design, the running stitch allows the surgeon to advance the suture faster than with the simple continuous suture (Knecht et al. 1975).

The simple continuous suture is useful in the closure of subcutaneous tissues and fascia in nontension planes. The knots are usually buried with simple continuous and running sutures (Knecht et al. 1975). It is also quite useful for tissues that require minimal holding strength but maximal tissue apposition (Knecht et al. 1975). For example, when simple continuous sutures are used to close the peritoneal cavity, they tend to create an

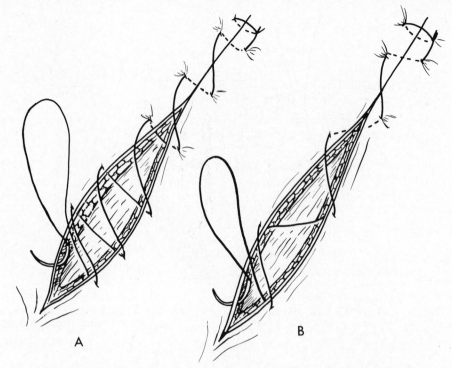

Figure 12–15 *A*, Simple continuous suture. *B*, A continuous running suture.

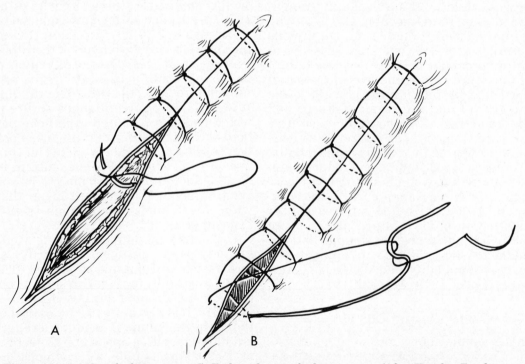

Figure 12–16 *A*, Interlocking suture. *B*, Ending the interlocking suture. (After Knecht: Fundamental Techniques in Veterinary Surgery. Philadelphia: W. B. Saunders, 1975, p. 44.)

air- and liquid-tight seal, which prevents passage of even minimal quantities of peritoneal fluid and/or omentum through the incision line (Knecht et al. 1975).

INTERLOCKING SUTURE

The interlocking suture is a modification of the simple continuous suture. The pattern is continuous, but each passage through the tissue is linked to the previously placed passage of the suture (Fig. 12–16) (Knecht et al. 1975). The advantage of the lock stitch is its greater stability in the event of partial failure of a knot or of a portion of the suture line. When failure occurs, it does not necessarily result in failure of the entire line (Knecht et al. 1975). In addition, a greater degree of tissue stability is achieved because sutured tissues have less tendency to slide (Knecht et al. 1975). The major disadvantages of the interlocking sutures are that a large amount of suture material is used, it is time-consuming to apply, and, if placed in the skin under tension, it frequently becomes buried in the skin, a result of pressure necrosis (Knecht et al. 1975).

CONTINUOUS HORIZONTAL MATTRESS SUTURE

The continuous horizontal mattress suture can be used for skin closure when a continuous suture is indicated and a degree of eversion is not objectionable (Knecht et al. 1975; Stashak 1977).

The suture pattern is begun with a simple interrupted suture; this suture is then tied, and the short end is cut (Knecht et al. 1975). The suture is advanced approximately 1 to 2 cm, and a second pass is made through the tissue perpendicular to the incision. Upon exiting from the tissue, the needle is advanced 1 to 2 cm and is reinserted perpendicular to the incision line in the opposite direction (Fig. 12–17A) (Knecht et al. 1975). Rapid closure is the major advantage to this pattern. An alternative to this is the continuous vertical mattress

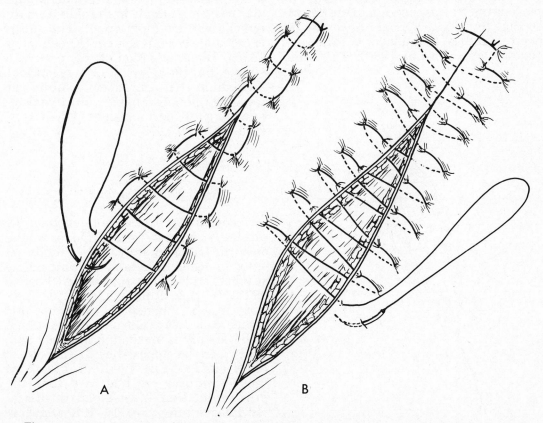

Figure 12–17 *A,* Continuous horizontal mattress suture. *B,* Continuous vertical mattress suture.

suture (Fig. 12–17B). Because of its geometric design, it causes minimal alteration in the blood supply. Its main disadvantage is that it takes longer to apply.

INTRADERMAL SUTURES

Intradermal sutures have often been incorrectly referred to as subcuticular sutures (Swaim 1980). However, as the names imply, intradermal sutures are placed in the dermis, whereas subcuticular sutures are placed under the dermis in the subcutaneous tissue.

Intradermal sutures are most frequently used in a continuous rather than an interrupted pattern (Knecht et al. 1975). Suturing is begun by passing the suture loop through the dermal tissues and tying the knot in a buried fashion in the subcutaneous tissue. The suture pattern is usually placed in a modified horizontal mattress design, with the needle crossing perpendicular to the incision but advancing in the dermis parallel to the incision (Knecht et al. 1973) (Fig. 12–18).

Ideally, intradermal sutures should be placed superficially enough in the dermis so that the skin edges are apposed, yet deep enough so that a layer of epidermis covers them (Swaim 1980). This mattress pattern is continued to the other end of the incision, and a knot is buried at the opposite end. Fine catgut or synthetic absorbable material is most frequently used when the suture is to be buried. Even though the skin edges appear well apposed after intradermal suturing, it is advisable to place a few fine skin sutures to help support the incision line (Swaim 1980). These support sutures are usually removed in about three to four days.

Intradermal closure can be attained with nonabsorbable suture material; however, an additional step is required to ensure the removal of the suture material. To start the pattern, a small simple interrupted suture is begun at one end of the incision, and the short end of the suture material is cut. The suture is inserted through the skin into the incision and applied in a modified continuous horizontal mattress pattern in the dermis as previously described. The passages of suture between bites in the dermis should be perpendicular (Knecht et al. 1975). At the end, the intradermal suture exits through the skin and another perpendicular passage is made in the skin from the outside surface (epidermis). The suture is tied and the ends are cut (Knecht et al. 1975). The application of this pattern is simple, but the removal may be difficult and painful. The intradermal suture pattern with nonabsorbable suture appears adequate for short incisions (2.5 to 5 cm) (Knecht et al. 1975).

Tension Sutures

Occasionally, excessive tension on the primary suture line is required for wound closure. Unfortunately, this usually results in local ischemia, cutting out of stitches, and wound disruption (Stashak 1977). In such situations, the use of tension sutures is beneficial. They are preplaced well away from skin edges so that blood supply is not compromised. Skin edges can be apposed with the aid of towel clamps (Fig. 12–19A). Preplaced tension sutures are tied, and then the primary incision line is apposed with interrupted sutures (Fig. 12–19B) (Stashak 1977).

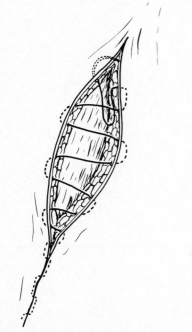

Figure 12–18 Continuous intradermal suture.

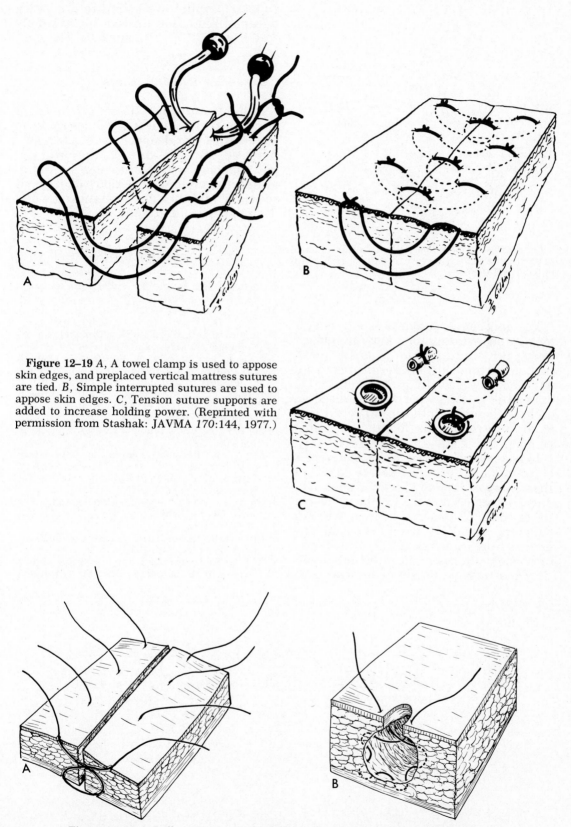

Figure 12–19 *A*, A towel clamp is used to appose skin edges, and preplaced vertical mattress sutures are tied. *B*, Simple interrupted sutures are used to appose skin edges. *C*, Tension suture supports are added to increase holding power. (Reprinted with permission from Stashak: JAVMA *170*:144, 1977.)

Figure 12–20 *A*, Pull-out suture. *B*, Modified pull-out suture to eliminate dead space.

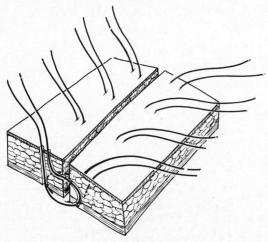

Figure 12–21 A modified pull-out suture is used to appose the underlying fascia. Skin sutures have to be placed to appose skin edges.

The addition of supports, such as buttons, rubber tubing, or gauze preplaced under the suture before it is tied, will reduce the tendency of the sutures to cut out. This method is frequently referred to as a quill pattern and is best used in areas with good soft tissue support (neck, trunk) where pressure bandages cannot be applied (Fig. 12–19C) (Stashak 1977). If bandages are applied, areas of necrosis corresponding to the surface area of these supports usually occur. Under bandages, it is preferable to place two or three rows of tension sutures without supports, to relieve the tension on any given suture (Stashak 1977). Application of tension sutures in an interrupted vertical mattress pattern will provide good support parallel to the suture line, with minimal reduction in local blood supply (see Fig. 12–19B) (Stashak 1977).

Pull-Out Sutures

Pull-out suture patterns are used in situations in which it is undesirable to bury sutures in deeper tissue. Their primary advantages are that they will appose deeper tissues, they can be maintained for prolonged periods of time, if required, and they can be removed when desired (Figs. 12–20 and 12–21).

REFERENCES

Forrester, J. C.: Suture Materials and their uses. Nurs. Mirror *140*:48, 1975.

Knecht, C. D., Welser, J. R., Allen, A. R., Williams, D. J., and Harris, N. N.: Fundamental Techniques in Veterinary Surgery. Philadelphia: W. B. Saunders, 1975, pp. 38–47.

Larsen, J. S., and Ulin, A. W.: Tensile strength advantage of the far-and-near suture technique. Surg. Gynecol. Obstet. *131*:123, 1970.

Menendez, C. V.: A technique of minor surgery: 125 consecutive cases without infection. Surgery *63*:890, 1968.

Price, P. B.: Stress, strain and sutures. Ann. Surg. *128*:408, 1948.

Pullen, C. M.: Reconstruction of the skin. *In* Current Techniques in Small Animal Surgery. Bojrab, M. J. (ed.). Philadelphia: Lea & Febiger, 1975, pp. 278–282.

Speer, D. P.: The influence of suture techniques on early wound healing. J. Surg. Res. *27*:385, 1979.

Stashak, T. S.: Reconstructive surgery in the horse. J.A.V.M.A. *170*:143, 1977.

Swaim, S. F.: Surgery of Traumatized Skin. Philadelphia: W. B. Saunders, 1980, pp. 165–168.

MOBILIZATION OF ADJACENT SKIN TO COVER FULL SURFACE DEFECTS

In situations in which skin defects cannot be closed by suturing techniques alone, mobilization of adjacent tissues should be considered (Stashak 1977; 1978). Fusiform defects usually require only local undermining of the adjacent skin to cover a full surface skin defect (Stashak 1977; 1978; Swaim 1980). Large rectangular, square, triangular, and circular defects more typically require a combination of strategically placed incisions and local undermining to form skin flaps capable of covering the wound (Stashak 1977; 1978; Swaim 1980). Additional skin tension relief can be obtained with a V-Y advancement flap or Z-plasty (Stashak 1977; 1978; Swaim 1980). A combination of skin mobilizations, tension relief, debulking procedures, and W-plasty is sometimes required for cosmetic reconstruction of large scars (Kirk 1976b; Stashak 1977; 1978). When indicated, mobilization of adjacent tissue is superior to skin grafts because it provides more reliable healing and better cosmetic and functional results (Cramer and Chase 1974).

GENERAL PRINCIPLES

Mobilization of adjacent tissue to cover full surface defects must be a series of planned events (Stashak 1977; 1978; Swaim 1980). Lines of skin tension are determined at rest and during dynamic movement of the affected part by puckering the skin adjacent to the defect with the thumb and forefinger. If performed in a systematic manner, this technique will define the area of available skin for skin mobilization or flap formation (Stashak 1977; 1978). A skin flap to cover the defect is selected based on available skin and the defect's configuration. A sterile ruler and a marking pen* or sterile methylene blue applied with sterile toothpicks is used to draw the pattern on the skin (Stashak 1977; 1978; Swaim 1980).

After making the appropriate skin incisions, the skin is mobilized. Flaps are created by separating tissues in their natural cleavage plane deep within the subcutaneous tissue (Fig. 12–22). Care must be taken to maintain available blood supply to the undermined skin (Stashak 1977; 1978). After sufficient undermining has taken place, tension is tested. If more undermining is needed, it should be performed at this time. A rubber drain† is placed under the flap and brought out through a stab incision ventral to the surgical site (Stashak 1977; 1978). If required, tension sutures are placed in strategic locations to reduce tension on the primary incision line, after which the skin is apposed with interrupted nonabsorbable sutures.

The choice of physical restraints (e.g., bandage, cast) is dictated by lesion location and the amount of primary suture-line tension. Stent bandages (tie-over bandages) are useful in areas not amenable to routine bandage or cast application (Fig. 12–23) (Stashak 1977; 1978). They protect the wound from external contamination, and, if secured tightly with sutures, they reduce the tension on the primary suture line and provide uniform pressure to the surgical site. Drains

---

*Skin Skribe, Hospital Marketing Services Co., Inc., Fairfield, CT.

†Penrose Drains, Davol, Inc., Providence, RI.

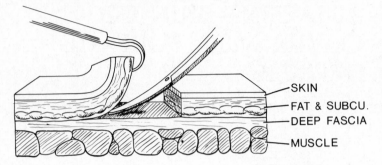

Figure 12–22 Mobilization of a skin flap by separating the subcutaneous tissue from deep fascia to maintain a good blood supply. (After Swaim: Surgery of Traumatized Skin. Philadelphia: W. B. Saunders, 1980, p. 242.)

Figure 12–23 *A,* Split thickness graft is covered by a sterile petroleum gauze. *B,* Preplacing the tie-over sutures. *C,* Cotton pack and gauze is placed over nonadherent dressing. *D,* Tie-over sutures are tied in an X pattern. (From Swaim: Surgery of Traumatized Skin. Philadelphia: W. B. Saunders, 1980, p. 420.)

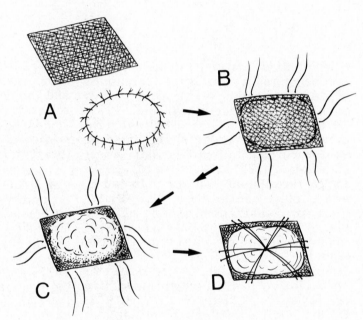

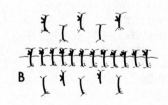

Figure 12–24 *A,* After fusiform excision, skin tension is reduced by undermining adjacent skin (dotted line). *B,* Tension suture closure. (Reprinted with permission from Stashak: JAVMA *170*:144, 1977.)

Figure 12–25 *A,* Top (correct). Incision ends are tapered. *B,* Top (correct). Skin closure without dog ears. *C,* Bottom (incorrect). Incision ends are blunted. *D,* Bottom (incorrect). Skin closure with dog ears. (Reprinted with permission from Stashak: JAVMA *170*:144, 1977.)

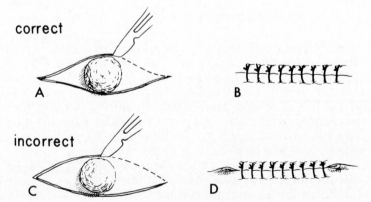

Figure 12–26 *A*, Excess skin is held to one side and the original incision is continued. *B*, The flap is held up and its base excised to remove excess skin. *C*, Closure with simple interrupted sutures. (Reprinted with permission from Stashak: JAVMA *170*: 144, 1977.)

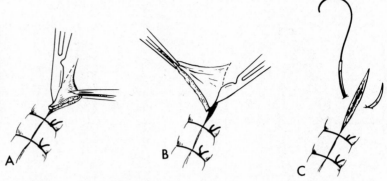

can be removed in two to three days unless drainage is still continuing, in which case they are left until drainage ceases. Casts are usually removed in from 14 to 21 days. The decision of when to remove a cast is dependent upon the amount of skin mobilization and the suture tension required to close the defect (Stashak 1977; 1978). Compress bandages are maintained from four to six weeks for the best cosmetic results. Tension sutures placed under a cast are removed at the time of cast removal; those under bandages are removed in from 4 to 10 days, depending on skin tension.

Elongated Defects. Elongated defects are best removed with a fusiform (elliptical) excision (Fig. 12–24) (Stashak 1977; 1978). The term fusiform is more correct, since the incision ends are tapered, whereas a true ellipse is oval (Swaim 1980). The correct axis for removal is determined by lesion position and tension lines. It is important to premark reference points before the incisions are made. Failure to do so may lead to excessive tissue removal and lack of mirror imagery and may result in difficult or unsightly closure (Stashak 1977; 1978). In some instances closure may require tension-suture support or tension-relieving procedures (see Fig. 12–24B). "Dog ears" frequently accompany skin closure after fusiform excision (Buntine 1969). They can be prevented, in part, by tapering rather than blunting the incision ends (Buntine 1969) (Fig. 12–25). When they do occur, however, they can be removed as shown in Figure 12–26 (Buntine 1969). Alternate methods for closure of fusiform defects are also illustrated (Figs. 12–27, 12–28, and 12–29) (Pick 1950).

Square Defects. Sliding "H" flaps are used for repair of square or rectangular defects (Stashak 1977; 1978; Swaim

Figure 12–27 Alternate method of suture closure of a fusiform defect.

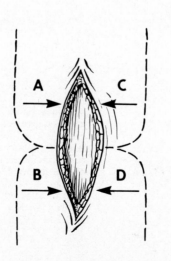

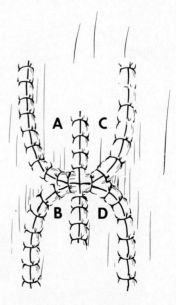

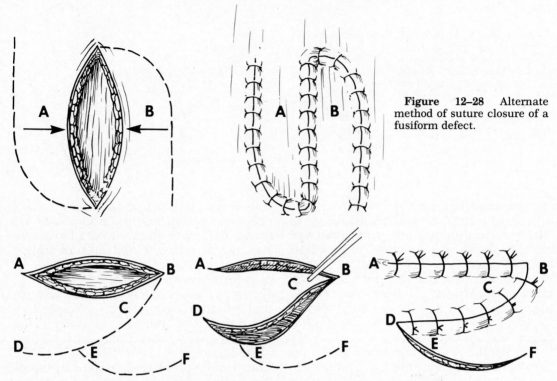

Figure 12–28 Alternate method of suture closure of a fusiform defect.

Figure 12–29 Alternate method of suture closure of a fusiform defect.

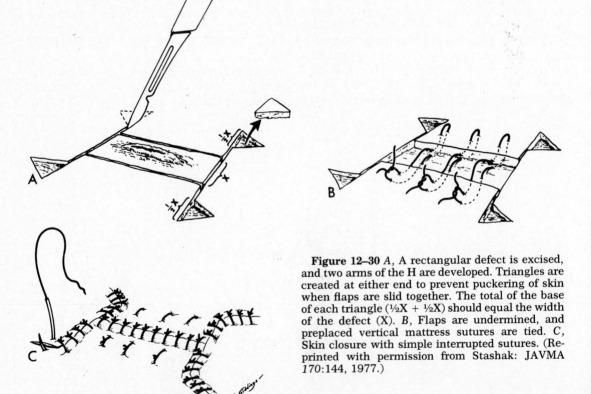

Figure 12–30 *A,* A rectangular defect is excised, and two arms of the H are developed. Triangles are created at either end to prevent puckering of skin when flaps are slid together. The total of the base of each triangle ($\frac{1}{2}$X + $\frac{1}{2}$X) should equal the width of the defect (X). *B,* Flaps are undermined, and preplaced vertical mattress sutures are tied. *C,* Skin closure with simple interrupted sutures. (Reprinted with permission from Stashak: JAVMA *170*:144, 1977.)

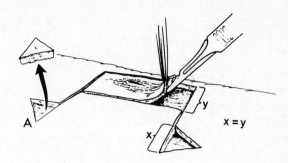

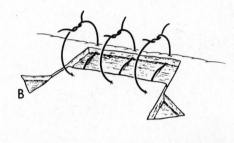

Figure 12–31 A, The width (Y) of the lesion is removed, and triangles with an (X) are made and removed. B, Skin flap is undermined, and simple interrupted sutures are placed. C, Closure with simple interrupted sutures. (Reprinted with permission from Stashak: JAVMA 170:144, 1977.)

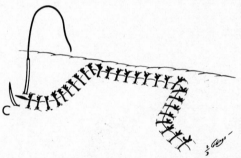

1980) (Fig. 12–30). Normally, two flaps are created; however, if skin is available on only three sides of a defect, half of the H-plasty is used (Fig. 12–31) (Pick 1950).

Triangular Defects. Adjacent tissue is used to cover triangular defects (Fig. 12–32). If there is excess tension, one or two inverted triangles are made, two to three triangle widths away from the lesion. Flaps are undermined, rotated into posi-

tion, and sutured (Figs. 12–33 and 12–34) (Stashak 1977; 1978; Swaim 1980). The decision to create one or two flaps is dictated by tension and available skin (Stashak 1977; 1978). In most cases, two inverted triangles, each with a base one-half the width of the original defect, relieves more tension than one large inverted triangle (Stashak 1977; 1978).

Circular Wounds. Rotation flaps or interpolated pedicle flaps can be used to

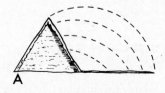

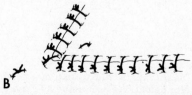

Figure 12–32 A, Triangular defect has been removed and an incision the length of which equals the base of the triangle is made. Dotted lines represent local undermining of skin to form a flap. B, Skin flap is slid into place and sutured. (Reprinted with permission from Stashak: JAVMA 170:144, 1977.)

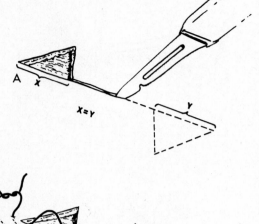

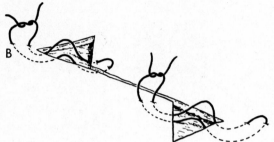

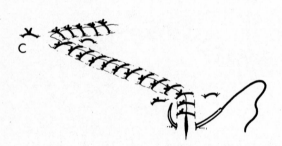

Figure 12–33 Diagrammatic illustration of a method for repair of triangular defects requiring moderate tension relief. *A*, Triangular defect has been removed and one inverted triangle of equal size is made two or three triangle widths away. *B*, Tissues are undermined, and vertical mattress tension sutures are placed. *C*, Tissues are slid into positions and secured with interrupted sutures. (Reprinted with permission from Stashak: JAVMA *170*:144, 1977.)

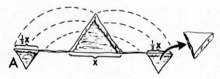

Figure 12–34 Diagrammatic illustration of a method for repair of triangular defects in tight-skinned areas. *A*, Triangular defect has been removed, and two inverted triangles are created one-half a triangle width away from the original defect. The total of the base of each inverted triangle (½X + ½X) should equal the width of the defect (X). Dotted lines represent undermining of the skin. (Reprinted with permission from Stashak: JAVMA *170*:144, 1977.)

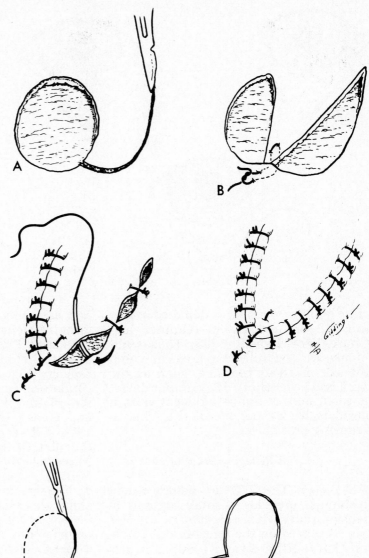

Figure 12–35 Diagrammatic illustration of rotation flaps used for repair of circular wounds in areas of loose skin. *A*, A skin incision is extended from the wound, and a flap is created by undermining. *B*, The flap bisects the circular defect and is held in place by a vertical mattress tension suture. *C*, Simple interrupted sutures are used for closure. *D*, Closure is complete. (Reprinted with permission from Stashak: JAVMA *170*:144, 1977.)

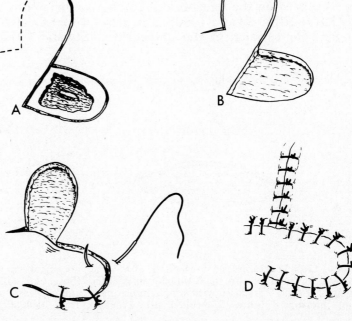

Figure 12–36 Diagrammatic illustration of interpolation flaps used for circular wound repair. *A*, The skin surrounding the defect is incised and the outline of a flap of equal size is drawn (dotted line) and incised. *B*, The defect is removed, and a flap is created. *C*, The flap is rotated into the site of the excised defect. *D*, Closure with simple interrupted sutures. (Reprinted with permission from Stashak: JAVMA *170*:144, 1977.)

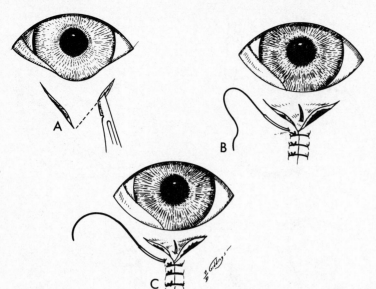

Figure 12–37 Diagrammatic illustration of the V-Y flap advancement technique used for scar revision of the palpebrum. *A,* Wound contracture and scar tissue formation resulted in a defect of the ventral palpebrum. A V incision is created just ventral to the defect, with the apex of the V on the tension axis. *B,* The V has been undermined and advanced toward the palpebrum. The apex of the V is closed with simple interrupted sutures to create a Y. *C,* Simple interrupted sutures are used to close the Y defect. (Reprinted with permission from Stashak: JAVMA *170*:144, 1977.)

close circular wounds, as depicted in Figures 12–35 and 12–36 (Cramer and Chase, 1974; Twaddle 1969). These techniques are best utilized in areas in which the skin is freely movable, such as the neck and lower trunk. If a circular defect is in an area of tightly adjacent skin, it is advisable to use one of the tension-relieving procedures.

Tension-Relieving Procedures

V-Y Flap. The V-Y flap advancement technique provides a small amount of tension relief when the apex of the V-Y flap is placed on the tension axis (Stashak 1977; 1978; Swaim 1980). It is useful for scar revision of the palpebrum

and as a relaxation procedure for fusiform incisions (Figs. 12–37 and 12–38).

Z-Plasty. Probably the most commonly used technique for tension relief is the Z-plasty (Fig. 12–39). Interchanging two equilateral triangular flaps will lengthen the original line by 50 per cent (Cramer and Chase 1974; Furnas and Fischer 1971). This is easily understood by noting that length (a–b) is exchanged for the transverse diagnosis (TD) (see Fig. 12–39B). This principle is used for excision of linear scars requiring tension relief along their longitudinal axis. It is also beneficial for relief of excessive tension associated with lesions requiring fusiform excision (Fig. 12–40) (Kirk 1976a; Stashak 1977; 1978).

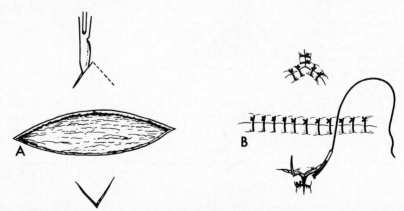

Figure 12–38 Diagrammatic illustrations of a V-Y advancement flap used for tension relief of elliptical incisions. *A,* V incisions are made on both sides of the ellipse. Skin flaps are created by undermining. *B,* The apex of each V is closed with simple interrupted sutures to form a Y, and the defect is closed with simple interrupted sutures. (Reprinted with permission from Stashak: JAVMA *170*:144, 1977.)

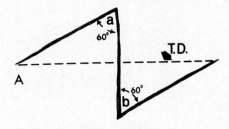

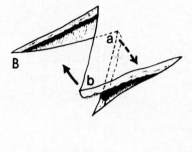

Figure 12–39 Diagrammatic illustration of Z-plasty used for excision of linear scars. A, The vertical line (a–b) represents excision of a linear scar. Two equilateral triangles are created by making incisions beginning at a 60-degree angle from the line (a–b) and extending to the ends of the horizontal transverse diagonal line (TD). Skin flaps are created by undermining the equilateral triangles. B, These flaps are interchanged. C, Line a–b is horizontal and line TD is vertical. This interchanging provides a 50 per cent gain in vertical length. Closure is performed with simple interrupted sutures. (Reprinted with permission from Stashak: JAVMA 170:144, 1977.)

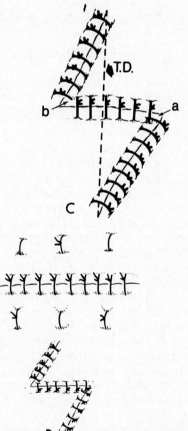

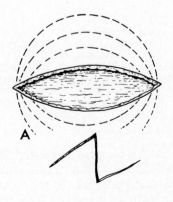

Figure 12–40 Diagrammatic illustration of Z-plasty used for relief tension associated with fusiform excisions. A, The fusiform excision is complete, and adjacent tissues are undermined (dotted lines). Z-plasty is created, with the vertical length placed perpendicular to the fusiform defect and parallel to the lines of tension. Skin flaps are created by undermining the equilateral triangles. Flaps are rotated. B, The excision is closed with vertical mattress tension sutures and simple interrupted sutures. Z-plasty is closed with simple interrupted sutures. (Reprinted with permission from Stashak: JAVMA 170:144, 1977.)

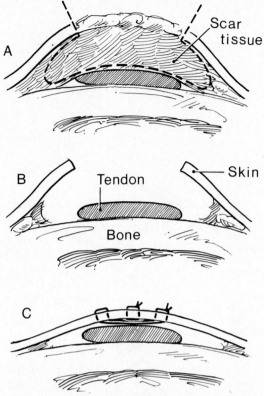

Figure 12–41 *A*, Dotted lines represent incisions made to remove granulation tissue or scar tissue. *B*, The abnormal tissue is removed down to normal tissue. *C*, Suture closure using vertical mattress suture to reduce tension.

Debulking

Tissue debulking can be helpful for cosmetic reconstructive surgery of mature wounds with excessive scar tissue formation or for exuberant granulating wounds in which delayed primary closure is being considered. It is also used in conjunction with tissue mobilization or tension-relieving and suturing techniques to aid in wound closure. The technique is illustrated in Figure 12–41.

Incisions for removal of unwanted tissue are extended slightly beyond the limits of the lesion (see Fig. 12–41A). This allows the surgeon to identify normal tissue planes for dissection and removal of this tissue. In situations in which small lesions are encountered, the entire lesion can be excised. On the other hand, larger raised lesions may require tissue debulking in conjunction with local undermining and skin flap formation (see Fig. 12–41).

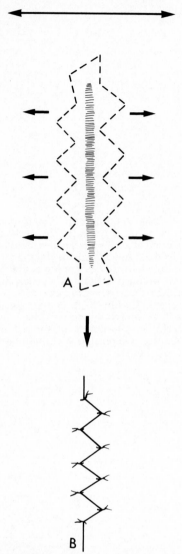

Figure 12–42 *A*, Arrows represent lines of tension. A scar tends to widen when it is oriented perpendicular to lines of tension. Dotted lines represent incision for W-plasty. *B*, Scar revision by W-plasty orients incision along lines of tension and reduces the tendency for the scar to widen. (After Swaim: Surgery of Traumatized Skin. Philadelphia: W. B. Saunders, 1980, p. 420.)

W-Plasty. The W-plasty technique was developed to overcome some of the disadvantages of Z-plasty in revising straight and curved hypertrophied scars (Kirk 1976a; Swaim 1980). These scars become converted into a zigzag pattern of interdigitating triangles that imparts an accordion-like elasticity to the incision and postoperative scar (Fig. 12–42A). The ideal scar for consideration of W-plasty is a linear scar, neither de-

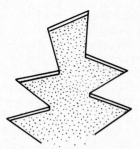

Figure 12–43 Incorporation of Ammon's triangle at either end of the W-plasty allows for smooth closure without dog ears. (After Swaim: Surgery of Traumatized Skin. Philadelphia, W. B. Saunders, 1980, p. 420.)

pressed nor raised, that crosses rather than follows lines of skin tension (Kirk 1976b; Swaim 1980). The triangular flaps are angled at 50 to 55° and are strategically placed so that they perfectly interdigitate when apposed with sutures (Fig. 12–42B). The number of Ws needed is dependent on the length of the scar. Incorporation of Ammon's triangle at either end of the running W-plasty allows for closure without formation of dog ears (Kirk 1976b; Swaim 1980) (Fig. 12–43).

REFERENCES

Buntine, J. A.: "Elliptical" excision and suture. Med. J. Aust. 2:449, 1969.

Cramer, L. M., and Chase, R. A.: Plastic and reconstructive surgery. In Principles of Surgery, 2nd ed. Schwartz, R. C., Lellehei, R. C., Shires, G. T., Spencer, F. C., and Storic, E. H. (eds.). New York: McGraw-Hill, 1974.

Furnas, D. W., and Fischer, G. W.: The Z-plasty: Biomechanics and mathematics. Br. J. Plast. Surg. 24:141, 1971.

Kirk, M. D.: Selective scar revision and elective incision techniques applicable to the legs of horses. VM/SAC 71:661, 1976a.

Kirk, M. D.: Selective scar revision and elective incision techniques applicable to the legs of horses. Part 2. VM/SAC 71:801, 1976b.

Pick, J. F.: Surgery of Repair: Principles, Problems, Procedures. Philadelphia: J. B. Lippincott, 1950.

Stashak, T. S.: Reconstructive surgery in the horse. JAVMA 170:143, 1977.

Stashak, T. S.: Full thickness sliding skin flaps for reconstructive surgery in the horse. Proceedings of the American Association of Equine Practitioners:396, 1978.

Swaim, S. F.: Moving local tissues to close surface defects. In Surgery of Traumatized Skin. Philadelphia: W. B. Saunders, 1980, pp. 297–320.

Twaddle, A. A.: Clinical communications, rotation flap skin graft. N.Z. Vet. J. 17:178, 1969.

FREE SKIN GRAFTING IN THE HORSE

Free skin grafting should be considered in situations in which full thickness skin defects exceed the capabilities of epithelialization, wound contraction, conventional suturing techniques, and sliding flaps to cover them. Large full thickness skin defects, located below the carpus and hock joint in the horse, frequently fall into this category (Boyd 1967). If these wounds go untreated, they usually heal unsatisfactorily, with formation of exuberant granulation tissue and/or a dense keloid (Boyd 1967). In addition to having the capabilities of covering the wound, skin grafts markedly reduce the time required to bring about a satisfactory result (MacKay-Smith and Marks 1968; Meagher and Adams 1970; 1971; Swaim 1980).

The purpose of this section is to review classification of grafts, describe the technique for graft bed preparation, and review types and techniques for free skin grafting that have been reported in the horse.

CLASSIFICATION OF SKIN GRAFTS

Skin grafts are conventionally classified according to donor-recipient relationship and thickness (Boyd and Hanselka 1971; Swaim 1980). An autograft (autogenous graft) is a transplant in which the donor and recipient are the same animal. An allograft (homograft) is a transplant between different individuals within the same species. A xenograft (heterograft) is a transplant between different species. Clinically, autografts are superior to other grafts because the donor and recipient are identical antigenically (Boyd 1967; Swaim 1980). Immunogenic rejection is a problem with the other grafting techniques.

When grafts are classified according to their thickness, they can be either split or full thickness grafts. As the name implies, split thickness grafts are created by splitting a full thickness of skin into various cleavage planes within the dermis (Swaim 1980). The depth of this cleavage plane determines whether the graft is considered a thin, intermediate, or thick split thickness graft (Obel 1951). Full thickness grafts are composed of all elements of the epidermis and dermis, exclusive of the attached subcutaneous tissue and fascia (Fig. 12–44) (Boyd 1967).

Because thicker grafts contain more glands and hair follicles, a better cosmetic, physiological, and functional end result is expected. Unfortunately, the thicker the graft, the more difficult it is to have it take (Swaim 1980).

GRAFT BEDS

Graft survival, referred to as graft take, is the establishment of adequate arterial and venous connections between the graft and the recipient bed (Swaim 1980). Grafts most frequently take when they are placed on healthy, noninfected, convexly shaped, immobile granulation tissue or on fresh wound surfaces that

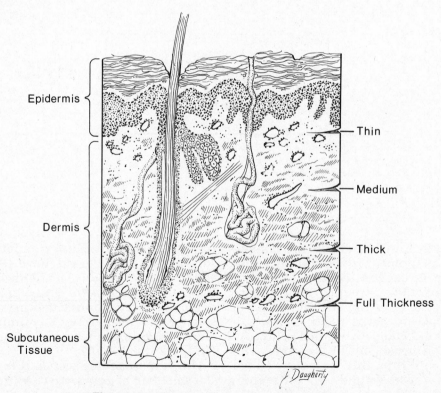

Figure 12–44 Various thicknesses of skin grafts.

have sufficient vascular supply to support them (Swaim 1980). Grafts will not take when placed on avascular sites such as stratified epithelial surfaces; denuded bone without its periosteum; bared tendons without their paratendon or sheath; or cartilage surfaces without a perichondrium. In certain situations, small avascular areas less than 1 cm in diameter or width may be bridged by adjacent vessels from healthy granulation tissue, thus allowing the graft to survive (Swaim 1980). Other poor recipient beds for grafts include fat, heavily irradiated tissue, old granulation tissue, irregular granulation tissue surfaces, and surfaces with chronic ulceration (Swaim 1980). The most common reasons for graft failure are infection, hematoma and seroma under the graft, and movement of the graft independent of the recipient bed (Boyd 1967; Meagher and Adams 1971; Swaim 1980).

Graft Bed Preparation

An absolute prerequisite for successful skin grafting of a contaminated wound is the preparation and formation of a healthy granulating bed that is free of infection. This is particularly important for full or split thickness sheet grafts and is less important for pinch and punch graft techniques. To achieve this goal, the wound edges should be widely clipped and shaved, followed by a thorough scrubbing with an antiseptic soap and a rinsing with physiological saline. In situations in which excessive granulation tissue is present, the wound is excised with a scalpel blade to just below the skin level, after which a sterile nonadherent dressing* and pressure bandage are applied (Meagher and Adams, 1970; 1971). The following day, the bandage is removed, and samples for culture and sensitivity are taken. Any coagulated blood is removed with sterile gauze soaked in physiological saline. An appropriate broad spectrum antibacterial or antiseptic ointment is selected and applied. A sterile bandage is then reapplied. Systemic antibiotics are indicated for all

---

*Non-Adherent Dressing, #1404, Minnesota Mining and Manufacturing Co., St. Paul, MN.

infected wounds. The wounds are treated in this manner, on a daily or alternate-day basis, until a smooth, pink, granulating bed that extends slightly above the skin surface is observed (Meagher and Adams 1971). This process takes a variable period of time and is obviously dependent upon the condition of the wound. In those cases in which depressions are present in the granulation tissue, several granulation tissue excisions may be required before depressions fill in (Meagher and Adams 1971). Lesions that are severely contaminated with large necrotic foci may require the addition of proteolytic enzymes to the antibacterial ointment or antiseptic agent selected, and systemic antibiotics may be required (Meagher and Adams 1971).

When a smooth bed of pink granulation tissue that protrudes slightly above the skin edge is present, final preparation for skin transplantation is begun. This involves reclipping, shaving, antiseptic scrubbing, and sterile bandaging of the wound. The following day, this wound should be ready for grafting.

Since infection developing under the graft signifies graft failure, some authors have recommended the use of quantitative bacterial analysis as a prognostic index (Bacchetta et al. 1975; Swaim 1980). This recommendation has developed as a result of some experimental studies that have correlated grafting success with bacterial quantification in the wound (Bacchetta et al. 1975). In cases in which bacterial counts were above 10^5 organisms per gram of tissue, less than a 20 per cent graft survival rate was expected, whereas wounds with less than 10^5 organisms per gram of tissue had a 94 per cent graft survival rate (Bacchetta et al. 1975). An alarming side light is that all wounds, no matter what their bacterial counts were, appeared clinically ready for grafting (Bacchetta et al. 1975). For more information regarding the techniques for quantitative bacterial analysis, the reader is referred to the works of Bacchetta and coworkers (1975) and Swaim (1980).

When noncontaminated incised wounds or freshly created, minimally contaminated traumatic wounds are encountered, they can be grafted immediately with full thickness or split thickness grafts (Meagher and Adams 1970; 1971). Strict asepsis and good hemostasis are required in both situations. Additionally, thorough debridement is required for the minimally contaminated traumatized wound.

SELECTION OF DONOR SITE

Since one of the objectives of skin grafting is to arrive at a cosmetically acceptable end result, the selection of the donor site warrants some comment. If possible, a donor site with similarly colored hair and a unidirectional hair pattern of the same texture as the recipient site is selected (Swaim 1980). In most instances, the ventral abdomen, lateral shoulder, and thigh area are used for selection of split thickness grafts, whereas the cranial pectoral area, lateral neck, or posterior thigh is selected for full thickness grafts (Boyd 1967; Hanselka 1974). The technique for obtaining these grafts will be covered in the discussion of specific types of grafting.

PHASES OF GRAFT ACCEPTANCE

The growth of the successful graft may be divided into three phases: the adherence phase; the phase of revascularization; and the phase of organic union (Boyd and Hanselka 1971; Swaim 1980). During the adherence phase, the graft is held in position by fibrin formed from the coagulation of plasma and is nourished by a to-and-fro exchange of fluids between the transplant tissue and the graft bed (Boyd and Hanselka 1971; Swaim 1980).

The second phase, revascularization, begins from about 24 to 48 hours postoperatively and is initiated by the formation of anastomotic vessels within the graft. Small vessels within the granulating bed are stimulated to grow toward the graft while preexisting vessels within the graft actively proliferate to help establish this host and graft interconnection. The development of a good anastomotic union is usually complete by about the tenth day after surgery and signifies a graft take.

During the third phase, organic union, a firm fibrous union forms between the graft and its bed. Wound contraction, pigmentation, and reinnervation occur during this period and may require up to 18 months for completion (Boyd and Hanselka 1971).

TYPES OF SKIN GRAFTS

Pinch Grafts (Seed Grafts)

Pinch grafts were developed to aid in the healing of large surface skin defects. They consist of thin, intermediate, and full thickness grafts that are placed in granulation tissue pockets at specific intervals in the granulating bed (MacKay-Smith and Marks 1968; Swaim 1980). These pockets provide an excellent protective, nutritive environment for graft acceptance (MacKay-Smith and Marks 1968).

Pinch grafts aid healing by providing a source of epithelium that spreads from each edge of the graft over the granulating bed until epithelial zones coalesce (MacKay-Smith and Marks 1968; Swaim 1980). They also are reported to stimulate the growth of epithelium from the recipient site's wound edges (MacKay-Smith and Marks 1968; Swaim 1980). As epithelium grows from the grafts, the cover of granulation tissue over the pockets begins to slough, and the graft appears as a dark spot on the wound surface.

The donor site most frequently used for pinch grafts in the horse is the ventral abdominal area. However, any thin-skinned, relatively hairless area near the wound is acceptable (MacKay-Smith and Marks 1968). After aseptic preparation of the donor and recipient sites, the donor site is anesthetized by a subcutaneous injection of a suitable local anesthetic agent. Since the recipient site is insensitive, it does not require local anesthesia. A parallel row of separate tissue pockets is created in the lower edge of the granulating bed with a #15 scalpel blade (Fig. 12–45B). These pockets are approximately 1 to 2 cm deep and 1 cm apart and open in an upward direction (MacKay-Smith and Marks 1968). Grafts are obtained by elevating (tenting) tissue with a fine tooth forceps, after which they are cut as thin as possible at right

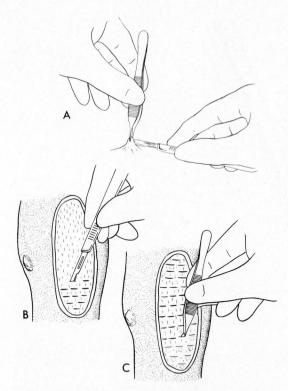

Figure 12–45 *A,* Technique for obtaining pinch grafts. *B,* The knife is pointing to parallel arranged pockets that are made in the recipient granulating bed. *C,* Pinch grafts are inserted downward into tissue pockets with the epithelial surface facing outward.

angles to the elevation so that grafts 2 to 3 mm in diameter are obtained (Fig. 12–45A) (MacKay-Smith and Marks 1968). These grafts are then flattened and inserted with their epithelial surface outward into the granulation tissue pockets (Frankland, Morris, and Spreull 1976; MacKay-Smith and Marks 1968) (Fig. 12–45C).

This technique is continued row by row from bottom to top until the entire wound surface is seeded with grafts (MacKay-Smith and Marks 1968). After all grafts are in place, a topical antibiotic spray is applied. MacKay-Smith and Marks have suggested the light application of steroid cream (1968). In situations in which bandages are employed, a sterile nonadherent pad is applied, followed with sterile gauze cotton supported with an elastic material.* MacKay-Smith and

Marks found that bandaging is only required to prevent self-mutilation (1968).

The advantage of pinch grafting is that it does not require general anesthesia. Pinch grafts are easy to apply, relatively resistant to infection, and can withstand some movement (MacKay-Smith and Marks 1968; Swaim 1980). The disadvantages include a poor cosmetic end result, leaving a cobblestone appearance, and poor quality healing of the skin with a tendency to bleed and crack with movement (Obel 1951).

Punch Grafting

Punch grafting was developed for use on horses with extensive lacerations of the lower part of the limbs (Boyd and Hanselka 1971). Full thickness donor tissue is obtained aseptically from the cranial portion of the pectoral region. A fusiform piece of skin 10 × 3.7 cm usually suffices for the graft and allows for easy skin closure of the donor site. The donor skin is placed hair side down on a sterilized polypropylene board and held in place by elastic hooks (Fig. 12–46B) (Boyd and Hanselka 1971). The underlying fat and fascia are trimmed from the donor tissue with the aid of thumb tissue forceps, scissors, and a #22 scalpel blade. A 7-mm skin biopsy punch† is used to cut small uniform donor grafts (see Fig. 12–46B). This cutting is continued until enough grafts have been harvested to cover the defect. Grafts are stored temporarily on sterile gauze soaked in saline.

Meagher (1981) described an alternative method for obtaining grafts. Instead of incising a full thickness piece of skin, grafts are obtained from the ventrolateral abdominal area in the standing horse with the 7-mm biopsy punch. This, of course, requires subcutaneous injections of local anesthetics. Subcutaneous tissue and fascia are removed from each graft before placement (Meagher 1981). This step can be eliminated if split thickness punch grafts are taken. Donor site holes are allowed to heal by second intention.

---

*Elasticon, Johnson & Johnson Co., New Brunswick, NJ.

†Keyes Skin Punch, Aloe Medical Instruments, Dallas, TX.

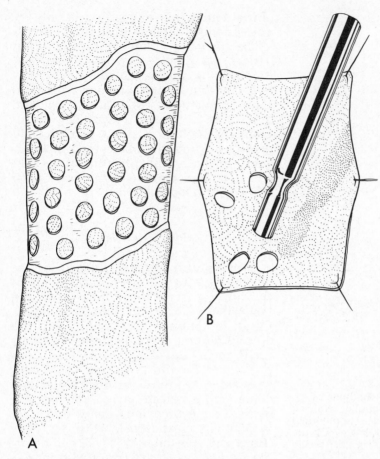

Figure 12–46 *A*, A 5-mm biopsy punch is used to make holes in the recipient bed to recover the 7-mm punch graft. *B*, A 7-mm biopsy punch is used to obtain punch grafts from donor skin.

After aseptic preparation of the recipient site, small circular holes are made in the granulating bed using a 5-mm biopsy punch (Fig. 12–46A). These recipient holes are spaced about 7 mm apart in every direction over the entire surface of the wound (Boyd and Hanselka 1971). Blood clots that form in the recipient areas are removed with a mosquito forceps and dry sterile gauze. The donor grafts are then placed, one by one, into the recipient sites (Boyd and Hanselka 1971). Since the 7-mm donor grafts have a tendency to contract, they fit snugly into the 5-mm–diameter recipient holes. After surgery, a sterile nonadherent dressing is applied to the wound with sterile gauze and held in place by an elastic support bandage. This bandage is left in place for 10 to 14 days. Sufficient bandage pressure is applied to keep the free grafts in their recipient beds (Boyd and Hanselka 1971). Aftercare consists of rebandaging as needed.

The advantages to punch grafting parallel those of pinch grafting. However, this procedure provides a better cosmetic end result because hair follicles and glands are transplanted with the full thickness of skin. It has also been reported to have a 75 to 95 per cent graft survival rate (Boyd and Hanselka 1971). The disadvantages include the requirement for general anesthesia in some cases and the unsightly multidirectional hair growth that occurs. Hair growth orientation can be improved by the proper alignment of grafts when they are placed in their recipient beds.

Tunnel Grafts

Tunnel grafts were developed to overcome graft displacement observed with other techniques (Obel 1951). Narrow strips of split thickness skin are applied, hair side down, to pieces of white adhesive tape of the same width. The grafts with attached adhesive tape are placed tape side up parallel to each other in the granulation tissue with the aid of a large needle (Obel 1951). Longitudinal displacement of the tunnel grafts is prevented by fixing the exposed ends with sutures. A sterile petroleum gauze is applied and held in place by bandaging. Bandages are changed as needed. After eight days, the grafts are exposed by excising the roof of granulation tissue overlaying them. The attached adhesive tape becomes separated from the grafts during this eight-day period and is usually easy to remove. Epithelialization of the wound usually occurs by 50 to 65 days (Obel 1951).

Split Thickness Skin Grafts

As the name implies, this type of graft is composed of epidermis and various thicknesses of dermal tissue (Meagher and Adams 1970; 1971; Swaim 1980). These grafts may be thin split thickness, intermediate split thickness, or thick split thickness, depending on the thickness of dermal tissue included (Swaim 1980) (see Fig. 12–44). The thicker the graft, the more closely its properties resemble those of full thickness transplants (Swaim 1980). The indications for this type of graft include reconstruction of large skin defects below the carpus and tarsus in the horse.

The donor site most frequently used to obtain split thickness grafts is the ventral abdominal area. This site is selected because it is relatively accessible in horses under general anesthesia and in lateral recumbency. It also represents a relatively large, flat skin surface with uniform hair direction, and any residual effects of healing go unnoticed because of the ventral location. Other donor sites for split thickness skin grafts include the lateral neck, lateral shoulder, and rump area (Boyd 1967; Frankland, Morris, and Spreull 1976). However, in the author's opinion, these are not as acceptable as the ventral abdominal area because of the location and the relative difficulty in obtaining these grafts with dermatomes.

There are three instruments designed to obtain split thickness grafts: free-hand instruments;* electric and pneumatic

dermatomes;† and drum-type dermatomes‡ (Frankland, Morris, and Spreull 1976; Meagher and Adams 1970; 1971; Swaim 1980). All three instruments have a sharp blade that moves back and forth to cut the split thickness grafts (Swaim 1980). The donor site must be relatively flat, dry, and immobile to obtain uniform grafts. Some authors have suggested that a subcutaneous injection of sterile saline may be beneficial because it places the skin under slight tension, making it relatively flat and easier to immobilize. Epinephrine can also be added to this fluid to provide hemostasis (Funquist and Obel 1979; Swaim 1980). The thickness of the graft can be controlled by calibrated settings on these instruments or by the surgeon's estimation (Swaim 1980). Most grafts usually vary from 0.625 to 0.1250 cm in thickness (Hanselka 1974; Meagher and Adams 1970; 1971). These grafts should be cut large enough to allow for overlapping of the skin graft over the recipient site (Meagher and Adams 1971; Swaim 1980).

Once the graft has been obtained, it is applied to the previously prepared recipient bed site so that there is a 1.5-cm overlap. Some surgeons recommend placing small holes or slits at equal distances over the entire graft to prevent the accumulation of blood or serum under the graft (Hanselka 1974; Fackelman 1973). These grafts are sutured to the overlapped skin with 3-0 monofilament nylon placed in a simple interrupted pattern (Meagher and Adams 1971; Swaim 1980). This placement prevents the sutures from passing through the vascular granulation tissue, which would increase the chances of bleeding underneath the graft (Meagher and Adams 1971; Swaim 1980).

If one graft is not large enough to cover the recipient site, another graft is taken and the two grafts are sutured together using simple interrupted 4-0 monofilament sutures. The united grafts are then applied and sutured to the recipient site as previously described. Funquist and

---

*Ferris-Smith Skin Graft Knife, Edward Weck, Co., Long Island City, NY.

†Striker Electric Dermatome, Striker Corp., Kalamazoo, MI.

‡Padgett-Hood Dermatome, Kansas City Assemblage Co., Kansas City, MO.

Obel have reported the use of stainless steel staples for graft fixation (1979). Stay sutures of 0 monofilament nylon are placed approximately 2.5 cm from the periphery of the recipient bed and about 5 cm apart around the entire grafted area. Suture ends are left about 20 to 25 cm long. The transplant is then covered with a single layer of sterile petroleum gauze, after which a sterile pack made of cotton surrounded by sterile gauze is applied and held in place by tying stay suture ends in an "X" pattern over the top (Meagher and Adams 1971) (see Fig. 12–23). This tie-over pack applies even, continuous, stable pressure to the skin transplant and, because it is sutured to the skin, reduces the influence of movement of the surrounding supporting bandage on the graft site (Funquist and Obel 1979). If skin transplants are placed over joints or areas of increased mobility, a plaster cast will be required. On the other hand, transplants placed in relatively immobile areas can be protected with a bulky cotton elastic supportive bandage* (Meagher and Adams 1971).

The donor site is protected with a sterile gauze applied after graft removal. It is held in place by coagulated blood on the surface of the wound. This protective gauze usually falls off the epithelialized wound in about 10 to 20 days (Meagher and Adams 1971). The dressings and casts are changed in about 12 to 14 days, and the tie-over bandage is removed at this time. The grafted area is then protected with a bandage until overlapped skin edges have sloughed and the transplant is healed.

Although all researchers do not agree, it is generally accepted that the major advantage of free split thickness grafts is that they take more successfully than do full thickness grafts (Swaim 1980). It is proposed that, since the denser capillary networks are located in the more superficial dermal areas, there is a better chance of capillaries from the graft uniting with capillaries from the graft bed (Swaim 1980). The thinner graft seems to have the ability to survive longer on plasmatic imbibition until revascularization occurs (Swaim 1980). Another ad-

vantage is that defects can be covered without disfigurement of the donor site (Swaim 1980). The major disadvantages of split thickness grafting are that general anesthesia is required and the equipment required to obtain these grafts is expensive. Also, a reduction in the number of hair follicles and sebaceous and sweat glands has been observed in split thickness grafts when compared with normal full thickness skin (Swaim 1980).

Mesh Grafts

Mesh skin grafts are grafts in which multiple small parallel staggered cuts are made to allow for expansion of the graft (Hanselka 1974; Swaim 1980). This grafting technique was developed to cover large skin defects in extensively burned human patients for whom insufficient donor skin was available (Hanselka 1974; Swaim 1980). It is also beneficial when grafting wounds that have very irregular surfaces that are difficult to immobilize (Swaim 1980). Mesh grafts can be made from either split thickness or full thickness grafts. Split thickness grafts have the advantage of covering greater surface areas and for that reason are used more frequently (Hanselka 1974).

Split thickness donor skin is obtained from the ventral abdominal area with the aid of the dermatome. The skin usually varies from 0.0625 to 0.1250 cm in thickness (Hanselka 1974; Meagher and Adams 1971). After harvesting, the donor skin is kept moist with sterile physiological saline. Expansion of the graft is accomplished by the use of the mesh graft dermatome.* This instrument is composed of a solid aluminum base into which multiple parallel staggered cutting edges fit. To mesh the graft, it is spread evenly, hair side up, on the dermatome, after which a Teflon roller is passed over the graft to perforate it. A 3:1 expansion ratio of available skin is produced (Fig. 12–47B) (Hanselka 1974; Swaim 1980). After the recipient bed is aseptically prepared for surgery, exces-

---

*Elasticon, Johnson & Johnson Co., New Brunswick, NJ.

*Mesh Skin Graft Expander, #P-160, Pagette Instrument Co., Kansas City, KS.

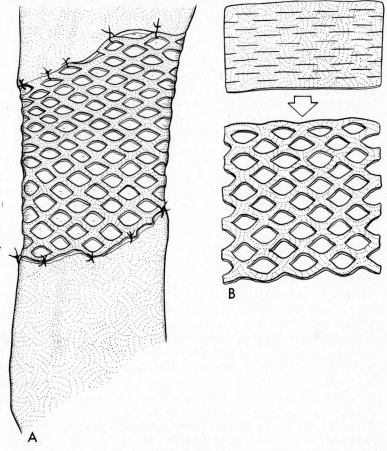

Figure 12–47 *A*, Simple interrupted sutures hold the mesh graft in place. *B*, Top: skin graft has been perforated with a mesh dermatome to form parallel incisions. Bottom: a 3:1 expansion ratio of the graft is achieved.

sive granulation tissue is trimmed. Hemorrhage is controlled with moist gauze sponges and pressure.

There are two factors to consider when making and placing a mesh graft (Swaim 1980). First, the graft should be slit so that when it is expanded, the hair direction of the graft aligns with that of the surrounding tissue. Second, healing is faster and more cosmetic if the mesh graft is not expanded to its full extent (Swaim 1980). Once placed, simple interrupted sutures are used at the periphery to hold the graft. Size 2-0 to 4-0 medium chromic gut has been used; (Hanselka 1974; Swaim 1980); however, the author prefers 3-0 monofilament nylon sutures.

After the graft is sutured, a nonadherent sterile dressing is applied and held in place by sterile bandages supported by an elastic adhesive bandage. Additional protection can be afforded by the inclusion of a foam pad (1.27 cm thick) over the original bandage. This is held in place by more elastic adhesive bandage (Hanselka 1974). Cast application is required for grafted wounds located over the dorsal surface of the carpus and tarsus. The first bandage is changed after four days. After examining and cleansing the graft with sterile physiological saline, another bandage is applied. Casts are left on 10 to 14 days, after which bandages are applied. Observation and rebandaging is performed on an alternate-day basis until the wound is entirely epithelialized (Hanselka 1974). The donor site is sprayed with antiseptic spray and allowed to heal by second intention healing.

The advantages of mesh grafts are: (1) they are easy to apply; (2) they are flexible enough to conform to almost any surface; (3) openings in the graft allow for drainage of blood, exudate, and serum away from the wound; (4) they can withstand a certain degree of movement; (5) small amounts of donor tissue can be used to cover large defects; (6)

and they increase the number of edges for healing and reduce the amount of wound contraction because of their geometric design. The major disadvantages include the following: (1) general anesthesia is required; (2) expensive mesh dermatomes are required; and (3) the cosmetic end result can be somewhat undesirable, taking on a diamond-shaped pattern initially; however, problems can be minimized by not maximally expanding the graft (Hanselka 1974; Swaim 1980). Long-term studies show that these grafts eventually become as cosmetically acceptable as split thickness sheet grafts.

Full Thickness Skin Grafts

This type of graft is composed of epidermis and full thickness dermis (see Fig. 12–44). The closely adherent subcutaneous tissue and fascia are removed from the underside of the dermis before grafting is performed (Boyd 1967). Since these grafts contain all of the tissue elements of normal skin, they most closely resemble it after healing (Swaim 1980). Unfortunately, they can only cover a limited area because of the limitation of the donor site. They also require optimal conditions for a take, since revascularization occurs more slowly than with other types of grafts (Swaim 1980).

Full thickness grafting of the horse is indicated for full thickness skin defects small enough so that the donor site can be effectively sutured. It is also indicated in situations in which the best cosmetic end result is required (Boyd 1967). Donor skin for full thickness grafts is most frequently obtained from the cranial pectoral region (Boyd 1967). Recipient sites are prepared according to the type of wound that the surgeon is confronted with. Grafting can be performed at the time of excision of a noncontaminated lesion (Boyd 1967; Meagher and Adams 1970; 1971). Traumatic contaminated wounds should be allowed to heal for 10 to 14 days or until healthy granulation tissue is observed before grafting is performed (Boyd 1967; Meagher and Adams 1971). In either case, it is beneficial to obtain measurements of the recipient site so that the same amount of tissue can be removed from the donor site.

An effective way to measure is to cut or outline the dimensions of the recipient site using a thin sheet of sterile nylon* or sterilized x-ray film. A sterilized, pointed toothpick dipped in methylene blue is excellent for outlining or drawing the dimensions of the lesions (Swaim 1980). This outline is then transferred and placed over the aseptically prepared donor site, and a full thickness skin graft is obtained. After graft retrieval, the edges of the donor site are incised, undermined, and sutured. Tension sutures may be required for closure.

Preparation of the donor skin for application consists of placing the tissue, hair side down, and surgically removing all subcutaneous fat and fascia down to glistening white dermis (Boyd 1967). The graft is kept moist by application of sterile physiological saline. Once prepared, the graft is placed in the recipient site, making sure that proper hair growth orientation is present. It is then sutured using 3-0 monofilament nylon in a simple interrupted suture pattern. Any blood that has accumulated under the graft is removed prior to placing the final sutures (Boyd 1967). A sterile nonadherent dressing is placed over the graft, after which a sterile tie-over pack is applied to provide constant pressure. Bandaging with cotton, gauze, and supportive elastic bandage is advised for areas with limited motion, whereas casts are used in highly mobile areas. Bandages and casts are changed in 12 to 14 days, after which cotton bandages are maintained as needed.

The advantage of a full thickness graft is that a functionally cosmetic end result is produced inexpensively with minimal graft contraction (Swaim 1980). The disadvantages include the following: (1) general anesthesia is required; (2) donor skin sites are limited; and (3) the take is not as good as that observed with split thickness grafting (Swaim 1980). However, Boyd (1967) has reported a success rate of 18 of 24 full thickness grafts as

---

*Nylon Film, Tubular Autoclavable, V. Mueller and Co., Chicago, IL.

compared with 16 of 24 for split thickness grafting techniques.

REFERENCES

Bacchetta, C. A., Magec, W., Rodehauer, G., Edgerton, M. T., and Edlich, R. F.: Biology of infections of split thickness skin grafts. Am. J. Surg. 130:63, 1975.

Boyd, C. L.: Equine skin autotransplant for wound healing. JAVMA 151:1618, 1967.

Boyd, C. L., and Hanselka, D. V.: A skin punch technique for equine skin grafting. JAVMA 158:82, 1971.

Fackelman, G. E.: A new technique of skin transplantation and a preliminary evaluation of the effects of solcoseryl on graft acceptance. Equine Vet. J. 5:105, 1973.

Frankland, A. L., Morris, P. D. G., and Spreull, J. S. A.: Free, autologous skin transplantation in the horse. Vet. Rec. 98:105, 1976.

Funquist, B., and Obel, N.: Fixation of skin grafts in the horse using stainless steel staples. Equine Vet. J. 11:117, 1979.

Hanselka, D. V.: Use of autogenous mesh grafts in equine wound managements. JAVMA 164:35, 1974.

MacKay-Smith, M. P., and Marks, D.: A skin grafting technique for horses. JAVMA 152:1633, 1968.

Meagher, D. M.: Wound management in horses. Proceedings of the 42nd Annual Conference for Veterinarians at Colorado State University, Fort Collins, 1981, pp. 23–26.

Meagher, D. M., and Adams, O. R.: Skin transplantation in horses. Can. Vet. J. 11:239, 1970.

Meagher, D. M., and Adams, O. R.: Split thickness autologous skin transplantation in horses. JAVMA 159:55, 1971.

Obel, A. N.: Tunnel plastik vid behandling AV caro luxurians hoshast. Nord. Vet. Med. 10:869, 1951.

Swaim, S. F.: Skin grafts. In Surgery of Traumatized Skin. Philadelphia: W. B. Saunders, 1980, pp. 423–476.

CHAPTER 13

THE RESPIRATORY SYSTEM

SURGICAL ANATOMY OF THE LARGE ANIMAL RESPIRATORY SYSTEM

CARLETON L. LOHSE, D.V.M.

The respiratory system consists of the conducting airways, lungs, pleural sacs, thoracic wall, circulatory vasculature, and other structural components involved in respiratory gas exchange. Many processes take place in these structures in addition to the exchange of gas between the animal and its environment. For example, heat loss due to evaporation from moist mucous membranes and vocalization take place. Insignificant-appearing structures, such as the hair surrounding nostril openings and the cilia of air passage epithelium, assist in removal of foreign matter from the air. Moisture on the surface of mucous membranes helps clear the air of chemicals as well as particles.

The continuous function of the respiratory system during surgery is crucial, yet ventilation, anesthesia, and the surgical procedure may take place simultaneously. A procedure such as endotracheal intubation makes an understanding of structures in the larynx a prerequisite for maintaining the animal on a gas anesthetic and initiating the surgery.

The functional anatomy of structures will be emphasized in this introduction. The following paragraphs apply in general to the five species under considera-tion and deal with normal structures that are similar among large animals. This is not intended to be an encyclopedic effort, and the introductory material is on common features or concepts relating to the respiratory apparatus. Unique or dissimilar features of the respiratory system of each species will be covered under separate headings.

Those passageways that conduct air into and out of the lungs may be divided at the thoracic inlet into upper and lower airways. The upper conducting airways are outside the thorax, and the lower conducting airways lie within the thoracic cavity. Problems altering mechanical aspects of respiration may affect the upper or lower airways independently or simultaneously. For the purposes of anatomical description, the upper airway structures will be considered first.

Upper Airways

The nostrils (nares)* open from the nasal cavity to the outside environment.

---

*When an important Anglicized term is used for the first time, the Nomina Anatomica Veterinaria (1973) form will follow it in parentheses. Thereafter, only the English term will be used.

Nostrils vary in size and shape from rather small and nondistensive to large, soft, and easily dilated. All species under consideration have a nasal vestibule (*vestibulum nasi*) immediately inside the nostril, but only the horse possesses a false nostril (*diverticulum nasi*) opening into the nasal vestibule. The topographical anatomy of the false nostril will be described in the section on the horse.

The nasal cavity is separated from the mouth by the hard palate. It is also divided into right and left halves by the nasal septum. Both halves of the nasal cavity open into the nasopharynx through the caudal nares (*choanae*). Each half of the nasal cavity is subdivided into five passageways. These are the dorsal nasal meatus, the middle nasal meatus, the ventral nasal meatus, the nasopharyngeal meatus, and the common nasal meatus. The first three are separated from one another by scrolls of bone covered with mucous membrane, whereas the common nasal meatus communicates with all five passageways. The medial boundary of the common nasal meatus is the nasal septum, and the structures projecting from the lateral side of the nasal cavity form most of the lateral boundary.

Paranasal sinuses are air-filled cavities in the bones of the head. They open into passageways leading either to another paranasal sinus or directly into the nasal cavity. The maxillary, frontal, sphenoid, and palatine sinuses are excavated within bones of the same name. The sphenoid and palatine sinuses may be fused to form the sphenopalatine sinus. In addition, a lacrimal sinus is located within the lacrimal bone of several species. Dorsal, middle, ventral, and ethmoidal conchal sinuses are described.

The pharynx is functionally part of both the digestive and respiratory systems and may be divided into an oral portion and the nasal pharynx. This discussion will focus on features of the nasal pharynx, which is located dorsal to the soft palate. Openings into the nasal pharynx are the caudal nares, the intrapharyngeal opening (*ostium intrapharyngeum*), the laryngeal pharynx (*pars laryngea*), and the pharyngeal openings of the auditory tubes (*ostium pharyngeum tubae auditivae*). Each auditory tube of the horse has a large diverticulum called the guttural pouch, which is closely related to the pharynx in that air normally passes from the nasal pharynx to the middle ear through the auditory tubes.

The larynx prevents the inhalation of most foreign objects and is essential for vocalization. It regulates air inspiration and expiration. There are several cartilages that help maintain the air passageway through the cavity of the larynx. Caudal to the base of the tongue is the unpaired epiglottic cartilage, which is attached to the thyroid cartilage of the larynx by the thyroepiglottic ligament. Supporting and maintaining the cavity of the larynx is the large thyroid cartilage, consisting of a body and two laminae. Several muscles and ligaments, notably the cricothyroid ligament, attach to the thyroid cartilage and subsequently to the cricoid cartilage. The cricoid cartilage lies caudal to the thyroid cartilage with a narrow portion ventrally and an enlarged ring-like part dorsally. Circular cricoid cartilage helps maintain the airway through the larynx and provides an attachment for laryngeal muscles. The cricotracheal ligament attaches the cricoid cartilage to the first tracheal ring. Arytenoid cartilages provide attachment for muscles that abduct the vocal folds and these cartilages form the dorsal boundary of the laryngeal opening (*aditus laryngis*). Vocal folds form the ventral aspect of the glottis. Paralysis of these muscles, because of recurrent laryngeal nerve disruption, results in laryngeal hemiplegia. Difficult and noisy breathing may result when the vocal folds flutter either unilaterally or bilaterally during exercise.

The trachea consists of a series of cartilage rings, which are either incomplete dorsally (Getty 1975) or overlapping. Attached to adjacent tracheal cartilages are the annular ligaments. Mucosa-containing tubuloalveolar glands cover the inner surface of the trachea. At the thoracic inlet the cervical trachea (upper airway) becomes the intrathoracic trachea, which is the first part of the lower airway.

Lower Airways

The cranial opening into the thorax, the thoracic inlet, is bounded by thoracic vertebrae dorsally, by the first pair of ribs laterally, and by the cranial sternum ventrally. Rib numbers vary between species as does the attachment of costal cartilages to the sternum. The thoracic outlet is closed in the living animal by the diaphragm.

Supporting bones and cartilages shown in Figure 13–1 maintain the general form of the thorax in spite of pressure changes within it. The thoracic vertebrae, ribs, costal cartilages, and sternum form a movable cage surrounding the thoracic cavity. Intrathoracic pressure changes are necessary for respiration, yet the mechanical support of bone and connective tissues is required to simultaneously protect the heart and lungs. The vertebrae have a typical vertebral structure, but their total number differs in the various species (Table 13–1). Sternal ribs have a head, neck, tubercle, costal groove, and costochondral junction. Ribs attached to the sternum by costal cartilage are termed sternal ribs. Their costal cartilage forms part of the costal arch. Sternebrae make up the body of the sternum with a cariniform cartilage on the cranial manubrium and the xiphoid cartilage located on the caudal extremity.

The rib articulates with the thoracic vertebrae by two diarthrotic joints. A diarthrodial joint is formed between the costal head and the spinal column; another lies between the rib tubercle and the transverse process of each respective vertebra. Ligaments reinforce the joint capsules of these joints. The costochondral articulations (synarthrodial joints)

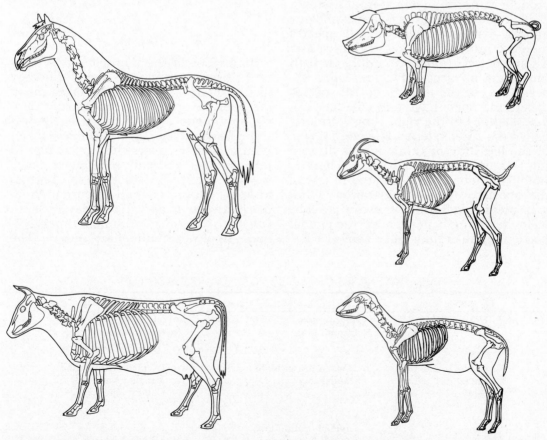

Figure 13–1 Shape of the thorax as outlined in large animal species varying from the elongated, conical form of the horse to the wedge-shaped chest of the cow. (After Getty, 1975.)

Table 13–1 NUMBER OF VERTEBRAE IN VARIOUS SPECIES

Species	Thoracic Vertebrae	Ribs		
		Sternal	Asternal	Total
Horse	18	8	10	18
Cow	13	8	5	13
Sheep/Goat	13	7	6	13
Pig	14–15	7	7–8	14–15

are fibrous in the horse. In cattle and sheep the second to eleventh joints are diarthroses. In the pig only the second to fifth joints are diarthrotic. The costosternal articulations are diarthroses and are supported by costosternal ligaments in all species under consideration.

Near the base of the heart the trachea divides into right and left principal bronchi. Lobar and segmental bronchi are the next lower divisions of the bronchial tree. Under a modern system of terminology (NAV 1973), the criterion for naming lung lobes is based on division of the bronchi rather than on external fissures. This provides the best possible homology among domestic animals. All species have a cranial lobe (lobus cranialis) and a caudal lobe (lobus caudalis) in both lungs and an accessory lobe (lobus accessorius) in the right lung. All species except the horse have a middle lobe (lobus medius) in the right lung (formerly called the cardiac lobe). The cranial lobe of the left lung of ruminants is divided into cranial and caudal parts. There is no middle lobe in the left lung in any of the species under consideration. What was previously termed the cardiac lobe of the left lung is now called the caudal portion of the cranial lobe (Table 13–2).

Bronchioles terminate as they form respiratory bronchioles. Air passageways from the respiratory bronchiole to the respiratory membrane are no longer tubular with walls but rather are spaces in a network of partitions. These spaces are named by their size and position as the respiratory bronchioles, alveolar ducts, alveolar sacs, and alveoli. The respiratory bronchioles and alveolar ducts are like hallways with doorless rooms opening into them from all sides (Julian and Tyler 1962). The partitions separating the alveoli are the respiratory membranes.

PLEURA

Both sides of the thoracic cavity contain closed membranous sacs formed by pleura. Pleura is a serosal membrane of mesodermal origin and consists of a simple squamous epithelium on a connective tissue layer, the lamina propria. Pleura closely covers the lungs (pleura pulmonalis), and only a capillary space (cavum pleurae), which in the normal animal contains a small amount of fluid, lies between it and the parietal pleura (pleura parietalis). Autonomic nerve fibers supply the pulmonary pleura. The

Table 13–2 LOBES OF THE LUNGS IN VARIOUS SPECIES

Species	Left Lung	Right Lung
Horse	Cranial lobe Caudal lobe	Cranial lobe Caudal lobe Accessory lobe
Cow Sheep Goat	Divided cranial lobe Caudal lobe	Divided cranial lobe Middle lobe Caudal lobe Accessory lobe
Pig	Divided cranial lobe Caudal lobe	Cranial lobe Middle lobe Caudal lobe Accessory lobe

blood supply to the pulmonary pleura is mainly from branches of the bronchial arteries, and venous drainage is through the pulmonary veins. The pleural cavity extends cranial to the first rib where it is called the pleural cupula.

Parietal pleura is attached to the inner aspects of the thorax, diaphragm, and mediastinum. It is attached to the deep surface of thoracic structures by endothoracic fascia, which is a sheet of fibroelastic connective tissue that lines the thoracic cavity. Medially over the mediastinal space, the two pleural sacs cover structures such as the great vessels, heart, and esophagus with serous membrane. When the mediastinum is covered with two complete layers of pleura, the right and left portions of the thoracic cavity do not communicate. The mediastinum is usually a complete partition at birth. Fat and connective tissue increase the thickness of the mediastinum in ruminants, making the division more substantial. The caudoventral mediastinum is usually incomplete in the horse and permits direct communication between the right and left pleural cavities.

On the right side, the caudal vena cava passes to the heart and is covered by a reflection of pleura called the plica vena cava. The portion of the pleural cavity situated between the mediastinum and the plica vena cava is called the mediastinal recess. The accessory lobe of the right lung fills this recess in all species under consideration.

RESPIRATORY STRUCTURES OF THE HORSE

Upper Airway

During normal breathing, the nostrils of the horse are semicircular openings bounded by relatively soft tissues. When the respiratory air volume increases, the nostrils are dilated and become more circular (Nickel et al. 1973). The dorsal aspect of the nostril opening leads into a blind pouch or false nostril (*diverticulum nasi*). Its topographical location beneath the skin of the nose is indicated by a broken line in Figure 13–2. Foerner reviewed false nostril anatomy as it re-

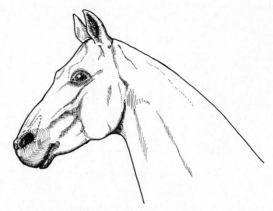

Figure 13–2 Surface anatomy of the horse head. Broken line indicates the topographical location of the diverticulum nasi in relation to the nostril.

lated to surgery and described how alar folds continue caudally to form the medial walls of the false nostrils (1967). Alar and accessory cartilages support the alar fold, which projects laterally. A cast of the left nostril drawn from a dorsal view shows the excursion into the airway created by the alar fold (Fig. 13–3). Robinson, Sorensen, and Goble reported that 80 to 90 per cent of resistance to air flow within the upper respiratory tract was in the nasal cavity at the level of the nostrils (1975). Normally the airway leads through the nostril, into the vestibule, and continues caudally through the ventral nasal meatus. The opening of the nasolacrimal duct lies on the floor of the nasal vestibule. Tears flowing from it often help determine its location. A view of the nasal cartilages of the horse is shown in Figure 13–4.

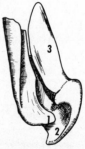

Figure 13–3 Dorsal view of a cast of the left nostril and nasal diverticulum of the horse showing the form of the nasal vestibule (*1*), the impression made by the alar fold (*2*), and the outline of the cast material replicating the nasal diverticulum (*3*). (After Getty, 1975.)

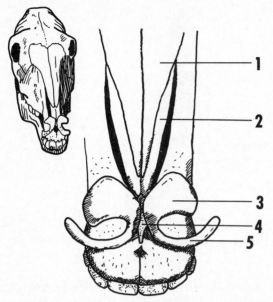

Figure 13–4 The skull of the horse with an isolated view of the nasal bone *(1)*, dorsal lateral cartilage *(2)*, lamina of the alar cartilage *(3)*, nasal septum *(4)*, and cornu of the alar cartilage *(5)*.

NASAL CAVITY

The median nasal septum is of interest, especially at the point at which it becomes widened dorsally to support the parietal cartilages *(cartilago nasi lateralis dorsalis)*. The bony septum is made up of the vomer ventrally and the perpendicular plate of the ethmoid bone caudally. The major part of the septum, however, is composed of hyaline cartilage (Getty 1975).

In the horse the dorsal nasal turbinate *(concha)* (Fig. 13–5) extends from the angle of the lip to the cribriform plate of the ethmoid bone. Ethmoidal turbinates *(conchae)* are found in the caudodorsal aspect of the nasal cavity. Together with the dorsal and ventral nasal turbinates

they divide the remaining parts of the nasal cavity into three passageways. The larger of these air-filled passages is the ventral nasal meatus. It is immediately above the floor of the nasal cavity and leads caudally into the nasopharyngeal meatus, which continues through the caudal nares to the nasal pharynx. A flexible probe entering the nostril and vestibule continues in the ventral nasal meatus to take the shortest course to the nasal pharynx. The caudal nares that connect the ventral nasal meatuses with the nasal pharynx are confluent at the nasopharyngeal meatus in the horse. The common nasal meatus communicates with the other meatuses, and it occupies the space between the floor and roof of the nasal cavity lateral to the nasal septum.

There are six pairs of diverticula leaving the nasal cavity; they are called the paranasal sinuses *(sinus paranasales)*. The largest and one of the most important surgically is the maxillary sinus, and it is contained within the maxilla, lacrimal, and zygomatic bones. A line drawn caudally from the **infraorbital foramen*** parallel to the **facial crest** of the maxilla marks the dorsal limit of the maxillary sinus. The rostral boundary may be determined by drawing a line from the rostral end of the facial crest to the infraorbital foramen. The maxillary sinus extends caudally to a transverse plane rostral to the root of the **zygomatic process.** Medially it is bounded by the maxilla, infraorbital canal, ventral nasal concha, and a small portion of the ethmoidal labyrinth.

The air-filled cavity of the maxillary sinus is divided into rostral and caudal

---

*The names of structures that are palpable anatomical landmarks are set in boldface type.

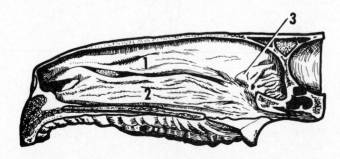

Figure 13–5 Sagittal section of the horse head showing the right side of the nasal cavity with the dorsal *(1)*, ventral *(2)*, and middle nasal turbinates (conchae) *(3)*. (After Getty, 1975.)

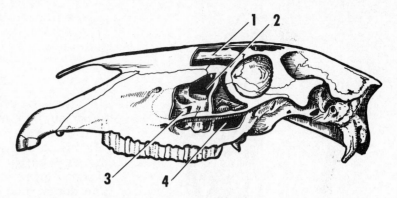

Figure 13–6 A horse skull opened to show the frontoturbinate (conchofrontal) sinus (*1*), the nasomaxillary opening (*2*), and the rostral (*3*) and caudal maxillary sinuses (*4*). (After Getty, 1975.)

portions by an oblique septum. Laterally, the margin of the septum is about 5 cm from the rostral end of the facial crest and it is oriented medially, caudally, and slightly dorsally. Getty points out that portions of the septum are delicate and variable in position, and in exceptional cases there is an opening in the dorsal portion of the septum (1975). Mucous membrane lining the paranasal sinuses and covering the septa is thin and relatively avascular in the horse.

The rostral maxillary sinus communicates with the middle nasal meatus by the nasomaxillary opening. It also opens dorsally to the osseous infraorbital canal through the conchomaxillary opening into the caudal portion of the ventral nasal concha as outlined in Figure 13–6.

The caudal maxillary sinus is larger than the rostral compartment, and it opens into the middle conchal sinus. It communicates directly with the spheno-

palatine sinus and the frontal sinus by way of the oval frontomaxillary opening. A nasomaxillary opening allows communication between the caudal maxillary sinus and the caudal part of the middle nasal meatus.

The frontal sinus is outlined in Figure 13–7. It is separated from the opposite side by a complete septum. The rostral limit of the frontal sinus may be determined by the point at which the nearly parallel **lateral edges of the nasal bones** diverge (Fig. 13–8). Caudally, the sinus extends to the level of a transverse plane placed slightly rostral to the **temporomandibular joint.** The ethmoidal turbinates project into the floor of the sinus, which is divided into a number of communicating diverticula. In the horse the frontal sinus communicates with the dorsal turbinate sinus; these two sinuses are collectively referred to as the conchofrontal sinus.

The sphenopalatine sinus is an air-

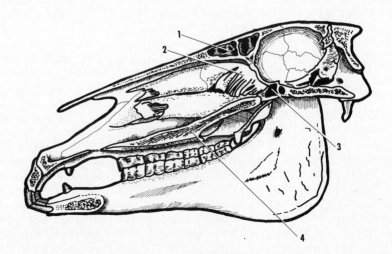

Figure 13–7 Sagittal section of the horse skull showing the frontal sinus (*1*), the ethmoidal turbinates (conchae) (*2*), the sphenopalatine sinus (*3*), and the osseous vomer (*4*), which supports the caudal nasal septum. (After Popesko, 1977.)

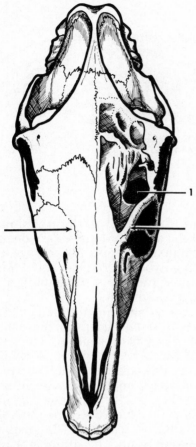

Figure 13–8 The external plate of bone covering the left frontal sinus of the horse has been removed to show the frontomaxillary opening (*1*). Arrows indicate the rostral limit of the frontal sinus. (After Popesko, 1977.)

filled cavity in the sphenoid and palatine bones. The sphenopalatine and caudal maxillary sinuses also communicate. The dorsal turbinate sinus is excavated within the dorsal nasal turbinate (Fig. 13–9). It has an extensive communication with the frontal sinus caudolaterally. A smaller middle nasal turbinate sinus communicates with the maxillary sinus laterally. The caudal part of the ventral nasal turbinate is air-filled, forming a ventral turbinate sinus, and it too has a common opening with the maxillary sinus. Ventral to its scroll-like wall is the floor of the nasal cavity, which makes the ventral nasal turbinate vulnerable to a stomach tube being passed through the ventral nasal meatus. Ventrally it is wide, but dorsally the ventral nasal meatus narrows. Inspired air

passes into the nasopharyngeal meatus after leaving the nasal cavity at the caudal nares.

PHARYNX

There is no pharyngeal septum in the horse, so the nasopharynx is not divided on the midline. Ventral to the nasopharynx is the soft palate, which separates the oral cavity from the nasopharynx except during swallowing (Getty 1975). The dorsal surface of the soft palate is covered by mucous membrane, and the free border is concave and thin. Folds of mucous membrane pass laterally to the tongue on both sides to form the palatoglossal arches of the soft palate. Another fold, called the palatopharyngeal arch of the soft palate, extends on each side on the ventral wall of the pharynx to unite with the opposite fold over the beginning of the esophagus. Within the space between the palatoglossal and palatopharyngeal arches is a series of lymphoid masses, which may become enlarged. The soft palate closes the caudal nares during swallowing; however, its caudal border is in contact with the ventral surface of the apex of the epiglottis as normal respiration resumes.

Cook observed the pharyngeal openings of the auditory tubes in the conscious patient (1974). Getty described how each auditory tube of the horse expands into a diverticulum called the gutteral pouch (*diverticulum tubae auditivae*) (1975). The right and left guttural pouches are in contact with one another on the midline where their mucous membranes lie on either side of a thin septa. They are related to the pharyngeal region in that air normally passes from their nasopharyngeal openings to the cavity of the middle ear. The guttural pouches affect vocalization to a degree, and they have complex anatomical relationships to other structures near the base of the cranium and the atlas of the neck. Habel discussed the applied anatomy of the guttural pouches, listed their capacity at about 300 ml each, and described how an endoscope may be passed into a guttural pouch by introducing it through the ventral nasal meatus (1978). Endoscopy of a guttural pouch shows that the stylohyoid bone invaginates the caudoven-

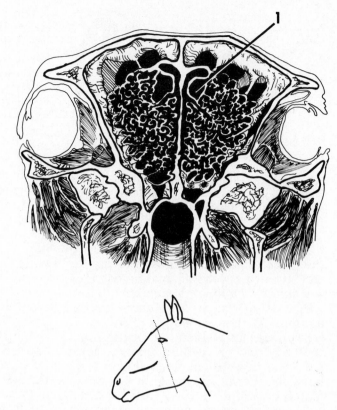

Figure 13–9 A section through the orbits of the eyes of the horse illustrates the sinuses of the dorsal nasal turbinates (1).

tral aspect of the pouch and divides it into a large medial and a smaller lateral compartment. The air passing through the guttural pouch equalizes the atmospheric pressure on the inner surface of the tympanum and the outside ambient atmospheric pressure. A guttural pouch may be approached from its lateral aspect through Viborg's triangle. This area is bounded on three sides by the **mandible,** the **tendon of the sterno-mandibularis muscle** dorsally, and the **linguofacial vein** ventrally.

LARYNX

This hollow organ is palpable at the point at which it normally lies between the rami of the mandible in a superficial position between the head and neck. It is covered ventrally by skin, subcutaneous tissues, and the sternohyoid and omohyoid muscles. Laterally the larynx is related to the pterygoidei, sternothyroideus, occipitomandibularis, and digastricus muscles. The **thyrohyoid bones** articulate with the larynx (Fig.

13–10) and support it like a sling. Intrinsic muscles move the cartilages of the larynx, whereas the extrinsic muscles pass from the larynx to other points of attachment.

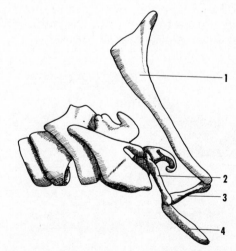

Figure 13–10 Lateral view from the right side of the equine hyoid apparatus, larynx, and first tracheal cartilage showing the stylohyoid bone (1), the thyrohyoid bone (2), the ceratohyoid bone (3), and the lingual process of the basihyoid bone (4).

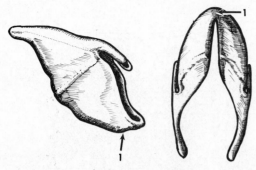

Figure 13–11 Right lateral and ventrocaudal views of the thyroid cartilage of the horse showing the laryngeal prominence (1), which is rostral to the caudal thyroid notch. (After Getty, 1975.)

The thyroid cartilage is the largest of the three unpaired cartilages of the larynx. It is composed of hyaline cartilage surrounded with connective tissue, which supports the extensive thyroid laminae. With advancing age this cartilage undergoes ossification, beginning in the body and proceeding into the laminae. The **thyroid cartilage** (Fig. 13–11) is palpable ventrally where it lies immediately caudal to the epiglottis. An extensive caudal thyroid notch permits incision through soft tissue to enter the cavity of the larynx.

A **cricothyroid ligament** is attached to the borders of the **caudal thyroid notch** and the ventral arch of the **cricoid cartilage.** These lines of attachment of the cricothyroid ligament are palpable and roughly form a triangle. When the cricothyroid ligament is incised and the cut edges are retracted from the midline incision the glottis can be viewed.

The structures of the glottis are the two vocal folds, arytenoid cartilages with vocal processes including their mucosal coverings. The glottis borders the glottic cleft (*rima glottidis*), which is the airway and which is of major importance. The vocal folds, ventricles, vestibular folds, and vestibule are surgically important structures (Fig. 13–12). Nickel and associates state that there is a median laryngeal ventricle in the floor of the vestibule of the horse (1973).

Recurrent laryngeal nerves innervate all the intrinsic muscles of the larynx except the cricothyroideus muscles. These muscles are supplied by the cranial laryngeal nerves (Getty 1975), which also innervate the laryngeal mucosa. Paralysis and atrophy of the cricoarytenoideus dorsalis muscle due to insufficiency of the recurrent laryngeal nerve allows the vocal fold to swing into the airway on inspiration. The lateral ventricle shown in Figure 13–13 affects air flow through the laryngeal portion of the upper airway. An endoscopic view obtained by passage of the endoscope through the ventral nasal meatus and nasopharynx to the laryngopharynx allows inspection of the vocal folds and the entrance to the larynx (Fig. 13–14).

The epiglottic cartilage is the second unpaired cartilage; however, in the horse it is fused with the two cuneiform cartilages rostral to the thyroid cartilage. It is composed entirely of elastic connective tissue and shows no ossification with increasing age. The outline of the epiglottis is shown in Figure 13–15, and its apex is pointed toward the caudal border of the soft palate. The aryepiglottic folds

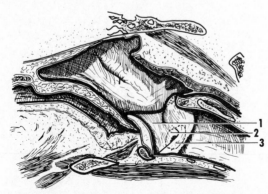

Figure 13–12 Sagittal section of the horse head showing, on the right side, the vestibule (1), vestibular fold (2), and vocal fold (3). The broken line indicates the outline of the lateral laryngeal ventricle. (After Getty, 1975.)

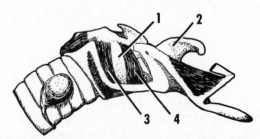

Figure 13–13 Right lateral view of the larynx and hyoid attachments of the horse showing the lateral ventricle (1), and the epiglottis (2). Part of the right lamina of the thyroid cartilage has been cut away exposing the vocal (3), and vestibular muscles (4). (After Getty, 1975.)

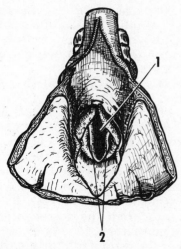

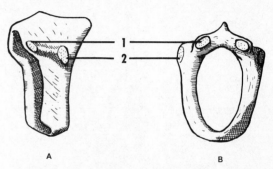

Figure 13–16 *A*, Lateral and (*B*) caudal views of the cricoid laryngeal cartilage of the horse. (*1*), Arytenoid articular surface; (*2*) oval facets for articulation with the thyroid cartilage. (After Getty, 1975.)

Figure 13–14 Dorsal view of the equine laryngopharynx with the esophagus opened to show the laryngeal aditus (*1*), and the vocal folds (*2*). (After Getty, 1975.)

(*plica aryepiglottica*) extend from the lateral borders of the epiglottic cartilage to the corniculate and arytenoid cartilages of the same side. Elastic fibers extend from the base of the epiglottic cartilage to the medial surfaces of the thyroid laminae and are termed thyroepiglottic ligaments.

Oehme and Prier describe a surgical approach through an incision in the cricothyroid ligament to reach the lateral ventricles of the roarer (1974). They also discuss surgical repositioning of the arytenoid cartilage of the horse.

The cricoid cartilage is the third unpaired cartilage of the larynx, and it lies between the thyroid laminae and the first cartilaginous tracheal ring (Fig. 13–16). The caudal cornua of the thyroid cartilage articulates at the oval, concave facets at the junction of the lamina and arch on both sides of the cricoid cartilage.

On the dorsal surface of the lamina are two shallow concave areas from which the cricoarytenoideus dorsalis muscles arise. Caudally the cricoid cartilage is attached to the first tracheal ring by the cricotracheal membrane. Mucous membrane continuous with the infraglottic and tracheal cavities covers the inner surface of the cricoid cartilage. Two areas on the rostral border of the cricoid lamina are convex and smooth and articulate with each of the arytenoid cartilages.

Rostral to the cricoid cartilage and somewhat medial to the laminae of the thyroid cartilage are the two arytenoid cartilages. Their shape has been described as somewhat pyramidal (Getty 1975) and has been outlined in Figure 13–17. Attachment of the vocal ligament

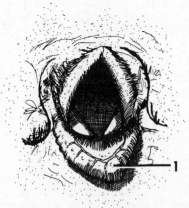

Figure 13–15 View of the equine epiglottis and laryngeal aditus obtained with an endoscope. (*1*), Apex of the epiglottis.

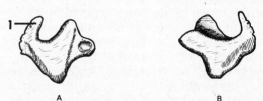

Figure 13–17 (*A*), Medial and (*B*) lateral views of the right arytenoid cartilage of the horse. The corniculate cartilage (*1*) is attached to the arytenoid cartilage. (After Getty, 1975.)

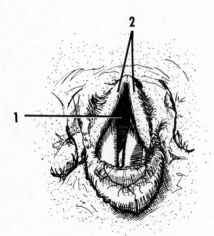

Figure 13–18 Dorsal endoscopic view of the laryngeal aditus of the horse (1) showing the paired corniculate cartilages meeting dorsally (2).

is at the vocal process where the rostral and caudal borders converge ventrally. The vocal muscle attaches at a rounded muscular process at the lateral angle of the base of each arytenoid cartilage. At the apex of each arytenoid cartilage is an area for attachment to the base of the respective corniculate cartilage. The corniculate cartilage is horn shaped and is shown attached to an arytenoid cartilage (Fig. 13–18). The two corniculate cartilages come quite close together dorsally. They are composed of elastic cartilage and form a distinctive anatomical landmark.

The strong cricoarytenoid ligament supports the ventromedial aspect of the cricoarytenoid joint. From the cricoid cartilage its fibers pass ventrally to attach to the medial surface of the arytenoid cartilages. The transverse arytenoid ligament is a narrow band that connects the dorsomedial angles of the opposing arytenoid cartilages.

There are eight pairs of intrinsic muscles of the equine larynx. The cricoarytenoideus dorsalis muscle is a paired intrinsic muscle and has been mentioned previously because of its importance in laryngeal dysfunction. Airflow is restricted by a flaccid vocal fold. The thyroarytenoideus muscle is composed of two parts, the rostral vestibular muscle and the vocalis muscle, which is located caudal to the lateral ventricle. The other paired muscles include the cricothyroideus, cricoarytenoideus lateralis, thyroarytenoideus accessorius, and tensor ventriculi lateralis. Finally, the unpaired arytenoideus transversus muscle attaches to the muscular processes of the arytenoid cartilages.

The most **cranial tracheal ring** (usually located ventral to the atlas) is nearly circular in cross section. The internal diameter of the upper trachea is about 5 cm. Between the larynx and thoracic inlet the trachea is called the cervical trachea. The shape of the tracheal cartilages changes to oval in the midcervical region, with the transverse distance being greater than the dorsoventral diameter. The thyroid gland is located superficial to the third and fourth cartilaginous rings, with the isthmus of this gland continuing around the ventral aspect of the trachea.

The wall of the equine trachea is composed of tracheal cartilage, mucosa, submucosa, and adventitia. The ends of the tracheal cartilages overlap dorsally in the caudal neck and thorax (Fig. 13–19).

In the upper cervical region the trachea is related dorsally to the esophagus; however, in the caudal cervical region it is beneath the longus colli muscles. Dorsolaterally the common carotid arteries, vagosympathetic nerve trunks, and recurrent laryngeal nerves are bound together by connective tissue into the carotid sheaths located superficial to the trachea.

The sternohyoideus muscles cover the trachea ventrally, with the medial borders of the right and left muscles meeting on the ventral midline. The sternomandibularis muscles are thick and fleshy at their origin from the sternum, and in the midcervical region they diverge from the ventral midline before continuing to their insertions on the mandible. Right and left **omohyoideus muscles** converge toward each other on

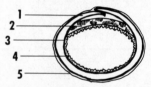

Figure 13–19 Cross section of the trachea of the horse through the tracheal cartilage (1) with the tracheal muscle (2), submucosal layer (3) beneath the mucosa (4), and the surrounding adventitia (5). (After Getty, 1975.)

the ventral midline cranial to where the **sternocephalicus muscles** diverge. The borders of the two pairs of muscles make a quadrilateral boundary, which may be palpated. A midventral tracheostomy can be performed at this boundary without penetrating either the sternomandibularis or the omohyoideus muscles.

In the midcervical region the esophagus is related to the left side of the trachea. Deep cervical lymph nodes, tracheal lymphatic ducts, and phrenic nerves lie in the neck near the trachea. The arterial blood supply to the tracheal wall is from the branches of the common carotid and bronchoesophageal arteries. Veins draining the trachea and associated structures are tributaries of the jugular and bronchoesophageal veins. Sympathetic and parasympathetic nerve fibers that supply the trachea originate from the sympathetic nerve trunks or the vagus nerves. Lymphatic drainage of the trachea is into the deep cervical, cranial, sternal, and mediastinal lymph centers.

Lower Airways

At the thoracic inlet the trachea continues within the mediastinum to the fifth or sixth intercostal space, where it terminates by dividing into the right and left principal bronchi. The tracheal bifurcation is dorsal to the heart, and the ridge formed between the principal bronchi is termed the carina. The esophagus lies on the dorsal surface at the carina after passing along the left lateral aspect of the trachea from the thoracic inlet to the third intercostal space. Considerable movement of the flexible trachea occurs with each breath and with the trachea's ventral association to the beating heart. The trachea passes dorsal to the cranial vena cava and the carotid and pulmonary arteries.

Tracheal muscle (*musculus trachealis*) extends between the inner surfaces of the ends of each cartilage. Tracheal muscle is composed of smooth muscle fibers. Negus reported that contraction of the tracheal muscles can reduce the diameter of the lumen, especially since the cartilages are not complete dorsally (1965).

In the horse the long thoracic cavity is like a cone that is compressed from either side with the narrowest portion at the thoracic inlet. The base is very oblique and is closed off from the abdominal cavity at the thoracic outlet by the diaphragm. The boundaries of the thorax and the components of the thoracic wall have been described.

The lateral attachments of the diaphragm, with its pleural covering, are along the eighth, ninth, and tenth costal cartilages to the sternal-costal articulation of the tenth rib. The diaphragm then continues in its attachment to the sternal ends of the eleventh, twelfth, and thirteenth ribs and then caudally to each rib at an increasing distance from their sternal ends until the line reaches the middle of the most caudal rib. The attachment of the diaphragm then follows the last rib dorsally to the area ventral to the vertebral end of the last intercostal space. Within the equine thoracic cavity the two pleural sacs are separated by a longitudinal septum, which lies somewhat to the left of midline. The heart is within this septum or mediastinum, as are all the organs in the thoracic cavity except the lungs, right phrenic nerve, and caudal vena cava.

PLEURA

The thick pulmonary pleura of the horse adheres closely to the lungs and is supplied by branches of the bronchial arteries. The deeper connective tissue layer of the pleura is drained by lymph channels and tributaries of the pulmonary veins. Lymph drains from the pulmonary pleura into the tracheobronchial lymph nodes (Smith 1979).

Parietal pleura adheres to the ribs (*pleura costalis*), diaphragm (*pleura diaphragmatica*), and mediastinum (*pleura mediastinalis*). In some horses the caudal mediastinum is very thin and appears to be incomplete. Intercostal arteries, the phrenic branches of the phrenicoabdominal arteries, and the mediastinal artery branches supply the parietal pleura. The venous drainage is via tributaries of regional vessels. Lymph from parietal pleura flows mainly into the sternal nodes except for mediastinal and diaphragmatic pleura, which flows into mediastinal lymph nodes. Parietal pleura is well supplied with receptor fibers from intercostal and phrenic nerves in addition to being autonomically innervated. In humans, diseases of the pleura can be very painful; the pain may be localized or it may be referred to the shoulder region.

There normally is a small amount of fluid in the pleural cavity, which allows the pulmonary pleura to slide freely over the parietal pleura. Pleural fluid is constantly being produced and resorbed at equal rates. In the horse, branches of systemic arteries supply both pulmonary and parietal pleura. There is probably no unidirectional resorption of fluid from one specific serosal surface relative to another surface of the pleura.

Parietal pleura is reflected along the sternum, thoracic vertebrae, and diaphragm in three clinically important "lines of pleural reflection." The sternal line of pleural reflection is where the costal pleura is reflected dorsally and becomes mediastinal pleura. The left and right sternal lines of pleural reflection are close together near the thoracic inlet, but they separate caudally on either side of the sternal attachment of the fibrous pericardium (sternopericardial ligament).

Along the bodies of the thoracic vertebrae the costal pleura turns ventrally to form the vertebral line of pleural reflection. It is continuous with the diaphragmatic pleura caudally. The costal pleura leaves the deep surface of the ribs and joins the diaphragmatic pleura along the diaphragmatic line of pleural reflection.

The diaphragmatic line of pleural reflection, with the costodiaphragmatic recess (recessus costodiaphragmaticus) lying immediately cranial to it, is important surgically. In paracentesis thoracis, the line is the demarcation between the thoracic and abdominal cavities. The diaphragmatic line of pleural reflection (Getty 1975) extends along the eighth and ninth costal cartilages, crosses the sternal end of the ninth rib, and passes caudad and dorsad in a gentle curve. It continues at a gradually increasing distance from the sternal ends of the ribs so that its most caudal part is at about the middle of the cranial border of the last rib. The middle of the cranial border of the last rib is the most caudal extent of

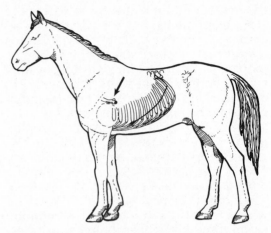

Figure 13–20 Surface features and palpable structures indicate the location of the carina and principal bronchi (near point of arrow). The topographical location of the heart is shown by a broken line, and the approximate position of the diaphragmatic line of pleural reflection is indicated by a solid line.

the pleural cavity, and here the diaphragmatic line curves medially and cranially and terminates near the vertebral end of the last intercostal space. A solid line in Figure 13–20 over the lateral surface of the caudal thorax illustrates the approximate position of the diaphragmatic line of pleural reflection. The costodiaphragmatic recess is located at that part of the pleural cavity within the acute angle formed by the reflection of pleura from ribs to diaphragm.

LUNGS

A horse lung has a caudal base (basis pulmonis) and apex (apex pulmonis), a costal surface (facies costalis), a medial surface (facies medialis), and three borders. An extensive and surgically important aspect of each lung is the costal surface. Pulmonary pleura closely covering the costal surface of the lung glides over the fluid-covered pleura on the ribs, which allows the lung to move easily during respiration. It is the costal surface of the lung that is seen by the surgeon as the costal pleura is incised and the pleural cavity is opened.

The three lung borders are the dorsal, ventral, and basal borders. The clinically important basal border is oval and bounds that portion of the lung directed toward the diaphragm (Fig. 13–21).

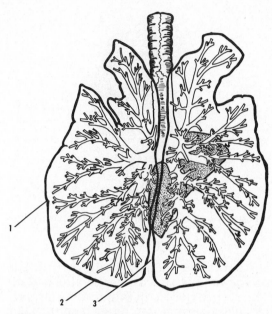

Figure 13–21 Dorsal view of the horse lungs showing the ventral (1), basal (2), and dorsal borders (3). (After Getty, 1975.)

The costal and medial surfaces of the lung are separated from the base of the lung by the basal border. That portion of the basal border between the diaphragmatic surface or base and the medial surface is broad and rounded. The lung is angular and the basal border is sharply defined between the base and the costal surface. The basal border extends into the costodiaphragmatic recess, although it does not usually fill the recess. Pleural fluid and small amounts of air are found in the costodiaphragmatic recess.

The lobules (*lobuli*) of the horse are incompletely separated by interlobular tissue (Tyler and Gillespie 1969). The lobule is the functional unit of the lung and is composed of a bronchiole, respiratory bronchioles, alveolar ducts, alveolar sacs, and alveoli. Division of the lung into small lobular units allows the changes in shape that the lungs make during respiratory movements.

Blood vessels of the lungs may be divided into those of the functional blood supply and those of the nutritional blood supply (Nickel et al. 1973). The functional blood supply comes from the pulmonary arteries, and it passes through the alveolar capillaries, leaving the lungs through the pulmonary veins. The functional blood supply nourishes the lung tissue distal to the bronchioles. The nutritional blood supply arises from the bronchoesophageal artery and follows as bronchial arteries along the branches of the bronchial tree. Bronchial arteries supply the bronchi proximal to the bronchioles. Since bronchial veins are absent, venous drainage is through the alveolar capillary networks and is returned by the pulmonary veins. In the horse, as in the human, the pulmonary arteries follow the bronchi distally, whereas tributaries of the pulmonary veins return intersegmentally as they collect blood from adjacent bronchopulmonary segments.

The hilus (*hilus pulmonis*) is located on the medial surface of the lung at the point at which the pulmonary pleura is reflected to the mediastinum. In this area the lung root (*radix pulmonis*) is composed of structures that enter or leave the lung. Three essential structures are found in the root—bronchus, pulmonary artery, and pulmonary vein. Associated with these are the bronchial vessels and nerves and the lymphatics. The principal bronchus is located dorsally in the roots of both lungs. Each bronchus has a bronchial artery near it, and the pulmonary veins usually lie ventral to the corresponding pulmonary arteries. A double layer of pleura, the pulmonary ligament (*ligamentum pulmonale*), leaves the lung caudal to the hilus.

RESPIRATORY STRUCTURES OF THE RUMINANT

Upper Airways

The nostril openings are bounded by epithelium, cartilage, and the bodies of the incisive bones. In cattle each nostril resembles an inverted comma (Fig. 13–22), with a lining of hairless integument continuing into the vestibule until it blends with nasal mucosa. Skin surrounding the nostrils is richly innervated with sensory fibers from the infraorbital nerve. Sheep (Fig. 13–23) and goats (Fig. 13–24) have slit-like nostril openings that are variable in size and shape. Contraction of muscles of the nose and face dilates the nostrils. The nostrils are fur-

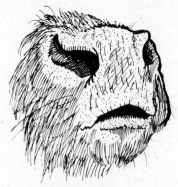

Figure 13–22 Dorsolateral view of the nasolabial plane and nostrils of the cow.

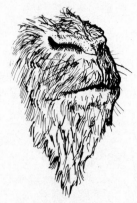

Figure 13–24 Dorsolateral view of the nasal plane and nostrils of the goat.

ther from each other dorsally than they are ventrally, and the **nasal septum** lies medial to them.

The nasal septum of older cattle may become ossified, especially ventrally where it articulates with the incisive bones. The median septum is relatively avascular; however, the mucosa covering it receives its blood supply from terminal branches of the palatine arteries.

Three cartilages support the nostrils and make them somewhat immobile. Medially, the hyaline cartilage of the nasal septum forms part of the skeleton of the nostrils. The rostral part of the dorsal lateral cartilage supports the medial aspect of the nostril and is separated from the remainder of the cartilage by a deep notch in cattle. The dorsal lateral cartilage extends further laterally in sheep and goats than in cattle. The third cartilage supporting the nostrils is the lateral accessory cartilage.

NASAL CAVITY

The opening of the nasolacrimal duct is in the vestibule of the nasal cavity immediately caudal to the nostril (about

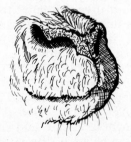

Figure 13–23 Dorsolateral view of the nasal plane and nostrils of the sheep.

2.5 cm). The opening is difficult to see on the medial surface of the alar fold, in contrast to horses in which the nasolacrimal duct orifice can be seen on the floor of the vestibule. Air passageways dorsal to the hard palate within the nasal cavity are smaller than would be supposed when examining the surface of the head. The walls of the bony skeleton of the ruminant face are thickened to contain sinus cavities, and the nasal cavity holds scrolls of turbinate bone, which further decrease the size of the airways. The passageways called meatuses are also reduced by thick mucous membranes that are heavily vascularized. The blood flow within the submucosa warms the air, but when vascular plexuses become congested the airways are decreased in size and interfere with nasal breathing.

Numerous plexuses, consisting mainly of veins, become engorged within nasal cavity submucosa and swell to reduce the flow of air. The vestibule of the nasal cavity is lined with stratified squamous epithelium, whereas the middle portion and nasal septum are covered with ciliated pseudostratified epithelium-containing serous glands. The lateral nasal gland lies close to the nasomaxillary opening in sheep and goats but is absent in cattle. Its duct, when present, runs along the middle meatus and opens into the vestibule so that secretions from the lateral nasal gland pass through the incisive duct into the oral cavity. The incisive duct (*ductus incisivus*) is a small tube opening on the floor of the ventral nasal meatus, which then passes ventrally into the oral cavity. It is about 6 cm long in cattle and 1 cm long in small ruminants, and it is lined with stratified epithelium. The mucosa contains olfactory nerve endings in the caudal part of the nasal cavity.

The ruminant nasal cavity is relatively long but becomes rather narrow caudally. The cavity is incompletely divided by the nasal septum, which fails to reach the floor caudoventrally. Therefore, a channel common to both halves of the nasal cavity is formed, called the nasopharyngeal meatus. A probe may be passed into the ventral nasal meatus, which then continues caudally through the nasopharyngeal meatus into the nasopharynx. The ventral and common nasal meatuses are the principal respiratory pathways. The middle nasal meatus communicates with the sinuses, and the dorsal meatus leads to the ethmoidal conchal spaces over mucosa involved with the sense of smell.

The dorsal nasal turbinate is widest in its middle part and tapers on either end. It is located in the dorsal part of the nasal cavity as shown in Figure 13–25 and extends from about the first cheek tooth to the cribriform plate of the ethmoid bone. The middle nasal turbinate is caudoventral to the dorsal nasal turbinate. Its rostral end is related ventrally to the ventral nasal turbinate at about the level of the last two cheek teeth. The broad ventral nasal turbinate extends from the notch formed by the articulation between the **incisive** and **nasal bones** to the level of the last cheek tooth. Continuing the ventral turbinate rostrally is the alar fold. There are differences among cattle, sheep, and goats in the ventral nasal turbinate that are described in detail by Nickel and associates (1973). The greater palatine, sphenopalatine, and ethmoidal arteries supply the nasal cavity, and venous drainage is through the corresponding regional veins. Innervation of the nasal cavity mucosa is from branches of the trigeminal and olfactory nerves with lymphatic drainage into the mandibular, parotid, and retropharyngeal lymph nodes.

PARANASAL SINUSES

Within the nasal turbinates are the dorsal, middle, and ventral turbinate sinuses. Sinuses, which are considered diverticula of the nasal cavity, extend into various parts of the skull so that ruminants have air spaces in the maxillary, palatine, lacrimal, frontal, and sphenoid bones.

The skull of the sheep with opened paranasal sinuses is outlined in Figure 13–26. Sheep have large lateral and small medial compartments of the frontal sinus. Openings from the nasal cavity allow *Oestrus ovis* larvae to enter the sinuses. Treatment may be given by puncturing the sinuses about 5 mm from the base of the horns or near the median line in polled sheep in a transverse plane through the middle of the orbit.

Right and left frontal sinuses of cattle are separated by a median septum. On both sides of the median septum there are venous tributaries draining laterally. Subcutaneously within the supraorbital groove the surgically important frontal vein is formed by several superficial veins. This large vein then enters the **supra-orbital foramen,** which may be palpated at the point at which the supraorbital canal originates, about 2 cm dorsocaudal to the lateral angles of the eyelids.

Mature cattle have a large caudal frontal sinus and three smaller rostral sinuses (Fig. 13–27). The caudal limit of the large part, which communicates with the cornual diverticulum in horned animals, is the occipital bone. The lateral limit of the frontal sinus is the **temporal**

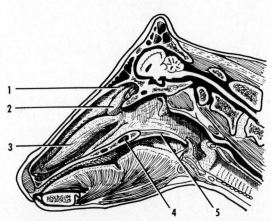

Figure 13–25 Sagittal section of the head of the cow made slightly to the right of the nasal septum. The dorsal (*1*), middle (*2*), and ventral nasal turbinates (*3*), palatine sinus (*4*), and soft palate (*5*), are outlined. (After Getty, 1975.)

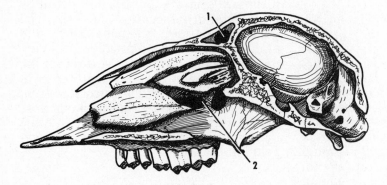

Figure 13–26 Sagittal section of the skull of the sheep showing the frontal (*1*) and the maxillary sinus (*2*). (After Popesko, 1977.)

Figure 13–27 Dorsal view of the skull of the cow with the external face of the frontal bone sculptured to expose the frontal paranasal sinus. (After Popesko, 1977.)

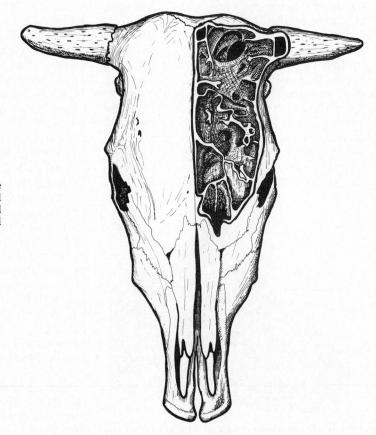

line, and the rostral limit is an oblique septum that passes from the middle of the orbit caudomedially to join the median septum.

Surgically important nuchal and postorbital diverticula of the frontal sinus lie caudal to the jugular process and orbit of the eye. A small opening to the caudal sinus from the nasal cavity passes through the ethmoid meatus. The three small rostal compartments lie between the rostral half of the orbit and the median septum. Each opens into the nasal cavity separately.

Topographical boundaries for the maxillary sinus extend from the orbit to a point slightly rostral to the **facial tuberosity.** The maxillary sinus is ventrally bounded by a line from the **zygomatic arch** to the facial tuberosity. The dorsal border is a line from the medial commissure of the eyes to the **infraorbital foramen.**

Most of the maxillary sinus (Fig. 13–28) is within the maxilla and zygomatic bones. It communicates with the caudal part of the nasal cavity through the nasomaxillary opening. In ruminants the maxillary sinus has a large common passageway with the palatine sinus over the infraorbital canal. A series of cross sections of an Angora goat head (Figs. 13–29, 13–30, and 13–31) illustrates the location of several paranasal sinuses. The cornual diverticulum of the frontal

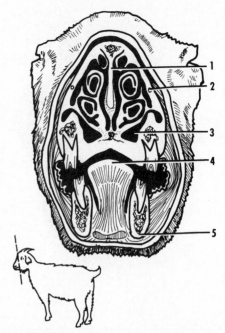

Figure 13–29 Cross section through the head of a goat viewed from the rostral aspect showing the nasal septum (*1*), infraorbital canal (*2*), palatine sinus (*3*), tongue (*4*), and mandible (*5*).

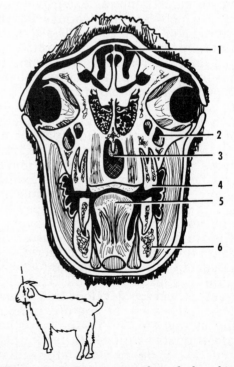

Figure 13–30 Cross section through the orbits of a goat's eyes viewed from the rostral aspect showing the frontal sinus (*1*), maxillary sinus (*2*), nasal septum (*3*), second molar (*4*), tongue (*5*), and mandible (*6*).

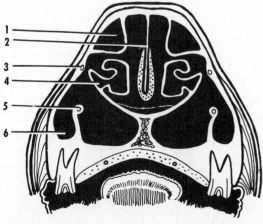

Figure 13–28 Cross section through the nasal cavity of the cow rostral to the orbits of the eyes showing dorsal turbinate sinus (*1*), nasal septum (*2*), nasolacriminal duct (*3*), ventral turbinate sinus (*4*), infraorbital canal (*5*), and maxillary sinus (*6*).

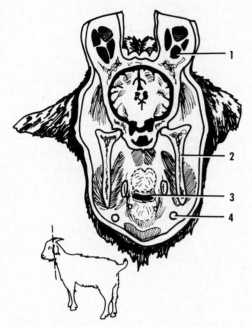

Figure 13–31 Cross section through the head of a goat viewed from the rostral aspect showing the cornual diverticulum of the frontal sinus (1), mandible (2), pharynx (3), and lingual vein (4).

sinus of goats is not as extensive as in cattle, which has implications for the dehorning of adult goats. The mucous membrane is especially sensitive to touch, and the remainder of the frontal sinus in goats is simply divided into medial and lateral compartments.

In cattle, the sinuses within bones surround the nasal cavity almost completely and extend into the caudal part of the skull. Maxillary, palatine, and lacrimal sinuses communicate with the middle nasal meatus through the nasomaxillary opening, whereas the frontal, sphenoidal, and conchal sinuses open separately in the caudal part of the nasal cavity.

The functions of the sinuses are thought to be protection and thermal insulation of the brain along with decreasing the weight of the skull. The sinus system is poorly developed in young calves, and even in mature animals some changes occur in the maxillary compartments as the cheek teeth erupt. Percussion of the frontal and maxillary sinuses may be done over the air-filled cavities; this procedure aids in locating the fluid levels following injury or dehorning.

PHARYNX

The pharyngeal septum, which continues caudally from the mid-dorsal line, divides the upper aspect of the nasopharynx into right and left parts. The septum is present in sheep, goats, and cattle projecting from the roof of the nasopharynx.

Lateral to the pharyngeal tonsil in the walls of the nasopharynx are two slits, the pharyngeal openings of the auditory tubes. They lie on a transverse plane passing just rostral to the level of the temporomandibular joints. A flap of mucosa covers each orifice. Caudodorsal to the orifice is a narrow, midline space termed the pharyngeal recess. The confluent choanae limit the nasopharynx toward the nasal cavity. Caudally the palatopharyngeal arches separate the nasopharynx from both the oropharynx and laryngopharynx as outlined in Figure 13–32.

The laryngopharynx lies lateral and dorsal to the larynx. Mucosa lining it continues without a visible demarcation line into the esophagus, and the pharyngoesophageal junction is arbitrarily located over the rostral portion of the lamina of the cricoid cartilage. In ruminants, the pyriform recesses remain open around the larynx during nasal breathing to allow saliva to flow into the esophagus without the swallowing movements that would disrupt breathing. There are

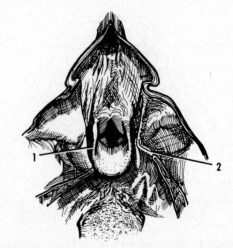

Figure 13–32 A view of the bovine larynx and esophagus obtained by cutting along the dorsal median line to show the epiglottis (1) and the palatopharyngeal arch (2). (After Getty, 1975.)

four muscles of the soft palate; they raise the palate to constrict the nasopharynx, flattening the soft palate and acting as a sphincter of the intrapharyngeal opening. The blood supply to the laryngopharynx is from branches of the ascending palatine and sphenopalatine arteries. A minor palatine vein that drains the soft palate and associated nasopharynx has been described in cattle.

LARYNX

On external palpation, the ruminant larynx feels rather short and wide. Orientation by finding the **mandibular rami,** the **body of the hyoid bone,** and the **thyroid** and **cricoid cartilages** is useful. Palpators who are accustomed to the topographical anatomy of the horse larynx may feel uncertain when first examining the ruminant because there is no caudal thyroid notch within the thyroid cartilage to separate it from the cricoid cartilage. Reduced space between the thyroid and cricoid cartilages makes the cricothyroid ligament much smaller than that of the horse. Tracheal cartilages palpable behind the cricoid cartilage assist in locating the caudal boundaries of the larynx.

Laterally, the constrictor, hyopharyngeus, cricopharyngeus, and thyropharyngeus muscles continue over the larynx to insert on the mid-dorsal raphe. The entrance to the esophagus also lies dorsal to the larynx. Caudally, the larynx is related to the rostral border of the thyroid gland, and ventrally the larynx is associated with the sternohyoideus muscle and the lingual tributary of the linguofacial vein.

The epiglottis projects above the floor of the laryngeal pharynx. This region may be examined with an endoscope, and the curled margins of the epiglottic cartilage and corniculate processes of the arytenoid cartilage are visible dorsal to the aryepiglottic folds.

The cavity of the larynx is distinguished by the absence of median and lateral ventricles. Vestibular walls continue with little irregularity to the glottic cleft, located where the infraglottic cavity begins. No vestibular folds are present; so the vocal folds together with the arytenoid cartilages form the glottis. The shape of the glottic opening varies.

During inspiration the vocal folds are drawn apart, whereas on expiration the glottis is narrowed by adduction of arytenoid cartilages and vocal folds. In ruminants the glottic cleft is never very wide, which places a limit on the outside diameter of an endotracheal tube used for inhalation anesthesia.

The laryngeal muscles are supplied by the recurrent laryngeal nerves, with the exception of the cricothyroideus muscles, which are innervated by the cranial laryngeal nerves. Section of the recurrent laryngeal nerves paralyzes both abductors and adductors of the vocal folds. The abductor effect of the dorsal cricoarytenoideus muscle is the more important to normal glottic movements, and after section of the nerve the vocal fold is held in partial adduction.

The cavity of the larynx is supported by the framework of cartilages and by the hyoid apparatus ventrolaterally. Intercartilaginous articulations between laryngeal cartilages allow movement between the parts of the larynx and between the organ and the supporting base of the hyoid bone with its attachments to the tongue. The thyroid and arytenoid cartilages of the goat are shown in Figure 13–33.

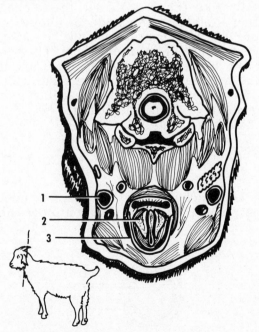

Figure 13–33 Cross section through the occipital bone of a goat showing the external jugular vein (*1*), an arytenoid cartilage (*2*), and the thyroid cartilage (*3*).

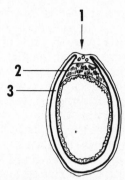

Figure 13–34 Cross section of the trachea of a cow showing lymphoid tissue *(1)* located dorsal to the tracheal muscle (2) and tracheal cartilage (3). (After Getty, 1975.)

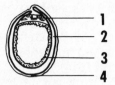

Figure 13–36 Cross section of the trachea of a goat showing the tracheal muscle *(1)*, tracheal cartilage (2), mucosa (3), and adventitia (4).

The trachea continues the upper airway caudal to the cricoid cartilage. Tracheal cartilages and spaces partially filled by annular ligaments are palpable near the rami of the mandible where the **sternomandibularis muscles** diverge to their mandibular insertions. The trachea is not subcutaneous between the larynx and thoracic inlet because the sternohyoideus muscles lie between it and the skin. Near the larynx the free ends of the tracheal cartilages are separated so that the airway is flattened, but further caudally the rings nearly come together dorsally. In cattle (Fig. 13–34), the trachea is of a relatively small outside diameter; the width is about 4 cm and the dorsoventral distance is about 5 cm. The trachea of sheep has overlapping ends of the tracheal cartilages as in Figure 13–35, whereas the tracheal cartilages of goats have a variable distance between their dorsal ends (Fig. 13–36).

Lower Airways

The trachea enters the thoracic inlet surrounded by fascia that continues the connective tissue of the neck. Loose fascia continuing into the thorax around the trachea provides a pathway for fluids and for the spread of infection. This is important, especially when there is a tear in the esophagus, which lies dorsal to the trachea within the thoracic inlet and mediastinum (Fig. 13–37). The overall length of the trachea in cattle is about 65 cm, and in sheep and goats the length is approximately 25 cm. The outside diameter of the trachea in smaller ruminants is about 2 cm.

The trachea lies dorsal to the tributaries of the cranial vena cava within the thoracic inlet and continues above the heart. During life the ruminant trachea lacks a dorsal ridge because of contraction of the trachealis muscle. Lymphoid

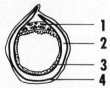

Figure 13–35 Cross section of the trachea of a sheep showing the tracheal muscle *(1)*, cartilage (2), mucosa (3), and adventitia (4). (After Getty, 1975.)

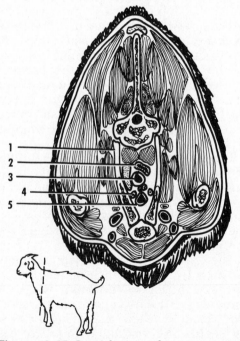

Figure 13–37 Cranial view of a cross section through the thoracic inlet of a goat showing the first rib *(1)*, esophagus (2), trachea (3), common carotid artery (4), and cranial vena cava (5).

tissue may be found in the space between the open ends of the bovine tracheal cartilages superficial to the trachealis muscle.

The trachea is related to the thymus; the lymphatics, and the sympathetic, vagal, phrenic, and recurrent laryngeal nerves. More caudally the aorta, azygos vein, and bronchopulmonary lymph nodes are also near the trachea, which adheres to the right lung from the third rib caudally. Before terminating at the carina opposite the fifth rib, the trachea gives off a tracheal bronchus, which goes to the cranial lobe of the right lung. In ruminants the cranial mediastinum is pushed across to the left side by the cranial part of the right lung. The ventral portion of the cranial mediastinum is thin and contains only a vestige of the thymus in older animals. Thoracic vertebrae approach the sternum near the thoracic inlet and in general reduce the mediastinum, although this is more obvious in the middle mediastinum, which contains the heart. Dorsally, the mediastinum contains the esophagus, pulmonary vessels, aortic arch, thoracic duct, large veins, lymph nodes, and vagal nerves. The septum is intact, although it may only be two sheets of pleura in some areas.

Caudal mediastinum is also generally thin and lengthens caudal to the heart. It contains the continuation of the aorta and vagal nerves. The mediastinum is pushed to the left by the large caudal lobe of the right lung.

THORACIC CAVITY

Compared with other species, the thoracic cavity of ruminants is short and wide. The thoracic inlet of the ox is about 22 to 25 cm in dorsoventral diameter, and in sheep or goats it is about 7.5 to 10 cm. The transverse diameter of the oval inlet in the ox is about 10 cm; its greatest width in sheep is approximately 5 cm.

The lateral walls of the thorax are flattened, giving a narrow outline to about the seventh intercostal space, where the ribs then arch outward rather evenly to the eleventh intercostal space, producing a more oval thoracic outlet. The thoracic outlet is closed by the diaphragm. The

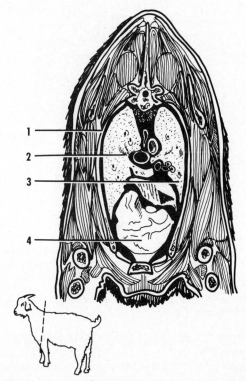

Figure 13–38 Cranial view of a cross section of the goat thorax through the fifth rib (1) showing that the right lung (2) is larger than the left lung (3). Outline of the left ventricle (4).

diaphragm extends further craniodorsal on the left side than it does on the right because the left half lies over the rumen and reticulum.

The thoracic cavity contains two pleural sacs separated on the median plane. Each pleural sac resembles half of a double-layered cone. The base of the cone is on the diaphragm. The apex reaches to the first rib and even beyond it on the right side, and the curved surface fits against the deep surface of the thorax. The pleura is relatively thick, and the two sacs are always completely separate. Because of the increased size of the right lung as opposed to the left (Fig. 13–38), the right pleural sac is larger than the left. On the right side the pleural sac extends cranially beyond the first rib deep to the scalenus muscle.

LUNGS

Each lung is invaginated within a pleural sac and is movable on its attachments at the hilus and pulmonary liga-

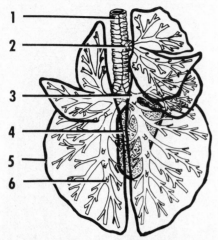

Figure 13–39 Dorsal view of the lungs of the cow showing the trachea (1), tracheal bronchus (2), right principal bronchus (3), accessory lobe of right lung (shaded) denoting interlobular septa (4), pulmonary pleura (5), and caudal lobar bronchus (6). (After Getty, 1975.)

ments. The lungs of the ox are relatively shorter in the craniocaudal axis than are those of the sheep and goat. The cranial apex, caudal base, and medial and costal surfaces are rather well defined, and the branching of the bronchial tree (Fig. 13–39) is similar to that outlined in the introduction. Large amounts of connective tissue form septae that demarcate areas of the lung surface and extend inward to divide the lung substance. These interlobular septae can be seen without magnification in cattle lungs as small polygonal areas on the lung surface. Interlobular septae become thickened during some disease processes and may help localize infection.

In Figure 13–40, the caudal vena cava is outlined as it passes to the heart within the caval fold of pleura. The right phrenic nerve passes from the base of the heart to the diaphragm, with the caudal vena cava within a separate fold of pleura, which is continuous with the plica vena cava. The mediastinal recess, which contains the accessory lobe of the right lung, is medial to the caval fold.

RESPIRATORY SYSTEM OF THE PIG

Upper Airways

The round nostrils open on the flattened surface (*planum rostrale*) of the

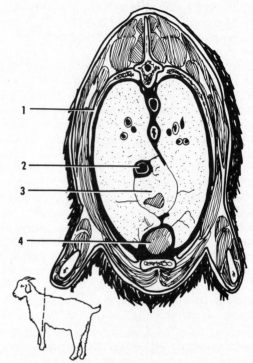

Figure 13–40 Cranial view of a cross section of the goat through the seventh rib (1) showing the caudal vena cava within the caval fold of pleura (2), the accessory lobe of the right lung lying in the mediastinal recess (3), and the apex of the heart (4).

snout. The openings are lined with epithelium and are supported by cartilage and bone (Fig. 13–41). A rostral bone (*os rostrale*) lies under the skin between the nostrils and is in the form of a transverse plate attached to the nasal septum. The rostral bone serves as a firm adaptation for digging, and the connective tissues

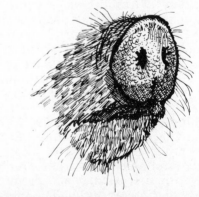

Figure 13–41 Dorsolateral view of the snout and nostrils of the pig.

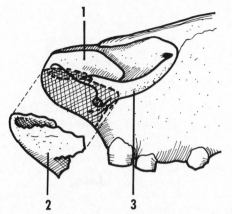

Figure 13–42 Lateral projection of the dorsal lateral nasal cartilage (*1*), rostral bone (*2*), and ventral lateral nasal cartilage (*3*). (After Getty, 1975.)

allow some mobility of the nostrils during inspiration and expiration.

The dorsal lateral cartilages shown in Figure 13–42 arise from the nasal septum and rostral bone. Projecting laterally from the ventral portion of the rostral bone is the lateral accessory cartilage (Fig. 13–43).

Sensory nerve impulses are carried from the nostrils by infraorbital nerve fibers. Muscles that move the nose and nostrils are innervated by the facial nerve. The nostrils and surrounding skin are supplied by terminal branches of the infraorbital and palatine arteries.

NASAL CAVITY

The nasal cavity of the pig is relatively long and narrow, although this depends

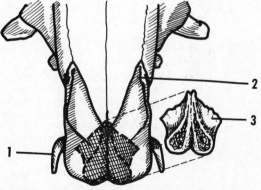

Figure 13–43 Dorsal views of the lateral accessory cartilage (*1*), dorsal lateral nasal cartilage (*2*), and rostral bone of the pig (*3*). (After Getty, 1975.)

to a degree on the shape of the head. The nasal septum is distinctive in that it has an osseous part, a cartilaginous part, and a membranous part. The perpendicular plate of the ethmoid bone and the vomer compose the bony portion. Hyaline cartilage makes up the central part, and the caudal nasal septum is composed of mucous membrane.

A transverse bony plate (*lamina transversalis*) covered with periosteum and mucous membrane divides the nasal cavity into a dorsal olfactory portion and a ventral respiratory portion. The respiratory portion surrounds the air passageway through the ventral nasal meatus and the caudal nares into the nasopharyngeal meatus. The crest of the midline vomer is continued caudally by a fold of mucous membrane, which forms the membranous part of the nasal septum and divides the dorsal aspect of the nasopharynx into right and left halves.

Much of the nasal cavity is filled with nasal conchae, and a relatively small amount of space remains for air to flow through. The long, narrow dorsal nasal concha extends from the cribriform plate of the ethmoid bone to the rostral portion of the nasal bone. A dorsal conchal sinus lies within the dorsal concha and communicates with the airspace within the caudal part of the nasal bone. The broad, ventral nasal concha, including its sinus, occupies the floor of the nasal cavity. Between the dorsal and ventral nasal conchae in the lateral wall of the nasal cavity are the nasofrontal and nasomaxillary apertures. The middle nasal concha lies ventral to the dorsal concha and also contains a conchal sinus. The conchae and meatuses of the pig are shown in Figure 13–44.

The ventral nasal meatus is located between the ventral nasal concha and the mucosa covering the floor of the nasal cavity. An opening of the nasolacrimal duct occurs in the caudal portion of the ventral meatus. The smaller dorsal nasal meatus lies between the mucosa covering the nasal bones and the dorsal nasal concha. A narrow, middle nasal meatus communicates with the nasomaxillary opening at about the level of the fifth or sixth cheek tooth. Connecting the dorsal, middle, and ventral meatuses is the common nasal meatus, which lies

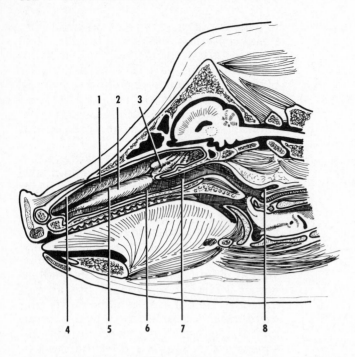

Figure 13–44 Lateral view of a sagittal section of the head of the pig showing the dorsal (*1*), ventral (*2*), and middle nasal turbinates (conchae) (*3*). Note the dorsal (*4*), middle (*5*), and ventral nasal meatuses (*6*), the nasopharyngeal meatus (*7*), and the pharyngeal diverticulum (*8*). (After Popesko, 1977.)

between the conchae and the nasal septum. Several air passageways lie between the ethmoid conchae; they lead to the openings into the frontal, lacrimal, and sphenoidal sinuses. Continuing the common nasal meatus into the nasopharynx is the nasopharyngeal meatus.

PARANASAL SINUSES

In adult pigs the frontal sinuses are extensive and compose the largest of paranasal sinuses. The internal and exter-

nal plates of the frontal bones are widely separated dorsal to the brain, and a transverse septum divides the air-filled cavity into rostral and caudal compartments as shown in Figure 13–45. The right and left frontal sinuses are separated by a septum.

The caudal frontal sinus is excavated within the occipital bones and may extend into parts of the temporal bones of adult animals. Two rostral frontal sinuses lie medial to the orbit. The lacrimal sinus, which is located between the frontal and maxillary sinuses, lies lateral

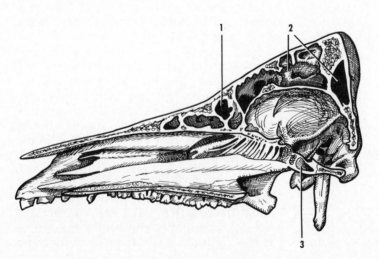

Figure 13–45 View of the right half of the skull of the pig showing the outline of a rostral portion of the frontal sinus (*1*), caudal parts of the frontal sinus (*2*), and the sphenoid sinus (*3*). (After Popesko, 1977.)

to the rostral compartments of the frontal sinuses.

Within the maxilla and to some degree within the zygomatic, lacrimal, and ethmoid bones is a well-developed maxillary sinus. A ridge or lamella divides the cavity into medial or lateral recesses, and deep to the lamella is the osseous portion of the infraorbital canal. The nasomaxillary opening connects the nasal cavity with the maxillary sinus.

In mature swine the sphenoid sinus has a large central cavity and three recesses. The location of this sinus is important because it is ventral to the optic chiasm within the presphenoid and basisphenoid bones. The largest sphenoid sinus recess is in the squamous part of the temporal bone.

NASOPHARYNX

Air passing through the caudal nares enters the relatively narrow nasopharynx. The thick soft palate continues the hard palate caudally for about 5 cm in the adult, and it usually has a small projection on its free border called a uvula. This projection, with the remainder of the free edge of the soft palate and the palatopharyngeal arches, borders the intrapharyngeal opening.

Caudal to the soft palate and dorsal to the esophagus is the median pharyngeal diverticulum. This blind pouch is lined with mucosa and is about 4 cm deep. It is dorsal to the esophagus and the caudal boundary of the intrapharyngeal opening. It may trap an endoscope intended for the trachea, and a vigorous push can send the tip of the tube through the mucosal lining of the pharyngeal diverticulum.

The pharyngeal septum extends caudally to the level at which the auditory tubes open into the pharynx. Ventrally the laryngopharynx surrounds the laryngeal opening.

LARYNX

Immediately caudal to the aperture into the pig larynx is a median laryngeal ventricle. It lies within the floor of the vestibule in a manner similar to that noted in the horse (Fig. 13–46). The aryepiglottic folds, which connect the bor-

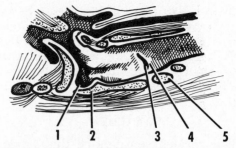

Figure 13–46 Sagittal section of the laryngeal region of the pig as viewed from the left side showing the median laryngeal ventricle (*1*), thyroid cartilage (*2*), lateral laryngeal ventricle (*3*), vocal fold (*4*), and arch of the cricoid cartilage (*5*). (After Popesko, 1977.)

ders of the epiglottis with the dorsal walls of the laryngopharynx, are the lateral boundaries of the laryngeal opening in swine. In horses the arytenoid cartilages provide dorsal points of attachment for right and left aryepiglottic folds.

No vestibular folds project into the cavity of the pig larynx, but lateral ventricles, which lie between the vocal ligaments, occur at the caudal aspect of the elongated vestibule. The caudal portion of the vocal ligament and the thyroarytenoideus muscle form the vocal folds.

Mucous membrane lining the cavity of the larynx is loosely attached except over the caudal aspect of the epiglottis, on the vocal ligaments, and over the medial aspect of the cricoid cartilage. Small amounts of lymphoid tissue may be present in the laryngeal mucosa. Muscles of the larynx are unusual because the thyroarytenoid muscle is not separated into ventricularis and vocalis portions.

The thyroid cartilage of the swine larynx is lengthy and has extensive laminae. Located on the ventral body of the thyroid cartilage is a thickened laryngeal prominence. The arch of the cricoid cartilage lies caudal to the body of the thyroid cartilage. The laryngeal cavity is an oval shape within the cricoid cartilage. Rostral to the lamina of the cricoid cartilage lie the arytenoid cartilages. They resemble a three-sided pyramid with the apex directed rostrally and the base caudally. Between the ventral border and the base is the vocal process where the dorsal aspect of the vocal fold attaches. Corniculate cartilages are fused with the arytenoid cartilages and project dorsally and medially. Several ligaments attach the laryngeal cartilages to each other, with the distinctive cricotracheal ligament attaching the caudal border of the cricoid cartilage to the cranial border of the first tracheal ring.

TRACHEA

The cervical portion of this flexible tube continues the upper airway to the thoracic inlet. The trachea is almost circular in cross section (Fig. 13–47) and has from 32 to 36 cartilages within the wall. Cranially in the neck the esophagus lies dorsal to the trachea, but as the trachea enters the thoracic inlet it comes in contact with vertebral muscles and the esophagus is displaced dorsolaterally to the left. The carotid sheath, which contains the common carotid artery, internal jugular vein, vagosympathetic trunk, and recurrent laryngeal nerve, crosses the lateral surface of the trachea in an oblique manner. Lobes of the thyroid gland extend from immediately caudal to the larynx over about the first six tracheal rings. Up to approximately one year of age the thymus gland is found in the neck ventral to the trachea.

Lower Airways

In mature pigs the length of the trachea from the first tracheal ring to its termination is about 15 to 20 cm, and it usually terminates at the level of the fifth thoracic vertebra. At that level the tracheal bifurcation lies to the right of the midline and on its left side is related to the arch of the aorta. Before dividing at the carina, the trachea courses within the craniodorsal region of the mediastinum.

The mediastinum is located in the mid-

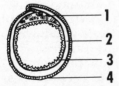

Figure 13–47 Cross section of the trachea of the pig showing the tracheal muscle (*1*), tracheal cartilage (*2*), mucosa (*3*), and adventitia (*4*). (After Getty, 1975.)

dle of the thorax except for the ventral portion of the cranial mediastinum, where it is deflected to the left by the cranial lobe of the right lung. This places the cranial mediastinal pleura in contact with the left costal parietal pleura. Ventral to the esophagus the caudal mediastinum is forced to the left by the accessory lobe of the right lung. Both pleural sacs are complete, and no communication exists through the caudal mediastinum.

The diaphragmatic line of pleural reflection can be traced along the eighth costal cartilage to the costochondral articulation of the eighth rib. It extends to the middle of the fourteenth rib in a curve, which turns toward the median plane dorsally. Fibroelastic endothoracic fascia attaches the pleura firmly to the inner surface of the thoracic cavity.

When sectioned transversely at the sixth intercostal space, the pig thorax is more cylindrical than that of the horse. The sixth interspace may be used as an example of intercostal blood supply for the pig chest wall where there may be 13 or 14 intercostal spaces. Dorsally, the aorta gives rise to the sixth intercostal artery, and because the aorta is to the left of the vertebral column, the right sixth intercostal artery is longer than the left. The artery continues ventrally behind the rib between the intercostal vein and nerve. Near the sternum the intercostal arteries anastomose with the internal thoracic arteries, which divide caudally to become the cranial superficial and deep epigastric arteries. Medial to the first two pairs of ribs and intercostal spaces, the internal thoracic arteries lie in contact with pleura before they dive beneath the transversus thoracis muscle. To avoid entering the pleural cavity to ligate an internal thoracic artery, the procedure should be done caudal to the third intercostal space.

LUNGS

The right lung of the pig is larger than the left, as it is composed of four lobes as compared with the two lobes of the left lung. Lobation of both lungs follows the pattern listed in Table 13–2. The tracheal bronchus provides an airway from the trachea for the undivided cra-

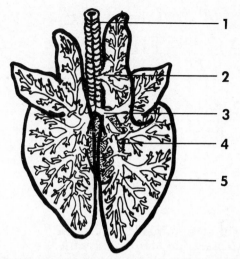

Figure 13–48 Dorsal view of the lungs of the pig showing the trachea (*1*), tracheal bronchus (*2*), right principal bronchus (*3*), accessory lobe of right lung (shaded) (*4*), and pulmonary pleura (*5*). (After Getty, 1975.)

nial lobe of the right lung as outlined in Figure 13–48. Pulmonary pleura adhering to all surfaces of the lungs gives them a glistening appearance over the normally pink-colored parenchyma.

The costal surfaces form the largest area over the lungs and can be approached surgically using the en bloc thoracotomy technique of Lumb and Butterfield (1977). This technique enables the surgeon to approach the costal surface of the right lung, which is larger than either the medial or diaphragmatic surface.

A principal bronchus enters each lung at the caudodorsal aspect of the hilus. Pulmonary artery branches form part of the lung root together with each principal bronchus. Generally, the pulmonary artery lies on the opposite side of the bronchus as does the lobar vein. The bronchial branch of the bronchoesophageal artery passes ventrally from the aorta to reach the dorsal aspect of the bifurcation of the trachea. The bronchial artery then divides into a separate vessel supplying the cranial lobe of the right lung and its terminal branches. Terminal bronchial branches end by surrounding the bronchioles in a capillary network, formed together with branches from the pulmonary arteries.

Afferent lymph channels leave the roots of the lungs as they pass to the thoracic duct on the left side. The tracheobronchial lymph nodes are associated with the lung roots, as are the bronchial nerves, and are of surgical significance in removing a lung. Intrapulmonary septae of the pig lungs are relatively heavy. They separate the boundaries of the lobules, which can be seen on close inspection of the lung surfaces.

REFERENCES

Cook, W. R.: Some observations on disease of the ear, nose and throat in the horse, and endoscopy using a flexible fiberoptic endoscope. Vet. Rec. *94*:533, 1974.

Foerner, J. R.: The diagnosis and correction of false nostril noises. *In* Proceedings of the American Association of Equine Practitioners *13*:315, 1967.

Getty, R.: Sisson and Grossman's The Anatomy of the Domestic Animals, 5th ed. Philadelphia: W. B. Saunders, 1975, pp. 104–1296.

Habel, R. E.: Applied Veterinary Anatomy, 2nd ed. Ithaca, NY: Robert E. Habel, 1978, pp. 175–179.

Julian, L. M., and Tyler, W. S.: Functional Comparative Anatomy of the Domestic Animals. Davis, CA: School of Vet. Med., U.C. Davis, 1962, pp. 172–187.

Lumb, W. V., and Butterfield, A. B.: En bloc thoracotomy in miniature swine. Am. J. Vet. Res., *38*:285, 1977.

Negus, V.: The Biology of Respiration. London: E. and S. Livingston, 1965, pp. 109–110.

Nickel, R., Schummer, A., Seiferle, E., and Sack, W. O.: The Viscera of the Domestic Mammals. Berlin: Verlag Paul Parey, 1973, pp. 211–279.

Nomina Anatomica Veterinaria, 2nd ed. Vienna: World Association of Veterinary Anatomists, 1973, pp. 51–56.

Oehme, F. W., and Prier, J. E.: Textbook of Large Animal Surgery. Baltimore: Williams & Wilkins, 1974, pp. 340–359.

Popesko, P.: Atlas of Topographical Anatomy of the Domestic Animals, Vol. 2, 2nd ed. Philadelphia: W. B. Saunders, 1977, pp. 12–161.

Robinson, N. E., Sorenson, P. R., and Goble, D. O.: Patterns of airflow in normal horses and horses with respiratory disease. *In* Proceedings of the American Association of Equine Practitioners *21*:11, 1975.

Smith, B. P.: Diseases of the pleura. Vet. Clin. North Am. *1*:197, 1979.

Tyler, W. S., and Gillespie, J. R.: Animal models for biomedical research II. Washington DC: Publication #1736 National Academy of Sciences, 1969, pp. 38–51.

RESPIRATORY PHYSIOLOGY OF THE SURGICAL PATIENT

J. R. GILLESPIE, D.V.M., Ph.D.,
AND T. C. AMIS, B.V.Sc., Ph.D.

INTRODUCTION

The aims of this section are (1) to present some of the newer, general knowledge of respiratory physiology of large domestic animals; and (2) to provide the reader with the opportunity to critically review and select that which he believes will improve the care of his surgical patients. New information about respiratory physiology of large domestic animals has come forth in recent years; however, it is all too often sparse for particular species and often nearly totally lacking for others. Of necessity, we will speak in general terms about most aspects of cardiopulmonary physiology and we will be specific only when good data exist on a particular species. We will be more interested in presenting a useful overall picture than in being rigorous in citing all the studies on detailed aspects of function in any one species.

The *respiratory system* is defined as all those body structures involved in the transport and exchange of respiratory gases between the animal's (organism's) environment and its metabolic machinery. The respiratory system of terrestrial mammals includes the *pulmonary* and *cardiovascular systems.*

The fact that the life of tissues or the animal cannot continue if there is respiratory failure for as little as a few minutes emphasizes the importance of this system to the surgical patient and the veterinary surgeon. Although animals have, in general, evolved with significant respiratory reserve, general anesthesia and surgical procedures cause significant dysfunction of this system. In addition, animals whose reserve has been compromised by disease processes are placed at significantly increased risk when subjected to the respiratory dysfunction associated with any surgical procedure. We will introduce some of these often interrelated problems in this section and then discuss them in more detail along with possible preventive measures in a section to follow.

Depressive Effects of General Anesthetic Agents upon Cardiopulmonary Function. Most general anesthetic agents, if used in sufficient dosages to produce analgesia in the patient, also produce some degree of respiratory dysfunction. These effects include central nervous system changes that affect cardiovascular and respiratory control and local effects on cardiac, vascular, and perhaps epithelial tissue (e.g., depression of cilia activity).

Position of Patient During Surgical Procedures. Surgical procedures frequently require particular positions and restraint procedures that compromise the normal movement and function of the respiratory system structures. These mechanical constraints can be serious and complex in their effects upon lung function.

Surgical Manipulation Around the Thoracic and/or Abdominal Compartments. Respiratory muscles include some of those in the thoracic and abdominal walls in domestic mammals. Cutting these muscles, applying pressure, and/or restraining their motion by putting them under stress or tension can limit their ability to do respiratory work. Certainly, opening the chest is a very serious and special case, in which surgical manipulation has very pronounced effects on respiratory function.

Blood-Loss Anemia with Surgery. Ane-

356

mia may be viewed as a special and very important consequence of surgical manipulation. Healthy blood, present in sufficient quantities and of adequate quality, is essential for the transport of respiratory gases and nutrients (including electrolytes and water) and the buffering of hydrogen ion (H^+) in the surgical patient.

Body Heat Regulation with Surgery. Depending on other heat loss and preservation mechanisms available to a particular species, the respiratory system plays a greater or lesser role in heat regulation for an animal. Most often there is a degree of hypothermia in surgical patients that may be complicated by various positive pressure ventilatory procedures.

Acid-Base Regulation During Surgery. The regulation of acid-base balance in the animal is as important as respiratory gas exchange to the life of the tissues and the whole animal. Intracellular, and ultimately extracellular, hydrogen ion concentration ($[H^+]$) must not vary too much from normal if the metabolic enzymes are to function properly and produce the energy required for life. A disturbance in respiratory function can perturb the normal acid-base regulation by compromising CO_2 removal. The resulting acidosis (CO_2 retention) can cause secondary disturbances of other body functions, e.g., gastrointestinal function and the body's electrolyte balance.

Problems Associated with Recovery from General Anesthesia. Several potentially serious problems can develop during the immediate postsurgical period and during recovery from general anesthesia. They include (1) adaptation to a new inspired gas mixture associated with no longer breathing from the closed circuit anesthesia machine; (2) pulmonary atelectasis and/or edema; (3) cardiovascular shock and pulmonary edema associated with recovery trauma and postsurgical pain; and/or (4) chest wall and/or abdominal pain.

Special Surgical Problems Associated with Patients with Cardiopulmonary Disease. The heart and lungs operate with significant margins of safety in healthy animals. However, if they are diseased and/or have additional stress, such as general anesthesia, they may precipitously fail.

Management of the patient with respiratory disease during general anesthesia is difficult, and surgery should be postponed, if possible, until the patient has recovered from the respiratory disease.

Special Cardiopulmonary Problems During Surgery in Particular Species. There are particular cardiopulmonary problems associated with surgery in ruminants and larger domestic animals. Most of these problems are caused by mechanical constraints to the free movement of the pulmonary system.

OVERVIEW OF RESPIRATORY FUNCTION

Before discussing in detail the respiratory problems associated with general anesthesia and surgical procedures, we will describe the divisions of respiratory function and their underlying mechanisms. We will emphasize those aspects of respiratory function that are known to be most affected by general anesthesia and surgical procedures and those that are newer and may not have been a part of your previous reading on the respiratory system.

The major function of the respiratory system is gas exchange between the environment and the intracellular metabolic machinery (IMM) of the organism. The respiratory system has two major divisions: *pulmonary* and *cardiovascular*. The detailed structural relationships of these two systems are beyond the scope of this section. It is essential that the reader have a knowledge of the structure of these systems and their relationships for a useful understanding of respiratory function.

Briefly, the pulmonary system includes all the conducting airways from the mouth or nares to the bronchioles entering the alveolar spaces, the alveolar-capillary membranes, the pulmonary circulation, the associated pulmonary nerves and lymphatics, the chest wall and diaphragm, and the associated neuromuscular systems that move the pulmonary structures during breathing. The cardiovascular system includes the heart, blood, the right (pulmonary) and left (systemic) side vascular systems, and the associated nervous and endocrine control systems (Fig. 13–49).

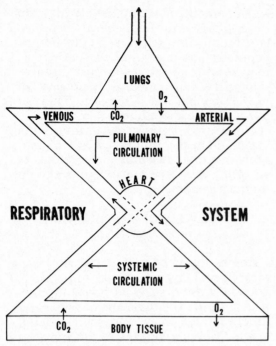

Figure 13–49 Model of respiratory system that includes schema of pulmonary system (lungs) at top of model and schemata of pulmonary and systemic circulations at bottom of model.

Pulmonary Respiratory Function

Two complex processes operate in the pulmonary system to bring about gas exchange between the environment and the pulmonary capillary blood (PCB): *ventilation* and *diffusion* of gas from the alveolar space to the PCB.

Ventilation. Ventilation (or total ventilation) ($\dot{V}$) is the process by which gas is pumped into (inspiration) and out of (expiration) the lung. It is measured as the volume of gas per minute (Vmin) entering or leaving the lungs and is the product of the breath size or *tidal volume* (VT) and number of breaths per minute or *frequency* (f). It follows that $\dot{V}$ = VT × f. VT has two parts: the *dead space volume* (VD) and the *alveolar volume* (VA), and VT = VD + VA (Fig. 13–50). Viewed anatomically, VD is that part of the VT going only to airways during the breath cycle and VA is that part going to the alveolar space. From this, we may write $\dot{V}$ = (VD + VA)f or $\dot{V}$ = fVD + fVA. The gas entering or leaving the VD per minute is f VD and is called *dead space ventilation* ($\dot{V}$D). Similarly, the gas entering the VA per minute is fVA and is the *alveolar ventilation* ($\dot{V}$A). We can write total ventilation ($\dot{V}$) as $\dot{V}$ = $\dot{V}$D + $\dot{V}$A. It should be noted that $\dot{V}$A is the *effective ventilation* in terms of respiratory gas exchange. If $\dot{V}$D becomes larger with certain pulmonary diseases or general anesthesia (e.g., very long endotracheal tube), then the effective ventilation ($\dot{V}$A) may well be decreased. We will discuss this point in more detail later.

Up to this point we have described $\dot{V}$D as occurring only in the airways and $\dot{V}$A as occurring in the anatomically defined alveolar spaces. It is important to define $\dot{V}$D and $\dot{V}$A functionally to appreciate abnormalities that occur during general

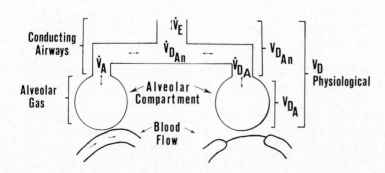

Figure 13–50 Model of the pulmonary system depicting the conducting airways in which the anatomical dead space (VD$_{An}$) and two alveoli are shown. The alveolus on the left receives pulmonary capillary blood flow; the one on the right does not. The gas in the alveolus on the right is alveolar dead space gas (VD$_A$). Physiological dead space (V$_D$) is the sum of the VD$_{An}$ and VD$_A$. Total ventilation ($\dot{V}$E) is the sum of the effective alveolar ventilation ($\dot{V}$A) (left alveolus), $\dot{V}$DA (right alveolus), and $\dot{V}$D$_{An}$.

anesthesia, surgical procedures, and/or pulmonary disease. Functionally, $\dot{V}_A$ is that part of the ventilated gas volume that takes part in respiratory gas exchange between the air spaces and the pulmonary capillary blood (PCB). In the healthy lung, gas exchange with the PCB takes place through most of the alveolar-capillary membranes and also through the walls of some of the adjoining, very small, airways. Even in the healthy lung, some alveolar spaces contribute very little or nothing to gas exchange because, for example, they have little or no blood flow in relation to their ventilation. Since respiratory gas exchange is not limited to alveolar-capillary membranes, the term *exchange area* is used to describe all of the surfaces in the lung where gas exchange occurs. Since the V_D is not only in the airways but also in the alveolar space, there are two dead space volumes: *anatomical dead space* (in the airways) and *alveolar dead space* (in the alveoli where gas exchange is absent or very small). Increases in V_D with pulmonary disease or general anesthesia occur most often because of increases in alveolar dead space. Again, note that since $\dot{V} = \dot{V}_D + \dot{V}_A$, at a constant $\dot{V}$, an increase in $\dot{V}_D$ requires a decrease in effective ventilation ($\dot{V}_A$) and a decrease in respiratory gas exchange (see Fig. 13–50).

An important part of pulmonary ventilation is the complex chest wall and diaphragmatic movements that cycle gas in and out of the exchange area. These movements involve muscle groups in the chest wall and abdominal wall in addition to the diaphragm. The complexity of the integration of the movement of these groups of muscles is only beginning to be understood in some animals. At least two very important features of the ventilatory motion (breathing) are modified by general anesthesia and/or some surgical procedures: (1) central respiratory neural drive and associated neuromuscular activity to the respiratory muscles; and (2) distribution of respiratory muscle work between the various respiratory muscle groups. Since control of breathing is associated with both the pulmonary and cardiovascular respiratory functions, we will describe this aspect after our discussion of the respiratory function of the cardiovascular system.

Pulmonary Diffusion. The second process of pulmonary gas exchange is diffusion from the alveolar space to the PCB. This is a passive process (requiring no metabolic energy) in which there is (1) a net transfer of oxygen (O_2) from the pulmonary gas space (PGS) through the pulmonary tissue membranes to the pulmonary capillary blood (PCB), where it is bound to hemoglobin (Hb); and (2) a net transfer of carbon dioxide (CO_2) from the PCB to the PGS. The force that drives the diffusion of O_2 and CO_2 is the concentration difference of these gases between the two spaces: PGS and PCB. Since the animal's tissues take up O_2 to produce high-energy compounds, there is a constant drain of the O_2 from the blood; the O_2 concentration in the PCB as it enters the pulmonary capillaries is less than in the PGS. On the other hand, since the animal's tissue forms CO_2 as a product of energy metabolism and since the fresh gas breathed in at the nose has only traces of CO_2 in it, the CO_2 concentration in the PCB as it enters the pulmonary capillaries exceeds that in the PGS.

To understand pulmonary diffusion more completely and to see what circumstances may affect O_2 and CO_2 exchange during surgical procedures, we will look at factors that influence the diffusion force or pressure for each gas and their relationships. We can express the diffusion force for O_2 and CO_2 as a function of the partial pressure differences for these gases between the PGS and PCB. We can write the partial pressure difference for O_2 as $P_{A_{O_2}} - P\bar{c}_{O_2}$ and for CO_2 as $P\bar{c}_{CO_2} - P_{A_{CO_2}}$ where $P_{A_{O_2}}$ is the partial pressure of O_2 in the PGS and $P\bar{c}_{O_2}$ is the mean partial pressure of O_2 in the blood along an average pulmonary capillary. $P\bar{c}_{CO_2}$ is the mean partial pressure of CO_2 in the PCB, and $P_{A_{CO_2}}$ is the partial pressure of CO_2 in the PGS. In general, the greater the $P_{A_{O_2}} - P\bar{c}_{O_2}$ or $P\bar{c}_{CO_2} - P_{A_{CO_2}}$, the greater will be the net transfer between the PGS and PCB for O_2 and CO_2, respectively.

Beginning with O_2 diffusion, we will examine first those factors that may determine $P_{A_{O_2}}$. Keeping $P\bar{c}_{O_2}$ constant, increasing $P_{A_{O_2}}$ will, in general, increase the net transfer of O_2 to the PCB. Three interrelated factors affect PA_{O_2}: (1) the O_2 concentration or partial pressure in the inspired gas (PI_{O_2}); (2) the level of alveolar ventilation ($\dot{V}A$); and (3) the rate of removal of O_2 from the PGS compared with its "renewal" by $\dot{V}A$.

The concentration of O_2 in the inspired gas is an important consideration during general anesthesia in which a closed circuit anesthesia machine is used and all the O_2 must be supplied to the machine and animal from an external O_2 supply. When the animal is breathing air at sea level, the O_2 concentration in the inspired gas is 20 per cent and the PI_{O_2} is about 150 torr. If the animal is breathing an O_2-enriched mixture, PI_{O_2} will be greater than 150 torr. At high altitudes or if insufficient O_2 is added to the closed-circuit anesthesia machine, PI_{O_2} will be less than 150 torr. In general, the greater the PI_{O_2}, the greater will be PA_{O_2}; the less PI_{O_2}, the less PA_{O_2}. A healthy animal breathing air at sea level will have a PA_{O_2} of about 100 torr. The difference between PI_{O_2} and PA_{O_2} is related to the addition of water vapor and CO_2 to the alveolar gas in the lungs and to the level

of alveolar ventilation ($\dot{V}A$). Figure 13–51 summarizes the partial pressure of O_2 and CO_2 normally found in the respiratory system.

Increasing $\dot{V}A$ above the normal level is called *hyperventilation* and occurs when greater amounts of CO_2 are removed from the gas exchange space and greater amounts of O_2 are added to the space than are required by the animal's metabolic needs. Since the animal is not taking up the excess O_2 in the exchange space nor adding additional CO_2, hyperventilation leads to high PA_{O_2} and low PA_{CO_2}. Conversely, lowering $\dot{V}A$ below the normal level, *hypoventilation*, causes inadequate amounts of CO_2 to be removed from the exchange space and inadequate amounts of O_2 to be added to the space to meet the metabolic needs of the animal. During hypoventilation, PA_{CO_2} will be high and PA_{O_2} will be low.

In steady state, the production of CO_2 by the body ($\dot{V}_{CO_2}$) is equal to the amount of CO_2 being eliminated by alveolar ventilation, which in turn is simply the difference between the volume of CO_2 entering and leaving the alveolar gas per unit time. Since only negligible amounts of CO_2 enter the alveoli in the inspired gas, then:

$$\dot{V}_{CO_2} = \dot{V}A \times FA_{CO_2} \qquad (1)$$

where FA_{CO_2} is the fractional concentration of CO_2 in the alveolar gas, i.e.,

$$\dot{V}A = \dot{V}_{CO_2}/FA_{CO_2} \qquad (2)$$

Now, if we convert FA_{CO_2} to PA_{CO_2}, i.e.,

$$PA_{CO_2} = FA_{CO_2} \times K$$

where K is a constant, then

$$\dot{V}A = \frac{\dot{V}_{CO_2}}{PA_{CO_2}} \times K \qquad (3)$$

This shows the close relationship between $\dot{V}A$ and PA_{CO_2} or, even more interestingly, between $\dot{V}A$ and Pa_{CO_2}, the partial pressure of CO_2 in the arterial blood. PA_{CO_2} is nearly equal to Pa_{CO_2} in healthy animals, i.e.,

$$\dot{V}A = \frac{\dot{V}_{CO_2}}{Pa_{CO_2}} \times K \qquad (4)$$

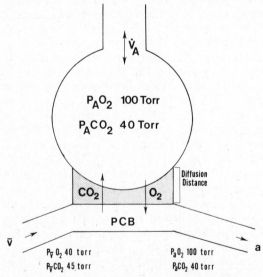

Figure 13–51 Model of the alveolar region of the lung showing the normal partial pressures for oxygen and carbon dioxide in the alveolus (PA_{O_2} and PA_{CO_2}, respectively), the mixed venous blood ($\bar{v}$) ($P\bar{v}_{O_2}$ and $P\bar{v}_{CO_2}$, respectively), and arterial blood (a) (Pa_{O_2} and Pa_{CO_2}, respectively) of an animal breathing air at sea level (barometric pressure 760 mm Hg). $\dot{V}A$ represents the alveolar ventilation and PCB represents the pulmonary capillary blood.

Thus, if alveolar ventilation ($\dot{V}A$) is halved, for example, the Pa_{CO_2} will double. This relationship is important in clinical practice when interpreting blood gas values. If alveolar hypoventilation is present, this will be shown by an abnormally high Pa_{CO_2} blood gas value.

The other major determinant of the O_2 diffusion pressure is $P\bar{c}_{O_2}$. The $P\bar{c}_{O_2}$ is determined by three major interrelated factors: (1) the partial pressure of the O_2 in the blood returning to the PCB from the body via the right heart and pulmonary circulation; (2) the rate at which O_2 is diffusing from the PGS into the PCB; and (3) the concentration of hemoglobin (Hb) in the PCB.

The O_2 concentration, or partial pressure ($P\bar{v}_{O_2}$), in the mixed venous blood varies, depending mainly on the level of metabolic activity of the body's tissues. During heavy muscular work, O_2 uptake by the tissues from the blood increases, and there will be a decrease in the P_{O_2} in the tissue capillaries and consequently the P_{O_2} of the blood entering the pulmonary capillaries ($P\bar{v}_{O_2}$). As the blood flows along the pulmonary capillaries in the walls of the exchange surface, O_2 diffuses from the PGS into the PCB until the P_{O_2} in the blood is in equilibrium with the PA_{O_2}. It follows, then, if the PA_{O_2} is 100 torr, that the blood in the pulmonary capillaries flowing out of the exchange surface should also have a P_{O_2} of 100 mm Hg, regardless of the $P\bar{v}_{O_2}$. The important difference between high and low $P\bar{v}_{O_2}$ as it relates to O_2 diffusion is this: when $P\bar{v}_{O_2}$ is low, the initial diffusion force ($PA_{O_2} - P\bar{c}_{O_2}$) will be great and a larger net transfer of O_2 will occur between the PGS and PCB to reach equilibrium than if $P\bar{v}_{O_2}$ is relatively high and the $PA_{O_2} - P\bar{c}_{O_2}$ is smaller.

The second factor affecting $P\bar{c}_{O_2}$ is the rate of transfer of O_2 from the PGS to the PCB. For our consideration here, the important factor is the tissue (and fluid) between the PGS and PCB (see Fig. 13–51). The greater the distance between the PGS and PCB, the greater the resistance will be to transfer O_2 between these compartments. One might imagine a lung with interstitial fibrosis or pulmonary edema in which fibrous tissue or edema fluid increased the distance between PGS and PCB and decreased O_2 diffusing rate. This is rarely a generalized problem in all of the units of the lung but can cause diffusion impairments in local areas of the lung. It is also possible that different tissue types (fibrous versus normal) may have different O_2 diffusion coefficients, which may change O_2 transfer. However, it should be emphasized that changes in tissue thickness or type between PGS and PCB rarely occur to the extent that they would adversely affect pulmonary diffusion for O_2 or CO_2.

The third factor that affects $P\bar{c}_{O_2}$, and thereby the net diffusion of O_2, is the hemoglobin (Hb) concentration of the blood. It is useful to think of Hb as a sink for O_2. Without Hb in the blood the plasma exposed to a P_{O_2} of 100 torr would hold less than 1 ml of O_2 per 100 ml of blood; whereas blood with normal amounts of Hb (approximately 15 gm Hb/100 ml of blood) can hold about 20 ml of O_2 per 100 ml blood. This point is emphasized in Figure 13–52. O_2 will continue to have a net movement from the PGS to the PCB as long as there is a PA_{O_2} greater than the $P\bar{c}_{O_2}$. If there is no (or only small amounts of) hemoglobin in the blood, relatively few molecules of O_2 moving from the PGS to the PCB will increase $P\bar{c}_{O_2}$ to equal PA_{O_2}, and no further net transfer of O_2 will occur. On the

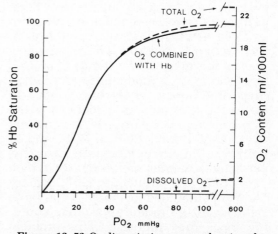

Figure 13–52 O_2 dissociation curve showing the general relationship between per cent hemoglobin (Hb) saturation (solid line), O_2 content (ml/100 ml) (upper broken line), and P_{O_2} (mm Hg). The lower broken line represents the O_2 content in the absence of Hb. (Reprinted with permission from West: Respiratory Physiology—The Essentials. Baltimore: Williams & Wilkins, 1974.)

other hand, if as O_2 molecules move from the PGS to the PCB they are bound to Hb to form oxyhemoglobin (HbO_2), the $P\bar{c}_{O_2}$ will rise to equal PA_{O_2} only after nearly all the O_2 sites on the Hb molecules are filled. Beside the Hb concentration (i.e., gm Hb/100 ml blood), the Hb available for O_2 uptake in the exchange area of the lung can be greatly varied, depending on the volume of blood in the pulmonary capillaries. The volume of the PCB is determined by (1) the density of capillaries (number per cm^2) in the pulmonary exchange surface; (2) the number of capillaries carrying blood; and (3) the amount of blood in each capillary (capillary distention). Increasing PCB volume and flow (PCB perfusion), as occurs with exercise or other circumstances in which there is an elevated pulmonary arterial pressure, will increase O_2 diffusion. In fact, PCB volume, under most circumstances, affects O_2 diffusion in the healthy lung more than any other factor.

CO$_2$ diffusion is less difficult to understand because it is less influenced by several of the mechanisms we have previously discussed for O_2 diffusion. CO_2 diffuses from the PCB to the PGS about 20 times more readily than O_2 diffuses from the PGS to the PCB. This is due mainly to its greater solubility in tissue fluid than O_2. CO_2 rapidly moves from the PCB to the PGS, and the partial pressure of CO_2 (P_{CO_2}) in the two compartments quickly reaches equilibrium as blood flows through the capillaries in the exchange surface. The most likely reason for inadequate removal of CO_2 from the PCB is inadequate ventilation (hypoventilation). Hypoventilation will cause PA_{CO_2} to increase, decreasing the CO_2 diffusing pressure, decreasing net CO_2 transfer from PCB to PGS, and finally resulting in an increased Pa_{CO_2} (hypercapnia). Under conditions in which ventilation and pulmonary perfusion are badly mismatched or there is a large right to left pulmonary vascular shunt, the $P\bar{a}_{CO_2}$ may increase. This problem will be taken up later.

Blood-Gas Analysis. A clinical test, blood-gas analysis, is a valuable clinical measurement of many aspects of pulmonary respiratory function. Because this test has been found very useful for evaluating the pulmonary respiratory function in animals and because the principles of the test enable us to describe important features of pulmonary function, we will discuss the physiologic meaning of the values from blood-gas analyses of arterial blood.

If one is to gain all of the advantages from using this test to evaluate patients, one must understand and adhere to the technical requirements of the test, understand the limits of the test, and know the physiologic meaning of each of the values. We will not discuss the technical basis and requirements for the test, as they are well described elsewhere (Siggaard-Anderson et al. 1960; Siggaard-Anderson 1961; Severinghaus 1959).

Blood-gas analysis usually gives three values: (1) partial pressure of O_2 (P_{O_2}); (2) partial pressure of CO_2 (P_{CO_2}); and (3) blood pH. If the analysis is done on systemic arterial blood, the results can be used to evaluate several important aspects of pulmonary function.

The P_{O_2}, P_{CO_2}, and pH values in blood in a systemic artery (e.g., carotid artery) are *nearly* identical to the blood flowing away from the exchange area of the lung and represent the end result of pulmonary respiratory function (see Fig. 13–51). Table 13–3 shows an approximate normal range of values for blood gases and pH for a typical terrestrial mammal breathing air at sea level. The values in this table do not apply precisely to the values in the different species. However, the range given does include the most accepted values reported for the large domestic mammals. The blood-gas values for the arterial blood are clinically most useful. Blood from the several millions of pulmonary capillaries from all of the millions of alveoli is collected in the pulmonary veins and mixed in the left heart chambers and aorta. Arterial blood composition represents an average of all the effects of the various pulmonary gas exchange units. If there are values for arterial P_{O_2} (Pa_{O_2}), P_{CO_2} (Pa_{CO_2}), and/or pH (pHa) outside the range given, one should expect some dysfunction of the pulmonary system. We will give possible deviations from normal for each of the three values and discuss their functional meaning.

Arterial Oxygen Pressure (Pa_{O_2}). There are three states of Pa_{O_2}: *normoxemia, hyperoxemia,* and *hypoxemia. Normox-*

Table 13–3 APPROXIMATE RANGE OF BLOOD-GAS AND pH VALUES IN VARIOUS COMPARTMENTS OF THE RESPIRATORY SYSTEM OF A TYPICAL TERRESTRIAL MAMMAL BREATHING AIR AT SEA LEVEL

	P_{O_2} (torr)	P_{CO_2} (torr)	pH
Inspired air	150	0	—
Alveolar gas	100–105	38–42	—
Av. PCB	95–105	38–42	7.38–7.44
Arterial blood	85–100	38–42	7.38–7.44
Av. TCB	40	42–46	7.35–7.40
Av. PAB	40	42–46	7.35–7.40

Notes: Av. PCB = average pulmonary capillary blood.
Av. TCB = average tissue capillary blood.
Av. PAB = average pulmonary arterial blood.

emia describes the condition of a healthy animal breathing air at sea level and with blood-gas values within the range given in Table 13–3. *Hyperoxemia* is the condition in which the Pa_{O_2} values exceed the normal range. This can occur in two circumstances in the healthy individual: hyperventilation and/or O_2-enriched inspired gas (elevated PI_{O_2}). An individual can elevate Pa_{O_2} slightly by hyperventilation with concurrent washout of CO_2 from the alveoli and blood. Breathing air, the maximum Pa_{O_2} an individual can achieve with hyperventilation is about 115 torr.

Giving O_2-enriched gas to breathe is a frequent clinical practice, particularly during general anesthesia and surgical procedures. In the ideal system, a high PI_{O_2} would lead to an elevated Pa_{O_2}; however, the increase in Pa_{O_2} is often less than anticipated despite the high PI_{O_2}. A lower than expected (predicted) Pa_{O_2} during O_2 breathing is called *relative hypoxemia*. It is caused by the same mechanisms that cause hypoxemia. The causes of hypoxemia are described hereafter.

If a subject's Pa_{O_2} value is lower than normal (or lower than predicted based on PI_{O_2}), the subject is *hypoxemic*. There are five causes of hypoxemia: (1) low PI_{O_2}; (2) hypoventilation; (3) low pulmonary diffusion from the alveolar space to the PCB; (4) mismatching of ventilation and perfusion; and/or (5) right to left pulmonary vascular shunt. The first cause of hypoxemia is associated with the O_2 concentration in the inspired air, and the last four are associated with *pulmonary respiratory dysfunction*. We have already described the first three mechanisms, and specific examples for

each are given in the section on respiratory dysfunction with general anesthesia and surgery to follow. The fourth and fifth mechanisms are similar; however, they are functionally quite distinct and it can be clinically important to distinguish them.

During the last 20 years, a good deal has been written about *mismatching of ventilation and perfusion* in humans and animals with respiratory disease and/or surgery. This area of respiratory function is superbly discussed by West (1977). In the ideal lung, $\dot{V}A$ would be evenly distributed throughout the lung and perfectly matched with evenly distributed PCB flow ($\dot{Q}$). This would lead to perfect gas exchange, and end-PCB P_{O_2} and P_{CO_2} would exactly equal the PA_{O_2} and PA_{CO_2}, respectively, assuming no barrier to diffusion. In humans and presumably also in domestic mammals, neither $\dot{V}A$ nor $\dot{Q}$ are evenly distributed nor are they matched everywhere in the lung (Fig. 13–53). This is thought to occur mainly because of the effects of gravity. The weight of the lung is suggested as the major factor that leads to a vertical gradient of pleural pressure within the chest, pleural pressure being more negative over the top of the lung than at the bottom. The negative pleural pressure expands alveoli in upper regions and makes them less distensible; hence ventilation is less at the top of the lung than at the bottom. Correspondingly, the weight of the column of blood within the pulmonary circulation leads to increased perfusion of dependent zones. The rate of increase of perfusion of blood is greater than that of ventilation at each lower zone in the lung, i.e., gravity af-

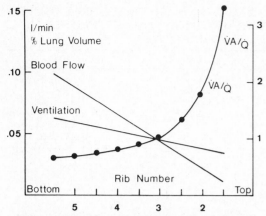

Figure 13–53 The approximate relation between ventilation and blood flow, and their ratio ($\dot{V}A/\dot{Q}$) from bottom to top of an adult human lung. (Reprinted with permission from West: Ventilation/Blood Flow and Gas Exchange. Oxford: Blackwell Scientific, 1970.)

fects the distribution of pulmonary capillary blood more than pleural pressure. Hence, $\dot{Q}$ is in excess of $\dot{V}A$ in most lower regions of the lungs.

Much of the theory concerning the distribution of $\dot{V}A$ and $\dot{Q}$ has been based on work in human subjects and has yet to be clearly demonstrated in large domestic animals (Fig. 13–54). However, evidence does exist that some of the components of the theory, such as the vertical pleural pressure gradient, are present in large domestic animals (Derksen and Robinson 1980). The result is less than ideal gas exchange, and, as a result, PA_{O_2} is always slightly greater than end-PĊB P_{O_2}.

The relationship between $\dot{V}A$ and $\dot{Q}$ is often expressed as a ratio ($\dot{V}A/\dot{Q}$) (see Fig. 13–53). The nearer the value for the $\dot{V}A/\dot{Q}$ ratio is to 1, the more ideal will be the gas exchange. If the ratio is above 1, that region of the lung has more $\dot{V}A$ than $\dot{Q}$ and there is *wasted ventilation* or high $\dot{V}D$ in that region. If the ratio is less than 1, that region of the lung has more $\dot{Q}$ than $\dot{V}A$ and there is *wasted perfusion*.

Figures 13–53 and 13–54 depict a lung in a normal human subject with the usual distribution of $\dot{V}A/\dot{Q}$ ratios from top to bottom. Such lungs cannot have ideal gas exchange, and end-PCB P_{O_2} will be less than PA_{O_2}. One may question why the high $\dot{V}A/\dot{Q}$ ratio at the top does not offset the low $\dot{V}A/\dot{Q}$ at the bottom and

lead to overall ideal gas exchange. The reason, of course, is that the small amount of blood at the top (see $\dot{Q}$ in Fig. 13–54) will be loaded with O_2 to essentially the same O_2 concentration as the region in the middle with a $\dot{V}A/\dot{Q}$ ratio of 1. In other words, it is not possible to superload the blood with O_2. At the bottom of the lung where the $\dot{V}A/\dot{Q}$ is lower than 1, there is simply not enough ventilation to supply enough O_2 to load all the Hb in this region. Blood flows away from the lower regions with inadequate O_2 and an end-PCB P_{O_2} less than PA_{O_2} (see P_{O_2} in Fig. 13–54). When the blood from the different regions of the lung is mixed in the left heart, some regions provide blood with near-ideal P_{O_2} and others provide blood with low P_{O_2}. The result is a mixture with a P_{O_2} value lower than ideal and between the highest and lowest P_{O_2} values flowing from the various regions. The effect of regional $\dot{V}A/\dot{Q}$ on regional gas tensions is exemplified in Figure 13–54.

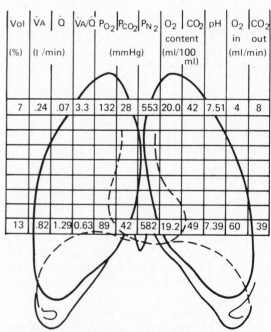

Vol (%)	$\dot{V}A$ (l/min)	$\dot{Q}$	$\dot{V}A/\dot{Q}$	P_{O_2}	P_{CO_2}	P_{N_2} (mmHg)	O_2 content (ml/100 ml)	CO_2	pH	O_2 in out (ml/min)	CO_2 in out (ml/min)
7	.24	.07	3.3	132	28	553	20.0	42	7.51	4	8
13	.82	1.29	0.63	89	42	582	19.2	49	7.39	60	39

Figure 13–54 Regional differences in respiratory gas exchange values from top to bottom of lung. Only the extremes are shown at the very top and bottom regions. Graduated intermediate values would be seen in the intermediate regions. (Reprinted with permission from West: Respiratory Physiology—The Essentials. Baltimore, Williams & Wilkins, 1974.)

General anesthesia and several surgical procedures can have adverse effects on the $\dot{V}A/\dot{Q}$ ratios throughout the patient's lungs, and this will contribute to a Pa_{O_2} much less than PA_{O_2} (*relative hypoxemia*). We will discuss specific examples in a later section. The reader is encouraged to consider examples of pulmonary airway or circulatory disease and their potential effects on regional $\dot{V}A/\dot{Q}$ ratios and gas exchange.

The fifth cause of hypoxemia is *right to left pulmonary vascular shunt* (RL/PVS). An RL/PVS is a vascular pathway for blood from the right ventricle to the left heart without passing through a functional, gas exchange area. It may be part of the normal structure; for example, the blood that supplies the metabolic needs of the pleura, airways, and other pulmonic structures and that flows to the pulmonary veins and left heart. This blood has relatively low P_{O_2} and will lower Pa_{O_2}. This blood flow is called *venous admixture* and is a major cause of PA_{O_2} being larger than Pa_{O_2} in the healthy individual. The difference between PA_{O_2} and Pa_{O_2} ($PA_{O_2} - Pa_{O_2}$ or $(A-a)O_2$) is often used as an index of the magnitude of venous admixture and the effectiveness of pulmonary respiratory function and will be discussed in more detail later.

There can be more severe RL/PVS associated with pulmonary abnormalities that occur with respiratory disease, general anesthesia, and certain surgical procedures. For example, it has been well documented that large RL/PVSs develop in horses breathing spontaneously under general anesthesia (Hall, Gillespie, and Tyler 1968; McDonell and Hall 1979). These horses were healthy prior to anesthesia but developed large areas of pulmonary atelectasis (no ventilation with PCB perfusion) during anesthesia, and these areas contributed to a large RL/PVS. Under these conditions there is a significant relative hypoxemia.

Arterial Carbon Dioxide Pressure. There are three states of Pa_{CO_2}: *normocapemia (normocapnia)*, *hypercapemia (hypercapnia)*, and *hypocapemia (hypocapnia)*. *Normocapemia* is the condition in which the Pa_{CO_2} values are within the normal range given in Table 13–3, or about 40 torr. There is an important

physiological difference in the regulation of the normal values of Pa_{O_2} and Pa_{CO_2}. Pa_{CO_2} is regulated by respiratory mechanisms within a much narrower range (38 to 42 torr) than is PA_{O_2} (85 to 100 torr). The tight regulation of the level of CO_2 in the arterial blood (and the body as a whole) is associated with the adverse effects of CO_2 and associated hydrogen ions (H^+) on metabolic processes. It is important to remember that CO_2 in water will be hydrated to carbonic acid (H_2CO_3), which almost completely dissociates to H^+ and bicarbonate (HCO_3^-):

$$CO_2 + H_2O \rightleftarrows H_2CO_3 \rightleftarrows H^+ + HCO_3^-$$

Failing to ventilate CO_2 from the body causes retention of CO_2 in the blood, which leads to *hypercapemia* (the condition of the body *hypercapnia*) because more and more CO_2 will be formed by metabolic processes as long as the animal lives. There are three causes of hypercapemia. The first, and most important, is *hypoventilation*. The other two are less usual causes and must be very severe to cause hypercapnia: mismatching of $\dot{V}A$ and $\dot{Q}$ and RL/PVS. With hypoventilation, $\dot{V}A$ is insufficient to wash the newly formed CO_2 out of the PGS; the PA_{CO_2} will increase and equilibrate with the Pa_{CO_2} at an abnormally high level. Elevated Pa_{CO_2} causes the formation of more H^+, resulting in acidosis in the animal. Since this acidosis is the result of hypoventilation (respiratory inadequacy), it is called *respiratory acidosis*.

The response of a healthy animal with a large ventilatory reserve to hypercapnia is to increase $\dot{V}A$ and re-establish normal levels of CO_2 and pH in the blood and tissue. In animals with depressed ventilatory drive (e.g., with general anesthetic depression) or with pulmonary obstructive disease, the animal may not be able to increase $\dot{V}A$ and the hypercapnia and acidosis will persist. Remember, *hypercapnia* should nearly always be associated with *hypoventilation*.

Why don't those pulmonary dysfunctions (diffusion impairment, mismatching of $\dot{V}A$ and $\dot{Q}$, and RL/PVS) that cause hypoxemia also cause significant hypercapnia? As we have seen, because of the relatively high solubility of CO_2 in body fluids, there is no diffusion impairment for CO_2 in the exchange area. Mismatching of $\dot{V}A$ and $\dot{Q}$ and RL/PVS may cause slight hypercapnia if they are very large. In such cases, one can expect to see a very severe hypoxemia. If CO_2 in the mixed venous blood from the right heart perfuses inadequately or to nonventilated gas exchange spaces in the lung, higher levels of CO_2 will appear in the systemic circulation and will cause a momentary elevation of Pa_{CO_2}. In response, the regulatory mechanisms of the body would cause an increased $\dot{V}A$ sufficient to cause Pa_{CO_2} to return to normal. If the abnormalities progressively worsened, $\dot{V}A$ would continue to compensate until all the ventilatory reserve were "used." If either abnormality increased in severity beyond this point, the animal would probably die of hypoxia. In other words, mismatching of $\dot{V}A$ and $\dot{Q}$ and RL/PVS have much greater adverse effects on O_2 exchange than on CO_2 exchange.

There are rather complex reasons why hypoxemia cannot be compensated for in the same way as hypercapemia. Basically, however, it is because of the different regulatory mechanisms for CO_2 and O_2 in the body and the way in which they are transported in the blood. Increasing Pa_{CO_2} is a far more powerful stimulation to respiration than decreasing Pa_{O_2}, and since CO_2 is very soluble and freely diffusible, it leaves the PCB and enters the PGS readily. Most of the oxygen in blood, however, is bound to hemoglobin, and once the available binding sites are occupied, increasing Pa_{O_2} through hyperventilation can add little to the oxygen content of the blood (see Fig. 13–52).

Hypocapemia (hypocapnia in body) occurs when CO_2 is being removed from the blood (or body) at a greater rate than it is being formed by metabolism. This occurs with *hyperventilation* (excess $\dot{V}A$). Because of the body's tight regulation of CO_2, this condition rarely occurs in the healthy, resting individual. It can occur when the individual is in severe pain and higher brain centers override the central involuntary control mechanisms of breathing. It is not unusual to find anesthetized patients with intermittent positive-pressure ventilation (IPPV) having a low Pa_{CO_2} because of the mechanically induced hyperventilation.

During hyperventilation, Pa_{CO_2} and body CO_2 are reduced and the CO_2-hydration reaction moves to the left, causing a low H^+ concentration and *respiratory alkalosis*.

$$CO_2 + H_2O \leftrightarrows H^+ + HCO_3^-$$

Arterial pH. The following possible *acid-base states* exist in an animal: (1) normal; (2) respiratory acidosis; (3) respiratory alkalosis; (4) metabolic acidosis; (5) metabolic alkalosis; (6) a combination of respiratory acidosis and metabolic acidosis; (7) a combination of respiratory acidosis and metabolic alkalosis; (8) a combination of respiratory alkalosis and metabolic acidosis; and (9) a combination of respiratory alkalosis and metabolic alkalosis. Respiratory acidosis and alkalosis have been defined previously. Since it is beyond the scope of this chapter to discuss all the physiological mechanisms involved in the regulation of H^+ concentration ([H^+]) or base concentration in the body, we will only give a functional definition of the other possible states. A *normal acid-base state* is more than a normal pH value; in addition, it means that the [H^+] and the concentration of all body bases are within normal limits. *Metabolic acidosis* is a deficiency of body base. *Metabolic alkalosis* is an excess of body base. In general, the kidneys regulate the conservation or excretion of body base and largely determine the body base level. Further, the kidneys may conserve excess base (metabolic alkalosis) to help compensate for respiratory acidosis (a combination of respiratory acidosis and metabolic alkalosis). Both the respiratory and renal systems may fail and one would have both respiratory and metabolic acidosis or, conversely, respiratory and metabolic alkalosis (a combination of respiratory acidosis and metabolic acidosis, and a combination of respiratory alkalosis and metabolic alkalosis, respectively).

It is worth noting that arterial blood pH (pHa) values give an excellent reading of the acid-base status of the body. Since blood from all the body tissues returns to the right heart and is then pumped through the lung, where the CO_2 level (and consequently the pH) is adjusted, the arterial blood pumped from the lung represents a final "averaging" of all the physiological mechanisms influencing pH and prepares the blood to "bathe" the body's cells. With a good medical history and Pa_{CO_2} and pHa values, one can make an assessment of the patient's acid-base status with confidence. A final word of caution: the definitions given here relating to acid-base status in animals cannot be expected to give a clinician all the physiological background needed to deal with acid-base disturbances that may arise in his patients. Acid-base balance is physiologically complex, involving nearly every body system in bringing about normal regulation. A clear understanding of acid-base status and fluid-electrolyte balance makes rational management of surgical (and other) patients possible (see Chap. 5).

Interpretation of Arterial Blood Gas Analysis Values. Having discussed the physiological meaning of values obtained from arterial blood gas analysis, we will now outline an approach for the use of these values to assess the effectiveness of gas exchange in the lung.

We shall be dealing with the fundamental manifestations and causes of *respiratory failure,* which is defined as the clinical syndrome in which there is inadequate respiratory gas exchange, causing hypoxemia and/or hypercapnia. The most frequent and often the earliest

arterial blood gas change in a patient with lung disease is hypoxemia. For that reason we will focus primarily on causes of abnormally low Pa_{O_2}, i.e., hypoxemia.

A mammal with hypoxemia will have one or more of the following conditions: (1) low inspired P_{O_2} ($\downarrow PI_{O_2}$); (2) hypoventilation ($\downarrow \dot{V}A$); (3) abnormally large pulmonary diffusion impairment ($\uparrow DI$); (4) abnormally large $\dot{V}A/\dot{Q}$ inequality ($\uparrow \dot{V} \neq \dot{Q}$); or (5) abnormally large RL/PVS ($\uparrow RL/PVS$). Because appropriate therapeutic response depends on the fundamental cause, the clinical problem is to determine how much each of these possible abnormalities contributes to the hypoxemia of a patient. Our intention is to approach this problem of assessing the hypoxemic patient in a step-by-step fashion. This will require an examination of some definitions and simple equations.

Table 13–4 shows a general schema of delivery of O_2 from the environment to the arterial blood and the five abnormalities that may disrupt O_2 transport to the arterial blood. The first two abnormalities, $\downarrow PI_{O_2}$ and $\downarrow \dot{V}A$, cause a decrease in PA_{O_2}, which in turn leads to a $\downarrow Pa_{O_2}$. The other three abnormalities, $\uparrow DI$, $\uparrow \dot{V}A \neq \dot{Q}$, and $\uparrow RL/PVS$, have their functional effect "downstream" from the alveolar compartment and cause an abnormally large difference between the PA_{O_2} and Pa_{O_2} [(A-a)O_2].

If PA_{O_2} and, consequently, Pa_{O_2} are ab-

Table 13–4 SCHEMA OF OXYGEN DELIVERY FROM THE ENVIRONMENT TO ARTERIAL BLOOD BY THE PULMONARY SYSTEM AND THE FIVE ABNORMALITIES (BOXED) THAT CAUSE HYPOXEMIA ($\downarrow Pa_{O_2}$)

		Cascade of Pulmonary Compartments			
	Environment	Airways (AO → A)	Alveolus	Exchange Surface	Arterial Blood
Normal P_{O_2}*	150 Torr		100 torr		85 to 100 torr
	$\boxed{\downarrow PI_{O_2}}$ ——————→		$\downarrow PA_{O_2}$ ——————————→		$\downarrow Pa_{O_2}$
		$\boxed{\downarrow \dot{V}A}$ →	$\downarrow PA_{O_2}$ ——————————→		$\downarrow Pa_{O_2}$
			PA_{O_2} ————	$\boxed{\uparrow DI}$ ——→	$\downarrow PA_{O_2}$
			PA_{O_2} ———	$\boxed{\uparrow \dot{V}A \neq \dot{Q}}$ ——→	$\downarrow PA_{O_2}$
			PA_{O_2} ———	$\boxed{\uparrow RL/PVS}$ ——→	$\downarrow PA_{O_2}$

*The values are expected values when an animal is breathing air at sea level.
Notes: AO = airways opening.
    A = alveolar space.
    Other symbols are given in the text.

normally low because of $\downarrow P_{I_{O_2}}$ and/or $\downarrow \dot{V}_A$, then any of the other three abnormalities will cause an additive effect and will lead to a further decline in Pa_{O_2}, depending on how greatly they disrupt the O_2 delivery between the alveolar and arterial blood compartments. To determine to what extent the last three abnormalities ($\uparrow DI$, $\uparrow \dot{V}_A \neq \dot{Q}$, and $\uparrow RL/PVS$) contribute to a hypoxemia, one must know (1) the $P_{I_{O_2}}$ and $\dot{V}_A$; and (2) the PA_{O_2}.

The $P_{I_{O_2}}$ is usually easy to calculate or estimate from the gas mixture the animal is breathing and the barometric pressure (PB). One can estimate if $\dot{V}_A$ is normal (Pa_{CO_2} approximately 40 torr), low ($Pa_{CO_2} > 41$ torr, hypoventilation), or high ($Pa_{CO_2} < 38$ torr, hyperventilation) with a measurement of Pa_{CO_2} or end-expired P_{CO_2}. A more precise value for $\dot{V}_A$ can be calculated with equation 4.

Because the abnormalities ($\uparrow DI$, $\uparrow \dot{V}_A \neq \dot{Q}$, and $\uparrow RL/PVS$) can potentiate a low PA_{O_2} and cause a dangerously low Pa_{O_2},

it is valuable to know the PA_{O_2}. This can be calculated from the following equation:

$$PA_{O_2} = F_{I_{O_2}}(P_B - 47) - PA_{CO_2}\left(F_{I_{O_2}} + \frac{I - F_{I_{O_2}}}{R}\right) \quad (5)$$

where $F_{I_{O_2}}$ is the fraction of O_2 in the inspired gas and R is the *respiratory exchange ratio*.

$$R = \frac{\dot{V}_{CO_2}}{\dot{V}_{O_2}} \quad (6)$$

where $\dot{V}_{CO_2}$ is the CO_2 output per minute and $\dot{V}_{O_2}$ is O_2 uptake per minute by the animal.

Table 13-5 gives an example of the conditions and blood gas values of a horse under general anesthesia. It also shows the steps one can take to determine the major abnormalities causing the large $(A-a)O_2$ in this horse. In this example the horse is breathing a high

---

Table 13-5 PROBLEM SET AND SOLUTIONS RELATED TO AN EXAMPLE OF A SURGICAL PATIENT WITH HYPOXEMIA

Conditions: Horse in lateral recumbency; general anesthesia closed circuit machine; 95% O_2 inspired gas; $P_B = 700$ torr

Blood gas values: $Pa_{O_2} = 131$ torr
$Pa_{CO_2} = 40$ torr
pH = 7.34

Problem 1: What is the PA_{O_2}?
Solution: Begin with equation 5.

$$PA_{O_2} = F_{I_{O_2}}(P_B - 47) - PA_{CO_2}\left(F_{I_{O_2}} + \frac{1 - F_{I_{O_2}}}{R}\right)$$

a. $F_{I_{O_2}} = 0.95$
b. $P_B = 700$ torr
c. Since $PA_{CO_2} = Pa_{CO_2}$, $PA_{CO_2} = 40$ torr
d. We assume R to be 0.85

Then: $PA_{O_2} = 0.95(700 - 47) - 40\left(0.95 + \dfrac{1 - 0.95}{0.85}\right) = 580$ torr

Problem 2: What is $(A-a)O_2$?
Solution:
$PA_{O_2} = 580$
$- Pa_{O_2} = 131$
_____
449 torr

Problem 3: What caused the relative hypoxemia or the large $(A-a)O_2$?
Solution:

$P_{I_{O_2}}$?	No, $P_{I_{O_2}} = 620$ torr
$\dot{V}_A$?	No, $Pa_{CO_2} = 40$ torr; normal
DI?	Perhaps, but not likely to be the only cause of a very large $(A-a)O_2$
$\dot{V}_A \neq \dot{Q}$	Perhaps, likely during surgery with animal in lateral recumbency
LR/PVS?	Yes, Pa_{O_2} less than 300 torr while animal is inspiring nearly 100% O_2

concentration of O_2 (95 per cent), which is usual if the horse is being given gas anesthesia. The horse at the time of the arterial blood sampling was normoventilating, since the Pa_{CO_2} was 40 torr. It would not have been unusual to have found a Pa_{CO_2} greater than 40 torr, indicating hypoventilation in the anesthetized patient. Based on these assessments we can conclude that $\downarrow PI_{O_2}$ and $\downarrow \dot{V}A$ are not the cause of the hypoxemia. Since Pa_{CO_2} is normal in our example, the acidosis (pH = 7.34) must be caused by a *metabolic acidosis*.

We are left with $\uparrow DI$, $\uparrow \dot{V}A \neq \dot{Q}$, and/or RL/PVS as possible causes of the hypoxemia. As we have seen, these abnormalities have their effect downstream of the alveolar space. The calculated PA_{O_2} is 580 torr, and the (A-a)O_2 is 449 torr. In the healthy, awake, upright horse the (A-a)O_2 value should not exceed 20 torr.

If the horse had a healthy respiratory system prior to the induction of general anesthesia, it is unlikely that there is a significant increase in DI. On the other hand, the effects of abnormal body position on respiratory system movement and gravitational forces on the lung and pulmonary circulation can cause $\uparrow \dot{V}A \neq \dot{Q}$ and $\uparrow RL/PVS$ during general anesthesia. It is very likely that both of these abnormalities contribute to the hypoxemia [and $\uparrow$(A-a)O_2]. Certainly, one can be quite sure there is a significantly large RL/PVS associated with a Pa_{O_2} less than 300 torr when the animal is inspiring a 95 per cent O_2 mixture.

Nonrespiratory Function of the Pulmonary System. Recently, more attention has been paid to the important nonrespiratory functions of the pulmonary system. Generally, nonrespiratory functions of the lung can be classified under four headings: (1) lung and body defense; (2) filtration of the circulating blood; (3) activation and inactivation of circulating substances; and (4) phonation. As we learn more about the metabolic functions of the lung, the list of nonrespiratory functions grows. We will list and describe some of those that we believe are particularly important to the surgeon in caring for his patients.

LUNG AND BODY DEFENSE. Since the gas exchange surface is second only to the skin in surface area exposed to the environment, it is in a position to be repeatedly challenged by significant concentrations of potentially toxic substances in the inspired air (e.g., anesthetic vapors). The system has evolved into a sophisticated defense to protect the exchange surface and the body from harmful substances. The *pulmonary defense system* can be divided into physical, cellular, and humoral mechanisms.

The *physical mechanisms for pulmonary defense* are (1) the physical shape of the airways; (2) the liquid lining; (3) the mucociliary escalator, and (4) cough. In most large domestic animals the nasal passages are very irregular and convoluted. This shape causes the inspiratory airflow stream to be very irregular. This forms turbulent air streams, which collide with the moist mucous membrane of the nostrils. There are three known physiologic benefits of the turbulent inspiratory flow and greater contact with the lining membranes of the nostrils: (1) warming of the inspired air to near body temperature; (2) humidification of the air (addition of water vapor); and (3) entrapment of inspired foreign particles in the fluid lining. These three mechanisms serve to protect the more fragile, deep pulmonary surfaces from cold, dryness, and/or foreign particles. The nasal passages are an avenue for the loss of excess body heat. During inspiration, heat is added to the respired gas as it is warmed and humidified. During expiration, an amount of heat nearly equivalent to that added during inspiration is exhausted from the body in the warm, moist expired gas. Under normal circumstances, the pulmonary heat loss is probably secondary to other avenues in large domestic mammals. For additional reading on heat loss in large animals, see the recent article by Schmidt-Nielsen (1981).

Because of the increased branching of the airways from nose to alveoli and the character and decreasing rate of inspired gas flow, there is a tendency for smaller and smaller particles to fall out of the air stream and be deposited on the moist mucous membranes of the airways. The larger and denser suspended particles (> 1 μ in diameter) are deposited in the upper airways, and very small particles (< 1 μ) travel to the small bronchioles and alveoli.

The entire lining of the air passages in

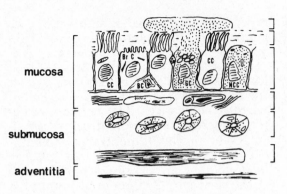

mucous layer
serous layer

epithelium

lamina propria

glands

cartilage

mucosa

submucosa

adventitia

Figure 13–55 Diagrammatic representation of the airway wall. The biphasic liquid layer of mucous islands floating on a serous subphase covers the epithelial lining cells and ciliated (CC), goblet (GC), nonciliated (NCC), brush (Br C), and basal cells (BC).

the pulmonary system is covered with a *biphase liquid lining* (Fig. 13–55). In the nasal area and in most airways it consists of a watery subphase and a mucoid surface phase; in the alveoli and the very small airways adjoining them it consists of a more watery subphase and a phospholipid, surfactant surface phase. The liquid serves to entrap, solubilize, and dilute particulate and gaseous agents inhaled with the inspired gas. The surface mucoid layer is produced by the goblet cells and mucous glands in the epithelial lining of the airways. The serous or watery layer is leaked into the airways from the adjoining capillaries and/or is produced by special submucosal glands in the airways. The alveolar, surfactant, surface layer is thought to be produced by large, round type II cells in the epithelial lining of the alveoli. It serves to stabilize the shape of the alveoli.

The mucoid layer floats on top of the serous layer and is propelled toward the throat by ciliated epithelial cells (see Fig. 13–55). Those cells in the nose move the mucous layer in waves caudad toward the throat; those in the airways move the mucous layer cephalad toward the throat. The composition of the mucous layer is important because (1) it floats on the surface of the airways; (2) it is sticky, entraps foreign material, and moves as a sheet; and (3) it forms a tenacious layer to protect the lower serous layer and epithelium. The composition of the serous subphase is important because (1) it allows free sweeping movements of the cilia; (2) it is present in sufficient quantity to dilute foreign substances; and (3) it is thought to contain locally produced

antibodies and other substances that kill or facilitate the killing of microorganisms.

Between the epithelial cells lining the larger airways that begin in the nose and continue down through several branches of bronchi, there are afferent nerve endings that, when stimulated by physical or chemical agents, initiate a rapid inspiration followed by an explosive, forced expiration called a sneeze (nose stimulation) or a cough (lower airway stimulation). There appears to be considerable variation in the strength of the cough (or sneeze) reflex of different species, but in all large domestic animals its presence helps clear airways of foreign particulate material and excess mucous (liquid) secretions in the lung (Leith 1977).

The *cellular defense mechanisms* of the lung refer mainly to the free (unattached) alveolar macrophages. These cells are sometimes called the lung's last line of defense. If a dangerous inhaled substance is not inactivated or removed by the physical processes previously described, then it is left to these cells to engulf and kill and/or detoxify the substance. These cells appear to move about the surface of the alveoli and adjoining small airways and are attracted to some foreign substances. They increase in numbers in response to many different lung irritants, presumably being produced from undifferentiated cells in the alveolar wall and from circulating lymphocytes in the blood. The complexity of these cells and their many functions are now under intense study. Of particular importance to the management of surgical patients are investigations studying inhibition of the pulmonary defense function of these cells by various inhaled substances (including gaseous anesthetics).

The phrase "humoral defense mechanism" is, no doubt, too nonspecific, and better terminology will be forthcoming as our understanding of these mechanisms improves. Our intention is to draw your attention to the intense research on solubilized antibacterial, antiviral, and smooth muscle active materials being identified in the fluid in the airways. It is becoming increasingly apparent that we can no longer view the liquid lining of the lung as a passive wash and diluting medium. (For further reading on this subject, see Brain, Proctor, and Reid 1977; Green et al. 1977; Schwartz and Christman 1979; and Brain 1977).

FILTRATION OF THE CIRCULATING BLOOD. Comroe (1966) described the important function the pulmonary circulation serves by filtering the circulating blood for the body. All the blood from the body tissues returns to the right heart and is then pumped to the lungs and the pulmonary capillary bed. All but about 1 per cent of the blood from the body must traverse the pulmonary capillaries before returning to the body tissues via the left heart and left-side arteries. Emboli or other "particles" in the blood that are of sufficient size to cause an infarct in a capillary bed are caught in the pulmonary capillary bed; the more vital capillary beds in the brain and heart are spared. The healthy lung has considerable pulmonary vascular reserve and anastomoses between capillaries so that many pulmonary capillaries can be blocked without significantly interfering with respiratory gas exchange. In time, the blocked capillaries are recannulated and return to carrying blood. In human medicine a very serious post-surgical problem is pulmonary embolism, in which large (or numerous) emboli break loose from the surgical site and embolize large pulmonary arteries. This can lead to severe pain, respiratory distress, and sudden death. To date, pulmonary embolism has not been reported as a major problem following surgery on domestic animals. However, it may be that the problem has just not been recognized. Pulmonary embolism unrelated to *Dirofi-*

laria immitis infestation was previously thought not to be a serious clinical problem in dogs; however, with the introduction of more sophisticated diagnostic techniques in small animal medicine it is becoming increasingly recognized.

ACTIVATION AND INACTIVATION OF CIRCULATING SUBSTANCES. We will not attempt to list all of the substances that have been shown to be activated or deactivated as they go through the pulmonary circulation. This is a relatively new area of study, and very few large domestic animals have been included in these studies. Perhaps the first physiologically important substance to be shown to be acted upon in the pulmonary circulation was the conversion of angiotensin I (less active) to angiotensin II (more active) (Ryan 1982). Also very important is the deactivation of histamine (Bergofsky 1980). The endothelial cells in the pulmonary capillaries are thought to be particularly important in the activation and deactivation of substances in the blood. The lung is also being increasingly recognized as a major site of prostaglandin metabolism in the body (Hymann, Spannhake, and Kadowitz 1978).

Cardiovascular Respiratory Function

After pulmonary respiration, there are three steps to complete respiration: (1) transport of O_2 from the PCB to the body tissues; (2) respiratory gas (O_2 and CO_2) diffusion between the tissue capillary blood (TCB) and the intracellular metabolic machinery (IMM); and (3) transport of CO_2 from the TCB to PCB.

O_2 Transport

O_2 CONCENTRATION IN BLOOD. The amount of O_2 transported per unit time from the PCB to the TCB depends on (1) O_2 concentration in the PCB leaving the lung and (2) the cardiac output (CO). We have described those factors that influence the delivery of O_2 from the PGS to the PCB and have emphasized the importance of Hb in determining the amount of O_2 that can be carried by the blood. To summarize, the *two most important factors* that determine the

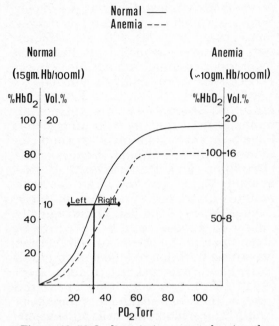

Normal ——
Anemia ---

Normal
(15gm. Hb/100ml)

Anemia
(~10gm. Hb/100ml)

Figure 13–56 O_2 dissociation curve showing the general relationship between per cent hemoglobin (% HbO_2), O_2 content (vol %), and P_{O_2} in conditions of normal (solid S-shaped curve and left Y axis) and anemia (broken S-shaped curve and right Y axis). The arrow on the P_{O_2} axis shows the P_{50} for the normal blood. The arrows on the solid line show the directions of shifts the curve may take under different local conditions in the blood.

amount of O_2 in a ml of blood are (1) the concentration of healthy Hb in the blood (gm/100 ml) and (2) the P_{O_2}.

Figures 13–52 and 13–56 show (solid lines) the classic relationship between per cent Hb saturation with O_2 (% HbO_2), O_2 concentration in the blood (O_2 vol %), and P_{O_2}. The exact shape and axis relationships of these curves vary slightly among species. These figures show that increasing P_{O_2} in the PCB (by increasing PA_{O_2}) leads to increasing amounts of O_2 loading onto Hb and that O_2 vol % in the blood goes up with % HbO_2. With increases in P_{O_2} above about 60 torr there is less increase in O_2 vol % in the blood as nearly all of the Hb sites for O_2 are filled. With a P_{O_2} below 60 torr, the Hb unloads (or loads) relatively large amounts of O_2 with each unit change in P_{O_2}.

The arrow in Figure 13–56 on the P_{O_2} axis (about 33 torr) represents the point

at which 50 per cent of the Hb is loaded with O_2 and is called the P_{50}. This expression is useful to describe some factors that influence the loading and unloading of O_2 on Hb. If the P_{50} goes up (e.g., to 40 torr), it is called a *right shift* of the % HbO_2-P_{O_2} dissociation curve and it represents situations in which O_2 is less tightly bound to Hb than normal. Conversely, when the P_{50} goes down (e.g., 25 torr), it is called a *left shift* of the % HbO_2-P_{O_2} dissociation curve and this represents situations in which O_2 is more tightly bound to Hb. The dissociation curve may be different (right or left shift) within different pools of blood within an individual depending on the local chemical and thermal environment. Increased heat, [H^+], CO_2, and some phosphate compounds (e.g., 2,3-diphosphoglycerate) cause a right shift, whereas decreases in these factors cause a left shift.

Also in Figure 13–56 is shown the approximate effect of a 20 per cent reduction in the Hb concentration on the % HbO_2-P_{O_2} dissociation curve (broken line). Note that the maximum O_2 vol % possible in this case is 16, regardless of the P_{O_2}; increasing PI_{O_2} and PA_{O_2} will not alleviate or compensate for the anemic condition.

CARDIAC OUTPUT. The second major determinant of the amount of O_2 transported from the PCB to the TCB is the cardiac output (CO). CO is the amount of blood pumped by the heart (leaving the heart) per minute. The right and left ventricles contract the same number of times per minute and deliver almost exactly the same amount of blood flow (ml/min). Increasing the output on one side of the heart will, in time, be matched with output on the other. In a healthy individual, increasing CO to the pulmonary circulation will not significantly change the amount of O_2 loaded in each ml of blood. At basal levels of CO the blood will leave the lung with about 20 ml O_2/100 ml of blood; at five times greater CO, the concentration of O_2 in the blood leaving the lung will be the same. The difference is that there is five times more blood being pumped away from the lung and therefore five times more oxygen going to the body tissues per minute. Similarly, decreasing CO does not substantially change O_2 concentration in the blood that is pumped away from the lung. However, the amount of O_2 delivered to the tissues per minute is decreased by a factor equivalent to the decrease in CO.

In an individual with a healthy pulmonary system, probably no other part of the environment-to-tissue pathway for O_2 can influence the rate of O_2 delivery more than CO. Again, since hyperventilation does not significantly increase O_2 content in the blood, the most ready means of increasing O_2 delivery to the tissues is by increasing the rate of blood flow to them.

CARDIOVASCULAR CONTROL. It is not the purpose of this chapter to discuss in detail all aspects of cardiovascular function; however, because of the important and tight link between cardiovascular control and respiratory function, a brief overview of cardiovascular control will be given here. Aortic pressure is the major control set point of the cardiovascular system, and it is monitored by two sets of receptors, the aortic and carotid sinus baroreceptors. In general, aortic pressure is influenced by two interacting phenomena: CO and peripheral resistance. CO, the volume of blood pumped from the heart per minute (ml/min), is the product of the stroke volume (SV) and frequency of the heart beat (beats per min [fH]). The peripheral resistance is the pressure in the vascular bed downstream from the aorta per unit flow (mm Hg/ml/sec) and is largely dependent upon the sum of the cross-sectional area of the arterioles in the systemic circulation. Aortic pressure can be increased by increasing CO and/or increasing total peripheral resistance and conversely decreased by decreasing one or both of these parameters.

CO is a function of heart performance (SV and fH), which is controlled by intrinsic and extrinsic control mechanisms. The *intrinsic* mechanisms are those phenomena of "self-control" in the myocardia; for example, when the ventricular myocardium is stretched with a large volume it contracts more forcibly and more completely empties the ventricle. There are other examples of intrinsic control of the heart related to its local chemical environment. *Extrinsic control* of the heart relates to the sympathetic and parasympathetic nervous control and circulating substances (e.g., catecholamines) that influence SV and/or fH. For example, the following occurs if aortic pressure falls below the set point: the baroreceptors produce afferent nerve activity, which excites the cardiovascular control center in the medulla; this in turn causes, in part, an inhibition of vagal (parasympathetic) efferent activity to the heart and fH increases, producing an increased CO and an associated increase in aortic pressure.

The peripheral resistance is also modified by sympathetic innervation from the central cardiovascular control centers. Using the same example, if aortic pressure falls, part of the response to reestablish aortic pressure is a sympathetic outflow, causing arteriolar constriction and an associated increase in peripheral vascular resistance. Sympathetic outflow also causes venous constriction, which effects a mobilization of pooled blood into the circulation and increases venous return to the heart, leading to an increased CO.

The *intrinsic control* (local) of peripheral resistance is very important and dominates, in most circumstances, other controller mechanisms. The local chemical environment determines the drive for intrinsic peripheral vascular resistance control. Substances such as O_2, CO_2, H^+, angiotensin, histamine, and other metabolic products influence the smooth muscle tone in the peripheral vascular bed. For example, in many body tissues, low levels of O_2, high levels of CO_2, and/or high levels of H^+ cause local vasodilatation, reduced peripheral resistance, and increased local blood flow (as long as adequate aortic pressure is maintained).

Important points concerning intrinsic peripheral vascular control follow. (1) Since it is the dominant controller of aortic pressure and thereby cardiovascular function, it follows that intrinsic peripheral vascular control is one of the major influences on respiratory function (i.e., the exchange of gases between lung and tissues). (2) Levels of respiratory gases and pH in the environment of the small vessels in the tissues have powerful effects on local peripheral vascular control. (3) All tissues of the body are not perfused equally with blood, and a tissue may change its requirements for perfusion depending on its metabolic activity from minute to minute. Local vascular control allows the body to distribute the blood perfusion based on metabolic requirements of tissues at different times. (4) Drugs, such as anesthetic agents, can depress or override both intrinsic and/or extrinsic heart and/or peripheral vascular control. The effects on the respiratory function of the animal can be disastrous.

Gas Exchange in the Tissues. The delivery of O_2 to the TCB is an active process requiring the active pumping of blood by the heart. Once the O_2 is in the TCB, its delivery to the intracellular metabolic machinery (IMM) is by the passive physical process of diffusion. Just as during gas exchange in the lung between the PGS and the PCB, O_2 and CO_2 move to and from the TCB and IMM in proportion to the difference in each of their partial pressures in the two compartments (P_{O_2} in TCB $-$ P_{O_2} in IMM, and P_{CO_2} in IMM $-$ P_{CO_2} in TCB).

The P_{O_2} and P_{CO_2} in the IMM are functions of their metabolic utilization and formation, respectively, and the rate of O_2 diffusion into and CO_2 diffusion out of the cells. The rate of diffusion is a function of the distance between the interior of the cell and the TCB and the P_{O_2} and P_{CO_2} in the TCB. Unlike the situation in the lung in which diffusion distance is relatively small and uniform, diffusion distance in the tissues can be limiting to gas exchange and varies, depending on the density of the perfused capillaries.

The P_{O_2} and P_{CO_2} in the TCB are largely a function of the rate of blood flow through the capillaries and their density in the tissue. A useful way of viewing respiratory gas exchange under most physiological circumstances at the tissue level is to begin with the metabolic demand for O_2 input and CO_2 output. If metabolism goes up, there will be a transient fall in the IMM P_{O_2} and a rise in the IMM P_{CO_2}. Assuming a constant flow of the TCB, there will be an increased diffusion pressure for both O_2 and CO_2 and a consequent increase in net movement of them between the IMM and TCB. The relatively low O_2 and high CO_2 in the local tissue environment will stimulate more blood perfusion (in most tissues) by decreasing local peripheral vascular resistance; this will increase the rate of delivery of O_2 and washout of CO_2 in the TCB.

CO_2 Transport. The third step in cardiovascular respiratory function is the delivery of CO_2 from the TCB to the PCB. This step is as important to the survival of the animal as is delivery of O_2 to the tissues. CO_2 is more soluble than O_2 and diffuses readily through body tissues. It exists in several forms in the body: CO_2 in solution, H_2CO_3, HCO_3^-, and in complex with proteins like Hb.

There is a greater concentration (mmole/liter) of total CO_2 in the body than of O_2. It plays an important role in the acid-base chemistry of the body and is the dominant chemical in respiratory control. As we have seen, CO_2 is delivered to the TCB in proportion to its formation in the IMM compartment. Part of the new CO_2 from the IMM stays in the plasma as free CO_2 in solution, part enters the red blood cell (RBC) and combines with H_2O to form HCO_3^-, and part combines with deoxygenated Hb. Much of the newly formed HCO_3^- diffuses out of the RBC and is transported in the plasma, and chloride ion (Cl^-) moves into the RBCs to re-establish electrical equilibrium.

The combination of CO_2 and Hb produces two favorable effects for gas exchange: (1) the pressure that enables CO_2 to combine with Hb forces O_2 off Hb and frees it to diffuse into the tissues; and (2) deoxygenated Hb can take up H^+ ions and help buffer the H^+ from the hydration of CO_2 and other fixed acids that are products of metabolism.

Control of Respiratory Function

Respiratory control physiology is a complex process, and there is much yet to be learned about it in large domestic animals. In considering its several divisions, we must not lose sight of the unifying strategies that operate in controlling respiratory function in both the pulmonary and cardiovascular systems.

The primary function of the respiratory system is to provide sufficient respiratory gas exchange between the environment and IMM to support the life of the animal. This function dictates the unifying strategy for control of the system; there must be mechanisms to sense the need for gas exchange for metabolism (input related to set point) and mechanisms to adjust respiration to meet the need (output related to set point). The major control mechanisms have detectors for the respiratory gases O_2 and CO_2 (and associated H^+) near the IMM in the tissues and downstream from the lung in the circulatory system. Both are ideally located to control both pulmonary and cardiovascular contributions to respiratory gas exchange.

We have, in the preceding section, discussed the most important control mechanisms for the respiratory function of the cardiovascular system. Next we will discuss the control systems for the pulmonary system.

Intrinsic Pulmonary Control. The intrinsic mechanisms are local reflex control mechanisms in the airways and pulmonary vasculature that respond to chemical changes in their environment and cause changes in local airway or pulmonary vascular resistance. The resistance changes are brought about by smooth muscle contraction in the walls of the airways or vessels (principally arterioles).

The most important chemical substances for the purpose of discussion are O_2, CO_2, and H^+, which act on the pulmonary smooth muscle. Low levels of O_2 and elevated levels of CO_2 and $[H^+]$ cause smooth muscle contraction in the walls of the airways and pulmonary arterioles (bronchial and arteriolar constriction). The local vasoconstriction in response to low regional PA_{O_2} levels in the lung is called "pulmonary hypoxic vasoconstriction" and is particularly important when patients travel to high altitudes or are under general anesthesia. If there is local hypoxia, hypercapnia, and/or acidosis in a region of the lung (e.g., caused by hypoventilation to the region), the reflex bronchial and pulmonary vascular constriction causes ventilation and perfusion to be shunted away from this region to one where ventilation and perfusion are more evenly matched and gas exchange is more effective. This reflex can be very important in supporting respiratory gas exchange in the anesthetized

patient, which will have a tendency for an increased number of regions with poor $\dot{V}A$-$\dot{Q}$ relationships. However, the reflex can complicate generalized pulmonary hypoxia, hypercapnia, and acidosis by increasing overall airway and pulmonary vascular resistance, leading to an associated increase in the work of breathing and in the work of the heart.

Two final points must be mentioned before leaving the intrinsic pulmonary control system: (1) enriching the O_2 in the lung and decreasing the CO_2 and $[H^+]$ with positive pressure ventilation will relax pulmonary smooth muscle and decrease airway and pulmonary vascular resistance, the work of breathing, and the work of the heart; and (2) hypoxia, hypercapnia, and acidosis cause vasodilatation in most of the systemic vascular beds, contrary to their effect of vasoconstriction in the pulmonary vascular bed.

Extrinsic Pulmonary Control. Extrinsic pulmonary control consists of two systems: mechanical control and chemical control. Figure 13–57 schematically shows the respiratory control units in the medulla (Fig. 13–57A) and its relation to mechanical and chemical control mechanisms (Fig. 13–57B). We have come to accept, perhaps too readily, the general principles of these two systems in applying them to all domestic animals. Unfortunately, there are very litte data on control of breathing in large domestic animals, and the literature is, to date, dominated by studies on anesthetized, decerebrate cats. This caution seems necessary, since the mechanical control system, which is often thought to be secondary, may have substantial effects on the breathing pattern of animals, particularly during general anesthesia.

MECHANICAL CONTROL. The mechanical control system (Fig. 13–57B) consists of (1) the pulmonary vagal afferents; and (2) the reflexes with receptors in the diaphragm, chest, and/or abdominal walls. There are three general types of pulmonary vagal afferents: (1) afferents from rapidly adapting *deflation receptors* (DN in Fig. 13–57B), predominantly in the airway epithelium of the trachea and larger airways; (2) afferents from slowly adapting *inflation (stretch) receptors* (IN in Fig. 13–57B) in the walls of small airways; and (3) afferents from receptors

Respiratory Control System

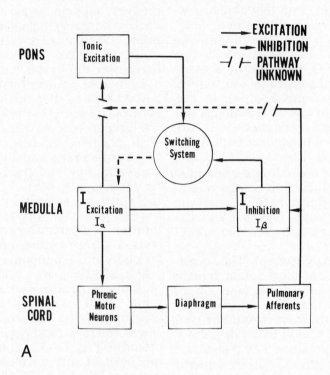

A

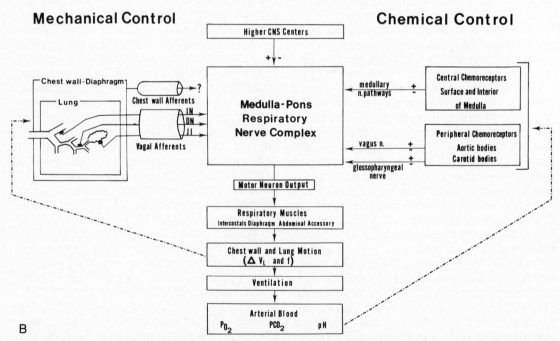

B

Figure 13–57 *A*, A proposed organization for the central neural complex and the generation of rhythmic breathing. *B*, The relation of the medulla-pons respiratory nerve complex to other breathing control mechanisms. The pulmonary mechanical afferents are inhalation (stretch) nerve fibers (IN), deflation nerve fibers (DN), and J fibers (JI).

in the intra-alveolar space (JI in Fig. 13–57B), which are sensitive to interstitial pressure of the lung. The last-named group has not been shown to have any effect on breathing, and we will not include it in our discussion.

Deflation receptors are part of the deflation limb of the Hering-Breuer reflex and under normal circumstances are not thought to affect breathing patterns in larger mammals. These receptors are distributed between epithelial cells near the airway surface of the trachea and larger airways. They respond to two stimuli, leading to two different responses: (1) airway irritation leading to coughing (Leith 1977) and; (2) lung deflation leading to a relatively short duration of strong inspiratory drive and a rapid breathing frequency (f). These receptors may cause periodic strong inspiratory effects to reverse regional atelectasis and/or decreases in lung volume that occur during general anesthesia.

The *inflation receptors* are part of the other limb of the Hering-Breuer reflex and are hypothesized to be an important control mechanism for breath size and f. The receptors for these slowly adapting vagal afferents are in the subepithelial layers of the bronchi and bronchioles. They increase firing in response to lung inflation. Their impulses reach the medullary respiratory centers, where they have an inhibitory effect on motor neurons to the inspiratory muscles (see Fig. 13–57A and B). During sustained lung inflation above the normal resting volume, this reflex causes slow, shallow breathing lasting for several minutes in some animals. During normal circumstances, it is hypothesized that excitation of these afferents progressively increases during inspiration until the intensity is sufficient to cause termination of motor nerve excitation to the inspiratory muscles. In this way, they affect the size of the tidal breath and the frequency of breathing. We will discuss their supposed integration with chemical control in the following section.

Little is known about the reflexes of the respiratory muscles (intercostal, diaphragmatic, abdominal, and accessory). In recent studies on mechanics and control of breathing in adult cattle, our data suggested a rather fine, integrated control of the different groups of inspiratory muscles. These initial studies suggested that more detailed studies of the control of activity of respiratory muscles might be important in part to (1) improve our understanding of the motion and work of breathing during different levels of physical activity; (2) know the effects of body position and general anesthesia on the motion and work of breathing; (3) predict the effects of cutting or injuring groups of muscles on the efficiency of breathing; and (4) know the factors that control lung volume in each species of large domestic mammals.

One of the reported effects of general anesthesia in humans and other animals is a regional and/or overall decrease in lung volume. If there is a regional decrease in lung volume, $\dot{V}A\text{-}\dot{Q}$, abnormalities are likely; if there is an overall decrease in lung volume, increase in the work of breathing is likely. To prevent these undesirable changes in lung volume, it would be useful to know what mechanisms set the normal end-expiratory volume or functional residual capacity (FRC). In humans, it is the stiff, passive, outward recoil of the chest wall that holds the lung volume, FRC, at about 45 per cent of the total lung capacity (TLC). Our measurements in conscious standing adult cows show that they use the same mechanism to set FRC at about 40 per cent TLC. It is not known if other large domestic animals use the same mechanism.

It may be that all large mammals depend on position (stretch) receptors in their respiratory muscles to sense their lung volume and to provide afferent information to adjust the proper tension and rate of contraction during the breathing cycle. Without a clearer knowledge of the existence and function of afferent nerves and reflexes in association with thoracic and abdominal muscles, it will be difficult to fully understand and appreciate the consequences of anesthesia, recumbency, and surgery on these large animals.

CHEMICAL CONTROL. Chemical control of breathing involves receptors for P_{O_2}, P_{CO_2}, and $[H^+]$ distributed centrally near or within the central nervous system (CNS) and peripherally in the walls of the aorta (aortic bodies) or carotid arteries (carotid bodies) (see Fig. 13–57B). The physiological schemata to be presented is a generalized picture. There simply is not sufficient data to justify discussion of chemical control in individual species (even groups of large domestic animals). In general, all of the chemical receptors, both central and peripheral, respond to changes in O_2, CO_2, and/or $[H^+]$ from set points (or ranges) for each. Decreases in P_{O_2} and increases in P_{CO_2} and $[H^+]$ cause an increase in ventilation (increase VT and f), and increases in P_{O_2} and decreases in P_{CO_2} and $[H^+]$ cause a decrease in ventilation.

There are central receptors that respond relatively strongly to small changes in CO_2 and/or $[H^+]$ from normal arterial values and for that reason are thought to have a predominant effect on breathing control. Central receptors respond less strongly to changes in P_{O_2}. In general, peripheral chemical receptors respond to changes in P_{O_2}, P_{CO_2}, and $[H^+]$ and are thought to be more responsive to changes in P_{O_2} than are central receptors. There are probably specific receptors for each of the chemical entities, P_{O_2}, P_{CO_2}, and $[H^+]$ centrally and peripherally, and their separate effects on breathing may be important under particular situations. However, it is not necessary for our discussion to identify and separate specific central or peripheral receptors. We will group the P_{CO_2} and $[H^+]$ effects and discuss them together

with our description of P_{CO_2} effect, which follows.

Figure 13–58 shows the general ventilatory response to changes in Pa_{CO_2} and Pa_{O_2}. The graph is meant to show the direction and relative magnitude of changes in ventilation in response to changes in arterial blood gas. For that reason, there are no units for ventilation. Zero on the Y axis represents normal ventilation when Pa_{O_2}, P_{CO_2}, and $[H^+]$ are within normal limits. Points above 0 on this axis represent increases in ventilation; points below represent decreases. The solid lines in graphs A and B represent the ventilatory response to changes in PA_{CO_2} and Pa_{O_2}, respectively. The normal ranges for Pa_{CO_2} and Pa_{O_2} are shown by a heavy line on the X axis; note that there is a narrower range for Pa_{CO_2} compared with that of Pa_{O_2}. In response to very small (3 to 5 torr) increases and decreases of Pa_{CO_2}, there are, respectively, increases and decreases in ventilation. In contrast, substantial changes must occur in Pa_{O_2} before changes follow in ventilation (see Fig. 13–58B). In Figure 13–58A, we represent the combined effects of low Pa_{O_2} (hypoxemia) and increasing Pa_{CO_2} on ventilation. Under these circumstances, the slope of $\dot{V}$-Pa_{CO_2} is steeper than normal. During general anesthesia, we can expect the $\dot{V}$-Pa_{CO_2} relationship to be depressed. This is shown by the broken line in Figure 13–58A.

Although decreases in Pa_{O_2} between

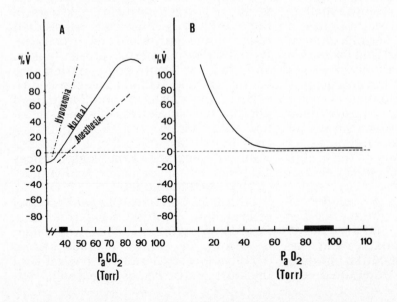

Figure 13–58 The general relationship between per cent of normal ventilation (% $\dot{V}$) in relation to Pa_{CO_2} (A) and Pa_{O_2} (B). The black boxes on the abscissa show the normal blood gas ranges (set points) for Pa_{CO_2} and Pa_{O_2}.

normal values and about 45 torr appear to have very little effect on ventilation in those animals studied (see Fig. 13–58B), there is evidence that there is increased afferent nerve activity from the aortic and carotid bodies with small decreases in P_{O_2} below 100 torr. These impulses increase in intensity as P_{O_2} decreases and reach a central threshold when Pa_{O_2} is about 45 torr and then have an effect on ventilation.

A general unifying hypothesis is helpful in giving us an overview of the control of breathing (see Fig. 13–57). There are groups of neurons in the medulla and pons that regularly fire and cause impulses to go via motor neurons (e.g., the phrenic) to the inspiratory muscles. If it were possible to completely isolate these respiratory neurons from outside depression or excitation, it is hypothesized that they would periodically fire at a basal rate, causing periodic inspiration. If we now add the afferent vagal nerves, which conduct impulses from the stretch receptors of the lung, we add a periodic depression to the central inspiratory neurons. During each inspiration there is an increased intensity of afferent vagal impulses arriving in the medulla, and their effect is to depress inspiratory drive. At some point during inspiration, depending on lung volume, rate of change of lung volume, and the level of central inspiratory excitation, the vagal afferent impulses will lead to a halt in further inspiratory motor impulses, and expiration will follow. Now, we add the chemical receptors and their afferents to the medulla. If there is a high chemical drive (e.g., low P_{O_2} and/or high P_{CO_2} and $[H^+]$), impulses arriving in the medulla from the chemical receptors will cause a heightened central inspiratory excitation. This will cause greater inspiratory motor neuron activity to the inspiratory muscles, the inspiratory period will be shortened, and inspiration will go to greater volumes before being shut off by vagal afferent impulses. This fits the picture we have of animals breathing deeper and faster during high chemical drive. For a more detailed discussion of this current control model, the reader might wish to read the series of articles from two recent symposia (Central mechanisms 1977; Recent advances 1980).

SPECIAL RESPIRATORY PROBLEMS DURING SURGICAL PROCEDURES

We will discuss in this section the problems listed in the introduction of the chapter. Our intention is to discuss these selected problems as they specifically relate to respiratory function and, when possible, suggest solutions for them. We acknowledge that the list might be lengthened and that our discussion too often oversimplifies the problems of surgery to only those considerations relating to the respiratory system. Nevertheless, an understanding of the mechanisms underlying these problems and the physiological principles applied in their solution should provide a sound basis with which the surgeon can better deal with the complexities of surgery.

Depressive Effects of General Anesthetic Agents upon Cardiopulmonary Function. To our knowledge, there is no perfect general anesthetic agent for large domestic animals. There are those that affect cardiovascular and/or pulmonary function less than others, yet all seem to have some adverse effects. The most common adverse effect is the depression thought to occur at the site of those medullary neurons that influence pulmonary and cardiovascular function. The pulmonary depression causes persistent hypoventilation and an associated respiratory and metabolic acidosis. The dangerous consequences of acute acidosis on the metabolism and life processes of body tissues and, in particular, the central nervous system and heart are well known. Patients with pre-existing heart disease or surgical injury are more susceptible to the physiological stress associated with hypoventilation, and cardiac arrhythmias and fibrillation are likely.

Hypoventilation can be reversed with various regimens of intermittent positive pressure ventilation (IPPV). Although IPPV will very likely improve PA_{O_2}, its principal purpose is to re-establish normal Pa_{CO_2} and pHa values. It is not wise to hyperventilate and cause the associated hypocapnia and respiratory alkalosis in order to raise PA_{O_2}. This can usually be accomplished by enriching the O_2 in the inspired gas mixture.

Some general anesthetics appear to directly affect the heart and/or the peripheral vascular system. Most general anesthetics decrease cardiac performance and thereby decrease aortic pressure. Profound decreases in peripheral vascular resistance caused by many anesthetics contribute to further decreases in aortic pressure and have profound adverse effects on local tissue metabolism and the overall distribution of systemic circulating blood.

The solutions to these drug-related problems are complex. The first step is to avoid, when possible, the use of anesthetics that cause profound cardiac or vascular effects. If combinations of anesthetics are used, special care must be exercised to avoid additive depressive cardiopulmonary effects. Cardiovascular stimulants in conjunction with general anesthetics are generally of no value and can cause severe adverse side and/or aftereffects. It is important to support the cardiovascular respiratory function by providing ventilatory support to the pulmonary system (enriching inspired O_2 and IPPV to remove CO_2) and fluid replacement to replenish volume and adjust acid-base balance. Acid-base balance is discussed in more detail in a section to follow. Monitor the respiratory (pulmonary and cardiovascular) function of your patient.

Position of Patients During Surgical Procedures. We know that changing the position of large animals can have profound adverse effects on the function of their respiratory system. When conscious cows go from the standing to the sternal-recumbent position there is a large increase in pulmonary work (Musewe, Gillespie, and Berry 1976). Anesthetized horses have a lesser degree of hypoxemia in the sternal-recumbent position than in the lateral recumbent position (Hall, Gillespie, and Tyler 1968). As a final example, awake cows restrained in dorsal recumbency during abdominal surgery with local anesthetic may have Pa_{O_2} values between 30 and 60 torr, i.e., severe hypoxemia.

The mechanisms that underlie respiratory dysfunction during prolonged abnormal body position are (1) unusual and uncompensated directions of the force of gravity acting on the circulatory and/or pulmonary system (Fig. 13–59). Gravitational force under these conditions causes uncompensated maldistribution of blood perfusion to the dependent regions of the pulmonary and systemic circulations and causes a substantial increase in the maldistribution of ventilation. These effects on the pulmonary system contribute to an abnormal $\dot{V}A/\dot{Q}$ distribution and a decreased efficiency of pulmonary gas exchange. (2) Mechanical restraint on the thoracic and/or the abdominal wall leading to constraint or immobilization of the breathing apparatus. For example, the weight of the body above the down rib cage can restrict its motion and contribution to breathing. (3) Stretching and/or distorting the thorax, diaphragm, and/or abdomen (e.g., head down suspension). This loads the respiratory muscles and reduces their efficiency and force of contraction.

The solution is complex. The surgeon must choose the best position for the patient to accomplish the surgical procedure. His choice of position must be based, in part, on the ease and efficiency of accomplishing his surgical task. Sacrificing these factors would certainly not

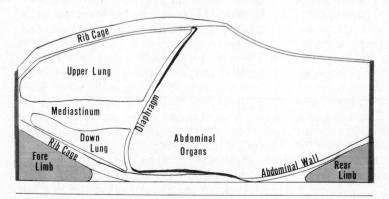

Figure 13–59 Diagram of the sagittal section of a large animal in lateral recumbency, with the general conformation and relationship of the thoracic and abdominal organs outlined.

be in the best interest of the patient. In addition, he must consider the effects of various positions on the function of the patient's respiratory system and its ability to support this function. The better prepared the surgeon is to monitor and support the patient's respiratory function, the greater number of choices he will have for positioning his patients and, it follows, the greater choice of surgical procedures.

Surgical Manipulation Around the Thoracic and/or Abdominal Compartments. The mechanisms underlying these problems are, for the most part, not different from those relating to body position. Special attention will be given to the following: (1) pneumothorax; (2) injury to the lungs; (3) pressure, tension, and/or bruising of the breathing apparatus; and/or (4) incision and/or injury to the respiratory muscles.

Pneumothorax (e.g., thoracotomy) can completely disrupt effective ventilatory motion, and IPPV must be provided to maintain respiratory function. The technical complexities of IPPV are beyond the scope of this chapter. It is important to mention that the physiological effects on the cardiovascular and pulmonary functioning of the various IPPV regimens must be understood to successfully support the patient with an open chest.

The second point, lung injury, can occur in two ways: (1) from ventilatory pressure being too high or too low; and (2) from manipulation of pulmonary tissue during the surgical process. In the first instance, we have discussed the desirability of ventilating as evenly as possible all regions of the lung. This is complicated by anesthetic depression of the ventilatory apparatus, body position restricting ventilatory motion, and gravitational force effects on the distribution of pulmonary blood perfusion. We have discussed the first two. The third can be described using the example of an anesthetized large animal in left lateral recumbency (see Fig. 13–59). In this case, the left lung is below the right lung and the heart and the pulmonary blood flowing into the left pulmonary artery has a greater pressure head than that flowing into the right pulmonary artery because of the additional force of gravity adding to the pressure on the blood as it flows

"downhill" to the lower lung. The greatest intra-capillary pressure will be in those capillaries at the very lowest point in the left lung in our example. The high intravascular pressure in the left lung causes fluid to leak out of the capillaries, causing extensive, regional pulmonary edema and atelectasis (Hall, Gillespie, and Tyler 1968). These lung lesions disrupt gas exchange and may be potential sites of pulmonary infections. The effect of regional pulmonary edema and atelectasis is to divert ventilation to other areas of the lung. One way of opening up atelectatic lower regions of the lung is to use regular or intermittent high ventilatory pressures (>30 cm H_2O). When using high ventilatory pressures, great care must be exercised not to cause lung injury, such as rupture, and/or compromise venous return and/or pulmonary capillary perfusion. The patient with old lung scars is more susceptible to lung injury or rupture from high ventilatory pressures.

Ventilatory injury or injury to the lung caused by surgical manipulation (e.g., palpation, clamping, packing, folding, or cutting) is very likely to cause injury to the lung tissue cells, vessels, nerves, and lymphatics, leading to edema, hemorrhage, and/or tearing or rupture. The immediate consequences are serious and often are complicated by post-surgical pulmonary edema and infection.

It is, perhaps, as important to protect the chest and abdominal walls from injury as it is to protect the lung. Pressure, tension, and/or other injury to these vital respiratory structures will compromise ventilation during and for various periods following surgery.

The solutions to these problems have been suggested in describing their underlying mechanisms. In sum, it is important to take care not to cause unnecessary injury to the pulmonary system in the course of surgery.

Blood-Loss Anemia and Volume Depletion with Surgery. Any type of anemia can cause serious dysfunction of respiration (see Fig. 13–56). This is especially true in surgical patients under general anesthesia. All major processes or respiratory functions of the cardiovascular system, i.e., O_2 transport, tissue gas exchange, CO_2 transport, and buffering of H^+, depend on an adequate amount of circulating Hb. There are several possible physiological responses and consequences of blood loss and to discuss each would be equivalent to discussing the whole area of vascular shock, which is beyond the scope of this chapter. There are different physiological sequelae to blood loss, depending on a variety of circumstances. We will limit our discussion to a single example of a chain of responses that occur with blood loss and that lead ultimately to (1) decreased circulating blood volume; (2) loss of peripheral vascular tone; and (3) decreased Hb concentration.

Briefly, in our example, blood loss before or during surgery will initially cause an increased fH and an increased peripheral vascular tone. Increased peripheral vascular tone helps maintain aortic pressure by decreasing central vascular runoff and increasing circulating blood volume by mobilizing blood from venous reservoirs throughout the body. If blood loss continues to the point where there is inadequate circulating blood volume to provide sufficient O_2 to the tissues, local factors cause a peripheral vascular relaxation and (1) blood pressure falls in the system and (2) *circulating* blood volume initially decreases. The low intravascular pressure promotes H_2O retention and re-absorption from the tissues into the vascular bed. This helps maintain circulating blood volume but also dilutes the blood, decreasing the Hb concentration. If the process is left unchecked, it will continue until there is vascular collapse or irreversible vascular shock. The adverse effects of anemia will be magnified in patients under general anesthesia during surgery. Anesthetized patients without IPPV will, very likely, be hypoventilating and have increased mismatching of $\dot{V}_A$ and $\dot{Q}$ and an increased RL/PVS. These abnormalities contribute to incomplete respiratory gas exchange betweeen the PGS and PCB. The consequences will be a low $P_{A_{O_2}}$ (unless supplemental O_2 is given in the inspired gas) and a high Pa_{CO_2} with an associated respiratory acidosis. If $P_{A_{O_2}}$ is low, each molecule of Hb leaving the lung will be incompletely saturated with O_2 (see Fig. 13–56). In our example of anemia, there are fewer molecules of Hb per ml of blood and each will be incom-

pletely saturated. The end result is substantially less O_2 per ml of blood in any part of the circulation. Depending on the stage of the vascular shock, the CO may be above or below normal. In either case, the amount of O_2 delivered to the tissues per minute will be less than normal, and there will be tissue hypoxia, hypercapnia, and acidosis.

Although our example is simplified and ignores many physiological responses possible during shock, it illustrates the fundamental and serious respiratory dysfunction that can occur with anemia. There are three general approaches in the treatment of vascular shock: indirect, direct, or both. In the indirect approach, various pharmacological circulatory stimulants are given. This approach by itself usually hastens the death of the patient. The direct approach involves replacing the blood lost and supporting the pulmonary function with increased PI_{O_2} and IPPV. Judicious (conservative) use of appropriate drugs along with the direct approach may be helpful, particularly if one is able to measure the patient's vascular pressures and Pa_{O_2}, Pa_{CO_2}, and pHa.

Body Heat Regulation with Surgery. Because of disturbances in the heat regulatory mechanisms associated with the effects of general anesthesia, patients may have hypo- or hyperthermia during surgery. Under normal circumstances, heat loss in large animals by way of the expired air is secondary to other mechanisms. When an animal is intubated, the inspired air bypasses the upper airways and, thereby, the important defense and conditioning functions of this part of the airways. The inspired air is not filtered, warmed, or humidified by the upper airways. These important functions are transferred to the lower airways, which are less well equipped to perform them. Ventilating animals by way of an endotracheal tube with dry gas from compressed gas tanks can dry and injure the airways near the end of the endotracheal tube. When high inspiratory flows are used with IPPV, any infectious agents or particulates present in the air stream will be propelled deep within the lung, particularly since the defense of the airways has been, in large part, bypassed and compromised by drying.

These adverse effects usually do not

cause major difficulties. However, they should be viewed as potential hazards and should be added to the list of possible sources of injury that can occur with general anesthesia and surgery. The following guidelines may be helpful in cases in which prolonged IPPV is required via an endotracheal tube during surgery. (1) Use only clean endotracheal tubes and ventilating equipment (e.g., avoid ventilating the talc used to preserve hoses on anesthetic machines into the airways). (2) Use a properly fitting endotracheal tube that will do the least amount of damage to the airway lining, being sure to keep the pressure in the endotracheal tube cuff at a minimum. (3) Do not ventilate with unnecessarily high inspiratory flow rates. (4) Humidify and warm inspired gas. This is usually difficult and would seem practical only in special circumstances. (5) Monitor deep body temperature and provide cooling and/or warming as required.

Acid-Base Regulation During Surgery. During induction of general anesthesia the patient develops metabolic acidosis, which is complicated by the concurrent hypoventilation with respiratory acidosis. The body can deal with this acidosis via three mechanisms: (1) buffer and dilute the excess H^+; (2) readjust the bicarbonate buffer system with increased $\dot{V}_A$; and/or (3) excrete the acid products and form increased amounts of base. The first mechanism is rapidly saturated. This is evident by the measured acidosis in the anesthetized patient. The second mechanism, increased $\dot{V}_A$, is prohibited by anesthetic depression, position of the patient, and physical constraints on breathing motion associated with restraint and position of the patient. The last mechanism, renal excretion, is relatively slow and requires hours to adjust acid-base disturbances back toward normal pH. Circulatory disturbances associated with general anesthesia and surgery may further depress renal function and slow its rate of correction of acidosis. If respiratory function is disrupted to the extent that the tissues are hypoxemic, metabolic acidosis will worsen during the course of surgery.

The result of all of these factors is that the surgical patient develops an acidosis without the respiratory, body buffer, or renal function to compensate or correct the disturbance. Three procedures will help the acidotic surgical patient; the most important and direct in their effects are the first two: (1) ventilatory support (e.g., IPPV); and (2) maintenance of a normal hemoglobin concentration to ensure adequate tissue gas exchange and blood buffering capacity. Dosages of base and level of ventilation can easily be established if the patient's Pa_{O_2}, Pa_{CO_2}, and pHa are known. The third procedure to help the acidotic surgical patient is (3) the intravenous provision of a base (e.g., sodium bicarbonate).

Problems Associated with Recovery from General Anesthesia. Serious respiratory problems may arise during the immediate postsurgical period that are the result of four related complications: (1) adaptation to a new inspired gas mixture; (2) pulmonary atelectasis and/or edema; (3) cardiovascular shock and pulmonary edema with recovery trauma and postsurgical pain; and (4) chest wall and/or abdominal pain.

If a patient has been breathing from an enriched O_2 gas supply during surgery, its O_2 requirements are usually met despite the existence of hypoventilation, mismatching of $\dot{V}_A$ and $\dot{Q}$, and/or RL/PVS. One point to note, however, is that high levels of inspired oxygen, especially if maintained for long periods of time, may have detrimental effects on the lung. This can include carbon dioxide retention associated with hypoventilation, toxic effects on alveolar epithelium and capillary endothelium, absorption atelectasis, and instability of low $\dot{V}_A/\dot{Q}$ units (oxygen is removed faster than it can be replaced in this situation). Although direct toxic damage to cells from administration of oxygen usually takes a number of days to develop, this is certainly not true of the other effects. The adverse effects of O_2 breathing are directly related to the concentration of O_2 in the inspired gas; i.e., the greater the O_2 concentration, the greater the adverse effects. The most prudent course would seem to be to use only as much oxygen in the inspired gas as is necessary to maintain adequate levels of PA_{O_2}. Furthermore, if the patient has been supported during surgery with IPPV, there may be compensation for, or correction of, the hypoventilation and associated hypercapnia and respiratory acidosis.

The problem then arises if, at the end of surgery, the anesthetized patient is abruptly disconnected from its O_2-enriched gas source and from the positive pressure ventilator. The PI_{O_2} will abruptly drop from greater than 200 torr to about 150 torr (P_{O_2} of air at sea level). Pulmonary dysfunction for which there was compensation during surgery (i.e., IPPV and high PI_{O_2}) is now manifested by very low Pa_{O_2} and pHa and high Pa_{CO_2}. How well the patient is able to cope with this respiratory failure is a function of (1) the depth of anesthesia and how rapidly it is reversed; and (2) the patient's ability to increase ventilatory efforts to correct hypoventilation and re-inflate atelectatic and edematous areas in its lungs.

The second respiratory problem, i.e., regional pulmonary atelectasis and edema, almost invariably occurs during general anesthesia in large domestic animals, particularly in their dependent lung regions. These abnormalities appear to be reversed during the recovery period if the animal has a calm, quick recovery from anesthesia and is able to make large inspiratory efforts. If the animal is unable to ventilate, the atelectasis and edema tend to worsen because of the adverse effects of (1) hypoxemia, hypercapnia, and acidosis, all of which cause local smooth muscle contraction and promote fluid leakage (edema) and the associated airway filling and atelectasis; and (2) gravitational forces acting on the pulmonary circulation, increasing vascular pressure in the dependent regions of the lung and causing greater vascular leakage (edema).

The third respiratory complication (cardiovascular shock and pulmonary edema with recovery trauma and postsurgical pain) is conceivable but to our knowledge has not been shown to occur in large domestic animals. The kinds of blows to the skull that may be self-inflicted by animals recovering from surgery have been shown to cause pulmonary congestion and edema. It remains to be shown if this phenomenon contributes to the pulmonary edema in large domestic animals that die during or following surgery.

The fourth complication (chest wall and/or abdominal pain) is a possible explanation for the failure of some animals to breathe (ventilate) properly following surgery. The pain associated with chest wall or abdominal movement or other postsurgical restrictions prevents adequate ventilatory motion. Ventilation during the postsurgical period was strikingly improved in a group of horses following the administration of meperidine to relieve some of the pain associated with the thoracotomy incision (Gillespie 1982). One of the advantages of early ambulation following surgery may be an improvement in ventilation.

Special Surgical Problems Associated with Patients with Cardiopulmonary Disease. Although special attention must be given to the respiratory systems of all mammals during general anesthesia and surgery, in general these problems are greatest in very small mammals (e.g., small rodents) at one extreme and very large mammals (e.g., adult horses and cows) at the other. The respiratory system of healthy large mammals has considerable functional reserve, and despite abnormalities that occur during the surgical and postsurgical periods, our patients most often survive these periods of respiratory dysfunction. The situation is not as favorable if there is pre-existing pulmonary and/or cardiovascular disease.

Two general points will be considered: (1) if a patient shows signs of respiratory disease, this suggests that there is dysfunction causing or contributing to the signs and that the subject has lost at least part of its respiratory reserve; and (2) the failing respiratory system is highly susceptible to cyclic, positive feedback phenomena, producing further degeneration of function and leading to complete failure.

Regarding this first point, the healthy respiratory system has considerable gas exchange reserve. Under normal circumstances this allows the system to accommodate large increases in demands for gas exchange during exercise or other physiological stresses. For example, it is not unusual to increase $\dot{V}_A$ and CO in excess of five times that of resting values during periods of exercise. Respiratory reserve allows compensation for the early physical or morphologic abnormalities of progressive respiratory disease. The disease process may advance to a considerable extent before intermittent and, finally, continuous signs of respiratory disease are seen. When signs of respiratory disease are seen, one can assume, as a general rule, that there has been significant physical and/or morphological change and that a substantial part of the respiratory reserve has been used. These patients are less able to tolerate the additional depressing effects of general anesthesia and surgery. In summary, we depend on respiratory reserve to help our healthy patients through our surgical procedures. If they have respiratory disease there is less reserve available and the margin of safety (for survival) is substantially reduced.

The second point, respiratory degeneration to failure, can be illustrated with an example of a patient with bronchitis. We will assume that this patient has widespread inflammation of its airways, with large amounts of exudate in the larger airways. There is sufficient hypoventilation in this patient to cause widespread pulmonary regions with hypoxia and hypercapnia and the associated vascular and airway smooth muscle contraction. Although our patient is upright and awake, the reflex vascular and airway constriction compensate in part for the abnormal $\dot{V}_A/\dot{Q}$; however, both ventilatory and heart work are above normal, increasing the need for tissue O_2. The problem is worsened during induction of anesthesia and intubation. The patient has a period of apnea, which causes an immediate worsening of the systemic and pulmonary hypoxemia, hypercapnia, and acidosis. These re-inforce the pulmonary vascular hypertension, further elevate the pulmonary airway resistance, cause a drop in peripheral vascular resistance (perhaps re-inforced by the general anesthetic), and lead to an associated increase in fH. When our patient requires increased ventilation, the respiratory muscles contract with less force and at a slower f because of anesthetic depression and/or body position. It is forced to work in a hypoxic, hypercapnic, and acidotic environment. The ventilatory problem is further complicated by laryngeal spasm, which occurs during efforts to pass an endotracheal tube. The spasm is promoted by the increased airway laryngeal irritation

brought on by the hypoxemia, hypercapnia, and acidosis. In the meantime the heart has been operating in an environment with only marginally sufficient O_2 and high CO_2 and $[H^+]$. It is reflexly stimulated to work harder, further adding to its stress. Local foci in the heart may become sufficiently hypoxemic and/or acidotic to cause ectopic beats, arrythmias progressing to fibrillation. A chain of events has been set into motion that will ultimately lead to respiratory failure and death of the patient. The patient can be saved only if one is able to re-establish respiratory function by (1) establishing an airway (perhaps by tracheostomy), (2) providing an enriched O_2 gas mixture to breathe, (3) giving IPPV, and (4) periodically cleaning the airways and endotracheal tube. In summary, the body tissues are "unforgiving" in their demand for a constant respiratory gas exchange. If pulmonary and/or cardiovascular disease and general anesthesia and/or surgical procedures disrupt respiratory function, the pulmonary and cardiovascular systems will be reflexly stimulated to increase their work to meet the tissues' demands for gas exchange, even after all cardiopulmonary reserve is gone. The respiratory system is driven to exhaustion and, ultimately, failure, having used all of its reserve to compensate for disease, anesthesia, and surgical stress.

Special Cardiopulmonary Problems During Surgery in Particular Species. We have attempted to discuss the major respiratory problems associated with general anesthesia and surgery for all large domestic mammals. There are special problems of some of these species that deserve special emphasis. In general, the larger the animal, the more serious the respiratory dysfunction during anesthesia. These problems have been discussed in previous sections and will not be taken up again here.

During surgery, ruminants are particularly susceptible to respiratory dysfunction because of the mechanical constraint the rumen and its contents place on the pulmonary and circulatory systems. Rumenal pressure on surrounding structures may lower lung volume, limit ventilation, and/or disrupt venous return to the heart. Several factors during anesthesia and surgery may increase the adverse effects of the rumen on the respiratory system.

First, when a ruminant is placed in recumbency during surgery, the opening of the esophagus into the rumen (cardia) may be submerged in the liquid of the rumen. The liquid blocks the esophageal exit for the gas forming in the rumen as a product of fermentation; the gas continues to form and distends the rumen (bloat), producing increased load on the breathing apparatus.

Second, when the ruminant is in recumbency the abdominal wall is forced against the rumen, which is displaced forward (in part) and occupies space previously available for the lungs. In addition to the reduction in lung volume and the available space for easy lung expansion, the abdomen is under greater tension and its displacement during inspiration requires greater inspiratory work (Musewe, Gillespie, and Berry 1976).

Third, relatively insoluble anesthetic gases will leave the blood and tissue space and move by diffusion into gas spaces in the gut until partial pressure of the anesthetic is equal in the blood and gas pockets in the gut. Considerable anesthetic gas can move into the voluminous rumen and cause substantial distension of the rumen before equilibrium occurs. The enlarged rumen will impinge upon the surrounding tissues (e.g., large veins, diaphragm, and lungs) and interfere with their normal function.

Attention to four techniques will help solve each of these problems. (1) It is important to pass a stomach tube prior to or soon after general anesthesia in a ruminant. This allows a passageway for gas (anesthetic and formed) from the rumen. The tip of the tube in the rumen must be kept clear of rumen liquid and food material. (2) Use an anesthetic that does not readily move into the gaseous phase of the rumen. (3) Intubate ruminants to prevent their inhalation of regurgitated ingesta. (4) When possible, avoid placing ruminants in positions that accentuate the rumen pressure on surrounding respiratory structures and/or limit its motion.

CONCLUSIONS

Immobilization, analgesia, and muscle relaxation are requirements for most major surgical procedures and necessitate the use of general anesthetics and, on occasion, additional muscle relaxants. These desirable factors for surgical procedures are antagonists to respiratory function and for that reason complicate the surgical procedures. The adverse effects are often complex and additive, and it seems impossible to us to develop a meaningful comprehensive list of the specific mechanisms involved.

Nevertheless, it may be useful to conclude by highlighting those pulmonary and cardiovascular functional mechanisms that are most frequently disrupted in large animals and about which today's large animal surgeon must have knowledge and a thorough understanding. Two cautions seem necessary. First, all aspects of respiratory function are interrelated; understanding any one part requires knowledge of all others. Second, any summary of this sort must emphasize the usual or most likely and must not be viewed as comprehensive. Instead, it may serve only as a reminder of the major problem areas for the respiratory system during general anesthesia and surgery.

During general anesthesia and surgery, respiratory function is disrupted in the pulmonary system by hypoventilation following central respiratory drive depression and loss of contractile strength and/or efficiency of respiratory muscles. Large increases in mismatching of $\dot{V}_A$ and $\dot{Q}$ and RL/PVS add to the inadequacy of pulmonary gas exchange manifested by hypoxemia, hypercapnia, and respiratory acidosis.

Dysfunction of the cardiovascular system caused by anesthetic effects, which are primarily on peripheral vascular control, complicate respiratory gas exchange with the body tissues. The system may be "overdriven" by control reflexes to adequately supply the body tissues with O_2 (and washout CO_2) at a time when the pulmonary system is failing to adequately oxygenate the blood or remove CO_2 from the body.

The respiratory system has a substantial reserve that enables the system to often compensate for the dysfunction imposed by general anesthesia and surgery. However, cardiovascular or pulmonary disease can substantially reduce the reserve and leave the system particularly vulnerable to the effects of anesthesia and surgical manipulation.

Essentially all surgical procedures on large animals that require general anesthesia and recumbency and that last for an hour or more will cause some pulmonary lesions. These and other factors make the patient particularly susceptible to complications during the postsurgical period.

The physiological reactions of any patient to a particular surgical procedure can be complex and are only predicated in a general way. To protect and care for each patient, one is well advised to monitor the cardiopulmonary function of the patient and support it according to each individual's specific need.

REFERENCES

Bergofsky, E. H.: Humoral control of the pulmonary circulation. Ann. Rev. Physiol. 42:221, 1980.

Brain, J. D.: Anesthesia and respiratory defense mechanisms. Int. Anesthesiol. Clin. 15:169, 1977.

Brain, J. D., Proctor, D. F., and Reid, L. M.: Respiratory Defense Mechanisms I and II. New York: Marcel Dekker, 1977.

Comroe, J. H.: The lung. Sci. Am. 214:56, 1966.

Derksen, F. J., and Robinson, N. E.: Esophageal and intrapleural pressures in the healthy conscious pony. Am. J. Vet. Res. 41:1756, 1980.

Gillespie, J. R.: Unpublished data, 1982.

Green, G. M., Jakab, G. J., Low, R. B., and Davis, G. S.: Defense mechanisms of the respiratory membrane. Am. Rev. Resp. Dis. 115:479, 1977.

Hall, L. W., Gillespie, J. R., and Tyler, W. S.: Alveolar-arterial oxygen tension differences in anesthetized horses. Br. J. Anaesth. 40:560, 1968.

Hymann, A. L., Spannhake, E. W., and Kadowitz, P. J.: Prostaglandins and the lung. Am. Rev. Resp. Dis. 117:111, 1978.

Kalia, M. (ed.): Central neural mechanisms of respiration. Fed. Proc. 36:2365, 1977.

Leith, D. E.: Cough. In Respiratory Defense Mechanisms II. New York: Marcel Dekker, 1977.

McDonell, W. N., and Hall, L. W.: Radiographic evidence of impaired pulmonary function in laterally recumbent anesthetized horses. Equine Vet. J. 11:24, 1979.

Musewe, V. O., Gillespie, J. R., and Berry, J. D.: Pulmonary mechanics and breathing patterns of cows in the standing and sternal-recumbent positions. Fed. Proc. 35:837, 1976.

Ryan, J. W.: Processing of endogenous polypeptides by the lungs. Ann. Rev. Physiol. 44:241, 1982.

Schmidt-Nielsen, K.: Countercurrent systems in animals. Sci. Am. 244:118, 1981.

Schwartz, L. W., and Christman, C. A.: Lung lining material as a chemotactant for alveolar macrophages. Chest 75S:284S, 1979.

Severinghaus, J. W.: Electrodes for P_{O_2} and P_{CO_2} in blood. In pH and Blood Gas Measurement. Boston: Little, Brown, 1959.

Siggaard-Anderson, O.: Sampling and storing of blood for determination of acid-base status. Scand. J. Clin. Lab. Invest. 13:196, 1961.

Siggaard-Anderson, O., Engel, K., Jorgensen, K., and Astrup, P.: A micro method for determination of pH, carbon dioxide tension, base excess and standard bicarbonate in capillary blood. Scand. J. Clin. Lab. Invest. 12:172, 1960.

Wasserman, K. (ed.): Recent advances in carotid body physiology. Fed. Proc. 39(9):1980.

West, J. B.: Ventilation/blood flow and gas exchange. Oxford: Blackwell, 1977.

SURGERY OF THE EQUINE RESPIRATORY TRACT

PETER F. HAYNES, D.V.M., M.S.

Recent advances in the diagnostic armamentarium of equine clinicians, combined with horsemens' improved awareness of the impact of respiratory diseases on equine performance, have markedly increased the incidence of surgical invasion of the respiratory tract. The vast majority of respiratory surgery involves the upper respiratory tract (URT) rostral to and including the larynx. Innovations and improvements in surgical technique and anesthetic regimens and a more thorough appreciation of pathophysiology have improved the postoperative prognosis of many conditions. Some disorders that were previously managed surgically are now managed conservatively, some previously managed conservatively are now more aggressively approached, and some previously considered hopeless may now improve following surgical intervention. In short, surgical intervention of the respiratory tract is more rewarding now than ever before. It is important to recognize that many procedures presently used have been in the profession for years and, with some modification of technique and our concurrent understanding of disease processes, are now enjoying increased efficacy.

ACKNOWLEDGEMENTS

The author wishes to acknowledge the contributions and efforts of the following people: Karen M. Short, medical illustrator, for the artwork; B. Scott Boatright, veterinary clinical technician, for photography; secretarial staff of the Veterinary Clinical Sciences Department; Instructional Resources Division; Dr. D. J. Hillman, Veterinary Anatomy Department, for his consultation and artistic efforts; and the faculty of the Veterinary Clinical Sciences Department, Louisiana State University, for their editorial efforts.

CLINICAL PERSPECTIVE AND DIAGNOSIS

Two hallmarks of respiratory disease indicate the need for surgical intervention: obstructive disease accompanied by abnormal respiratory noise and/or exercise intolerance, and chronic nasal discharge. Obstructive diseases may either be organic space-occupying lesions or functional abnormalities. Lesions that distort the respiratory tract include alterations of the external nares, nasal septum, paranasal sinuses, pharynx, larynx, and trachea. Abnormalities of function include dorsal displacement of the soft palate and laryngeal hemiplegia. Dynamic collapse, described as a reduction in airway diameter by soft tissues due to negative pressure during inspiration, frequently attends obstructive upper respiratory disease (Robinson and Sorenson 1978). Dynamic collapse or any space-occupying lesions can cause increased resistance to airflow, turbulence of airflow and abnormal respiratory noises, especially during periods of rapid and deep respiration.

Chronic nasal discharge frequently suggests empyema of the paranasal sinuses or the guttural pouch(es). Unilateral sinus infections are characterized by discharge on the involved side, whereas unilateral guttural pouch infections are typically accompanied by bilateral nasal discharge, *dominant* on the involved side. Either of these infectious diseases may require surgical intervention for resolution.

The decision to surgically intervene can only be based on sound diagnostic evaluation of the patient. Diagnostic evaluation starts with a thorough physical examination and should include endoscopy, radiography (plain and contrast), centesis procedures, and microbial culture and sensitivity. Attention should be given to asymmetry of the head and cranial cervical area, external nares including airflow and discharges, signs of cranial nerve dysfunction including dysphagia, oral cavity, nasal passages including nasogastric intubation, percussion of paranasal sinuses and thorax, and auscultation of the respiratory tract, especially after exercise or breath holding.

Endoscopic evaluation and appreciation of URT disease have dramatically improved in the last decade. Flexible fiberoptic endoscopes have markedly increased the clinician's understanding of respiratory tract structure and function and its relation to disease. Although rigid endoscopic systems remain as useful diagnostic instruments, fiberoptic endoscopes have exceeded them in popularity (Fig. 13–60). Detailed descriptions of these instruments and their use are contained in several excellent references (Cook 1965; 1970a; 1974; Johnson and Merriam 1975; Johnson et al. 1978; Marks et al. 1970b; Raker 1978b). A brief checklist of observations and considerations during endoscopy includes the following:

1. Documentation of observations can be very useful, especially when sequential examinations are conducted; in this regard an endoscopic examination form is suggested (Appendix A, see end of this section).

2. Tranquilization of the patient may cause relaxation of soft tissues and may thereby alter the movement of laryngeal cartilages, leading to misdiagnosis. Tranquilization should be avoided when evaluating functional abnormalities.

3. General features of the examination include observation for abnormal fluids (exudate, blood) and of the shape, position, and function of structures.

4. Sequential examination proceeds from the external nares to the cervical trachea and may be done bilaterally, especially if lesions of the nasal passages or sinus cavities are suspected. The following areas (structures) should be examined:

   a. Nasal passages including ethmoid turbinate area

   b. Pharyngeal orifice of guttural pouches (Fig. 13–61)

   c. Pharyngeal mucosa including dorsal pharyngeal recess (Fig. 13–61; see also Fig. 13–81)

   d. Soft palate: free border not normally visualized (Fig. 13–62A and B)

   e. Epiglottis: size and shape (see Fig. 13–62A and B)

   f. Larynx, including focal lesions or

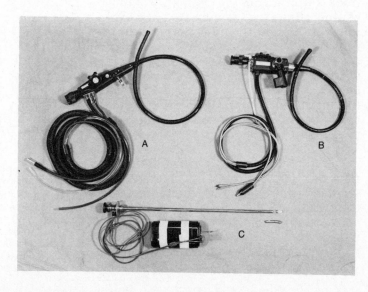

Figure 13–60 Endoscopic instrumentation. Flexible systems are demonstrated in *A* (American Optical) and *B* (American Cystoscope Makers Inc.). The battery-powered rigid endoscope (American Cystoscope Makers Inc.) is shown with the straight and curved tips (*C*).

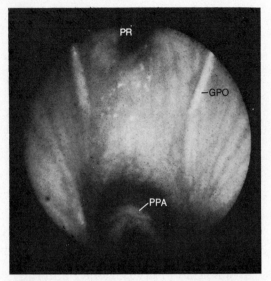

Figure 13–61 Endoscopic view of normal naso-pharynx. Dorsal aspect demonstrating the pharyngeal recess (PR) and pharyngeal orifices of the guttural pouch (GPO). Minimal pharyngeal lymphoid hyperplasia is seen in the dorsal pharyngeal mucosa. The "skull-cap" of the palatopharyngeal arches (PPA) is visible dorsal to the arytenoid cartilages in this three-year-old Thoroughbred.

of the procedures will be discussed with diseases of the individual structures.

Exercise intolerance is so often an admitting complaint that may be related to obstructive disease of the URT that an introduction would not be complete without expanding upon the nature of this complaint. Exercise intolerance resulting from obstructive disease is frequently associated with a respiratory noise, although this noise may go unnoticed by the owner or trainer. The epitome of this complaint is seen in the Thoroughbred racehorse that is incapable of extended exercise beyond 3/8 to 1/2 mile. Such horses frequently produce an abnormal noise referred to as a "whistle," "roar," "rattle," or "gurgle;" in racing vernacu-

abnormal function (Fig. 13–63A and B; see also Fig. 13–62A and B)

    g. Proximal cervical trachea (see Fig. 13–118)

5. Endoscopic examination following exercise may allow a better appreciation of URT function, especially of the larynx.

Radiography of the upper respiratory tract is well within the capability of most equine clinicians. It appears, however, that this diagnostic aid is not used to its full capacity. Radiography is useful in assessing the nasal cavities, paranasal sinuses, guttural pouches, nasopharynx, larynx, and trachea. Contrast material can be utilized to outline structures of the upper respiratory tract and may be a useful adjunct (see Figs. 13–82, 13–87, and 13–104).

Percutaneous centesis is a valuable diagnostic (and potentially therapeutic) technique for evaluating the respiratory tract (Fig. 13–64). Specimens may be obtained for cytological examination and microbial culture and sensitivity from the paranasal sinuses, guttural pouches, trachea, and pleural space. The details

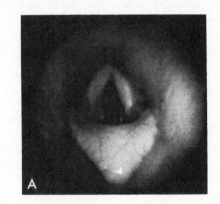

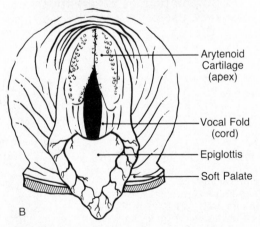

Figure 13–62 *A,* Caudal endoscopic view of normal nasopharynx. Posterior aspect of nasopharynx demonstrates normal anatomical relationships. The outline of the epiglottis is clearly visible, and the soft palate is in a subepiglottic position. (Patient was affected with left laryngeal hemiplegia.) *B,* Diagram of caudal nasopharynx and rostral larynx. Note the serrated margin of the epiglottis and its vascular pattern.

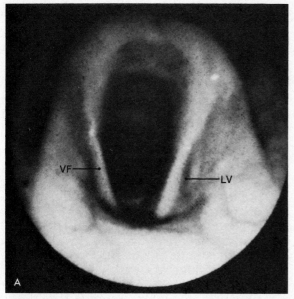

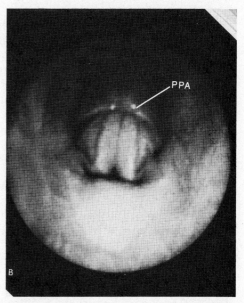

Figure 13–63 *A*, Endoscopic view of normal larynx. View during inspiration demonstrating near maximal abduction of the arytenoid cartilages. This degree of abduction is visualized following induction of the swallowing reflex. The vocal folds (VF) and openings to the lateral ventricles (LV) can be seen. *B*, Endoscopic view of closed larynx (adducted arytenoid cartilages). The palatopharyngeal arch (PPA) is more prominent.

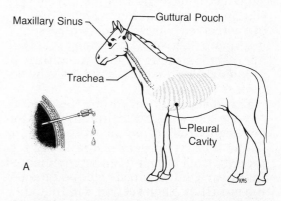

Figure 13–64 Percutaneous centesis. *A*, Location of sites for collection of samples from the equine respiratory tract. The procedures are described in discussion of the regional diseases. *B*, Instruments for centesis. *1*, Styletted needle, 14 gauge × 3½ inches; *2*, intravenous catheter, 14 gauge × 2¼ inches; *3*, mammary infusion tube; *4*, Oshner trocar, improved Philadelphia pattern, 10 gauge × 4 inches (Miltex Co.) with 8F canine urinary catheter.

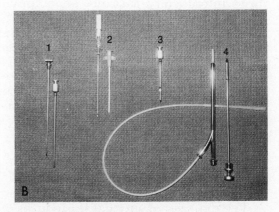

lar, they "stop" or "choke down." Although the diagnosis is often straightforward, occasionally it may be difficult to definitively identify the lesion responsible for the apparent complaint. Thus, a thorough patient history should be obtained including the following:

1. Duration of the problem
2. How much exercise can be tolerated?
3. How much exercise was tolerated prior to production of the noise?
4. Characterize the noise: "whistle," "gurgle"; continual, intermittent?
5. Has the problem worsened?
6. Any previous respiratory disease? Treatment? Results?
7. Has epistaxis been observed following exercise?

Figure 13–65A provides a brief overview of common diseases capable of contributing to exercise intolerance as well as directives for establishing a diagnosis. Figure 13–65B emphasizes that a thorough assessment of the patient should be performed before the respiratory system is incriminated as the only source of the problem. Disease of the musculoskeletal system may be overlooked as a cause of exercise intolerance; this is very common in the equine athlete. Finally, the perceived complaint may represent a mismatch between training management and athletic ability, resulting in greater athletic expectations than the patient is capable of.

The discussion of equine respiratory disease and surgical techniques will follow sequentially from the external nares to the thorax. Surgery of the lower respiratory tract is so infrequently indicated that nearly all emphasis will be directed toward URT. Each section will include a brief introductory passage, an abbreviated synopsis of pathophysiology, pertinent diagnostic criteria, and surgical indications. The reader will be referred to key literature sources, with an emphasis on review articles. Thus, the reference list is not intended to be a complete and all-inclusive summary of published information.

PERIOPERATIVE MANAGEMENT AND ANESTHESIA

The majority of surgical procedures of the respiratory tract are elective and are performed on patients in good physical condition. This allows for adequate patient preparation or a delay of surgery if circumstances are not ideal. The following brief discussion is intended to focus on elective procedures of the URT to prevent repetition of the material when each disease or procedure is subsequently described. This protocol may be altered as necessary, and other regimens may be equally effective.

Dietary regulation is of initial concern when patients have been consuming large concentrate rations. Reduction of the concentrate ration to 2 to 4 lbs daily in advance of surgery (three to five days) appears to decrease the incidence of postanesthetic myopathies. Concentrate and roughage are withheld for 12 to 18 hours prior to surgery, but water is continuously available. Tetanus toxoid and a loading dose of antibiotics (usually procaine penicillin) are administered the day before surgery. The surgical site is liberally clipped at that time. Phenylbutazone is administered orally the night prior to surgery and again intravenously four to six hours preoperatively.

The choice of anesthetic regimen is dependent upon the procedure performed. The patient is tranquilized with 25 to 30 mg of acetylpromazine maleate intravenously, and an indwelling catheter (see Fig. 13–64B) is placed in the jugular vein and secured to the skin with sutures. Five per cent guaifenesin containing 3 gm of a thiobarbiturate, administered intravenously to effect, is selected for most ventral laryngotomy procedures including ventriculectomy, soft palate resection, arytenoepiglottic fold resection, and pharyngeal cautery. These procedures each take 30 to 40 minutes and can usually be accomplished with 1 liter of anesthetic solution. If additional anesthesia is required, a second liter of guaifenesin is used (containing 1 gm of thiobarbiturate).

Inhalation anesthesia is used for extended procedures (e.g., prosthetic laryngoplasty) following induction with the guaifenesin/thiobarbiturate combination. Careful attention is given to patient positioning to avoid postanesthetic myopathy and neuropathy complications. An air-filled mattress* is used to

---

*Dunnage bag, Goodyear Tire and Rubber Co., Industrial Products, Akron, OH 44316.

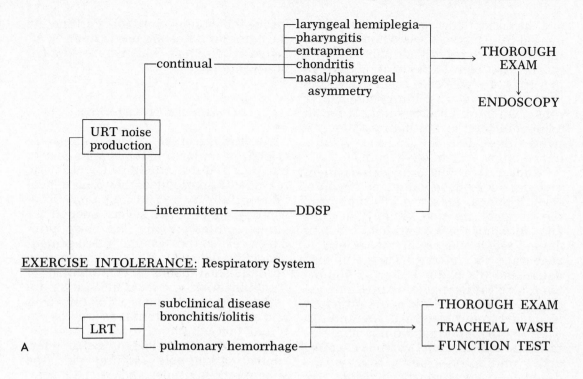

EXERCISE INTOLERANCE: Respiratory System

A

EXERCISE INTOLERANCE: Additional Causes

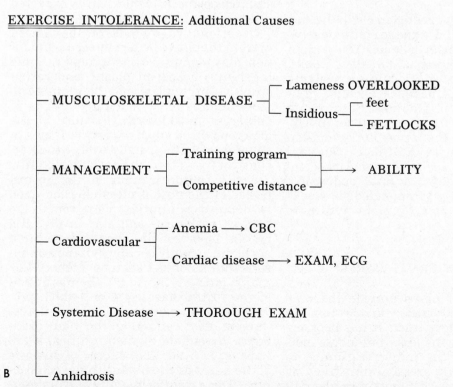

B

Figure 13–65 Exercise intolerance. *A*, Typical disease entities and diagnostic directives for exercise intolerance related to the respiratory system. *B*, Additional causes of exercise intolerance not related to the respiratory system. A thorough physical examination and data base are required to fully characterize these disorders. *URT*, Upper respiratory tract; *DDSP*, dorsal displacement of the soft palate; *LRT*, lower respiratory tract.

pad the patient and appears to be instrumental in reducing these complications. Intravenous fluids are administered at a rate of 3 ml/lb/hr. Patients are recovered in a 10′ × 10′ padded recovery stall, and intranasal oxygen is administered at a rate of 5 L/min. Feed is withheld for an additional four to six hours postoperatively; thereafter the routine maintenance ration schedule is resumed.

Postoperative monitoring of the patient includes close observation of appetite, stool, dyspnea, presence of cough, and the surgical incision. Phenylbutazone and antibiotics are continued for four days. Feed is placed on the ground to encourage the rostral drainage of exudates, and the halter is left off the patient. Ventral laryngotomy incisions are cleaned daily, and white petrolatum jelly is applied to the incisional site and rostrally in the intermandibular space to facilitate subsequent wound cleaning and to minimize scalding from wound drainage. Laryngoplasty incisions are kept dry and clean, and attention is given to preventing contamination of the incision with exudate from the laryngotomy site.

Owners are instructed to clean the surgical incisions daily and to continue feeding the horse at floor level. The patient is to be confined to a stall for 30 days, then allowed 14 to 21 days of "walking wheel" or small paddock exercise prior to resumption of training. Sutures are removed 10 to 12 days postoperatively. Drainage from the laryngotomy incision should cease in 14 to 21 days. Outward healing of the incision should be completed by 30 days. A final endoscopic examination is recommended six weeks after surgery, preceding the return to training.

THE EXTERNAL NARES

The external nares provide the only normal portal for airflow to and from the equine respiratory tract. It has been established that the external nares normally provide the major resistance to airflow in the *upper* respiratory tract; as such, alterations in function or obstruction to airflow through the nares can lead to dyspnea and respiratory distress (Robinson and Sorenson 1978). Fortunately the external nares are not frequently affected by diseases that require surgical intervention.

Trauma and Reconstruction

Lacerations of the external nares are seldom of major functional significance but may require attention for cosmetic reasons. If unattended, they tend to heal uneventfully by second intention. Occasionally, defects are severe enough for surgical intervention. The basic principles of sound wound management should be followed. Most repairs may be accomplished using a combination of tranquilization and local infiltration anesthesia. If the wound is of full thickness and involves the internal as well as external epithelium, a three-layered closure may be considered using interrupted absorbable sutures in the subcutaneous tissues and a nonabsorbable appositional closure of both the inner and outer epithelial surfaces. Such wounds usually heal uneventfully, and suitable cosmetic results can be expected if tissue loss is minimal.

Occasionally, wounds of the nostril margin that have healed by second intention may require cosmetic repair. Some ingenuity, based on plastic and reconstructive principles, may be required to move approximate adjoining tissues to obliterate the blemish. Because of the generous blood supply to facial tissues in general, one can usually expect such reconstructive efforts to heal satisfactorily.

Severe blunt trauma to the rostral bridge of the nose is often characterized by depression injuries of the soft tissue support structures and may involve the rostral aspect of the nasal bones. Such accidents usually occur when the animal runs into an object such as a fence. The major problem is usually the disruption of the rostral nasal septum, which provides axial support to the external nares, immediately caudal to the alar cartilages. A sequela of such injuries, if extensive, is a variable degree of stenosis of the nares due to fibrous tissue contracture. The extent of the injury will determine the selection of procedures to correct the nasal stenosis.

The primary goal of immediate therapy following severe depression injuries of the external nares is to ensure a patent airway. A midcervical tracheostomy should be considered if the animal is dyspneic. Considerations for repair of the collapsed rostral septum may include (1) a stent on either side of the septum, anchored together by through-and-through sutures of the damaged septum, extending from the floor of the nasal cavity to its normal height, (2) elevation and support of the depressed nasal bones by open reduction and support of an axially positioned bone plate, (3) circular stents (e.g., soft garden hose) placed through the external nares beyond the area of stenosis, and (4) appropriately placed drains to reduce soft tissue distension due to hemorrhage and edema. Antimicrobial and nonsteroidal anti-inflammatory agents are indicated in the postoperative period. The prognosis for such injuries and surgical procedures must be considered guarded. Subsequent surgical intervention may be elected to improve the rostral airway once the initial repair attempts have healed and matured.

Reconstructive surgery may be required following extirpation or cryotherapy of neoplastic or granulomatous lesions in or about the external nares. Neoplasia is uncommon; equine sarcoids and carcinomas may be the most frequent lesions in occurrence. Evaluation of the presence of local or regional metastasis (lymph nodes) by fine-needle aspiration should precede surgical intervention. The prognosis is guarded, except in the case of focal noninvasive lesions.

Epidermal Inclusion Cysts

Epidermal inclusion cysts (atheroma) of the respiratory system are almost exclusively located in the posterodorsal aspect of the nasal diverticulum (false nostril). These spherical enlargements usually range from 2 to 5 cm in diameter, although occasionally they may be larger. The cysts are typically soft and fluctuant, nonpainful, and relatively mobile in the subcutaneous tissue. The major concern is a cosmetic one since the airway is seldom compromised by their size or location. Unilateral involvement is most frequently seen. The lesions usually increase in size at a relatively slow rate and may remain as incidental findings. Definitive diagnosis may be established by needle aspiration of the cyst and microscopic visualization of nonkeratinized and keratinized squamous cells using a cellular stain (Gordon 1978). The fluid in the cyst is usually whitish-gray and odorless; it may be thick and tenacious.

These lesions were traditionally considered sebaceous cysts. However, this is a misnomer since the cyst wall does not have a sebaceous gland component (Gordon 1978). These lesions are likely to be a congenital disorder resulting from the aberrant location of epithelial tissue (Kelly and Watson 1976).

SURGICAL MANAGEMENT

Two approaches may be considered for management of epidermal inclusion cysts of the false nostril: drainage from within the false nostril and surgical extirpation.

Surgical drainage is established through the rostral and ventral aspects of the cyst from within the false nostril by local infiltration of anesthesia into the selected site followed by a 1-cm incision into the cyst with a scalpel. The contents are expressed and the cyst is subsequently swabbed or flushed daily with tamed iodine until obliteration of the cyst by granulation tissue and subsequent contracture results. Occasionally the cyst may recur when this technique is used.

Although more invasive, surgical extirpation offers a more assured resolution of the lesion. The procedure may be performed under tranquilization and local infiltration anesthesia. Following preparation of the surgical site, the skin and subcutaneous tissues are incised immediately over the cyst (Fig. 13–66). Dissection is continued around the cyst using scissors, taking care not to penetrate the cyst wall. These cysts are located very close to the epithelial lining of the false nostril, and occasionally the epithelium is penetrated. Once the cyst is delivered from the incision, the subcu-

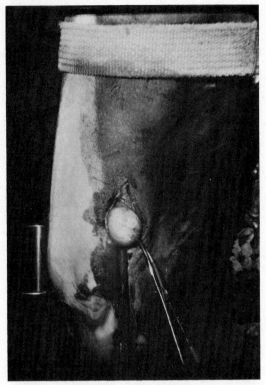

Figure 13–66 Epidermal inclusion cyst (atheroma). The intact cyst associated with the nasal diverticulum (false nostril) is being removed by surgical incision under local anesthesia.

Alteration in either the structure or function of the alar fold–false nostril relationship may be responsible for the production of a respiratory noise. The noise produced by the vibration of these structures has been described primarily as an expiratory noise or flutter and was originally reported in American Saddlebreds as an objectionable noise produced during exercise (Foerner 1967).

Occasionally, a horse may have external nares or rostral nasal cavities that are smaller than normal, and thus the alar fold may be a space-occupying lesion in a relative sense and may cause an abnormal noise even at rest. Unerupted canine teeth in young male horses (younger than three years) have been incriminated as a cause of a relative enlargement of the nasal process of the premaxilla resulting in a decreased diameter of the nasal passage (Boles 1979a). Such horses may exhibit a noise related to the alar fold that may decrease when the canine teeth have erupted.

Generally speaking, alar fold–false nostril abnormalities are uncommon, and alterations that cause dyspnea are even more unusual. The noise caused by vibration of the alar fold and false nostril

taneous space is obliterated with simple interrupted absorbable sutures (00 chromic gut). Skin apposition follows (00 nylon, horizontal mattress sutures). Healing is generally uneventful, and specific aftercare is not necessary. Skin sutures are removed 10 to 14 days later, and the prognosis is excellent.

Alar Folds

The alar folds are mucocutaneous structures located in the dorsal rostral aspect of the nasal cavity and extend caudally from the laminar portion of the alar cartilage to the rostral aspect of the ventral nasal concha. In their caudal extension, they form the ventral and medial aspects of the false nostril (Figs. 13–67 and 13–68). Tension placed on the alar fold during nostril dilation reduces the diameter of the false nostril, thus increasing the cross-sectional area of the rostral nasal cavity.

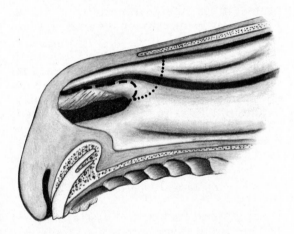

·········· Extent of diverticulum

▬ ▬ ▬ Plane of division, resection, alar fold

Figure 13–67 Anatomy of the nasal diverticulum (false nostril). Diagram of the right nasal diverticulum from its axial surface. The dotted line indicates the extent of the diverticulum. The dashed line indicates the plane of division for resection of the alar fold, which is the dorsal and rostral continuations of the ventral nasal concha.

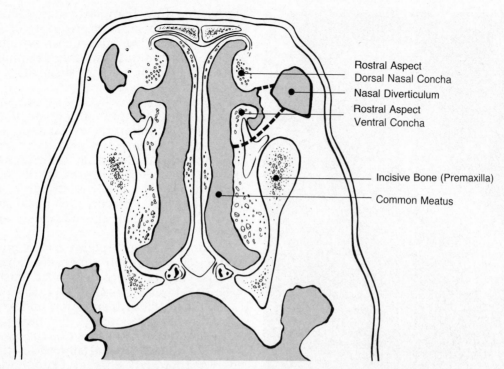

Rostral Aspect
Dorsal Nasal Concha

Nasal Diverticulum

Rostral Aspect
Ventral Concha

Incisive Bone (Premaxilla)

Common Meatus

Figure 13–68 Anatomy of the nasal diverticulum (false nostril). Transverse section through the nasal cavities, demonstrating the relationship of the nasal conchae to the nasal diverticulum. The dashed lines indicate the plane of division for resection of the alar fold. Note: Refer to Figure 13–73 for additional appreciation of these structures.

is usually of concern only to the owner and does not compromise airflow. Many Thoroughbreds normally produce an expiratory "blowing" or "fluttering" sound related to their external nares when they gallop.

Although the noise produced from soft tissue vibration of these structures sounds external in origin, it is necessary to distinguish it from the noise produced by other obstructive airway diseases. To establish whether a noise is produced by the alar fold–false nostril vibration, the nostrils should be temporarily sutured in a dilated position. A horizontal mattress pattern with heavy suture material is placed through each alar fold, within the external nares, and is tied on the midline over a gauze roll (Fig. 13–69). Infiltration of local anesthesia where the suture penetrates the alar fold will facilitate placement of these sutures. If the noise disappears following this technique, the alar folds may be incriminated and surgical intervention should be contemplated.

RESECTION OF THE ALAR FOLDS

Resection of the alar folds was originally described to eliminate noise from vibration of these structures (Foerner 1967). Bilateral resection is usually performed unless a specific unilateral lesion is present. The patient is positioned in dorsal recumbency under general anesthesia for access to both external nares. The external nares and alar folds are thoroughly prepared with a tamed iodine antiseptic.

The alar fold is grasped with an Allis tissue forceps. Scissors are used to divide the fold from the alar cartilage dorsally to the roof of the nasal passage and caudally through the medial wall of the false nostril, including approximately 2 cm of the rostral aspect of the ventral turbinate. Figures 13–67 and 13–68 demonstrate the lines of division for removal of the alar fold. The incision is closed with a simple continuous pattern of absorbable suture (0 chromic gut). Healing should be complete in 10 to 14 days, at

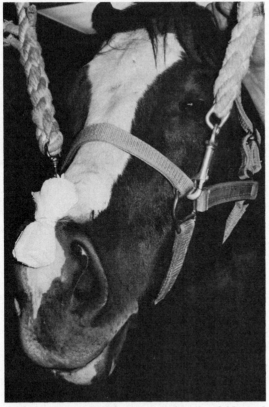

Figure 13–69 Stabilization of the alar folds and false nostrils. A mattress-type suture is used as a diagnostic technique in patients suspected of having a respiratory noise during exercise caused by vibration of these soft tissue structures.

which time the patient may return to exercise. Specific aftercare is not necessary.

The procedure can be accomplished on the standing tranquilized patient with the aid of local infiltration anesthesia. The planes of tissue dissection are identical, although it is more difficult to remove the posterior aspect of the fold. The incision is not sutured.

The prognosis in the patient that produces noise without dyspnea is favorable. If the patient is dyspneic and/or produces a noise at rest because of inadequate size of the rostral nasal cavities, the procedure may provide some relief but should not be expected to totally relieve the signs.

THE NASAL CAVITY

The nasal cavities of the horse are long and narrow, and their major portions are enclosed within bony structures. These factors limit surgical accessibility to the nasal cavities. The submucosa is richly endowed with a diffuse vascular supply, which further complicates surgical intervention of this region.

Typically, diseases of this region that require surgical intervention are characterized by unilateral or bilateral obstruction to airflow and may be accompanied by nasal discharge. Obstructions may be caused by diseases of the mucosal surface (e.g., polyps, granulomas, neoplasia), nasal conchae, or nasal septum or distortion of the paranasal sinuses.

The presenting complaint is most often production of a respiratory noise during exercise or, in more advanced cases, dyspnea at rest. Noise is typically produced during both inspiration and expiration. Unilateral nasal discharge is pathognomonic for disease of the nasal cavity or the paranasal sinuses of that side. A thorough clinical examination should be conducted to rule out other causes of URT obstruction.

Airflow from the external nares should be assessed relative to volume and symmetry. Holding the hands or a light pledget of cotton 4 to 6 inches in front of each nostril will readily allow evaluation of airflow. If a nasal cavity is obstructed to the extent that noise is produced by turbulent airflow through that structure, occlusion of the external nares on the involved side should eliminate the noise. The rostral 4 to 5 inches of nasal septum and nasal cavities can normally be visualized directly by dilating the external nares (sometimes with the assistance of digital examination). Passage of a nasogastric tube through the ventral nasal meatus may indicate narrowing of that structure, although dorsal septal lesions may be overlooked by this technique. Endoscopic examination of the nasal cavities should be conducted to help establish a diagnosis.

Radiographic examination of nasal cavities is the most effective method of evaluating lesions that cannot be thoroughly examined visually or digitally. The dorsoventral projection is very helpful in determining the location and extent of space-occupying lesions and those that cause increased thickness or abnormal positioning of the septum. It is imperative to achieve proper positioning during radiographic exposure so that a true dorsoventral view is obtained.

The following discussion refers to problems primary to the nasal cavities including the nasal septum. Diseases of the paranasal sinuses will be discussed in the next section.

Trauma and Reconstruction

External traumatic insults that result in distortion of the nasal cavity must first fracture facial bones, specifically the nasal bone (with the exception of trauma to the rostral nasal cavity, which is not supported by bony skeleton). Depression fractures of the nasal bone result from accidents such as running into objects, rearing into beams, and kicks. Profuse bleeding from the nares may occur, and subcutaneous emphysema may result if the respiratory mucosa is penetrated by fracture fragments. Such insults seldom result in airway obstruction, and the primary concerns are often the cosmetic appearance of an altered facial profile and the potential for the development of osteomyelitis and/sequestration of fracture fragments. Radiography should be utilized to determine the extent of bony disruption.

It is important to evaluate the neurological status of the patient when extensive injury to the frontal bones also involves the cranial vault. An ophthalmic examination is indicated as well, particularly if the zygomatic process of the frontal bone has been fractured, distorting the bony orbit.

The acutely injured patient should be thoroughly examined and should receive supportive therapy as indicated in the preoperative period (Levine 1979). Broad spectrum antimicrobials and tetanus toxoid should be administered and phenylbutazone used to reduce post-traumatic swelling. Superficial facial wounds should be treated and a compression bandage applied to the region. A delay of 1 to 2 days prior to surgery will likely be in the patient's best interests.

If depression fractures are not extensive, facial contour may be restored in the standing tranquilized patient by elevation of depressed fragments using local anesthetic infiltration. Such fractures frequently have irregular edges, and once elevation has been accomplished, using a narrow periosteal elevator or comparable instrument, additional stabilization of the fracture is seldom indicated.

Extensive depression fractures of the facial bone may require more aggressive surgical management. Fractures of this type most often involve the nasal and/or frontal bones; occasionally the maxillary bone may also be affected. General anesthesia is required to accomplish the extensive reconstructive effort. The patient should be positioned with the affected side uppermost. A wide skin incision (curvilinear or S-shaped) is made to expose the traumatized area and is extended an additional 3 to 5 cm in each direction over the normal perilesional structures. Bleeding can be controlled by electrocoagulation, and suction facilitates the careful removal of blood clots and small loose bone fragments. The periosteum should be spared. If paranasal sinuses are exposed, they may be thoroughly lavaged with sterile solutions to remove blood clots, small bone fragments, or other debris. Elevation of depressed fragments can usually be accomplished with a narrow periosteal elevator. Larger fragments that cannot be suitably elevated may be approached in one of two ways. If the fragment is stable, an orthopedic screw may be inserted at one or more strategic locations to assist appropriate elevation. An alternate technique involves drilling a hole in the bone peripheral to the depressed area and using a Langenbeck retractor to elevate the fragments from underneath, upward (Turner 1979; Wheat 1975). This technique may also assist in stabilizing fragments if transosseous wiring is used.

Whether or not wire sutures are necessary in the repair depends on fracture stability. Because there normally is no movement in the involved bones, those fragments that are wedged back in place need not be additionally stabilized. If stability is inadequate, the fragments are drilled with a Kirschner wire, bone drill, or pneumatic-powered burr and fixed with 18- to 24-gauge stainless steel wire.

The periosteum should be apposed in a simple interrupted suture pattern (00 chromic catgut) when possible. A drain may be placed in the subcutaneous space. Apposition of the skin edges with an intradermal pattern using fine non-absorbable suture material may provide a superior cosmetic appearance (Turner 1979). A pressure bandage should be applied over a nonadherent dressing for three to four days. Antimicrobial therapy should be continued for four to six postoperative days. Sutures can be removed in 7 to 10 days. The prognosis, including cosmetic appearance, is generally good if satisfactory alignment was achieved at the time of surgery.

Repair of fractures into the paranasal sinuses in which a septic sinusitis has become established will require a sinus lavage system at the time of surgery.

Nasal Septum Disease

Abnormalities of the nasal septum characterized by an increase in thickness or a deviation from normal position may potentially cause obstruction to airflow. Such abnormalities may be developmental, traumatic, or neoplastic in etiology. Developmental conditions include cystic dilations of the septum and deviations of the incisive bones (premaxilla) including the nasal septum. Severe traumatic injuries to the nostrils or nasal bones may result in fracture of the septal cartilage with subsequent thickening and distortion. Occasionally a chondroma will develop within the septum, resulting in airflow distortion (Fig. 13–70).

Primary disease of the nasal septum is seldom attended by external asymmetry of facial contour. Generally, diseases of the nasal septum do not resolve once they have become clinically evident, although seldom do they advance to the point of being life threatening. Thus, the decision of whether surgical intervention is necessary is based on the intended use of the patient.

RESECTION OF THE NASAL SEPTUM

Subtotal resection of the nasal septum is indicated for space-occupying lesions or distortions of the nasal septum that markedly alter airflow through the nasal cavities (Frank 1964). Because septal surgery may be accompanied by consid-erable blood loss, it may be advisable to have blood available for transfusion, particularly if the procedure is expected to take an extended time. A suitable donor may be identified and 4 to 6 liters of blood collected in an appropriate anticoagulant. If the surgery is elective and can be delayed for two to three weeks, blood may be obtained from the patient and stored for subsequent autotransfusion. Prophylactic antimicrobial therapy should be instituted preoperatively and tetanus toxoid administered.

General anesthesia is required, and the patient is positioned in lateral recumbency and intubated. A suitable aperture (2 cm) is created on the dorsal midline through the nasal bones at the caudal aspect of the lesion. It is preferable not to enter the frontal sinus. Thus, the most caudal site is at the divergence of the nasal bones, slightly caudal to the level of the rostral aspect of the facial crest (see Fig. 13–74).

A cruciate incision is made in the skin over the selected site. The skin is reflected and the periosteum similarly incised. The periosteum is reflected and a trephine or bone gouge used to create the desired opening through the nasal bones. The nasal septum is readily identified as it courses axially through the aperture. The mucosa on either side of the septum is divided longitudinally, providing access to both dorsal nasal meatuses. A Doyen intestinal forceps or suitable alternative is passed vertically through the caudal aspect of the aperture to the floor of the ventral meatus, engaging the nasal septum (Fig. 13–71).

The rostral aspect of the nasal septum is exposed by dilation of the uppermost nostril. An incision is made through the rostral aspect of the septum using electrosurgery. The incision should be curved caudodorsally and should extend from the ventral aspect of the nasal septum to its dorsal attachment (see Fig. 13–71). It is important that a sufficient amount of rostral septum remain (at least 3 to 4 cm) to provide support for the alar cartilages and external nares. An osteotome is then used to divide the nasal septum dorsoventrally to the floor of the ventral meatus through the caudal aperture immediately ahead of the positioned forceps. The septum is then di-

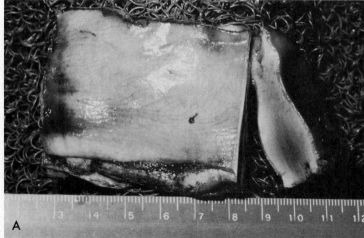

Figure 13–70 Chondroma of the nasal septum. *A,* The resected portion of the rostral nasal septum has been transversely divided, demonstrating its thickness and irregularity. Patient was a three-year-old Thoroughbred. *B,* Endoscopic view of nasal cavity 120 days postoperatively. The rostral edge of the remaining septum (arrows) is thickened and caused airflow obstruction. The horse was unable to withstand sustained exercise.

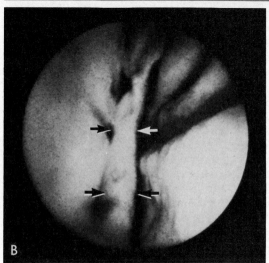

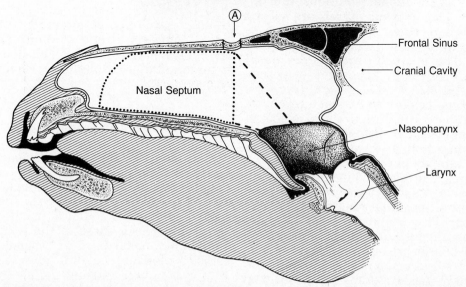

Figure 13–71 Resection of the nasal septum. The dotted lines indicate the planes of division for subtotal resection of the nasal septum via creation of an aperture on the dorsal midline (A). The dashed lines indicate the oblique division of the entire caudal ventral septum when obstetrical wire is used for near total removal of the septum. See Figure 13–74 for additional landmarks.

vided from its dorsal and ventral attachments by extending the rostral incision caudally to the forceps. A guarded chisel is suggested (Frank 1964), although an osteotome or bone gouge is an adequate substitute. By this time, hemorrhage is copious and the resection should proceed without delay. Traction should be applied to the loosened septum by grasping it at the external nares, and any remaining attachments should be severed. The resected section is then delivered through the nostril.

An alternate resection technique is to divide the septum at an angle of approximately 45° in a caudoventral direction, rather than vertically (Flynn 1978; Tulleners 1981), extending caudal to its ventral attachment on the hard palate (see Fig. 13–71). Obstetrical wire is threaded through each ventral nasal meatus and retrieved through the oval cavity after extubation. This maneuver will require a small hand or a pair of long forceps. The ends are secured together and the wire adjusted (threaded through the nasal cavities) so that a single strand enters one nostril and exits the opposite nostril, encircling the ventral aspect of the septum. Obstetrical wire can also be used to divide the septum from its dorsal attachment by threading it through the aperture created in the nasal bones.

Following septal resection, the nasal cavity should be tightly packed with gauze (antimicrobial solutions are optional). The external nares are closed with two to three mattress sutures to ensure that the packing remains in place. The aperture through the nasal bones is closed by apposition of periosteum and skin. A midcervical tracheostomy must be performed and a tracheostomy tube sutured securely in place. If the tube becomes dislodged, the patient will expire from asphyxia because of the gauze tampon in the nasal passages.

Aftercare involves continuation of antimicrobial therapy for four to six days. The nasal packing and tracheostomy tube should be removed 24 to 48 hours postoperatively. Subsequent hemorrhage and discharge are minimal, and the benefits of surgery should be apparent immediately. Local therapy of the surgical site is not necessary.

The prognosis for improving airway obstruction is guarded to good if the entire portion of the diseased septum was removed. The rostral edge of the remaining caudal segment of the septum tends to thicken following resection (see Fig. 13–70B). Thus, although airflow may be improved it may not be adequate for full exercise capacity. It is suggested that dividing the caudal septum at an angle places this thickened area more caudally so that the airway is wider at this site than at the level of the more rostral vertical site (see Fig. 13–71), where the nasal conchae are in closer proximity to the septum (Tulleners 1981). If neoplastic disease is present, recurrence of the primary lesion is possible. Healing should be complete in 30 days, and return to exercise should follow physical and endoscopic examination.

CORRECTION OF NASAL SEPTUM AND INCISIVE BONE DEVIATIONS

Developmental deviation of the incisive bones (premaxilla) and nasal septum is an uncommon occurrence. These patients, referred to as having a "wry nose," have severe obstruction of the nasal cavity on the convex side of the deviation and malocclusion of the incisors (Fig. 13–72). Correction of this defect has been reported using a two-stage operation (Valdez et al. 1978). Wedge osteotomy and an autogenous bone graft (rib) were used to reconstruct the incisive bones, followed by subtotal nasal septal resection and alignment of the nasal bones. A strong commitment on the client's part must be established prior to undertaking this extensive reconstructive surgery.

Other Space-Occupying Lesions

Additional lesions that occasionally cause obstructive disease of the nasal cavities include fungal granulomas (Fig. 13–73), neoplasia, nasal polyps, and ethmoid hematomas. Patients usually present with one or more of the following complaints: nasal discharge (purulent or serosanguineous), necrotic odor, and airway obstruction causing noise. The diagnosis of such lesions is established by techniques previously described. In ad-

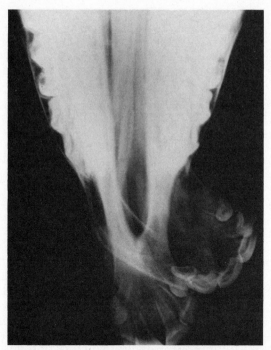

Figure 13–72 Congenital deviation of the incisive bones (premaxilla). Dorsoventral radiographic projection demonstrates severe deviation, which caused occlusion of the right nostril.

dition, biopsy of such lesions is important for definitive diagnosis. If lesions are located near the external nares, biopsy may be obtained under direct visualization by surgical incision, punch biopsy, or biopsy forceps. If the lesion is located in the caudal nasal cavity, biopsy may be obtained during endoscopic visualization, using either the biopsy system of the flexible fiberoptic instrument or biopsy forceps. Typically, the basket of an endoscopic biopsy forceps is too small to provide an informative tissue specimen because the surface of such lesions is often merely inflammatory tissue.

The most frequent cause of fungal granuloma of the upper respiratory tract is *Entomophthera coronata* (Hanselka 1977). Such lesions usually present a granulating surface and are frequently associated with a bloody nasal discharge. The lesions usually have a broad base of attachment and may be multifocal. Diagnosis may be established by direct or endoscopic visualization of the lesion and confirmed by histopathology and fungal culture. Excision of the lesion in

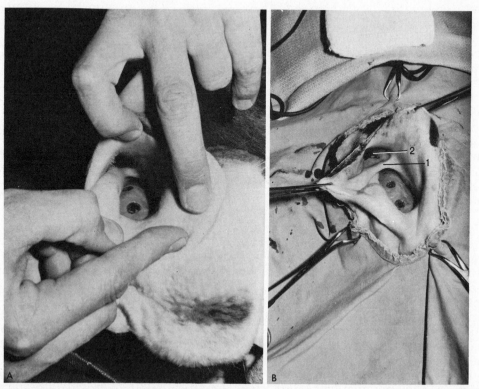

Figure 13–73 Fungal granuloma, nasal septum. *A*, A mucosal-covered space-occupying lesion is seen just caudal to the left external nares on the nasal septum. The two circular lesions are the result of biopsy techniques. Patient is in right lateral recumbency. *B*, Longitudinal division of the external nares was used to expose and excise the lesion. The cut edges of the nostril are retracted with Allis forceps, exposing the alar fold (*1*) and the medial wall of the nasal diverticulum behind it (*2*).

its entirety should be the primary goal of treatment, although this is seldom accomplished because of the lesion's location. The reported infiltration of lesions with amphotericin B is suggested as the treatment of choice (Hanselka 1977). Lesions of 10 to 15 cc volume should be infiltrated with 40 to 50 mg of the antifungal agent. If the lesion can be partially or totally removed, infiltration of the base of attachment is recommended. Daily topical therapy for 14 to 21 days with a 0.05% solution of amphotericin B in DMSO (100 mg in 200 cc) should be used as adjunctive therapy. Lesions should begin regression within 14 days, and total remission of lesions has been observed. The prognosis for combined therapy should be guarded, depending on the extent of the lesion.

Neoplasms of the nasal passage, although not commonly encountered, most often include squamous cell carcinoma and fibromas (Madewell et al. 1976). Such lesions are usually accompanied by odorous serosanguineous or mucopurulent nasal discharge related to tissue necrosis. Their infrequent occurrence precludes adequate description of their clinical management. If surgically accessible, excision is recommended, followed by cryosurgery of the base of attachment. If inaccessible to surgical removal, extensive cryosurgery of the tissue mass may be attempted. The prognosis in any regard must be considered guarded.

Nasal polyps are pedunculated growths usually considered inflammatory and consisting of loosely arranged fibrous tissue covered by epithelium (Moulton 1961). According to one report, the base of attachment is most often to the lateral aspect of the nasal cavity from one of the nasal conchae (Frank 1964). Surgical excision is the therapy of choice and may be accomplished by snare or direct extirpation at the base of attachment. The latter approach may require surgical invasion through the nasal or frontal bones to gain access to the involved nasal cavity (Berge and Westhues 1966).

Ethmoid hematoma has been described as a progressive expansile lesion usually originating from the ethmoid labyrinth or sphenopalatine sinus (Cook and Littlewort 1974). The disease is clinically characterized by spontaneous hemorrhagic nasal discharge and may cause nasal cavity obstruction. The etiology remains obscure, although it may be neoplastic (hemangioma-hemangiosarcoma). The lesion is composed of an encapsulated hematoma covered by respiratory epithelium, which may ulcerate focally. Expansion of the lesion may occur rostrally into the nasal cavity and caudally into the nasopharynx. Presumptive diagnosis is based on endoscopic recognition of a dark (bluish to blue-green) lesion in the caudodorsal aspect of the involved nasal cavity. Radiography may support the diagnosis of a space-occupying lesion.

Aggressive therapy is required for this lesion, and cryosurgery is reported to be the treatment of choice, as it apparently reduces the rate of recurrence (Cook and Littlewort 1974; Wheat 1980). The base of attachment is exposed by an approach through the conchofrontal sinus. A thorough double freeze-thaw cycle should be performed and may require 20 to 30 minutes, using a continuous source probe system. The prognosis is guarded to good.

SURGICAL APPROACH TO THE NASAL CAVITY

Surgical access to the nasal cavity to explore, excise, or cryosurgically manage lesions previously described can be achieved through a dorsal approach (Berge and Westhues 1966). A more extensive approach involves creating a bone flap (Wheat 1973) to gain a wider operative field and will be discussed under diseases of the paranasal sinuses (see Fig. 13–77).

The surgical approach to the nasal cavity is similar to that performed for the caudal division of the septum in subtotal resection of the nasal septum (Frank 1964). In this case, however, the aperture through the nasal bone is made lateral to the midline, allowing access into the nasal cavity on that side. The window created may be enlarged with a bone gouge or rongeurs or it may be extended longitudinally to provide greater exposure. This approach appears most suited to removing the base of attachment of pedunculated lesions such as polyps or fungal granulomas. Such lesions could then be delivered through the external nares.

When surgical access to the caudal nasal cavity or ethmoid labyrinth is required (e.g., ethmoid hematomas), exposure of the conchofrontal sinus is necessary. The bone flap technique is most applicable for suitable exposure of this region (see Fig. 13–77). The floor of the sinus is removed to form a window over the rostral aspect of the ethmoid labyrinth. Surgical excision or cryotherapy of the hematomas may then be performed.

THE PARANASAL SINUSES

The paranasal sinuses represent an evagination of respiratory mucosa into bony cavities of the skull and are at risk for diseases affecting the mucosa of the more axially related respiratory tract. This is particularly important in relation to infectious processes, as the sinuses may be overlooked in differential diagnoses rather than considered as reflecting the mucosal response to disease that occurs in the remaining respiratory epithelium.

The paranasal sinus most often diseased is the maxillary sinus, predisposed because of its association with dental structures and its dependent (ventral) location. The nasomaxillary opening provides the communication between the frontal, sphenopalatine, and maxillary sinuses and the nasal cavity. It is located immediately above the ventral nasal concha in the middle nasal meatus, at approximately the level of the fifth cheek tooth (M-2) (Fig. 13–75; see also Fig. 13–74). Because the maxillary sinuses are

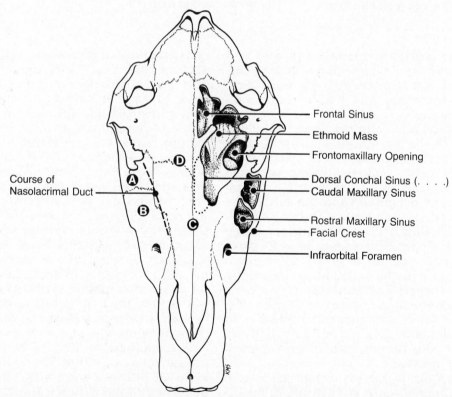

Figure 13–74 Trephination of the paranasal sinuses. Diagram of skull demonstrating location of frontal and maxillary sinuses and sites for trephination. The maxillary compartment is entered above the facial crest and below the nasolacrimal duct (dashed line) at (A) for the caudal compartment and (B) for the rostral compartment. The site for exposure of the nasal septum (e.g., septal resection) is located at the level where the nasal bones diverge (C). The frontal sinus may be entered at (D), and access to the nasal cavity on that side is obtained by removal of the floor of the dorsal conchal sinus.

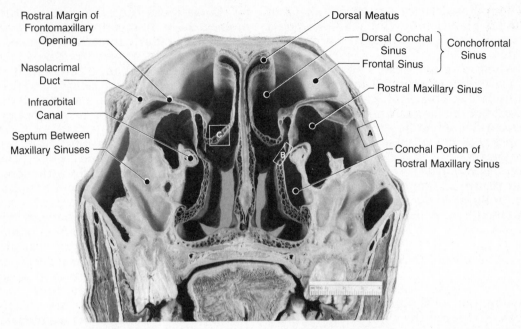

Figure 13–75 Trephination of the paranasal sinuses. Cross-section of skull at the level of the second molar (aged horse). Exposure of the rostral maxillary sinus by trephination (*A*). The turbinate portion of the sinus may be fenestrated (*B*) by passing dorsal and medial to the infraorbital canal. The caudal nasal cavity may be exposed by fenestration of the dorsal conchal sinus (*C*).

located rostral to the other sinuses and the nasomaxillary opening is located dorsally, there is a tendency for fluid (exudate) to accumulate within these compartments.

The primary clinical features of disease of the paranasal sinuses include nasal discharge, bony distortion, obstruction to airflow, and ocular discharge on the involved side (Mason 1975). Nasal discharge occurs only on the side of the involved sinus, because the nasomaxillary opening is located within the nasal cavity. Typically, exudate is mucopurulent, may contain a bloody component, and may even be malodorous (indicating tissue necrosis). Hemorrhage suggests granulomatous or neoplastic lesions. Necrosis may accompany neoplastic or granulomatous lesions and frequently involves bony tissues when alveolar periostitis is present.

External facial distortion associated with sinus disease is a feature of space-occupying lesions (neoplasms, cysts), alveolar periostitis, or fluid accumulations within a closed sinus compartment. As long as the nasomaxillary opening is patent, exudative processes usually do not cause facial distortion. However, chronic accumulations of inspissated exudate may cause distortion due to a reduced tendency to drain naturally. External distortion caused by space-occupying lesions or closed compartment distension usually causes a comparable internal distortion of the nasal cavity and subsequent obstruction to airflow. Bony distortion and nasal cavity obstruction secondary to alveolar periostitis are usually the result of tissue reaction surrounding the dental alveolus and are seldom associated with obstruction of the nasomaxillary opening. The tooth most often diseased, resulting in secondary sinusitis, is the first molar (Mason 1975).

A presumptive diagnosis of disease of the paranasal sinuses can be made from clinical symptoms and findings at physical examination. Percussion with simultaneous auscultation may identify areas of dullness suggestive of fluid or abnormal tissue within a sinus. The oral cavity should be examined for the presence of dental abnormalities or other conditions that may involve the sinus secondarily. Endoscopic examination of the nasal cavities may reveal exudate from the nasomaxillary opening or, in advanced cases, distortion secondary to sinus enlargement.

Radiography is a particularly useful method to evaluate the location and extent of paranasal sinus disease. Radiographic findings that may be seen include fluid lines within the sinus, space-occupying soft tissue densities including multicystic structures, decreased areas of bone density, abnormalities of teeth or dental alveoli, and fractures. The standing lateral and dorsoventral views may be augmented by oblique views. The radiographic film should be positioned on the side of suspected involvement to improve radiographic detail and reduce magnification.

Percutaneous Centesis

Percutaneous catheterization of sinus cavities can be both a diagnostic and a therapeutic procedure. The technique is performed by infiltrating local anesthesia (5 to 6 ml) subcutaneously over the center of the suspected sinus (see Figs. 13–74 and 13–75). A stab incision is made through the skin, and a trocar-tipped Steinmann pin and a Jacobs pin chuck are used to bore into the sinus. The pin should only extend 1 cm from the chuck to prevent damage to deeper structures once the sinus is entered. The size of the pin should be slightly larger than the catheter or needle selected to withdraw the sample. An intravenous catheter, canine urinary catheter, or mammary infusion tube is suggested for this purpose (see Fig. 13–64B). Retrieval of exudate by direct aspiration or by aspiration following a 20- to 30-ml saline flush establishes a diagnosis of sinusitis. Direct microscopic examination, a Gram stain, and culture and sensitivity tests should be carried out on the sample obtained.

If abnormal fluid is not recovered, the sinus should be lavaged with 250 ml of sterile saline. This fluid will enter the nasal cavity and will be voided from the nostril. If it does not contain any exudate, sinusitis is an unlikely diagnosis.

The skin incision can be sutured if further access to the sinus is not necessary. If subsequent local therapy is indicated, an indwelling catheter may be sutured in the sinus or the site can be left open for repeated introduction of a flushing device.

Surgical Approaches to the Paranasal Sinuses

Trephination is the traditional approach for surgical access to the paranasal sinuses. The bone flap technique was developed to allow greater exposure of sinus cavities than that achieved with trephination and is superior in that regard (Wheat 1973). The reader should review the landmarks of the maxillary and frontal sinuses and is reminded that the alveoli of the upper third through sixth cheek teeth comprise the ventrolateral floor of the maxillary sinuses. These sinus compartments enlarge as the teeth become shorter. Thus, the patient's age must be taken into consideration when planning the site of surgical intervention. Radiographs taken for preoperative evaluation will demonstrate the location of dental structures.

TREPHINATION

Figures 13–74 and 13–75 demonstrate the appropriate sites for trephination of the rostral and caudal maxillary sinuses and frontal sinuses. A trephine or bone gouge can be used to create the opening into the involved sinus following the removal of a circular piece of skin over the selected site. Local hemorrhage is controlled by direct ligation or electrocautery. When the rostral maxillary sinus is approached, the levator nasolabialis and levator labii maxillaris muscles are retracted dorsally to expose the periosteum. The periosteum is reflected using a cruciate incision, and a 2-cm diameter hole is made through the bone. Bone roungeurs may be used to enlarge the original opening if necessary.

Additional techniques can be used if the objective of surgery is to improve drainage beyond that accomplished by simple trephination. To establish drainage from the rostral maxillary sinus, its conchal (medial) wall is perforated to allow additional communication with the nasal cavity. A finger is inserted through the trephine opening and dorsally over the infraorbital canal (which divides the ventral conchal sinus from the rostral maxillary sinus) to palpate the most rostral aspect of the ventral conchal sinus (see Figs. 13–74 and 13–75). The thin bony wall at that site is subsequently broken down by forcing a rigid mare catheter (or other appropriate instrument) through it from within the nasal cavity. A gauze seton can then be guided through the sinuses into the nasal cavity and nares and tied back to the trailing end, which emerges from the trephine opening (Frank 1964).

If both caudal and rostral maxillary sinuses contain exudate, the thin bony plate dividing them may be disrupted to allow rostral (ventral) drainage into the latter. This may be accomplished by digital manipulation through the rostral trephine approach. The bony fragments should be removed and a lavage system established in the caudal maxillary sinus for subsequent therapy.

A seton can be placed through the floor of the conchal portion of the conchofrontal sinus in a manner similar to that described for the inferior maxillary sinus. The conchal portion is exposed by trephination on the involved side, immediately caudal to the divergence of the nasal bones and just lateral to the midline (see Figs. 13–74 and 13–75).

The objective of seton placement is to maintain a patent opening into the nasal cavity to facilitate drainage. To maintain effective drainage in the postoperative period, the seton should be manipulated (to-and-fro action) daily to dislodge the fibrin seal that develops. The seton may be changed at 5- to 7-day intervals by attaching a clean gauze to the cut end of the positioned seton and drawing an entire new seton into place. The length of time the seton should remain in place depends on the underlying problem. Removal of the seton may be followed by natural closure of the created conchal aperture, or it may remain as a permanent window.

The trephination site usually closes within 21 to 30 days with little, if any, blemish. Daily care should include cleaning and topical wound therapy. If setons are exposed or if insects are bothersome, the head may be protectively covered

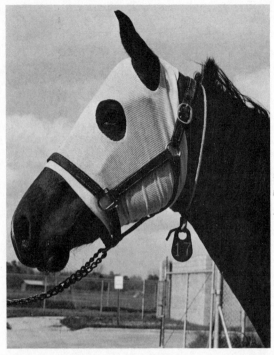

Figure 13–76 Protective head dressing. Six-inch stockinette can be used to protect surgical sites of the facial area.

during the postoperative course by a 6-in diameter stockinette with apertures for the eyes and ears (Fig. 13–76). The skin ventral to the site should be protected with a light coat of petrolatum to prevent scalding.

BONE FLAPS

Surgical exposure of the maxillary and frontal sinuses by creating bone flaps increases the surgical exposure without causing the postoperative blemishes that may attend larger trephine approaches. The improved surgical exposure allows superior assessment and manipulation of lesions and is particularly useful in revealing space-occupying lesions such as cysts and neoplasms. This technique can also be used to expose the nasal cavity.

The limits of the desired exposure are determined, and a three-sided rectangular skin incision is made with its base medially (Fig. 13–77). The skin and subcutaneous tissue are divided, and deep structures are reflected medially (i.e., levator labii maxillaris and levator nasolabialis muscles in a maxillary sinus approach). The periosteum is similarly

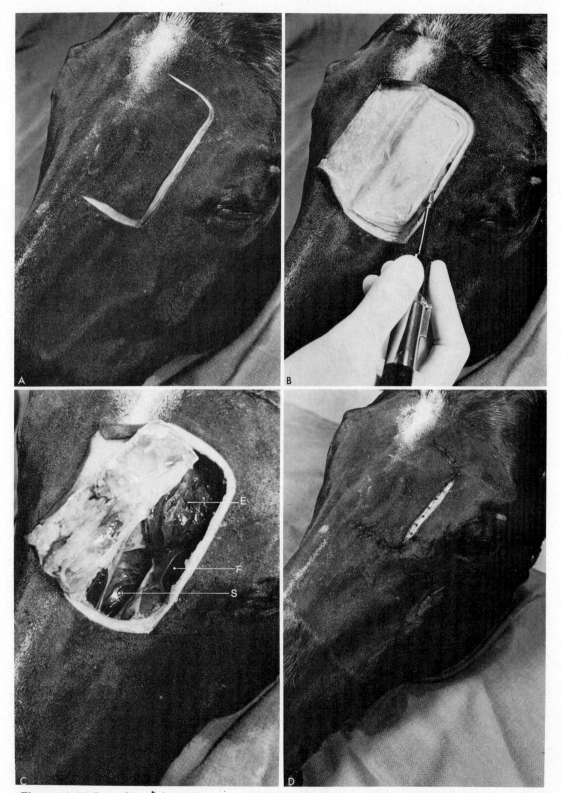

Figure 13–77 Bone flap technique to expose left frontal sinus. *A,* The skin and subcutaneous tissues are incised and reflected to expose the frontal bone. *B,* The frontal bone is divided with a pneumatic drill. *C,* The frontal and conchofrontal sinuses are exposed and the ethmoid mass (*E*), frontomaxillary opening (*F*), and floor of the conchofrontal sinus (*S*) are visible. Removal of the medial wall or floor of the chonchofrontal sinus allows entry into the common or middle meatus. *D,* Closure of the surgical approach is accomplished by apposition of the deep fascia and skin.

incised and reflected from the margin of the intended flap. A Hall air drill with a tapered burr or an oscillating bone saw can be used to divide the bone along the periosteal incision (Boles 1979b; Wheat 1973). It may be helpful to transect the bone at an angle so that the external surface of the flap is slightly larger than the deep margin of the defect into the sinus. The flap is then carefully elevated, exposing the underlying compartment. The intact margin of the rectangle acts as a hinge, creating an incomplete fracture.

Upon completion of intraoperative objectives, the flap is pressed back into place. Stainless steel wire sutures may be placed through drilled holes to secure the flap, although they are seldom necessary. The periosteum is sutured with absorbable suture material (0 chromic catgut). Subcutaneous tissue is similarly closed and the skin sutured with a nonabsorbable material. An indwelling lavage system may be secured in place to allow local therapy as needed to treat the underlying disease process. The incisions usually heal without complication or facial defect.

Sinusitis

Bacterial infection of the paranasal sinuses is the most frequently encountered disease process of these structures. Fluid accumulation is referred to as empyema and most commonly involves the rostral maxillary sinus when associated with dental disease (Cook 1965–1966; Mason 1975). Such infections may reflect a primary respiratory tract infection, or they may be secondary to facial bone fractures, dental abscessation, granulomatous lesions, or neoplasia.

Primary sinusitis is usually caused by *Streptococcus* sp. and may be an acute or chronic manifestation of respiratory disease complicated by that organism (Wheat 1973). It is suspected that subclinical disease occurs more often than is appreciated and resolves spontaneously. The usual history reveals a chronic unilateral mucopurulent nasal discharge that responds to antimicrobial therapy but that recurs when treatment is stopped. The patient is usually asymptomatic except for the nasal discharge and does not have facial distortion. A definitive diagnosis may be made by percutaneous centesis of the involved cavity and may be supported by radiographic examination. The suggested therapy is daily lavage of the sinus with 500 ml of saline including a broad spectrum antimicrobial or antiseptic until the definitive organism(s) are known and the sensitivity established. Systemic antimicrobials should support local therapy. Daily treatment should continue until the discharge is markedly reduced, at which time local treatment may be continued for an additional three to four treatments every other day. If this approach is unsuccessful after 14 days or if the condition recurs, trephination and the establishment of improved drainage into the nasal cavity may be considered. The prognosis is favorable.

Secondary sinusitis may be more difficult to manage and more frequently requires surgical intervention for treatment of the primary condition and improved drainage. Sinus infections secondary to facial fractures that are not associated with sequestration of bony fragments are exceptions to this generalization. Such cases should be managed by lavage initially, and surgery should be considered only if the medical approach is ineffective. If sequestration accompanies the sinus infection, surgical excision of the involved bone combined with sinus lavage should lead to an uneventful recovery.

The objective of therapeutic treatment of secondary sinusitis is removal of the inciting cause: diseased teeth, granulomas, or neoplasms. Invariably, surgical access to the involved sinus is required. The prognosis depends on the underlying lesion. It is usually favorable when sinusitis is secondary to dental disease. Management of cases that require either extraction or trephination and repulsion of the involved tooth or teeth are discussed in the section on equine colic surgery (Chap. 15).

Granulomatous and neoplastic lesions of the paranasal sinuses are generally difficult to manage successfully. Granulomatous lesions are usually caused by a variety of mycotic agents, including those of the Phycomycetes group, and

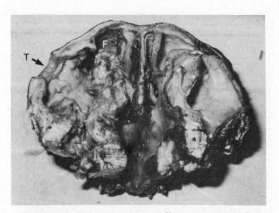

Figure 13–78 Squamous cell carcinoma, sinus. Clinical signs suggestive of sinusitis secondary to dental disease preceded removal of the second and third molars in this 20-year-old horse. The trephination site into the caudal maxillary sinus is evident (*T*). The lesion extended from the maxillary sinus into the frontal sinus (*F*), and the patient was euthanatized.

Cryptococcus sp. (Hanselka 1977; Scott, Duncan, and McCormack 1974). Successful management has been reported following the use of excision, cryotherapy, and local antifungal agents such as amphotericin B. The prognosis is generally guarded, however, and is dependent on surgical accessibility and the extent of the lesion.

Osteoma, osteosarcoma, squamous cell carcinoma, lymphosarcoma, and adenocarcinoma occur in the paranasal sinuses (Fig. 13–78) (Boles 1979a; Leyland and Baker 1975; Madewell et al. 1976; Reynolds et al. 1979). Neoplastic lesions are usually well established and have achieved local and regional metastases by the time they become clinically evident. Cryotherapy may be considered in the management of some neoplastic conditions, but the prognosis is generally guarded to poor.

Maxillary Cysts

Multiloculated cystic disease has been recognized as a cause of maxillary sinus enlargement and partial to complete nasal cavity obstruction (Cannon, Grant, and Sande 1976; Cook 1970b; Leyland and Baker 1975). Affected patients are usually one to two years of age, although the lesion can occur in older horses. Although clinical signs may suggest dental

disease, oral examination is generally unremarkable.

Percutaneous centesis typically yields a relatively acellular yellow or pink fluid unless the lesion has become secondarily infected. One or more permanent tooth germs may be absent on lateral or oblique radiographic views (Cook 1970b) (Fig. 13–79A). Dorsoventral views demonstrate that the rostral and/or caudal maxillary sinus is distended both axially and abaxially and may displace the nasal septum (Fig. 13–79B). Occasionally the cysts may extend into the conchofrontal sinus. The etiology remains unclear, although the cysts may be developmental and may arise from embryonic structures of the tooth root. Spontaneous resolution has not been reported. The objectives of therapy are to remove cystic structures and establish drainage of the sinus into the nasal cavity. The prognosis with surgical intervention is guarded since internal distortion of the nasal passage may not resolve, even if the cyst is successfully treated. The bone flap technique appears superior to trephination in accomplishing these objectives.

The area of cystic involvement is typically composed of a spongy membrane and may be rather extensive. This tissue is removed, as completely as possible, by blunt dissection or curettage. Involved teeth may be repelled. Additional drainage may be established into the nasal cavity by enlarging the nasomaxillary opening or breaking through the conchal portion of the involved sinus. To maintain these drainage avenues, gauze setons are positioned and exit through the external nares. Postoperative therapy should include lavage of the involved cavity through an indwelling system with antimicrobials or dilute povidone iodine (5 to 10 per cent of stock solution). The duration of this treatment is determined by exudate production, although it should be continued for at least 10 to 14 days. The setons should be manipulated to maintain drainage and are removed when lavage therapy is no longer necessary.

PHARYNX

The nasopharynx extends from the caudal nares to the intrapharyngeal os-

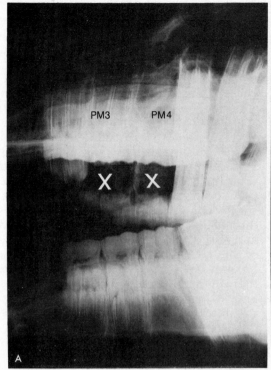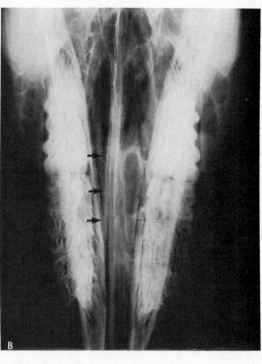

Figure 13–79 Right maxillary cyst. *A*, The ventrodorsal oblique view (taken from the left side) demonstrates that the permanent tooth germs for PM3 and PM4 are missing (Xs) on the right side. Compare the right with the left dental arcades, where the tooth germs are present (*PM3* and *PM4*). Deciduous premolars ("caps") are seen on both arcades. The patient was a 2-year-old Thoroughbred with an obstructed right nasal cavity. *B*, The ventrodorsal projection demonstrates expansion of the lesion into the nasal cavity and displacement of the nasal septum to the left (arrows).

tium, the aperture through which the rostral laryngeal cartilages project (Fig. 13–80). The nasopharynx is relatively unsupported by rigid structures and is therefore susceptible to distortion from the guttural pouches and functional obstruction by the soft palate in addition to focal or diffuse space-occupying lesions. The membranous lining of the nasopharynx is typical respiratory epithelium with diffusely distributed submucosal lymphoid aggregates (Fig. 13–81; see also Fig. 13–61). The nasopharynx may also undergo dynamic collapse secondary to obstructive lesions located rostral to it. Thus, pharyngeal obstruction may be either primary or secondary and is a potential cause for dyspnea and exercise intolerance because the horse is nearly an obligate nose-breather.

Clinical signs suggestive of pharyngeal disease include coughing, nasal discharge, dysphagia, and mild to marked obstruction of airflow. Coughing and na-

sal discharge, frequently associated with viral and bacterial infections of the respiratory tract, are reflections of generalized mucosal inflammation and are a common occurrence in the young horse population. Focal or diffuse respiratory mucosal lesions may result in comparable clinical signs. Neoplastic and granulomatous lesions are often attended by blood in the nasal discharge.

Dysphagia may be characterized by a reduction or inability to swallow, discharge of ingesta from the external nares, and aspiration pneumonia. Causes of dysphagia include pharyngeal paralysis from dysfunction of the glossopharyngeal and vagus nerves (IX and X), focal space-occupying lesions that interfere with palatal function, and palatal incontinence resulting from congenital cleft of the soft palate or excessive resection of the caudal free margin.

Obstructive conditions of the pharynx may be characterized by dyspnea or ster-

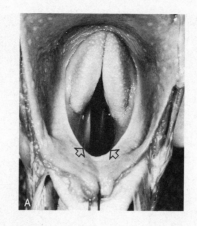

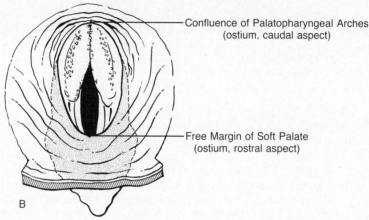

Confluence of Palatopharyngeal Arches
(ostium, caudal aspect)

Free Margin of Soft Palate
(ostium, rostral aspect)

B

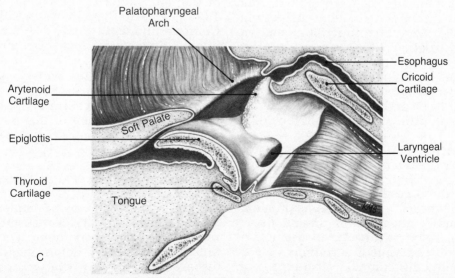

Palatopharyngeal
Arch

Esophagus

Cricoid
Cartilage

Arytenoid
Cartilage

Soft Palate

Epiglottis

Laryngeal
Ventricle

Thyroid
Cartilage

Tongue

C

Figure 13–80 Intrapharyngeal ostium and its relationship to dorsal displacement of the soft palate. *A,* Specimen of caudal nasopharynx with the soft palate divided transversely rostral to the ostium. The rostral aspect of the intrapharyngeal ostium (arrows) is visible because the soft palate has been displaced dorsal to the epiglottis (DDSP). The caudal aspect of the ostium (palatopharyngeal arches) is visible immediately dorsal to the apices of the arytenoid cartilages. *B,* Diagram of tissue specimen in *A* consistent with endoscopic view of DDSP. *C,* Diagram of a sagittal section of the pharynx and larynx with DDSP. The palatopharyngeal arch has been elevated rostrodorsally from the arytenoids to demonstrate a sagittal view of the intrapharyngeal ostium.

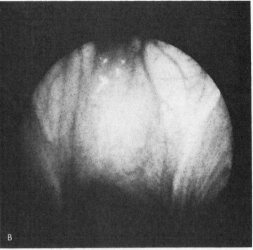

Figure 13–81 Pharyngeal lymphoid hyperplasia (PLH). *A,* Endoscopic view of two-year-old Thoroughbred with grade III PLH. *B,* Endoscopic view of mature horse. The pharyngeal mucosa is smooth and the submucosal vessels are visible in this four-year-old Thoroughbred.

torous breathing at rest, or they may only become apparent during exercise with maximal airflow through the nasopharynx. Those diseases evident in the resting patient usually represent marked distortion of the pharynx by space-occupying lesions including distension of the guttural pouch. Those that are evident only during exercise include mild lesions, minimal reductions in pharyngeal diameter, and functional pharyngeal obstruction (FPO) as a result of dorsal displacement of the soft palate (Heffron and Baker 1979). These "lesions," associated with exercise intolerance, may be quite subtle and are among the most difficult to definitively diagnose.

A presumptive diagnosis of disease of the pharynx is based on a detailed history and clinical signs. Endoscopic examination is the procedure of choice for definitive diagnosis. Although some problems are readily apparent, it should be re-emphasized that functional obstructions and mild pharyngeal variations may be extremely difficult to substantiate or quantitate. Endoscopic assessment may reveal a normal-appearing pharynx or one with mild inflammation (lymphoid hyperplasia). False negative and false positive evaluations are possible and contribute to the uncertainty of patient management and subsequent prognosis.

Radiographic evaluation of the pharyngeal region may suggest abnormalities of the nasopharynx or guttural pouch (see Fig. 13–112). Contrast pharyngography may enhance appreciation of tissue profiles and may aid in quantitation of space-occupying lesions, pharyngeal distortion, and the positional relationship of the soft palate to the epiglottis (Fig. 13–82; see also Figs. 13–87 and 13–104). Contrast fluoroscopy may document dysphagia and aspiration of ingesta into the respiratory tract.

Surgical intervention for lesions of the nasopharynx is most frequently performed through a ventral laryngotomy incision. A description of this and other approaches to the pharynx follows.

Surgical Approaches to the Pharynx

Four approaches can be made to the equine pharynx to perform surgical correction of various conditions. The selection of approach is determined by the disease present, the type or method of correction planned for the disease, and the surgical exposure required. Although each procedure has its advantages and disadvantages, the ventral laryngotomy or translaryngeal approach is used most often for surgery of the pharynx and larynx.

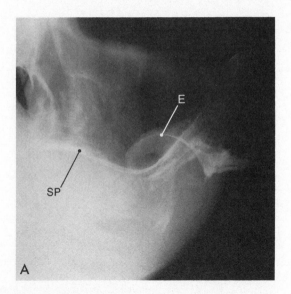

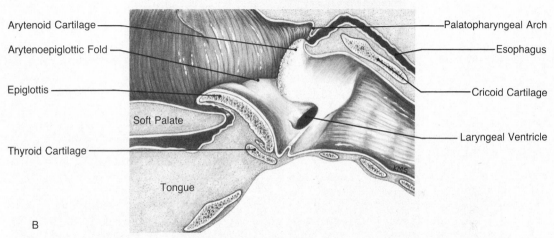

Arytenoid Cartilage

Arytenoepiglottic Fold

Epiglottis

Soft Palate

Thyroid Cartilage

Tongue

Palatopharyngeal Arch

Esophagus

Cricoid Cartilage

Laryngeal Ventricle

B

Figure 13–82 Contrast pharyngogram. *A*, Lateral radiographic view following deposition of contrast material in the nasopharynx of a normal horse. The dorsal surface of the soft palate (SP) and epiglottis (E) is outlined with contrast media, which has also entered the larynx. *B*, Diagram of sagittal section of normal pharynx and larynx.

VENTRAL LARYNGOTOMY

The ventral laryngotomy has been used since the turn of the century to provide exposure for pharyngeal and laryngeal surgical techniques. Although this procedure can be accomplished under local anesthesia with the patient standing, general anesthesia with the patient in dorsal recumbency is the method of choice. Precise patient positioning in dorsal recumbency will allow the easiest definition of the midline and thus the most direct, atraumatic approach. Because the patient's head is extended while in dorsal recumbency

and the ventral cervical muscles are under tension, the median muscular septum can be palpated immediately ventral to the larynx. The center of the incision should be at the point where a line continues from the caudal aspect of the vertical ramus of the mandible across the ventral midline (Fig. 13–83A). This prevents "exploring" anterior to the larynx or in the cricotracheal space.

A 10-cm incision is made through the skin and subcutaneous tissues, exposing the paired hyoideus muscles. Cutaneous and subcutaneous hemorrhage is controlled by electrocoagulation. Blunt scissor dissection is used to axially divide the

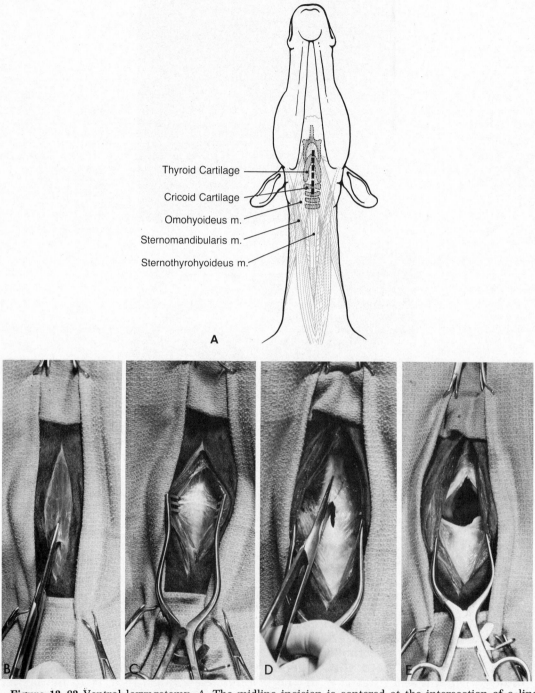

Thyroid Cartilage

Cricoid Cartilage

Omohyoideus m.

Sternomandibularis m.

Sternothyrohyoideus m.

A

Figure 13–83 Ventral laryngotomy. *A,* The midline incision is centered at the intersection of a line continued ventrally from the vertical ramus of the mandible. *B,* Scissors are used to divide the sternohyoideus and omohyoideus muscles. *C,* Self-retaining retractors are used to facilitate the deep dissection. *D,* The laryngeal lumen is entered through the cricothyroid ligament with a stab incision extended with scissors. *E,* Retraction allows visualization of the laryngeal lumen.

paired muscles, and a self-retaining retractor is inserted to expose the perilaryngeal fascia (Fig. 13–83B and C). Division of this fascia with a scalpel exposes a small fat pad immediately superficial to the cricothyroid ligament. The ventral aspects of the thyroid cartilages (which converge rostrally) are palpated and the fat pad divided on the midline. A medium sized vessel, located in the caudal aspect of the cricothyroid space, will require attention to control hemorrhage. The laryngeal lumen is penetrated by a quick stab incision through the cricothyroid ligament with a scalpel (Fig. 13–83D). This incision is extended with scissors rostrally to the body of the thyroid cartilage. The scissors should enter the lumen and divide the laryngeal mucosa and cricothyroid ligament simultaneously to prevent undermining the mucosa. The retractors are then repositioned to retract the wings of the thyroid cartilage and expose the lumen (Fig. 13–83E). If an endotracheal tube was utilized during anesthesia, it is withdrawn to reveal the laryngeal structures and caudal nasopharynx. This midline entry to the larynx enhances postoperative drainage, and minimal trauma reduces postoperative swelling.

The thyroid cartilage may be divided for an additional 1 to 1.5 cm rostrally on the ventral midline with a bone-cutting forceps to gain additional exposure to the pharynx if necessary. However, surgically divided cartilages may calcify postoperatively (Boles, Raker, and Wheat 1978; Raker and Boles 1978). Therefore, this procedure should be reserved for those few cases requiring greater exposure. In young horses, the cricoid cartilage may mistakenly be transected while extending the laryngotomy incision caudally. However, ventral division of the cricoid cartilage may be elective if additional laryngeal exposure is required (e.g., subtotal arytenoidectomy). Surgical apposition of the divided thyroid or cricoid cartilages is not necessary.

Properly executed, this surgical incision closes uneventfully in 21 to 30 days by second intention. Although it is unnecessary, some surgeons elect to totally or selectively reappose the tissue layers of a ventral laryngotomy incision. The inherent contamination present increases the frequency of wound sepsis and dehiscence. It is difficult to achieve an airtight closure to prevent the spread of pathogens into the reapposed tissues, and local sepsis may progress to cellulitis. Furthermore, the convenient portal for tracheostomy tube placement to alleviate occasional postoperative dyspnea may outweigh the indications for primary closure. In short, second intention healing is without complications and is difficult to improve upon.

The surgical site is cleansed daily during the postoperative period and white petrolatum jelly applied around the incision and in the intermandibular space. Drainage from the incision and postoperative swelling are markedly reduced in 10 to 14 days. Complete healing is achieved in 30 to 45 days.

ORAL APPROACH

Occasionally lesions of the nasopharynx may be approached orally. Diseases successfully managed by this technique include epiglottic entrapment and nasopharyngeal polyps (Boles, Raker and Wheat 1978; Speirs 1977; Stickle and Jones 1976). Intravenous anesthesia is utilized, although inhalation anesthesia may be administered by nasotracheal intubation (10- to 25-mm tube size) if it does not interfere with surgical manipulation (Steffey 1979).

The oral cavity is held open with a mouth speculum or dental wedge. The accessibility of the caudal pharynx is governed by the patient's size and the size of the surgeon's hand. In general, the horse must be of adequate size (1000 lb), and the surgeon must have a small enough hand to reach lesions caudal to the soft palate. Division of the rostral soft palate on the midline to manipulate a nasopharyngeal polyp for snare removal (through the nasal cavity) has been reported (Stickle and Jones 1976). Endoscopy through the nasal passage may facilitate surgical manipulation of a lesion in the nasopharynx. In summary, although the oral approach may be difficult to achieve because of the physical limitations of the patient and surgeon, it does have the advantage of not requiring more extensive surgical approaches.

MANDIBULAR SYMPHYSIOTOMY

Division of the mandibular symphysis has been reported as a method to provide adequate surgical exposure of the oral cavity and pharynx (Nelson, Curley, and Kainer 1971). This approach is indicated for diseases of the hard or soft palate, oropharynx, and caudal nasopharynx that require extensive exposure. This approach is most frequently used for congenital cleft of the soft palate, although it could be considered for any space-occupying lesion (neoplasia, granuloma, polyp). This surgical approach, combined with surgical division of the soft palate, allows generous exposure of the nasopharynx.

The surgical approach involves axial division of the ventral lip and mandibular symphysis. The incision is carried caudally between the horizontal ramus of the mandible and the tongue and associated muscles. A thorough review of the described technique and associated anatomy will prevent damage to vital structures. Surgical closure of the incision involves anatomical tissue apposition and stabilization of the mandibular symphysis. Internal fixation using the lag-screw technique is the procedure of choice. External fixation with a Kirschner fixation splint and Steinmann pins can be used. In addition, the incisor teeth may be wired together.

The major problem encountered with this approach is dehiscence of the lower lip incision. This closure may be supported by through-and-through fixation of the lip to the lower incisors. A suggested alternative is to leave the lower lip intact at its free margin. The intact margin can be drawn dorsal and caudal to the lower incisors and can still allow adequate reflection of the mandibular rami (Shires 1980). This alternative eliminates the need for secondary support of the lip incision and its dehiscence.

PHARYNGOTOMY

Ventral pharyngotomy has been reported to provide surgical access to the pharynx, particularly the oropharynx. Its use has been described for surgical manipulation of epiglottic entrapment and cleft of the soft palate (Cook 1974; Speirs 1977). The ventral midline incision is made rostral to the body of the thyroid cartilage (i.e., rostral to the site for ventral laryngotomy incision) between the paired thyrohyoid bones (Fig. 13–84A). The paired sternohyoideus muscles are divided, exposing the deeper omohyoideus muscles. The omohyoideus muscles are separated, and the thyrohyoid ligament is divided axially. The hyoepiglotticus muscle is divided on the midline, and the oropharynx is entered through the glossoepiglottic fold (Fig. 13–84B through D). The rostral extent of the incision is limited by the basihyoid bone, although reportedly this may be divided (Cook 1974). Neither vital structures nor extensive hemorrhage is encountered. Disadvantages of the approach are the depth of incision and limited visibility. Tissue planes may be surgically apposed, or the incision may be left to heal by second intention. The anticipated postoperative course is uncomplicated.

Pharyngeal Lymphoid Hyperplasia (PLH)

Pharyngeal lymphoid hyperplasia (PLH) is primarily a disease of the young athletic horse and is characterized by diffuse hyperplasia of lymphoid aggregates in the nasopharynx. PLH is reportedly the most common cause of partial obstruction of the URT in the young Thoroughbred and Standardbred (Raker and Boles 1978). This disease has been referred to by numerous names including follicular pharyngitis, pharyngeal follicular lymphoid hyperplasia, chronic lymphoid follicular hyperplasia (CLFH), and chronic pharyngitis. This syndrome should be differentiated from acute inflammatory pharyngitis (Boles 1979a).

The etiology of PLH has not been established. It has been recognized that young horses (two to three years old) have a normal population of lymphoid follicles distributed primarily over the dorsal and dorsolateral pharyngeal walls including the dorsal pharyngeal recess (see Fig. 13–61). These follicles usually regress to small white plaques by four years of age (see Fig. 13–81B), and thus their presence may be considered a normal phenomenon in the maturing horse (Boles 1975; 1979a). The number and size of these lymphoid aggregates appear

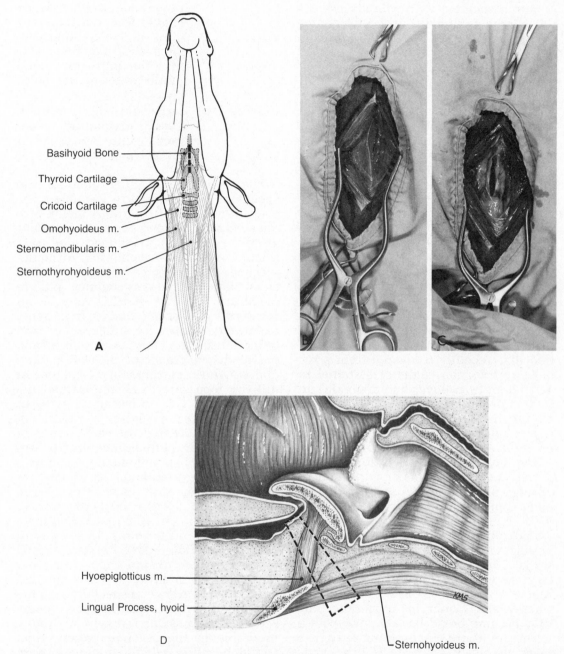

Basihyoid Bone

Thyroid Cartilage

Cricoid Cartilage

Omohyoideus m.

Sternomandibularis m.

Sternothyrohyoideus m.

A

Hyoepiglotticus m.

Lingual Process, hyoid

D

Sternohyoideus m.

Figure 13–84 Ventral pharyngotomy approach. *A,* Diagram indicating landmarks for the midline incision between the thyroid cartilage and the basihyoid bone. *B,* The sternohyoideus muscle and omohyoideus muscles are separated axially. *C,* The thyrohoid membrane is divided, followed by the hyoepiglotticus muscle and oral mucous membrane. *D,* Diagram demonstrating plane of tissue division and anatomy of the surgical field.

to increase in response to various stimuli, the most frequent of which is infectious agents (McAllister and Blakeslee 1977; Proceedings 1980). The infectious agents associated with this disease are the equine influenza virus and equine herpesvirus Types 1 and 2 (McAllister and Blakeslee 1977; Montgomery 1981). This nonspecific inflammatory response is histologically characterized in the initial phases by necrosis and inflammation and, more chronically, by fibrosis and lymphoid proliferation (McAllister and Blakeslee 1977). Environmental factors such as inhaled irritants or allergens may contribute to the multifactorial origin of this syndrome. Furthermore, subclinical lower respiratory tract disease following respiratory infections may contribute to exercise intolerance in these patients.

The primary presenting complaint for horses with PLH is exercise intolerance, frequently associated with a harsh inspiratory and expiratory noise during extended exercise. Cooling out following exercise may be prolonged. Although the history frequently reveals that the patient has recently recovered from a respiratory infection, signs of systemic involvement (e.g., fever and anorexia) are seldom present. A mild serous nasal discharge may be present, and an intermittent cough may occur during or following exercise.

The diagnosis of PLH is supported by a well-documented history, the general absence of systemic signs of disease, and endoscopic examination (see Fig. 13–81A). Early evidence of PLH includes visualization of small, nearly translucent vesicles raised from the pharyngeal walls. Central necrosis, hyperemia, and edema suggest an ongoing inflammatory reaction. Clinically, the nodules become thicker and firmer in appearance and may become broad based or polypoid in nature. A four-point grading system to more precisely characterize the endoscopic findings has been reported (Raker and Boles 1978).

Grade I: A few small inactive whitish follicles over the dorsal walls: normal.

Grade II: Numerous small inactive follicles, with the occasional hyperemic one, extending downward over the lateral pharyngeal walls. May cause exercise intolerance if pharynx is smaller than normal.

Grade III: More active follicles located close together, covering the entire dorsal and lateral walls of the pharynx.

Grade IV: Large and edematous follicles, frequently coalesced into broad-based and polypoid structures.

The syndrome of PLH includes the spectrum from normal to variable exercise intolerance. Respiratory noise produced during exercise suggests turbulent airflow related to a reduced cross-sectional area of the nasopharynx. Although marked PLH may be recognized as a cause of decreased performance, mild to moderate evidence of PLH may be an incidental endoscopic finding in patients experiencing exercise intolerance from other causes (e.g, laryngeal hemiplegia, dorsal displacement of the soft palate, and epiglottic entrapment). Evidence of mild to moderate PLH may attend apparent exercise intolerance without causing respiratory noise. The clinician must appreciate that the contribution of PLH to exercise intolerance may be difficult to establish and should continue a systematic examination to recognize other diseases that caused decreased work capacity. As previously mentioned, the patient's age is important, and moderate lesions in the young horse without noise production during exercise should prompt further examination. Inactivity for five to seven days will allow the pharyngeal appearance (especially hyperemia) to improve, and, therefore, endoscopic impressions may be more favorable in the inactive patient than would be observed if the patient were actively training. In summary, the pathogenicity of PLH remains unclear and deserves further evaluation.

MANAGEMENT

The traditional approach to management has included extended inactivity combined with systemic and/or local therapy. Inactivity should range from 30 to 60 days duration, with resumption of training based on regression of the lymphoid follicles. Systemic therapy most frequently includes steroids and antimicrobials. Local therapy may be administered either by nasopharyngeal spray with a catheter or by an indwelling catheter system, usually positioned in the guttural pouches. A variety of medicaments are used, including DMSO, steroids, and antibacterials one to two times daily for 10 to 14 days. Systemic therapy may provide satisfactory relief for mild cases maintained in reduced training, or it may be combined with rest. Spontaneous regression of the lymphoid follicles usually occurs with rest and may be quite dramatic within 10 to 14 days, apparently the result of reduced airway turbulence and irritation. Therefore, the actual effect of local and systemic therapy is difficult to evaluate.

The results of inactivity and medical therapy may be disappointing. It is not uncommon for the clinical symptoms to recur following return to training, especially when intense training schedules are achieved. Often this represents a loss of 90 to 120 days of competitive status. The uncertainty regarding the length of required inactivity has prompted more aggressive approaches to resolve the condition.

CHEMICAL CAUTERY

Chemical cautery of the pharynx with 50% trichloroacetic acid has been reported as a successful alternative to the more conservative management methods (McAllister and Blakeslee 1977). The procedure is performed with the patient sedated during endoscopic visualization of the pharynx. A cannula-protected catheter system (similar to uterine culturettes) is utilized. The cotton tip of the catheter is soaked with trichloroacetic acid and is protected with the cannula during passage through the contralateral nasal passage. All visible pharyngeal follicles and nodules are thoroughly swabbed. The pharyngeal openings of the guttural pouch, the epiglottis, and the arytenoid cartilages should be avoided. The procedure is repeated daily for three to five days until the involved mucosal surface has sloughed. Followup examination 30 to 45 days after cautery precedes the return to exercise. Normal function or marked improvement in exercise tolerance frequently results from this therapeutic technique.

Recently, cryotherapy has been utilized to manage PLH in an effort to reduce the convalescent period in athletic horses (Johnson 1980). Liquid nitrogen is applied to the pharyngeal surface of the anesthetized horse per nasum with an insulated spray system. Concurrent visualization of the pharynx is accomplished by endoscopy through the contralateral nasal passage. The brief application of the cryogen to the mucosal surface causes minimal tissue destruction and results in the reduction of edema and regression of the lymphoid follicles. The anticipated convalescent period is from two to four weeks. Although the procedure has not gained widespread acceptance, thorough evaluation of its efficacy may establish it as a viable therapeutic procedure for PLH.

PHARYNGEAL CAUTERY

Electrocautery (fulguration) has been used to successfully manage PLH (Boles 1975; Raker and Boles 1978) and appears to be particularly effective in refractory or relapsing cases. This procedure is convenient for concurrent PLH when surgical exposure of the larynx and pharynx is required for surgical management of other lesions including excision of larger lymphoid masses or polyps, epiglottic entrapment, and ventriculectomy. The procedure is not generally recommended for management of patients during the initial episode of PLH, as fulguration requires general anesthesia and a ventral laryngotomy approach. Surgery may be the initial treatment of choice if reduced convalescence is desired.

Following preoperative preparation, intravenous anesthesia is administered and the patient is positioned in dorsal recumbency. A ventral laryngotomy is performed, which allows direct visualization of the posterior and dorsal pharynx. A suction tube is placed into the rostral pharynx via the nasal cavity to remove the smoke resulting from fulguration. A fiberoptic endoscope placed through the contralateral nasal cavity provides more light within the nasopharynx. This also allows the surgeon to evaluate the effectiveness and thoroughness of the procedure.

Surgical exposure is increased by using hand-held retractors (Fig. 13–85A) in the rostral aspect of the incision; division of the thyroid cartilage is unnecessary. The soft palate, when displaced dorsal to the epiglottis, will obscure the operative field and should be repositioned ventral to the epiglottis. The finger is manipulated under the posterolateral margin of the epiglottis in a hook-like fashion and is used to raise the epiglottis over the posterior free margin of the soft palate. Upon release of the epiglottis, the soft palate should be forced ventrally. A curved instrument, such as a vascular clamp (Fig. 13–85B), can be similarly used to elevate the epiglottis for this maneuver.

A long, insulated, ball-tipped electrode is used to cauterize the involved mucosa (Fig. 13–85C). The electrocautery unit is set at a reasonably high coagulation setting. The involved mucosa is systemati-cally stroked in a manner similar to painting until the mucosa becomes whitish-gray. The mucosal surface must be repeatedly swabbed during the procedure to remove mucus accumulations. Mucus tends to ahdere to and insulate the instrument tip, preventing it from being an effective cautery instrument. It should be cleaned off frequently. Contact with the laryngeal cartilages and the pharyngeal openings of the guttural pouches should be avoided. The ventrolateral pharyngeal walls are difficult to visualize directly, and directions from an individual viewing the pharynx endoscopically will be necessary. Any lymphoid aggregates that require surgical excision are removed with long, curved scissors. Their removal should be delayed until the cautery has been completed, as hemorrhage may not only obscure vision but may make cautery very difficult.

Postoperative management includes allowing hay consumption six hours postoperatively and the maintenance grain ration in 12 hours. Phenylbutazone and antimicrobial therapy are continued for three and five days, respectively. The

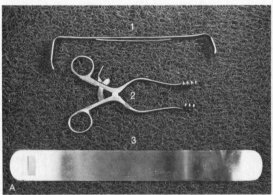

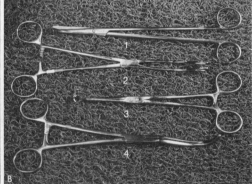

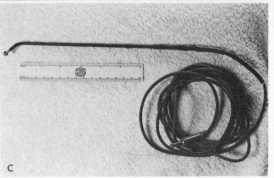

Figure 13–85 Instruments for laryngeal and pharyngeal surgery. A, Retractors: Army-Navy retractor (1), Weitlaner retractor (2), malleable (ribbon) retractor (3). B, Scissors and forceps: Long-handled Metzenbaum scissors (1), sponge forceps (2), Babcock forceps (3), and Stille vessel clamp (4). C, Pharyngeal cautery electrode. The instrument was fashioned from a stainless steel automobile antenna and insulated. Its length allows access to the pharynx through a ventral laryngotomy incision. (Courtesy Dr. J. R. McClure, Louisiana State University.)

ventral laryngotomy incision is treated in a routine manner. Patients experience little discomfort, and an uneventful recovery is the rule. Postoperative endoscopy demonstrates a yellow-white coagulum in the treated areas, which should slough in 10 to 14 days. Rest is recommended until endoscopic examination is performed at 45 days. Follicular regression, leaving a normal-appearing pharyngeal mucosa, is typically observed. Complications, including focal granuloma (polyp), pharyngeal–guttural pouch fistula, and disfigurement of the pharyngeal orifice of the guttural pouch, have been reported, although they are infrequent (Raker and Boles 1978). The complications did not cause any reduction of respiratory function, and the granulomas resolved spontaneously.

PROPHYLAXIS

Because viral agents are repeatedly suggested as components in the pathogenesis of this disorder, repeated inoculation with equine influenza and equine herpesvirus Type 1 vaccines has been recommended (Montgomery 1981; Proceedings 1980). It is important to have susceptible horses protected well in advance of the potential exposure to viral respiratory disease, and vaccination programs should be initiated in yearlings. It appears that repeated inoculation is necessary, and a 60-day interval is suggested following the initial vaccination series. Emphasis should be given to use of the equine influenza vaccines, as this disease is most troublesome in congregations of young (two- to three-year-old) horses. Although this program is not well-documented in the literature, it appears to be supported by the clinical observations of numerous practicing veterinarians.

Dorsal Displacement of the Soft Palate

Dorsal displacement of the soft palate (DDSP) describes the intermittent or persistent malpositioning of the caudal free margin of the soft palate dorsal to the epiglottis (Fig. 13–86). This terminology more appropriately defines what has been traditionally described as soft pal-

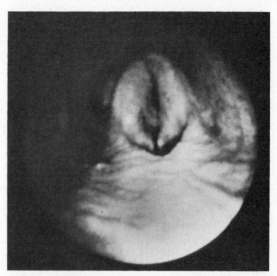

Figure 13–86 Dorsal displacement of the soft palate (DDSP). Endoscopic view that shows the rostral margin of the intrapharyngeal ostium below the arytenoid cartilages. The soft palate obscures appreciation of the epiglottis (see Fig. 13–80). This condition should be differentiated from epiglottic entrapment (see Fig. 13–103). Chondritis lesion of right arytenoid is visible.

ate paresis and/or elongation (Cook 1962; 1965; Quinlan, Van Rensburg, and Starke 1949). This syndrome, which is a cause of URT obstructive disease and exercise intolerance, should be differentiated from soft palate (pharyngeal) paralysis, which is caused by deficits of cranial nerves IX and X (Cook 1966a; Heffron and Baker 1979; Raker 1977). Palatal paralysis is characterized by dysphagia and regurgitation of food and water from the nostrils and is frequently complicated by aspiration pneumonia, whereas DDSP is typically asymptomatic in horses at rest.

The usual complaint in horses with DDSP is exercise intolerance and intermittent noise production (more often expiratory) associated with "choking down." The initial phases of exercise are often asymptomatic, but when stress and increased apprehension accompany an increased level of exercise intensity, respiratory distress becomes apparent. Such horses in racing terminology are said to "swallow their tongues" or "choke down," creating a gurgling noise. When the intensity of exercise is slowed and if the horse swallows, it may be reported that such horses "get their second wind."

This historical observation is of paramount importance in supporting a diagnosis of DDSP and is in marked contrast to those obstructive diseases that cause continual noise production during exercise (e.g., laryngeal hemiplegia). If patients are closely observed during the occurrence of displacement, mouth breathing (primarily expiratory) may be observed and is characterized by excessive salivation and bulging of the cheeks.

The etiology of DDSP remains unclear. DDSP may be an intermittent occurrence secondary to other disease of the URT including any URT inflammatory disease (e.g., guttural pouch empyema), pharyngeal lymphoid hyperplasia (PLH), obstructive lesions anterior to the rima glottidis that may cause dynamic collapse of the soft tissue structures during inspiration, entrapment of the epiglottis by the arytenoepiglottic fold (AEF), epiglottic abnormalities characterized by reduced size or lack of adequate substance (flaccid), and laryngeal hemiplegia (Cook 1965; Boles 1975; Boles, Raker, and Wheat 1978; Robinson and Sorenson 1978). DDSP may be a persistent finding secondary to marked hypoplasia or shortening of the epiglottis or following surgery for resection of an AEF entrapment of the epiglottis (Haynes 1978; 1981). In the past, DDSP has been considered a primary lesion. However, there is no evidence to support intrinsic lesions (hypertrophy, elongation) of the soft palate other than neurogenic muscle atrophy associated with pharyngeal paralysis.

Recently, functional pharyngeal obstruction (FPO) was described as a syndrome of DDSP unassociated with other substantial lesions of the URT (Heffron and Baker 1979). This disease is better defined as a laryngopalatal subluxation (Cook 1979; Heffron and Baker 1977) and has been attributed to caudal retraction of the larynx, which disengages the laryngeal cartilages, particularly the epiglottis, from the intrapharyngeal ostium (see Fig. 13–80). The intrapharyngeal ostium is the aperture bounded rostrally by the caudal free margin of the soft palate and caudally by the confluence of the palatopharyngeal arches (Getty 1975). The paired corniculate cartilages (apex of arytenoids) and the epiglottis protrude through this aperture

into the nasopharynx. In DDSP the epiglottis becomes unhooked from the caudal free border of the soft palate, disrupting the airtight seal and allowing the soft palate to displace dorsally into the nasopharynx, becoming a functional obstruction. This innovative concept provides a rational explanation for those patients previously considered affected with DDSP of idiopathic origin.

Functional pharyngeal obstruction may result from the action of the omohyoideus and sternothyrohyoideus muscles, both of which cause laryngeal retraction (Cook 1979; Heffron and Baker 1977). Proposed reasons for such retraction include apprehension, respiratory pain, and lower respiratory tract disease. Other interrelated causes of DDSP include caudal retraction of the tongue, excessive flexion of the poll, and contraction of the levator palatini muscles (Cook 1965; 1979). Tongue retraction may force the soft palate dorsally and the larynx caudally, increasing the predisposition for laryngopalatal subluxation. Excessive poll flexion reduces the cross-sectional diameter of the nasopharynx, thus increasing negative pressure with resultant dynamic collapse. The levator palatini muscles may contract owing to pharyngeal irritation or pain.

Dorsal displacement of the soft palate reduces the cross-sectional area of the nasopharynx, increasing airflow resistance and causing turbulence. Therefore, dynamic collapse is potentiated, especially since the soft palate is not maintained in its normal subepiglottic position. One might appreciate that the caudal free margin of the soft palate flutters immediately rostral to the laryngeal opening on inspiration and that during expiration a portion of the airflow is diverted through the oral cavity.

Endoscopically, DDSP is characterized by the intermittent or continued inability to visualize the epiglottis. The caudal free margin of the soft palate is clearly visible immediately below the arytenoid cartilages at the laryngeal opening (see Fig. 13–86). The shape of the epiglottis is not visible, which distinguishes this disease from epiglottis entrapment (see Fig. 13–103). It is important to differentiate the two conditions, and, in addition, to appreciate that they may occur simultaneously. During endoscopy, the patient should be stimulated to swallow by contacting the pharyngeal wall with the endoscope or by administering 2 to 3 cc of water through the flexible endoscope. Repositioning of the soft palate to its normal subepiglottic position is an important event to observe, as it will assist in distinguishing the normal variations from the abnormal.

Although the previous comments may appear to make the diagnosis rather straightforward, DDSP presently remains one of the major diagnostic challenges of obstructive URT diseases in the horse. Although the use of flexible fiberoptic equipment has markedly increased the recognition of this syndrome, differentiation between variations of normal and abnormal presents a diagnostic dilemma. It is not unusual to observe transient DDSP during endoscopy of the URT and to interpret it as a casual finding in horses without a supportive history. The patient frequently swallows, and the soft palate becomes repositioned. On the other hand, if the patient appears unaware of the DDSP and it remains after swallowing, it may substantiate a valid concern. The ease with which the soft palate can be displaced by manual nostril obstruction may further support the diagnosis (Heffron and Baker 1979). Finally, there are horses presented with a history very suggestive of a DDSP problem during exercise that, upon endoscopic examination, do not exhibit any abnormal findings. Observation of such horses during exercise and endoscopic examination immediately following stressful exercise may provide valuable diagnostic insight.

In addition to obtaining a thorough and detailed history, observing the horse during exercise, and conducting an endoscopic examination, pharyngeal radiography may provide valuable information regarding the etiology of DDSP. The lateral radiograph should be evaluated, specifically to measure the length of the epiglottis. Normal measurements should be in the 8- to 9-cm range from the apex to the base at the thyroid articulation. Horses with an epiglottis reduced in size to 6 to 7 cm in length appear more prone to DDSP. Thus, some prognostic insight may be provided by this procedure. Figures 13–82, 13–87, and 13–104 demonstrate contrast pharyngograms, which facilitate identification of anatomical structures.

Persistent DDSP has been associated with shortening of the epiglottis (Haynes 1981). Affected horses had a reduced capacity for exercise, produced a noise during exercise, and were not dysphagic. The epiglottis in reported cases was of inadequate length to maintain the soft palate in its normal subepiglottic position and measured approximately two-thirds of normal length (Fig. 13–88). The diagnosis of persistent DDSP secondary to epiglottic shortening is suspected following endoscopic examination of the

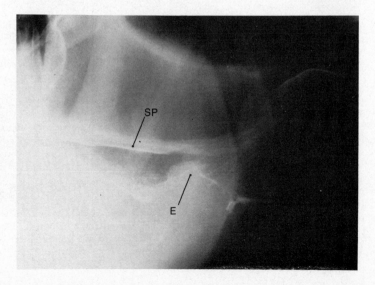

Figure 13–87 Persistent dorsal displacement of the soft palate. Contrast pharyngogram demonstrating the soft palate (SP) positioned dorsal to the epiglottis (E).

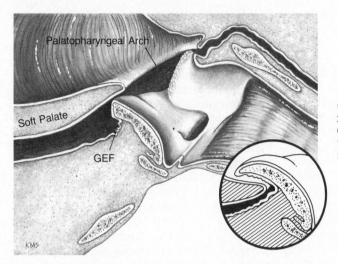

Figure 13–88 Diagrammatic representation of the right hemilarynx demonstrating epiglottic shortening and the normal (inset). The glossoepiglottic fold (GEF) attaches to the lingual surface of the epiglottis.

nasopharynx and may be confirmed by pharyngeal radiography (see Fig. 13–87) and endoscopy of the oropharynx (Fig. 13–89). The etiology is obscure, although developmental and acquired origins have been postulated. Surgical intervention (staphylectomy and resection of the sternothyrohyoideus muscles) did not appreciably alter the capacity for exercise.

In summary, the majority of DDSP cases are intermittent and idiopathic and may be considered functional pharyngeal obstructions. However, the patient should be examined carefully for lesions that may predispose to the occurrence of this syndrome, and DDSP must be differentiated from epiglottic entrapment. Because it is difficult to establish a definitive diagnosis in many cases, management of DDSP can be frustrating. One should be cautious in developing enthusiastic prognoses in such cases.

MANAGEMENT

If DDSP is secondary to other conditions of the URT, the primary therapy should be directed at the underlying

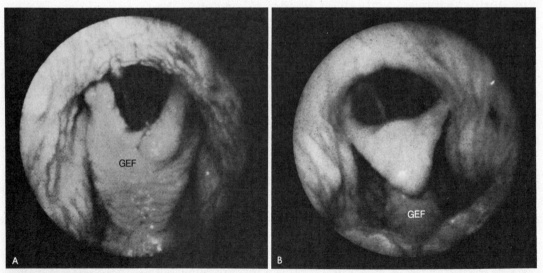

Figure 13–89 Persistent dorsal displacement of the soft palate. Endoscopic view of the epiglottis *per os* in affected horse (*A*) and normal horse (*B*). The soft palate is located dorsally and the glossoepiglottic fold (GEF) is more visible in the affected patient. (Reprinted with permission from Haynes: JAVMA, *179*:677, 1981.)

cause. It is common, for example, for DDSP and pharyngeal lymphoid hyperplasia to resolve simultaneously when they are interrelated.

The use of a tongue tie is a reasonably effective method to reduce the frequency of DDSP, particularly in mild and intermittent cases. A strap of cloth or other material is used to secure the tongue to the mandible in the interdental space. Preceding exercise, the strap is tied around the tongue immediately rostral to the frenulum, then to the mandible. This is a frequent practice in racehorses of all breeds, and the results can be quite dramatic. The procedure reduces retraction of the tongue and elevation of the soft palate by the base of the tongue and decreases the caudal movement of the larynx transmitted via the hyoid apparatus.

PARTIAL RESECTION OF THE SOFT PALATE (STAPHYLECTOMY)

Partial resection of the soft palate was first described in 1949 (Quinlan, Van Rensburg, and Starke 1949). The objective of this procedure is to resect redundant tissue, based on the concept of hypertrophy or elongation of the soft palate, allowing it to maintain its normal subepiglottic position. Although this procedure enjoys widespread use, it should be recognized that it enlarges the intrapharyngeal ostium and thus is contrary to recent thoughts on laryngopalatal subluxation. Partial resection of the soft palate has greater application for patients that experience intermittent rather than persistent DDSP. The latter group of patients usually has an irreversible reduction of epiglottis size with the resultant inability to maintain the soft palate ventrally.

Partial resection of the soft palate is performed through a ventral laryngotomy incision with the horse positioned in dorsal recumbency. Intravenous anesthesia is adequate for this relatively short procedure. The caudal free margin of the soft palate can be visualized in the posterior pharynx if it is dorsally displaced (i.e., the palate will be displaced if an endotracheal tube was utilized during anesthesia and withdrawn). If the soft palate is positioned normally, the index finger can be introduced under the caudolateral margin of the epiglottis to elevate the epiglottis and allow the palate to displace dorsally.

Traditionally, a crescentic piece of tissue, 4 to 6 cm in transverse length by 1 to 2 cm in axial width, is removed from the visible free margin of the soft palate (Fig. 13–90). The edge of the palate is grasped on the midline with a pair of long tissue forceps. A second forceps is placed 2 to 3 cm lateral to the first one. A curved Metzenbaum scissors is used to divide the palate, starting immediately lateral (and caudal) to the second forceps and continuing rostral and somewhat parallel to the palatal margin to just ahead of the axially placed forceps. The line of division (excision) should start close to the margin of the palate and should reach its maximum width at the midline. The amount of palate to resect (i.e., the width of the tissue removed from the midline) is arbitrary. The suggested maximal depth of incision at the midline is 2 cm, removed under tension. Thus, the piece of tissue removed would actually represent an in situ tissue width of approximately 1.5 cm. The opposite side of the palatal margin is incised in a similar fashion so that the two incisions meet on the midline. Hemorrhage is usually minimal, and the incision is left to heal by second intention.

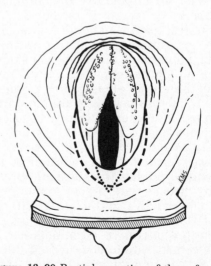

Figure 13–90 Partial resection of the soft palate (staphylectomy). The caudal free margin of the soft palate may be notched axially (dotted lines), or a more extensive piece of tissue may be resected along the dashed lines. Both techniques increase the aperture of the intrapharyngeal ostium.

An alternate method of partial resection of the soft palate margin is to notch it axially (Boles 1979b; Haynes 1978; Raker 1978). A triangular piece of tissue 1.5 to 2 cm in transverse and axial dimensions is resected (see Fig. 13–90). A convenient way to perform this notching is to precisely position a sponge forceps over the edge of the palate that includes approximately 1 cm of tissue. Scissors are used to symmetrically resect the tissue held within the forceps, creating a notch of the desired dimensions. A two-layer closure with absorbable suture has been described to increase the transverse tension of the palate (Roberts 1964). Although this technique may have merits, it does not seem well accepted. With either procedure, the incised palate should be closely examined to ensure that the remaining tissue contours are smooth and confluent and that any tissue tags or asymmetries are appropriately trimmed. Figure 13–90 diagrammatically represents the planes of surgical incision for both techniques. The laryngotomy incision is allowed to heal by second intention.

Postoperative management includes resumption of the hay ration in 6 hours and the maintenance concentrate ration in 12 hours. Antimicrobial therapy should continue for three to five days. The laryngotomy incision is managed as previously discussed. An uncomplicated postoperative course is expected. A return to full exercise should follow endoscopic examination, and the continued use of a tongue tie should be considered.

The prognosis following partial resection of the soft palate is guarded. Approximately 50 per cent of patients can be expected to successfully return to competitive exercise if DDSP was not secondary to other unresolved obstructive disease. As previously mentioned, it is difficult to predict the surgical outcome of any disease with a poorly understood pathophysiology, and clearly intermittent DDSP is frequently in this category.

Two postoperative circumstances deserve consideration as causes of failure. The first is palatal incontinence subsequent to excess removal of tissue, resulting in ingesta being voided through the nostrils. This sequela of partial resection is an irreversible disaster; however, it is seldom encountered if resection has been conservative. It is far better to remove too little tissue than to remove too much.

The second and by far more frequent circumstance is failure to achieve repositioning of the soft palate. Either the animal continues to displace the shortened palate, obscuring vision of the anterior epiglottis, or the epiglottis is visible in the surgically created defect although not positioned above the palate. Two explanations are proposed: (1) the normal relationship cannot be established, regardless of the length of the soft palate and/or (2) either too much or too little tissue was resected. Such cases clearly present a dilemma, and any subsequent resection efforts will in all likelihood be unsuccessful. It is likely that the size and function of the intrapharyngeal ostium and epiglottis contribute to such failures.

RESECTION OF THE STERNOTHYROHYOIDEUS MUSCLE

Laryngopalatal subluxation has been described as an innovative concept for the pathogenesis of DDSP (Cook 1979; Heffron and Baker 1979). Caudal retraction of the larynx is considered the basic mechanism, and thus resection of the sternothyrohyoideus muscle has been suggested (Cook 1979). This procedure is simple to perform and is presently endorsed as the initial treatment of choice for idiopathic and intermittent DDSP. The technique can be readily accomplished in the standing sedated patient with the use of local anesthesia. If general anesthesia is used to perform other surgical procedures on the URT, the myectomy can be performed while the patient is positioned in dorsal recumbency.

When performed on the standing patient, the head should be elevated to place the ventral cervical muscles under tension, making the sternothyrohyoideus muscle readily apparent on palpation. The surgical site is on the ventral midline, at approximately the midcervical level, where the paired muscle bellies are of the smallest diameter and are most superficial (Fig. 13–91A). Local anesthesia is infiltrated on the midline for 8 cm to the depth of the trachea. A 6- to 8-

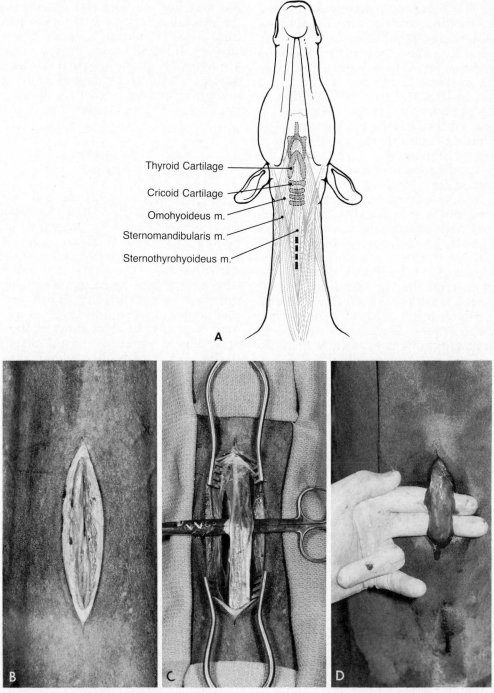

Figure 13–91 Resection of the sternothyrohyoideus muscle. *A,* The landmarks for the midcervical midline incision. *B,* The incision exposes the superficial cutaneous colli muscle. *C,* The sternothyrohyoideus muscle is elevated for partial resection in this cadaver specimen positioned in dorsal recumbency. *D,* The muscle may be exteriorized for resection in the standing patient, using local anesthesia.

cm incision is continued through the skin and subcutaneous tissue, exposing the thin cutaneous colli muscle (Fig. 13–91B). The cutaneous muscle is divided on the midline, and the fascia surrounding the sternothyrohyoideus muscle is visualized. The sternothyrohyoideus muscle is very mobile within the loose fascia superficial to the trachea and should be stabilized on the midline to divide the overlying fascia. The muscle is elevated through the incision, and the deep fascia is bluntly removed over a 5- to 6-cm distance (Fig. 13–91C and D). The exposed section of muscle should be examined for vessels that deserve ligation, usually located on its deep surface. The muscle is stabilized and transected distally with scissors. Proximal transection results in the removal of a 4- to 5-cm section of the paired muscle bellies. The free ends of the muscle retract from the incisional site; the minimal hemorrhage that results is, therefore, difficult to control. Closure of the incision is done in three layers. Absorbable suture (0 chromic catgut) is used to close the deep fascia and cutaneous colli muscle in a simple interrupted and space-obliterating suture pattern. A simple interrupted subcutaneous closure (00 chromic gut) is followed by interrupted skin closure (00 nylon). Mild to moderate postoperative swelling may result, although healing is uneventful. The patient may be returned to work within 7 to 10 days, as incisional swelling resolves. The sutures are removed 10 to 12 days after surgery.

Although this technique has not been extensively evaluated, it appears to be at least as effective as partial resection of the soft palate. Advantages of the procedure are that it can be performed on the standing patient and the results of the procedure can be evaluated upon return to work within 10 days following surgery. If DDSP occurs during exercise, a tongue tie should be tried. If the condition persists as a cause of exercise intolerance, partial resection of the soft palate should be considered.

Rostral Displacement of the Palatopharyngeal Arch

Rostral displacement of the palatopharyngeal arch (PPA) has been reported as a cause of exercise intolerance in the horse (Cook 1974; Goulden et al. 1976). This disease is discussed in conjunction with diseases of the pharynx because the PPA constitutes the caudal aspect of the intrapharyngeal ostium. However, the production of noise and exercise intolerance appear to be related to a restriction of arytenoid abduction by the displaced tissue and may be associated with laryngeal paralysis.

In addition to an inspiratory noise and an inability to tolerate exercise, rostral displacement of the PPA has been characterized by dysphagia, discharge of ingesta from the nostrils, persistent coughing, and, occasionally, noise at rest or during eating (Goulden et al. 1976).

Endoscopy of the nasopharynx reveals a fold of tissue covering the apex of one or both arytenoid cartilages (Fig. 13–92). The fold of tissue appears to limit the

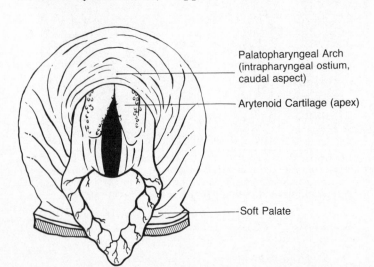

Palatopharyngeal Arch (intrapharyngeal ostium, caudal aspect)

Arytenoid Cartilage (apex)

Soft Palate

Figure 13–92 Rostral displacement of the palatopharyngeal arch. Diagrammatic representation that demonstrates the apices of the arytenoid cartilages partially obscured by the fold of the palatopharyngeal arch. Radiographic demonstration of this condition is seen in Figure 13–112.

range of abduction of the arytenoid cartilage, and such patients appear to have laryngeal hemiplegia if the malpositioned tissue is unilateral. Radiography may help demonstrate the displaced fold of tissue rostral to the apices of the arytenoid cartilages (see Fig. 13–112).

The etiology of rostral displacement of the PPA remains unclear, although a developmental origin has been suggested (Cook 1974) and subsequently described in one case (Goulden et al. 1976). In the latter report, the abnormality was associated with a grossly misshapen thyroid cartilage, bilateral absence of the cricopharyngeus muscles, and hypoplasia of the thyropharyngeus muscles. It was suggested that the anomaly may have resulted from aberrant development of the fourth branchial arch. Abduction of arytenoid cartilages was reduced, although the abductor muscles were unaffected, and thus may have been related to the abnormality of the thyroid cartilage.

The occasional patient may possess a slight fold of PPA over the arytenoid apices without experiencing any clinical abnormality (see Fig. 13–62). This incidental finding occurs more commonly than does the clinically apparent displacement previously described and should not be misinterpreted as a cause of decreased laryngeal function.

SURGICAL CORRECTION

Resection of a wedge of tissue from the rostrally displaced PPA has been considered as a potential method of correction for this abnormality (Goulden et al. 1976). It should be recognized, however, that this disease may be associated with developmental abnormalities of the larynx and that relief of the displaced tissue may not result in normal laryngeal function.

The pharynx is approached through a ventral laryngotomy incision while the horse is positioned in dorsal recumbency. The displaced PPA is readily visible immediately ahead of the arytenoid apices. If the tissue displacement is symmetrical (covering both apices), an axial wedge is removed. The free margin is grasped with forceps and a 1- to 1½-cm triangular wedge is removed by scissor incision,

similar to the incision used when notching the free margin of the soft palate. An alternate approach is to remove a crescentic piece of tissue from the free margin of the PPA, 4 to 6 cm in length and 1 to 1 ½ cm in width. If the PPA covers only one arytenoid, the notch should be centered at the site where the arytenoid is maximally covered. The surgical site and laryngotomy incision are allowed to heal by second intention. Aftercare is identical to that suggested for partial resection of the soft palate. The arytenoid cartilage should become fully visible endoscopically within a few days postoperatively. The prognosis for return to full function depends on the initial extent of compromise but should be considered guarded.

Pharyngeal Cysts

Pharyngeal cysts are space-occupying lesions of the pharynx that are capable of causing clinical signs related to airway obstruction or dysphagia (Koch and Tate 1978; Stick and Boles 1977). The most frequent location of these structures, ranging in size from 1 to 5 cm in diameter, is beneath the epiglottis. An occasional cyst may be located in the mucosa of the dorsal nasopharynx. Typically, a cyst most frequently becomes apparent in horses less than three to four years of age.

Pharyngeal cysts in the adult horse are most often characterized by respiratory noise production during exercise and cause exercise intolerance. Occasionally the primary complaint may be coughing, nasal discharge, and dysphagia or dyspnea at rest, particularly if a sizeable lesion involves the subepiglottic tissue.

In foals, the primary clinical signs associated with subepiglottic cysts are chronic cough, nasal discharge, and pneumonia. Such patients may be recognized because of refractory lower respiratory tract disease secondary to dysphagia and aspiration of ingesta caused by the space-occupying cyst (Stick and Boles 1977).

The etiology of pharyngeal cysts may be either developmental or acquired. It has been suggested that the subepiglottic cysts may be a remnant of the embryonic thyroglossal duct or a post-traumatic inflammatory lesion (Harvey, Raker, and O'Brien 1973; Koch and Tate 1978; Raker 1976; Stick and Boles 1977). Those of the dorsal nasopharynx may be remnants of Rathke's pouch (Raker 1976). The smooth-walled and fluctuant cysts usually contain a thick viscous mucus and are lined by stratified squamous, pseudo stratified columnar, or cuboidal epithelium (Koch and Tate 1978).

The diagnosis of pharyngeal cysts is confirmed by endoscopic examination (Fig. 13–93A). Those that protrude from the nasopharyngeal surface are readily apparent. Cysts located in the subepiglottic tissue may not be readily visible when the soft palate is properly positioned (Fig. 13–93B). The patient should be stimulated to swallow and subsequently observed for the emergence of a cystic structure from beneath the epiglottis. Dorsal displacement of the soft palate may be observed, obscuring both the epiglottis and the subepiglottic cyst. This occurs owing to an inadequate length of free rostral epiglottis to maintain the soft palate in its normal position.

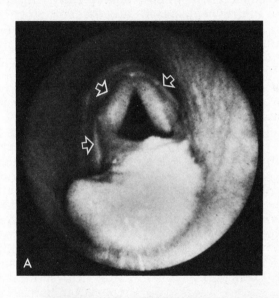

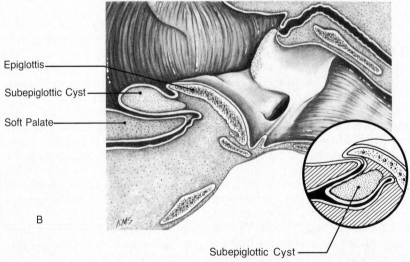

Epiglottis

Subepiglottic Cyst

Soft Palate

B

Subepiglottic Cyst

Figure 13–93 Subepiglottic cyst. *A,* Endoscopic view of subepiglottic cyst positioned dorsal to the soft palate. The palatopharyngeal arch (arrows) in this case is seen lateral and dorsal to the arytenoid cartilages. *B,* Diagrammatic representation of subepiglottic cyst positioned dorsal to the soft palate, drawn from a sagittal section. Inset demonstrates cyst positioned beneath the soft palate. An endoscopic view of this patient would appear normal.

SURGICAL RESECTION

Resection of pharyngeal cystic structures is accomplished through a ventral laryngotomy approach with the patient in dorsal recumbency. Intravenous anesthesia is usually adequate for this relatively short procedure. It is seldom necessary to divide the body of the thyroid cartilage for additional exposure. The passage of an endoscope through the ventral nasal meatus may be considered to provide additional illumination of the pharynx and to enhance visibility.

Cystic structures located on the dorsal pharyngeal surface can be grasped with long forceps (see Fig. 13–85B) and stabilized during division of the base of attachment with scissors or an electroscalpel. Hemorrhage following scissor dissection may be controlled by electrocoagulation. It is unnecessary to appose the edges of the mucosal defect with sutures. The occasional pedunculated cyst may be removed from the conscious patient by an improvised snare passed through the ventral meatus while being visualized endoscopically through the opposite nostril.

Cystic structures located in the subepiglottic tissue become readily apparent with the epiglottis in a retroverted position. The index finger is introduced beneath the epiglottis from its caudolateral margin. As the epiglottis is elevated and drawn caudally, the subepiglottic mass becomes visible and should be grasped with a pair of tissue forceps. Caudal traction on the cyst continues to retrovert the epiglottis until the entire cyst can be appreciated. The tip of the epiglottis should be stabilized caudally with sponge forceps. An endotracheal tube may be inserted through the oral cavity and oropharynx and pushed up against the retroverted epiglottis to assist positioning. Large quantities of cystic fluid may be aspirated to aid manipulation.

The cyst should be elevated and dissection initiated by dividing the mucosa with scissors close to the cyst, nearest the tip of the epiglottis. Elevation and traction on the cyst allow continued mucosal division close to the cyst wall. Thus, adequate perilesional mucosa is left intact to allow closure of the defect by second intention. An alternate procedure is to divide the mucosa over the cyst and dissect it free without removing any mucosa. Closure of the mucosal defect with buried absorbable sutures (00 chromic catgut) has been described but is considered optional.

Removal of pedunculated subepiglottic cysts has been described by the oral approach (Boles 1979b). A mouth speculum is used to fully dilate the oral cavity of the anesthetized patient. A snare may be placed over the cyst and its position confirmed by nasopharyngeal endoscopy. Manual access of the posterior oropharynx is limited to personnel with small hands and may be a determining factor in the success of the procedure.

The expected postoperative course is uncomplicated. Aftercare involves the resumption of hay in 6 hours and the maintenance concentrate ration 12 hours postoperatively. The patient should be confined until the ventral laryngotomy is healed (30 days). Endoscopy should be performed prior to returning the patient to work. The prognosis is favorable, and recurrence is uncommon.

Cleft Soft Palate

Cleft palate in the horse is characterized by the discharge of ingesta through the external nares. The defect is usually recognized soon after birth because milk runs from the nostrils during nursing. Affected foals tend to be unthrifty, owing to the reduced efficiency in nursing. Aspiration pneumonia may be a sequela and may attract the owner's attention when dyspnea develops. Occasionally, affected animals grow to maturity and appear asymptomatic with the exception of the nasal discharge.

The etiology of cleft palate is unknown. Some process interrupts the orderly rostrocaudal fusion of the palatal folds in the embryo. Thus, any variation of a midline defect, from a complete cleft of the hard and soft palates to that which involves only the caudal part of the soft palate, is possible (Jones et al. 1975). The most common defect is an incomplete cleft of the soft palate, involving the caudal half to two-thirds of that structure. Entrapment of the epiglottis by the arytenoepiglottic fold may be seen

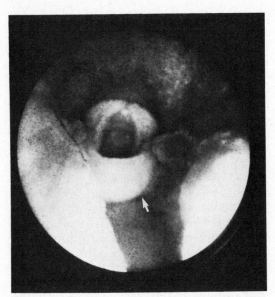

Figure 13–94 Cleft of the soft palate. This endoscopic view demonstrates an entrapped epiglottis (arrow) visible in the posterior oropharynx between the margins of the cleft. The patient was a two-year-old Thoroughbred in race training. (Reprinted with permission from Haynes and Qualls: JAVMA *179:*910, 1981.)

in association with this congenital defect (Fig. 13–94).

The diagnosis of cleft soft palate may be confirmed by endoscopic examination of the nasopharynx (see Fig. 13–94). The epiglottis will be visualized immediately above the base of the tongue, within the defect. The axial margins of the cleft continue caudally into the corresponding palatopharyngeal arches. More extensive clefts may be visualized during oral examination.

Repair of cleft palate has been successfully described (Cook 1974; Jones et al. 1975; Nelson, Curley, and Kainer 1971; Schneider 1974; Stickle, Goble, and Braden 1973). Because there is an implication of heredity in the etiology of cleft palate in the horse, the owner should be appropriately advised and may consider subsequent neutering of the patient. Preoperative assessment of the patient should include thorough evaluation of the lower respiratory tract. Extensive coexisting pulmonary disease will markedly increase the risks of general anesthesia and may even be the limiting factor in the patient's future use.

SURGICAL CORRECTION

Three approaches to expose the pharynx have been described to repair cleft palate in the horse: oral, pharyngotomy, and mandibular symphysiotomy (Jones et al. 1975). The oral approach may be used for foals less than 30 days old. The oropharynx is more accessible at this age, in contrast to older patients, as subsequent growth of the head makes it relatively narrower (Schneider 1974). The pharyngotomy approach may be effective in repairing limited defects in the caudal soft palate, although surgical exposure is limited. The surgical approach used most often is the mandibular symphysiotomy (see previous discussion). Although this is a rather extensive and invasive approach, it allows full visualization of the hard and soft palates and is suggested as the procedure of choice.

Once the palatal defect has been exposed, the free edges are carefully divided along the junction of oral and nasal mucosa. The mucosa is undermined for 4 to 5 mm to readily separate the edge of the shelf into two layers. The soft palate is reapposed in two layers with absorbable suture (0 or 00 chromic catgut or polyglycolic acid) in a simple interrupted suture pattern. Suturing should start with precise apposition of the caudal margin of the soft palate and should progress rostrally. Lateral relaxing incisions are seldom needed to reduce tension on the suture line, although additional horizontal mattress sutures are placed to reinforce the primary suture line. If the defect involves the hard palate as well, a mucoperiosteal flap technique is suggested (Sinibaldi 1979).

Postoperatively, foals are allowed to resume nursing immediately, although solid food is withheld. In weaned horses, a limited ration of moistened pelletized feed (gruel form) is offered for 7 to 10 days. If the patient does not eat this, nasogastric intubation should be performed to administer feed four times daily. The prognosis is guarded to good.

Space-Occupying Lesions of the Nasopharynx

A variety of acquired space-occupying lesions of the nasopharynx may cause signs associated with disease of the upper respiratory tract: nasal discharge, airway obstruction, noise production, and even dysphagia. The presenting clinical signs will depend on the location and extent of the lesion. Early signs may consist of recurrent nasal discharge and may include blood if the lesion has a granulating or ulcerating surface. As lesions enlarge, exercise intolerance and noise production may become apparent. Marked enlargements will ultimately cause severe airway obstruction, which may cause the patient to mouth breathe. Lesions of the soft palate may cause dysphagia, resulting in the reflux of ingesta through the nasal cavities and, possibly, inhalation pneumonia.

The most frequent causes of nasopharyngeal lesions include neoplastic disease and fungal granulomas. Parasitic lesions caused by *Habronema* sp. have also been reported (Johnson and Merriam 1975). The majority of neoplastic processes are malignant, with squamous cell carcinoma and fibroma or fibrosarcoma predominating (Dorn and Priester 1976). Fungal granulomas are most often caused by *Enthomopthera* sp. (Fig. 13–95).

The diagnosis of space-occupying lesions can be confirmed by endoscopy and a definitive diagnosis established by histological examination of biopsy specimens. Radiographic evaluation, including contrast pharyngograms, should be considered to determine the extent of the process. Regional lymph nodes should be carefully evaluated and a fine-needle aspiration performed if any evidence of enlargement is present.

TREATMENT

Treatment of space-occupying lesions depends on the cause, location, and extent of the lesion. Localized neoplastic lesions may be managed by direct excision in conjunction with cryosurgery. Fungal and parasitic granulomas may be excised, if localized, and treated with topical amphotericin B and organophosphate, respectively. The surgical approach required may vary from a ventral laryngotomy to a mandibular symphysiotomy. The prognosis depends on the nature of the lesion and would likely be guarded to poor, especially with neoplastic conditions.

LARYNX

The larynx plays a very important role in the function of the respiratory tract. Laryngeal closure protects the lower respiratory tract from aspiration of ingesta during deglutition and also participates in phonation. Laryngeal dilation is necessary during inspiration, especially during exercise, to allow unobstructed airflow from the pharynx into the trachea. Mild decreases of the laryngeal aperture may be tolerated, because the size of the lumen on maximal dilation exceeds that of the trachea (Marks et al. 1970a).

Diseases of the larynx produce typical signs of URT obstruction: production of noise associated with air movement and exercise intolerance. Severe compromise of the laryngeal lumen may cause signs in the resting horse; however, most horses with laryngeal disease only show signs during exercise. The arytenoid cartilages are abducted during inspiration; if this function is reduced, dynamic collapse results in an inspiratory obstruction.

Endoscopic examination is the most

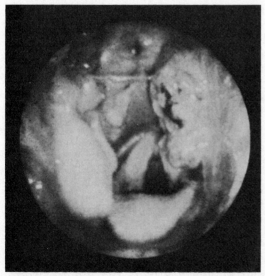

Figure 13–95 Diffuse fungal granulomas of the pharynx. Endoscopic view of a patient in which lesions were excised through a ventral laryngotomy approach and treated successfully with local amphotericin B.

definitive method of diagnosing laryngeal disease. The larynx should be closely observed for symmetry of abduction. If movement of the arytenoids is minimal, the patient should be stimulated to swallow. Near maximal abduction of the arytenoids occurs immediately after swallowing when the patient takes a deep breath (see Fig. 13–63A). Swallowing may be induced by the administration of a few milliliters of water into the pharynx through the flexible endoscope or by touching the soft palate or epiglottis with the endoscope. Endoscopy immediately after exercise will also allow assessment of abductor ability. The least amount of physical or chemical restraint necessary for endoscopic examination is ideal for evaluating normal laryngeal function. Chemical restraint or sedatives should be avoided because they may alter laryngeal activity. Phenothiazine tranquilizers tend to reduce spontaneous arytenoid abduction, and xylazine may produce asynchrony of movement.

Radiographic examination of the larynx may provide valuable supportive evidence of laryngeal disease (see Figs. 13–82, 13–87, 13–102, 13–104, and 13–112). It is especially applicable for evaluation of the epiglottis (size and/or presence of entrapment), mineralization of the laryngeal cartilages (associated with chondritis or hypertrophic ossification), the dorsoventral diameter of the laryngeal lumen, and whether a ventriculectomy has been previously performed (Cook 1974; Haynes et al. 1980; Shapiro et al. 1979). Standing lateral views are suggested and are within the capabilities of portable radiographic equipment.

Laryngeal Hemiplegia

Laryngeal paralysis is most often a unilateral disease and involves the left hemilarynx more than 95 per cent of the time. This disease has been recognized as a frequent cause of upper airway obstruction since the mid 1800s. Affected horses are referred to as roarers because of the classic inspiratory noise produced during exercise. The primary signs of laryngeal hemiplegia are inspiratory noise production during galloping and decreased ability to tolerate high-intensity exercise over a distance. Respiratory distress usually commences after $3/8$ to $1/2$ mile of extended galloping. As the depth of respiration increases with exertion, the inspiratory noise becomes increasingly evident. The noise is synchronized with the gait and occurs as the forelimbs leave the ground in extension.

Laryngeal hemiplegia may be either a complete paralysis of the involved cartilage or a partial reduction in abductor function. Laryngeal hemiplegia results from decreased motor activity of the cricoarytenoideus dorsalis muscle, the primary dilator of the rima glottidis, due to loss of innervation through the recurrent laryngeal nerve. Constrictors (adductors) of the rima glottidis share the same innervation and are also affected. The disease is considered a peripheral neuropathy (Duncan and Griffiths 1973). The paralyzed arytenoid cartilage and vocal fold collapse into the laryngeal lumen, causing a reduction in its cross-sectional area. Negative pressure created in the upper respiratory tract during inspiration causes additional dynamic collapse of the arytenoid cartilage into the lumen. Without abduction of the arytenoid cartilage, the vocal fold is relaxed. As a result, the lateral ventricle on the involved side tends to fill with air, further displacing the vocal fold axially and narrowing the laryngeal lumen (Marks et al. 1970b; Williams 1945). In cases of partial paralysis, some abductor function is present, but the abductor muscle fatigues, allowing the arytenoid to displace axially, causing a progressive compromise of the airway during exercise (Marks et al. 1970b).

Numerous theories have been suggested to explain the etiology of the nerve damage including respiratory infections, toxicity, "physiologic" trauma, and heredity (Cook 1965; 1966a; Marks et al. 1970b; Mason 1973; Rooney and Delaney 1970). The observations that the disease is found primarily in large horses (in excess of 16 hands at the withers) and nearly always affects the left recurrent laryngeal nerve suggest that certain anatomical relationships may be important. The disease may be related to specific diseases, such as guttural pouch

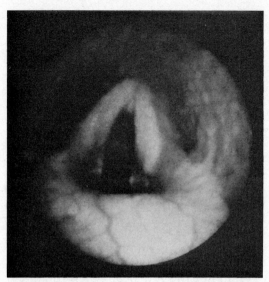

Figure 13–96 Left laryngeal hemiplegia. This endoscopic view demonstrates the left arytenoid in a near vertical position. The palatopharyngeal arch is more prominent on the left side. Note the vascular pattern on the dorsal surface of the epiglottis.

mycosis, or to accidental perivascular injection of irritant drugs, but the majority of cases are considered idiopathic at this time (Cook 1966a; Marks et al. 1970b).

A definitive diagnosis of laryngeal hemiplegia can best be established by endoscopy (Fig. 13–96). Movement (or lack thereof) of the arytenoid cartilages must be visualized. When completely paralyzed, the involved arytenoid stays in a vertical or paramedian position (Johnson et al. 1977) and does not abduct with the contralateral cartilage during inspiration. Partial paralysis is characterized by reduced range of abduction and, often, a more rapid dropping of the affected cartilage into the laryngeal lumen than that of the contralateral cartilage. This should be differentiated from asynchronous laryngeal abduction, which is characterized by discordant timing of abduction but does not affect the maximal degree of abduction that can be achieved. Asynchronous laryngeal abduction may be a normal variation, whereas partial paralysis may precede total paralysis.

Additional techniques have been employed to diagnose laryngeal hemiplegia. The muscular process of the arytenoid cartilage (see Fig. 13–101) becomes palpable when atrophy of the cricoarytenoideus dorsalis muscle is marked (Cook 1965). By external digital compression of the muscular process toward the laryngeal lumen, a vibrating inspiratory sound may be produced when the affected side is manipulated. This is referred to as the arytenoid depression maneuver (McKay-Smith and Marks 1968; Marks et al. 1970b). Two techniques have been described to evaluate adductor function of the larynx: "grunting to the stick" (Cook 1965) and the slap test (Greet et al. 1980). Both techniques are based on the lack of spontaneous adduction of the affected arytenoid cartilage following an external stimulus to the thorax. A prolonged grunt may indicate inability to fully close the larynx. The results of the slap test are assessed by endoscopic visualization of laryngeal function.

It is imperative to differentiate reduced arytenoid abduction due to paralysis from that caused by chronic chondritis of the arytenoid cartilage. This is particularly true when a right-sided "paralysis" is observed, since the idiopathic disease rarely affects the right hemilarynx. Both diseases may be characterized by reduced arytenoid abduction; however, management is distinctly different.

Surgical intervention in cases of laryngeal hemiplegia is only necessary if the patient is unable to attain the desired degree of exercise tolerance. The sedentary horse is relatively unaffected by the disease and does not require surgery. The traditional procedure suggested for laryngeal hemiplegia is the ventriculectomy (Berge and Westhues 1966; Hobday 1936; O'Connor 1965; Williams 1907; 1945). Since 1970, prosthetic laryngoplasty has improved the prognosis for affected patients and is suggested as the optimal procedure for maximal exercise potential (Marks et al. 1970a).

VENTRICULECTOMY

Removal of the mucosal lining of the lateral ventricle of the larynx was introduced in the 1800s to improve the exercise potential of patients affected with laryngeal hemiplegia. The objective of the procedure was to produce abduction of the arytenoid cartilage by formation of

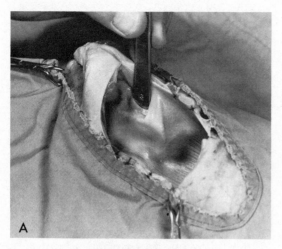

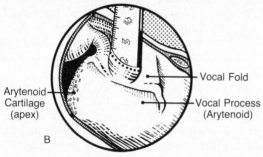

Arytenoid
Cartilage
(apex)

Vocal Fold

Vocal Process
(Arytenoid)

B

Figure 13–97 Incision along the vestibular fold. *A*, A window has been created in the lateral aspect of the larynx specimen to demonstrate axial displacement of the arytenoid cartilage by placing scalpel handle in the laryngeal ventricle. *B*, A mucosal incision (dotted line) along the vestibular fold allows submucosal undermining of the ventricle with a finger prior to mucosal eversion with a burr. The patient is in dorsal recumbency with the rostral aspect to the left.

adhesions between the arytenoid and thyroid cartilages and to reduce filling of the ventricle during inspiration (Williams 1907; 1945). The latter objective appears to be the primary reason for improvement, since abduction and fixation of the arytenoid cartilage are not effectively accomplished by this procedure (Cook 1965). This procedure is not as effective as prosthetic laryngoplasty and is suggested for patients with partial hemiplegia and those with complete hemiplegia when the arytenoid is in the paramedian (resting) position. The procedure may also be considered in those patients that do not economically justify the more invasive and expensive laryngoplasty. Ventriculectomy may improve exercise capacity but usually does not

eliminate noise production during exercise.

Ventriculectomy is performed through a ventral laryngotomy incision. The procedure may be performed on the standing patient under local anesthesia, although it is usually performed under general anesthesia with the patient positioned in dorsal recumbency. Upon entry into the larynx (Fig. 13–97; see also Fig. 13–83), the lateral ventricle on the involved side is identified. The objective of the procedure is complete removal of the mucosal lining of the lateral ventricle. This is most readily performed by insertion of a burr (Fig. 13–98) into the ventricle, engagement of the mucosa under rotational tension, and subsequent eversion of the mucosa. When the entire mucosal lining is everted, it is clamped at the ventricular orifice with a curved forceps (see Fig. 13–85) and excised. Suturing of the ventricular orifice has been described (Pouret 1966), although it is not considered necessary. Bilateral ventriculectomy is frequently done, even in cases of unilateral involvement. However, there is no evidence to support that this is more effective than ventriculectomy on the involved side alone.

Removal of the ventricular mucosa may be facilitated by first making an incision along the vestibular fold of the ventricle and accomplishing submucosal elevation prior to mucosal eversion (Hobday 1936; Vaughan 1962) (see Fig. 13–

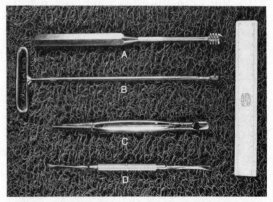

Figure 13–98 Instruments for ventriculectomy and arytenoidectomy. *A*, Roaring burr, Blattenburg model; *B*, Roaring burr, French model; *C*, Sayre periosteal elevator; *D*, Freer nasal septal elevator. *C* and *D* may be used to elevate mucosa during subtotal arytenoidectomy.

97). This is especially useful if a suitable burr is unavailable. The Blattenburg burr is most suited to ventricular eversion, whereas other types tend to fragment the mucosa and make eversion difficult. These may be covered by a gauze sponge to increase surface contact with the mucosa and facilitate complete eversion. The ventral laryngotomy incision is not closed and heals by second intention.

Postoperatively, roughage is withheld for 4 to 6 hours and grain for 12 hours. The use of postoperative antimicrobials is optional. The laryngotomy incision is cleaned daily, and petroleum jelly is liberally applied around the surgical site and intermandibular space. Stall confinement for 30 days followed by limited exercise for 14 days is recommended. Endoscopic examination is advised prior to resuming training. If any abnormalities are observed endoscopically (incomplete healing or granuloma formation), limited exercise should be extended for an additional 14 to 30 days.

Complications following ventriculectomy are uncommon. Postoperative swelling in the laryngeal lumen is usually minimal, although it is good practice to have a tracheostomy tube available for 24 to 48 hours following surgery. If needed, the tube can be inserted through the ventral laryngotomy incision. Granuloma formation at the surgical site may result from removal of too much laryngeal mucosa (Haynes 1978).

The prognosis for improvement in exercise capacity is approximately 50 per cent, although this depends on the extent of laryngeal paralysis. In horses with total paralysis and a vertically positioned arytenoid cartilage, the prognosis is poor. If partial paralysis is present and the involved cartilage is in a paramedian position, the prognosis may be improved. However, improvement may only be transient (one to two years) because the cartilage will "relax" further into the larynx with the progression of muscular paralysis (Marks et al. 1970a). The prognosis for elimination of noise during extended exercise is poor, and clients should be made aware of this. Airflow turbulence and the resultant inspiratory noise are due to a failure of the technique to adequately stabilize the arytenoid cartilage in an abducted position.

PROSTHETIC LARYNGOPLASTY

The technique for performing a prosthetic laryngoplasty was first described in 1970 and has markedly improved the postoperative performance for laryngeal hemiplegics (Johnson 1970; Marks et al. 1970a; Speirs 1972). Laryngoplasty is currently suggested as the best procedure to alleviate exercise intolerance and eliminate inspiratory noise, particularly for patients with complete paralysis. The placement of an extraluminal suture between the axial caudodorsal aspect of the cricoid cartilage and the muscular process of the arytenoid cartilage simulates the action of the paralyzed cricoarytenoideus dorsalis muscle and abducts the arytenoid, enlarging the rima glottidis.

Laryngoplasty is combined with a ventriculectomy on the involved side of the larynx. There is an increased incidence of failure when laryngoplasty is performed without the concurrent ventriculectomy (MacKay-Smith, Johnson, and Baker 1973). The extraluminal aseptic procedure is performed prior to the ventriculectomy. Horses that have previously had a ventriculectomy should have the ventricle reopened to allow the development of an arytenoid-thyroid adhesion with the arytenoid in the abducted position.

It is imperative that the surgeon become completely familiarized with laryngeal anatomy and the surgical approach to successfully perform this procedure. Dissection of cadaver specimens is quite helpful.

The original technique described (Marks et al. 1970a) remains well accepted, although modifications have been added (Johnson 1970; Speirs 1972). The patient is positioned in lateral recumbency with the affected side uppermost and the head and neck extended. A 10- to 12-cm skin incision is made immediately below the linguofacial vein extending from the sternomandibularis muscle rostrally (Fig. 13–99). Hemorrhage is controlled by vascular ligation and electrocautery. A plane of dissection is established over the exposed omohyoideus muscle and deep to the linguofacial vein. The fascia and connective tissue around the vein should be spared by dissection close to the omohyoideus muscle.

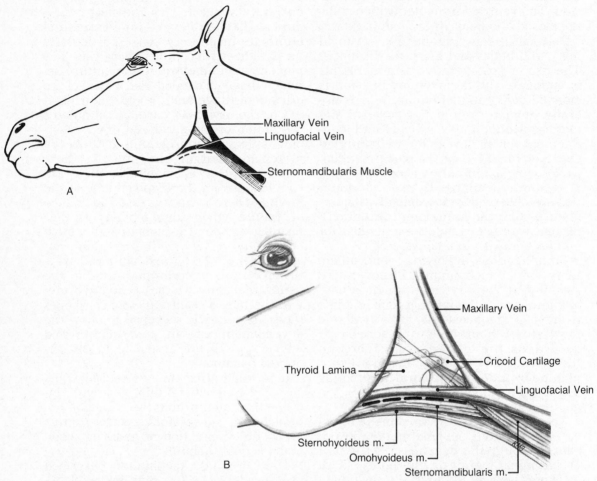

Figure 13–99 Prosthetic laryngoplasty. *A,* Landmarks for surgical incision. *B,* Superficial anatomy of surgical site. *C,* Laryngeal anatomy and exposure of the muscular process. *D,* Anchoring the prosthesis in the cricoid cartilage. Axial positioning is imperative to achieve desired direction of traction on muscular process (see Fig. 13–101). *E,* Retrieval of prosthesis under the cricopharyngeus muscle using a curved forceps (Stille vessel clamp). The site for anchoring the prosthesis through the muscular process is indicated by the dot. *F,* Diagram of technique for threading prosthesis through muscular process in a medial to lateral direction. This is an anterior-to-posterior view of a transverse section of the larynx at the level of the muscular process. *G* and *H,* Endoscopic view of left laryngeal hemiplegic cases following prosthetic laryngoplasty. Optimal abduction has been achieved in *G.* The maximal abduction achieved in *H* may predispose patient to coughing by allowing ingesta to enter the larynx.

Illustration continued on opposite page

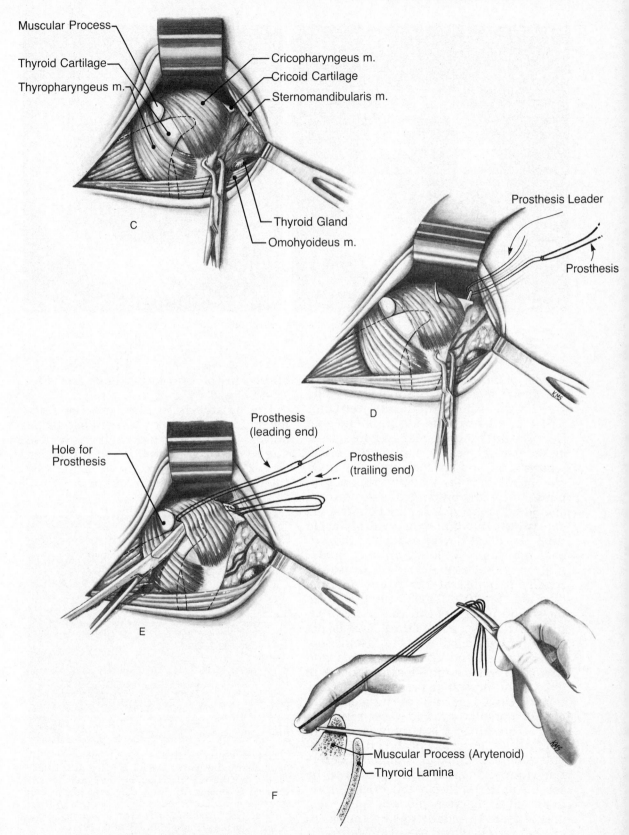

Muscular Process

Thyroid Cartilage

Thyropharyngeus m.

Cricopharyngeus m.

Cricoid Cartilage

Sternomandibularis m.

Thyroid Gland

Omohyoideus m.

C

Prosthesis Leader

Prosthesis

D

Hole for Prosthesis

Prosthesis (leading end)

Prosthesis (trailing end)

E

Muscular Process (Arytenoid)

Thyroid Lamina

F

Figure 13–99 *Continued. Illustration continued on following page*

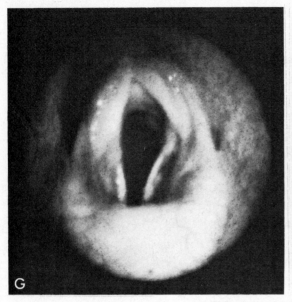

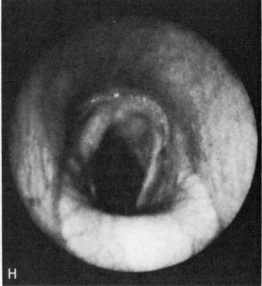

Figure 13–99 *Continued*

As the plane of dissection is expanded, the dorsal aspect of the incision is elevated with a broad malleable retractor (see Fig. 13–85). The fascia is elevated from the lateral laryngeal area by scissor dissection to clearly expose the cricopharyngeus and thyropharyngeus muscles. The vascular pedicle, which supplies the thyrolaryngeal structures, should be preserved. It may be retracted caudally to facilitate removal of fascia from the caudodorsal aspect of the cricoid cartilage. A notch on the caudal margin of the cricoid cartilage is usually readily palpable at the dorsal midline (see Fig. 13–101). This is the landmark for suture placement in the cricoid cartilage. After exposure of the dorsal aspect of the cricoid cartilage, the fascial septum between the cricopharyngeus and thyropharyngeus muscles is divided to expose the muscular process of the arytenoid cartilage and the cricoarytenoideus dorsalis muscle (see Fig. 13–99C). This process is very prominent in patients with atrophy of the cricoarytenoideus dorsalis muscle. A plane of dissection (tunnel) is made with forceps in the fascial plane between the cricopharyngeus and cricoarytenoideus dorsalis muscles, directed caudally toward the notch of the cricoid cartilage. The suture is drawn through this tunnel once an-chored in the cricoid cartilage (see Fig. 13–99D and E).

The prosthesis (suture) may be fashioned from a variety of nonabsorbable suture materials, although a double strand of No. 5 Dacron is recommended (Fig. 13–100). The prosthesis is made by folding a 24- to 30-inch length of suture

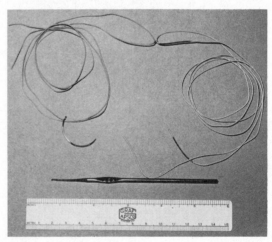

Figure 13–100 Abductor muscle prosthesis. A double strand of No. 1 Dacron is used as a leader for the prosthesis (No. 5 Dacron). The prosthesis is marked to ensure that the proper ends are tied together once the strand is divided in two. A Martin's uterine needle (#3) is used to penetrate the cricoid cartilage, and the crochet hook (#10) is used to thread the leader through the muscular process.

material in half and attaching a leader of No. 1 Dacron at the fold. One side of the prosthesis is marked with a permanent marker to facilitate appropriate knot placement later. A Martin's uterine needle (No. 3) is used to place the suture through the cricoid cartilage.

To improve exposure of the dorsal aspect of the cricoid cartilage for prosthesis placement, the caudolateral margin of the cricoid cartilage can be grasped with a towel clamp and simultaneously elevated and rotated outward (see Fig. 13–99D). The needle is inserted behind the caudal margin of the cricoid cartilage as close to the midline as possible and is advanced submucosally along the inner surface of the cricoid cartilage to prevent penetration into the laryngeal lumen. Removal of the endotracheal tube during placement of the suture increases the submucosal space between the cricoid cartilage and the first tracheal ring. The needle should be drawn through the cricoid cartilage on its circular arc to prevent the needle from breaking and should include a bite of at least 1.5 cm of cartilage. The carotid artery and esophagus are in close proximity to the dorsal aspect of the cricoid cartilage, and care must be taken to ensure that they are retracted to prevent penetration during withdrawal of the needle through the cricoid cartilage. Occasionally, a thyrolaryngeal vessel is penetrated during prosthesis placement. Bleeding from this vessel is difficult to control because it is located deep in the incision. The easiest method to control the bleeding is to pack the area with sponges, which can be removed after the procedure is completed. A pair of curved forceps is passed caudally through the tunnel between the cricopharyngeus and cricoarytenoideus dorsalis muscles, and the leading and trailing ends of the prosthesis are drawn rostrally (see Fig. 13–99E).

The fascia covering the muscular process is elevated and undermined by a finger passed under it close to the axial surface of the process. A 16-gauge needle is used to drill a hole in the process from the lateral side. The hole should enter the muscular process immediately dorsal to the thyroid lamina and should be positioned rostrally to ensure adequate holding power for the prosthesis. After the hole is drilled, a No. 10 crochet hook is inserted into the hole and digitally palpated on the axial surface of the muscular process. The leader for the prosthesis is positioned over the index finger of the left hand under tension and is carried over the axial surface of the muscular process deep to the point of the crochet hook (see Fig. 13–99F). It is then slipped off the finger and secured under the crochet hook. Tension is maintained on the leader as the crochet hook is used to draw the prosthesis through the muscular process. After retrieval of the end of the prosthesis through the process, the leader is cut off, leaving two separate prosthesis sutures. Tension is applied to each strand to evenly distribute the suture. The strands are tied individually with maximum tension using an instrument or hand tie. Endoscopic evaluation may be considered after removing the endotracheal tube to determine the optimum tension to achieve the desired degree of abduction. Greater tension is usually required to abduct the arytenoid cartilage in older patients (Boles 1979b).

The fascial plane between the cricopharyngeus and thyropharyngeus muscles is apposed with absorbable suture (00 chromic catgut). The paralaryngeal fascia is sutured to the laryngeal fascia as necessary to obliterate space. The fascia adjacent to the linguofacial vein should be apposed to that of the omohyoideus muscle with deep and superficial rows. Absorbable suture (00 chromic catgut) is used in a simple interrupted pattern. The subcutaneous tissues are apposed, and the skin is sutured with a nonabsorbable suture (00 nylon), using a simple interrupted pattern.

After completion of the prosthetic laryngoplasty, the patient is repositioned in dorsal recumbency and a ventral laryngotomy performed. After the larynx is entered, the endotracheal tube is removed. The laryngeal mucosa should be examined to determine whether penetration with the prosthesis occurred at the caudal aspect of the cricoid cartilage. If penetration occurred, the mucosa under the prosthesis is incised, elevated to cover the prosthesis, and sutured with a simple interrupted pattern using 000 polyglactin. The arytenoid cartilage on the involved side should be markedly abducted. The laryngeal ventricle will be difficult to enter if the prosthesis has effectively abducted the cartilage. Ventriculectomy is performed as previously described. If a previous ventriculectomy has been performed, an incision is made at the ventricular orifice, and the ventricular mucosa is bluntly elevated by finger manipulation and excessive mucosa removed. The ventral laryngotomy is allowed to heal by second intention.

Postoperative management is identical to that suggested for ventriculectomy. Postoperative endoscopic examination should reveal a marked abduction of the arytenoid cartilage on the involved side (see Fig. 13–99G and H). The surgical sites should be cleaned daily. Contamination of the laryngoplasty incision with exudates from the ventral laryngotomy should be avoided. Endoscopic examination at 45 days postoperatively should precede return to work.

One of the most important aspects of positioning the prosthesis successfully is the dorsal and axial placement of the suture in the cricoid cartilage. The cricoarytenoideus dorsalis muscle fibers extend from the dorsal, caudal, and axial regions of the cricoid cartilage to the muscular process in a rostrolateral direction. The fibers of the cricoarytenoideus dorsalis muscle attach perpendicularly to the axis of the cricoarytenoid articular surfaces, and the prosthesis should be placed in a similar direction (Fig. 13–101). Traction on the muscular process by the cricoarytenoideus dorsalis muscle elevates the arytenoid cartilage and also rotates it outwardly. If the caudal placement of the prosthesis is positioned too far laterally from the dorsal midline, some elevation of the cartilage will be produced but not adequate abduction (outward rotation). If the prosthesis is not positioned to include adequate substance of the cricoid cartilage or muscular process of the arytenoid cartilage, the cartilage may relax into the airway 30 to 60 days postoperatively as the suture cuts through the cartilage.

Potential complications of the prosthetic laryngoplasty procedure include wound dehiscence, infection of the synthetic implant, and development of a chronic cough. The frequency of dehiscence and infection can be reduced if hemorrhaging is adequately controlled, soft tissue spaces are properly obliterated, and aseptic technique is strictly followed. Saline and antimicrobial lavage of the surgical field prior to closure may also be beneficial. Early signs of incisional complications are swelling and serum exudation through the suture line. A sequela of incisional dehiscence and infection is the development of a chronic sinus tract associated with infection around the suture (Fig. 13–102).

Some horses will cough following prosthetic laryngoplasty. Clients should be informed of this possibility prior to surgery. Coughing appears to be related to the lateral fixation of the arytenoid and the larynx's inability to protect the trachea from the aspiration of ingesta (Greet, Baker, and Lee 1979; Johnson 1975; MacKay-Smith, Johnson, and Baker 1973; Marks et al. 1970a; Raker 1975a). Abduction of the arytenoid cartilage reduces the size of the pyriform recess (lateral food channel from oropharynx to esophageal orifice). Coughing may also be associated with granuloma formation resulting from intraluminal penetration of the prosthesis.

The prognosis following prosthetic laryngoplasty/ventriculectomy is favorable. Eighty-five to ninety per cent of the cases will demonstrate a marked improvement in respiratory capacity, and the majority of these will not produce noise during exercise. Even if the arytenoid cartilage is abducted less than desired, the success rate exceeds that of ventriculectomy alone. It is suggested that the fixation of the arytenoid cartilage by the prosthesis prevents its collapse into the airway during high-volume inspiratory efforts.

Epiglottic Entrapment

Epiglottic entrapment is the envelopment of the apex and lateral margins of the epiglottis by the arytenoepiglottic fold (Fig. 13–103). The disease is characterized by exercise intolerance, respiratory noise production, and occasionally, coughing (Boles 1975; Boles, Raker, and Wheat 1978; Cook 1974; Fretz, 1977; Speirs 1977). Noise production may be produced during inspiration, ex-

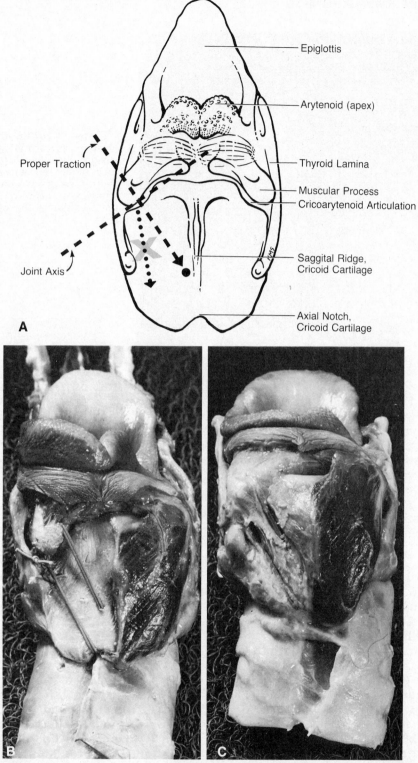

Labels in figure A:
- Epiglottis
- Arytenoid (apex)
- Proper Traction
- Thyroid Lamina
- Muscular Process
- Cricoarytenoid Articulation
- Joint Axis
- Saggital Ridge, Cricoid Cartilage
- Axial Notch, Cricoid Cartilage
- A
- B
- C

Figure 13–101 Placement of abductor muscle prosthesis. *A,* Diagram demonstrating dorsal aspect of laryngeal cartilages following removal of extrinsic and intrinsic musculature. Traction should be caudomedial, perpendicular to the axis of the cricoarytenoid articulation to simulate the function of the cricoarytenoideus dorsalis muscle (CAD). Traction in a caudal direction elevates, although it does not adequately abduct, the arytenoid. Furthermore, if the suture is not positioned in the axial notch, it tends to displace laterally and become loose. *B,* Laryngeal specimen with the left CAD removed, showing correct placement of the prosthesis. *C,* Laryngeal specimen of horse with left hemiplegia. The prosthesis had been implanted 12 months earlier, and it can be seen where the soft tissues were removed. Note the atrophy of the left CAD muscle. (Courtesy of Dr. J. R. McClure, Louisiana State University.)

445

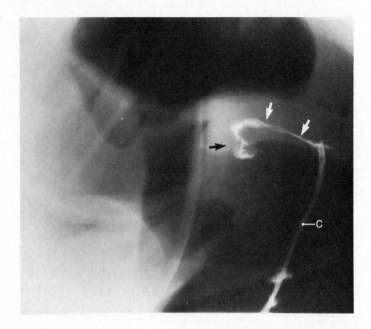

Figure 13–102 Prosthetic laryngoplasty. Contrast radiograph demonstrating an infected prosthesis site four months postoperatively. The contrast media was introduced with a flexible catheter (C) and identifies the location of the prosthesis (arrows).

piration, or both (Boles, Raker, and Wheat, 1978). Epiglottic entrapment may be an incidental finding in some horses and may not markedly interfere with exercise potential.

Epiglottic entrapment appears to fall into two categories: those with congenital defects of the epiglottis and those with a normal epiglottis. Entrapment is often a sequela to congenital epiglottic hypoplasia, particularly in young Standardbreds, and thus becomes apparent soon after training is initiated (Boles 1975; Boles, Raker, and Wheat 1978). Epiglottic entrapment has been recognized concurrently with congenital cleft of the soft palate (Cook 1974; Haynes and Qualls 1981). The condition is more often acquired in Thoroughbreds since epiglottic abnormalities are seldom present with entrapment and since the age for the onset of signs is variable. Ulcers are frequently located on the arytenoepiglottic fold in patients with entrapment. It is not known whether the ulcers play a primary role in the development of the condition or whether they occur secondary to entrapment.

The arytenoepiglottic fold (AEF) is a membranous fold of respiratory epithelium extending from the lateral aspect of the arytenoid cartilage to the ventrolateral aspect of the epiglottis. This fold of respiratory mucosa is continuous with the squamous epithelium covered glossoepiglottic fold of the oral cavity in the subepiglottic area (see Fig. 13–88). The subepiglottic epithelium is folded in an accordion fashion, providing a reserve of tissue that can expand when the epiglottis is elevated during deglutination. In entrapment, the subepiglottic and arytenoepiglottic tissues protrude upward to cover the periphery of the epiglottis or envelop the total rostral aspect of the epiglottis. The entrapping tissue is therefore a fold of tissue with a mucosal surface that is both superficial and deep and is seldom adherent to the dorsal surface of the epiglottis (see Fig. 13–103C). This condition may be intermittent and occasionally allows unobstructed visualization of a normal epiglottis.

Dorsal displacement of the soft palate may be associated with epiglottic entrapment. If the entrapment is due to hypoplasia of the epiglottis, the reduced epiglottic size may be inadequate to maintain the soft palate in a subepiglottic position. When the epiglottis is of normal size, the entrapment may hinder epiglottic function and may decrease the ability of the epiglottis to maintain the soft palate ventrally (Boles, Raker, and Wheat 1978).

The definitive diagnosis of epiglottic

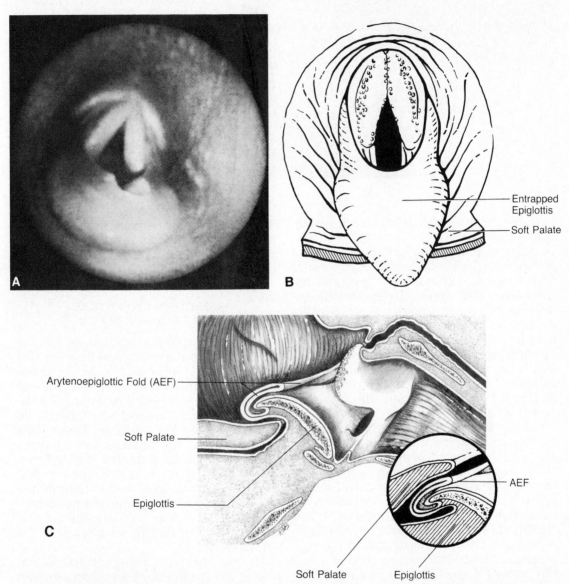

Figure 13–103 Epiglottic entrapment. *A*, Endoscopic view that demonstrates that the shape of the epiglottis can be appreciated, although the margin detail is obscured by the arytenoepiglottic fold. The caudal free margin of the entrapment is seen below the arytenoid cartilages. This condition must be differentiated from DDSP (see Figs. 13–80 and 13–86). *B*, Diagrammatic representation of epiglottic entrapment. The soft palate continues caudally, ventral to the entrapped epiglottis. The intrapharyngeal ostium cannot be visualized. *C*, Diagram of sagittal section of larynx with epiglottic entrapment. Note that the arytenoepiglottic fold is more prominent. Inset diagram demonstrates concurrent DDSP. The presence of both lesions may create confusion from diagnostic and surgical standpoints.

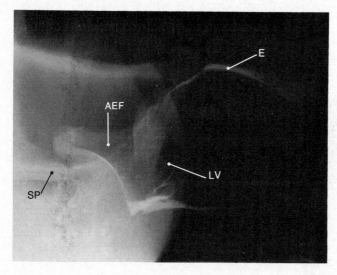

Figure 13–104 Contrast pharyngogram of patient affected with epiglottic entrapment. The rostral profile of the epiglottis is rounded, and the aryteno-epiglottic fold (AEF) is well visualized. The soft palate (SP) is positioned ventral to the epiglottis. Contrast medium is present in the esophagus (E) and ventral larynx. The laryngeal ventricles (LV) are recognized by their air density. Compare this lateral view with that in Figure 13–82.

entrapment is established by endoscopic examination (see Fig. 13–103). The general shape of the epiglottis can be visualized, although its serrated margin and dorsal vascular pattern are obscured by the entrapping tissue. An area of ulceration is frequently present on the visible surface of the entrapping tissue. This may be mistakenly diagnosed as an epiglottic ulcer. Pressure necrosis may result in formation of a fistula in the entrapping tissue and may allow the epiglottic apex to protrude through the entrapping tissue.

Confusion may exist in differentiating epiglottic entrapment from a dorsally displaced soft palate (DDSP). Both conditions present a free margin of tissue at the ventral aspect of the arytenoid cartilages, although DDSP also obscures visualization of the epiglottic shape. Both conditions may exist concurrently, and it may not be possible to appreciate the presence of an entrapment endoscopically unless the soft palate resumes normal position (see Fig. 13–103C). Repeated stimulation of swallowing may be necessary to facilitate understanding of the conditions present. Radiography, including contrast pharyngography, can be used to further assess the area and will allow evaluation of epiglottic length (Fig. 13–104).

Surgical resection, notching, and splitting of the abnormally placed tissue are used to relieve the entrapment in horses that experience exercise intolerance.

The surgery may be performed through the oral cavity or a ventral laryngotomy or ventral pharyngotomy incision (Boles, Raker, and Wheat 1978; Speirs 1977).

RESECTION BY VENTRAL LARYNGOTOMY

Surgical exposure of the entrapped epiglottis is readily obtained by a ventral laryngotomy approach. Intravenous anesthesia is used for the procedure, and the patient is positioned in dorsal recumbency. It is not necessary to divide the body of the thyroid cartilage. The caudal margin of the entrapment can be visualized or digitally palpated through the cricothyroid space dorsal to the epiglottis. It is imperative to distinguish between the caudal free margin of the entrapment and that of the soft palate, which may be dorsally displaced at the time of surgery.

The free margin of the entrapping tissue is grasped with tissue forceps and retracted caudally into the laryngeal lumen. This causes the epiglottis to be retroverted into the lumen. An atraumatic forceps (sponge forceps) is used to grasp the apex of the epiglottis. An endotracheal tube can be placed in the caudal oropharynx and used as a buttress to stabilize the retroverted epiglottis caudally to minimize direct trauma to that structure. A crescentic piece of tissue is excised to within 3 to 4 mm of the epiglottic margin in a fashion similar to

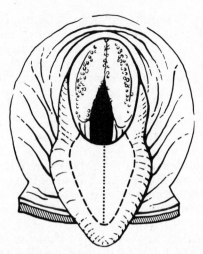

Figure 13–105 Resection of the arytenoepiglottic fold. The envelope of entrapping tissue may be resected peripherally, near the margin of the epiglottis (dashed line), or it may be divided axially (dotted line).

that described for resection of the caudal free margin of the soft palate (Fig. 13–105). Tissue forceps are used to grasp the caudal aspect of the AEF, and it is divided with scissors to just rostral to an axially placed forceps. This is repeated on the opposite side so that the two incisions meet at the midline of the entrapment. The resected piece of AEF may approach 8 cm in transverse length by 2 cm in anteroposterior length. One should be careful not to cut the epiglottic cartilage. The site is allowed to heal by second intention.

Alternative surgical procedures include removing a triangular notch in the entrapping tissue about 2 cm on a side over the tip of the epiglottis and dividing the entrapment on the midline without removing any tissue (see Fig. 13–105). Both have been suggested to reduce postoperative complications. It should be noted, however, that the occasional case in which axial division of the entrapment is performed may heal in a fashion that allows re-entrapment by the AEF because no tissue was removed.

The postoperative management following AEF resection is identical to that used for laryngeal ventriculectomy. The desired postoperative course includes 45 days of inactivity followed by endoscopic examination and a subsequent return to work if the condition is resolved.

The most significant postoperative complication associated with resection of the entrapping AEF is the development of DDSP (Haynes 1978). The relationship of DDSP to epiglottic hypoplasia has been mentioned, and DDSP will occur with higher frequency in these cases. For those patients in which DDSP was recognized preoperatively, the incidence of postoperative DDSP will likely be increased and might suggest the concurrent need for myectomy of the sternothyrohyoideus muscle. Persistent DDSP has developed in patients without any preoperative evidence of its presence. A causative factor may include iatrogenic epiglottic dysfunction from epiglottic retroversion, although the etiology of this complication is unknown. Postoperative DDSP may resolve spontaneously in 10 to 14 days or it may persist. In those patients in which DDSP remains as a persistent finding, surgical intervention to manage the palatal condition is generally unrewarding.

The association of epiglottic entrapment with DDSP reduces the prognosis following surgery for this disease. If DDSP is present preoperatively, the success rate is about 50 per cent. When entrapment alone is present, the success rate may approach 75 per cent, although the presence of epiglottic hypoplasia and postoperative DDSP are potential complications.

Granuloma formation at the site of removal can complicate the postoperative course. Fibrous tissue proliferation in the subepiglottic area may become covered by mucous membrane and may be visualized as an enlargement on the ventral surface of the epiglottis. Occasionally these soft tissue masses may be incorrectly interpreted as re-entrapment of the epiglottis. Resection of these masses is sometimes indicated, although the prognosis is guarded. Such cases seem particularly prone to persistent DDSP postoperatively.

ALTERNATIVE SURGICAL APPROACHES

Two other surgical approaches have been used to manage epiglottic entrapment (Boles, Raker, and Wheat 1978; Speirs 1977). The entrapping tissue may be resected, notched, or axially split by a pharyngotomy approach or by an oral approach. One potential advantage of these techniques may be that retroversion of the epiglottis into the laryngeal lumen is not required. Thus, if retroversion contributes to the postoperative development of DDSP, then its incidence may be reduced. The disadvantage of the pharyngotomy approach is the limited surgical exposure compared with that of ventral laryngotomy.

The oral approach is performed under general anesthesia. The oral cavity is opened with either a mouth wedge or dental speculum. The selected procedure can be done digitally if the surgeon's hand is small or with special long instruments through a tubular speculum. Because of limited access, the entrapment is usually either notched with a long biopsy forceps (equine uterine biopsy forceps) or split with an improvised long-handled scalpel while stabilized with long-handled forceps. The surgical manipulation can be visualized by oral endoscopy through a speculum. Although

the oral approach may be difficult, it does provide the advantage of being less invasive than laryngotomy or pharyngotomy. The postoperative convalescent period may be reduced by two to three weeks.

Arytenoid Chondritis

Chondritis of the arytenoid cartilage is a chronic disease that results in progressive exercise intolerance and inspiratory noise produced during exercise (Haynes et al. 1980). The initial signs of arytenoid chondritis are similar to those of laryngeal hemiplegia; in both conditions the range of abduction of the involved arytenoid cartilage is reduced. The disease may progress until it produces dyspnea in the resting horse. Marked distortion of the rima glottidis may occur and may cause laryngeal stenosis, particularly in patients with bilateral involvement (Fig. 13–106A).

The pathogenesis of chronic chondritis

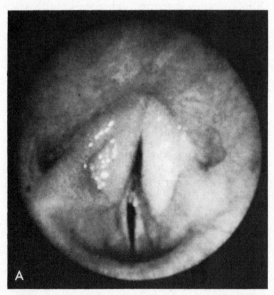
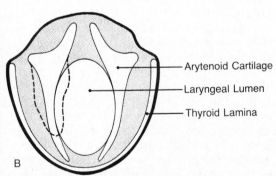

Arytenoid Cartilage

Laryngeal Lumen

Thyroid Lamina

Figure 13–106 Arytenoid chondritis. *A*, Endoscopic view of horse with bilateral chondritis and laryngeal stenosis, which caused dyspnea at rest. *B*, Diagram of cross section of larynx that demonstrates the space-occuping effect of chondritis. *C*, Cross section of arytenoid cartilages affected with chondritis (N = normal cartilage). *D*, Endoscopic view of larynx with chondritis of left arytenoid in a horse that was dyspneic following light exercise. The axially protruding lesion distinguishes this disease from laryngeal hemiplegia. *E*, Intraoperative view of horse via ventral laryngotomy exposure with division of the thyroid and cricoid cartilages revealing exudate and granuloma (GR) associated with the left arytenoid. *F*, Endoscopic view of horse in *D* 120 days following left subtotal arytenoidectomy. *G*, Axial view of left arytenoid cartilage removed from *A*. *H*, Normal left cartilage for comparison (note that articular facet [AF] was removed with both cartilages). (*B* reprinted with permission from Haynes et al.: JAVMA 177:1135, 1980.)

Illustration continued on opposite page

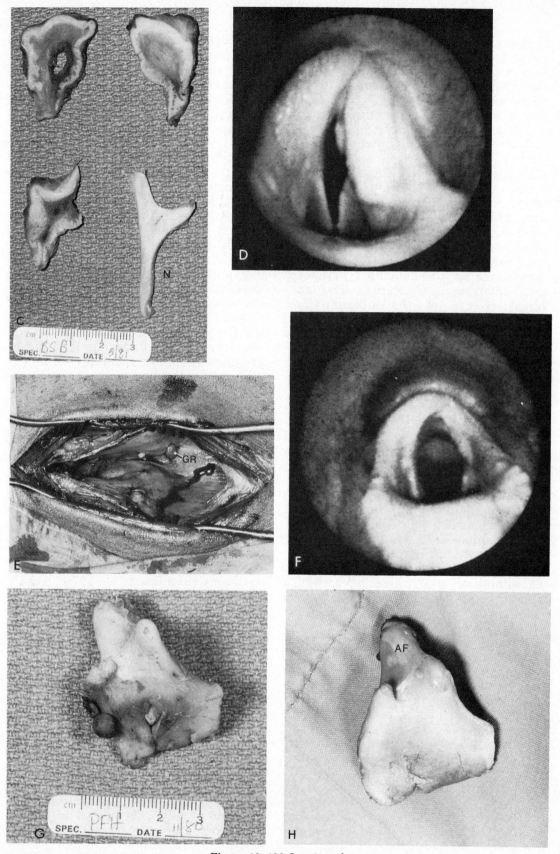

Figure 13–106 *Continued*

remains speculative. A septic process involving the body of the arytenoid cartilage results in sinus tracts that open into the laryngeal lumen and may recurrently drain and heal, causing fibrous tissue lamination and distortion of the involved cartilage. The cartilage becomes irregularly enlarged and the mucosal surface scarred and adherent to the cartilage. Enlargement of the cartilage may cause contact erosions on the contralateral cartilage, resulting in granuloma formation and predisposing to the development of septic involvement of that cartilage. The septic process of the hyaline cartilage may extend into the intrinsic musculature of the larynx, causing a perilaryngeal inflammatory response. The combined effects of the inflammation, thickening of the arytenoid cartilage (Fig. 13–106), and involvement of the cricoarytenoid articulation result in a reduced range of abduction. The disease appears to be progressive, and spontaneous resolution has not been reported. This disease is seen most often in patients over four years of age.

The hyaline cartilage is disrupted by a fibrous tissue infiltrate. Central necrosis and fibrosis are surrounded by fibrocartilage at the interface of normal and abnormal tissue. Osseous metaplasia of the cartilage, including the surrounding soft tissue or cartilage (cricoid), may occur. Cross sections of diseased cartilage are demonstrated in Figure 13–106C.

Diagnosis is established by endoscopic examination. Mild cases of arytenoid chondritis appear similar to laryngeal hemiplegia, i.e., axial displacement of the involved cartilage with limited abduction during laryngeal dilation. However, close examination of the luminal surface of the rima glottidis reveals roughening and projections from the affected cartilage (Fig. 13–106D). The firm, mucous-covered projection of one cartilage may be associated with a granulating lesion of the contralateral cartilage in a symmetrical position (contact lesion). The apex of the arytenoid cartilage (corniculate cartilage) is not involved, although its position may be distorted by the irregular shape of the body of the arytenoid. The palatopharyngeal arch on the involved side is usually more prominent, as the arytenoid apex is forced into an axial position. In advanced cases, the involved arytenoid may be displaced across the midline, resulting in marked obstruction of the rima glottidis. In patients with bilateral involvement, the rima glottidis may be nearly occluded and may prevent the visualization of luminal lesions (see Fig. 13–106A). Whenever laryngeal obstruction and reduced abduction of the arytenoid cartilages occur, particularly on the right side, chondritis should be a primary differential diagnosis. Intermittent DDSP may be seen as a concurrent condition and should be recognized.

Laryngeal palpation and radiography may support a diagnosis of arytenoid chondritis. External compression of the larynx may markedly increase laryngeal stenosis and dyspnea and may reveal that the larynx is not as resilient as normal. In advanced cases the larynx may be quite firm and noncompressible. Osseous metaplasia may occur with this condition and can be assessed radiographically.

The differential diagnosis includes any cause of reduced rima glottidis diameter. Foremost among these is laryngeal hemiplegia, as mentioned previously. Other less frequent space-occupying lesions of the rima glottidis include chondroma of the arytenoid cartilage (Cook 1974; Trotter, Aanes, and Snyder 1981), granuloma formation following intraluminal surgery of the larynx (Haynes 1978), and hypertrophic ossification of the laryngeal cartilages (Shapiro et al. 1979). Differentiation between these lesions and arytenoid chondritis can be difficult and may only be established during surgical intervention and histological examination.

Management of arytenoid chondritis depends on the extent of the disease and the intended use of the patient. Surgical intervention may be delayed in mild cases that do not require extended exercise capacity. Two techniques are described for the surgical management of chronic chondritis. One technique involves merely excision of the projecting lesions into the lumen and curettage of any sinus tracts (Haynes et al. 1980). The more extensive technique is described as a subtotal or partial arytenoidectomy (Haynes et al. 1980; White and

Blackwell 1980). Both techniques include a ventriculectomy on the involved side.

VENTRICULECTOMY AND FOCAL EXCISION OF INTRALUMINAL LESIONS

The combined procedure is moderately successful and transiently effective on mildly affected patients. Patients that experience dyspnea only during exercise, have a limited compromise of the rima glottidis, and have only partially reduced arytenoid function are candidates for this combined procedure.

The laryngeal lumen is exposed by a ventral laryngotomy incision with the horse maintained under intravenous anesthesia and positioned in dorsal recumbency. Firm focal projections of cartilage are excised by sharp dissection with a No. 15 scalpel to a level below the mucosal surface. Granulating lesions are examined for sinus tracts. Tracts in the cartilage are curetted with a small bone curette, and the surrounding granulation tissue is removed. A ventriculectomy is performed on the involved side.

A prosthetic laryngoplasty does not improve the surgical prognosis because the axial position of the arytenoid cartilage is a function of an increase in its transverse thickness and pericartilaginous inflammation. Arytenoid chondritis is an occasional cause for the poor abduction following laryngoplasty if the primary disease has not been recognized.

Postoperative management is similar to that following ventriculectomy for management of laryngeal hemiplegia. Endoscopy should be performed between the forty fifth and sixtieth postoperative days and the patient returned to exercise if the surgical sites are healed. This procedure is expected to be about 50 per cent successful on selected cases with mild obstruction of the larynx. It is suggested, however, that the technique is only transiently effective, since the course of arytenoid chondritis is usually progressive, although marked compromise of the rima glottidis may take an extended period of time to develop (in excess of 6 to 12 months).

SUBTOTAL ARYTENOIDECTOMY

Subtotal arytenoidectomy is indicated in cases of advanced arytenoid chondritis characterized by marked compromise of the rima glottidis. Bilateral subtotal arytenoidectomy may be performed simultaneously. Although subtotal arytenoidectomy should be considered a salvage procedure, it may allow return of exercise capacity in some patients (Haynes et al. 1980; White and Blackwell 1980). Arytenoidectomy was originally described for surgical relief of laryngeal hemiplegia (Cadiot 1901; Fleming 1903). More recently, arytenoidectomy has been used to increase the rima glottidis diameter in patients compromised by chondritis or chondroma of the arytenoid cartilage, laryngeal hemiplegia refractory to prosthetic laryngoplasty and ventriculectomy techniques, and ossification of the laryngeal cartilages (White and Blackwell 1980). Partial arytenoidectomy is described as a modification of the original arytenoidectomy procedure (White and Blackwell 1980).

Arytenoid chondritis involves the hyaline portion of the arytenoid cartilage. The object of subtotal arytenoidectomy is to remove that portion, leaving the corniculate cartilage (apex of the arytenoid, which is elastic cartilage) to protect the laryngeal lumen from aspiration of ingesta. The muscular process of the arytenoid may be left in situ, depending on the ease of its removal.

Subtotal arytenoidectomy is performed through a laryngotomy incision with the horse positioned in dorsal recumbency and maintained on inhalation anesthesia. Inhalation anesthesia is administered by an endotracheal tube placed in a midcervical tracheostomy incision. In cases of severe stenosis of the rima glottidis, preoperative placement of a tracheostomy tube may be necessary to relieve dyspnea. In patients without respiratory compromise at rest, the tracheostomy may be performed either prior to general anesthesia or immediately following the administration of the intravenous agents used for induction.

The laryngeal lumen is exposed by performing a ventral laryngotomy. To increase exposure, the body of the thyroid and cricoid cartilages may be divided on the ventral midline. Bone-cutting forceps are often required to divide the body of the thyroid cartilage because of the normal osseous metaplasia of that structure.

Two pairs of self-retaining retractors are used to widely retract the incisional margins. Examination of the laryngeal lumen should reveal the axial lesions of the arytenoid cartilages, which often drain exudate when compressed (see Fig. 13–106E). Figure 13–107 demonstrates the subtotal arytenoidectomy technique.

Sterile saline may be injected submucosally on the axial surface of the arytenoid cartilage to help elevate the mucosa. The arytenoid cartilage is exposed by an incision extending from immediately below the articular facet dorsally, to the vocal process ventrally, and rostrally along its ventral margin to the level of the corniculate cartilage. The mucosa is elevated from the axial surface by blunt dissection utilizing a nasal septal elevator or a narrow periosteal elevator (see Fig. 13–98). An effort should be made to keep the mucosa intact, although it is frequently disrupted in the area of luminal projection. Once the mucosa has been freed from the axial surface of the involved arytenoid cartilage, the abaxial (lateral) surface of the cartilage is dissected free of its surrounding tissues with scissors. These tissues include the vestibularis, vocalis, and cricoarytenoideus lateralis muscles and the lateral ventricle. The corniculate cartilage is divided along its attachment to the body of the arytenoid cartilage with scissors. The arytenoid cartilage is grasped with towel forceps and retracted axially and rostrally. The arytenoid cartilage may be either disarticulated at the cricoarytenoid joint or transected, leaving the muscular process and articular facet in place (Fig. 13–107E). Heavy scissors can be used to divide this cartilage if its disarticulation is difficult. The muscular attachments on the dorsal surface of the cartilage (deep in the incision) are divided with scissors as close to the cartilage as possible. Once the involved cartilage is removed, the lateral ventricle on that side is removed by incising along the laryngeal orifice. The mucosal incision is closed with a simple interrupted suture pattern (000 polyglactin). The ventral laryngotomy is allowed to heal by second intention. A tracheostomy tube is secured in place during recovery.

The postoperative course is characterized by laryngeal swelling, which requires that the tracheostomy tube be cleaned and maintained patent. Antimicrobials and phenylbutazone are administered for five days postoperatively. The patient is returned to a normal ration 12 hours postoperatively and the tracheostomy tube removed in three to five days, depending on the patency of the laryngeal airway.

Few postoperative complications have been reported. Dysphagia and aspiration pneumonia are not common postoperative sequelae inasmuch as the corniculate cartilage provides some protection for the laryngeal opening. It would be anticipated, however, that were such complications to develop, they would be seen more frequently when bilateral subtotal arytenoidectomy is performed. Endoscopic examination at 60 to 90 days postoperatively should reveal that the surgical site has healed (see Fig. 13–106F). Training may be resumed at that time. If DDSP had been a frequent preoperative observation, myectomy of the sternothyrohyoideus muscle would be suggested at the time of surgery and could be achieved at the tracheostomy site.

The prognosis for improvement of the laryngeal diameter is favorable. The prognosis for resumption of full exercise capacity is guarded to good.

Cricotracheal Eversion

Eversion of the cricotracheal membrane has been reported to cause obstruction of the URT during exercise (Pouret 1966;1967). Clinically, the condition is similar to other obstructive diseases associated with dynamic collapse during inspiration and is characterized by exercise intolerance and inspiratory noise. A flaccid or elongated cricotracheal membrane protrudes into the airway during inspiration. The condition is uncommon and is most often associated with obstructive disease rostral to the cervical trachea.

The definitive diagnosis is established by palpation of a larger than normal cricotracheal space. Indentation of the space by external manipulation may cause slight noise production at rest. Si-

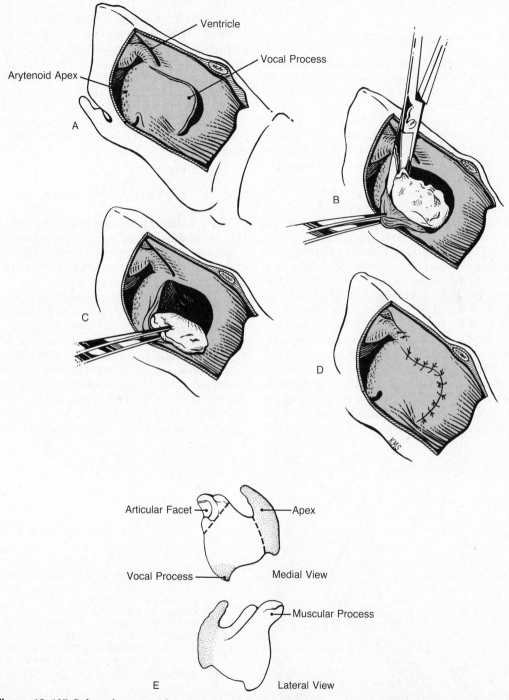

Figure 13–107 Subtotal arytenoidectomy. Diagram of laryngeal specimen (Figure 13–97A) in dorsal recumbency with the rostral aspect to the left and with a window in the right aspect of the larynx, exposing left arytenoid for diagrammatic purposes. *A*, Mucosal incision along the caudal and ventral margins of the cartilage. *B*, Division of cartilage to leave apex in situ. *C*, Lateral soft tissue dissection accomplished to deliver cartilage. *D*, Closure of the surgical site. *E*, Diagram of the left arytenoid cartilage with dotted lines indicating planes of division (division of muscular process is optional).

multaneous palpation and endoscopic examination will reveal a bulging of the cricotracheal mucosa into the airway.

SURGICAL TECHNIQUE

Surgical management of cricotracheal eversion involves resection and apposition of the membrane in the ventral aspect of the space. The surgery is performed through a ventral midline incision over the cricotracheal space (slightly caudal to the approach used for ventral laryngotomy) with the horse positioned in dorsal recumbency and maintained on intravenous anesthesia. The cricotracheal space is exposed and divided on the midline between the cricoid cartilage and the first tracheal ring, exposing the tracheal lumen. The cricoid cartilage is apposed to the first tracheal ring with stainless steel sutures, thus reducing the axial length of the cricotracheal space. The incision into the lumen is closed with absorbable sutures and the skin edges apposed. The patient may resume exercise within 30 days.

An imbricating technique has been described as an alternative approach (Wheat 1979). The same surgical exposure is required, although rather than dividing the ligament and mucosa in the cricotracheal space, horizontal mattress sutures (No. 2–3 chromic catgut) are placed through the cricotracheal ligament without penetrating the tracheal lumen. This reduces the space without entering the tracheal lumen. In summary, this condition may be secondary to obstructive lesions further rostral in the respiratory tract, and treatment of the primary condition may reduce the effect of cricotracheal eversion on upper airway obstruction without the need for surgery.

GUTTURAL POUCHES

The guttural pouches are paired diverticula of the eustachian tubes extending from the nasopharynx to the middle ear. Each pouch has a potential volume of approximately 300 cc. They contact one another axially immediately below the longus capitus muscle, at the base of the skull dorsally, and at the wing of the atlas caudally. The greater cornu of each stylohyoid bone courses through the posterolateral aspect of each pouch, dividing it into a lateral compartment that communicates rostrally with a medial compartment (Fig. 13–108). The medial aspect of the pouch is approximately three

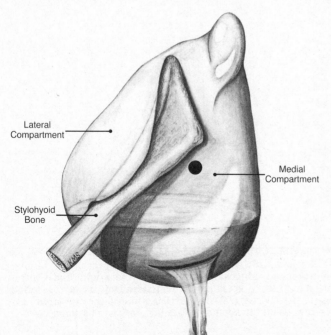

Lateral Compartment

Stylohyoid Bone

Medial Compartment

Figure 13–108 Lateral view of the left guttural pouch. The diagram demonstrates the relationship of the lateral compartment to the medial compartment. The black dot indicates the site of percutaneous centesis. The incision is located in the ventrolateral aspect of the medial compartment, the site for drainage of guttural pouch empyema.

times the size of the lateral compartment and extends more ventrally. The mucosal lining of the guttural pouches is typical respiratory epithelium.

A number of vital structures are intimately associated with the guttural pouch and should be considered in their relationship to the symptoms of guttural pouch disease and their location during surgical intervention. The internal carotid artery; cranial nerves VII (facial), IX (glossopharyngeal), X (vagus), XI (spinal accessory), and XII (hypoglossal); and the cranial sympathetic nerve trunks are associated with the dorsal and caudomedial aspects of the guttural pouch. The internal maxillary artery and vein and cranial nerves XI and XII are associated with the posterolateral aspect of the pouch. The location of the arterial branches associated with the guttural pouch can be appreciated by angiography (Fig. 13–109). Retropharyngeal lymph nodes are associated with the ventral medial aspect of the pouch.

The function of the guttural pouches remains unclear. It has been suggested that they provide a mechanism for warming inspired air by filling during expiration and swallowing and subsequently emptying during inspiration, contributing warm air during inspiration (Cook, 1966b; Heffron, Baker, and Lee 1979). The function of the eustachian tube structure, as in other species, is to equalize pressure between the pharynx and the middle ear.

The location, configuration, and anatomical associations of the guttural pouches contribute to the variety of clinical signs demonstrated when diseased. Chronic nasal discharge is often associated with guttural pouch disease. Because the pharyngeal orifice of the guttural pouch is located caudal to the nasal septum, drainage of exudate into the pharynx causes a bilateral nasal discharge, although it is *dominant* through the nostril on the involved side. The pharyngeal orifice of the guttural pouch enters the rostrodorsal aspect of the pouch well above its ventral extent, and this relationship predisposes to retention of fluid (exudate, blood) within the diseased pouch. When the head is lowered, drainage from the pouch is facilitated and may be quite copious. Accumulations of exudate or air within the guttural pouch that cannot be expelled through the pharyngeal orifice will cause distension of the pouch. Distension may be characterized by external distortion deep to the parotid salivary gland and by pharyngeal compression, which may cause dyspnea. The majority of guttural pouch diseases, however, do not cause external distortion.

The intimate relationship of vascular and nervous structures within the guttural pouch predicates that epistaxis and cranial nerve dysfunction are also suggestive of guttural pouch disease.

A tentative diagnosis of guttural pouch disease may be suggested by a history and clinical observations including chronic nasal discharge (mucopurulent and/or serosanguineous), pharyngeal distortion and dyspnea, and cranial nerve dysfunction. The definitive diagnosis can be supported by pharyngeal endoscopy, direct endoscopic examination of the guttural pouch, centesis and lavage of the pouch, and radiographic examination.

Endoscopic visualization of the pharyngeal openings to the guttural pouch (see Fig. 13–61) should be routine in respiratory tract endoscopy. The visual-

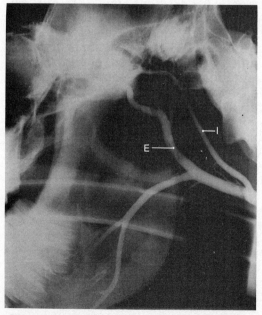

Figure 13–109 Carotid angiogram. Angiography performed on anesthetized horse in right lateral recumbency and maintained on inhalation anesthesia (note endotracheal tube). The internal carotid artery (I) courses along the posteromedial aspect of the guttural pouch, and the external carotid artery (E) is located rostral and lateral to it.

ization of exudate or blood from the orifice should suggest guttural pouch disease and the need for direct endoscopy of the guttural pouch. Direct visualization of the guttural pouch endoscopically can be done with a rigid endoscope using the curved tip or with flexible fiberoptic instrumentation (see Fig. 13–60). The cartilaginous flap of the guttural pouch orifice may be elevated with a rigid endoscope, a curved-tip catheter, with a wedge-shaped tip over the end of the flexible endoscope (tip of canine endotracheal tube), or by using the flexible biopsy device of fiberoptic systems (Fig. 13–110).

Catheterization of the guttural pouch may be accomplished either through the pharyngeal orifice or by a percutaneous technique. The pharyngeal orifice can be entered with a rigid curved-tip catheter (Fig. 13–111). A Chamber's uterine catheter or an artificial insemination pipette may be used to elevate the cartilaginous orifice and allow entry into the pouch. The pharyngeal orifice is most patent dorsally, and thus catheterization techniques should concentrate on entry into that aspect of the opening. Aspirated exudate should be examined cytologically and microbiologically by culture and sensitivity. If aspiration fails, lavage of the pouch with sterile fluids (500 ml) may yield a productive sample.

Percutaneous centesis is considered an alternative procedure when direct endoscopic visualization or catheterization of the pouch cannot be accomplished. A site is selected approximately 2 to 3 inches below the base of the ear midway between the mandible and the wing of the atlas. This space may be enlarged by elevating the chin of the horse, facilitating entry into the pouch. The site is aseptically prepared, and a trocar, catheter, or needle at least 2 inches in length is inserted at right angles to the midline (see Fig. 13–64). When the stylohyoid bone is contacted, the needle is directed off the posterior and ventral aspects of the bone to enter the pouch (see Fig. 13–108). Aspiration of fluid or air establishes that the pouch has been entered. If aspiration of a sample is unsuccessful, lavage of the pouch may confirm that either exudative or serosanguinous fluids are present.

Radiography of the guttural pouch is very useful in providing supportive information about the guttural pouch disease (Cook 1973). The guttural pouch may be characterized as an air-filled density within the osseous and soft tissue densities of the skull. A standing lateral view is suggested as the first projection to obtain when evaluating the size and shape (profile) of the pouch. Radiographic signs that suggest guttural pouch disease include distension of the pouch and the observation of a fluid line within it (Figs. 13–112 and 13–113). Clinical evaluation and endoscopic examination may be necessary to identify the involved pouch, as they are superimposed upon each other in the lateral projection. Contrast media instilled into the pouch may facilitate identification of the involved pouch and may contribute to the appreciation of space-occupying lesions.

The most frequently observed diseases of the guttural pouch include empyema, mycotic infection, and tympany, Each disease will be characterized and therapeutic approaches suggested. Specific surgical approaches, including their advantages and disadvantages, will be discussed separately.

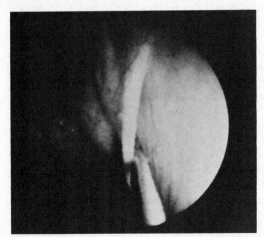

Figure 13–110 Catheterization of the left guttural pouch. The biopsy forceps are advanced from the tip of the fiberoptic endoscope through the dorsal aspect of the pharyngeal orifice. Rotation of the endoscope may facilitate its entry into the pouch.

Guttural Pouch Empyema

Empyema of the guttural pouch refers to the accumulation of exudate within a

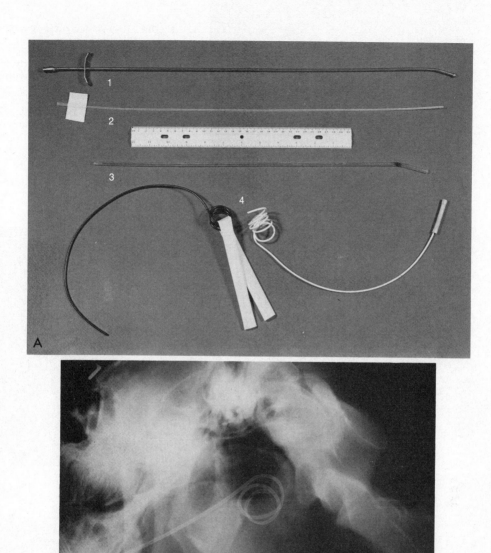

Figure 13–111 Guttural pouch catheters. *A*, Chambers intrauterine infusion catheter (*1*), or artificial insemination pipette with a bent tip (*3*) can be used to collect guttural pouch contents or for lavage. The canine urinary catheter (*2*) or angiography catheter (*4*), coiled by heating, may be used as indwelling systems. They can be sutured to the external nares to keep them in place. *B*, Self-retaining guttural pouch catheter in place. Lateral radiographs of yearling presented with dyspnea and nasal discharge due to retropharyngeal lymph node abscessation and subsequent guttural pouch empyema. A modified Whitehouse approach was performed to establish ventral drainage and the catheter was placed in the pouch for postoperative lavage. Note the restricted nasopharyngeal airway (arrows) due to guttural pouch distention.

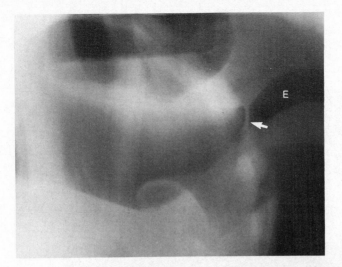

Figure 13–112 Guttural pouch empyema. Bilateral. The lateral radiographic projection demonstrates a fluid line within the pouches (nearly superimposed). The patient was also affected with rostral displacement of the palatopharyngeal arch and that fold of tissue (arrow) is seen just rostral to the profile of the arytenoid cartilages. The esophagus (*E*) is air filled.

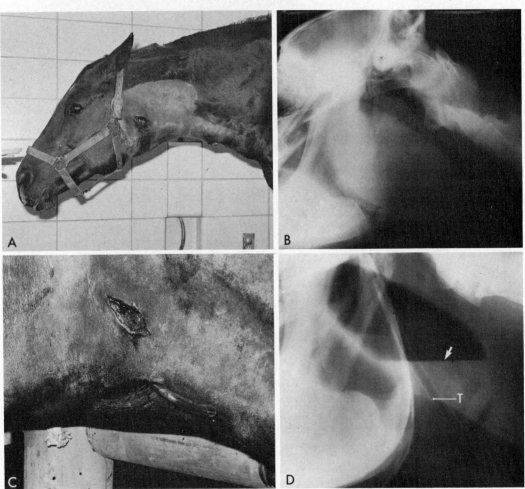

Figure 13–113 Guttural pouch empyema. *A,* Photograph of eight-year-old quarter horse mare affected with marked swelling of the rostral cervical area, dyspnea, dysphagia, and nasal discharge. Note tracheostomy tube in place and that a previous attempt had been made to drain the involved pouch. *B,* Lateral radiographic projection of the guttural pouch. Note the mottled character of the guttural pouch contents, indicative of inspissated exudate, and the marked dorsoventral compression of the nasopharynx. *C,* Drainage was established, with the aid of local anesthesia, through a modified Whitehouse approach, and a tube was sutured in place to flush the involved pouch. *D,* Lateral radiographic projection taken seven days following surgery. Fluid line is visible in the affected pouch (arrow) and contralateral pouch. The dorsoventral dimension of the nasopharynx has been markedly increased. The radiopaque tube into the pouch is visible (*T*).

pouch. Guttural pouch empyema should be considered whenever a patient is affected with a chronic mucopurulent nasal discharge. Guttural pouch empyema most often occurs unilaterally and produces an asymmetrical bilateral nasal discharge that is *dominant* on the involved side. Pharyngeal irritation and inflammation, secondary to the presence of exudate in the pharynx, may stimulate coughing, and DDSP is frequently observed. As long as the inflammatory process produces only a liquid exudate, external swelling and nasopharyngeal swelling are uncommon. Pharyngeal paralysis and dysphagia may be complications of an advanced disease process (McAllister 1977).

Guttural pouch empyema (GPE) is most often secondary to other disease processes. The majority of patients with GPE have a history of respiratory tract infection caused by viral agents, bacterial agents, or a combination of both. It is quite likely in patients with infectious disease of the URT that the mucous membrane of the pouches is involved, comparable to the mucosa of the paranasal sinuses and the pharynx. Accumulation of exudate or mucus within the pouches is transient, however, and resolves concurrently with the recovery of the patient.

The most frequent cause of chronic GPE is respiratory tract infection initiated by beta-hemolytic streptococci (Cook 1971; Knight et al. 1975; Mansmann and Wheat 1972; McAllister 1977). A typical history in such patients is a continued nasal discharge following recovery from the streptococcal infection. Systemic antimicrobial therapy may reduce the quantity of the discharge, although relapse often follows cessation of treatment. Frequently with streptococcal infections, the retropharyngeal lymph nodes become abscessed and spontaneously drain into the guttural pouch (Knight et al. 1975). Occasionally the inflammatory process within the pouch becomes well established and will not respond to systemic therapy alone.

Any disease process that alters the function or patency of the pharyngeal opening of the guttural pouch or that is located within the guttural pouch may cause a secondary septic process of this structure. Examples of such processes include neoplasia and fungal granulomas. Gram-negative organisms (especially *Pasteurella* sp.) are often involved.

In long-standing cases of GPE, especially those that have been neglected or that have gone unrecognized, it is not uncommon for the exudate to become inspissated (see Fig. 13–113). The septic products will assume the consistency of cottage cheese or scrambled eggs and will not drain freely through the pharyngeal orifice. This process is self-perpetuating and is the primary cause of marked distension of the guttural pouch (into the nasopharyngeal lumen and evident externally) and may cause dyspnea and dysphagia. Occasionally the exudate may form firm ovoid concretions referred to as chondroids (Fig. 13–114) (Fleming 1903). These concretions may be rather numerous but do not always cause outward evidence of pouch distension.

The diagnosis of GPE should be considered in any patient with a chronic and nonresponsive nasal discharge. The techniques to confirm the diagnosis include endoscopy, catheterization, lavage, and radiography. The endoscopic visualization of a stream of mucopurulent exudate from the pharyngeal orifice of the guttural pouch should be supportive of a definitive diagnosis. However, false negative and false positive

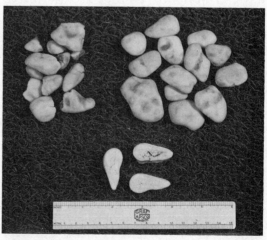

Figure 13–114 Chondroids from guttural pouch. These inspissated concretions were removed from a patient affected with nasal discharge due to a chronic guttural pouch infection. Guttural pouch distention was not clinically apparent. (Courtesy of Dr. Y. L. Lindsay, Louisiana State University.)

impressions are possible. The failure to observe exudate from the pouch opening does not eliminate the presence of GPE, especially if the exudate has become inspissated. Intradiverticular endoscopy should be performed in such cases. On the other hand, visualization of a slight mucoid exudate from the pouch does not confirm established disease within that structure (McAllister 1977). It is not uncommon to observe a slight amount of discharge in patients with marked pharyngeal inflammation, and in such cases the guttural pouch inflammation is merely a manifestation of inflammation of the respiratory mucosa.

In patients with exudate draining from the guttural pouch, catheterization and collection of the exudate should be conducted to identify the incriminated organism and its antimicrobial sensitivity.

Radiographic evidence of GPE includes the demonstration of a fluid line within the pouch, distension of the pouch, or the presence of a fluid-dense material suggestive of inspissated exudate (see Fig. 13–113). The lateral radiographic projection is most useful in this regard, and the size and shape of the pouches may also be determined.

In patients with acute GPE, systemic antimicrobial therapy (penicillin, ampicillin, or sulfas) may enhance the resolution of the condition within 10 to 14 days. If systemic therapy is ineffective or if the disease is chronic, the pouch may be treated locally by utilizing an indwelling catheter (see Fig. 13–110). Daily lavage of the pouch with 500 ml of antiseptic or antimicrobial solution should be accomplished until the nasal discharge abates. A variety of solutions can be used including 5 to 10% povidone iodine or a dilute solution of antimicrobials based on sensitivity testing. Concurrent systemic antimicrobial therapy is useful. When infections are refractory to systemic and local therapy, ventral drainage of the pouch should be established surgically. In patients with inspissations or chondroids of the guttural pouch, medical management of the disease will usually be ineffective until the incriminated material is removed from the pouch. Once the pouch has been entered surgically, a spoon can be used to remove the foreign material, followed by copious lavage. Failure to remove all the semisolid material from the pouch will predispose to recurrence of the condition.

The prognosis for guttural pouch empyema is favorable with early and vigorous treatment. Pouches distended with inspissations usually respond favorably, although the occasional case may be affected with an irreversible neurogenic dysfunction of the pharynx. This complication is characterized by the reflux of water and ingesta from the nasal cavities through the external nares. Although not usually a complete pharyngeal paralysis, this condition may contribute to recurrent infection of the guttural pouches and chronic weight loss.

Tympany of the Guttural Pouch

Tympany of the guttural pouch is characterized by an abnormal filling and distension of the guttural pouch with air (Cook 1966b; 1971; 1973; Wheat 1962). The disease usually becomes apparent within the first few months following birth, and is a result of a malfunctioning pharyngeal orifice of the guttural pouch. The typical swelling of the parotid area may extend ventrally over the lateral aspect of the larynx and is fluctuant, nonpainful, and resonant to percussion. In mild cases, affected patients may be otherwise asymptomatic. In advanced cases with extreme distension, both dyspnea and dysphagia may be evident owing to pharyngeal collapse and ventral displacement of the larynx and rostral cervical trachea. Although the condition is most often unilateral, bilateral involvement has been reported (Johnson and Raker 1970).

The pathological lesion responsible for the air-distended pouch has not been well characterized. Excessive mucous membrane may be attached to the medial lamina of the eustachian tube cartilage or the salpingopharyngeal fold may be abnormally large and redundant (Cook 1971; Freeman 1980a). The resultant effect is that air, which normally enters the guttural pouch, is trapped within by a one-way valve effect. Continued distension occurs and is recognized clinically. It is not uncommon for secondary infection to occur, as the normal mucous secretions of the guttural pouch mucous membrane are also sequestered within the pouch. The disease is usually seen in the young horse, supporting its congenital occurrence, and appears to affect females more than males (Cook 1971). It is conceivable that acquired inflammatory disease of the guttural pouch could cause a similar phenomenon.

The diagnosis of guttural pouch tympany is based on clinical signs. Although the disease is most often unilateral, extreme distortion of a single pouch may appear to be nearly bilaterally symmetrical. Endoscopy, pharyngeal catheterization of the guttural pouches, and radiography are used to confirm which pouch is involved. Endoscopic examination should suggest that the nasopharynx is more compressed by expansion of the guttural pouch on the involved side. Catheterization of the guttural pouch orifice on the involved side should allow decompression of the distended pouch. Selective instillation of contrast material into the guttural pouch will demonstrate radiographically whether it is located within the distended or normal pouch margins. Radiographic visualization of a normal pouch outline may be appreciated in cases of unilateral involvement. If distortion is extreme, the uninvolved pouch may be compressed by the distended pouch, obscuring its outline. A fluid line in the ventral aspect of the involved pouch is frequently seen. In patients with extreme distension, the silhouette of the nasopharynx is markedly compressed and the larynx and proximal cervical trachea displaced ventrally.

MANAGEMENT

Effective management of tympany of the guttural pouch requires surgical intervention. Two techniques have been described for resolution of this condition. The original technique (Wheat 1962) involves surgical exposure of the guttural pouch and liberal resection of the membranous flap of the pharyngeal orifice within the pouch. With the patient under general anesthesia, the redundant tissue is grasped with a pair of forceps and dissected free with a pair of long-handled scissors. The second, and reportedly more effective, technique involves the fenestration of the medial septum, which permits communication of the involved pouch with the normal one (Cook 1966b; 1971). The window created between the two pouches should be liberal and at least 3 cm in rectangular or circular dimension. Care should be taken to ensure that the windows in each membranous surface are identical in location and size. A ventral approach is suggested for either technique. When the disease is bilateral, resection of the redundant mucous membrane from the pharyngeal orifice within the pouch should be performed on at least one side, with concurrent septal fenestration. Fenestration of the septum has been done electrosurgically utilizing endoscopic instrumentation and has eliminated the need for surgical exposure (Cook 1971).

The prognosis following surgical intervention is favorable if involvement is unilateral. If resection of the membranous flap is performed or if the disease is bilateral, there is a greater tendency for recurrence and a second surgical intervention may be necessary. The surgical approach to the guttural pouch is left to heal by second intention, and the pouch should be lavaged with antiseptic or antibiotic solutions on a daily basis until the drainage site becomes occluded (10 to 14 days). Primary closure may be considered if infection within the pouch is not well established. Follow-up examination endoscopically and radiographically should demonstrate that the involved pouch resumes a near-normal dimension.

Guttural Pouch Mycosis

Guttural pouch mycosis is described as a fungal disease of the guttural pouch that may invade the neurovascular structures in the immediate vicinity (Cook 1966a; 1968a; 1968b; 1971). The most frequent clinical signs include intermittent spontaneous epistaxis and cranial nerve dysfunction, most notably characterized by dysphagia. Although reported as the most common disease of the guttural pouch in the United Kingdom (Cook 1971), the disease is sporadic and infrequent in occurrence in the United States.

The variation in clinical signs is predicated by which vital structures are involved by the disease process. Epistaxis is the most frequent sign associated with this disease and is usually the result of disruption of the internal carotid artery. Pharyngeal paralysis, the next most frequently observed sign, is related to dysfunction of cranial nerves IX (glossopharyngeal) and X (the pharyngeal branch of the vagus nerve). Other signs in decreasing order of occurrence include laryngeal hemiplegia, nasal discharge, Horner's syndrome, dorsal displacement of the soft palate, abnormal head posture and incoordination of limbs, mild colic, and subparotid abscess formation and facial paralysis (Cook 1966a).

The extent of the epistaxis can be quite variable. Fresh blood may be visualized at the external nares (in greater amounts on the involved side) or dark clotted blood may be voided, particularly when the patient lowers its head. The large amount of hemorrhage into the guttural pouch may be reflected by profound decreases in the packed cell volume (10 to 15 per cent PCV is not uncommon in severe cases) or hemorrhagic shock followed by death.

Because of the variable clinical signs associated with this disease, guttural pouch mycosis should be considered in the differential diagnosis of numerous diseases capable of causing comparable symptomology. This would include a disease as common as laryngeal hemiplegia and may be particularly considered when a right-sided laryngeal paralysis is observed.

The lesion, most often unilateral, is located in the dorsal and medial aspects of the guttural pouch, closely associated with the base of the skull. A predilection to the right or left side has not been recognized. The lesion grossly resembles a brownish diphtheretic membrane elevated from the mucosal surface. The lesion may vary in size from 1 cm in diameter to one that covers the entire dorsal surface of the guttural pouch (Cook 1966a). *Aspergillus* sp. is the most commonly incriminated organism.

The pathogenesis of this condition remains unclear. Current information suggests that the invasive process is secondary to an aneurysm of the internal carotid artery immediately before it enters the base of the skull (Cook 1978). Although this concept appears to explain the rather consistent location of the lesion, the pathogenesis of the aneurysm is not well appreciated.

The diagnosis of guttural pouch mycosis may be suggested by clinical signs including epistaxis and/or cranial nerve dysfunction. Direct visualization of the mycotic lesion during endoscopy of the guttural pouch is diagnostic. Radiography of the guttural pouch may demonstrate a granular or ground-glass appearance of the dorsal aspect of the guttural pouch. Carotid angiography can be used to demonstrate aneurysms of the internal and external carotid arteries (Cook 1978).

Because of the potentially fatal implication associated with this disease, aggressive therapy should be instituted. The local instillation of antifungal agents into the involved pouch has been described (Cook 1971), and amphotericin B is the current drug of choice. Additional local therapy may include enzymes and antiseptics. Because the lesion is located in the dorsal aspect of the pouch, general anesthesia and positioning of the patient in dorsal recumbency have been suggested at four- to seven-day intervals to allow prolonged contact (30 minutes) of the medication with the involved lesion (Cook 1971). Direct nebulization of medication into the guttural pouch may be considered as an alternative approach. The results of medical therapy to date have not been very rewarding.

Surgical intervention for management of this mycotic lesion has also been reported (Cook 1971; Johnson and Merriam 1973; Owen 1974). Vascular ligation of the internal carotid artery on the cardiac side of the lesion as a prophylactic technique to prevent fatal hemorrhage was originally considered unsuccessful (Cook 1971). It was thought that the circle of Willis provided enough retrograde blood flow so that continued hemorrhage from the lesion would occur. Surgical removal of the diphtheritic membrane through a ventral approach to the guttural pouch was considered hazardous and capable of causing a fatal hemorrhagic episode (Cook 1971; Johnson, Merriam, and Attleberger 1973). However, surgical removal of the lesion has been successfully reported with concurrent ligation of the internal carotid on the cardiac and cranial sides of the lesion (Owen 1974).

Because it is difficult to expose the lesion and vasculature within the pouch and because vascular ligation may be traumatic to the closely associated cranial nerves, an extradiverticular (not invading the pouch) ligation technique has been suggested (Cook 1978). It is currently proposed that ligation of the internal carotid artery on the cardiac side of the lesion will ultimately cause the formation of a thrombus that extends to the cranial side of the lesion, thus preventing retrograde bleeding from the circle of Willis.

Most recently, occlusion of the internal carotid artery by means of a balloon-tipped catheter has been described (Freeman and Donawick 1980a; 1980b). The internal carotid artery was located through an incision comparable to that of the hyovertebrotomy approach, although positioned to expose the ventral half of the wing of the atlas. A balloon-tipped catheter was introduced through an incision into the arterial lumen and advanced cranially to a predetermined distance above the lesion based on assessment of the lesion's location radiographically. The artery was ligated around the catheter as well as double ligated at its origin. Thrombosis of the internal carotid artery resulted, and the catheter was removed in approximately 14 days. Medical therapy of the lesion was subsequently carried out.

The prognosis of guttural pouch mycosis is guarded. Although spontaneous recovery has been reported (Cook 1968a), the possibility of a prolonged course of intermittent and spontaneous epistaxis does exist as well as the potential for a fatal hemorrhagic episode. In those patients that exhibit signs of cranial nerve dysfunction associated with the presence of mycotic invasion of the guttural pouch, the prognosis is poor, as the neurogenic lesions are seldom reversible. If pharyngeal paralysis develops, emacia-tion, aspiration pneumonia, and death are likely sequelae. It is suggested that thrombosis of the involved artery be achieved surgically, either by the more simple extradiverticular ligation of the artery or by introduction of a balloon-tipped catheter as described previously.

EXTRADIVERTICULAR LIGATION OF THE INTERNAL CAROTID ARTERY

Surgical exposure of the internal carotid artery at its origin from the common carotid artery has been described (Cook 1978; Freeman and Donawick 1980a; 1980b). An 8- to 10-cm curvilinear incision is made through the skin immediately rostral to the ventral aspect of the wing of the atlas. The parotid salivary gland is reflected rostrally, and the internal carotid artery is located deep and caudal to the occipitomandibular portion of the digastricus muscle. The vessel is freed from the surrounding fascia and double ligated (No. 2 chromic catgut) immediately above its origin. The surgically divided tissue can be reapposed with an interrupted suture pattern (00 chromic catgut) and the skin closed with nonabsorbable suture (00 nylon). Healing by first intention should be expected. The advantage of extradiverticular ligation is that a septic and contaminated guttural pouch is not penetrated, thereby allowing the surgical site to heal without complication.

Surgical Approaches to the Guttural Pouch

Three basic surgical approaches to the guttural pouch have been described. These include a dorsal approach, an approach through Viborg's triangle, and a ventral approach. The dorsal approach is referred to as the hyovertebrotomy approach and was originally described by Chabert and Dieterich (Berge and Westhues 1966; Fleming 1903; O'Connor 1965). Dieterich described the combined use of the dorsal approach and ventral drainage through Viborg's triangle (Berge and Westhues 1966; O'Connor 1965). The ventral approach was described by Whitehouse (O'Connor 1965) and may be accomplished through a ventral midline or paramedian incision (Guard 1953). The approach selected for surgical invasion of the guttural pouch should be based on the disease present, the therapeutic objective, and the extent of guttural pouch distension. Figure 13–115 demonstrates the landmarks for the surgical approaches to the guttural pouch.

The most common reason for surgical invasion of the guttural pouch is to establish drainage of septic accumulations within the pouch. The modified Whitehouse approach is suggested as the procedure of choice for this objective. The greater surgical exposure compared with Viborg's approach makes it preferable. The ventral midline approach may be suggested if entry into both pouches is required; however, the cervical muscles (sternohyoideus and omohyoideus) make adequate exposure more difficult. In the author's opinion, the hyovertebrotomy approach is seldom indicated. The modified Whitehouse approach is suggested for ventral drainage associated with empyema and exudative inspissations as well as for septal fenestration for treatment of guttural pouch tympany. Extradiverticular ligation of the internal carotid artery is suggested for treatment of guttural pouch mycosis and subsequent epistaxis and is performed through a modified (more ventral) hyovertebrotomy approach.

Any patient that is dyspneic during the preoperative period should have a tracheostomy tube inserted before surgery. This precaution should avoid complications due to asphyxia during anesthetic induction prior to endotracheal intubation.

An endoscope may be passed through the pharyngeal orifice into the involved guttural pouch intraoperatively to assist in the visualization of surgical manipulations and to provide illumination within the surgical field. When a nondistended pouch is surgically invaded, an endoscope or rigid catheter within the pouch may facilitate its identification. The close proximity of vital neural and vascular structures within the guttural pouch necessitates a thorough knowledge of the involved anatomy prior to surgical intervention (Figs. 13–116 and 13–117).

MODIFIED WHITEHOUSE APPROACH

The modified Whitehouse approach is suggested to be a superior ventral approach to expose the guttural pouch (Guard 1953). The surgical approach is identical to that for prosthetic laryngoplasty, i.e., immediately below the linguofacial vein (see Figs. 13–115 and 13–117). The major advantage of this approach over that on the ventral midline is that lateral soft tissue retraction does not involve the sternohyoideus or omohyoideus muscles and is thus more efficient in allowing surgical visualization of the involved pouch. This approach may be performed under local or general anesthesia. When the involved pouch is markedly distended, the procedure may be done in the standing patient if the objective is merely to establish ventral drainage. However, if visual assessment of the pouch is necessary or if the pouch is not distended, general anesthesia is preferred and the patient is positioned in lateral recumbency.

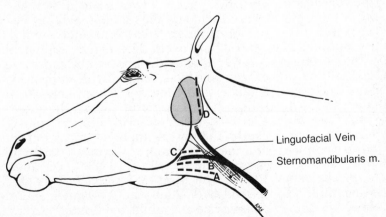

Linguofacial Vein

Sternomandibularis m.

Figure 13–115 Landmarks for surgical approaches to the guttural pouch. The Whitehouse approach (A) is ventral, the modified Whitehouse (B) is paramedian, Viborg's approach (C) is ventrolateral, and the hyovertebrotomy approach (D) is dorsolateral.

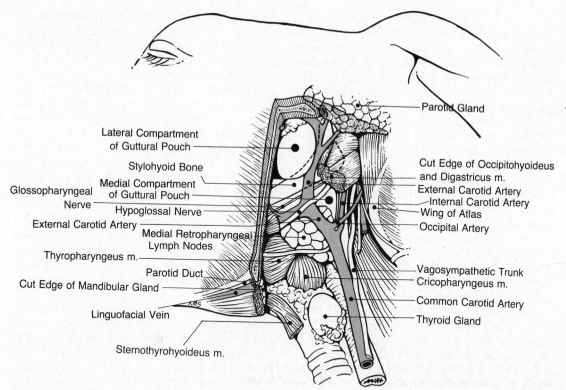

Figure 13–116 Surgical anatomy of lateral guttural pouch area. Dissection reveals lateral and deep anatomy.

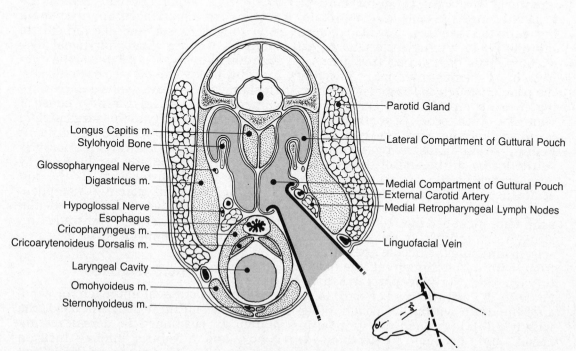

Figure 13–117 Anatomy of the modified Whitehouse approach. The diagram is of a transverse section taken with the head and neck extended, just caudal to the mandible (inset). The structures encountered in a modified Whitehouse approach to the medial compartment of the guttural pouch are identified.

A 10-cm skin incision is made lateral to the larynx immediately below the linguofacial vein, dividing the skin and subcutaneous tissues. A plane of dissection is established between the omohyoideus muscle and the linguofacial vein to expose the lateral laryngeal fascia and is continued by blunt dissection toward the ventral aspect of the pouch. At a depth of approximately 6 to 8 cm, the retropharyngeal lymph nodes can be visualized overlying the ventral lateral aspect of the medial compartment of the guttural pouch (see Fig. 13–116). If the pouch is distended, palpation or needle aspiration can be used to identify its location. Once the ventral aspect of the medial compartment is penetrated with a pair of scissors, the jaws of the scissors are opened and retracted to enlarge the opening into the pouch. A broad band malleable retractor (see Fig. 13–85) is used for retraction so that the pouch can be examined internally. The dorsal aspect of the guttural pouch can be visualized, and the medial septum can be seen.

A drain should be positioned through the incision into the pouch, and the surgical incision is allowed to heal by second intention. The Penrose drain may be looped through the coils of a self-retaining catheter (see Fig. 13–111) placed into the pouch through the pharyngeal opening. This system can then be used in an ingress-egress manner by lavaging the pouch through the catheter and having it drain around the Penrose drain ventrally. An alternative method would be to anchor the proximal end of the Penrose drain in place by securing a suture leader to the end of the drain. A large-curved needle can be used to penetrate the pouch from within through the superficial structures to secure it to the skin. Care must be taken to palpate vital structures (particularly the carotid vessels) in directing the needle's penetration from within the lumen of the pouch through the overlying parotid salivary gland to the skin. It is necessary to secure the drain within the pouch, otherwise it will fall through the surgical incision and become ineffective. An alternative to a Penrose drain would be installation of a semirigid rubber tubing (e.g., canine endotracheal tube), which can be used to maintain the patency of the ventral incision and also as an avenue for postoperative flushing of the pouch (see Fig. 13–113C).

The pouch should be flushed daily, and the catheters may be withdrawn 7 to 10 days postoperatively, depending on the degree of drainage at that time. The surgical site should be cleaned daily and petrolatum jelly liberally applied to the paraincisional area to prevent scalding from the drainage products. Healing should be uneventful, and the surgical site should close within 21 days.

One potential complication of any surgical approach to drain the medial compartment ventrally is damage to the innervation of the pharynx (glossopharyngeal nerve and pharyngeal branch of the vagus nerve). This complication has been reported following Viborg's approach (Mansmann and Wheat 1972) and has been seen by the author following a modified Whitehouse approach (patient in Fig. 13–113). The clinical signs associated with this complication included the reflux of water and ingesta through the nostrils, although the patient was capable of swallowing enough food and water to maintain an adequate level of nourishment. If the patient had experienced any dysphagia prior to surgery, it would be difficult to establish whether this pharyngeal dysfunction (paresis) was related to the original guttural pouch disease or to the surgical procedure. The involved nerves are vulnerable to surgical trauma because of their close proximity to the surgical field and because they are small and difficult to identify intraoperatively, particularly if the normal anatomy is obscured by guttural pouch distension. In the author's opinion, this potential complication is unavoidable when the medial compartment is invaded ventrally, regardless of the approach used.

VENTRAL APPROACH

When this surgical approach for exposure of the guttural pouch is used, the patient is positioned in dorsal recumbency, and a ventral midline incision (see Fig. 13–115) is made similar to that for a ventral laryngotomy. The sternohyoideus muscles are separated on the midline and liberally retracted laterally. Deep dissection extends around the lateral aspect of the larynx and is continued on an axial plane deep to the carotid vasculature. The ventral margin of the medial compartment of the guttural pouch is identified either because it is distended or because it presents a hollow void in the soft tissue dissection. Needle aspiration of the pouch will establish its location by aspiration of either exudate or air (if the pouch is not distended by exudate). The ventral aspect may also be identified by palpating a rigid catheter placed within the pouch through the pharyngeal orifice.

The advantage of this approach is that it allows access to both the right and left pouches through a common skin incision. The contralateral pouch can be approached by dissection along the opposite aspect of the larynx. The disadvantage of the approach is that the sternohyoideus and omohyoideus muscles present a significant muscle mass to retract laterally; this reduces visual assessment of the pouch. The ability to visualize the inner aspect of the pouch is poor at best and is determined by its degree of distension, being most limited when the pouch being entered is of normal size. Aftercare is identical to that for the modified Whitehouse approach.

VIBORG'S APPROACH

Viborg's triangle is bounded dorsally by the tendinous insertion of the sternomandibularis muscle, ventrally by the linguofacial vein, and rostrally by the vertical ramus of the mandible. This surgical approach is typically described as one that is relatively free of vital neurovascular structures and therefore without much hazard of postoperative complication. It should be noted, however, that the establishment of drainage through this approach into the ventral aspect of the medial compartment of the guttural pouch is basically identical to that of the Whitehouse or modified Whitehouse approach except that the incision is above the linguofacial vein. If the involved pouch is markedly distended, this approach may be performed under local anesthesia in the standing patient. In patients without significant

distension of the pouch, which therefore requires more definitive dissection of the tissue, the patient should be restrained in lateral recumbency under general anesthesia.

A 6- to 8-cm incision is made through the skin immediately dorsal to the linguofacial vein (see Fig. 13–115). Careful dissection of the soft tissues should be performed to reflect the parotid salivary gland and salivary duct (if visible) dorsally and rostrally. A deep plane of dissection is established immediately ventral to the external carotid artery until the guttural pouch is encountered. Needle aspiration of the pouch can be accomplished to locate it. The pouch may be entered by bluntly penetrating its wall with a pair of scissors, opening the jaws of the scissors, and retracting them to enlarge the ventral opening. A drain (Penrose or self-retaining) or seton should be positioned within the pouch to maintain the patency of the surgical site during the postoperative period. The aftercare is identical to that suggested for the modified Whitehouse approach.

When this surgical approach is used in conjunction with a dorsal approach (hyovertebrotomy) to the guttural pouch, it is referred to as the Dieterich approach (Berge and Westhues 1966; O'Connor 1965).

HYOVERTEBROTOMY APPROACH

The hyovertebrotomy approach involves entry into the dorsal and lateral aspects of the medial compartment of the guttural pouch. It is referred to as the hyovertebrotomy approach because it is performed between the hyoid apparatus (greater cornua of the stylohyoid bone) and the vertebral column (wing of the atlas). It was described particularly for the removal of chondroids and inspissated pus from the involved pouch. Because the procedure exposes the vital structures of the caudomedial aspect of the guttural pouch, it should be accomplished under general anesthesia with the patient restrained in lateral recumbency and with the head and neck extended.

A 10- to 12-cm skin incision is initiated approximately 4 cm below the base of the ear and midway between the vertical ramus of the mandible and the wing of the atlas. The auriculocutaneous muscle and the parotid salivary gland are exposed and reflected rostrally. The posterior auricular nerve in the caudal and dorsal aspects of the incision should be preserved. The deeper dissection is continued with scissors immediately rostral to the wing of the atlas. The dorsal aspect of this plane of dissection will be limited by the obliquus capitus cranialis muscle. The glistening fascia of the occipitomandibularis muscle becomes visible in the rostral aspect of the incision. The occipitomandibularis muscle may be divided on the long axis of the muscle fibers (O'Connor 1965) although it is suggested that the muscle be retracted rostrally. Immediately deep to the caudal aspect of the muscle are the internal carotid artery and its associated nerves including the glossopharyngeal, hypoglossal, and vagus. Careful dissection should be achieved into the caudolateral aspect of the medial pouch immediately rostral to these structures.

It is difficult to visualize the dorsal aspect of the pouch because of the anatomical limitations imposed by the presence of the stylohyoid bone and the obliquus capitus cranialis muscle. The medial septum between the adjacent pouches can be directly visualized.

Although this approach is commonly described in the literature, it appears to have two major disadvantages: the close proximity of the aforementioned neurovascular structures and the fact that it does not allow ventral drainage of the involved pouch. Thus, in the majority of circumstances, it is combined with a procedure that does allow ventral drainage (Dieterich approach). When combined with a procedure that establishes ventral drainage, the hyovertebrotomy incision may be closed by appositional suturing of the divided structures including the skin (00 chromic catgut and nylon).

Aftercare depends on whether or not drainage through a ventral approach was established. In either case, an indwelling catheter system is indicated for postoperative lavage of the pouch. The hyovertebrotomy incision should heal by first intention without complication. If a ventral approach was used as well, aftercare includes daily wound care as previously described.

TRACHEA AND LOWER RESPIRATORY TRACT

Surgically correctable disorders of the lower respiratory tract (trachea, bronchial tree, pulmonary parenchyma) are relatively infrequent in occurrence, in contrast to surgically correctable diseases of the upper respiratory tract. The trachea serves as a conduit for air transport from the upper respiratory tract to the pulmonary parenchyma. The total cross-sectional area of the trachea is much smaller than the total cross-sectional area of the pulmonary bronchi. Thus, any reduction in the diameter of the trachea caused by either extraluminal compression or an intraluminal space-occupying lesion will markedly reduce the efficiency of airflow through that system. The trachea is supported by relatively rigid rings of hyaline cartilage and therefore is infrequently affected by the phenomenon of dynamic collapse. Lesions that interfere (encroach) with normal airflow are usually characterized by both inspiratory and expiratory noise production and even dyspnea in advanced cases. Lesions that restrict the tracheal airflow may result from congenital abnormalities (scabbard trachea), traumatic lesions (fractured tracheal rings), infectious disease (peritracheal abscess), or postsurgical stenosis.

Specific diagnostic techniques that can be utilized for the assessment of tracheal or pulmonary disease include endoscopy, radiography, transtracheal aspiration, and thoracocentesis.

Endoscopy of the cervical trachea may be accomplished by passing a flexible fiberoptic endoscope through the nasal cavity and larynx into the cervical trachea (Cook 1974) (Fig. 13–118). Visualization of the distal trachea including the carina (tracheal bifurcation) requires endoscopic equipment in excess of 110 cm and may be accomplished via a cervical tracheostomy. In the unanesthetized patient, parenteral narcotic agents or the instillation of local anesthetic into the trachea may reduce the cough reflex and eliminate patient apprehension. Rigid endoscopic equipment can be utilized for visualization of the cervical or proximal thoracic trachea when introduced by tracheotomy (Cook 1965).

Radiography of the cervical trachea is

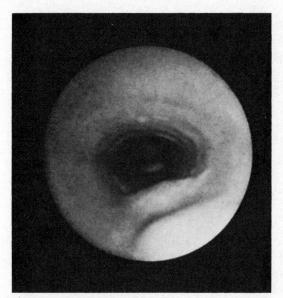

Figure 13–118 Tracheoscopy. A flexible endoscope was passed through the nasopharynx and larynx into the trachea, and this view is at approximately the midcervical level. Exudate from lower respiratory tract disease is visible in the ventral aspect of the trachea.

well within the capabilities of portable radiographic equipment. Although the usual assessment of the cervical trachea includes the lateral view (Fig. 13–119), the ventrodorsal view becomes more difficult with portable equipment owing to superimposition of the cervical spine and soft tissues. However, most space-occupying lesions of the cervical trachea can be identified by the lateral view alone. Evaluation of the thorax has become increasingly available at referral centers with the appropriate equipment.

Techniques that should be included for diagnosis of lower respiratory tract disease include transtracheal aspiration and thoracocentesis. Both techniques are intended to assess disease of the thoracic respiratory viscera and, more specifically, disease of the pulmonary parenchyma and/or the pleural surface of the thoracic cavity.

Transtracheal Aspiration

Transtracheal aspiration in horses was originally described for obtaining specimens for bacteriological culturing of the lower respiratory tract (Mansmann and Knight 1972). The technique involves penetration of the tracheal lumen in the lower cervical area with a trocar through which a catheter is introduced caudally into the trachea for retrieval of a specimen. A variety of instruments and catheters can be adapted for this procedure. The ventral midline of the lower cervical trachea is liberally clipped and prepared for aseptic technique. The site selected should be at the approximate junction of the middle and lower thirds of the cervical trachea where it is relatively superficial and palpable without interference from the ventral cervical musculature. Local anesthesia is infiltrated subcutaneously and along the intended tract of penetration for the trocar. An Oschner trocar will conveniently allow the passage of a No. 8 French canine urinary catheter into the caudal trachea (Fig. 13–64B). A stab incision is made through the skin at the intended site, and the trocar is introduced until the tracheal cartilages are contacted. The trachea should be manually stabilized while the trocar penetrates the annular ligament between consecutive tracheal rings. Once the lumen has been entered, the trocar should be directed caudally and the catheter introduced to its maximal extent (40 cm). A large syringe (35 ml or greater) should be used to rapidly aspirate any tracheal fluids that may be available. If aspiration does not yield a sample, 30 ml of sterile saline should be introduced through the catheter and immediately withdrawn to wash the trachea and provide a sample for cytological analysis. The volume introduced may be repeated if the initial aspiration is unproductive, and lowering the head may enhance retrieval of a specimen. The sample retrieved should be evaluated cytologically (Beech 1975) and submitted for aerobic and anaerobic culture and antimicrobial sensitivity. The catheter should be slowly withdrawn, followed by removal of the trocar, to minimize contamination of the peritracheal tissues with organisms from the respiratory tract. Complications of transtracheal aspiration include local abscess formation, local emphysema if a plug of tracheal cartilage has been removed, trauma to the carotid sheath structures if the trachea was not stabilized during introduction of the trocar, and pneumomedias-

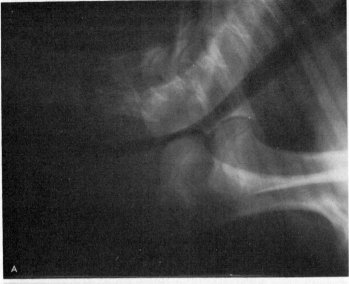
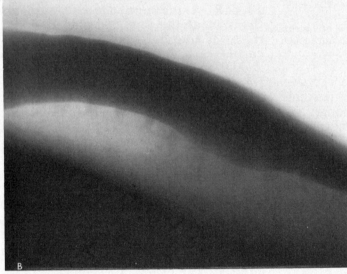

Figure 13–119. Tracheal radiography. *A,* Dorsoventral flattening of the trachea. A miniature pony foal was presented because of dyspnea, and this lateral radiograph confirmed a flattened trachea in its caudal cervical and rostral thoracic portions. *B,* Tracheal collapse following ventral longitudinal division of three tracheal rings for relief of postoperative laryngeal swelling. The dorsoventral dimension is increased owing to the lateral collapse of the trachea.

tinum (Farrow 1976). Peritracheal emphysema is usually self-limiting and is of minimal consequence. Local abscess formation typically responds to systemic antimicrobial therapy. The potential hazards of transtracheal aspiration are far outweighed by the information gained from the cytological and bacteriological examinations of the samples retrieved.

Thoracocentesis

The collection of pleural fluid by thoracocentesis may be equally important in evaluating lower respiratory tract dis-

ease. Furthermore, the combined use of transtracheal aspiration and thoracocentesis will give the clinician the best opportunity to define disease within the thoracic cavity caused by bacterial infections (Smith 1979). The collection site through the sixth or seventh intercostal space is identified immediately above the lateral thoracic vein (spur vein) or on the line drawn between the point of the elbow (olecranon) and the tuber coxae. A variety of instruments can be used for retrieval of pleural fluid including a mammary infusion tube, an intravenous catheter, and a trocar (see Fig. 13–64B). The selected site should be infiltrated subcutaneously and along the intended tract of penetration with local anesthesia. If a blunt instrument is used, a stab incision through the skin with a scalpel is necessary. Penetration through the intercostal space should favor the anterior aspect of the caudal rib of the space to avoid the intercostal vasculature. The pleural cavity should be penetrated to a depth of approximately 4 to 6 cm. Complications of the technique are few and may include seeding of the site with a septic process extended from the pleural cavity. Samples retrieved from the pleural space should be evaluated for cytology, including total and differential counts of WBCs, total protein, and culture and antimicrobial sensitivity.

Trachea

Disease of the equine trachea is uncommon. Those conditions that affect the trachea include space-occupying lesions within the tracheal lumen, diseases of the cartilaginous tracheal rings that fail to maintain the tubular tracheal structure, and peritracheal lesions that compress the trachea.

Diseases of the trachea may interfere with efficient air flow, causing noise production, exercise intolerance, or even dyspnea. Most lesions that cause a reduction in the luminal diameter of the trachea create air flow turbulence, particularly on inspiration, although this turbulence may affect the expiratory phase as well.

Diseases of the cervical trachea may be readily appreciated by external palpation, auscultation with a stethoscope, endoscopy, and radiography. The use of a stethoscope should allow one to identify the site of maximal airflow turbulence, particularly in patients breathing rapidly or deeply. Further diagnostic evaluation can then be conducted once the major site of involvement is suggested.

The most frequent cause of intraluminal tracheal lesions appears to be stenotic cicatrix formation or granuloma formation following tracheostomy (Tate et al. 1981). Other possible causes of intraluminal lesions include penetrating lesions into the tracheal lumen and neoplastic disease.

Tracheal collapse (flattening) may occur from external traumatic insults or as a sequela of tracheostomy techniques that totally divide a tracheal ring or it may be developmental in origin. Trauma may fracture a tracheal ring, which may subsequently heal in malalignment, resulting in a reduction in the diameter of the tracheal lumen. Tracheostomy performed by the division of one or more tracheal rings on the ventral midline may result in a reduction of the transverse width of the trachea because the rings are not complete dorsally (Fig. 13–120A). Extensive tracheal collapse characterized by a marked dorsoventral flattening of the tracheal lumen has been described (Carrig, Groenendyk, and Seawright 1973; Hanselka 1973). The lesion may involve both the cervical and thoracic tracheae and is the result of cartilage rings that form shallow arcs with a stretched and thinned dorsal fibroelastic membrane (Fig. 13–119A). As in the canine tracheal collapse syndrome (Vasseur 1979), this condition is characterized by inspiratory dyspnea if the cervical trachea is involved and by expiratory dyspnea if the thoracic trachea is involved. It would appear, however, that the condition usually involves both the cervical and thoracic tracheae (Boyd and Hanselka 1976).

Any disease that causes swelling or distortion of the tissues surrounding the trachea may compress (collapse) the trachea. Tracheal compression has been reportedly associated with mediastinal lymph node abscessation (Randall and Myers 1973) and can cause tracheal compression at the thoracic inlet. Suggestive signs include inflammation of the tissues at the thoracic inlet and the presence of a compressive lesion, identified by radiography of the area. Although uneventful recovery may follow careful drainage of the abscess cavity, it has been suggested that the tracheal deformity may be permanent.

The need for surgical intervention for diseases of the trachea may be related to primary disease of the trachea as described previously or may provide temporary or permanent relief from upper airway obstructive disease rostral to the cervical trachea. Although tracheostomy is the most frequently performed surgical technique, the following descriptions include tracheal anastomosis and prosthetic repair.

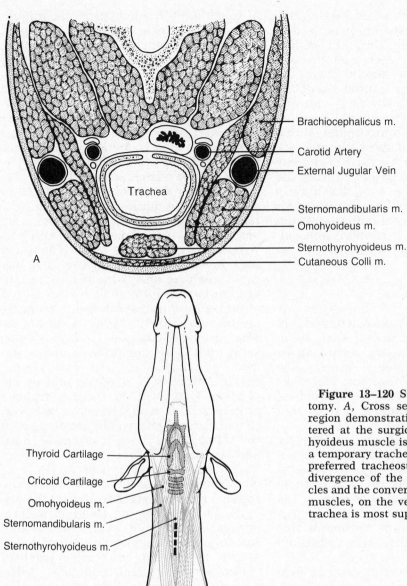

Brachiocephalicus m.

Carotid Artery

External Jugular Vein

Trachea

Sternomandibularis m.

Omohyoideus m.

Sternothyrohyoideus m.

Cutaneous Colli m.

A

Thyroid Cartilage

Cricoid Cartilage

Omohyoideus m.

Sternomandibularis m.

Sternothyrohyoideus m.

B

Figure 13–120 Surgical site for tracheostomy. *A,* Cross section of the midcervical region demonstrating the anatomy encountered at the surgical site. The sternothyrohyoideus muscle is reflected laterally during a temporary tracheostomy procedure. *B,* The preferred tracheostomy site is between the divergence of the sternomandibularis muscles and the convergence of the omohyoideus muscles, on the ventral midline, where the trachea is most superficial.

TEMPORARY TRACHEOSTOMY

The indications for temporary tracheostomy include obstructive disease of the upper respiratory tract and tracheal intubation for inhalation anesthesia and to divert airflow postoperatively. Causes of obstructive URT disease that may require a temporary tracheostomy include nasal obstruction due to post-traumatic swelling or snake bite, regional lymph node abscessation and cellulitis caused by *Streptococcus equi* infections, and guttural pouch distentions from either tympany or inspissated empyema. In considering the temporary tracheostomy for these conditions, it is assumed that the primary disease will respond to therapy and allow the re-establishment of a patent rostral airway.

A temporary tracheostomy may be used as a portal for endotracheal intubation and the administration of inhalation anesthetics (Steffey 1979). Examples of such conditions include surgical techniques of the URT that could not be performed with an endotracheal tube in normal position (e.g., subtotal arytenoidectomy).

A temporary tracheostomy may also be indicated in the postoperative period when surgical techniques have the potential to markedly reduce or obliterate the lumen of the URT. Examples of such techniques include resection of the nasal septum when packing of the surgical site is necessary to control hemorrhage and subtotal arytenoidectomy wherein postoperative swelling within the laryngeal lumen may cause respiratory embarrassment. Temporary tracheostomy is not considered necessary in cases of routine laryngeal surgery: i.e., prosthetic laryngoplasty and/or ventriculectomy. In these cases, if significant swelling within the laryngeal lumen follows surgical intervention, a tracheostomy tube can be placed through the ventral laryngotomy incision into the larynx and lumen of the rostral cervical trachea.

Temporary tracheostomy may be performed under local anesthesia in the standing patient or in the anesthetized patient, depending on the disease condition for which it is indicated. The surgical site is on the ventral midline in the middle to upper-middle third of the neck, where the trachea is most palpable and superficial in location. When performed on either the standing or recumbent patient, it is useful to have the head and neck extended (the recumbent patient in a dorsal recumbency position) to facilitate identification of the ventral peritracheal structures (see Fig. 13–119).

Local anesthesia should be infiltrated at the midline surgical site over a distance of approximately 8 cm. The skin is incised on the ventral midline and the incision carried through the superficial cutaneous colli muscle. Deep to this cutaneous muscle, the paired bellies of the sternothyrohyoideus muscle are visualized. The muscle should be displaced laterally and the annular ligament between consecutive tracheal cartilages identified. The tracheal lumen should be penetrated with a scalpel and the incision extended laterally with scissors to include approximately one-fourth to one-third of the luminal diameter. Removal of an elliptical piece of tracheal cartilage from the ring above and below the surgical site (Fig. 13–121) has been suggested if a longer-term temporary tracheostomy is required (Berge and Westhues 1966; O'Connor 1965). Although longer-term temporary tracheostomy may be interpreted as that required for two to four weeks, obstructive lesions of the URT seldom require that length of time for resolution. If they do, a permanent tracheostomy should be considered. Longitudinal (axial) division of tracheal cartilages is contraindicated. This technique frequently results in lateral collapse of the incised tracheal cartilages and contributes to tracheal stenosis (see Figs. 13–119B and 13–121D).

Temporary tracheostomy incisions require a tracheostomy tube, either commercially available or improvised, to allow continued patency of the stoma created. Figure 13–122 demonstrates examples of some available tracheostomy tubes. It is important to ensure that tracheostomy tubes are secured in place when they are the only airway portal of

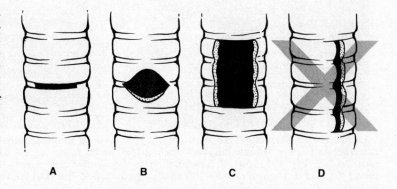

Figure 13–121 Tracheostomy techniques. Division of annular ligament for short-term tracheostomy (A). Removal of an elliptical segment of cartilage from consecutive rings to facilitate long-term use of a tracheostomy tube (B). Removal of tracheal cartilages for permanent tracheostomy (C). Longitudinal division of tracheal cartilages, contraindicated, and predisposing to tracheal collapse (D) (see Fig. 13–119A).

A   B   C   D

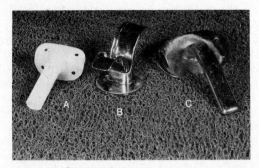

Figure 13–122 Tracheostomy tubes. (A) Small tube improvised from handle of a 1-gallon plastic container (courtesy of Dr. D. Hanselka, Texas A & M University). (B) Self-retaining tube. (C) The frequently used "J" tube.

the respiratory tract (e.g., packing of the nasal passages following septal resection).

The surgical site should be cleaned daily, and the tracheostomy tube should be cleared of dried, potentially occluding mucus accumulations. Most tracheostomy tubes are removed within 7 to 10 days. The surgical site is allowed to heal by second intention and usually does so without complication.

The major complication of temporary tracheostomy is tracheal stenosis (Tate et al. 1981). The incidence of stenotic scarring or granuloma formation follow-

ing temporary tracheostomy will increase in relation to the time the tracheostomy tube is left in place. Such complications may require a second surgical intervention to restore maximal patency of the trachea.

PERMANENT TRACHEOSTOMY

The indication for permanent tracheostomy is irreversible or refractory obstructive disease of the URT. Examples may include severe obstructive disease following trauma to the rostral nasal passages, neoplasia of the URT, or laryngeal stenosis caused by mineralization of the laryngeal cartilages.

The surgical site for permanent tracheostomy is identical to that used for the temporary technique. The skin, subcutaneous tissues, and cutaneous colli muscles are incised on the midline over a distance of approximately 12 to 15 cm (Hanselka 1980). The exposed sternothyrohyoideus muscle is resected at the proximal and distal aspects of the incision, clearly exposing the ventral aspect of the trachea (Fig. 13–123A). The ventral one-fourth to one-third of three consecutive tracheal rings is removed. To accomplish this, the annular ligament immediately above the rostral ring and

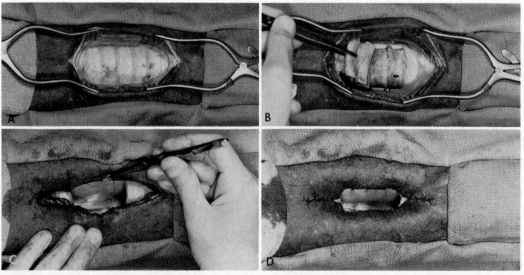

Figure 13–123 Permanent tracheostomy. *A,* The ventral midline, midcervical incision is made where the trachea is most superficial. The trachea is exposed following excision of the sternothyrohyoideus muscles (see Fig. 13–120*B*). *B,* Tracheal rings are divided and removed, leaving the tracheal mucosa intact. *C,* The tracheal mucosa is divided and sutured to the skin following local excision of the axial margins of the sternomandibularis muscles. *D,* Completed stoma.

immediately below the caudal ring is transversely incised, then extended laterally to connect both incisions through the tracheal rings (Fig. 13–123B). Care must be taken not to penetrate the tracheal mucosa. Scissors are used to elevate the incised portions of the tracheal rings. Once the tracheal rings have been removed, the tracheal mucosa is divided on the midline in the central half of the surgical site, then continued to the corners of the exposed tracheal mucosa in an H-shaped pattern. The axial margin of the omohyoideus muscle on either side of the incision is removed by a crescentic incision. This reduces the depth of tissue between the tracheal lumen and the skin. Once hemorrhage has been appropriately controlled, the margin of the incised tracheal mucosa is sutured to the skin with a nonabsorbable suture (00 nylon) (Fig. 13–123C). The stoma created will be approximately 4 cm in axial length by 2 to 3 cm in transverse width (Fig. 13–123D). A tracheostomy tube may be positioned through the cervical site to maintain patency of the airway during the ensuing postoperative swelling. The tracheostomy tube may be removed in 7 to 10 days, and the stoma should mature to its anticipated size within 21 days.

Because the permanent tracheostomy stoma creates an airway that is unprotected by the defense mechanisms of the upper respiratory mucosa, such patients may be predisposed to lower respiratory tract infections. Furthermore, because the stoma is on the ventral aspect of the cervical trachea, the mucociliary escalator will dispose of its products at the ventral aspect of the incision. Thus, a permanent tracheostomy is a surgical technique that requires continued maintenance and observation for maximal efficiency. Although published reports of the longevity of patients with a permanent tracheostomy are unavailable, it seems reasonable to expect that the majority of patients could survive for at least 12 months, depending on the nature of the disease for which the permanent tracheostomy was required.

TRACHEAL ANASTOMOSIS

Tracheal reconstruction by resection and end-to-end anastomosis may be indicated for focal stenotic lesions involving the cervical trachea. A technique for resection of three to five consecutive tracheal rings has been developed and used successfully (Tate et al. 1981). The most common cause of a narrowed tracheal airway in that report was postoperative stenosis following tracheostomy performed by longitudinal division of one or more tracheal cartilages.

Prior to performing tracheal resection and anastomosis, the patient should be conditioned to the use of a martingale-type harness, which maintains the head and neck in a flexed position with an adjustable extension from the halter to a thoracic girth. The use of this harness is very important in the postoperative period to minimize tension at the anastomosis site.

The patient is positioned in dorsal recumbency and maintained on halothane anesthesia. The trachea is exposed through a 40-cm ventral midline incision centered over the intended site of resection. The trachea is mobilized by dissecting it free from the adjacent adventitia. Traction sutures can be placed around a tracheal cartilage (normal) above and below the resection site (two to three cartilages away in either direction) to facilitate subsequent manipulation. The first normal tracheal ring above and below the lesion is longitudinally divided ventrally and removed by blunt dissection, sparing the tracheal mucosa. The exposed mucosa is then divided circumferentially closest to the diseased tracheal cartilages to be removed. At this time the endotracheal tube is withdrawn and a sterile endotracheal tube positioned through the surgical field and into the distal airway.

The tracheal mucosa is everted over the edge of the exposed tracheal rings and is sutured circumferentially with a simple continuous pattern (00 chromic gut) to the adventitia adhering to that cartilage. The endotracheal tube is removed from the surgical field, and that in the proximal segment is again passed into the distal segment. The horse's neck and head should be flexed into a near vertical position to reduce tension for the ensuing anastomosis.

Interrupted sutures with 25-gauge stainless steel wire are used in a simple interrupted pattern (Fig. 13–124). The

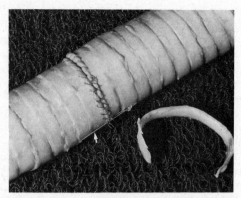

Figure 13–124 Tracheal anastomosis. Ventral view of a tracheal specimen demonstrating technique of tracheal anastomosis. Following mucosal eversion with a simple continuous pattern, the tracheal rings are apposed with a split-thickness interrupted pattern using surgical stainless steel. A tension suture is demonstrated (arrow). The tracheal cartilage removed submucosally demonstrates that the rings are incomplete dorsally.

full thickness of the cartilage is not penetrated to prevent exposure of the suture material to the tracheal lumen. Preplacement of the sutures in the dorsal aspect of the trachea may facilitate the technique. The previously positioned traction sutures can be utilized to stabilize the trachea, and towel clamps can be modified to be of assistance as well. The anastomotic site is checked for leaks by withdrawing the endotracheal tube to the proximal trachea, applying positive pressure, and observing for bubbles in the surgical field following the instillation of a saline and antibiotic solution (500 ml). A continuous suction drain can be placed in a peritracheal position prior to appositional closure of the surgical site.

The Martingale apparatus should be maintained in position for approximately three weeks following surgery, and the patient is given systemic antimicrobials for 7 to 10 days. If the tension across the anastomotic site can be maintained at a minimum by using the martingale-type harness, postoperative complications are limited. The tracheal lumen diameter was reduced by approximately 10 per cent in the experimental series (Tate et al. 1981).

PROSTHETIC IMPLANTS FOR TRACHEAL DISEASE

Prosthetic implants have been used in the surgical management of tracheal disease. A soft polyvinyl chloride wire-reinforced corrugated hose was used to replace the cervical trachea in a horse affected with dorsoventral flattening (Carrig, Groenendyk, and Seawright 1973). The patient was destroyed nine months after the prosthesis was inserted because of obstructive granuloma formation at the proximal end of the prosthesis.

Prosthetic implants have been used to support and dilate segmental collapse of the trachea (Boyd and Hanselka 1976; Horney 1975). The most appropriate use of this technique appears to be in those patients with collapse of two to three tracheal cartilages (e.g., following trauma or longitudinal tracheostomy) and involves the use of an appropriately sized half cylindrical implant. The use of a polypropylene syringe casing has been reported (Boyd and Hanselka 1976). Other semirigid materials could be used as well. Prosthetic implants are most appropriate for those cases of segmental collapse without intraluminal lesions.

The segment of involved trachea is exposed by ventral midline incision, similar to but more extensive than that used for tracheostomy. The involved trachea is mobilized and freed of its adventitia. The prosthesis should be long enough to extend over one normal ring on either side of the collapsed segment. It is positioned so that it extends circumferentially to an equal extent on either side of the apex of the tracheal deformity. A partial chondrotomy (Boyd and Hanselka 1976) may be necessary at the site of deformity to allow circular expansion of the tracheal lumen. The prosthesis is anchored to the trachea with nonabsorbable suture that surrounds the tracheal rings but does not penetrate the tracheal lumen (Fig. 13–125). Intraoperative endoscopic examination of the tracheal lumen may assist in the placing of the sutures to ensure that the lumen is not penetrated and that the trachea is expanded appropriately. The surgical site

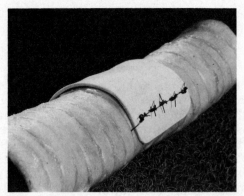

Figure 13–125 Tracheal stent. Ventral view of a tracheal specimen with a stent anchored in place with nylon sutures. This technique would be indicated for tracheal collapse following trauma or errantly divided tracheal cartilages (see Figs. 13–119 and 13–121).

should be appropriately closed and the patient placed on systemic antimicrobials postoperatively. The prognosis may be guarded to good and depends on the extent of the original injury, the success of enlarging the tracheal lumen, and postoperative sepsis.

Thorax

The thoracic cavity of horses is seldom invaded surgically because of the low incidence of surgical diseases of the thorax, the prognosis attending such diseases, and economic considerations. The size of the patient and the substantial substance of the rib cage markedly limit surgical accessibility to thoracic organs in contrast to that enjoyed by the small animal surgeon. Indications for thoracotomy include repair of diaphragmatic hernias and closure of penetrating wounds (Fowler 1963; 1973), drainage of an intrathoracic abscess (Ferguson, Boyd, and Morris 1970; Colahan and Knight 1979), implantation of electromagnetic flow probes to monitor cardiovascular function experimentally (Waugh et al. 1980), and repair of rib fractures (Fowler 1973). Other indications include partial lobectomy for neoplastic or septic conditions (Fowler 1973), correction of congenital cardiovascular anomalies, and exposure of the thoracic esophagus.

The techniques necessary to support the diagnosis of thoracic disease that may require surgical intervention include thoracocentesis, thoracic radiography, and possibly contrast radiography (angiograms and barium swallow). The efficacy of thoracic radiography and contrast studies depends on both the size of the patient and the capabilities of the radiographic equipment.

The most frequent approach used for exposure of the thoracic cavity is a lateral thoracotomy (Fowler 1973). A transsternal or ventral splitting procedure may be adapted from techniques used in the dog and applied for use in smaller patients such as foals and ponies.

LATERAL THORACOTOMY

The lateral thoracotomy approach may be made through an intercostal space or in conjunction with resection of a rib. The surgical site selected depends on the requirements for exposure. The rib resection technique provides superior exposure to the intercostal technique and is suggested. The most frequent incision site is over the sixth rib, immediately caudal to the border of the triceps brachii muscle. Specialized instrumentation and equipment include a large rib retractor (commercially available or improvised) and a means for positive pressure ventilation during surgery.

The patient is positioned in lateral recumbency under general anesthesia with the uppermost leg in extension. A 40- to 50-cm skin incision is made directly over the sixth rib, extending from the caudal aspect of the scapular cartilage. The cutaneous trunci muscle is exposed and divided along the incisional plane. The latissimus dorsi muscle is similarly transected in the upper aspect of the incision. The serratus ventralis muscle is exposed and its fibers divided on the long axis of the muscle parallel to the rib. The adherent intercostal fascia and periosteum are divided longitudinally with a scalpel on the long axis of the rib. The periosteum is reflected from the rib, which is subsequently divided dorsally using obstetrical wire, and ventrally disarticulated at the costochondral junction. The pleural cavity is then invaded by incising the exposed periosteum and pleura deep to it.

Following the intrathoracic procedures, an indwelling drain tube may be positioned prior to closure. A 24 to 30 French sized catheter should be used, and it should have three or four side fenestrations on its proximal end. The drain should be placed in the lower thorax in the seventh or eighth intercostal space. It should enter the pleural cavity after being·drawn through a stab incision and tunneled obliquely through the body wall. The 8 to 10 cm in distance between the site of pleural entry and that of cutaneous exit will help delay retrograde contamination of the pleural space. The drain should be secured to the skin with a purse-string suture. The first layer of wound closure should include the pleura and deep periosteum in a simple interrupted suture pattern (No. 2 chromic catgut). The second layer includes the superficial periosteum, intercostal muscles, and intercostal fascia, using the same suture pattern. An alternative would be to use a heavier suture material (No. 3 chromic catgut) and combine the suturing of all the layers. Prior to sealing the thorax with the last suture, the lungs should be maximally inflated to expel air and fluid from the thoracic cavity. The serratus ventralis and latissimus dorsi muscles can be reapposed with an interrupted suture pattern. A Penrose drain (optional) may be placed in the wound prior to closure of the cutaneous trunci muscle and subcutaneous tissues. The skin should be sutured with an interrupted pattern using nonabsorbable suture.

The surgical site may be protected by a body bandage. The chest drain should be protected and packed off with an antibacterial ointment. The drain should be checked daily and aspirated to remove any intrapleural air or fluid. It can be removed approximately three days postoperatively. Fluid accumulation within the thorax may be treated by percutaneous needle aspiration on the same side. A course of postoperative antimicrobial therapy should be continued for five to seven days. Postoperative complications may include sepsis of the incision and/or pleural cavity; thus, the procedure should not be taken lightly.

DIAPHRAGMATIC HERNIA

Diaphragmatic hernias in the horse are infrequently encountered and usually cause signs suggestive of abdominal disease. Diaphragmatic hernias may be either congenital or acquired in origin (Firth 1976; Wimberly, Andrews, and Haschek, 1977). Congenital diaphragmatic hernias have been observed in the left dorsal quadrant of the diaphragm (Firth 1976). Acquired hernias most frequently occur in the tendinous portion of the diaphragm as it blends into the more peripheral muscular portion (Wimberly, Andrews, and Haschek, 1977). Increased intra-abdominal pressure resulting from external trauma, violent exercise, falling, and even parturition may contribute to the development of the hernia (Firth 1976; Scott and Fishback 1976; Wimberly, Andrews, and Haschek 1977).

The most frequent complaint associated with diaphragmatic hernia is abdominal distress. The clinical course of the digestive disturbance may vary from low-grade, recurrent colic responsive to medical therapy to a fulminating crisis requiring surgical intervention. Visceral pain is related to the displacement of abdominal organs into the thoracic cavity. Reportedly, the organs herniated in descending order of occurrence are the small intestine, stomach, large colon, spleen, and cecum (Wimberly, Andrews, and Haschek 1977).

The diagnosis of diaphragmatic hernia may be difficult to make and may only be recognized in some cases at the time of surgery. Systematic examination of patients with acute abdominal distress may fail to suggest a diaphragmatic hernia. Although the majority of patients reported had tachypnea and painful or forced respirations, such symptoms may be consistent with a severe abdominal crisis. Smaller hernial rings favor the entry of small intestine, especially the jejunum, into the thorax, whereas larger and more ventral defects are prone to large intestinal displacement.

Borborygmi or fluid sounds in the caudal and ventral thorax may suggest diaphragmatic hernia, although they are frequently heard in normal horses. A more suggestive sign is an increased area of dullness or reduced cardiac sounds on the involved side in the ventral to caudoventral thorax. Thoracic radiography is the primary definitive method used to diagnose diaphragmatic hernia.

Successful surgical repair of diaphragmatic hernia has been reported in two cases (Scott and Fishback 1976; Verschooten et al. 1977). The surgical approach in both cases was a ventral midline incision immediately caudal to the xiphoid cartilage. A defect 25 cm in length with smooth edges was closed by interrupted sutures of heavy suture (No. 4 nonabsorbable) in one case (Verschooten et al. 1977). In the other case a 20 × 25 cm defect was repaired using a synthetic mesh (Scott and Fishback 1976).

Both horses made uneventful recoveries. The success of surgical intervention is dependent on the surgical accessibility of the diaphragmatic hernia and whether or not herniated viscera can be replaced into the abdominal cavity. Adhesions may prevent successful replacement and thus dictate termination of the case. It is suspected that repair of hernial defects through a lateral thoracotomy may be quite difficult in the adult horse. Because it may be difficult to determine exactly where the hernia is located, it is conceivable that the surgical incision may be on the wrong side of the chest. The extent and location of a diaphragmatic hernia in a foal should be easier to characterize radiographically, and thus a thoracotomy approach may provide better surgical accessibility.

Appendix A. Equine respiratory exam form.

Clinician: _____

Student: _____

Date: _____

PERTINENT HISTORY: Duration of condition: _____ Present contact: _____

   Complaint: _____

   _____

   _____

   Class/Use of animal: _____

   Training methods: _____

   Racing distance: _____

   Record: Starts _____; Win _____; Second _____; Third _____

YES   NO   COMMENTS (by number):

_____ _____ 1. Nasal discharge _____

_____ _____ 2. Cough _____

_____ _____ 3. Noise production _____

_____ _____   continuous _____

_____ _____   intermittent _____

_____ _____ 4. Exercise intolerance _____

_____ _____ 5. Previous therapy:

            antimicrobials _____ , steroids _____ , furosemide _____ ,

            bronchodilators _____ , tongue-tie _____ , other _____ : _____

PHYSICAL EXAMINATION: Height: _____ Weight: _____ Condition: _____

   Temperature: _____ Heart rate: _____ Respiratory rate/character: _____

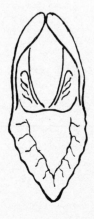 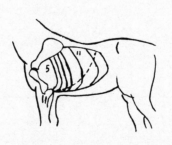 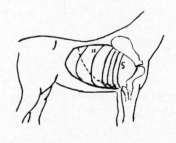

Normal	Abnormal	Not examined		Comments (by number):
____	____	____	1. Nares	_____
			Airflow	_____
____	____	____	2. Sinuses	_____
			Percussion	_____
____	____	____	3. Facial symmetry	_____
____	____	____	4. Regional symmetry	_____
____	____	____	5. Laryngeal palpation	_____
____	____	____	6. Tracheal compression	_____
____	____	____	7. Lung fields	_____
			auscultation	_____
			percussion	_____
____	____	____	ENDOSCOPY: R__ , L__	_____
____	____	____	8. Nasal passages	_____
____	____	____	9. Ethmoid area	_____
____	____	____	10. Pharynx	_____
____	____	____	11. G.P. openings	_____
____	____	____	12. Soft palate	_____
____	____	____	13. Epiglottis	_____
____	____	____	14. Arytenoids	_____
____	____	____	15. Ventricles	_____
____	____	____	16. Trachea	_____
____	____	____	17. Guttural pouches	_____
____	____	____	OTHER Dx PROCEDURES	_____
____	____	____	18. Exercise evaluation	_____
____	____	____	19. Post-ex. endoscopy	_____
____	____	____	20. Radiography	_____
____	____	____	21. Tracheal wash	_____
____	____	____	22. Thoracocentesis	_____
____	____	____	23. Other	_____

MISCELLANEOUS COMMENTS:

_____

_____

_____

REFERENCES

Beech, J.: Cytology of tracheobronchial aspirates in horses. Vet. Pathol. *12*:157, 1975.

Berge, E., and Westhues, M.: Veterinary Operative Surgery. Baltimore: Williams & Wilkins, 1966, pp. 61–66, 135–140, 159–160, 167–168.

Boles, C. L.: Abnormalities of the upper respiratory tract. Vet. Clin. North Am. *1*:89, 1979a.

Boles, C. L.: Treatment of upper airway abnormalities. Vet. Clin. North Am. *1*:127, 1979b.

Boles, C. L.: Epiglottic entrapment and follicular pharyngitis: diagnosis and treatment. *In* Proceedings of the American Association of Equine Practitioners: 29, 1975.

Boles, C. L., Raker, C. W., and Wheat, J. D.: Epiglottic entrapment by arytenoepiglottic folds in the horse. JAVMA *172*:338, 1978.

Boyd, C. L., and Hanselka, D. V.: Prosthesis for correction of collapsed trachea. J. Am. Anim. Hosp. Assoc. *12*:829, 1976.

Cadiot, P. J.: Clinical Veterinary Medicine and Surgery. New York: William R. Jenkins, 1901, pp. 30–34.

Cannon, J. H., Grant, B. D., and Sande, R. D.: Diagnosis and surgical treatment of cyst-like lesions of the equine paranasal sinuses. JAVMA *169*:610, 1976.

Carrig, C. B., Groenendyk, S., and Seawright, A. A.: Dorsoventral flattening of the trachea in a horse and its attempted surgical correction: A case report. J. Am. Vet. Radiol. Soc. *14*:32, 1973.

Colahan, P. T., and Knight, H. D.: Drainage of an intrathoracic abscess in a horse via thoracotomy. JAVMA *174*:1231, 1979.

Cook, W. R.: Biomechanics of the pharynx. Paper presented at A.C.V.S. Surgical Forum, Chicago, 1979.

Cook, W. R.: Carotid angiography. Paper presented at A.C.V.S. Surgical Forum, Chicago, 1978.

Cook, W. R.: Some observations on diseases of the ear, nose and throat in the horse, and endoscopy using a flexible fiberoptic endoscope. Vet. Rec. *94*:533, 1974.

Cook, W. R.: The auditory tube diverticulum (guttural pouch) in the horse: its radiographic examination. J. Am. Vet. Rad. Soc. *XIV*(2):51, 1973.

Cook, W. R.: Diseases of the ear, nose and throat in the horse. Part I: The ear. *In* The Vet Annual. Grunsell, C. S. G. (ed.). Bristol: John Wright and Sons Ltd, 1971, pp. 12–43.

Cook, W. R.: Procedure and technique for endoscopy of the equine respiratory tract and eustachian tube diverticulum. Equine Vet. J. *2*:137, 1970a.

Cook, W. R.: Skeletal radiology of the equine head. J. Am. Vet. Radiol. *11*:35, 1970b.

Cook, W. R.: The clinical features of guttural pouch mycosis in the horse. Vet. Rec. *83*:336, 1968a.

Cook, W. R.: The pathology and aetiology of guttural pouch mycosis in the horse. Vet. Rec. *83*:422, 1968b.

Cook, W. R.: Observations on the aetiology of epistaxis and cranial nerve paralysis in the horse. Vet. Rec. *78*:396, 1966a.

Cook, W. R.: Clinical observations on the anatomy and physiology of the upper respiratory tract. Vet. Rec. *79*:440, 1966b.

Cook, W. R.: Dental surgery in the horse. *In* General Proceedings of the British Equine Veterinary Association: 34, 1965–66.

Cook, W. R.: The diagnosis of respiratory unsoundness in the horse. Vet. Rec. *77*:516, 1965.

Cook, W. R.: Clinical observations on the equine soft palate. *In* Proceedings of the British Equine Veterinary Association: 5, 1962.

Cook, W. R., and Littlewort, M. C. G.: Progressive haematoma of the ethmoid region in the horse. Equine Vet. J. *6*:101, 1974.

Dorn, C. R., and Priester, W. A.: Epidemiologic analysis of oral and pharyngeal cancer in dogs, cats, horses and cattle. JAVMA Assoc *169*:1202, 1976.

Duncan, I. D., and Griffiths, I. R.: Pathological changes in equine laryngeal muscles and nerves. *In* Proceedings of the American Association of Equine Practitioners: 97, 1973.

Farrow, C. S.: Pneumomediastinum in the horse: A complication of transtracheal aspiration. J. Am. Vet. Radiol. *27*:192, 1976.

Ferguson, H. R., Boyd, C. L., and Morris, E. L.: Surgical correction of a thoracic abscess in a colt. JAVMA *156*:868, 1970.

Firth, E. C.: Diaphragmatic hernia in horses. Cornell Vet. *66*:353, 1976.

Flemming, G.: A Textbook of Operative Veterinary Surgery. New York: William R. Jenkins, 1903, pp. 406, 411–427.

Flynn, D.: Corrective facial osteotomy with submucosal resection of the nasal septum. Paper presented at A.C.V.S. Surgical Forum, Chicago, 1978.

Foerner, J. J.: The diagnosis and correction of false nostril noises. *In* Proceedings of the American Association of Equine Practitioners: 315, 1967.

Fowler, M. E.: Intrathoracic surgery in large animals. JAVMA *162*:967, 1973.

Fowler, M. E.: Intrathoracic surgery in the horse. Am. J. Vet. Res. *24*:766, 1963.

Frank, E. R.: Veterinary Surgery, 7th ed. Minneapolis: Bergess Publishing Co., 1964, pp. 83–84, 85–88.

Freeman, D. E.: Diagnosis and Treatment of Diseases of the Guttural Pouch (Part I). The Compendium on Continuing Education. Lg. An. Suppl. I:S3, 1980a.

Freeman, D. E.: Diagnosis and Treatment of Diseases of the Guttural Pouch (Part II). The Compendium on Continuing Education. Lg. An. Suppl. II:S25, 1980b.

Freeman, D. E., and Donawick, W. J.: Occlusion of internal carotid artery in the horse by means of a balloon-tipped catheter: evaluation of a method designed to prevent epistaxis caused by guttural pouch mycosis. JAVMA *176*:232, 1980a.

Freeman, D. E., and Donawick, W. J.: Occlusion of internal carotid artery by means of a balloon-tipped catheter: clinical use of a method to prevent epistaxis caused by guttural pouch mycosis. JAVMA *176*:236, 1980b.

Fretz, P. B.: Case report: endoscopic differentiation

of epiglottic entrapment and elongation of the soft palate: including surgical correction of epiglottic entrapment. Can. Vet. J. 18(12):352, 1977.

Getty, R. (ed.): Sisson and Grossman's The Anatomy of the Domestic Animals. Philadelphia: W. B. Saunders, 1975, p. 475.

Gordon, L. R.: The cytology and histology of epidermal inclusion cysts in the horse. J. Eq. Med. Surg. 2:371, 1978.

Goulden, B. E., Anderson, L. J., Davies, A. S., et al.: Rostral displacement of the palatopharyngeal arch: a case report. Equine Vet. J. 8:95, 1976.

Greet, T. R. C., Baker, G. J., and Lee, R.: The effect of laryngoplasty on pharyngeal function in the horse. Equine Vet. J. 11:153, 1979.

Greet, T. R. C., Jeffcott, L. B., Whitwell, K. E., et al.: The slap test for laryngeal adduction function in horses with suspected cervical spinal cord damage. Equine Vet. J. 12:127, 1980.

Guard, W. F.: Surgical Principles and Technics. Columbus, OH: W. F. Guard, 1953, pp. 92–93.

Hanselka, D. V.: Surgery of the trachea. Paper presented at A.C.V.S. Surgical Forum, Chicago, 1980.

Hanselka, D. V.: Equine nasal phycomycosis. VM/SAC 72:251, 1977.

Hanselka, D. V.: Tracheal collapse and laryngeal hemiplegia in the horse: A case report. VM/SAC 68:859, 1973.

Harvey, C. E., Raker, C. W., and O'Brien, J. A.: Pharyngeal and laryngeal diseases causing airway obstruction in the dog and horse. Arch. Am. Coll. Vet. Surg. 2:15, 1973.

Haynes, P. F.: Persistent dorsal displacement of the soft palate associated with epiglottic shortening in two horses. JAVMA 179:677, 1981.

Haynes, P. F.: Surgical failures in upper respiratory surgery. In Proceedings of the American Association of Equine Practitioners:223, 1978.

Haynes, P. F., and Qualls, C. W.: Cleft soft palate, nasal septal deviation and epiglottic entrapment in a Thoroughbred filly. JAVMA, 179:910, 1981.

Haynes, P. F., Snider, T. G., McClure, J. R., et al.: Chronic chondritis of the equine arytenoid cartilage. JAVMA 177:1135, 1980.

Heffron, C. J., and Baker, G. J.: Observations on the mechanism of functional obstruction of the nasopharyngeal airway in the horse. Equine Vet. J. 11:142, 1979.

Heffron, C. J., Baker, G. J., and Lee, R.: Fluoroscopic investigation of pharyngeal function in the horse. Equine Vet. J. 11(3):148, 1979.

Hobday, F.: The surgical treatment of roaring in horses. North Am. Vet. 17:17, 1936.

Horney, F. D.: Tracheal prosthesis in a calf. JAVMA 167:463, 1975.

Johnson, J.: Pharyngitis syndrome—past, present, and future. Paper presented at A.C.V.S. Surgical Forum, Chicago, 1980.

Johnson, J. H., and Raker, C. W.: The relationship of the guttural pouch to upper respiratory conditions. In Proceedings of the American Association of Equine Practitioners:247, 1970.

Johnson, J. H., Moore, J. N., Garner, H. E., et al.: Clinical characterization of the larynx hemiplegia. In Proceedings of the American Association of Equine Practitioners:259, 1977.

Johnson, J. H.: Complications in equine laryngeal surgery. Arch. Am. Coll. Vet. Surg. 4(1):9, 1975.

Johnson, J. H.: Laryngoplasty for advanced laryngeal hemiplegia. VM/SAC 65:347, 1970.

Johnson, J. H., and Merriam, J. G.: Equine endoscopy. Vet. Scope XIX:2, 1975.

Johnson, J. H., Merriam, J. G., and Attleberger, M.: A case of guttural pouch mycosis caused by Aspergillus nedulans. VM/SAC 68:771, 1973.

Johnson, J. H., Moore, J. N., Coffman, J. R., Garner, H. E., Tritschler, L. G., and Traver, D. S.: Selection, care and maintenance of endoscopic equipment for use in horses. JAVMA 172:2, 1978.

Jones, R. S., Maisels, D. O., DeGeus, J. J., et al.: Surgical repair of cleft palate in the horse. Equine Vet. J. 7:86, 1975.

Kelly, D. F., and Watson, W. B. J.: Epidermoid cyst of the brain in a horse. Equine Vet. J. 8:110, 1976.

Knight, A. P., Voss, J. L., McChesney, A. E., et al.: Experimentally-induced Streptococcus equi infection in horses with resultant guttural pouch empyema. VM/SAC 70:1194, 1975.

Koch, D. B., and Tate, L. P.: Pharyngeal cysts in horses. JAVMA 173:858, 1978.

Levine, S. B.: Depression fractures of the nasal and frontal bones of the horse. J. Eq. Med. Surg. 3:186, 1979.

Leyland, A., and Baker, J. R.: Lesions of the nasal and paranasal sinuses of the horse causing dyspnoea. Br. Vet. J. 131:339, 1975.

MacKay-Smith, M. P., Johnson, J. G., and Baker, R. H.: Laryngoplasty—a progress report. In Proceedings of the American Association of Equine Practitioners:133, 1973.

MacKay-Smith, M. P., and Marks, D.: Clinical diagnosis of laryngeal hemiplegia in horses. In Proceedings of the American Association of Equine Practitioners:227, 1968.

Madewell, B. R., Priester, W. A., Gillette, E. L., and Snyder, S. P.: Neoplasms of the nasal passages and paranasal sinuses in domesticated animals as reported by 13 veterinary colleges. Am. J. Vet. Res. 37:851, 1976.

Mansmann, R. A., and Knight, H. D.: Transtracheal aspiration in the horse. JAVMA 160:1527, 1972.

Mansmann, R. A., and Wheat, J. D.: The diagnosis and treatment of equine upper respiratory disease. In Proceedings of the American Association of Equine Practitioners:375, 1972.

Marks, D., MacKay-Smith, M. P., Cushing, L. S., et al.: Use of prosthetic device for surgical correction of laryngeal hemiplegia in horses. JAVMA 157:157, 1970a.

Marks, D., MacKay-Smith, M. P., Cushing, L. S., and Leslie, J. A.: Etiology and diagnosis of laryngeal hemiplegia in horses. JAVMA 157:429, 1970b.

Mason, J. E.: Empyema of the equine paranasal sinuses. JAVMA 167:727, 1975.

Mason, J. E.: Laryngeal hemiplegia: a further look at Haslam's anomaly of the left recurrent nerve. Equine Vet. J. 5(4):150, 1973.

McAllister, E. S.: Guttural pouch disease. In Proceedings of the American Association of Equine Practitioners:251, 1977.

McAllister, E. S., and Blakeslee, J. R.: Clinical observations of pharyngitis in the horse. JAVMA 170:739, 1977.

Montgomery, T.: A clinical consideration of the causes of chronic pharyngitis in the equine. Equine Pract. 3:26, 1981.

Moulton, J. E.: Tumors in Domestic Animals. Berkeley and Los Angeles: University of California Press, 1961, pp. 115–116.

Nelson, A. E., Curley, B. M., and Kainer, R. A.: Mandibular symphysiotomy to provide adequate exposure for intra-oral surgery in the horse. JAVMA 159:1025, 1971.

O'Connor, J. J. (ed.): Dollar's Veterinary Surgery, 4th ed. London: Bailliere, Tindall and Co., 1965, pp. 296–298, 302–307, 308–314.

Owen, R. R.: Epistaxis prevented by ligation of the internal carotid artery in the guttural pouch. Equine Vet. J. 6(4):143, 1974.

Pouret, E.: Modification of the technique of laryngeal ventriculectomy described in 1966. In Proceedings of the American Association of Equine Practitioners:379, 1967.

Pouret, E.: Laryngeal ventriculectomy with stitching of the laryngeal saccules. In Proceedings of the American Association of Equine Practitioners:207, 1966.

Proceedings of the 1980 Invitational Workshop on Equine Viral Respiratory Disease and Complications. AAEP Newsletter No. 2:92, 1980.

Quinlan, J., Van Rensburg, S. W. J., and Starke, N. C.: The soft palate (palatinum molle) as a cause of dyspnoae in two racehorses. J. SA Vet. Med. Assoc. 20:125, 1949.

Raker, C. W.: Pathology and related surgery of the pharynx. Paper presented at A.C.V.S. Surgical Forum, Chicago, 1978.

Raker, C. W.: Clinical characterization of the larynx in laryngeal hemiplegia. In Proceedings of the American Association of Equine Practitioners:263, 1977.

Raker, C. W.: Diseases of the pharynx. Mod. Vet. Pract. 57:396, 1976.

Raker, C. W.: Complications related to the insertion of a suture to retract the arytenoid cartilage to correct laryngeal hemiplegia in the horse. Arch. Am. Coll. Vet. Surg. 4(2):64, 1975a.

Raker, C. W.: Endoscopy of the upper respiratory tract of the horse. In Proceedings of the American Association of Equine Practitioners:3, 1975b.

Raker, C. W., and Boles, C. L.: Pharyngeal lymphoid hyperplasia in the horse. J. Eq. Med. Surg. 2:202, 1978.

Randall, R. W., and Myers, V. S., Jr.: Partial tracheal stenosis in a horse. VM/SAC 68:264, 1973.

Reynolds, B. L., Stedham, A. M., Lawrence, J. M., et al.: Adenocarcinoma of the frontal sinus with extension to the brain in a horse. JAVMA 174:734, 1979.

Roberts, E. J.: Some modern surgical operations applicable to the horse. Vet. Rec. 76:137, 1964.

Robinson, N. E., and Sorenson, P. R.: Pathophysiology of airway obstruction in horses: A review. JAVMA 172:299, 1978.

Rooney, J. R., and Delaney, F. M.: An hypothesis on the causation of laryngeal hemiplegia in horses. Equine Vet. J. 2:35, 1970.

Schneider, J. E.: The Respiratory System. In Textbook of Large Animal Surgery. Oehme, F. W., and Prier, J. E. (eds.). Baltimore: Williams & Wilkins, 1974, pp. 340–359.

Scott, E. A., Duncan, J. R., and McCormack, J. E.: Cryptococcosis involving the postorbital area and frontal sinus in a horse. JAVMA 165:626, 1974.

Scott, E. A., and Fishback, W. A.: Surgical repair of diaphragmatic hernia in a horse. JAVMA 168:45, 1976.

Shapiro, J., White, N. A., Schafler, D. H., et al.: Hypertrophic ossification of the laryngeal cartilages of a horse. J. Eq. Med. Surg. 3(8):320, 1979.

Shires, G. M. H.: Cleft palate surgery. Paper presented at A.C.V.S. Annual Meeting Knoxville, 1980.

Sinibaldi, K. R.: Cleft palate. Vet. Clin. North Am. 9:245, 1979.

Smith, B. P.: Diseases of the pleura. Vet. Clin. North. Am. Large Anim. Pract. 1:197, 1979.

Speirs, V. C.: Entrapment of the epiglottis in horses. J. Eq. Med. Surg. 1:267, 1977.

Speirs, V. C.: Abductor muscle prostheses in the treatment of laryngeal hemiplegia in the horse. Austr. Vet. J. 48:251, 1972.

Steffey, E. P.: Anesthetic management of the horse with respiratory disease. Vet. Clin. North Am. 1:113, 1979.

Stick, J. A., and Boles, C.: Subepiglottic cyst in three foals. JAVMA 177:62, 1977.

Stickle, R. L., Goble, D. O., and Braden, T. D.: Surgical repair of cleft soft palate in a foal. VM/SAC 68:159, 1973.

Stickle, R. L., and Jones, R. D.: Nasal polyp in a horse. VM/SAC 17:1453, 1976.

Tate, L. P., Jr., et al.: Tracheal reconstruction by resection and end-to-end anastomosis in the horse. JAVMA 178:253, 1981.

Trotter, G. W., Aanes, W. A., and Snyder, S. P.: Laryngeal chondroma in a horse. JAVMA 178:829, 1981.

Tulleners, E. P.: Nasal septum resection in the horse. Paper presented at A.C.V.S. Annual Meeting, New Orleans, 1981.

Turner, A. S.: Surgical management of depression fractures of the equine skull. Vet. Surg. 8:29, 1979.

Valdez, H., McMullan, W. C., Hobson, H. P., and Hanselka, D. V.: Surgical correction of deviated nasal septum and premaxilla in a colt. JAVMA 173:1001, 1978.

Vasseur, P.: Surgery of the trachea. Vet. Clin. North Am. 9:231, 1979.

Vaughan, J. T.: The "roaring" operation (modified index finger technique). Auburn Vet. 18:78, 1962.

Verschooten, F., Oyaert, W., Huylle, E., DeMoor, A., Steenhaut, M., and Moens, Y.: Diaphragmatic hernia in the horse: four case reports. J. Am. Vet. Radiol. 18:45, 1977.

Waugh, S. L., Campbell, K. B., Klavano, P. A., and Grant, B. D.: Surgical implantation of cardiovascular devices in the thorax of the horse. Am. J. Vet. Res. 41:816, 1980.

Wheat, J. D.: Surgery of the paranasal sinuses. Paper presented at ACVS Surgical Forum, Chicago, 1980.

Wheat, J. D.: Surgery of the larynx. Paper presented at A.C.V.S Surgical Forum, Chicago, 1979.

Wheat, J. D.: Fractures of the head and mandible of the horse. In Proceedings of the American Association of Equine Practitioners:223, 1975.

Wheat, J. D.: Sinus drainage and tooth repulsion in the horse. In Proceedings of the American Association of Equine Practitioners:171, 1973.

Wheat, J. D.: Selected clinical cases. In Proceedings of the British Equine Veterinary Association:62, 1966.

Wheat, J. D.: Tympanites of the guttural pouch of the horse. JAVMA 140:453, 1962.

White, N. A., and Blackwell, R. B.: Partial arytenoidectomy in the horse. Vet. Surg. 9:5, 1980.

Williams, W. L.: Recollections of and reflections upon sixty-five years in the veterinary profession. Cornell Vet. XXXV(3):231, 1945.

Williams, W. L.: The surgical relief of roaring. Am. Vet. Rev. 32:333, 1907–1908.

Wimberly, H. C., Andrews, E. J., and Haschek, W. M.: Diaphragmatic hernias in the horse: a review of the literature and an analysis of six additional cases. JAVMA 170:1404, 1977.

CHAPTER 14

THE CARDIOVASCULAR SYSTEM

G. FREDERICK FREGIN, V.M.D.

Cardiovascular problems requiring surgical intervention are uncommon in large domestic animals. Since cardiac disease more commonly involves individual animals, abnormalities of the heart and vessels are usually economically less important than are diseases of other body systems that have a higher incidence and affect groups of animals. Exceptions include the presence of congenital or acquired cardiovascular disease in valuable blood stock that requires specific diagnosis and therapy. Congenital defects of the cardiovascular system pose still another problem because of their potential inheritability.

CONGENITAL CARDIOVASCULAR DISEASE

The true incidence of congenital heart disease in large domestic animals is difficult to accurately determine. It has been estimated to be 0.11 per cent in lambs (Dennis and Leipold 1968), 0.7 per cent in bovine fetuses (Kemler and Martin 1972), 0.17 per cent in cattle, and 0.16 per cent in swine (VanNie 1966). The prevelance of congenital cardiovascular disease among horses has not been determined; however, the interventricular septal defect, alone or in combination with other malformations, appears to occur most frequently, as has been reported for other domestic animals.

PATENT DUCTUS ARTERIOSUS

Although less commonly reported in large domestic animals than in dogs or humans, patent ductus arteriosus occurs as an isolated lesion and in combination with other cardiac malformations (Rooney and Franks 1964; Fregin 1982). Affected animals may develop signs of congestive failure within the first few days of life or by four to eight weeks of age, whereas some may reach maturity before signs develop (Buergelt et al. 1970; Fregin, Donawick, and Buchanan 1981).

In young animals without significant pulmonary hypertension, palpation of the thorax should reveal the characteristic continuous thrill over the third and fourth left intercostal spaces just ventral to the level of the point of the shoulder. A thrill may not always be evident in adult animals. As with other arteriovenous fistulas, the arterial pulse usually has a rapid rise and decline similar to the characteristic water-hammer pulse described for aortic insufficiency.

A grade 3 (out of 5) or greater continuous, machinery-like murmur is usually heard best over the aortic-pulmonic valve areas and must be distinguished from innocent systolic flow murmurs, which may be heard in some young animals. The diastolic component of the continuous murmur may be sharply localized at the level of the point of the shoulder to the third to fourth left intercostal space in the horse and to the second to third left intercostal space in the ruminant. The diastolic component may be diminished in intensity with the onset of pulmonary hypertension and only a systolic murmur may be heard (Carmichael et al. 1971; Glazier, Farrelly, and Neylon 1974). Severe pulmonary hypertension may be associated with accentuation and splitting of S_2 and no audible murmur.

Insufficient data are available to describe any characteristic electrocardiographic or radiographic changes for large domestic animals with patent ductus arteriosus. Aortography in foals (Scott, Kneller, and Witherspoon 1975) and calves (Fregin, Tennant, and Rendano 1982) can reveal opacifications of the ductus and pulmonary artery. Since other congenital defects might also be present, atrial and ventricular injection of radiopaque dye may also be of value.

Cardiac catheterization of domestic animals with a left-to-right shunt should demonstrate an increased right ventricular and pulmonary arterial pressure and elevated pulmonary arterial O_2 saturation (Critchley 1976). If pulmonary hypertension develops, the pulmonary arterial pressure may be similar to the aortic pressure. Long-term survival of affected animals is unusual, although one affected 6-year-old horse has been seen by the author, and 8-month-old and 3- and 20-year-old survivors have been reported (Buergelt et al., 1970; Carmichael et al. 1971; Hare 1931; Glazier, Farrelly, and Neylon 1974; Fregin, Donawick, and Buchanan 1981).

Surgery

Although thoracotomy is not a common clinical procedure in large domestic animals, both clinical and experimental applications have been described (Peyton, Hoffer, and Calahan 1976; Fowler 1973; Waugh et al. 1980; Tranquilli et al. 1981). The principles involved in thoracotomy are similar for small and large animals and are covered in Chapter 13. Surgical interruption of the patent ductus arteriosus is possible in young domestic animals and has been accomplished in an adult horse, although there are no published reports of this (Fregin, Donawick, and Buchanan 1981). Similar surgical approaches, however, have been described for implantation of electromagnetic flow probes onto the coronary arteries in the calf and pony (Tranquilli et al. 1981) and around the ascending aorta in the adult horse (Waugh et al. 1980).

Surgical Preparation

One day prior to surgery, the hair should be clipped over the left side of the thorax from the sternum to the dorsal midline beginning at the spine of the scapula caudally to the tenth to fifteenth rib. The animal should be bathed and the surgical field scrubbed with a disinfectant solution. The surgical site should be covered with a sterile gauze pad held in position by a self-adherent bandage* placed around the thorax. Horses should be medicated on the day prior to surgery by intramuscular injection of 20,000 U/kg of procaine penicillin G (b.i.d.) and 7.7 mg/kg of dihydrostreptomycin (t.i.d.). Calves may be medicated with penicillin, although treatment with a sulfonamide solution (70 mg of sulfamethazine and 65 mg of sulfathiazole per ml) administered intravenously at a dose rate of 1.6 ml/kg has also been described (Tranquilli et al. 1981).

Anesthesia, Monitoring, and Support

The general principles for anesthesia of the large animal patient are described in Chapter 8. Calves are premedicated with atropine (0.06 mg/kg, IM) and anesthesia is induced with an IV bolus of thiamylal sodium† (10 mg/kg). Horses may be premedicated with IV acepromazine‡ (0.66 mg/kg). A plane of anesthesia sufficient to allow intubation in horses is induced with 5% glyceryl guaiacolate§ and 0.2% thiamylal sodium by rapid intravenous infusion to effect.

---

*Elastikon, Johnson & Johnson, New Brunswick, NJ.

†Surital, Parke-Davis, Morris Plains, NJ.

‡Acepromazine, Ayerst Laboratories, New York, NY.

§Glycodex, Burns-Biotic Laboratories Div., Oakland, CA.

Anesthesia is maintained with halothane in oxygen using positive pressure ventilation at a rate of 7 to 12 breaths per minute. Arterial and central venous blood pressures should be recorded along with the electrocardiogram. A balanced electrolyte solution should be administered through an indwelling venous catheter during the procedure to assist in maintaining arterial blood pressure should hypotension occur. Cardiac antiarrhythmic agents, such as lidocaine (0.02%) in a drip or as a bolus (20 to 30 ml), may be administered IV to aid in the control of ventricular dysrhythmia provided hypotension, hypoxemia, or hyperkalemia has been corrected. Atrial arrhythmias are not uncommon even in halothane-anesthetized normal animals and, with the exception of atrial fibrillation, rarely require treatment. Spontaneously occurring atrial fibrillation may be accompanied by hypotension and decreased cardiac output if the ventricular rate is rapid. Digoxin administered IV at a dose of 2.5 to 5.0 µg/kg may be used to slow the ventricular rate and improve cardiac output. Treatment may be repeated in 10 to 15 minutes if a favorable response is not achieved. Since the maximum effect of digoxin may not occur for 60 minutes or more, further treatment may result in toxicity before marked slowing is noted.

The patient is positioned in right lateral recumbency on a partially inflated air mattress with the left foreleg fully extended to expose the operative site, which has been shaved and then scrubbed surgically. In horses, the right foreleg may be extended and the left hind leg elevated to help prevent postoperative myositis. The hooves should be covered with surgical gloves or other suitable material. The fore- and hind quarters are covered with sterile drapes and the operative site with an adherent surgical drape.*

In young animals and lean adults, the high surface-to–body weight ratio and low body fat content make heat conservation more difficult. Foals and calves should be insulated from the operating table, exposed areas covered, and a

warm circulating blanket placed in contact with the body if hypothermia is not desired. Scrubbing, irrigating, and intravenous solutions should be warmed and the operating room temperature raised to 75°F.

Surgical Technique

The surgical approach for a lateral thoracotomy has been described in Chapter 13. The skin is incised caudal to the border of the long head of the triceps brachii muscle over the fourth intercostal space. The incision begins near the posterior angle of the scapula and extends ventrally 40 to 50 cm to the level of the costochondral junction. The cutaneous trunci, latissimus dorsi, serratus ventralis, and a portion of the deep pectoral muscle fibers are transected or divided as previously described. The thoracodorsal artery and external thoracic vein should be transfixed and double ligated. The periosteum is incised and then removed from the fourth or fifth rib with periosteal elevators. A portion of the rib is excised by cutting dorsally with an obstetrical wire and ventrally by disarticulation at the costochondral junction. Hemorrhage should be controlled by ligation of the vessels with 00 silk. The rough edges of the bone should be removed with rongeurs and bone wax or Gelfoam placed over the fractured cortical surfaces.

Pneumothroax frequently occurs during rib resection, requiring positive pressure ventilation. The pleural cavity is invaded by extending the incision through the periosteum and pleura deep to it, exposing the thoracic cavity for palpation and visual inspection. A modified Finochietto rib retractor is then placed between the ribs, the lungs packed off with sterile saline–moistened towels, and the retractors spread to obtain maximum exposure. The pericardium may be sprayed with 2% lidocaine HCl to help prevent cardiac arrhythmias. The left phrenic, vagus, and left recurrent laryngeal nerves should be carefully isolated and retracted from the operative site. A horizontal incision through the pericardium at the level of the left atrium is made and the epicardium irrigated

---

*Vi-Drape Instant Surgical Film, Parke-Davis, Morris Plains, NJ.

with 2% lidocaine HCl. The main pulmonary artery, which is frequently dilated and thin-walled, may then be visualized and palpated.

The aorta and pulmonary artery at the heart base are covered by the visceral layer of the serous pericardium. In most instances an extrapericardial approach is sufficient for exposure of the operative site (Fig. 14–1). Careful medial blunt dissection between the main pulmonary artery and the ascending aorta may be accomplished using a curved hemostat or long vascular clamp. The left recurrent laryngeal nerve, which had been isolated along with the vagus, should be retracted from the operative site to avoid left laryngeal hemiplegia. In young animals the aorta may be dissected free to allow cross-clamping should injury to the ductus or great vessels occur. This procedure is difficult to impossible in the adult.

If ligation is selected as the method of interruption, a long right-angle Mixter or Satinsky forceps is placed deep into the

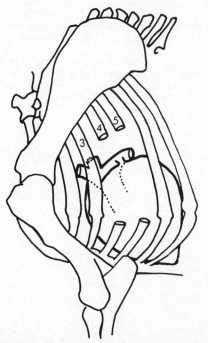

Figure 14–1 Extrapericardial approach for exposure of the operative site. The fourth and fifth rib sections have been removed for diagrammatic purposes. (Redrawn from Waugh, S. L., Campbell, J. B., Klavano, P. A., and Grant, B. D.: Surgical implantation of cardiovascular devices in the thorax of the horse. Am. J. Vet. Res. *41*:816, 1980.)

dissected area caudal to the ductus and then carefully advanced until the tips of the forceps can be visualized. Excess tissue should be incised or bluntly dissected before the ligatures are grasped and the forceps slowly retracted. Ligation with two silk sutures (young animals) or heavy umbilical tape (adult) with a fold of ductus tissue between the ligatures is recommended.

Pulmonary artery pressure (Ppa) should be recorded while the ductus is temporarily occluded. If the Ppa remains high or is increased, successful ligation with survival of the patient may not be achieved. A fall in Ppa during temporary occlusion of the ductus suggests a more favorable prognosis. In the absence of other cardiac defects, a normal physiological state should be achieved following successful closure of the patent ductus arteriosus.

Before closure, as described in Chapter 13, the thorax may be flushed with 10^6 U K^+ penicillin G in a liter of normal saline solution. The intercostal muscles and pleura are approximated using a nonabsorbable suture* encircling the third and fifth ribs in a horizontal mattress pattern. The sutures may be preplaced while suction is maintained to drain the thorax. Before tying the last suture, the lungs are maximally expanded to expel air and fluid from the thoracic cavity. An indwelling thoracic drain may be placed prior to closure; however, unless it is removed quickly after the animal is standing it may serve as a source of infection (Waugh et al. 1980; Fregin et al. 1981).

Simple continuous sutures are placed along the tendinous layer to complete the airtight seal. The transected edges of the deep pectoral and serratus ventralis muscles are apposed with horizontal mattress sutures. An 18-gauge Penrose drain may be placed between the serratus ventralis and the latissimus dorsi or between the latissimus dorsi and the cutaneous trunci before closure with simple interrupted sutures. The subcuticular tissues are then approximated with a continuous suture and the skin closed using a vertical mattress suture of heavy Vetafil.

---

*Vetafil, Look Inc., Boston, MA.

Recovery and Postoperative Care

The patient is placed in lateral recumbency with oxygen administered through an indwelling nasal tube until the animal is standing. A self-adherent bandage is then placed around the thorax to prevent contamination of the wound site and seroma formation. On the second to fourth postoperative day, the bandage and the Penrose drains may be removed. The incision is covered with an antibacterial dressing on a nonadherent pad that may be changed as needed. The skin sutures may be removed on the tenth to fourteenth postoperative day.

REFERENCES

Buergelt, C. D., Carmichael, J. A., Tashjian, R. J., and Das, K. M.: Spontaneous rupture of the left pulmonary artery in a horse with patent ductus arteriosus. JAVMA 157:313, 1970.

Carmichael, J. A., Buergelt, C. D., Lord, P. F., and Tashjian, R. J.: Diagnosis of patent ductus arteriosus in a horse. JAVMA 158:767, 1971.

Critchely, K. L.: The importance of blood gas measurement in the diagnosis of an intraventricular septal defect in a horse: A case report. Equine Vet. J. 8:128, 1976.

Dennis, S. M., and Leipold, H. W.: Congenital cardiac defects in lambs. Am. J. Vet. Res. 29:2337, 1968.

Fowler, M. E.: Intrathoracic surgery in large animals. JAVMA 162:967, 1973.

Fregin, G. F.: The cardiovascular system. In Equine Medicine and Surgery, Vol. 1, 3rd ed. Mansmann, R. A., and McAllister, S. (eds.). American Veterinary Publications, Inc., Santa Barbara, CA, 1982, pp. 645–701.

Fregin, G. F., Donawick, W. J., and Buchanan, J. W.: Surgical correction of patent ductus arteriosus in an adult horse. Unpublished data, 1981.

Fregin, G. F., Tennant, B. C., and Rendano, V. T.: Patent ductus arteriosus in a calf. Unpublished data, 1982.

Glazier, D. B., Farrelly, B. T., and Neylon, J. F.: Patent ductus arteriosus in eight-month-old foal. Irish Vet. J. 28:12, 1974.

Hare, T. J.: Patent ductus arteriosus in a horse. J. Pathol. 34:124, 1931.

Kemler, A. G., and Martin, J. E.: Incidence of congenital cardiac defects in bovine fetuses. Am. J. Vet. Res. 33:249, 1972.

Peyton, L. C., Hoffer, R., and Calahan, P.: Intrathoracic surgery in the horse with a pictorial guide to partial lobectomy. VM/SAC 71:1190, 1976.

Rooney, J. R., and Franks, W. C.: Congenital cardiac abnormalies in horses. Pathol. Vet. 1:454, 1964.

Scott, E. A., Kneller, S. K., and Witherspoon, D. M.: Closure of ductus arteriosus determined by cardiac catheterization and angiography in newborn foals. Am. J. Vet. Res. 36:1021, 1975.

Tranquilli, W. J., Manohar, M., Thurmon, J. C., Benson, G. J., Shawley, R. V., and Feller, D. L.: Surgical technique and considerations for implantation of electromagnetic blood flow transducer and occluder onto the coronary arteries. Am. J. Vet. Res. 42:893, 1981.

VanNie, C. J.: Congenital malformations of the heart in cattle and swine. A survey of a collection. Acta Morphol. Neerl. Scand. VI:387, 1966.

Waugh, S. L., Campbell, K. R., Klavano, P. A., and Grant, B. D.: Surgical implantation of cardiovascular devices in the thorax of the horse. Am. J. Vet. Res. 41:816, 1980.

CHAPTER 15

THE DIGESTIVE SYSTEM

SURGERY OF THE BOVINE DIGESTIVE TRACT

F. D. HORNEY, D.V.M.,
AND CHARLES E. WALLACE, D.V.M.

The diseases of the bovine digestive system and the differential diagnosis of some of these complex problems are of great importance to the bovine surgeon. Generally, one must obtain an adequate history of the case being examined. Then, one must stand back and look at the animal while recording all observations of the animal and its environment, at least mentally.

Basically, the functions of the digestive tract are movement (prehension, mastication, swallowing, churning), secretion, digestion, and absorption. One can focus on abnormalities of these functions and look for manifestations of disease when examining a patient. Manifestations of disease include abnormalities of prehension, mastication, or swallowing; vomition; salivation; fever; colic; change in nature of the feces; abdominal distension; tenesmus; and abnormalities of hunger and thirst.

Methods of diagnosis used in cattle are abdominal palpation, oral examination, rectal palpation, percussion, and auscultation. Sampling and analysis of saliva, stomach contents, feces, or abdominal fluid may yield information of importance in the differential diagnosis. Hematological examination for complete blood count and determination of chemical components is also of use in the differential diagnosis.

DIFFERENTIAL DIAGNOSIS OF DIGESTIVE DISEASES

The diagnosis of digestive disorders in cattle can be a very complex and difficult task. The surgeon must learn to read the signs and become expert in physical examination. Laboratory tests may be very useful in diagnosis. They should be used to confirm suspicions rather than relied upon to prove a case without a good physical examination. Laboratory test results can help provide a diagnosis and may guide one in choosing the time for surgical intervention. Knowing when to operate is as important as knowing why, how, and where. The book *Clinical Examination of Cattle* by Rosenberger provides a storehouse of information on diagnosis.

One or more signs of digestive disturbance may be noted initially, depending on the class of livestock involved. For example, in stabled cattle anorexia or a change in feces is easily noted, whereas in loose-housed cattle depression or separation from the herd is more noticeable. With dairy cattle a decrease in milk pro-

493

duction, although a vague sign in itself, often alerts the handler to observe a particular animal more closely for other signs of disease, such as decreased appetite, change in fecal or urinary excrement, or change in social behavior.

Some signs indicative of digestive disorders that may require surgical intervention include vomition, salivation, fever, expiratory grunt, colic, abdominal distension, tenesmus, change in feces, and change in appetite.

Vomition. The projectile vomition is a rarely observed sign in cattle (Fig. 15–1). In some cases animals may have sharp enamel points on the teeth or loose, missing, or broken teeth. This leads to ineffective chewing of roughage and, in some cases, a balling of the roughage in the cheek. These animals might then lose a cud, and this might be mistaken for vomiting. The vomition in cattle is usually associated with a disturbance of the forestomachs, as in traumatic gastritis, or blockage of the digestive tract, as in torsion of the mesentery. In rare instances it will be observed in animals with left abomasal displacement.

Salivation. The drooling of saliva can be associated with stomatitis of any cause. Also, foreign bodies lodged in the mouth or pharynx will stimulate excessive salivation. Rabies should be considered as a differential diagnosis in some cases because of its zoonotic importance.

Fever. Fever may be related to a concurrent disease such as mastitis or endometritis rather than a digestive disease. A localized infection, such as an abscess or a focal peritonitis or hepatitis, may cause fever. Septicemia may cause fever also.

Expiratory Grunt—Shallow Breathing. These signs may accompany a respiratory disease such as pleuritis or atypical interstitial emphysema. They may also accompany peritonitis of any origin, such as perforation of an infected uterus, or an abomasal ulcer, traumatic reticulitis, or liver abscessation.

Colic. Colic is a sign of abdominal pain and can be caused by tension on the mesentery or by stretching or tearing of adhesions between the visceral peritoneum or abdominal organs and the parietal peritoneum lining the abdominal cavity. This sign can accompany such diseases as abomasal displacements; torsions or volvulus of colon, intestines, or uterus; dilatations or displacements of organs; foreign body penetration of the digestive tract; and urethral calculus.

Abdominal Distension. This is an important sign of abdominal disease in cattle and may aid a keen observer in reaching a diagnosis or forming a differential diagnosis. With gaseous distension of the rumen (tympany or rumen bloat), the left paralumbar fossa will be distended. With tympany of the abomasum there will be distension under the last rib bulging into the paralumbar fossa on either the right or left side. When displaced, a distended abomasum may be palpable occasionally on the left side and usually on the right side by rectal examination. Rumen distension that accompanies vagal indigestion or outflow obstruction, such as with partial or complete abomasal or intestinal obstruction, may manifest as a bilateral abdominal distension, mostly on the left side. The right ventral aspect of the abdomen may become distended if abomasal atony or impaction is also present. Hydrops of the fetal membranes or an accumulation of ascitic fluid within the abdomen will cause bilateral distension, often in the lower part of the abdomen unless an advanced disease is pres-

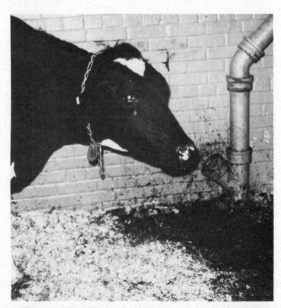

Figure 15–1 Clinical appearance of a cow suffering with projectile vomition as a result of traumatic gastritis.

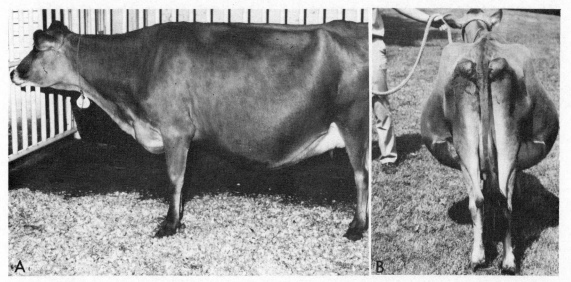

Figure 15–2 *A*, Clinical appearance of a cow with bilateral abdominal distension due to hydrops of the fetal membranes. *B*, Posterior view.

ent (Fig. 15–2). Herniation of the reticulum through a diaphragmatic hernia is also a cause of bloat. Rupture of the urinay bladder may also cause abdominal distension (Fig. 15–3).

Tenesmus. Straining may accompany rectal irritation, as from excessive trauma during rectal examination. Another cause is absence of negative pressure within the abdomen following surgery. Constipation and diarrhea are also possibilities. Further causes include urethral obstruction in steers or bulls, cystitis or urinary bladder disease, vaginal irritation, and dystocia.

Change in Feces. Examination of the feces can be a very important part of physical examination when disease of the digestive tract is suspected. The consistency, quantity, color, and odor are all important. Diarrhea, an apparently increased amount of feces with increased fluidity, accompanied by a normal odor may indicate parasitism, simple indigestion, renal insufficiency, or congestion of the systemic circulatory system. Diarrhea accompanied by an abnormal odor may indicate enteritis (fetid odor), salmonellosis (sweet odor), Johne's disease, or complex indigestion.

The size of particles in the feces may give a clue to the nature of the digestive upset. The duration and thoroughness of rumination are primary influences on the

appearance of poorly digested particles in feces. Thus, failure of rumination or accelerated passage of ingesta through the forestomachs results in increased amounts of poorly digested particles. Sometimes cattle with acute traumatic reticuloperitonitis may excrete a clump

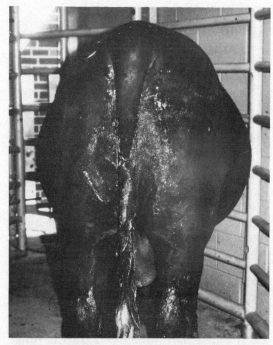

Figure 15–3 Posterior view of a bull with abdominal distension due to rupture of the urinary bladder.

of undigested fiber in otherwise normal-appearing feces. Abnormally well-digested particles are observed in feces with a delayed passage of ingesta, which allows more frequent and thorough rumination than normal.

The presence of fresh blood in the feces may indicate disease of the colon or rectum or may follow an irritating rectal examination. Dark, tarry, or sticky feces (which may be loose occasionally) may indicate blood loss into the stomach or high intestinal tract such as with abomasal or rumen ulcers or some intestinal foreign bodies (trichobezoars, phytobezoars). A decreased rate of passage of feces may be associated with a darker color and more pungent odor. In cases of complete obstruction, as with an intussusception, only a mucous plug may be found on rectal examination. Fibrin strands are associated with enteritis.

Change in Appetite. This clinical sign may be rather vague. In some cases appetite may go unnoticed unless the animal is closely observed. Appetite is decreased with infection, pain, or obstruction of the digestive tract. In the case of left abomasal displacement there is usually a preference for forage rather than concentrates.

PREOPERATIVE GOALS IN THE TREATMENT OF DIGESTIVE DISORDERS IN CATTLE

The major preoperative goal in the surgical treatment of digestive disorders in cattle is adequate and correct assessment of the clinical situation. As previously stated, this involves identification of the problem with which the animal is presented together with physical examination to confirm the presence and degree of severity of the problem along with other abnormalities that might not be as readily apparent. Confirmation of the diagnosis should be made using appropriate laboratory tests. However, in a (clinical) practice situation there often is not adequate time to submit samples for analysis and wait for a report. Many situations require more urgent therapeutic attention. Therefore, the surgeon must draw on his knowledge of the common or usual laboratory findings associated with various disease processes.

There are some problems that require immediate intervention, such as omasalabomasal, cecal, or intestinal volvulus; intestinal displacements accompanied by colic; and some dystocias. There are other problems that may allow some degree of preoperative assessment with laboratory parameters and preoperative therapy to stabilize or improve the animal's condition prior to surgery. Examples of such problems might include left abomasal displacement, traumatic reticulitis, intussusception, and some types of dystocia. Cattle that fall into the last-named category often can be effectively treated prior to surgery so that an improved prognosis for return to function can be achieved.

To illustrate such preoperative measures, consider a cow with left abomasal displacement accompanied by ketosis, endometritis, and mastitis. Sometimes obvious sepsis and septicemia accompanied by diarrhea are evident. A hemogram will often show a total white blood cell count below 4000 cells/mm.^{3} Treatment aimed at controlling the septic process, re-establishing hydration, and correcting concurrent ketosis will allow the cow to improve, as often noted in her attitude and in an increased total white blood cell count. If the count rises to above 4000 cells/mm^3 and the sepsis is partially or completely controlled, a much improved surgical prognosis can be given. If the cow fails to improve or dies, one has saved the client the expense of surgery and oneself some time as well as the embarrassment of a "surgical" death.

Another obvious goal of preoperative assessment is to determine whether or not the function of the animal can be restored by reversal of the disease process. The physical examination should aid in this determination. Sometimes the initial response to medical therapy will be a determinant in this regard. In food animal surgery, sometimes even the temporary restoration of normal function is desirable so that the animal may be salvaged for slaughter later.

Goals of Surgical Therapy in the Treatment of Digestive Disorders

Basically, the objectives of therapy in our cases are as follows:

1. Restore normal anatomical relationships,
2. Restore normal motility of the digestive tract,
3. Restore normal flora of the digestive tract,
4. Restore acid-base balance,
5. Prevent sepsis,
6. Treat other concurrent diseases,
7. Provide a comfortable environment during recovery, and
8. Provide adequate nutrition parenterally or free choice.

Let us consider each of these points in relation to surgical intervention. First, it is obvious that with many disorders of the digestive tract there are abnormal anatomical relationships that develop because of displacement, compression, volvulus, torsion, herniation, impaction, and so on. Unless or until these physical abnormalities can be corrected, the animal will continue to have abnormal digestion or may even die. The various abdominal surgical sites in cattle usually allow only limited visual inspection of the viscera. Therefore, the surgeon must develop ambidextrous skill in manual palpation of the abdominal contents. Such skill can be obtained only through the palpation of many cattle during abdominal surgery, although a basic knowledge of visceral anatomy is imperative. Once normal anatomical relationships and their variations can be recognized, the surgeon will more easily be able to determine abnormal relationships and correct them, if possible. If they cannot be corrected, the prognosis will be unfavorable.

If the surgeon is able to restore the anatomy, he can focus his attention on the restoration of normal physiological function including the restoration of normal motility, flora, and acid-base balance. In some cases even though the normal anatomical relationships have been restored, a poor functional result follows because of circulatory disturbances to the organs involved. Specifically, thrombosis of larger or smaller vessels will cause hypoxic changes within the muscular or mucosal portions of those organs. Sometimes such changes are visibly or palpably apparent, but occasionally they are not. A poorer prognosis can be given if changes are observed; otherwise, a guarded prognosis should be offered.

Frequently for the first day or two after abdominal surgery the animal will have some degree of inappetence and may have loose feces or diarrhea. The diarrhea may result from the peritoneal irritation of the operation or from the release of trapped gastric or intestinal contents. Constipation may follow this phase, particularly if the air has not been completely evacuated from the abdominal cavity so as to restore the normal negative pressure and allow an abdominal press to cause evacuation of the rectum in defecation.

Water is an important nutrient for the maintenance of both hydration and a normal fecal consistency. Water should be offered free choice with or without electrolytes as deemed appropriate by the nature of the disease process.

Restoration of normal microbial flora can be accomplished by offering a variety of palatable, wholesome foodstuffs to encourage feed intake. An alternative method is transfaunation or the administration of rumen liquor from a normal animal. This procedure is especially indicated and desirable in cases in which there has been prolonged antimicrobial therapy with antibiotics or sulfonamides.

Simultaneous improvement in acid-base balance may occur in cases in which the disease process has been mild or minor. In other cases homeostasis will need to be evaluated and monitored periodically by laboratory tests so that appropriate therapy can be instituted. For example, alkalosis is sometimes present prior to correction of abomasal displacement and is usually present in cases of abomasal volvulus; however, the alkalosis will often shift toward normalcy spontaneously after surgery, even to the point of slight acidosis.

Water is usually given by stomach tube if the animal will not drink. Electrolytes can be added to warm water. Sometimes a sick animal will not drink even if dehydrated. Contraindications to oral fluid therapy include disease of the forestomachs in which pooling of water and electrolytes within the lumen of the stomachs is common and further forced oral fluid therapy will not help to restore hydration.

The prevention of sepsis can be aided by antibacterial therapy as indicated for concurrent diseases or to guard against abscess formation, which might result from leakage of abomasal or intestinal contents prior to or during surgery.

Ketosis is a common concurrent disease in lactating or pregnant cattle. Intravenous solutions of glucose or glucose/fructose can be given to provide energy in such cases. Vitamin and mineral supplementation may be necessary, depending on the cow's condition and degree of anemia. Comfortable surroundings should be provided postoperatively. A salt block and good diet also should be provided. Isolation of an animal from the group should be avoided, but the animal should not be pushed around by the other, more aggressive, normal animals. Some degree of exercise is important.

If the animal refuses to eat even after correction of acid-base balance and offering of free choice quality foodstuffs, it may be fed a gruel of pelleted feed via stomach pump. Rumen transfaunation may help. If the animal still does not improve, the situation has to be re-assessed.

THE ORAL CAVITY

One of the most important parts of the animal is the oral cavity, particularly the teeth. Although the surgical treatment of diseases of the teeth does not occupy much of the veterinarian's time, there are certain points worthy of mention.

Anatomy

The mouth and dental structures of cattle are well designed for ingesting large quantities of roughage. This material is initially poorly masticated. The muscular and rough tongue and the palate and dental pad play a more important role than the teeth in the prehension and preliminary preparation of the fibrous diet for digestion.

Although deglutition is comparable in all domestic animals, the ruminant needs to regurgitate and ruminate to initially prepare the digesta before passing it along to the abomasum and intestines.

Tremendous quantities of saliva are continuously secreted, but the rate and quantity vary, depending on the diet, the act of eating, and whether the animal is ruminating or resting. Although dental disease may interfere with eating, viral and bacterial infections acting centrally or peripherally result in deglutition and prehension disorders that more seriously interfere with ingestion.

Examination

Examination of the teeth not only is important for determining age but also helps to identify abnormalities that might be present such as prognathism, brachygnathism (Fig. 15–4), stomatitis, fractured teeth, sharp enamel points, oral tumors, and other problems (Figs. 15–5 and 15–6).

Good light, a suitable mouth speculum,

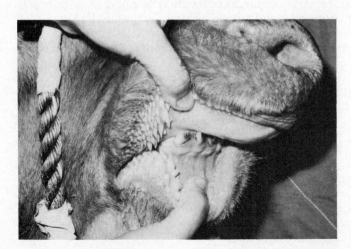

Figure 15–4 Brachygnathism or "parrot mouth" in a Guernsey cow.

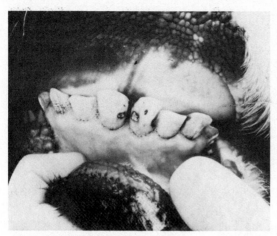

Figure 15–5 Pitting of the dental enamel as seen in fluorosis.

and adequate restraint are essential for proper examination. Particulate matter may be present, obscuring the view of the oral cavity; some means of flushing this debris from the mouth is, therefore, needed. The veterinarian should protect himself by wearing gloves in areas where rabies is endemic.

Age can be determined by examination of the incisors. Grazing on pastures with sandy soil may increase wear on the teeth. The permanent central incisors erupt at about 18 months of age and are in full wear at about two years of age. By five years of age all of the permanent teeth are in wear. Occasionally, retained caps on any of the teeth may cause prob-

lems, as in the horse. This might be characterized by difficult chewing. Another problem is periodontitis caused by breaks in the mucous membrane and lodging of food particles alongside the tooth roots. Periodontitis is also associated with broken teeth. Physical examination with the aid of a mouth speculum assists diagnosis. In some cases radiography is useful in determining the extent of involvement and aiding in prognosis. If a periodontal abscess can be drained satisfactorily or if broken teeth can be removed, the prognosis should be good. If extensive lysis of the mandible or maxilla has occurred, the prognosis will be guarded to unfavorable. Sometimes abscesses of the oral cavity are associated with actinomycosis or actinobacillosis infection. Maxillary sinusitis may be a clinical sign. Bacteriological examination is needed to confirm a diagnosis so that appropriate medical therapy can be undertaken. The surgical curettage and drainage of bone abscesses of the maxillary sinus can be useful adjunctive treatment (Fig. 15–7).

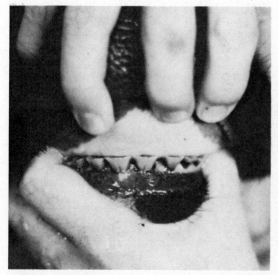

Figure 15–6 Discoloration of the teeth as seen in congenital porphyria.

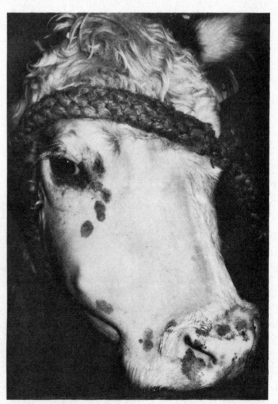

Figure 15–7 A cow with osteomyelitis of the maxillary sinus.

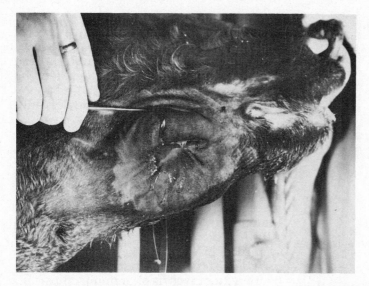

Figure 15–8 Actinomycosis involving the ramus of the mandible.

Trauma

Injury is always possible owing to incomplete mastication and the tendency of cattle to pick up metallic foreign material. Various oral lesions are associated with viral diseases and may take the form of small mucosal erosions or deeper ulcers with secondary bacterial contamination. Objects may wedge between the posterior molars and interfere with rumination. Alveolar periostitis and osteomyelitis associated with actinomycosis as well as soft tissue lesions of the tongue in actinobacillosis are more commonly associated with problems of prehension and mastication (Fig. 15–8).

Direct trauma can involve both the mandible and the maxilla. Pathological fractures of both jaws can be seen following extensive infection with actinomycosis. Reduction and immobilization of traumatic fractures is usually achieved by the use of transverse pins, bone plates, or a combination of both with wiring and external fixation. Neoplasms of the pharyngeal mucosa may be encountered during examination of the oral cavity of anorectic cows (Fig. 15–9). These neoplasms are usually pedunculated and may result in intermittent blockage of the oral or nasal pharynx. In most instances they are not detected until well advanced. Although some neoplasms may be excised by wire snare, salvage of the animal for slaughter is more frequently advised.

Aging and wear of the teeth in some areas has prompted the capping of incisor teeth that are prematurely worn down, but this is not a common procedure (Newcomb 1961).

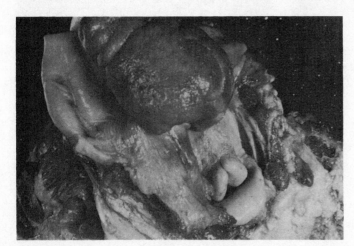

Figure 15–9 Pharyngeal polyp.

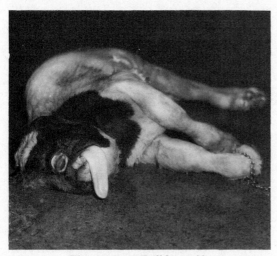

Figure 15–10 Bulldog calf.

Congenital conditions are self-limiting. Brachygnathism (bulldog) calves are usually culled rather than raised (Fig. 15–10). Cleft palate (Fig. 15–11), because of its frequent association with other congenital anomalies (arthrogryposis), also results in the elimination of these animals, rather than keeping them as replacement stock.

Foreign bodies lodged in the oral cavity or pharynx are common problems. Cattle seem to eat or try to eat or chew on almost anything. Foreign bodies range from sticks and stalks to twine and string. The most noted signs are salivation and drooling. The animal will try to eat but will not be able to. If the foreign body has been present for some time, the animal will be very thin. A good oral examination is required to verify the diagnosis. The method of removal depends on the type of foreign body encountered. Again, one should always consider the possibility of rabies when examining cattle with the aforementioned symptoms.

The tongue is subject to penetration by foreign bodies and laceration. Foreign bodies can be removed without too much difficulty. Small lacerations will usually heal satisfactorily, whereas larger ones will benefit from partial to complete closure with sutures.

Self-Sucking

In ruminants kept for milk production, the occasional animal learns to self-suck.

This is a difficult problem to control with mechanical contrivances designed either to keep the animal from reaching the udder or to create sufficient difficulties in removing milk from the udder. This can also be a very serious problem, especially among bucket-reared calves. Individual confinement helps to limit the problem. Some mechanical devices have been used to help break calves of the nursing habit, but the results are variable. The reason for breaking calves of this vice is that a high incidence of mastitis or blind quarters will be found in these animals when they freshen later.

The use of Elizabethan or cradle-type collars is not advisable for animals on pasture because of the possibility of the animal becoming entangled in fencing. Metallic tags, rings, and so on are sometimes inserted in the frenulum of the tongue to discourage self-sucking.

The most successful technique for dealing with this problem is to surgically alter the contour of the tongue by removing a wedge-shaped segment from the ventral surface (Fig. 15–12) (Wright 1953). Sedation with xylazine supple-

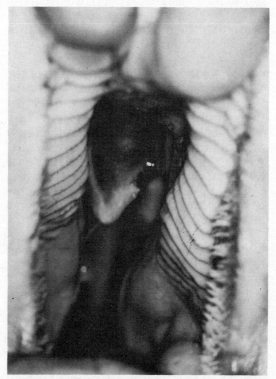

Figure 15–11 Cleft palate in a neonate. This animal also had arthrogryposis.

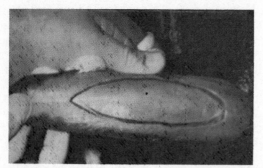

Figure 15–12 The ventral surface of the tongue is scrubbed with Betadine. An elliptical incision is begun just anterior to the attachment of the frenulum. This incision should penetrate only through the thick mucosa, be approximately 2 inches wide at the widest point (depending on the size of the animal), and extend to about 1 inch from the tip of the tongue. (Reprinted with permission from McCormack: VM/SAC 71:681, 1976.)

mented by local anesthesia is sufficient for this surgery. The tongue is best immobilized by an assistant. A mouth gag, such as a wedge speculum or a Drinkwater gag, facilitates manipulation of the tongue. Gauze bandaging may be used to encircle and stabilize the tongue as well as to provide a tourniquet effect to minimize hemorrhage. Various configurations of wedge resection are used, but a simple elliptical wedge is adequate. A triangular segment of tongue substance is removed from the ventral surface, creating a more rounded contour on the dorsal surface, which then prevents the animal from cupping the tongue around the teat (McCormack 1976).

To minimize blood loss, start the suturing before removing the full ellipse and alternately cut and suture as the wedge resection is performed. Simple interrupted sutures of nonabsorbable material are adequate for closure. Some postoperative discomfort can be expected but is minimal.

Partial glossectomy is another technique that can be effective as a surgical treatment for self-sucking. This involves good restraint of the animal and sedation with a drug such as xylazine. The goal of the procedure is to remove a portion of the tip of the tongue in a diagonal manner to prevent the animal from curling the tongue to nurse. Of course, the postoperative pain associated with this procedure also dissuades the animal

from nursing. The tongue can be grasped with a tenaculum forceps and withdrawn from the mouth. A strip of gauze bandage can be wrapped around the base of the tongue both to act as a tourniquet and to aid in restraint for surgery. Large hemostatic forceps can be placed across the tongue from either side in a diagonal manner. Stay sutures can be used to hold the tongue behind these forceps, or the gauze can be used. Local analgesia is given caudal to the proposed surgical excision site. A scalpel can be used to sever the tip of the tongue. The edges can be brought together with absorbable interrupted sutures to appose the edges of the mucous membrane and aid in controlling hemorrhage. The animal may have some difficulty eating for a few days, but the operation site heals well, and the operation usually is successful in controlling nursing.

Abscessation

Pharyngeal or retropharyngeal abscessation is commonly encountered. Sometimes abscesses develop in calves as a result of septicemia. More frequently these are the result of trauma to the pharyngeal mucosa from sharp objects. In fact, a number of these cases result from too vigorous use of balling guns or dose syringes, particularly during deworming. An animal restrained in a chute for deworming may suddenly lunge forward during the treatment, causing the instrument to injure the pharynx. In most instances the animal will show little discomfort at the time of injury. Some days or even weeks later a swelling will be noted in the pharyngeal area as an abscess develops. The mucous membrane of the pharynx seems to heal rapidly, allowing infection to develop and sometimes even trapping medication within a cavity. These abscesses are usually slow in developing, as in the case of a six-month-old calf presented for bloat because the abscess enlarged internally, compressing the trachea and esophagus. Most animals show signs of slobbering or drooling saliva, anorexia, slight fever, cough, or nasal discharge in addition to an enlargement of the pharyngeal area caudal to the jaw. Some animals will show few outward signs, even absence of pain in the pharyngeal area. One cow had three large boluses of medication lodged in a submucosal pharyngeal pouch with no signs except depression and anorexia.

Diagnosis must be made based on the history and a good physical examination. Radiography may be useful in a few cases. Certainly a sample obtained from the swelling using a syringe and needle is most useful. Caution must be used in restraining animals with respiratory conditions, as overrestraint or undue excitement will cause severe hypoxia, leading to death.

Once the abscess is located and more or less defined, surgical drainage is the therapy of choice. The abscess may be drained internally, if that is feasible; however, access for the treatment of an abscess through the oral cavity is limited. Therefore, external drainage is probably the method of choice. If the abscess is located using a needle, a stab incision with the scalpel can be made along the shaft of the needle into the abscess. Sometimes the abscesses point and their location can be found more easily. Once an opening is established, it can be enlarged safely if internal palpation of the cavity shows that vital structures such as the jugular vein or carotid artery are not close.

More than one opening is advised. Then, rubber Penrose drainage tubing can be inserted. The abscess should be flushed thoroughly with water or saline solution. The cavity can be packed with a gauze soaked in antibacterial solution or mild iodine tincture. Daily flushing of the abscess will speed recovery. The abscess cavity must heal from the inside out, so the skin incisions must be kept open. Treatment with systemic antibiotics for several days is advised. The prognosis is good in most cases.

Abscesses may also occur in the parotid lymph node or salivary glands. A differential diagnosis in these cases must include lymphosarcoma. Needle aspiration will help establish a diagnosis. Drainage of such abscesses may not effect a cure in this area. Resection of the encapsulated abscess or lymph node may

be necessary. Prognosis in such cases must be guarded, as it is difficult to resect these masses without complications such as hemorrhage or infection.

ESOPHAGUS

Physiology of Esophagus and Stomach

The rate of passage of ingested food material is dependent on the ability of the animal to get the food first to the stomach and then from the stomach to the outside in the form of feces. The first stage is prolonged in ruminants by the time required for fermentation and digestion by grinding, mixing, and protozoal activity in the rumen. In addition to rumination, a synchronized motility pattern is required to selectively move the material through the various compartments. The omasum acts essentially as a pump, supplying the abomasum with digesta for further processing.

Eructation and regurgitation rely on a patent passage between the reticulum and mouth, a well-synchronized sphincter, and a pressure mechanism for propelling boluses of gas and semifluid digesta to the mouth. Any problem with this mechanism, whether neurogenic or physical, will delay or inhibit the digestive process. All may be in vain if the animal is unable to remasticate and return the cud to the rumen. In some conditions the animal is unable to prevent the reflux of abomasal contents into an atonic rumen; the resulting sequestration of hydrogen and chloride ions in the rumen leads to metabolic alkalosis (Gingerich and Murdick 1975).

Foremost in importance in the physiology of digestion in a healthy animal is gastrointestinal motility. Excess fermentation in overload results in rumen acidosis. In traumatic reticuloperitonitis, circumscribed peritonitis occurs following perforation by foreign bodies, resulting in irregular or ineffective rumen motility. Some undetermined factor, most recently believed to be influenced in part by volatile fatty acid concentrations (Svendsen 1969), leads to stasis of the abomasum with subsequent dilatation, displacement, or torsion, which can be disastrous to normal gastric function (Svendsen 1969). Important in the understanding of the displacement is the arrangement of the parietal and visceral peritoneum with their interconnecting omental and ligamentous attachments.

Surgical Conditions

ESOPHAGUS

The most important surgical problem involving the esophagus is choke or obstruction caused by foreign objects. In the adult ruminant this problem may require immediate attention, as blockage of the esophagus will limit or prevent the eructation of gases produced by fermentation in the rumen. A delay in treatment may lead to death from the respiratory embarrassment of tympany.

Some of the more common objects causing choke in cattle include potatoes, fruits, beets, and other vegetable roots. In some instances the cattle are being fed these foodstuffs, whereas in other cases the cattle may be scavenging these objects while grazing. Cattle may choke on ground feed if they eat too rapidly, but in this case they usually have the capacity to cough and thus expel the feed from the pharyngeal area.

Compression of the lumen of the esophagus by space-occupying lesions, such as the thymic form of lymphosarcoma or in mediastinal lymphadenopathy, also causes obstruction. Trauma may be caused by stomach tube passage, chemical irritation from medicated boluses that lodge in the esophagus, damage caused by the lesions of migrating *Hypoderma* larvae, or the disintegration of these larvae in the submucosa of the esophagus. All cattle exhibiting signs or symptoms of choke must be classified as having rabies until proved otherwise.

Alimentation is only possible if a patent route or entry to the stomach is established. In situations other than complete obstruction, stomach tubes may be passed to place liquids and gruels in the rumen and to relieve rumen bloat (tympany), if necessary.

If the animal is choked, the diagnosis can usually be made from a history of eating a particular foodstuff together with a physical examination showing bloat, tenesmus, urine dribbling, retching, and salivation. If the object can be palpated in the cervical area it may be possible to restrain the animal and retrieve the object manually from the esophagus. If it cannot be reached, one may pass a stomach tube and try to push the object into the stomach. If the object lodges at the cardia, a rumenotomy may have to be performed to allow the surgeon to reach through the cardia and retrieve the obstructing object, thereby allowing gas to escape. An alternative to surgery is slaughter of the animal, especially if it is not possible to economically treat the case.

Esophagotomy has been performed in cattle for cases of choke.

Surgical intervention for esophageal obstructions is necessary, especially for those in the cervical region that are not relieved by conservative treatment. Direct esophagotomy over the obstructing mass is advised. If the esophageal wall is healthy, primary suturing may be performed. If the esophagus shows evidence of pressure necrosis, primary suturing should not be attempted. It is preferable to leave the esophageal wound as an open fistula, which of course risks postoperative stricture formation. In cases of neurogenic dysphagia, such as in listeriosis, rumen fistulation is employed as a temporary means of alimentation.

Recent papers comment on the success of incision into and anastomosis of the esophagus; removal of foreign bodies and alleviation of stricture were the indications. This tends to dispel the fear that surgeons once had of esophageal surgery. The wise application of surgical principles, including the inversion of mucous membrane while closing the structure, no doubt accounts for success. Formerly, wound dehiscence and esophageal fistulization were common complications of such procedures.

Sometimes smaller nonobstructing objects become lodged within the esophagus. Such items have included fishhooks attached to fishing lines. In these cases esophagotomy must be performed.

Although it is necessary to insert a tube into the rumen for feeding some anorectic ruminants or during convalescence in certain procedures, it is also possible to insert a feeding tube into the esophagus for forced feeding. Such a technique has been described for horses. With such a procedure an incision is made in the lower middle third of the neck. The esophagus is located and brought to the level of the skin incision. Then its wall is tensed over a stomach tube already in place within the lumen. The muscular layer is incised longitudinally until the submucosal and mucosal layers can be identified and everted through the incision. A small transverse incision is made to allow for the fitting of the indwelling tube. The tube is inserted through the mucosal incision and secured by sutures to the animal so that it will not slip out. This method is probably only good for relatively short-term placement in larger ruminants because of interference with regurgitation. The wounds will heal spontaneously following removal of the indwelling tube.

STOMACH

The rumen, reticulum, and omasum are sometimes regarded as esophageal dilatations. This view is considered erroneous, since these compartments develop from the embryonic stomach and not from the esophagus. Generalization of surgical conditions involving the stomach of the ruminant is hampered by the fact that, depending on the age of the animal, there are differences in the development and function of this organ. Cattle fall into two general classes, pre-

ruminant and ruminant, and the complex transition of the stomach from one to the other creates many problems. In spite of the marked differences in structure and function, many of the surgical conditions that present in the ruminant are encountered in simple-stomached animals.

The ingestion of foreign objects is common to both ruminant and nonruminant. Penetration of the wall of the reticulum in the ruminant was frequently a cause of digestive disturbances in the past. Since large animal practitioners and owners have been introducing rumen magnets, the incidence of foreign body penetration has decreased but still cannot be overlooked as a cause of digestive disturbance. Suspected foreign body penetration remains an indication for medical or surgical intervention.

Diagnosis can be confirmed by radiography (Fig. 15–13) in exceptional cases, but when clinical signs are vague, the diagnosis is more commonly confirmed by exploratory laparotomy under paravertebral block (Fig. 15–14). Although many animals respond to conservative treatment, the following are considered indications for surgical intervention: traumatic reticuloperitonitis not responding to conservative treatment; animals affected by penetrating foreign bodies during the last three months of gestation; animals suffering from recurrent attacks of traumatic reticuloperitonitis; and overloading of the rumen.

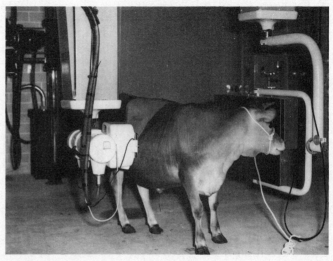

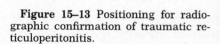
Figure 15–13 Positioning for radiographic confirmation of traumatic reticuloperitonitis.

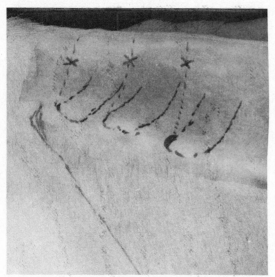

Figure 15–14 Sites for paravertebral anesthesia for exploratory laparotomy and rumenotomy.

OMASUM

This organ has not received a great deal of attention in relation to digestive disturbances. Since its location in the abdominal cavity hampers definitive palpation, examination most frequently is carried out by direct palpation during exploratory laparotomy or indirectly through the right rumen wall while doing an exploratory rumenotomy. Although the omasum can be the primary site of digestive disturbances, most authorities consider this organ to be involved only secondarily to some other digestive upset in the other compartments of the stomach. There is difficulty in establishing what is the normal size and consistency of the omasum; there is great variation among animals. If exploratory rumenotomy findings are negative, it is wise to closely examine the esophageal groove and the leaves of the omasum adjacent to the omasal sulcus for irregularities such as abnormal mucous membrane and inadequate patency of the omasal sulcus.

Anatomy of the Peritoneum

The embryonic development and postnatal enlargement of the anterior compartments of the stomach as the animal starts to ruminate create a marked change in the structure of the mesentery and omentum. The dorsal attachment of the greater omentum and mesoduodenum suspends the stomach from the esophagus to the end of the descending portion of duodenum. A sling of omentum is thus formed as the rumen and abomasum enlarge, which fixes them more securely than in the simple-stomached animal. The abomasum is effectively suspended, interposed between the lesser and greater omenta. These omenta are important in determining movement in abomasal displacement.

Initially, the duodenum is also suspended by the greater and lesser omenta, then by the greater omentum and mesoduodenum. Access to the anterior duodenum is restricted by the rib cage. Only the descending part of the anterior duodenum can be surgically approached from the right paralumbar fossa.

The mesentery of the small intestine is a fan-like arrangement of mesenteric root fused, in part, with the mesocolon at the turning point of the duodenum so that the free edge of the combined superficial and deep omenta, mesocolon, and mesoduodenum limits the exposure of viscera at this point. The uniformity of the fan shape of the mesentery is altered by an indentation and by the added length in the segment accommodating the distal jejunum and proximal ileum. Caudal to this point the ileum is attached to the cecum by the ileocecal mesentery.

The spiral colon and cecum, with the intervening large colon, are unstable except at the attachment in the region of the caudal flexure of the duodenum. Kinking of the colon at this point may obstruct the flow of digesta. The free apex of the cecum beyond the ileocecal mesentery may also kink on itself.

Preoperative Preparation for Abdominal Surgery in Cattle

The preoperative preparation of cattle for abdominal surgery has been mentioned briefly in reference to the preoperative treatment of some disease conditions to improve the prognosis.

In a more general sense we will consider the principles of surgical preparation. For most conditions that are encountered there is little time for specific preparation. The exception is the case of

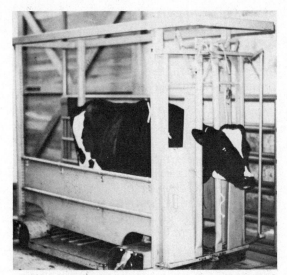

Figure 15–15 A movable restraining chute used for standing surgical procedures.

elective surgery for either exploratory laparotomy or rumenotomy (Fig. 15–15). In these cases the animal may already be inappetent; otherwise, deprivation of food for 12 to 24 hours may help to decrease the volume of gastric contents and thus facilitate exploratory surgery (Fig. 15–16). In some cases deprivation of water may also be desirable but is usually not necessary. However, if general anesthesia is involved, water and food deprivation is desirable to decrease gastric contents and reduce fermentation (which causes tympany), both of which may exert pressure on the thorax or induce regurgitation and possible sub-

sequent aspiration of gastric contents into the lungs.

The surgical site should be clipped, preferably before the animal is taken to the surgical area. Preliminary skin preparation and induction of local analgesia should also be performed outside the surgical area. However, availability and limitation of facilities in field situations often dictate the extent of preparation. The surgical area itself should be clean and dust-free and should include an adequate means of restraining the animal for the operation, whether it be standing or recumbent, under local or general anesthesia.

Equipment should be available for the administration of intravenous fluids during the procedure. Also, a few drugs should be kept nearby for emergency situations that might arise during the procedure. Surgical equipment and supplies should be available in an area adjacent to the operating site in case they are needed during surgery. Complications should be anticipated and plans developed to cope with them prior to the start of the procedure to minimize surgical time and maximize the efficiency of the surgeon.

Basic Procedures of Abdominal Digestive Surgery

The basic bovine digestive surgical procedures performed include incision (rumenotomy, abomasotomy), excision

Figure 15–16 Surgical correction of left abomasal displacement being performed in a portable restraining chute within the surgical suite.

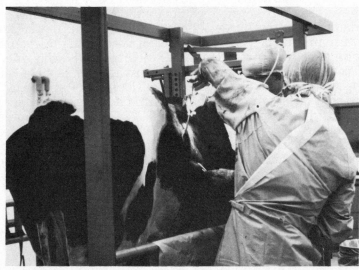

(enterectomy), fistulization (rumenostomy), stabilization (abomasopexy), decompression (centesis, trocarization), and derotation (of volvulus). The principles involved in the performance of these techniques in cattle are the same as those in other species. Some specific comments will be made about the problems of applying basic surgical principles to the specific problems encountered in bovine digestive surgery.

Incision is performed to allow exploration of the cavity of an organ, to evacuate the stomach contents, or to retrieve an object. In cattle this procedure may be complicated because surgery is often performed with the animal standing and locally anesthetized. This usually allows the animal some freedom of movement and the possibility of lying down, even though the animal may not feel pain. The intravenous administration of 5% glucose solution may help keep the animal standing for the duration of the surgery. The use of sedatives and tranquilizers cannot be recommended, as this may result in the animal going down during the procedure. It is especially important to isolate the organ being entered from the rest of the abdominal cavity during the procedure to prevent contamination. The organ must be held securely while open; the sudden cough of the animal may cause gastric contents to explode onto the surgeon and his equipment and may cause contamination of the abdominal cavity. Or worse, the organ may herniate through the abdominal incision onto the floor.

Several retraction or retaining devices have been developed specifically for rumenotomy procedures. The rumen ring with an attached shroud has been used, but only to supplement other devices. Procedures involving incision into the other organs usually require an assistant to hold the organ while the surgeon completes the procedure.

In the bovine, excisional procedures usually involve enterectomy. The same principles should be followed as for incisional procedures. If the procedure involves an intestinal tract that is heavily distended with fluid or gas, decompression of the organ is advised prior to continuing with the corrective surgery. Many surgeons prefer to operate on animals with intestinal problems with the animal in recumbency, as tension on the mesentery may cause pain and may induce the animal to go down during the procedure. Otherwise, the principles of enterotomy followed in other species apply in the bovine.

Fistulization of the rumen (rumenostomy) as a treatment for chronic ruminal tympany is the only commonly performed procedure of this type. No special precautions need be taken except those used to ensure a good seal between the rumen and the peritoneal cavity to avoid leakage of ingesta and ensuing peritonitis. Abomasal fistula is sometimes a complication of abomasopexy procedures. Usually they can be closed surgically if the fistula is large; however, small fistulae may not affect the function of the animal.

Stabilization procedures (-pexy) usually apply to the rumen, abomasum, cecum, or omentum. Since these procedures are used as corrective treatment for varying degrees of displacement of digestive organs, permanent fixation of an organ is usually the desired goal. To achieve this, a firm adhesion must be developed. In most cases this involves passing sutures through the serosa, muscularis, and mucosa into the lumen and out. Perhaps a small amount of ingesta will leak around the suture and thus cause a focal peritonitis, which leads to the development of a firm fibrous adhesion to hold the organ in a fixed position. In the case of omentopexy the sutures should not be pulled so tightly as to disturb the circulation within the omentum; strangulation may result in dehiscence at a later date. Too large a bite of tissue in the abomasum coupled with too much tension on the tied sutures may be responsible for the eventual development of abomasal fistula as a complication of abomasopexy.

Decompression may involve incision and evacuation of the contents of an organ prior to a manipulative procedure. However, decompression of gas only involves percutaneous centesis or trocarization of an organ with a needle. In the case of rumen tympany the procedure is performed with a trocar usually larger than 10 gauge. Such a needle must be of sufficient length to pass through the thickness of the abdominal wall in the paralumbar fossa and extend into the lumen for several centimeters. If a needle of insufficient diameter is used, clogging will be a problem. If a needle of insufficient length is used, contraction of the deflating organ away from the needle may cause it to be pulled out or may result in leakage of gastric contents into the peritoneal cavity. A similar percutaneous technique using a smaller gauge needle at least 15 cm in length can be applied to the distended abomasum or cecum.

Decompression of gas from an organ during a surgical procedure when the abdomen is open usually involves using a 13- to 15-gauge needle. In most cases centesis can be performed without taking any special precautions to guard against leakage subsequent to the withdrawal of the needle from the organ. However, the surgeon may want to prepare a small purse-string suture around the site of centesis so that the opening into the lumen made by the needle can be firmly closed following its withdrawal. Alternatively, he may want to use a smaller gauge needle.

Derotation or replacement of displaced abdominal viscera usually requires the removal of accumulated gas from the organ involved and often necessitates the removal of an abnormal accumulation of fluid within the lumen of the organ. These are prerequisites for successful manipulation of often friable organs while decreasing the possibility of spontaneous or accidental rupture of the organ during manipulation.

Successful repositioning of organs requires a knowledge of normal anatomic relationships. Sometimes organs that have been filled with fluid or gas to an abnormal degree may move a considerable distance from their normal position while not being involved in a torsion or volvulus themselves. If an organ is involved, there will be a twisting or kinking at its origin or attachment. The direction of the displacement must be determined by the surgeon before he can proceed. Then the palm of the hand is used to push the organ around and back into normal alignment. The forearm and upper arm are sometimes used as levers in performing the procedure. The surgeon

should avoid pulling on organs or their attachments, as they tear or rupture. Rather, they should be pushed as gently as possible. In some cases it may be difficult for the surgeon to be sure of the outcome. Rotation of the structure in the opposite direction may help to determine which way feels and looks normal.

Some Guidelines for Laparotomy

The basic criteria used for decision making in laparotomy include assessment of the history and clinical signs together with physical findings and confirmation of suspicions using laboratory tests. The history usually indicates a sudden onset of illness, and observation of the surroundings of the animal and its diet, together with herd history, may be suggestive of a problem amenable to surgical correction.

Although the body temperature may be an unreliable indicator, a pulse rate near 100/min suggests a serious problem. Progressive dehydration, weakness, or recumbency indicates deterioration of the situation and carries a poorer prognosis. Gradually progressive abdominal distension, especially if the abomasum, cecum, or intestines seem involved, suggests laparotomy.

Diminished or scant fecal passage is suggestive of functional obstruction, as in vagal indigestion, or physical obstruction, as in abomasal volvulus. Often an abnormality can be tentatively diagnosed by rectal palpation. The feel of fibrinous adhesions pulling apart during rectal examination suggests peritonitis and possibly indicates a poor prognosis. Colic implies pain due to tension on the mesenteric root or uterine ligaments and is a good indication for surgery.

Specific laboratory tests that may assist in surgical decision making include peritoneal fluid analysis, hemogram, and serum electrolyte determination.

Left-side exploratory laparotomy is undertaken when one suspects traumatic gastritis, vagal indigestion, or disease of any organ easily reached from the left side. Incisions can be made as noted in Figure 15–17, depending on what the surgeon expects to find.

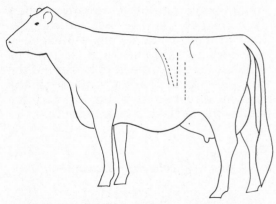

Figure 15–17 Left side of a dairy cow, showing sites for surgical incision.

Exploratory laparotomy from the right paralumbar fossa is performed for evaluation of the liver, gallbladder and bile duct, pancreas, intestinal tract, genital tract, and kidneys. Specifically, this approach may facilitate examination of the abomasum for diseases such as impaction, volvulus, and displacement.

Surgical Approaches in the Treatment of Abdominal Disease

There are several approaches to the surgical exploration of the bovine abdomen and the treatment of abdominal diseases. These approaches are illustrated in Figures 15–17 and 15–18: right or left flank approach—paralumbar fossa; right or left flank approach—low flank; right or left flank approach—low, above udder; right or left paramedian approach (per rectus); and midline approach. The indications for these approaches and the surgical techniques are described.

Right or Left Flank Approach—Paralumbar Fossa (Fig. 15–17). This method is useful for diagnostic laparotomy (right or left), rumenotomy (left), replacement of abomasal displacements (right or left), therapy of intestinal disorders (right), caesarean section (right or left), and therapy of urogenital diseases (right or left). The approach can be made in any part of the paralumbar fossa, depending on the task and the disease being treated.

In most cases the skin incision will be 20 to 30 cm in length. An incisional approach is made through the muscles, one layer at a time. When the transversus abdominis muscle is reached, a small opening can be made in its center using a Metzenbaum scissors. When the peritoneum is located, it can be grasped, lifted away from underlying abdominal organs, and incised. Then the peritoneum and muscle can be incised together. This method avoids accidental incision of underlying abdominal organs and facilitates closure of the peritoneum after the operation.

The surgeon should develop a routine method of examination of the abdomen for abnormalities even if the diagnosis is apparently obvious, such as might be the case with an abomasal displacement. For example, from the left flank the surgeon should examine the rumen, spleen, reticulum, sublumbar lymph nodes, kidneys, genital tract, urinary bladder, intestinal tract, omentum, liver, and abomasum. The presence or absence of fluid or fibrin can be visualized before palpation of the organs. The authors prefer to use the right arm for palpation of the abdomen from the left side. From the right side the order of inspection is the

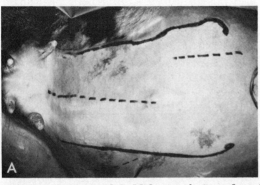

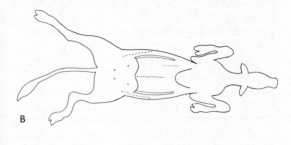

Figure 15–18 A and B, Mid-ventral view of cow's abdomen showing the right paramedian approach, the mid-ventral approach, and the low flank approach.

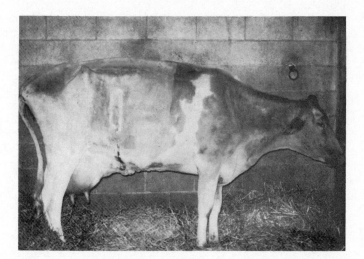

Figure 15–19 Right flank approach, low flank, in standing animal.

omentum, pancreas, liver, gallbladder, omasum, abomasum, reticulum, diaphragm, intestinal tract, kidneys, sublumbar nodes, genital tract, and urinary bladder.

Closure of the abdominal cavity in an adult animal is usually accomplished by using a simple continuous suture pattern with #3 chromic catgut in the transversus abdominis muscle and peritoneum, closing these as one layer from top to bottom. The remaining two muscle layers can be closed as one unless they are rather thick; if they are thick, then two layers should be used. A simple continuous pattern as previously mentioned is used. Normally, a subcutaneous suture is not required. The skin can be closed with a continuous pattern unless sepsis has been encountered; in such cases, a simple interrupted pattern should be employed in case a subcutaneous infection should develop.

Other methods of closure have been used. The technique of choice is the decision of the surgeon.

Right or Left Flank Approach—Low Flank (Figs. 15–19 and 15–20). This approach is used in standing animals for some cases of caesarean section or in recumbent animals for exploratory laparotomy or therapy of some gastrointestinal disorders. Basically, the surgical technique for this approach is the same as that for the paralumbar approach. Occasionally, some difficulty may arise in closing the abdominal incision and extra tension may be required.

Right or Left Flank Approach—Low,

Above the Udder (Fig. 15–18). This approach is used in the recumbent animal as an approach for caesarean section. Incision should be made carefully, one layer at a time. The approach provides good access for examination of the gravid uterus but offers limited access to the rest of the abdominal cavity.

Right or Left Paramedian Approach (Per Rectus) (Fig. 15–18). This procedure is used on the right side for access to the abomasum and omasum and is primarily used for therapy of abomasal disease. A 20- to 30-cm incision is made with the animal in dorsal recumbency. The abomasum is normally just beneath the surgical site. A three-layer closure is made,

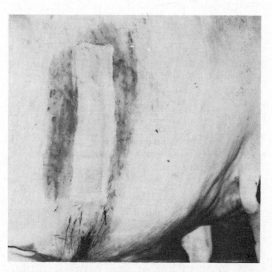

Figure 15–20 A colloidion bandage in place over a surgical incision site on the flank of a cow.

Table 15–1 SURGICAL APPROACHES TO THE ABDOMEN

Approach	Advantages	Disadvantages
Paralumbar fossa	1. Performed on standing animal 2. Ease of exploration of entire abdomen	Animal may go down if adhesions are encountered or if tension is applied to mesentery
Low flank	1. Performed on standing animal 2. Good access to intestines and genital tract	Potential for spillage of organs during surgery is increased
Low flank, above udder	Good access to caudal abdomen and uterus	1. Requires good restraint in recumbency 2. Incision difficult to extend
Paramedian (per rectus)	Good access to forestomachs and abomasum on right side	1. Requires good restraint in recumbency 2. May be difficult to extend incision 3. Access to caudal abdomen is poor
Midline	Incision can be easily enlarged for more access	Requires good restraint in recumbency

using catgut in the fascia and muscle and a nonabsorbable suture in the skin.

Midline Approach. The ventral midline approach is used with the animal in dorsal recumbency or tipped slightly. The usual indication for this approach is caesarean section, but this approach can be used for treatment of some intestinal disorders.

The advantages and disadvantages of the approaches to the abdomen are summarized in Table 15–1.

Diseases of the Rumen and Reticulum

Diseases of these parts of the ruminant digestive tract are very common. Tympanitis, rumenitis, ruminal acidosis, rumen impaction, foreign body obstruction, foreign body penetration, and focal peritonitis are everyday problems in bovine practice. In many cases medical therapy will help to restore function, but in other cases surgical intervention is needed to speed recovery.

Tympany. Rumen tympany may have several basic causes. These are disturbances of eructation of the gas associated with obstructions, pain, herniation, and frothy rumen contents. More specific examples include the following:

1. Foreign body obstruction of the esophagus or cardia.

2. Pain in the diaphragmatic area due to pneumonia; focal peritonitis; extensive fibrous adhesions of the anterior abdomen; liver abscessation; or foreign body penetration of the rumen, reticulum, or pericardium.

3. Diaphragmatic herniation of the reticulum; presence of abscess or tumor.

4. Left abomasal displacement or abomasal volvulus involving the omasum and/or reticulum.

5. Frothy bloat associated with dietary changes.

Tympany can be relieved by passing a stomach tube and/or administering surfactant. The primary cause should be determined so that corrective action can be taken. If the inciting cause cannot be found, rumenostomy may be indicated.

Acidosis. There is a tendency in some areas of the world to confine ruminants for beef or dairy production and feed them for maximum rate of gain or lactation. Sometimes they are fed more like monogastrics than ruminants. Such feeding practices may lead to ruminal acidosis or related digestive disorders, which cause many diagnostic problems for the practitioner. Many of these problems require surgery.

Acidosis usually results from sudden dietary changes, especially a change from a high forage to a high energy ration. Some diets are too finely chopped or too wet, thus discouraging chewing and the production of saliva, one of the best natural buffers. If acidosis is a problem based on diagnosis of individual animal problems, some recommendations for correction and prevention include the following:

1. Increasing the level of forages in the ration.

2. Increasing the fiber level of the grain mixture.

3. Feeding the same amount of grain

divided into smaller portions fed more frequently.

4. Changing the texture of the grain from finely ground to coarse or rolled.

5. Chopping forages such as corn silage in larger pieces and ensiling at less than 65 per cent moisture.

6. Ensuring that the total ration fed offers a minimum crude fiber level between 13 and 17 per cent.

Traumatic Gastritis. The penetration of the ruminant forestomachs by foreign objects has been recognized and treated for many years. Cattle are inquisitive and tend to consume all sorts of objects while foraging (Fig. 15–21). In more recent times some management problems, such as feeding ground or pelleted feeds or chopped hay or silage, have contributed to the presence of foreign objects in feeds. The objects most commonly contributing to traumatic puncture of the stomach are metallic: wires, nails, needles, and staples.

The syndrome shown by any one animal affected with a foreign body puncture of the stomach may be quite variable and depends on a number of factors, including (1) size, shape, and nature of the foreign body; (2) location and degree of damage at the puncture site; and (3) degree of contamination at the time of and subsequent to puncture. Thus, an animal may show signs varying from mild pain, listlessness, and anorexia to severe pain, recumbency, and severe depression. Common signs of traumatic gastritis include anorexia, depression, fever, decreased milk production in lactating cattle, pain in the anterior abdomen, expiratory grunt, stiffened gait, and constipation.

The condition may occur in any animal. Although a case has been reported in a one-month-old calf, most cases occur in adults. Cows may be affected in late pregnancy or at parturition, especially.

The laboratory confirmation of the disease may also perplex the practitioner. Neutrophilic leukocytosis with a left shift is common. But in severe cases with overwhelming sepsis a leukopenia is present.

CASE HISTORY. A six-year-old Holstein cow had recently calved and had a poor appetite. She walked with an arched back. There was a mucoid nasal discharge. No rumination had been seen. On physical examination the temperature was 101.4° F. The respiratory rate was 32/min with slightly harsh lung sounds.

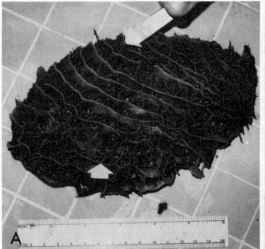

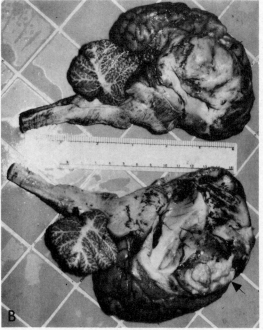

Figure 15–21 A, Necropsy specimen showing penetration of a wire through the folds of the reticulum. B, The brain from the cow in A. This cow had recurrent bouts of nervous disease, which was at first thought to be nervous ketosis.

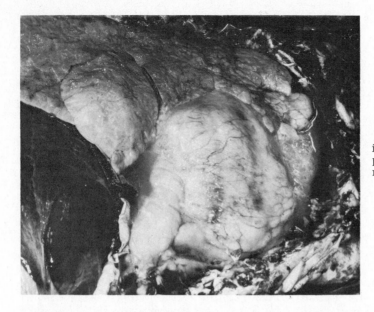

Figure 15-22 Fibrinous pleuritis in a cow that died as a result of a penetrating foreign body from the reticulum to the thorax.

The heart rate was 84/min. On examination, the rectum seemed adherent to surrounding structures.

The hemogram yielded the following information: hemoglobin 11.6; PCV 33 per cent; white blood cells 16,300; segmented neutrophils 67 per cent, 10,921; nonsegmented neutrophils 19 per cent, 3,097; lymphocytes 12 per cent, 1,956; eosinophils 2 per cent, 326. Diagnosis: traumatic reticuloperitonitis. Prognosis: poor.

Some of the common complications of traumatic gastritis include traumatic pericarditis and vagus indigestion. Traumatic pericarditis is usually associated with foreign body puncture of the reticulum, diaphragm, and pericardium. If the heart is punctured, death may be sudden. Otherwise, infection develops within the pericardium, resulting in a tamponade and signs of heart failure and sepsis (Fig. 15-22). Some animals may respond to conservative therapy of pericardial drainage and/or antibiotic instillation but may later develop constrictive pericardial adhesions. Some serious cases may require pericardiotomy, pericardiostomy, or partial pericardectomy. Prognosis in most cases is guarded to poor for return of function.

CASE HISTORY. A Holstein cow was admitted for examination with a vague history of inappetence. The cow was pregnant and due to calve shortly. Temperature was 103° F. The respiratory rate was 56/min with some open-mouth breathing related to tenesmus. The heart rate was 132/min. No brisket edema or jugular vein distension was noticed. Splashing sounds were heard over the heart. There was no rumen motility, and feces were loose and scant in quantity. Hemogram showed anemia and neutrophilia with electrolytes normal except for low bicarbonate and high phosphate values.

The cow was in labor, but the owner did not realize it. A live calf was delivered. Pericarditis was treated medically, with some improvement noted. However, the cow was destroyed subsequently because of its deteriorating condition.

Vagal Indigestion. Another consequence of traumatic gastritis may be the development of vagal indigestion. However, other causes of vagal indigestion syndromes include peritonitis from various causes such as perforating abomasal ulcers or abomasal volvulus, interference with normal digestion from fat necrosis lesions or lymphosarcoma neoplasms, and occlusion of the omasal orifice with tumors or neoplasms.

The right vagal nerve (ventral) mainly innervates the reticulum, omasum, and abomasum, whereas the left vagal nerve (dorsal) serves the rumen with branches to the other areas. The physiological importance of the vagal nerves can be demonstrated by their role in rumen and reticular contractility, transport of ingesta from the reticulum to the abomasum, eructation, regurgitation, closure of the esophageal groove during suckling, abomasal motility, and abomasal secretion.

Hoflund described four types of functional disturbances associated with sectioning of the vagal nerves in different areas.

1. Functional stenosis between the reticulum and omasum with atony of the rumen and reticulum.

2. Functional stenosis between the reticulum and omasum with normal or hyperactive ruminal and reticular motility.

3. Permanent functional stenosis of the pylorus with atony or normal activity of the reticulum.

4. Incomplete pyloric stenosis.

CONSERVATIVE TREATMENT FOR SUSPECTED CASES OF TRAUMATIC GASTRITIS

Stober advises that the basis for non-surgical therapy in traumatic gastritis is that many metallic foreign bodies eventually return to the reticulum and often corrode until they can no longer be found when the cavity is explored. Such treatment methods have included the following:

1. External massage of the xiphoid process.

2. Administration of purges orally.

3. Elevation of the forequarters of the animal.

4. Fasting.

5. Intraperitoneal antibiotic therapy.

6. Search with a retriever magnet.

7. Administration of a magnet or a cage magnet.

The first two methods are not helpful. Elevation of the forequarters may help to relieve pressure from the diaphragmatic area and when combined with antibiotic therapy and administration of a magnet may be of some use. The use of antibiotics alone sometimes is useful, but the degree of the problem cannot be ascertained without surgery. Therefore, the prognosis with antibiotic therapy cannot be accurate.

The magnetic retriever was at first thought to be a great advance in therapy. It was subsequently shown to be effective in only 20 per cent of cases as well as being time-consuming in its use.

Since most foreign bodies are metallic, such as wires and nails, the use of magnets as therapeutic and preventive measures was instituted. With the commonly used round or I-shaped bar magnets, some odd-shaped wire objects were still capable of penetration. Therefore, caged magnets or magnets with plastic flanges have been introduced to overcome the problem.

The success of magnets in retrieving embedded or offending foreign objects ranges from 20 to 80 per cent. The early administration of a magnet, particularly a caged magnet, is the most promising conservative treatment available for traumatic gastritis. Of course, accurate diagnosis and conscientious follow-up treatment of the patient, as noted by Stober, are important in successful therapy.

The decision to operate should be based on diagnosis and the economics of the situation. Some cattle may not be valuable enough to warrant the cost of surgery. In some instances antibiotics may have been given already, thus precluding slaughter for some withdrawal time. Surgery allows for removal of the offending object and exploration to determine the degree of involvement, thus offering at least a stabilization of the disease process and an opportunity to give a more educated prognosis in each case.

Surgery of the Rumen and Reticulum

RUMENOTOMY

Rumenotomy is a useful procedure both diagnostically and therapeutically. Many times cattle present with a vague set of clinical symptoms from which one cannot make a definite diagnosis or confirm a diagnosis with laboratory tests. Such animals are candidates for exploratory laparotomy in the left paralumbar fossa and possible rumenotomy to explore for abnormalities within the stomach.

Many alternatives to the standard rumenotomy procedure have been suggested but unfortunately do not lend themselves to adequate exploration because of interference with other organs or because of the walling-off process that may have already commenced. The direct approach to the reticulum is a midline incision immediately posterior to the xiphoid of sufficient length to insert a

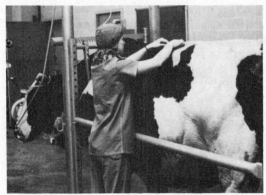

Figure 15–23 Because of their size, dairy bulls pose problems in exploratory examination of the reticulum.

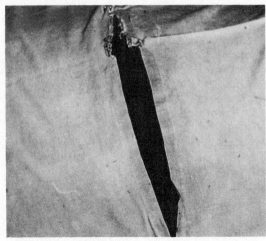

Figure 15–24 Oblique incision close to the last rib to give extra reach.

hand. To approach the reticulum from the ventral aspect, it is necessary to break down adhesions that may have formed to prevent the spread of infection. This would permit a more diffuse spread of infection and is, therefore, contraindicated.

The indirect approach necessitates entering the reticulum via the rumen. Because of the bulk of the ingesta that is normally present in this organ and the difficulty in manipulating such a large organ, a standing laparotomy is desirable. The operator must be able to reach the reticulum to carry out a thorough examination of its inner aspect. The factors that must be taken into consideration in accomplishing this include the site of the laparotomy incision, the size of the animal, and the length of the operator's arm (Fig. 15–23).

The laparotomy incision must be of adequate size to permit the insertion of a hand and arm, and it must be close enough to the paracostal border to permit the operator to reach the reticulum (Fig. 15–24). Sufficient flank wall caudal to the ribs must be left to suture the wound, and the opening must be high enough in the flank to expose the rumen above the left longitudinal groove and its attached superficial fold of greater omentum.

It is necessary to consider a means of preventing gross contamination of the peritoneal cavity once the rumen is opened. This may be done in a number of ways, and although most surgeons have preferences, such preferences should not become hard-and-fast rules. The character of the rumen contents rather than the preference of the operator should dictate the method used (Noordsy 1980).

Consider the case of an adult Charolais bull presented with vague signs of listlessness, weight loss, and abdominal distension (Fig. 15–25). Physical examination did not confirm a diagnosis of peritonitis, nor did laboratory tests. Left flank diagnostic exploratory laparotomy was performed but did not reveal any abnormalities. Only when the rumen was opened and evacuated was the problem discerned. Many keratinized papillomata were acting to obstruct outflow from the reticulum and rumen into the omasum and abomasum (Fig. 15–26).

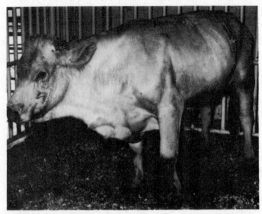

Figure 15–25 A bull with symptoms of vagus indigestion. In this case exploratory laparotomy did not reveal peritonitis. Exploratory rumenotomy revealed blockage of the omasal orifice with cornified papillomas.

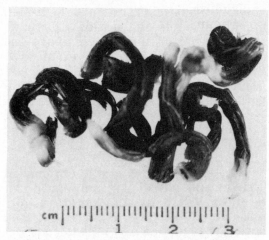

Figure 15–26 Cornified papillomas removed from the omasal orifice in a bull with symptoms of vagus indigestion.

When these were removed, the bull's condition was improved.

Care must be taken in making the incision through the peritoneum, as sometimes the rumen is directly adherent to the abdominal wall or is sometimes very full and easily accidentally punctured. Exploratory laparotomy is performed before the rumenotomy procedure. This allows the surgeon to evaluate the presence or absence of suspected abnormalities and may aid in establishing a prognosis.

Several techniques are available for performing rumenotomy. In general, it is necessary to use some method whereby the rumen wall is temporarily secured firmly against the flank wall so that contamination of the muscles and peritoneal cavity is avoided. These methods include suturing the rumen to the skin before incision, the use of a rumen ring and shroud inserted into a rumenotomy incision, and the use of a self-retaining rumen retractor employing large vulsellum forceps and hooks. All of these techniques aim to avoid contamination of the peritoneal cavity by isolating the rumen before opening it or as it is opened. Regardless of the method used, a rubber shroud should be added to complement the retention device and thus avoid excessive gross contamination of the surgical field by the rumen contents (Fig. 15–27).

The self-retaining rumen retractor is held in place with Merillat vulsellum forceps and stainless steel hooks (Fig. 15–28). The forceps are used to grasp the rumen in an area of relative avascularity. Then the rumenotomy incision is started ventrally and continued dorsally, with the hooks applied as required (Fig. 15–29). This technique helps to avoid contamination of the musculature and abdomen from dribbling rumen ingesta (Fig. 15–30). In cases in which the rumen is full of very liquid, finely digested material, as in vagal indigestion, a very large diameter rubber stomach tube can be used to siphon off the contents to allow exploration of the chambers. In the case of coarse material, manual removal of the contents will have to be performed to a point at which the cavity can be explored.

The search of the reticulum will necessitate either removing some ingesta or

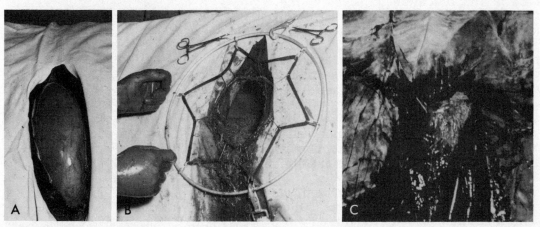

Figure 15–27 *A*, Temporary stay suture, rumen to skin. *B*, Michael and McKinley rumenotomy ring. *C*, Rubber rumenotomy shroud.

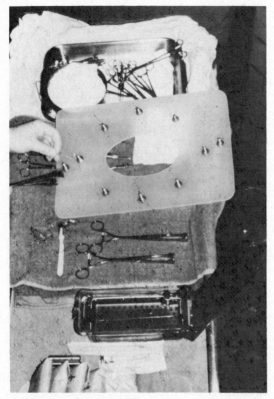

Figure 15–28 Equipment for rumenotomy including the Gabel rumen retractor board and Merillat vulsellum forceps.

forcing an arm through the ingesta in the direction of the reticulum, since the solid phase in the stratification of the rumen contents is such that it interferes with the approach to the reticulum. A thorough search of the interior of this compartment is then conducted. The anteromedial wall, the ventral wall beneath the esophageal groove, and the area of the reticulum adjacent to the rumenoreticular fold should not be overlooked. The cardia and the esophageal groove should be examined by direct palpation. An indirect assessment of other parts of the stomach can be made through the right wall of the rumen. This is usually carried out when the ventral aspect of the rumen is examined. By palpation through the right rumen wall, one can identify and to a certain extent assess the condition of the abomasum and omasum.

The incision in the rumen should be made in the dorsal compartment. After some ingesta is removed, the rumen wall collapses in against the remaining in-

gesta. Although this portion of the rumen quickly distends again with a gas cap, rumen incisions made well above the groove are not in contact with the left flank wall for a short period and are less likely to become adherent to the parietal peritoneum.

Next, a magnet can be introduced and swept over the surface of the rumen and reticulum to retrieve metal objects (Figs. 15–31 and 15–32).

The motility of the cardia, esophageal groove, and reticulo-omasal orifice can be checked digitally. A rather grave prognosis should be given if the last-named structure is dilated and fails to constrict as the fingers probe.

Before the rumenotomy incision is closed, a magnet can be left in the reticulum if desired. Mineral oil or lubricant can be pumped through a tube placed in the reticulo-omasal orifice into the omasum and abomasum for the treatment of impaction. As an alternative, an indwelling nasogastric tube can be left in the reticulo-omasal orifice for repeated postoperative treatment. The rumen can be re-inoculated with normal flora, or some fresh coarse hay can be placed within the cavity before closure.

Regardless of the method used to retain the rumen, some means of temporary control must be available until the first row of rumen sutures is applied for closure. A temporary stay suture technique (temporary rumenostomy) can be

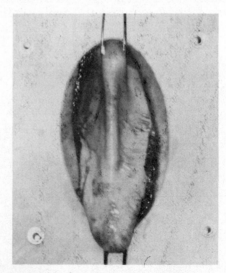

Figure 15–29 The rumen retractor in place prior to opening the rumen.

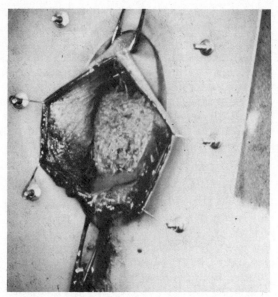

Figure 15–30 Opening the rumen and holding it in place with hooks. The rumen fluid flows out onto the board and does not contaminate the abdominal cavity.

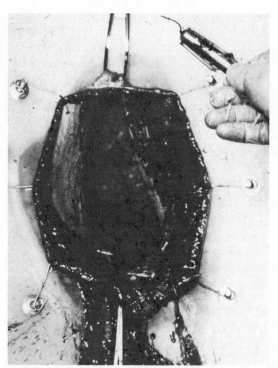

Figure 15–31 A wire and a nail have been removed from the reticulum with the aid of a magnet.

used; temporary control is often not possible with many of the mechanical contrivances mentioned previously that hook into the incised edge of the rumen incision. After adequate cleansing to remove gross contamination, a reinforcing second row of sutures is placed. It is enlightening to observe the force of rumen motility during surgery. These movements will pull the rumen away from the laparotomy incision if haphazard methods of control are used when the organ is open; this will result in contamination of the cavity. The dangers inherent in trocarization of the rumen should also be realized. This procedure should only be carried out in life-saving emergencies, fully realizing that sequelae to this approach may necessitate sacrificing the animal for slaughter. Since no one method is suitable for all circumstances, it is wise to familiarize oneself with several methods of avoiding contamination during this procedure.

Closure of the rumenotomy incision involves an inverting type of suture pattern such as Cushing, Lembert, or modified Cushing (Guard's rumen stitch). Closure should be started at the dorsal part of the incision and should progress downward, removing the hooks as needed. After the rumen incision is closed, dry swabs can

be used to remove any debris or fibrin from the wound margins before the rumen is replaced into the abdominal cavity. Washing with saline is generally avoided to prevent contamination of the peritoneal cavity.

The abdominal musculature can be flushed with an antibiotic solution before closure if some contamination is suspected. Skin closure should be performed with some form of interrupted suture pattern in case one or more sutures have

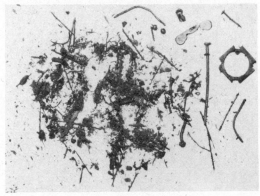

Figure 15–32. This photograph shows the wide array of metallic objects removed from a magnet in an old cow. None of these objects was penetrating the reticulum.

to be removed because of abscess development.

The complications of rumenotomy include peritonitis, abdominal wound dehiscence, and abscess formation in the abdominal musculature. All of these complications result from contamination of tissue with rumen ingesta. Mild cases of peritonitis result in the development of a few adhesions within the abdominal cavity, often causing the rumen to adhere to the body wall.

More severe peritonitis almost always results from imperfect closure of the rumenotomy incision and a resulting gross leak of ingesta. This may cause death in the immediate postoperative period, or a large abscess may form between the rumen and the laterodorsal abdominal wall, causing an accumulation of a great amount of fibrin and gas. Such cases may respond to treatment, but it will be very prolonged and thus probably not an economically feasible solution.

Abdominal wound dehiscence may accompany a gross leak of contents from the rumen. However, more often it is the result of a failure to isolate the rumen sufficiently from the body during the procedure or from a break in technique during surgery. Contamination of the musculature with ingesta is a difficult problem to solve because of the many fascial planes involved and the fact that plant fibers tend to adhere to tissue and are difficult to remove.

An abscess that develops postoperatively in the subcutaneous tissues or the abdominal wall usually results from a break in technique, allowing a small amount of contamination, and/or arises from an inadequate postoperative course of antibacterial therapy.

Abnormal distension may arise in the course of many disease conditions; the distension may be the result of fluid, gas, or grain overload. Surgical intervention, although possible in situations in which

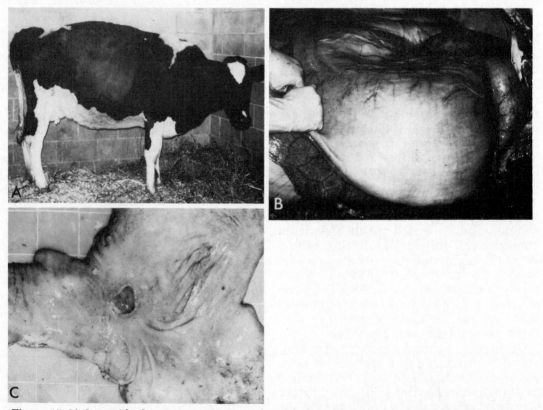

Figure 15–33 Cow with chronic inappetence and weight loss following surgical correction of omasal-abomasal torsion. *A,* This cow has all of the symptoms of vagus indigestion: bilateral abdominal distension, bloat, hypermotility of the rumen, and scant passage of feces. *B,* Huge distension of the abomasum. *C,* An abomasal ulcer in the abomasum.

one or two animals are involved, may not be feasible when a number of animals require attention, such as in herd or feedlot situations of grain overload. In some cases of traumatic reticuloperitonitis, a syndrome commonly referred to as vagus indigestion is encountered. The rumen may become distended and hypermotile, resulting in an intermix of ingesta and gas (frothy bloat), or there may be rumen atony and the rumen may be fluid filled (Fig. 15–33). It has been shown that a fasting animal or an animal off feed has a greater amount of fluid than an animal on full feed, and in some digestive disturbances excess water intake may add to the amount of fluid present. These cases pose problems during rumenotomy procedures because of the increased risk of contamination.

Tympany may be acute or chronic, and, although acute cases do respond to medical therapy, chronic cases are often resistant to treatment and must be handled by rumenostomy techniques (rumen fistulization) to avoid economic loss to the owner. Rumen fistulization can be performed by either surgical incision or a screw-type trocar technique.

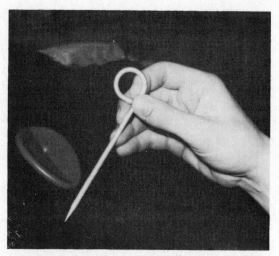

Figure 15–34 Insertion of a plastic screw cannula into the rumen in a case of chronic bloat. The trocar can be used for insertion and also for unblocking the cannula.

RUMENOSTOMY

Rumenostomy is a procedure performed for temporary or permanent alleviation of chronic rumen tympany of any cause. There are at least three methods of solving this problem. One involves suturing the rumen to the skin in the midparalumbar fossa area and making a fistula. Another involves placement of a large screw-type trocar and cannula. Also, a disposable plastic cannula is available for insertion into a rumen incision (Fig. 15–34).

The first technique involves making a small 5-cm incision vertically in the upper middle portion of the left paralumbar fossa. Local analgesia is used for this technique. The muscles and peritoneum can be separated with the use of scissors to allow the rumen to be grasped. The rumen is then sutured to either the skin or the abdominal musculature before a small incision is made to allow gas to escape. Usually the intermittent escape of gas will prevent closure of the fistula, but occasionally fibrous connective tis-

sue may cause a stenosis or closure of the opening. Some leakage of rumen contents may occur from this aperture, even though it is made in the dorsal part of the flank. The procedure is most useful in feedlot steers that have become chronic bloaters.

A second technique involves the temporary placement of a large plastic screw into the rumen through a skin incision. The screw-type cannula and its trocar are introduced into the rumen via a small incision through the skin and musculature. It is then screwed into place and left for as long as desired but usually only for a brief period of days. The disadvantage of this technique is that normal motility or hypermotility of the rumen may cause the stomach to become disconnected from the cannula. This could lead to peritonitis or death.

A third method, also temporary in nature, involves the placement of a plastic indwelling cannula called a bloat whistle* into the rumen. An incision is made in the upper portion of the paralumbar fossa. The rumen can be grasped and incised. One-half of the cylinder portion of the cannula can be slipped into the rumen. Then the second half can be slipped into position and snapped to the first, forming a hollow tube. A circular

---

*Bloat whistle (McVet, Inc., 102 Sunset Street, Waverly, IA 50677).

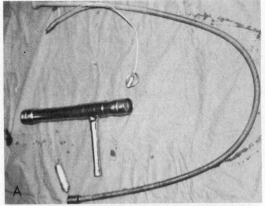

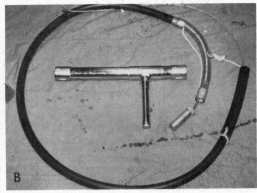

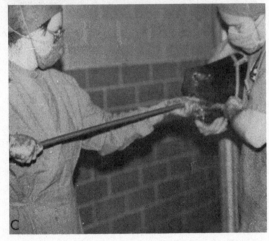

Figure 15–35 *A*, Muffly metal retriever. *B*, Modified Muffly metal retriever. *C*, Passing a metal retriever.

collar is slid over the two halves and is locked in place to form a secure fistula. The device reportedly can be left in place for a long period of time.

Grain overload and even some cases of vagal indigestion may best be handled by rumen lavage. Mechanical irrigation to relieve rumenal distension is carried out with a Kingman tube (oversized garden hose), more recently reviewed and reported with some modification (Radostits and Magnusson 1971). A similar approach has been used in the oral retrieval of foreign bodies and is still practiced by some veterinarians using a Muffly or modified Muffly retrieval device (Fig. 15–35). There are several modifications of this technique, one of which includes the flank approach through a trocar wound (Carlson 1958).

Neoplasms, abscesses, and trauma may involve the rumen and reticulum, but surgical correction is feasible only when there is minor involvement. Partial resection of the rumen and reticulum, although feasible experimentally, is not a procedure that is carried out in clinical situations. Surgical drainage of abscesses is possible when these are located and identified (Fig. 15–36), most frequently during exploratory rumenotomy procedures. Lancing and drainage

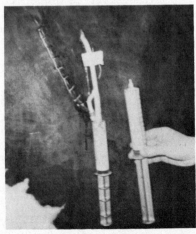

Figure 15–36 Surgical drainage of an abdominal abscess in a cow.

into the reticulum or rumen are possible with minimal risk of peritonitis because such abscesses are usually walled off.

DIAPHRAGMATIC HERNIATION

Chronic ruminal distension has many causes as previously described. This is also the most consistent clinical sign in diaphragmatic herniation. The most frequently herniated organ is the reticulum.

Since the incidence of diaphragmatic herniation is greatest secondary to traumatic reticuloperitonitis, most diaphragmatic defects are identified during rumenotomy procedures. If surgery is contemplated for diaphragmatic hernia, a second operation through a midline approach is preferred.

Congenital defects in the diaphragm have been encountered in calves (Fig. 15–37). They usually conform to the defect described as peritoneo-pericardial-diaphragmatic hernia. Although surgical repair is occasionally successful in calves, the economics of cattle practice preclude surgical intervention. Traumatic injuries causing diaphragmatic hernia in neonates can usually be corrected surgically.

Although the problem of herniation is infrequently reported in cattle, the incidence in buffalo seems to be increasing. The hernia in buffalo occurs at the musculotendinous junction of the diaphragm, ventral to the foramen vena cava and slightly lateral to the median plane. Often adhesions form between the reticulum and hernia ring, pleura, lung, pericardium, or thoracic wall. Diagnosis of this problem may be difficult without exploratory laparotomy. Recently, radiographic techniques have been used as an aid in diagnosis.

Once a diagnosis has been established, surgical therapy can be applied. Paracostal, paramedian, and lateral thoracic approaches have been used. A post-xiphoid approach, with the animal in dorsal recumbency, employing a curvilinear incision was applied with a reported 80 per cent success rate in more than 200 cases. Of course, general anesthesia is required for restraint and positive pressure ventilation must be maintained.

Abomasum

This compartment of the ruminant's stomach has in recent years been incriminated as a source of both acute and chronic indigestion. The range of surgical conditions includes distension, displacement, torsion, ulceration, impaction, neoplasia, and, probably, pylorospasm. Unlike its counterpart, the simple stomach, foreign bodies are uncommon in the abomasum but have been observed. In the preruminant calf, ingested food enters the abomasum via the esophageal groove. On farms where husbandry is poor, coarse fiber and ingested hair will collect and may obstruct the pylorus. Improved husbandry will eliminate most of these cases. However, those so affected usually require surgical treatment. In one case an Anico magnet was found in the abomasum of a mature cow. In equally rare circumstances, penetrating foreign bodies have been found involving the abomasal wall.

ABOMASAL DISPLACEMENT

Certainly the incidence of left abomasal displacement seems to have increased in the last 20 to 30 years. Perhaps previous to this time the condition was not recognized accurately (Fig. 15–38), or perhaps management has

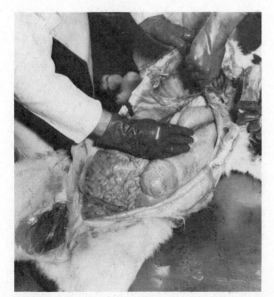

Figure 15–37 Peritoneo-pericardial-diaphragmatic hernia in a calf.

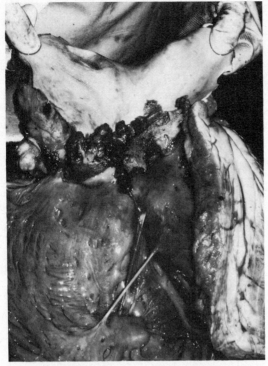

Figure 15–38 Chronic valvular endocarditis in a cow that was presented with a tentative diagnosis of abomasal displacement.

changed to bring about the apparent increase. Indeed, the problem has grown to the point where some veterinarians are advocating prophylactic surgery.

For years there has been considerable research on the subject of abomasal displacement involving epidemiological surveys, studies of the pathophysiology, examination of embalmed specimens, and pedigree analysis, to mention only a few investigations. A single cause for the problem seems to have been sought, yet a combination of factors seems to be more logical in explaining the development of the disease. Basically, genetic, mechanical, and physiological factors tend to be involved in the development of abomasal displacement.

The breeding of more productive dairy cattle has sometimes brought about the development of larger and deeper abdominal cavities, which might allow for more movement of the relatively free abomasum. Research supports this with the fact that cows with left abomasal displacement do have larger and deeper abdomens. In addition, the condition oc-

curs with more frequency in certain cow families or lines of cattle than in others.

Mechanical factors that favor the development of the condition include the shift or displacement of the abomasum brought about by the enlarging gravid uterus during pregnancy. There is an increased incidence of displacement in cows bearing twins or triplets. Confinement and/or the lack of exercise probably is another significant factor in the development of the disease. In a study conducted in 1974, an increased incidence of displacements was noticed in herds in which the dry cows were confined to free stall or cubicle housing as opposed to those herds in which the dry cows were housed loosely. In one very highly productive Jersey herd with a small incidence of this problem, forced exercise was probably preventive; it forced the cows to go down a rather steep hill, cross under a road, and climb another hill to the forage feeding area after milking and concentrate feeding.

Other mechanical factors may be dystocias, lameness of the left front or rear leg (Fig. 15–39), pain or swelling in the left half of the udder, and placement of animals in right lateral recumbency for hoof trimming (Fig. 15–40).

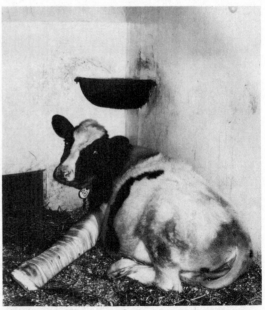

Figure 15–39 A six-month-old heifer with a comminuted open fracture of the metacarpus treated by external fixation. This calf always reclined on its right side and developed left abomasal displacement.

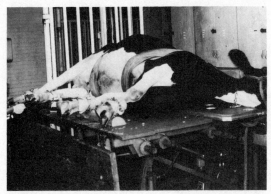

Figure 15–40 Positioning of a dairy cow on her left side on the operating table for foot trimming. Positioning of the cow on her right side has frequently resulted in subsequent left abomasal displacement.

The physiological factors that seem to be important in the pathogenesis of this disease include atony or hypomotility of the abomasum with delayed passage of ingesta and increased gas accumulation (Fig. 15–41), metabolic alkalosis, which may occur during the winter feeding period, and increased concentrate feeding or decreased crude fiber intake. Previous or concurrent diseases such as metritis, mastitis, and toxemia also seem to influence the development of the disease.

The diagnosis of left abomasal displacement can be ascertained in most cases from the history and physical examination (Fig. 15–42). Although there is no breed predisposition for the disease, the typical cow affected with abomasal displacement is four to six years old and develops signs of the condition within the first six weeks post partum. The disease seems to be more prevalent in the late winter and early spring. Commonly there is a history of concurrent disease or a stressful condition such as dystocia, multiple birth, transport, and so on shortly before signs develop.

Diagnosis can be confirmed by auscultation and percussion of the left side of the abdominal cavity. The differential diagnosis of gas sounds heard in the left flank should include rumen tympany, intraperitoneal abscesses dorsal to the rumen, and free gas in the peritoneal cavity. The laboratory data in uncomplicated cases will show a normal hemogram and normal acid-base balance. With severe concurrent diseases either leukopenia or leukocytosis may result. Stasis of the digestive tract may result in hypochloremic or hypokalemic metabolic alkalosis.

A classic sign of abomasal displacement is the selective appetite for forages but not concentrates. Other signs may be quite variable and may be related to the concurrent disease state. Some cows

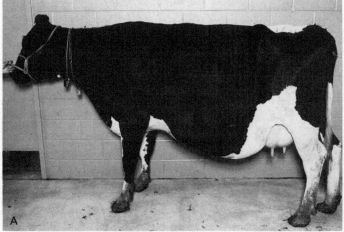

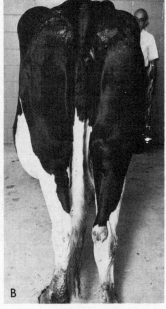

Figure 15–41 *A,* Hematoma as a result of rupture of an abdominal blood vessel. This cow reclined on her right side and developed left abomasal displacement. *B,* Posterior view.

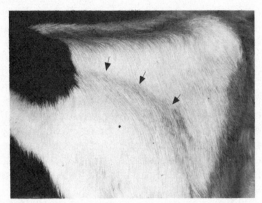

Figure 15–42 A dairy cow with left abomasal displacement showing a typical bulge of a gas distended organ under and behind the last rib on the left side.

may even have the disease for a long time and not show any signs.

The prognosis for conservative treatment of abomasal displacement is variable. Frequently, the condition recurs, probably because the omentum has been stretched and allows more freedom of movement of the abomasum. Rolling may lead to abomasal volvulus. Volvulus may also occur as a sequela spontaneously while cows are waiting for surgical treatment. Although abomasal displacement is not considered an emergency, prompt surgical correction is advisable. The corrective procedures will be detailed hereafter. The prognosis is usually quite favorable unless complications from concurrent disease interfere with return to function.

The abomasum can be easily reached from laparotomy incisions used in simple-stomached animals. Paracostal, ventral midline, or per rectus approaches may be used, depending on available facilities and operator preference. Surgical procedures carried out may involve pexis (fixation), incision, partial excision, decompression, and detorsion.

To provide stability and avoid recurrent displacement, various suturing procedures have been devised to anchor the organ to the abdominal wall or to anchor adjacent structures to prevent abnormal range of motion in the abomasum. The fear that such interference would inhibit normal function has been dispelled, and the fear that accidental penetration of the lumen in suturing would initiate diffuse peritonitis has not been warranted. The procedure is therefore acceptable, and the success rate is high.

Simple interrupted, simple continuous, or mattress sutures may be used. It is important to include more than the parietal peritoneum, otherwise the pexis may fail owing to the motility of the organ stripping the peritoneum from the abdominal wall at the site of attachment. In ventral approaches, the wall of the abomasum close to the attachment of the greater omentum may be sutured to the peritoneum and internal sheath of the rectus abdominis muscle. Suture bites should penetrate to the submucosal level of the abomasum. In the right flank omentopexy, the fold of greater omentum dorsocaudal to the pylorus is secured with mattress sutures to the peritoneum and fascia or muscle of the transverse abdominal muscle.

For left flank approaches, the greater omentum close to its attachment to the greater curvature of the abomasum is transfixed with a heavy suture, which is carried ventrally, keeping the anterior and posterior relationship of the suture strand constant. At the midline, anterior to the umbilicus, the full thickness of the abdominal wall is transfixed to secure these suture strands in mattress-suture fashion to the abdominal wall. Early North American reports included one series of 100 cases in which rumenopexy was performed, establishing a barrier to left displacement (Moore et al. 1955). This has been discarded, and other approaches are now used.

ABOMASAL VOLVULUS

Right-sided dilatation of the abomasum occurs in cattle. This may resolve spontaneously or may lead to the development of left abomasal displacement or abomasal volvulus. In the past the literature has referred to right-sided displacement of the abomasum and abomasal torsion. Since the term "torsion" implies the twisting of a body about its longitudinal axis, "volvulus" may be a better term, but both appear.

From a practical point of view, volvulus of the abomasum occurs in a counterclockwise direction as viewed from the right flank area (Fig. 15–43) (Gabel

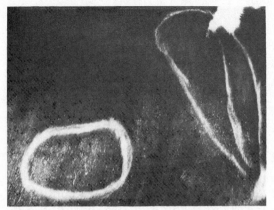

Figure 15–43 A dairy cow with abomasal volvulus. The area circled had the resonance of gas trapped within an organ.

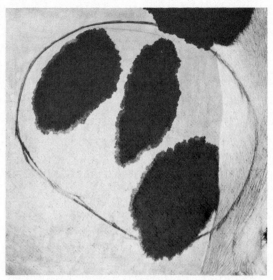

Figure 15–45 A Holstein cow with abomasal torsion. The area circled has gaseous resonance.

and Heath 1969b). Clockwise volvulus has been reported but is rare in the authors' experience. Varying degrees of volvulus seem to occur, including (1) volvulus of the abomasum in varying degrees, (2) volvulus of both the omasum and abomasum, and (3) volvulus of the reticulum, omasum, and abomasum. Without surgical intervention, the degree of volvulus cannot be ascertained, although one can predict that a more serious degree exists if there is a sudden onset with a severe degree of abdominal distension, anorexia, and cessation of lactation (Fig. 15–44).

Studies have shown that the severity of the condition is related to the amount of fluid sequestered in the abomasum. The most severely affected cows were markedly hypochloremic and hypoka-

lemic (Fig. 15–45). Packed cell volume, plasma protein concentration, and pulse rate increase with the severity of volvulus.

A significant correlation exists between the severity of the condition, serum chloride concentration, pulse rate, and the postsurgical outcome. The more severe types of volvulus exert great tension and pressure on the vagus nerve and the gastric blood vessels (Fig. 15–46). Thrombosis of these vessels occurs in some cases, so that even when the volvulus has been corrected, resulting infarction will lead to vagal indigestion syndrome and a nonfunctional animal.

ABOMASAL IMPACTION

Abomasal impaction may result from any of several causes. Traumatic gastritis and subsequent peritonitis or vagal involvement were mentioned previously. In these cases the motility of the abomasum is affected, usually causing it to gradually distend with ingesta. Other causes of impaction that affect motility include infiltration of the abomasum with lymphosarcoma and the development of large fat necrosis lesions adjacent to the abomasum.

An abomasal impaction can also occur through obstruction of outflow from the stomach. Causes of such obstruction might include neoplasia, fat necrosis, ab-

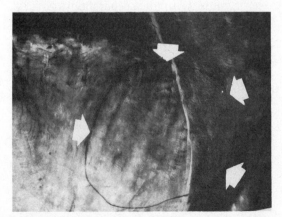

Figure 15–44 A Jersey cow with abomasal volvulus. The area outlined contained gas trapped within the organ.

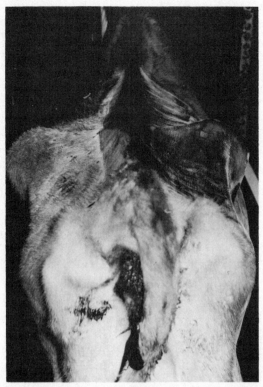

Figure 15–46 Clinical appearance of a cow chronically infected with incomplete abomasal torsion on the right side of the abdomen. Following surgical correction and fixation the cow returned to production and performed satisfactorily.

scessation, or stricture associated with adhesions.

Yet another, though perhaps infrequent, cause of impaction arises from the presence of foreign bodies in the abomasal lumen—sand accumulation, trichobezoars, phytobezoars, or other foreign objects that have been ingested.

The diagnosis is usually made from history, physical examination, and laparotomy. The abdomen of the cow will gradually enlarge on the right side, and the animal may become anorectic. Laboratory data may show hypochloremic alkalosis and dehydration.

The surgical approach to the treatment involves a flank or paramedian laparotomy, massage of the contents if possible, pyloromyotomy if appropriate, or abomasotomy. The prognosis depends on finding and treating the primary cause of the impaction. Some cases will have a hopeless prognosis, whereas the prognosis for others may be very good.

ABOMASAL ULCERS

Abomasal ulceration may be fairly common in cattle but yet subclinical. Diffuse ulceration may be present, or a single large ulcer or ulcers may develop. Nonperforating ulcers are difficult to diagnose. The affected animal may show few signs except for melena. Larger single ulcers may occur. These may be associated with the presence of another disease such as lymphosarcoma or abomasal displacement. If perforation occurs, focal or generalized peritonitis will result. In such cases the signs may vary from slight anterior abdominal pain and anorexia to severe shock and sudden death.

Most ulcers seem to occur in the fundic part of the abomasum. Occasionally, an ulcer will perforate through the abdominal wall and form a fistula. Although unsightly, the fistula may not interfere with function. However, it can be closed. First, the fistulous tract of the abomasum is resected from the skin. Then the organ is brought out so that the ulcer can be resected. Closure of the abomasum and abdominal wall is routine.

The prognosis for resection of a perforated ulcer in a cow or calf is poor. Accompanying peritonitis and toxemia are usually too severe to be reversed, even if the ulcer can be found and the defect repaired.

CASE HISTORY. A four-year-old Guernsey cow was presented with inappetence, depression, and roached back. The cow had been shown at an exposition the previous week. Temperature was 102.6° F. Respiratory rate was 72/min, with moist harshness of lung sounds. There was a mucoid nasal discharge and lack of motility in a rather full rumen. Feces were fluid in consistency. The hemogram yielded the following information: hemoglobin 13.0 gm/dl; PCV 42 per cent; white blood cell count 2,010; segmented neutrophils 10 per cent, 201; nonsegmented neutrophils 10 per cent, 201; lymphocytes 80 per cent, 1,608. The cow died, and post-mortem examination showed a perforating abomasal ulcer with generalized peritonitis, the perforation being through the diaphragm, and pleuritis.

CASE HISTORY. A Holstein cow was seen with a vague history of inappetence and weight loss. There had been a gradual distension of the abdomen. The cow was pregnant.

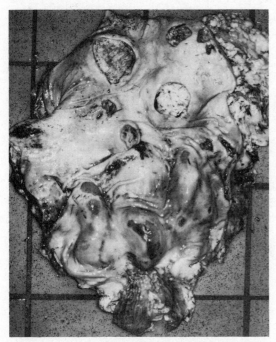

Figure 15–47 Multiple abomasal ulcers in the case of a cow with malignant lymphoma.

Heart rate was 100/min. No brisket edema was noted. The prefemoral lymph nodes were slightly enlarged. No intestinal motility was detected, nor were there any gas caps. The feces were scant, tarry, and black. Ketonuria was present. The hemogram yielded the following information: hemoglobin 9.1 gm/dl; PCV 25.5 per cent; white blood cell count 44,500; segmented neutrophils 8.5 per cent, 3,782; lymphocytes 91.5 per cent, 40,718. Lymphosarcoma was confirmed by laparotomy, and the cow was destroyed. Many large abomasal ulcers associated with neoplasia were present (Fig. 15–47).

SURGICAL CONSIDERATIONS IN ABOMASAL DISEASE

With abomasal displacement, care must be exercised in manipulating the abomasum and omental tissue regardless of the route of approach. Decompression is frequently necessary. The pylorus and omasal-abomasal junction should be palpated after decompression. The direction of the twist or kink, particularly as it involves the greater curvature, can be identified even if this was not possible prior to decompression.

Fluid sequestered in the abomasum will be difficult to remove if suction or other methods are not available. Abomasotomy and decompression of the abomasum via a standing right flank laparotomy are sometimes preferable in these shocked animals. Gross contamination of the cavity is less likely to occur with a right flank approach than with a ventral approach. In situations of extreme distension (fluid or impacted contents), avoiding gross contamination of the cavity is of major importance (Fig. 15–48).

Pulling on the greater omentum will frequently cause extensive damage to the vessels and omental attachment along the greater curvature. This could result in considerable hemorrhage and therefore should be avoided. The tendency to pull on the greater omentum is especially prevalent when attempting replacement from a right flank approach.

METHODS FOR SURGICAL CORRECTION OF ABOMASAL DISPLACEMENT

Several methods are available for the treatment of left abomasal displacement. All of them are highly successful in terms of recovery and nonrecurrence. These methods are as follows: left paralumbar fossa—omentopexy or abomasopexy; right paralumbar fossa—omentopexy; right paramedian—abomasopexy.

Abomasopexy and Omentopexy

Fixation of the replaced abomasum is advisable to prevent redisplacement. Recurrence is unfortunately still possible following the conservative rolling technique. This is not a condemnation of the conservative approach; for economic reasons, there is still a place for this approach and for the roll and blind suture technique described later. Of the numerous approaches and methods described over the years, three have remained in common use. Which technique is used depends on operator preference and the condition of the patient.

LEFT PARALUMBAR FOSSA—OMENTOPEXY

Utrecht Method (Fig. 15–49). This method was developed in the early 1960s specifically for those displacements in which a positive "ping" could be identified high in the left flank region. A left paralumbar fossa incision is made. The

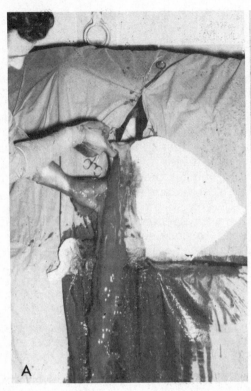

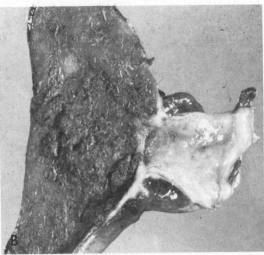

Figure 15–48 *A*, Fluid-filled abomasum. *B*, Necropsy view of impacted abomasum.

greater curvature of the displaced abomasum can be seen when the abdomen is opened (Fig. 15–50). The attachment of the greater omentum along the abomasum is easily located, and several bites are taken through this omentum as a long piece (60 cm) of nonabsorbable suture material is threaded through the

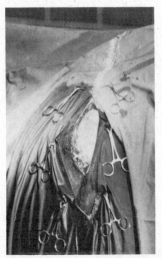

Figure 15–49 Mature bull with abomasal displacement. Utrecht method of fixation.

tissue. After this has been done the abomasum is decompressed using a 14- or 15-gauge, 5-cm needle and a piece of flexible rubber tubing. After the abomasum has been decompressed, it is carefully pushed to the bottom of the abdominal cavity so that the ends of the suture are not lost (Fig. 15–51). A cutting needle is placed on the anterior end of the suture and is then forced through the ventral midline 10 to 15 cm cranial to the umbilicus. An assistant can grasp the needle as it passes through the abdominal wall. A second cutting needle can then be threaded onto the caudal suture and similarly passed through the abdominal wall 5 to 10 cm cranial to the umbilicus. When the sutures have been placed, the assistant can pull them up tightly on the outside and tie them as the surgeon palpates the omentum on the inside of the abdomen to assure that the slack has been taken up in the sutures and that no other structures are caught between the sutures and the abdominal wall (Figs. 15–52 and 15–53). The object of the procedure is to create an adhesion between the omentum and abdominal wall to fix the abomasum into position

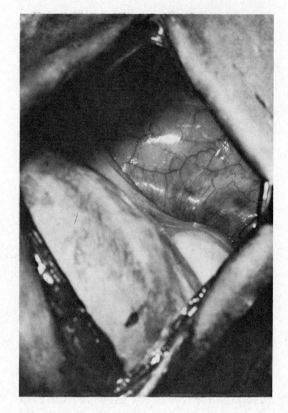

Figure 15–50 View from the left side of the abdominal cavity showing displaced abomasum in foreground and rumen behind it (the smaller organ).

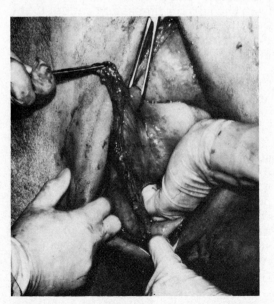

Figure 15–51 An adhesion that had to be severed to allow correction of left abomasal displacement. The adhesion was between the abomasum and the left abdominal wall.

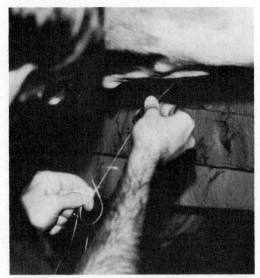

Figure 15–52 Ligature being tied on ventral abdomen to hold abomasum or omentum in position.

on the ventral floor. Some surgeons may prefer to bury the suture subcutaneously beneath a skin incision.

LEFT PARALUMBAR FOSSA—ABOMASOPEXY

Basically, this procedure is identical to the omentopexy. However, with this method the suture material is placed into the muscular wall of the abomasum or into the lumen of the abomasum using a single bite. The suture may be brought through the abdominal wall or in the right paramedian area, provided care is taken to avoid subcutaneous abdominal veins.

Both of the aforementioned procedures have the advantage of allowing some visual inspection of the abomasum as

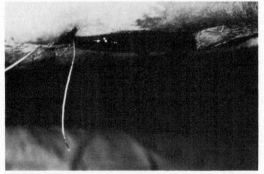

Figure 15–53 Ligature tied on ventral abdomen for holding abomasum in position.

well as good exploration of the rest of the abdominal cavity. If adhesions are present between the abomasum and the abdominal wall, these can be inspected and perhaps freed to allow replacement.

RIGHT PARALUMBAR FOSSA—OMENTOPEXY

Hanover Method. In this procedure the abdominal incision is made in the right flank. The abdomen can be explored before correction. When the abdomen is opened the duodenum is observed to be pulled downward and forward if the abomasum is displaced to the left. When the abomasum is located on the left side of the abdominal cavity it can be decompressed using a needle and tubing. Replacement can be accomplished by the surgeon using the left arm to go down along the abdominal wall from the right side, passing above the udder and under the ventral sac of the rumen. The surgeon can reach the abomasum, cup it in his hand, and push it downward to the right and back to its normal position on the right ventral floor of the abdomen. The surgeon can then grasp the greater omentum, pulling it up into the surgical incision until the pylorus and duodenum are located. An area on the surface of the superficial fold of the greater omentum, referred to by a variety of terms but essentially flange-like and protruding from the surface dorsal and caudal to the pylorus, is used to fix the omental curtain to the flank wall in the vicinity of the laparotomy incision.

The double fold of the greater omentum can be grasped caudal to the pylorus and held with vulsellum forceps. The omentum is sutured between the transversus muscle–peritoneal layer as it is closed. Usually, closure of this first layer starts ventrally and proceeds dorsally, fixing the omentum into position. The goal is an adhesion between the parietal peritoneum and the visceral peritoneum, covering the greater omentum to permanently hold the abomasum in position so that the pylorus rests several centimeters below the distal end of the twelfth rib.

The success rate of the Hanover method equals that of the Utrecht method. Care should be taken to avoid the temptation to apply traction on the greater omentum while reducing the displacement. Small plastic units were initially used to help avoid suture cutout of the omentopexy. Since there is some difficulty in replacing the abomasum, some veterinarians prefer rolling the cow first, hoping to correct the displacement prior to surgery.

RIGHT PARAMEDIAN—ABOMASOPEXY

The arguments against a ventral approach under field conditions are obvious, but with the introduction of newer chemical restraining agents such arguments may no longer be valid. Since it is a direct approach, minimal manipulation and damage to viscera is occasioned because the abomasum is frequently replaced when the animal is positioned in dorsal recumbency (Fig. 15–54). The animal is restrained in a variety of ways. A field block is necessary if tranquilizers, neuroleptics, or sedatives are used.

A right paramedian approach is performed with the animal rolled into dorsal recumbency and restrained (Fig. 15–55).

This method has the distinct advantage of causing the abomasum to return to a near-normal position because of the buoyancy of the gas trapped within, provided no adhesions are holding it in an abnormal location. A disadvantage of this approach is that it does not allow as thorough an exploration of the abdominal cavity as some other methods of correction.

As the greater curvature of the abomasum is usually just beneath the incision site, one can easily grasp the abomasum with vulsellum forceps and hold it while it is fixed to the abdominal wall with sutures. Replacement is facilitated because the rumen drops away from the abdominal floor. If gas is still present in the abomasum, the organ remains against the ventral incision, making abomasopexy easy.

Some practitioners prefer to use an absorbable suture and a continuous pattern to suture the greater curvature of the abomasum to the peritoneum. Others prefer to use a nonabsorbable suture and

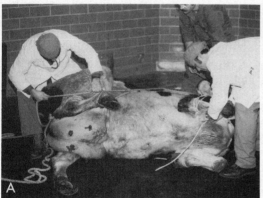

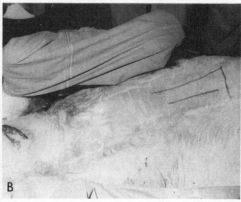

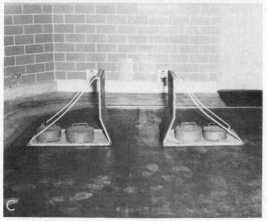

Figure 15–54 A, Double sideline rope restraint. B, Restraint in dorsal recumbency. The incision and inverted L block are marked. C, One method of keeping a cow in dorsal recumbency.

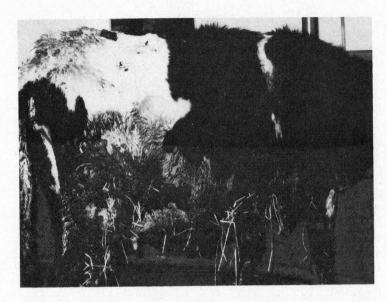

Figure 15–55 A cow presented for surgical correction of left abomasal displacement. The matting of feces on the hide makes aseptic surgery difficult if not impossible, especially by a ventral approach.

penetrate the lumen of the organ when suturing. The latter method will result in a localized peritonitis, which will create a more extensive adhesion but will also add the risk of abscessation.

In fixing the abomasum to the ventral abdominal wall, the peritoneum and internal rectus sheath should be included to avoid having the peritoneum strip away and the pexis fail. Routine closure of the celiotomy is performed.

A complication of this procedure is the development of an abomasal fistula or chronic abscessation at the surgical site. An abomasal fistula is sometimes caused by the surgeon taking too large a bite with the sutures in the abomasum, which will cause necrosis when the sutures are tightened. Chronic infection or the development of a small hernia in the muscle wall of the abdomen has been associated with the use of a nonsterilized, nonabsorbable suture material.

CONSERVATIVE THERAPY IN ABOMASAL DISPLACEMENT

Rolling. This is a conservative technique of correcting abomasal displacement and also may be part of the surgical therapy when a ventral paramedian surgical approach is used. The cow can be cast using a rope so that she goes down onto the right side. This allows the gas-filled abomasum, which was trapped on the left side because of the buoyancy of the gas, to move toward the midline. As the animal is further rotated into dorsal recumbency, the abomasum continues to float back toward a normal position. The animal can be held in dorsal recumbency for a few minutes to allow passage of gas through the pylorus to the intestinal tract. In some cases treatment with calcium or gastric stimulants may facilitate the emptying of gas from the abomasum. The cow should be rolled onto the left side then and allowed to rise from that position.

Tacking. This procedure is a closed method of suturing the abomasum to the abdominal wall used to create fixation and prevent redisplacement. The cow is restrained and rolled into dorsal recumbency as previously mentioned. The dilated abomasum can be auscultated by percussion in the right paramedian area, and a large curved needle threaded with nonabsorbable suture can be forced directly through the skin, hooked into the abomasum, and directed outward, thus fixing the stomach into position. The procedure has the advantage of being quick and economical and therefore is possibly useful in an animal of marginal economic value. However, it has the disadvantage of not allowing the surgeon visible or palpable access to the tissue being sutured. Therefore, mistakes can occur. Another disadvantage is possible abscessation.

Paracostal Approach. As indicated pre-

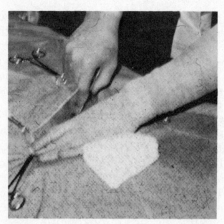

Figure 15–56 A right paracostal incision.

viously, when cattle are positioned in lateral recumbency, variations in the direction of the celiotomy incision can be made quite easily. Usually oblique incisions are designed to follow one or another of the oblique muscles so that a partial muscle separation technique may be employed (Fig. 15–56). In calves and occasionally in mature subjects, a paracostal incision will be more easily performed than a ventral incision, especially for procedures that require adequate exposure of the abomasum.

PYLORIC STENOSIS

This is usually considered a congenital problem but has been suggested as a possible contributing etiological factor in abomasal impaction. Pylorospasm or functional inadequacy due to ulceration, positioning, kinking, and so on may be more prevalent than muscular hypertrophy. External compression by space-occupying lesions of abdominal fat necrosis and visceral lymphosarcoma will frequently reduce the size of the lumen of the pyloric antrum and pylorus, causing partial obstruction (Fig. 15–57).

COMPLICATIONS OF ABDOMINAL SURGERY

Gross contamination may occur when rumen fixation devices fail and when rumen contents enter the abdominal cavity. Extensive adhesions and abscessation may result. The ability of cattle to wall off infection, although remarkable, cannot be expected to cope with extensive leakage from a rumenotomy incision, whether resulting from inadequate suturing during rumenotomy, accidental incision of the rumen during a caesarean section, or emergency trocarization as a life-saving measure. The area of infected pocketing between the flank wall and rumen may be extensive, and one or more tortuous sinus tracts may lead to the exterior.

Abomasopexy and omentopexy, if not performed carefully, can cause malpositioning of the abomasum. This is best prevented by having a thorough topo-

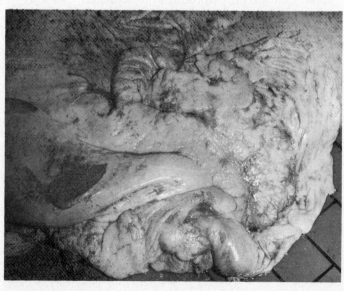

Figure 15–57 Partial obstruction of the pylorus owing to lymphosarcoma.

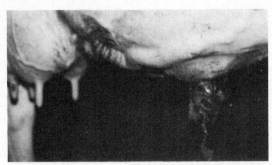

Figure 15–58 Abomasal fistula with mucosal prolapse.

graphical knowledge of the normal position of the viscera and by repositioning it accordingly. Wound dehiscence is not a problem except in situations of gross contamination, bloat during surgical intervention, or postoperative incisional abscess or herniation. In ventral abomasopexy either of the latter two may result in abomasal fistulation (Fig. 15–58). This, although rare, is a serious complication and must be corrected early. If extensive debridement is required, partial resection of the abomasum can be carried out without too much difficulty. When extensive debridement of the ventral abdominal wall is required, mesh repair of the ventral wall may be necessary.

SPECIAL PROBLEMS ENCOUNTERED IN THE CORRECTION OF LEFT ABOMASAL DISPLACEMENT

The concurrent problems associated with left abomasal displacement as well as the clinical laboratory findings have been previously discussed. The special problems encountered in the surgical correction of this disease will be discussed. Sometimes laboratory values are not available and clinical judgement must be used to determine whether surgery should be performed.

Metritis. Metritis and pyometra are the most common diseases found concurrently with left abomasal displacement. If the condition is very active with serosanguineous discharge from the uterus or if the cow is septic (Fig. 15–59), chances are good that the cow has a fever and perhaps a leukopenia. Metritis and pyometra should be treated medically until the cow's condition has improved and stabilized.

Enteritis. Cows with left abomasal displacement frequently have loose stools. Sometimes diarrhea and enteritis are real problems. They may accompany a septic condition such as metritis or mastitis and may not be related directly to the left abomasal displacement. In one series, surgery on cows with left abomasal displacement and concurrent diarrhea resulted in a much worse prognosis and a higher death rate. If the diarrhea is concurrent with another systemic or septic disease, surgery should probably be delayed.

Lameness Due to Hoof Disease. If lameness associated with overgrown hooves, abscesses, or ulcers accompanies the displacement, the hooves should be trimmed or treated before surgical correction of the displacement. This will make the cow feel better and will avoid stress on a surgical site postoperatively.

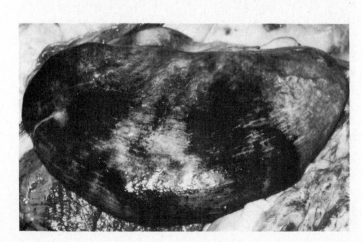

Figure 15–59 Severe necrosis of the uterus in a cow presented for correction of abomasal disease.

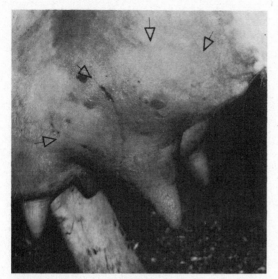

Figure 15-60 Gangrenous mastitis as a post-surgical sequela to correction of abomasal displacement. Note the sloughing of the epidermis and the discoloration.

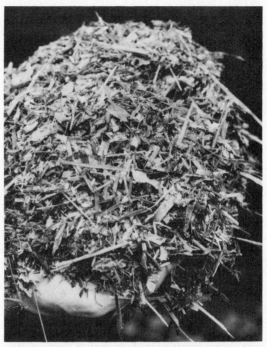

Figure 15-62 Corn silage, a major component of the diet of dairy cows in many parts of North America.

Leukopenia. If a cow with abomasal displacement is known to have leukopenia, a septic disease should be suspected, found, and treated before surgery (Fig. 15-60).

Obesity (Fig. 15-61). The extremely obese cow, which often has been fed a high carbohydrate/low protein diet such as corn silage (Fig. 15-62), is best treated by ventral abomasopexy. The extremely fat omentum may not allow good replacement from a left flank approach or may not facilitate an omentopexy from the right flank (Fig. 15-63).

Emaciation. The thin cow may be chronically ill or even cachectic from the abomasal displacement or complications. In these cases body fat is depleted and often the omentum is very thin and transparent. This tissue may not be sufficiently strong to work with in an omentopexy.

Pregnancy. Sometimes abomasal displacement is encountered when the cow

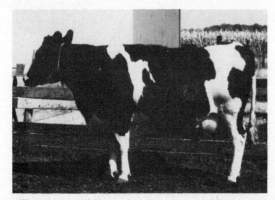

Figure 15-61 Typical appearance of a fat cow, i.e., one fed corn silage, high moisture corn, and protein supplement, and from a herd with a high incidence of fatty liver disease and abomasal displacement.

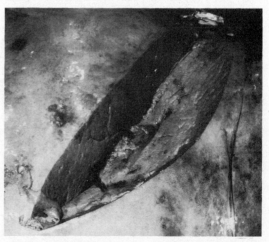

Figure 15-63 Severe case of fatty infiltration of the liver in a dairy cow.

is several months pregnant or even in the last trimester. If the cow is near term, it may be best to nurse her along until she calves or induce parturition. Surgery in a heavily pregnant cow via a paramedian or flank approach can be difficult because of increased abdominal tension or, as in the case of a right flank omentopexy, because of the uterus lying within the stretched omental sac.

Abdominal Fat Necrosis. Often small flecks of abdominal fat necrosis are found at surgery and are of little consequence. Sometimes large tumors of necrotic fat are found along the greater curvature of the abomasum or in the greater omentum near the pylorus. Omentopexy may be difficult in some cases.

Abomasal Adhesions. In 1 to 2 per cent of cases of left abomasal displacement, adhesions are found anchoring the abomasum into a position in the left anterior quadrant of the abdominal cavity. There is no way of diagnosing this problem before the operation. Sometimes these are small fibrinous or fibrous adhesions, which may be torn or incised to allow replacement. Extensive peritonitis or adhesions of the entire stomach cannot be effectively treated. The cow should be salvaged for slaughter.

CORRECTION OF ABOMASAL VOLVULUS

Gastrocentesis. Gastrocentesis is a technique that has recently been developed and employed as an emergency treatment for some cases of abomasal volvulus (Fig. 15–64). This technique has been used on animals that the authors would have normally operated on as quickly as possible but for some reason (time, assistance, or equipment deficit) were not able to. Centesis is performed to evacuate the gas from the abomasum and buy time before operating (Fig. 15–65). Surprisingly, this technique has resulted in effective correction of the abomasal volvulus even though surgery was subsequently performed to fix the abomasum into position. Apparently once the gas has been evacuated, the abomasum returns to a normal position if there is not an excessive amount of fluid present. In one case the abomasum

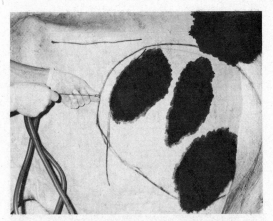

Figure 15–64 Aspiration of gas from abomasum using a 14-gauge, ½-inch cannula and an 18-gauge, 4- to 6-inch needle inserted behind the last rib.

became displaced to the left following decompression.

The procedure is performed with the cow restrained in a standing position (Fig. 15–66). Often the abomasum can be seen bulging behind the last rib on the right side. A small area is clipped and surgically prepared. A 14-gauge, ½-cm needle is used as a cannula (Fig. 15–67), through which an 18-gauge, 15-cm needle is passed to trocarize the abomasum. Suction is then applied to decompress the abomasum (Figs. 15–68 through 15–71).

In severe cases of abomasal or omasal/abomasal volvulus accompanied by excessive pooling of fluid in the abomasum,

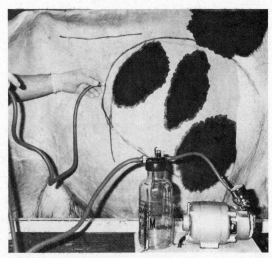

Figure 15–65 Aspiration of gas from abomasum using a portable suction unit.

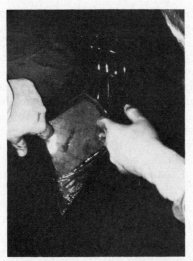

Figure 15–66 Standing right flank laparatomy in a case of abomasal torsion. The abomasum often lies directly under the incision site, and care must be taken to avoid accidental puncture.

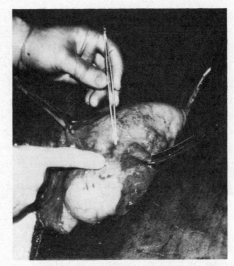

Figure 15–68 After detorsion of the abomasum, the organ can be replaced and the pyloric area can be elevated to the incision site and identified.

this technique will not work. Unfortunately, one cannot be certain of the degree of volvulus in any particular case; but generally speaking, animals with volvulus of 180 degrees or greater have a more severe illness with a more sudden onset and extreme depression and suppression of milk production, greater degree of abdominal distension because of sequestration of ingesta and fluid in the stomachs, and very scant or absent passage of feces.

RIGHT PARAMEDIAN APPROACH. The surgical approach is the same as that for left abomasal displacement. However, a slightly larger incision may be necessary to allow entrance of the entire arm for exploration of the abnormal anatomical relationships and to allow for the manip-

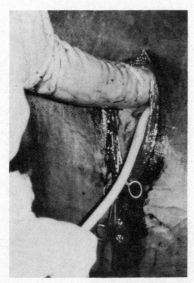

Fgiure 15–67 Decompression of the distended abomasum using a 14-gauge needle and rubber tubing connected to a suction device.

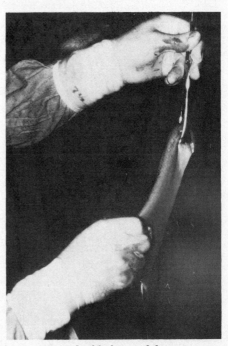

Figure 15–69 A double layer of the greater omentum is grasped through the incision and will be sutured in place to form an omentopexy, which tends to hold the abomasum in position.

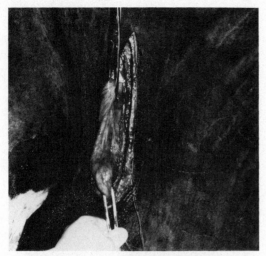

Figure 15–70 The omentum is held in position while stay sutures are placed on either side of the incision site.

ulative effort to replace the abomasum. The surgeon should work from the right side of the cow with the cow restrained in dorsal recumbency. Exploration can be done with either arm, although the authors prefer to use the left arm. In only a few cases will it be necessary to decompress both fluid and gas before untwist-

ing the organ. In most cases removal of gas by suction is all that is necessary.

The surgeon can evaluate the degree of volvulus, whether or not other organs (reticulum, omasum) are involved, and whether or not thrombosis may exist in the large gastric blood vessels in the area of the twist. The surgeon can usually expect to find a counterclockwise twist of the abomasum (as viewed from the rear). Therefore, he can reach on the medial aspect of the twisted abomasum and to the dorsal part (bottom) of the abdominal cavity, grasp the abomasum gently, and roll it upward and over into a normal position.

RIGHT PARALUMBAR APPROACH. The authors prefer this approach for most cases because the cow can be restrained in a more normal manner. This is important because it stresses the animal less. Another advantage is the surgeon's ability to more adequately explore the abdominal cavity and to appreciate the abnormal anatomical relationships more astutely.

The greater curvature of the abomasum is visible as soon as the abdomen is opened. In fact, added caution is important in opening the abdominal incision, since the abomasum is directly beneath (Fig. 15–72). In most cases, especially severe ones, the abomasum has risen into the upper right dorsal

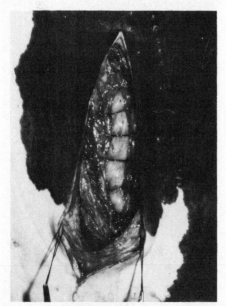

Figure 15–71 The omentum has been sutured into place with the closure of the transversus muscle and peritoneum. The stay sutures will be tied on either side as the closure of the abdominal muscles continues.

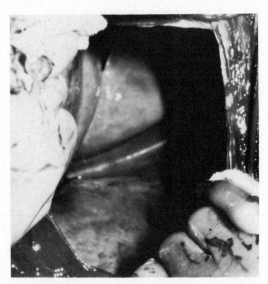

Figure 15–72 View from the right side of the abdominal cavity showing abomasal torsion displacing the liver medially.

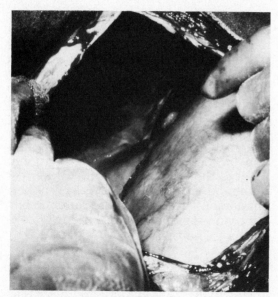

Figure 15–73 Another view of abomasal torsion from the right side.

quadrant of the abdominal cavity and displaces the liver to the left (Fig. 15–73). The volvulus can be palpated by passing the left hand and arm over the top of the abomasum, downward, and forward on the medial side. There the volvulus can usually be palpated in a counterclockwise direction between the omasum and abomasum or between the reticulum and omasum. Rarely, the reticulum will also be involved. When the omasum is involved it is located up behind the liver rather than on the ventral floor of the abdomen.

Three steps are involved in correction of this problem: decompression, detorsion, and fixation. Usually, only the gas has to be evacuated. In some cases the fluid may also have to be evacuated, using a sterile tube inserted into a small abomasal incision surrounded by a pre-placed purse-string suture. When the gas has been evacuated, the left forearm can be used to push the abomasum downward to the floor of the abdominal cavity and slightly to the left. Usually this will allow the abomasum to be untwisted. If the omasum is twisted, it can be untwisted by reaching under it with the palm of the hand and pulling it backward, simultaneously lifting it and rotating it upward. The third objective of the procedure, fixation, can be accomplished with an omentopexy in the right para-

lumbar fossa. Although this may not prevent subsequent dilatation and partial twisting of the abomasum, experience has shown this to be a rare occurrence.

ABOMASOTOMY

Abomasotomy is indicated in the therapy of impactions, for retrieval of foreign objects, and for decompression in some cases of abomasal volvulus. The safest approach is usually from the right paramedian area, with the cow tipped slightly so that the abomasum can be brought up to the incision and isolated before being opened. Occasionally, the abomasum can be drained by insertion of a stomach tube through a small stab incision in the paralumbar fossa approach in cases of volvulus.

PYLOROMYOTOMY

Pyloromyotomy is indicated in some cases of abomasal impaction or volvulus to assist in the emptying of the stomach. The value of this procedure is questionable; however, it does not seem harmful.

The technique involves identification and isolation of the pyloric area. A sharp scalpel blade can be used to incise the serosa and muscularis of the pylorus until the mucosa bulges through into the incision site. This must be carefully performed; there is a risk of perforation of the pylorus, which may lead to contamination of the abdominal cavity.

Simple Stomach—Preruminating Calf

Although most ingested foreign bodies, particularly heavy metallic objects, are deposited in the reticulum or the anterior dorsal sac of the rumen in the adult cow, the esophageal groove in the preruminant calf conveys most of the ingested material into the abomasum after first pooling it in the anterior dorsal sac. Heavy metallic objects are unlikely to be ingested by the calf; however, materials such as coarse fiber and hair sucked from other calves or from the dam may collect and mix with the milk curd in the abomasum. Such hairball obstruction is not common and can be almost entirely eliminated with proper husbandry procedures or individual holding pens for calves.

When the hairball obstruction remains in the abomasum as an intermittent ball valve type of impediment to the outflow of digesta, surgical removal by abomasotomy is necessary. In umbilical herniation in calves, a portion of the abomasum occasionally enters the hernial sac. This may become an identifiable diverticulum and may even become entrapped and adherent within the pouch of the hernia. Aspiration of the contents from such an irreducible hernia will identify the presence of ingesta. Exploratory surgery permits identification of an outpouching of the abomasum if present. Correction is by resection of the involved portion of the abomasum, followed by routine closure of the hernia.

GASTRIC RESECTION

There has always been a great deal of interest as to whether or not the preruminating calf can be continued as a nonruminant. To this end, removal of the forestomachs has been attempted in both sheep and calves. Survival is possible after surgical bypass of the reticulum, rumen, and omasum in young three- to four-week-old calves (Church 1975).

LIVER, GALLBLADDER, AND PANCREAS

Anatomy

The liver in ruminants is positioned almost entirely to the right of the median plane. This results from the development of the forestomachs of the embryo and neonatal calf. The progressive and remarkable development of the stomach on the left side of the abdominal cavity causes the left lobe of the liver to be dorsal to the right lobe. The association between the pancreas and the liver is intimate because of the incorporation between the layers of the mesoduodenum and the enclosure in the dorsal attachment of the greater omentum at the root of the mesentery. The pancreas is adherent dorsally to the liver, the common bile duct, and the duodenum.

Surgical Conditions

The liver, gallbladder, and pancreas are relatively inaccessible surgically. Fortunately, there are relatively few surgical conditions affecting these organs in cattle.

Liver Abscess

Spontaneous, primary, and secondary abscessation occur in the liver and may reach tremendous proportions (Fig. 15–74). Very little can be done for animals so affected. Those abscesses that are secondary to traumatic reticuloperitonitis, if well circumscribed with adhesions between the pyogenic capsule of the abscess and the reticular wall, may be drained by lancing. Drainage is into the reticulum, and its success is dependent

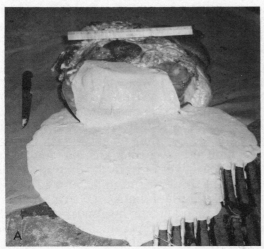 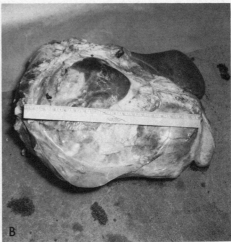

Figure 15–74 *A* and *B*, Liver abscess.

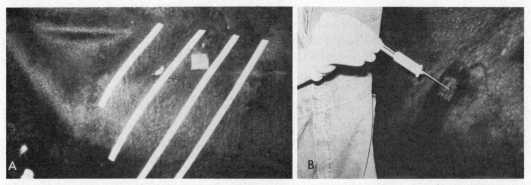

Figure 15–75 *A* and *B*, Percutaneous liver biopsy. (Courtesy of Dr. J. Baird.)

upon the degree of adhesion between the abscess and the wall of the reticulum.

Liver Biopsy

Liver biopsy is a procedure of great diagnostic value; it can be carried out percutaneously or directly during laparotomy. Some risks are associated with percutaneous liver biopsy, but economically, when such liver biopsy is needed, the value of the animal and the prognosis seldom warrant laparotomy (Fig. 15–75).

Gallbladder

Biliary stasis and colic have been diagnosed in cattle and can be relieved by choloduodenostomy (Hofmeyr 1955; Verine 1968). To eliminate an obstruction, the gallbladder is anastomosed to the duodenum where they are in close apposition, using an Eck fistula suture-cutting technique to establish patency after joining the wall of the gallbladder and the duodenum.

Pancreas

Experimentally, the bovine pancreatic ducts, which enter the duodenum and occasionally with an accessory duct enter the common bile duct, make cannulation more difficult than in sheep, in which the pancreas drains into the common bile duct and then into the duodenum.

It has been suggested that inflammatory states in the pancreas may be responsible for the escape of pancreatic enzymes and that abdominal fat necrosis may in fact be due to the enzymatic activity on the peritoneal fat, or that there could well be a dietary influence (Williams, Tyler, and Papp 1969). Fat necrosis can result in space-occupying masses that assume tremendous proportions but generally remain subclinical (Fig. 15–76). They can certainly be observed fairly frequently during abdominal surgery as multiple small foci in areas of fat deposition. External pressure on the viscera by such masses may cause progressive obstruction to the passage of digesta.

SMALL AND LARGE INTESTINES, RECTUM, AND ANUS

Anatomy

The unique arrangement of the bovine viscera and the secondary adhesions that lend support to the bulk of the compo-

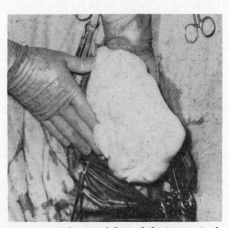

Figure 15–76 Omental fat exhibiting typical cauliflower-like mass of fat necrosis.

nents of the viscera, combined with the fusion between the mesenteric suspension of the small and large intestines, imposes limitations on the mobility and the extent to which exposure of any one portion of the viscera can be achieved. In large animal surgery the size of the abdominal cavity is such that any one incision will not provide access to all areas. Experience is necessary in the localization of the lesion to increase the chance of choosing the proper laparotomy incision. When care and respect for tissue have been carefully attended to by the surgeon, minimal functional impairment will be experienced in the postoperative period.

Physiology

It is generally agreed that there is no sensation of pain when crushing, cutting, or burning the intestinal wall. However, the intestinal wall is sensitive to stretching. With intestinal obstruction, peristaltic waves bring fluid and gas to the site of obstruction, distending this portion. In most animals propulsive activity is greater in the anterior segments of the small intestine than in the posterior portions lower down the tract. Persistent pain in man, according to Dennis (1954), is the result of distension. Diffuse pain, as opposed to crampy pain, is considered to be associated with edema and hemorrhage in the mesentery, causing tension on its root. This is especially the case when there is some degree of strangulation. Borborygmus (any intestinal sound due to gas and fluid propelled along the gut) increases in pitch in clinically established obstruction.

The classification of intestinal obstruction should be quite easy, since, broadly speaking, it can only imply blockage; the blockage may be partial or complete. The systemic effects of obstruction may, however, vary markedly, depending on the site of obstruction and the impairment of vascular supply by strangulation. Electrolyte imbalances, pain, and sequestration of fluid will all vary, depending on the species and the extent of the involvement. The outcome (survival or death) will be determined by the extent of fluid and electrolyte loss and the escape of intestinal contents (whether fluid, bacteria, or toxin) through a devitalized bowel wall into the peritoneal cavity or the circulation.

Surgical Considerations

Until quite recently, serosa-to-serosa apposition was thought to be necessary for proper union following intestinal resection. Since Armistead's work (1956) with experimental anastomosis in the dog, several comparison trials have been carried out involving nearly every possible method of uniting bowel ends. As a result of this experimentation, it has been shown that serosa-to-serosa apposition is not required for adequate healing in gut anastomosis.

The submucosa has the holding power in the intestinal wall and must be included in the suture pattern. The omentum aids healing of the intestinal anastomosis by covering the suture line and aiding in the revascularization of the anastomosis. The serosal surface heals quickly regardless of the technique used. However, mucosal continuity may not be established for considerable periods postoperatively, especially when the inverting techinque has been employed. Bennett and Zydeck have compared the lumenal size following three methods of end-to-end anastomosis and rate them as follows (1970):

1. With an interrupted end-to-end crushing pattern there is greater lumen size and better mucosal healing. Sutures usually slough into the intestinal lumen.

2. With an interrupted inverting Connell closure there is a greater degree of stenosis, more extensive omental adhesions, and a longer period of incomplete mucosal healing.

3. With an interrupted everting mattress closure there is a greater degree of fibrosis in the anastomosis, the sutures remain embedded in the wall, and there is incomplete healing of the mucosa.

The difficulty with this type of comparison became apparent in a similar trial on calves (Horney 1978). When two anastomoses were performed, separated as in the trial of Bennett and Zydeck (1976) by approximately 45 cm, the lumen size of the anterior anastomosis was increased by the distension of the intestine anterior to the more caudal anastomosis.

Although all anastomoses may be carried out using a single-layer closure, an oversew usually provides the safety factor that is preferred by most surgeons. Both open and closed techniques of intestinal anastomosis are employed, and although gross contamination is minimal with a properly applied open technique, temporary basting stitch closures will eliminate this contamination. In recent years autostapling equipment and techniques have been used to reduce gross contamination and surgery time.

All nonviable tissue should be removed in any resection, and the mesentery should be sutured to close any opening that might predispose postoperatively to internal hernia. Ligation of the mesenteric blood supply, although straightforward in small animals, sheep, pigs, and horses, presents a problem in cattle because of the heavy fat deposits present in the mesentery, obscuring these vessels. It is therefore necessary to carry out blind mass ligation in the bovine species. The usual technique is to stagger interrupted mattress sutures across the segment of mesentery of the portion to be resected.

Surgical Conditions of the Small Intestine

OBSTRUCTION

Probably the most frequently encountered surgical problems of the small intestine are obstruction of intraluminal or extraluminal origin and intussusception.

Intraluminal obstruction is usually associated with foreign bodies such as phytobezoars that may have entered the small intestine from the abomasum. In one case a bull had obstruction of the duodenum associated with intraluminal hemorrhage and intramural hemorrhage. Extraluminal obstruction is associated with constrictive fat necrosis lesions, abscesses, or adhesions that may result from faulty intraperitoneal injections. In one heifer, signs of intestinal obstruction were associated with acute enlargement of lymphatic tissue and in another case with hemorrhage in the mesentery as a result of external trauma.

The signs of obstruction usually occur acutely and consist of failure to pass feces, anorexia, depression, and abdominal enlargement. Some animals will exhibit colic or abdominal pain as well. Other signs vary with the type of obstruction. For example, some animals may be able to live well with a chronic progressive disease such as lymphosarcoma or abdominal fat necrosis (Fig. 15–77) until the lesions suddenly become large enough to interfere with normal function.

INTUSSUSCEPTION

This is a condition that primarily affects young cattle. In mature and aged animals intraluminal lesions or polyps may occasionally initiate telescoping of one segment of bowel into another. In cattle more so than in other large animal species, it would appear that double intussusceptions are commonly observed (Fig. 15–78). Intussusception is associated with a lesion in the bowel adjacent to the area of invagination, although diet may be a factor in some cases.

Two types of situations may be observed (Fig. 15–79). If the animal is closely observed, usually there is colic in the early stages. This may be followed by a stretching posture, failure to defecate, and anorexia. However, in some cases the animal may not be noticed to be in discomfort for days or even weeks. Advice is sought only when the abdomen becomes greatly distended. The diagno-

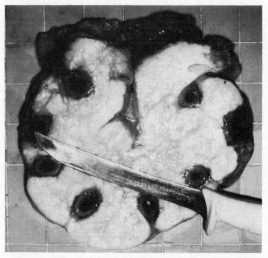

Figure 15–77 Abdominal fat necrosis around the intestines of a cow.

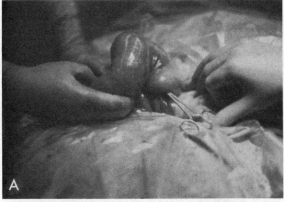
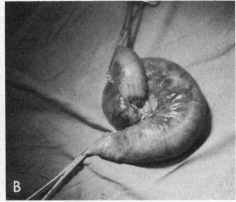
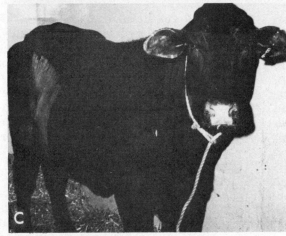

Figure 15–78 *A*, Right flank laparotomy with exposure of the double intussusception. *B*, Resected bowel. *C*, The animal postoperatively.

sis of intussusception is usually made by rectal palpation.

Surgical therapy involves laparotomy and usually enterectomy of the affected part of the bowel. Surgery may be carried out on the standing patient through a right flank approach. However, the pain resulting from the tension applied to the mesenteric root causes the animal to move or even lie down, making suturing difficult. It is therefore recommended that when resection and anastomosis are required, the animal should be restrained in left lateral recumbency.

MESENTERIC ROOT TORSION

Torsion of the mesentery of the small intestine occurs in both young and old of the bovine species and may involve all or part of the mesentery. Partial involvement appears to commence with the distal jejunal and proximal ileal segment, when there is a pronounced indentation of the mesentery. The twist may involve only one of these segments (Fig. 15–80),

or it may become more extensive and include all of the mesenteric root.

Once the problem has been identified, surgical therapy involves decompression of gas and sometimes fluid, followed by manipulative repositioning so that normal anatomical relationships are established. This may be difficult to accomplish, since needle punctures in this area of the bowel often plug with ingesta when aspiration is applied. Also, as the intestinal tract is manipulated trapped gases will shift from one segment of bowel to another, thus necessitating repeated puncture. Sometimes the bowel may have to be exteriorized and opened for adequate drainage and decompression.

Fibrous bands may result from adhesions in circumscribed peritonitis, and these may be strong enough to cause a fluid-filled segment of gut to be suspended over the adhesion, thus creating an obstruction. The same pathogenesis applies when congenital remnants of the vitelloumbilical band persist and cause

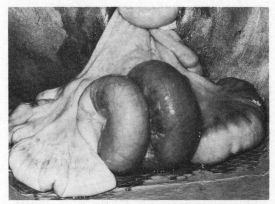

Figure 15–79 Intussusception in the jejunum of a bull.

a small intestinal strangulation (Koch, Robertson, and Donawick 1978). This type of involvement is less frequently seen in cattle than are obstructions caused by mesodiverticular bands in the horse.

Large Intestinal Disorders

Basically, the surgical problems of the large intestine are the same as those of the small intestine. The cecum may become dilated and may possibly undergo volvulus, either clockwise or counterclockwise. The colon may also undergo volvulus. Obstruction may also result from constriction of the lumen from fat necrosis lesions or bands of fibrous tissue resulting from peritonitis.

The diagnosis of these conditions rests on the history and thorough physical examination. Three basic signs present in large intestinal problems: colic, reduced fecal throughput, and postural abnormalities. Many other diseases can be considered as differential diagnoses. Auscultation and percussion of the abdomen, together with rectal palpation and possibly exploratory laparotomy, aid in confirming a diagnosis, alleviating abnormalities if possible, and restoring function.

When surgical disorders of the large intestine have been diagnosed, right flank laparotomy usually is the best approach to the problem. The cow may not stand up for the surgery because of mesenteric pain. The surgeon should develop a logical sequence of abdominal examination. Dilated loops of intestine and taut mesentery can be misdiagnosed as volvulus, when in fact only displacement exists because of the gas or fluid accumulation. Examination should include checking for full loops of bowel as opposed to empty loops. This helps to pinpoint the site of obstruction or abnormality.

CECAL DILATATION AND VOLVULUS

Dilatation of the cecum may not be pathological; in fact, this is a rather common incidental finding during routine rectal palpation in cattle that are eating normally, especially high grain rations. The dilatation is almost certain to be a prerequisite to displacement or volvulus. A common historical finding is unusual movement, such as the cow being in estrus or riding other cows in estrus. During such movements the cecum may flip over and become trapped in an abnormal position. As gaseous distension or fluid accumulation increases, the animal becomes painful and other signs develop, e.g., anorexia, decreased milk production, and so on.

The diagnosis is usually based on clinical findings such as auscultation and percussion of a filled organ on the right

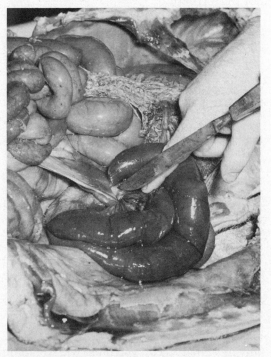

Figure 15–80 Torsion of the mesentery involving only a segment of the small intestine.

side, bulge in the right flank, and rectal palpation of the large organ.

It would appear that atony plays a part in volvulus of this portion of the alimentary tract, as it does in volvulus of the abomasum. There may be compression of the ileum or colon as a result of the volvulus, with resulting partial or complete obstruction. Volvulus in the cecum may involve only the apex, in which case the compression may or may not impede the passage of ingesta from the ileum into the colon but may interfere with the blood supply to the apex of the cecum and thus necessitate partial cecectomy. In other cases the mesocolon may be involved, which could result in the involvement of both the spiral colon and the cecum. The fixation of the anterior portion of colon to the greater omentum and mesoduodenum can predispose to obstruction by having a fluid-filled cecum and/or colon weighing down this segment, causing kinking and obstruction to the movement of digesta.

Surgically, therapy involves right flank laparotomy, decompression, and derotation of the organ. Occasionally typhlectomy may be indicated if there is necrosis of the organ. Sometimes the volvulus will recur; however, cecopexy usually is not performed.

Sometimes the condition will have gone unnoticed for so long that the cecum becomes necrotic and peritonitis develops. Some animals have lived for weeks with this problem before diagnosis. Therapy for chronic cases is hopeless, as peritonitis is too extensive.

CASE HISTORY. A Senepol bull was examined because of progressive anorexia and listlessness of three weeks duration. The temperature was 101.4° F. Pulse rate was 92/min. Respiratory rate was 24/min. Rumen contractions were 2/min. Peritonitis was tentatively diagnosed by rectal palpation of a full abdomen. The hemogram yielded the following information: hemoglobin 15.2; PCV 42 per cent; plasma protein 9.2; fibrinogen 1,300; white blood count 8,415; segmented neutrophils 5,385; nonsegmented neutrophils 1,683; lymphocytes 1,178; monocytes 168. Blood chemistry was as follows: BUN 256; creatinine 12.9; chloride 51; sodium 130; potassium 3.2; calcium 7.6; phosphates 15.6; bicarbonate 46.3; blood pH 7.430. Laparotomy revealed cecal volvulus with chronic peritonitis and adhesions. The bull was euthanized and surgical findings were confirmed.

Diagnostic Biopsies of the Cecum. There appears to be sufficient justification to perform such biopsies to confirm a diagnosis in suspected cases of Johne's disease when it is impossible to confirm the diagnosis by other diagnostic procedures.

SPIRAL COLON

Obstruction to the passage of digesta through this segment of the bowel may occur because of intraluminal lesions that block the flow of ingesta. Severe inflammatory changes in the bowel wall may result in a diphtheritic membrane, which will tend to occlude the lumen, as will blood clots following extensive hemorrhage. In abdominal fat necrosis, mentioned previously, involvement of the fat deposit in the regions of the spiral colon (Fig. 15–81A) and rectum (Fig. 15–81B) decreases the size of the gut lumen by external compression (Fig. 15–81C). Depending on the extent of involvement, the condition may require resection and anastomosis or a bypass as described by Smith and Donawick (1979). In most cases, however, decompression of the cecum will permit either spontaneous or surgical reduction of a simple torsion without the need for resection or bypass.

In Holstein calves there is a high incidence of segmental aplasia involving primarily the colon, rectum, and anus (Figs. 15–82 and 15–83). Animals with segmental aplasia show lack of continuity in the centrifugal segments of the spiral colon and an incomplete or hypoplastic gut from the spiral colon to the rectum (Fig. 15–84). There may be a relatively normal anus and rectum, which causes some problem in the identification of such cases on early neonatal inspection. Re-establishment of patency of the gut is achieved by anastomosis between the terminal part of the anterior segment as identified on exploratory laparotomy and the most anterior portion of what appears to be normal rectum or colon. This is frequently not possible, and cecostomy or colostomy may be required to salvage the animal for slaughter.

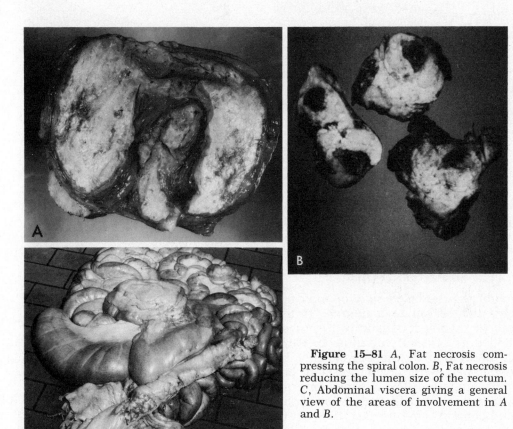

Figure 15–81 *A*, Fat necrosis compressing the spiral colon. *B*, Fat necrosis reducing the lumen size of the rectum. *C*, Abdominal viscera giving a general view of the areas of involvement in *A* and *B*.

Figure 15–82 Ventral midline approach in a heifer with segmental aplasia.

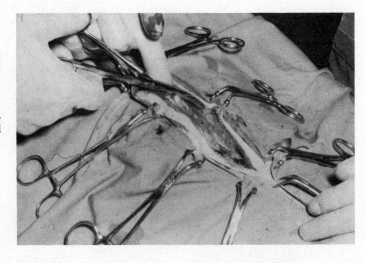

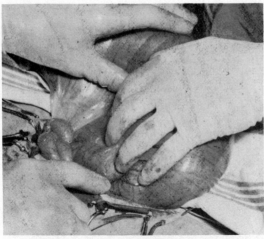

Figure 15–83 Cecal dilatation in segmental aplasia.

VOLVULUS OF THE COLON OR MESENTERIC STALK

Volvulus of the colon may or may not involve the cecum to a degree. If the cecum is involved it usually is not as distended as in cecal volvulus. In early cases derotation of the organ may be accomplished with decompression but without enterotomy. Sometimes enterotomy at the cecum will allow evacuation of fluid contents. In one case the cecum had to be emptied four times, as it filled on manipulation of the colon during derotation.

If the entire mesentery is twisted, the condition is acute and very serious (Fig. 15–85). In one case a yearling dairy bull had been observed to be tossed through

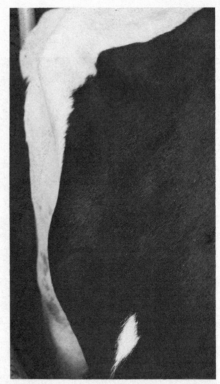

Figure 15–85 Bulge in the lower right flank of a cow with torsion of the colon.

the air and rolled over by an older bull. A couple of days later he was brought to the authors' attention and had extreme abdominal distension. He began to vomit in a projectile manner. Then he aspirated rumen contents and died.

Obstruction of the colon by neoplasia or a degenerative process such as fat necrosis carries a poor prognosis, as it is not usually amenable to therapy (Fig. 15–86).

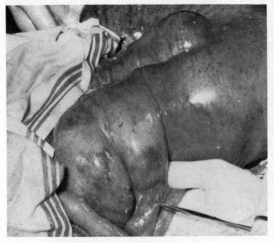

Figure 15–84 Blind end in centrifugal loop of spiral colon in segmental aplasia.

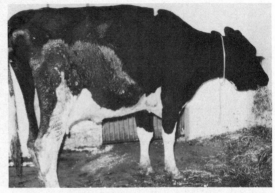

Figure 15–86 Clinical appearance of a cow with Johne's disease. Such animals sometimes are presented with pockets of gas in the colon, which can be mistaken for intestinal displacements.

Obstruction of the ascending colon as a result of localized peritonitis following faulty intraperitoneal injections has been reported. A reported surgical treatment for this problem involves side-to-side anastomosis of the ileum to the centrifugal spiral colon or descending colon following removal of digesta from the cecum and proximal loop of ascending colon. Stoma 5 to 6 cm long were created in each segment after uniting the seromuscular layers on the far side with 0 chromic continuous Lembert suture. The far side and near side cut edges were sutured together with 00 chromic catgut in a Connell pattern. The fourth row of sutures continued the first row and brought together the seromuscular layers of the near side. Three of four cows recovered.

Colonic atresia is recognized in calves, but attempts at surgical correction of the problem are not often successful.

Rectal and Anal Problems

Atresia of the anus sometimes occurs. If the space between the anus and rectum is small, it is possible to exteriorize the rectum and make an artificial anus. Radiography is helpful in making this determination, but exploratory surgery may be necessary. If the gap between where the normal anal opening should be and the existing rectum is great, a colostomy procedure could be considered. In most cases this procedure is not economically justified.

Tears in the rectal mucosa occur as a result of rough rectal palpation during examination or artificial breeding. Sometimes even the serosa may be perforated. If perforation occurs into the abdominal cavity, peritonitis of varying degrees may result and the animal will succumb or should be salvaged for slaughter. If the perforation occurs retroperitoneally, the lesion will heal but fibrosis will occur in the area adjacent to the perforation.

Third degree perineal lacerations involving the anus and rectum occur during forced extraction of fetuses at parturition. This phenomenon can be prevented by episiotomy techniques appropriately applied at calving. The procedure for surgical repair is the same as that in the mare.

Another common rectal problem is rectal prolapse. This can be a sequela to tenesmus of many causes. If the condition is recognized early, replacement of the rectum and a purse-string suture around the anus may help to solve the problem. However, the initiating cause must not be overlooked and must be treated to effect a cure.

Amputation of the rectum becomes necessary in prolonged cases of prolapse with severe necrosis or damage of rectal tissues, as in the case of swine chewing on exposed tissue of the rectum in a feedlot steer. The procedure involves placing horizontal mattress sutures around the site of the amputation before excision of the prolapsed tissue. The surgical complications may include dehiscence of the suture line and resultant peritonitis and death. Alternatively, a small stricture may develop at the surgical site and may interfere with defecation.

Some cattle with *Bos indicus* blood may develop hypersensitivity and chronic fibromas of the anus. These may not interfere with function unless they become large. In such cases resection of the fibroma is possible.

UMBILICAL HERNIAS

Umbilical herniation is fairly commonly observed in young calves. The differential diagnosis must include omphalophlebitis and abscessation due to foreign body penetration of the skin. Umbilical herniation is rarely a cause of intestinal obstruction in cattle. The omentum is the tissue usually found in the hernia. Although the majority of hernias are small, some are very large and are probably related to lack of development of normal abdominal musculature.

An uncomplicated umbilical hernia can be treated in a small calf by pressure bandaging around the middle part of the abdomen for a few weeks. In older calves surgical reduction is required. Surgery should also be performed when there are both an abscess and a hernia present concurrently.

ABDOMINAL HERNIAS

The large abdominal hernias of cattle are sometimes a sequela to trauma dur-

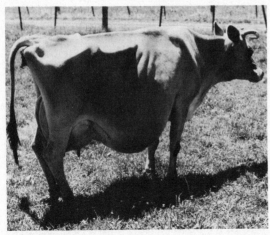

Figure 15–87 Abdominal hernia in a Jersey cow.

ing late pregnancy, with a resulting tear in the abdominal musculature (Fig. 15–87). Although it is possible to repair such hernias, this surgery is not practical economically. Usually these animals will be salvaged.

INGUINAL/SCROTAL HERNIAS

Inguinal/scrotal hernias are sometimes seen in breeding-age bulls. These defects may have a hereditary basis, although this has not been proved. The bull may not show any signs of intestinal obstruction, as would a stallion. Usually mesentery and intestines or omentum are herniated. Adhesions seem to de-

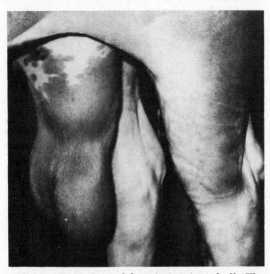

Figure 15–88 Scrotal herniation in a bull. The intestine was adhered within the hernia sac.

velop if the hernia is not reduced soon after occurrence (Fig. 15–88). The bull should be checked for fertility before surgery is contemplated. The swelling and inflammation associated with the hernia may induce testicular damage.

Surgery can be done from either of two approaches: left or right paralumbar fossa, or left or right inguinal. With the flank approach the surgeon must work primarily with one hand to free the contents of the hernia sac, replace them into the abdomen, and suture the inguinal ring with a large curved needle and interlocking suture pattern.

Although the flank approach can be performed with local analgesia, the inguinal approach requires general anesthesia. Incision can be made directly over the inguinal ring to gain access to the hernia sac, reduce the hernia, and suture the ring.

With both approaches the inguinal ring must not be closed so tightly as to impede the venous drainage of the testicle. Postoperative swelling should be expected and may require hydrotherapy.

REFERENCES

Armistead, W. W.: An experimental method for intestinal anastomosis in small animals. North Am. Vet. 37:968, 1956.

Baker, J. S.: Abomasal impaction and related obstructions of the forestomachs in cattle. JAVMA 175:1250, 1979.

Baker, J. S.: Displacement of the abomasum in dairy cows. Pract. Vet. 45:8, 16, 1973.

Bennett, R. R., and Zydeck, F. H.: A comparison of single layer suture patterns for intestinal anastomosis. JAVMA 157:2075, 1970.

Bose, S. S., Ramakrishna, O., and Krishnamurthy, N. T.: Surgical repair of a rectal fibroma in a bull. VM/SAC 76:1349, 1981.

Breukink, H. J., and Kuiper, R.: Digestive disorders following obstruction of flow of ingesta through the abomasum and small intestine. Bovine Pract. 15:139, 1980.

Carlson, V. A.: Removal of magnetic foreign bodies by paracentesis. JAVMA 133:261, 1958.

Church, D. C.: Digestive Physiology and Nutrition of Ruminants, Vol. 1, 1975, p. 43.

Dennis, C.: Current procedure in management of obstruction of the small intestine. JAMA 154:463, 1954.

Deshpande, K. S., Krishnamurthy, D., Nigam, J. M., and Sharma, D. N.: Patho-anatomy of herniation of the reticulum through the diaphragm in the bovine. Can. Vet. J. 22:234, 1981.

Divers, T. J., and Smith, B. P.: Diaphragmatic hernia in a cow. JAVMA 175:1099, 1979.

Edmiston, L. K.: An indwelling instrument for

relief of chronic bloat in cattle. VM/SAC 74:1497, 1979.

Freeman, D. E., and Naylor, J. M.: Cervical esophagostomy to permit extraoral feeding of the horse. JAVMA 172:314, 1978.

Gabel, A. A., and Heath, R. B.: Correction and right-sided omentopexy in treatment of left-sided displacement of the abomasum in dairy cattle. JAVMA 155:632, 1969a.

Gabel, A. A., and Heath, R. B.: Treatment of right-sided torsion of the abomasum in cattle. JAVMA 155:642, 1969b.

Gingerich, D. A., and Murdick, P. W.: Paradoxic aciduria in bovine metabolic alkalosis. JAVMA 166:227, 1975.

Grymer, J.: Venstresidig Løbedislokation. Thesis. Institut for Kirurgi, Copenhagen, 1979.

Habel, R. E., and Smith, D. F.: Volvulus of the bovine abomasum and omasum. JAVMA 179:447, 1981.

Hamilton, G. F., and Tulleners, E. P.: Intussusception involving the spiral colon in a calf. Can. Vet. J. 21:32, 1980.

Hemmingsen, I.: Ulcus Perforans Abomasi Bovis. Nord. Vet. Med. 19:17, 1967.

Hofmeyr, C. F. B.: Cholecystoduodenostomy in the cow. JAVMA 126:459, 1955.

Holmes, J. R.: Some observations on traumatic pericarditis in cattle. Vet. Rec. 72:355, 1960.

Horney, F. D.: Unpublished data, 1978.

Hull, B. L.: Closed suturing technique for correction of left abomasal displacement. Iowa State Univ. Vet. 3:142, 1972.

Ingling, A. L., Albert, T. F., and Schueler, R. L.: Left displacement of the abomasum in a clinically normal cow. JAVMA 166:601, 1975.

King, R. G.: Left-displaced abomasum in a 48-day-old calf. VM/SAC 74:1659, 1979.

Koch, D. B., Robertson, J. T., and Donawick, W. J.: Small intestinal obstruction due to persistent vitelloumbilical band in a cow. JAVMA 173:197, 1978.

Krishnamurthy, D., Nigam, J. M., Peshin, P. K., and Kharole, M. U.: Thoracopericardiotomy and pericardiectomy in cattle. JAVMA 175:714, 1979.

Kumar, R., Kohli, R. N., Prasad, B., Singh, J., and Sharma, S. N.: Diagnosis of diaphragmatic hernia in cattle. VM/SAC 75:305, 1980.

Leman, J.: Acidosis. Harvestore System Farming 20:20, 1981.

Little, P. B.: Surgical treatment of traumatic pericarditis in the cow. JAVMA 144:374, 1964.

McCormack, J.: Surgical procedure for prevention of self-sucking in cattle. VM/SAC 71:681, 1976.

Meagher, D. M., and Mayhew, I. G.: The surgical treatment of upper esophageal obstruction in the bovine. Can. Vet. J. 19:128, 1978.

Moore, G. R., Clark, C. F., Riley, W. F., Conner, G. H., and Rines, M.: Displacement of the bovine abomasum—its diagnosis and surgical correction. In Proceedings of the American Veterinary Medical Association:385, 1955.

Neal, P. A., and Edwards, G. B.: Vagus indigestion in cattle. Vet. Rec. 82:396, 1968.

Newcomb, W. C.: Bovine crowns introduce new professional service. Vet. Med. 56:56, 1961.

Nigam, J. M., and Manohar, M.: Pericardectomy as treatment for constrictive pericarditis in a cow. Vet. Rec. 92:202, 1973.

Noordsy, J. L.: Surgical preconditioning of potentially high-producing dairy heifers. VM/SAC 76:1778, 1981.

Noordsy, J. L.: Diagnostic and prognostic considerations related to exploratory laparorumenotomy in the bovine species. VM/SAC 75:862, 1980.

Pearson, H.: Intussusception in cattle. Vet. Rec. 89:426, 1971.

Pearson, H., and Pinsent, P. J. N.: Intestinal obstruction in cattle. Vet. Rec. 101:162, 1977.

Petty, R. D.: Surgical correction of left displaced abomasum in cattle: A retrospective study of 143 cases. JAVMA 178:1274, 1981.

Pinsent, P. J. N.: The diagnosis of the surgical disorders of the bovine abdomen. Bovine Pract. 12–13:40, 45, 1977–1978.

Poulsen, J. S. D.: Right-sided abomasal displacement in dairy cows: Pre- and postoperative clinical chemical findings. Nord. Vet. Med. 26:65, 1974.

Poulsen, J. S. D.: Clinical chemical examination of a case of left-sided abomasal displacement, changing to right-sided abomasal displacement. Nord. Vet. Med. 26:91, 1974.

Poulsen, J. S. D.: Abomasal displacement in dairy cows—clinical chemistry and studies on the aetiology. Thesis. Stockholm, 1973.

Prasad, B., Singh, J., Khanna, A. K., Khianey, N. K., and Kohli, R. N.: Abomasal involvement in bovine disphragmatic hernia and surgical management. Can. Vet. J. 20:26, 1979.

Radostits, O. M., and Magnusson, R. A.: A modification of an old method for emptying the rumen of cattle. Can. Vet. J. 12:150, 1971.

Radostits, O. S.: Diseases of the ruminant stomachs and intestines of cattle. Proceedings of the American Association of Bovine Practitioners 13:63, 1980.

Ramakrishna, O., Bose, A. S., and Chandrababu, P.: Traumatic reticulitis in a calf. JAVMA 178:1068, 1981.

Rebhun, W. C.: Vagus indigestion in cattle. JAVMA 176:506, 1980.

Rosenberger, G.: Clinical Examination of Cattle. Philadelphia: W. B. Saunders, 1979.

Rosenberger, G.: Krankheiten des Rindes. Berlin: Paul Parey, 1970.

Ruben, J. M. S.: Surgical removal of a foreign body from the bovine oesophagus. Vet. Rec. 100:220, 1977.

Singh, J., Kumar, R., Kohli, R. N., Prasad, B., Khianey, N. K., and Sharma, S. N.: Postxiphoid surgical approach for repair of bovine draphragmatic hernia. VM/SAC 75:106, 1980.

Smith, D. F.: Right-side torsion of the abomasum in dairy cows: Classification of severity and evaluation of outcome. JAVMA 173:108, 1978.

Smith, D. F., and Donawick, W. J.: Obstruction of the ascending colon in cattle. I. Clinical presentation and surgical management. Vet. Surg. 8:93, 1979.

Smith, D. F., and Donawick, W. J.: Obstruction of the ascending colon in cattle. II. An experimental model of partial bypass of the large intestine. Vet. Surg. 8:98, 1979.

Steenhaut, M., DeMoor, A., Verschooten, F., Desmet, P., and DeLey, G.: Surgical treatment of left abomasal displacement. VM/SAC 69:161, 1974.

Steere, J. H.: The wandering abomasum. Mod. Vet. Pract. 42:45–50, 1961.

Stober, M., Wegner, W., and Lunebrink, J.: Research on the familial occurrence of left side displacement of the abomasum in cattle. Bovine Pract. 10:59, 1975.

Svendsen, P.: Etiology and pathogenesis of abomasal displacement in cattle. Nord. Vet. Med. (Suppl. I) 21:1, 1969.

Tadmor, A., and Ayalon, N.: Surgical treatment of sucking in cows. Refuah Veterinarith 29:169, 1972.

Tulleners, E. P., and Hamilton, G. F.: Surgical resection of perforated abomasal ulcers in calves. Can. Vet. J. 21:262, 1980.

Verine, H.: Researches on lithic ailments in cattle. In Proceedings of the Fifth International Meeting on Diseases of Cattle:589, 1968.

Wallace, C. E.: Prognostic significance of diarrhea in cows with left displacement of the abomasum. Bovine Pract. 11:62, 1976.

Wallace, C. E.: Left abomasal displacement—a retrospective study of 315 cases. Bovine Pract. 10:50, 1975.

Wensvoort, P., and Van der Velden, M. A.: Torsion of the abomasum in ruminants: Diagrammatic representation of rotary movements based on post mortem findings. Vet. Q. 2(3):125, 1980.

Williams, D. J., Tyler, D. E., and Papp, E. P.: Abdominal fat necrosis as a herd problem in Georgia cattle. JAVMA 154:1017, 1969.

Wright, E. D.: Television—Bovine antisucking operation. In Proceedings of the American Association of Equine Practitioners:64, 1953.

EQUINE DIGESTIVE SYSTEM

C. Wayne McIlwraith, B.V.Sc., M.S., Ph.D., M.R.C.V.S.

MOUTH, TEETH, AND PHARYNX

Anatomy

Considerations of relevant anatomy of the oral part of the equine digestive tract (Getty 1975) must also necessarily include some anatomy of adjacent areas of the respiratory tract because of its involvement in some conditions of the oral cavity (e.g., cleft palate and paranasal sinusitis secondary to tooth disease).

The mouth is bounded laterally by the cheeks, dorsally by the palate, ventrally by the body of the mandible and the mylohyoid muscles, and caudally by the soft palate. The cheeks form the sides of the mouth; they are continuous in front with the lips and are attached to the alveolar borders of the bones of the jaw. They consist of skin, muscular and glandular layers, and mucous membrane. The muscular tissue is formed mainly by the buccinator muscle, but also by parts of the cutaneous, zygomaticus, dilatator naris lateralis, levator nasolabialis, and depressor labi inferioris muscles. The buccal glands are in two rows, the superior and inferior buccal glands. The mucous membrane is reflected upon the gums. The gums are composed of dense fibrous tissue, which blends at the edges of the alveoli with the alveolar periosteum. The gums are covered by smooth mucous membrane, are devoid of glands, and have a low degree of sensitivity.

The osseous base of the hard palate is formed by the premaxilla, maxilla, and palatine bones, and its borders are the alveolar arches. The mucous membrane is smooth and is attached to the bone by a submucosa with a rich venous plexus in its cranial part. The surface is corrugated with a central raphe and about 18 transverse ridges, which curve caudad. There are no glands in the submucosa. The blood supply is derived chiefly from the palatine arteries.

The soft palate is a musculomembranous fold that separates the cavity of the mouth from that of the pharynx. The oral surface faces cranioventrad. Numerous small ducts of the palatine ducts open on its surface. On each side a short, thick fold passes to the lateral border of the tongue (anterior pillar of the soft palate). The free border of the soft palate is concave and thin and is continued by a fold of mucous membrane, which passes on each side along the lower part of the lateral wall of the pharynx and unites with the opposite fold over the beginning of the esophagus (posterior pillar of soft palate). The soft palate consists of oral mucous membrane (continuous with that of hard palate), palatine glands, the aponeurotic and muscular layers (palatinus, levator palati, and tensor palatini muscles), and the pharyngeal mucous membrane (continuous with that of the nasal cavity).

The tongue is supported in a sling formed by the mylohyoid muscles. Its caudal part, the root, is attached to the hyoid bone, soft palate, and pharynx. The tongue consists of mucous membrane, glands, muscles, nerves, and vessels. The mucous membrane differs in thickness in various areas and presents numerous papillae. The lingual muscles may be divided into intrinsic and extrinsic groups. The intrinsic musculature is a system of fibers running in various directions and blending with the extrinsic muscles. The extrinsic muscles consist of the styloglossus (retracts tongue), hyoglossus (retracts and depresses tongue), and genioglossus (caudal part protrudes tongue, middle part depresses tongue, and cranial part retracts tip of tongue). A fold of mucous membrane, the frenulum linguae, passes from the lower surface of the free part of the tongue to the floor of the mouth.

The dental formula for the permanent teeth of the horse is:

$$2 \ (I\tfrac{3}{3} C\tfrac{1}{1} P\,^{3\,or\,4}_{\ \ 3} M\tfrac{3}{3}) = 40 \ or \ 42$$

There are four canine teeth in the male; they are usually absent or rudimentary in the mare. The premolars and molars make up the cheek teeth, and the constant number of these is 24 (12 in each jaw). An additional variant is the vestigial first upper premolar, or wolf tooth. If present, it is situated just cranial to the first properly developed maxillary cheek tooth (second premolar). The wolf tooth may erupt in the first six months and is often shed at about the same time as the deciduous tooth behind it, but it may remain indefinitely.

The cheek teeth are very large and quadrilateral in cross section, except for the first and last, which are three sided. The crown is very long, most of it being embedded in the bone or projecting into the maxillary sinus in the young horse. As the exposed part wears away, the embedded part erupts to replace it, so that a functional crown of about 2 cm is maintained. The root begins to grow at about five years of age and is complete at 12 to 14 years of age. The individual teeth differ in length. Their angulation increases with the more caudal teeth. The last three maxillary cheek teeth project into the maxillary sinus; the third may or may not. Other anatomic peculiarities are discussed under cheek tooth removal.

The deciduous teeth are smaller and fewer than the permanent set. The dental formula for the deciduous teeth is:

$$2 \ (Di\tfrac{3}{3} \ Dc\tfrac{0}{0} \ Dp\tfrac{3}{3}) = 24$$

The deciduous canines are vestigial and do not erupt. There are no deciduous molars.

Knowledge of normal eruption dates (Getty 1975) is pertinent to both aging of the horse and recognition of abnormalities (Table 15–2).

A consideration of the anatomy of the maxillary sinus and its relationships is relevant to disease of the maxillary cheek teeth. The boundaries of the maxillary sinus are as follows (Getty 1975): cranially—a line between the cranial end of the facial crest and the infraorbital foramen; caudally—cranial border of supraorbital process; dorsally—a line from the infraorbital foramen caudal and parallel to the facial crest; ventrally—alveo-

Table 15–2 ERUPTION TIMES FOR EQUINE TEETH

Tooth	Eruption Time
Deciduous	
Di1	Birth or first week
Di2	4 to 6 weeks
Di3	6 to 9 months
Dp2 ⎫	
Dp3 ⎬	Birth or first 2 weeks
Dp4 ⎭	
Permanent	
I1	2½ years
I1	3½ years
I3	4½ years
C	4 to 5 years
P1	5 to 6 months
P2	2½ years
P3	3 years
P4	4 years
M1	9 to 12 months
M2	2 years
M3	3½ to 4 years

Note: Eruption times for P3 and P4 are maxillary teeth. Mandibular teeth may erupt six months earlier.

lar part of maxilla bone; laterally—malar, lacrimal, and maxilla bones; medially—maxilla, ventral turbinate, and lateral mass of the ethmoid bone.

The maxillary sinus is divided into rostral (cranial) and caudal compartments by an oblique septum, which may be positioned anywhere from the rostral limit of the facial crest to 3 to 5 cm caudal to it. The rostral compartment is divided by the infraorbital canal into lateral maxillary and medial turbinate parts. The caudal compartment of the maxillary sinus is single and much larger.

The turbinate part of the rostral compartment communicates with the middle nasal meatus by a narrow slit situated at its dorsal aspect. The caudal compartment communicates with the sphenopalatine sinus caudomedially, with the frontal sinus dorsally via the large oval frontomaxillary opening, and with the caudal part of the middle nasal meatus through the narrow nasomaxillary opening.

The fifth and sixth cheek teeth lie in the caudal compartment; the fourth cheek tooth usually lies in the rostral compartment but the septum may lie over the root; the third cheek tooth may be within or cranial to the rostral compartment. In young horses, the tooth roots project higher into the maxillary sinus; for tooth repulsion, the trephine openings need to be as high as possible. In older horses the teeth grow out and sinuses enlarge. Consequently, trephine openings can be lower.

The parotid salivary gland is the largest salivary gland and is situated chiefly in the space between the ramus of the mandible and the wing of the atlas. The parotid duct leaves the parotid gland about 2 cm above the external maxillary vein and opens into the mouth in the area of the third maxillary cheek tooth. The mandibular or submaxillary gland is small, long, and narrow; lies beneath the parotid gland; and extends from the atlas to the hyoid bone. The mandibular duct enters the mouth ventrally over the body of the mandible at the level of the canine tooth. The sublingual gland is situated beneath the mucous membrane of the mouth, between the body of the tongue and the ramus of the mandible, and extends from the symphysis to the fourth or fifth mandibular cheek tooth. The sublingual ducts, about 30 in number, open on small papillae on the sublingual fold.

Physiology

The physiologic activities of this area of the digestive tract include prehension, mastication, salivation, and deglutition. In the horse, the lips are the major prehensile organ (Argenzio 1980). Mastication breaks the food down to expose a greater surface area for digestive enzymes and also permits the admixture of saliva, which lubricates the bolus in preparation for swallowing. Salivation itself facilitates mastication as well as swallowing, a function that is important in the horse on a roughage diet. Secretory flows as high as 50 ml/min have been recorded in a 150-kg pony during mastication (Alexander and Hickson 1970).

Deglutition begins as a voluntary act but becomes automatic when the bolus is delivered to the pharynx. Pharyngeal receptors send afferent impulses to the swallowing center in the medulla via the glossopharyngeal, vagus, and trigeminal nerves. Efferent impulses are conducted to the tongue, floor of the mouth, fauces, and laryngeal muscles via cranial nerves V through XII (Argenzio 1980). During the pharyngeal stage of swallowing, contraction of the laryngeal muscle closes the glottis, and the epiglottis is deflected caudally to cover the laryngeal orifice completely as the larynx is drawn rostrally by the hyoid apparatus. The nasopharynx is closed by elevation of the palate assisted by elevation of the pharynx. The swallowing center inhibits the respiratory center of the medulla during this stage so that respiration is suspended to allow swallowing to proceed.

Conditions of the Lips, Cheeks, and Tongue

Traumatic injury is the usual clinical problem of these areas. These injuries usually take the form of lacerations sustained from sharp objects. Minor abrasions and lacerations that are not significant cosmetically or functionally are not treated surgically. The lips, cheeks, and tongue possess a good blood supply, and rapid healing that is cosmetically and functionally acceptable is usually anticipated. However, in severe lacerations, reconstructive surgery is indicated. This can be problematical because of the high muscular content and movement in the lips and tongue. Careful attention should be paid to normal principles of wound cleansing and debridement. Tension sutures should be tied on the skin surface rather than over the mucous membrane (Fig. 15–89).

Spontaneous healing can occur even with very severe lacerations of the tongue (Fig. 15–90), but there may be cosmetic and functional compromise. It is recommended that suturing of severe lacerations be attempted (Adams and Becht 1978). Even if some dehiscence does occur, the end result may still be an improvement over what can be anticipated with spontaneous healing. Suturing should involve obliteration of dead space within the tongue substance, a surface layer of nonabsorbable sutures, and the use of tension sutures (vertical mattress) to minimize dehiscence. Tension sutures on the dorsum of the tongue are more effective than sutures placed on the ventral muscular portion, where the surface membrane is thin. Partial glossectomy should only be performed as a last resort.

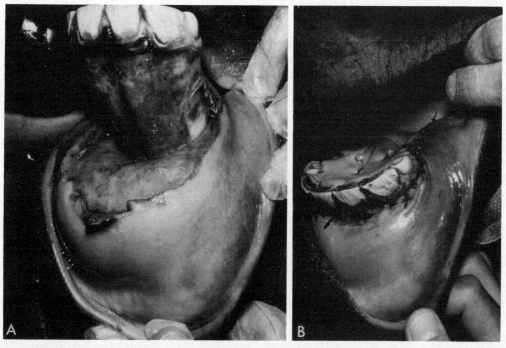

Figure 15–89 *A,* Avulsion of the lower lip from the gingival margin. *B,* Tension sutures were used to hold the lip in position.

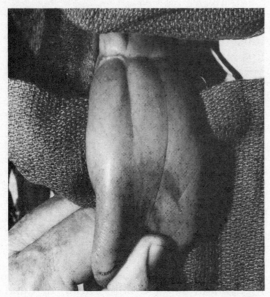

Figure 15–90 Natural healing of a severe laceration of the tongue. (Courtesy of Dr. W. A. Aanes.)

Lacerations of the frenulum linguae may occur in association with excessive tension during oral examination. They are left to heal spontaneously. Excessive pulling on the tongue may also cause a fracture of the hyoid bone. Protrusion of the tongue and dysphagia may be observed. This condition is treated conservatively, but stomach tube administration of water and nutrients may be necessary for a variable period of time.

Tumors of the cheeks occasionally occur and may present special management problems because of oral fistulation associated with the lesion itself as a result of therapy. A fibrosarcoma of the cheek is illustrated in Figure 15–91. The owners requested that any possible treatment be attempted. Cryosurgery was used, leaving a large defect in the cheek. The horse needed a deep bucket to drink out of in the postoperative period while healing of the defect occurred.

Pharyngeal Conditions Associated with Dysphagia

Various conditions of the pharynx need to be considered when the clinician encounters dysphagia in a horse. Pain, swelling, obstruction, or disturbances in motor function of the pharynx constitute reasons for dysphagia. Causes include pharyngeal injuries associated with improper administration of medicinal agents by dose syringe, balling guns, or stomach tube; foreign body penetration (Fig. 15–92); and retropharyngeal abscessation due to *Streptococcus equi* infection or secondary to trauma (Knight 1977; Scott 1975). Guttural pouch mycosis can cause neurologic dysfunction of the pharynx. Pharyngeal paralysis may also be caused by central nervous system disease, toxic agents (e.g., moldy corn poisoning, yellow star thistle poisoning, botulism), and hypocalcemia. Dysphagia resulting from unilateral rupture of the rectus capitis ventralis muscles has been reported (Knight 1977). Dysphagia associated with fracture of the hyoid bone has been mentioned previously. Pharyngeal polyps or subepiglottic cysts may also cause dysphagia. Some of these conditions will respond to conservative management. In appropriate instances surgical manipulation (foreign body removal, polyp removal, cyst enucleation, or abscess drainage) is indicated. The prognosis is poor for dysphagia due to guttural pouch mycosis.

Brachygnathia (Parrot Mouth)

This condition is thought to be inherited and is manifested as a shortened lower jaw with an overbite (Fig. 15–93). The condition may be seen in association with other problems including ruptured common digital extensor tendons, poorly developed pectoral muscles (Myers and Gordon 1975), and goiter (McLaughlin and Doige 1981). The ability of the animal to eat may be compromised, but usually the defect is merely cosmetic.

Before five to six months of age it is possible to improve the condition by placing wire braces from the incisors to the first maxillary cheek tooth to delay growth (Fig. 15–94). A Steinmann pin is used to place a hole dorsal to the gum line between the first and second upper cheek teeth. Cerclage wire (1.2 mm) is then placed through the hole and twisted around the first maxillary cheek tooth. The wire is then passed craniad and around the incisors to the opposite side, where it is wired to the second deciduous

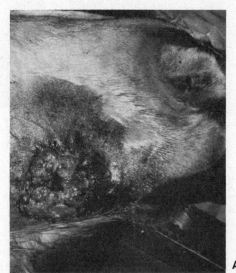

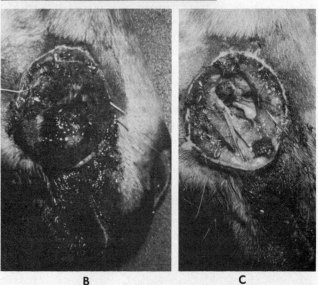

Figure 15–91 Fibrosarcoma of the cheek that was treated with cryosurgery. *A*, The lesion prior to treatment. There was diffuse involvement of the oral mucosa, and a fistula was present centrally. *B*, Nine days following cryosurgery. *C*, Fifteen days following cryosurgery.

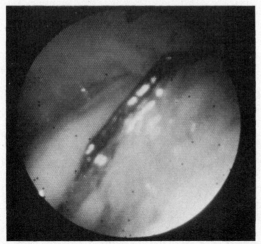

Figure 15–92 Endoscopic view of piece of wire lodged in the pharynx.

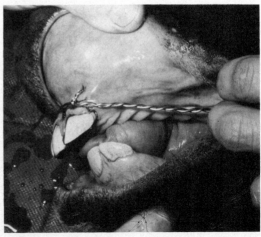

Figure 15–94 Wire braces placed between incisors and first maxillary cheek teeth in an attempt to help correct parrot mouth.

incisor (this operation cannot be performed until this tooth is present). The wires should be regularly checked by the owner for loosening or breakage. The wires are removed when the alignment is corrected or when no further improvement is attained.

The ethics of performing the surgery are predictably controversial. The hereditary nature of the disease is generally acknowledged, and correction of the problem and subsequent showing are unacceptable. However, if castration can be performed or assurance given that showing or breeding is not planned, the performance of the surgery is probably justified, particularly if the patient's eating is compromised.

Facial (Buccal) Nerve Paralysis

This condition does not have a surgical treatment but most commonly arises as a consequence of general anesthesia. Failure to remove the halter during anesthesia can cause local pressure in the buccal nerves. The clinical signs include hanging of the lower lip on the affected side, drooping of the upper lip, and collapse of the nostril. Feed may collect between the cheek and teeth on the affected side. The condition usually resolves spontaneously.

Cleft Palate

Cleft palate (palatoschisis) is a congenital defect, but the hereditary basis of the anomaly is less well defined. Fusion of the palatal folds in the fetus takes place rostrocaudad from the incisive foramen like a zipper. An interruption may occur in the process of normal fusion at any stage so that it is possible to have any degree of cleft, from a complete cleft of both the hard and soft palates to a small cleft of the caudal part of the soft palate only. Factors that are considered important in the condition in man include gene mutations, chromosomal aberrations, environmental teratogens, and multifac-

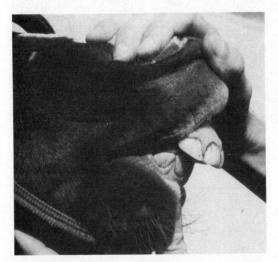

Figure 15–93 Parrot mouth in a four-month-old foal.

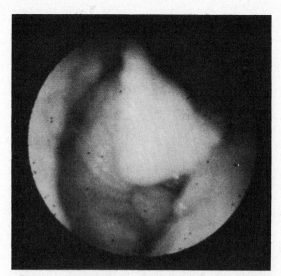

Figure 15–95 Endoscopic view of a cleft palate. The epiglottis is positioned within the cleft.

torial inheritance (Scott 1982). Further study is needed before the disease in foals is generally classified as hereditary, but at the same time clinicians must remain cognizant of the possible effects of breeding affected animals.

The presenting clinical signs include dysphagia with reflux of milk or food material through the nostrils. The presence of a cleft palate is confirmed by direct visual or endoscopic examination or both (Fig. 15–95). Epiglottic entrapment may accompany the condition (Fig. 15–96). Aspiration pneumonia is also commonly present owing to inhalation of milk that has passed from the oral cavity to the nasal cavity. Foals affected with a cleft palate may have received inadequate amounts of colostral antibody; therefore, evaluation of immunoglobulin levels is appropriate.

The presence of a cleft palate is usually obvious in the young animal, as there is some degree of compromise. However, the condition has been described in a two-year-old horse that was race training (Haynes and Qualls 1981). It did, however, later die of pulmonary complications.

The ethics of performing surgery for repair of cleft palate and possible potentiation of an inheritable defect are debatable as previously discussed. In addition, various complications are associated with palatoplasty, and, despite implications in the literature that results are

uniformly good (Jones et al. 1975), complete dehiscence of repairs is not uncommon (Bowman et al. 1982). Most surgeons agree that better and more predictable techniques are needed.

Palatoplasty is performed with the animal under general anesthesia in dorsal recumbency. The foal is intubated through a tracheotomy. An oral approach has been used (Kendrick 1950), but mandibular symphysiotomy gives the best exposure of the entire palate (Nelson, Curley, and Kainer 1971; Stickle, Goble, and Braden 1973). However, surgical exposure of the caudal soft palate is still poor with this approach, and the supplemental use of a midline pharyngotomy splitting the body of the hyoid has been described (Mason et al. 1971).

MANDIBULAR SYMPHYSIOTOMY APPROACH TO PALATE

A midline skin incision is made from the mandibular symphysis to the caudal aspect of the ventral ramus. An incision is then made in the buccal-lingual junction of the lower lip to permit inversion of the lower lip into the oral cavity and splitting of the mandible (Fig. 15–97A). This modification of the original technique (Shires 1980) eliminates incisional dehiscence of the lip, a complication of the original technique. The mylohyoideus muscle is incised along its midline insertion from the level of the symphysis to the level of the lingual process of the

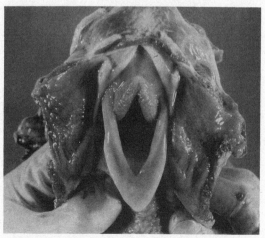

Figure 15–96 Entrapment of the epiglottis by the arytenoepiglottic folds in association with a case of cleft palate.

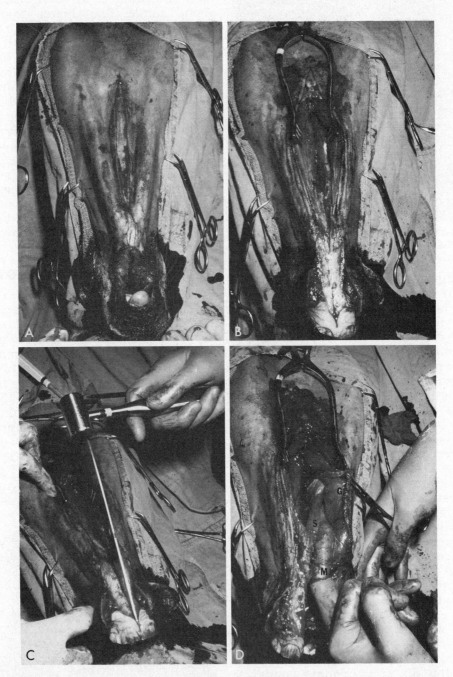

Figure 15–97 Transsymphysiotomy approach to hard and soft palate of the horse. *A,* Skin incision, including incision in lower lip (finger through incision) to permit inversion of lower lip into the oral cavity. *B,* Incision continued with retractors placed in incision through mylohyoideus muscle, and mandibular symphysis exposed. *C,* Splitting of mandibular symphysis. *D,* Identification of oral mucosa (M) prior to cutting it. The genioglossus muscle (G) has been incised and reflected. Styloglossus muscle (S.)

Illustration continued on opposite page

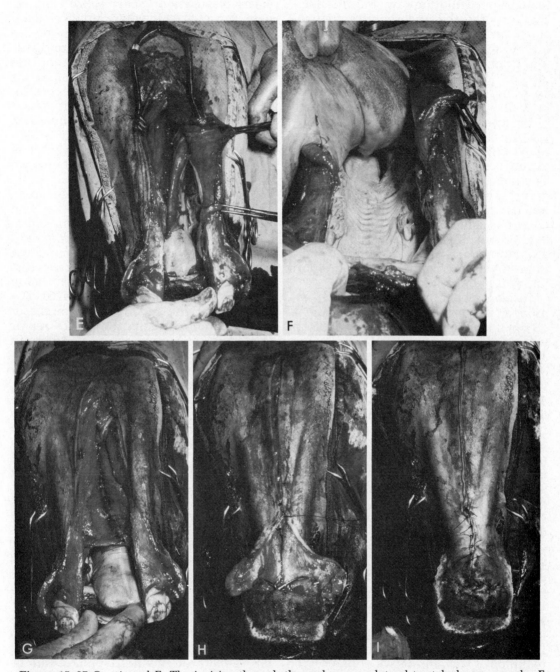

Figure 15–97 *Continued E*, The incision through the oral mucosa lateral to styloglossus muscle. *F*, Exposure of hard and soft palate. There is a cleft in the soft palate. Exposure can be improved with further retraction. *G*, Closure of oral mucosa prior to fixation of mandibular symphysiotomy. *H*, The mandibular symphysis has been closed using wire and Steinmann pins, the lip replaced, and all muscle layers closed. *I*, Skin closure in progress.

hyoid bone (Fig. 15–97B). The mandibular symphysis is separated using an osteotome or oscillating saw (Fig. 15–97C). This exposes the underlying geniohyoideus and genioglossus muscles; these are incised 1 to 2 cm from their mandibular origins. Care is taken to avoid damage to the sublingual salivary gland tissue and the sublingual salivary duct laterally. The incision is deepened by blunt dissection lateral to the styloglossus muscle. By spreading the mandibular rami, the oral mucosa can be visualized prior to incision (Fig. 15–97D). The hypoglossal and lingual nerves medially should also be avoided. The oral mucosa is incised so that flaps are left on either side for later closure (Fig. 15–97E). The tongue is reflected laterally and retraction of the mandibular rami maintained for visualization of the hard and soft palates (Fig. 15–97F).

To close the transsymphysiotomy approach, the oral mucous membrane is closed in a simple continuous pattern using 00 polyglactin 910 (Vicryl) (Fig. 15–97G). The mandibular symphysis is closed using a combination of lag screw, wire, and Steinmann pin (Fig. 15–97H). The deep tissue planes are closed with polyglactin 910 to obliterate dead space; the geniohyoideus and genioglossus muscle separations are also sutured. The mylohyoideus and subcutaneous incision is closed with another continuous row of sutures and the skin incision closed with nonabsorbable sutures (Fig. 15–97I).

Possible complications of this procedure include infection and drainage as well as osteomyelitis and loosening of the symphysiotomy site. It has already been stated that exposure of the caudal soft palate is not always entirely satisfactory. It should also be noted that the usefulness of the symphysiotomy technique is limited to foals. The length of the head in older animals prohibits the use of this technique. The alternative of pharyngotomy gives very limited exposure.

PALATOPLASTY

There are a number of ways to close a cleft hard or soft palate. Principles that should be aimed at include adequate mobilization of the tissues to be sutured,

apposition of fresh wound edges, and anatomical closure of the defect without excessive tension (Scott 1982). The repair of a cleft soft palate involves excision of the mucosal edge surrounding the cleft followed by a two- or three-layer closure (Fig. 15–98). Because of the loose nature of the border of the soft palate, determination of the exact caudal limit of the cleft can be difficult. There is some argument for not burying knots in the muscle. Absorbable suture material should be used for this layer. It is most convenient to appose nasal mucosa and the muscular layer with a simple continuous pattern, but an interrupted pattern (mattress preferred) is used on the oral mucosa. The use of monofilament nonabsorbable suture is theoretically ideal in terms of strength and low reactivity, but some of the more successful results have been reported using chromic catgut (Jones et al. 1975). Dehiscence of the repair is still a major complication of cleft soft palate repair (Batstone 1966; Bowman et al. 1982). In a recent report complete or partial dehiscence occurred in seven of eight soft palate repairs that were followed up postoperatively (Bowman et al. 1982). These experiences are not unique. Laterally placed relief incisions may be used in soft palate repairs, but there are no data to document that their use enhances the success rate (Bowman et al. 1982). It has been suggested that in some clefts the flaps of the soft palate contain a relative excess of glandular tissue and poor musculature (Jones et al. 1975). Such deviations from normal structure could potentially have an effect on healing. It has also been suggested that burying knots in the muscular layer is inappropriate (Bowman et al. 1982).

When repairing hard palate clefts, closure of defects without excessive tension requires tissue mobilization. Small caudal defects of the hard palate can be repaired using a mucoperiosteal sliding-flap technique combined with soft palate repair (Fig. 15–99). Large clefts of the hard palate may be best repaired by the mucoperiosteal reflected-flap technique, which has been used successfully in dogs (similar to vomer flap technique) (Howard et al. 1974) (Fig. 15–100). Partial

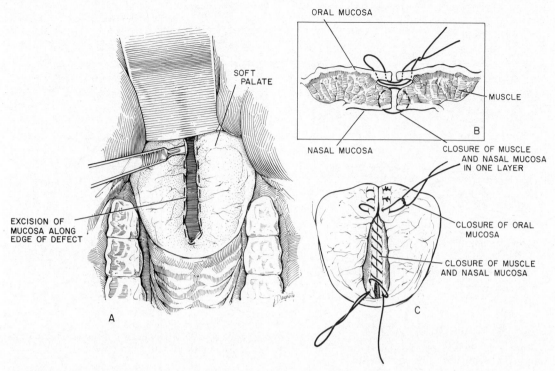

Figure 15–98 Repair of a cleft soft palate. *A*, Debridement of the edge of the cleft palate. *B*, Cross-sectional diagram of closure of the defect. *C*, Closure of the defect in 2 layers.

success has been reported in one case using the double vomer bone flap method in a horse (Tolksdorff 1966). One problem with using the mucoperiosteal reflected-flap technique is in the area of transition from hard to soft palate when the surgeon has to then repair the soft palate defect. The surgeon has the choice of either reverting to a simple apposition technique, which can leave a potentially defective area at the junction, or attempting to make a reflected flap in the soft palate. The latter is difficult to perform, and there is a risk of leaving further defects in the soft palate.

Because of poor results with cleft palate repair, an improved technique would still be most acceptable. An internal prosthesis to protect palatal healing has been used in the dog (Thoday et al. 1975), but it is not known whether such a device could be used in the horse.

There is no evidence that palatoplasty results are affected by the varying use of stomach tube, pharyngostomy, or esophagostomy postoperatively.

Fractures of the Mandible and Premaxilla

Fractures of the mandible or premaxilla are either due to kicks or are self-inflicted in association with catching the teeth on objects in the stall. The incisors will be involved, and avulsion of one or more teeth can occur (Fig. 15–101). Radiographs are used to confirm the extent of the fractures (Fig. 15–102) even though many are self-evident at clinical examination. Fixation with wire is a highly satisfactory method of repairing these fractures in many instances (Figs. 15–103 and 15–104). The teeth can be used for fixing the wire. Holes drilled through the bone may be necessary in other instances. Fixation is preceded by thorough cleansing and debridement of the mandible and premaxilla. Fractures of this area can heal well despite infection and some motion (wire does not provide absolutely rigid fixation); this is considered to be associated with the excellent blood supply to the area. In selected situations intramedullary pins,

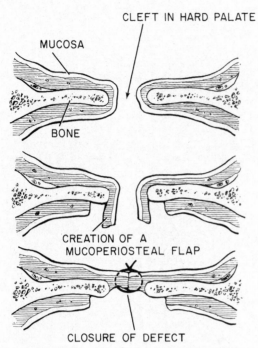

Figure 15–99 Mucoperiosteal sliding flap technique for repair of a cleft hard palate.

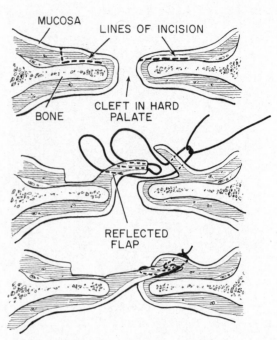

Figure 15–100 Mucoperiosteal reflected flap technique for repair of cleft hard palate.

compression screws, bone plating (Fig. 15–105), and splint assemblies (Gabel 1969) may be used.

Dental Disease and Its Diagnosis

Dental problems constitute the major problems of the oral cavity for which surgery is indicated. Various clinical signs may be present, depending on the individual problem, including (Scott et al. 1977):

1. Difficulty in mastication;
2. Quidding (i.e., when a horse drops food material out of its mouth in the process of mastication);
3. Weight loss as a result of anorexia and/or improper mastication;
4. Unilateral or bilateral nasal discharge;
5. Malodorous breath;
6. Swelling over the dental area;
7. Drainage from a fistula or sinus;
8. Sinusitis;
9. Reluctance to drink water;
10. Refractoriness to bit or adverse reaction to bit pressure;
11. Chewing of food on one side with tilting of the head;
12. Passage of unmasticated food in feces.

Initially, a careful oral examination should be performed. This will aid in identifying the presence of "caps," supernumerary teeth, wolf teeth, periodontal disease, or overgrown or projecting teeth. Such an examination will also help to eliminate the possibility of other oral problems. The presence of a patent infundibulum in a suspect tooth may be identified by examining the tooth surface with a pick or probe.

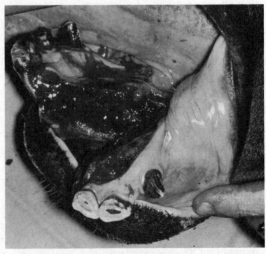

Figure 15–101 Fracture of the mandible with the intermediate and corner incisors and canine tooth contained in the fractured portion.

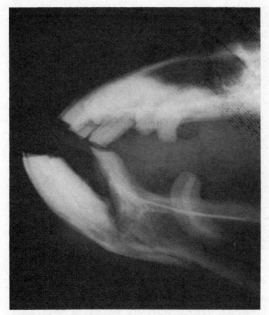

Figure 15–102 Radiograph of a fractured mandible involving the incisors. (Courtesy of Dr. W. A. Aanes.)

Radiography is an important part of the oral examination and is used to confirm the presence of abnormal eruption or supernumerary teeth, apical infection or alveolar periostitis, fractures, and associated sinusitis and its degree. Lateral and oblique radiographs are made. In most instances root and reserve crown detail rather than exposed crown detail is needed. This detail is achieved by using a 30° oblique beam to project the image of the normal arcade away from the diseased area (Baker 1971). In selected cases, greater detail may be ob-

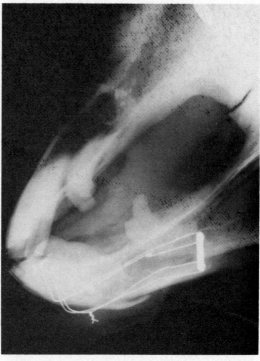

Figure 15–104 Radiograph of the repair of the fracture in Figure 15–102 using wire and a Steinmann pin. (Courtesy of Dr. W. A. Aanes.)

tained with the use of intraoral dental films (Baker 1971).

As with all clinical exercises, experience with the normal appearance is essential. The lamina dura (a radiographic white line representing the interface of the periodontal ligament and alveolar bone) is used to delineate a normal root apex. It must be noted, however, that eruption of the teeth is brought about by an increase in pulp vascularity and is

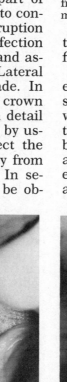

Figure 15–103 Fixation of fracture depicted in Figure 15–101 using wire. The soft tissue defects are being sutured.

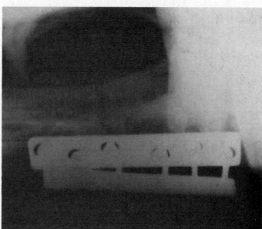

Figure 15–105 Repair of a mandibular fracture using bone plates.

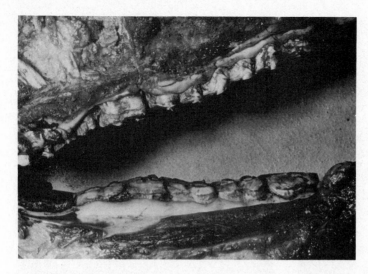

Figure 15–106 Necropsy specimen of a case of wave mouth.

seen radiographically as an apparent cystic distension of the lamina dura. These cystic distensions around erupting teeth can also be palpated in the normal horse as regular, symmetrical, nonpainful swellings along the ventral border of the mandible and sometimes on the maxilla rostral to the facial crest.

Additional diagnostic aids used in assessing the presence of sinusitis include endoscopic examination and, using local anesthesia, aspiration of the sinus contents through a small drilled hole (Kral 1954).

Abnormalities of Dental Wear

In its mildest and most common form, irregular dental wear is evidenced by excessive enamel points or edges that develop on the buccal aspect of the maxillary arcade and the lingual aspect of the mandibular arcade. The maxillary cheek teeth are set more laterally than the mandible cheek teeth, and ridges and points consequently form. These ridges and points are the main reason for regular rasping (floating of teeth). Malocclusions in the craniocaudal direction may also occur, and these lead to hooks in the rostral aspect of the first maxillary cheek tooth and the caudal aspect of the last mandibular cheek tooth. Most ridges can be eliminated with tooth rasping; larger hooks require the use of dental cutters.

Another abnormality of wear is wave mouth, in which the cheek teeth form an uneven or undulating arcade (Fig. 15–106). If clinically significant, rasping and cutting of the teeth can be performed; treatment of severe cases may not be very rewarding.

In step mouth there is an abrupt variation in the height of adjacent teeth. This is commonly due to defective growth or extraction of a tooth or consequent overgrowth of opposing teeth. This condition can severely compromise chewing, and the overgrown tooth needs to be rasped or cut back as soon as possible.

Cutting of teeth is performed with special dental cutters. The cutters are placed at the desired site and cutting performed with a sharp blow to the handle. Slow squeezing of the handles increases the risk of splitting the tooth.

Supernumerary Teeth

These are uncommon congenital problems associated with splitting of the dental bud. In the incisors, the condition is most commonly seen in the upper arcade. Dental crowding can result. Gingivitis or prehension difficulties may result, or there may be no clinical signs. Extraction is indicated in some cases; in others malocclusion may be controlled by rasping. The most common site for a supernumerary tooth in the cheek teeth is behind the last mandibular molar. Clinical signs will not be apparent until malocclusion occurs and the tooth grows up into the soft palate or causes ulceration of the tongue. If the tooth is loose, extraction can be performed; otherwise regular control of the tooth's growth with dental cutters is the preferred treatment.

Retained Deciduous Premolars

Retained deciduous premolars or "caps" are identified by examination of the teeth of horses with signs of mastication difficulties. A tooth crown is seen projecting about the level of the occlusal surface of the adjacent tooth. The cap is removed using leverage or molar extractors (Fig. 15–107).

Wolf Teeth

As described previously, wolf teeth are the first premolar teeth and typically are found in the maxillary arcade; in rare instances they may appear in the man-dibular arcade. The presence of wolf teeth has been associated with bitting problems, and for this reason removal of these teeth is often requested. They are of primary concern in harness horses and are associated with the wearing of a cheek bit or overcheck. Surgical correction is minor and is performed with the animal standing. Sedation may be used; local analgesia is not routinely necessary. The tooth is freed from its periodontal and alveolar attachments using a curved chisel or an instrument designed specifically for the purpose. The second premolar is used as a fulcrum to try and elevate the tooth, as this separation is performed on the caudal aspect of the wolf tooth. The tooth is removed with dental forceps. The surgeon should attempt to remove all the root; it is of little consequence if this is not done unless the retained portion is sharp and protrudes from the gum.

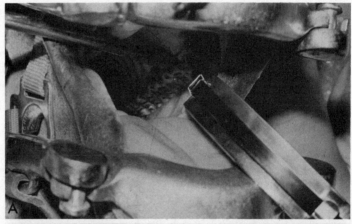
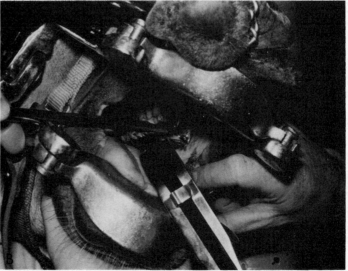

Figure 15–107 Removal of a retained deciduous premolar tooth (cap). *A*, A screwdriver is inserted under the edge of the cap. *B*, The cap is lifted off the permanent premolar. (Courtesy of Dr. W. A. Aanes.)

Elongated Tooth (Exsuperantia dentium)

If a tooth is missing, the opposite tooth will become longer than the other teeth because it is not worn away. It also grows faster because of the lack of masticating pressure (Hofmeyr 1974). This problem should always be explained to the owner whenever the decision is being made to remove a cheek tooth.

Treatment for an elongated tooth involves cutting the tooth back to the level of the remainder of the arcade or regular rasping to control overgrowth.

Alveolar Periostitis and Associated Manifestations

DEFINITION

The alveolar periosteum is a vascular layer of connective tissue that attaches the embedded part of the cheek tooth to the alveolus. The term *alveolar periostitis* includes the various conditions that cause inflammatory changes in this area of the cheek teeth with secondary bony enlargement, fistulation, or sinusitis and that necessitate removal of the teeth. Infection is involved in most cases but not necessarily in all. The exact pathogenesis of some entities is difficult to define, and the term alveolar periostitis is used to classify an entity with typical clinical and radiographic manifestations and a common treatment. It is the most common and problematical surgical disease of equine teeth.

PATHOGENESIS

Infectious alveolar periostitis is the typical presentation. The most common routes of infection include entrance of food material and resultant infection through a patent infundibulum (Frank 1964), between the gum and tooth (paradontal disease) (Baker 1970; Hofmeyr 1974), or in association with fracture of the tooth (Coffman 1969). The infundibuli are normally filled with cement; when they are not, food material can become impacted in the pulp cavity, and the subsequent decay can lead to continued necrosis and tooth infection. The deficit in the infundibulum may be a developmental problem associated with hypoplasia of the cement, or it may be caused by cemental necrosis in association with dental caries (Hofmeyr 1960). Either situation can probably exist in individual cases. Pulpitis and alveolar sepsis will lead to osteitis and osteomyelitis. Dental disease of the fourth through the sixth maxillary cheek teeth (also the third in some instances) that progresses through alveolar bone will produce sinusitis. Dental disease was considered the cause of 50 per cent of one series of cases of sinusitis (Mason et al. 1977). The most commonly affected tooth was the first maxillary molar, and infundibular necrosis was the most common dental disease associated with sinusitis in this survey (Mason et al. 1977). There is a predilection in young horses; this implies a developmental cause rather than infundibular problems associated with necrosis. However, it should also be noted that the first maxillary molar erupts at 9 to 12 months, which is much earlier than the other cheek teeth. Consequently, there is plenty of time for infundibular cemental necrosis to develop and subsequent tooth infection to become clinically manifest in the young horse. It can also be argued that cemental hypoplasia may be more of a problem in this tooth because it erupts much earlier than the other teeth and could be immature.

Chronic ossifying alveolar periostitis is a term used to describe a specific condition in two- to three-year-old horses (occasionally four to five years old); infection may or may not be in evidence, but there is productive osteitis and periostitis (Frank 1964). The exact etiology is unknown, but it has been noted that there may be an associated impaction of the corresponding developing permanent premolars (Hofmeyr 1960). Failure to remove deciduous teeth or caps has also been incriminated in that the retained caps could irritate the tooth and the alveolar periosteum. A variable amount of bone forms over the affected alveolus. The tooth most commonly involved is the third upper cheek tooth (fourth premolar), sometimes the second, and very occasionally the first. The bony enlargement is a serious blemish and may also cause severe compromise of the nasal cavity. There may be interference to the nutrition of the tooth, with consequent compromise in its development. Tooth removal is indicated if the disease state is causing a clinical problem. Gradual spontaneous regression of maxillary swelling due to diffuse ossifying alveolar periostitis may occur as the horse matures; therefore, the conservative route is probably preferable if the situation is purely one of cosmetics.

A third condition of alveolar periostitis that affects the mandibular premolars and first molar has been described (Hofmeyr 1960). It is common in two to four year olds and presents as swelling over the roots of the teeth. The enlargements are formed by dental sacs at the roots, contain a serum-like substance, and have been associated with overcrowding (Hofmeyr 1960). The swellings appear in association with eruption of the appropriate permanent teeth; if no fistulation develops, the swellings may disappear when the horse is six to eight years old. These cystic distensions are generally considered normal processes associated with eruption and should not be considered as disease. However, it is also noted that if there is overcrowding and consequent abnormal resistance to eruption, there may be pathological exacerbation of this pseudocyst, with formation of a painful swelling or a dental sinus (Baker 1971). In these instances surgical intervention (curettage or removal) may be indicated.

CLINICAL SIGNS AND DIAGNOSIS

Various signs of dental disease have been described previously. When the alveolar periosteum of the cheek teeth is affected, the clinical signs typically consist of firm circumscribed swelling on the side of the face or the ventrolateral surface of the mandible (Figs. 15–108 and 15–109), which may or may not be associated with a draining tract or unilateral or bilateral nasal discharge, and sinus enlargement. The clinical features of sinusitis (or empyema of the sinuses) include chronic purulent nasal discharge (usually unilateral), facial swelling over the sinus, respiratory noise and ocular discharge (only in cases with facial swelling), and dullness on percussion (negative result does not preclude sinus-

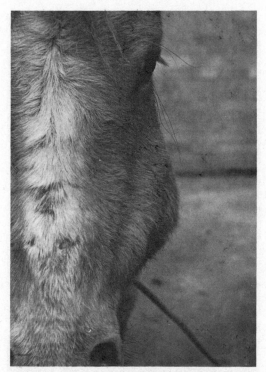

Figure 15–108 Facial swelling associated with a diseased maxillary tooth. (Courtesy of Dr. W. A. Aanes.)

itis) (Fig. 15–110) (Mason 1975). Definitive confirmation of the diagnosis can be made by radiographic demonstration of a fluid line (Fig. 15–111) or abnormal mass in the sinus and percutaneous aspiration of abnormal fluid from the sinus. For the latter procedure a Steinmann pin is introduced into the sinus under local analgesia (Kral 1954). If fluid cannot be aspirated, flushing with sterile saline will cause purulent material to be

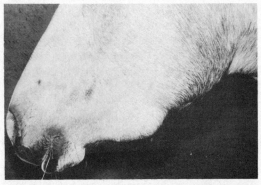

Figure 15–109 Swelling over the mandible associated with a diseased mandibular tooth. (Courtesy of Dr. W. A. Aanes.)

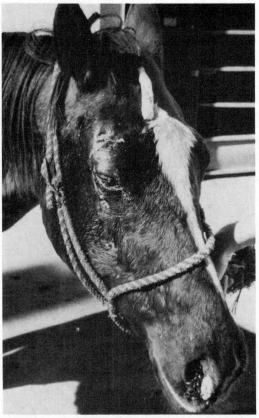

Figure 15–110 Facial swelling and nasal and ocular discharge with empyema of maxillary and frontal sinuses secondary to septic alveolar periostitis of PM4 and M1.

washed out the nostril via the nasomaxillary opening. Because the septum between the rostral and caudal compartments of the maxillary sinus may be complete, separate entry into each compartment is sometimes appropriate. More problems are anticipated in the rostral compartment because of the predilection for the first molar to be affected (Mason 1975). Radiography is also used to identify specific changes associated with the teeth. It is also to be noted that cystic lesions that are probably congenital in origin and that may or may not be associated with teeth cause nasal discharge and sinus swelling (Cannon, Grant, and Sande 1976). These need to be differentiated from alveolar periostitis and empyema.

Radiographic interpretation of tooth abnormalities requires a working knowledge of the normal radiographic appearance of the teeth and their location (Baker 1971; Scott 1982). The root of the

third upper cheek tooth (PM4) is variably located in the nasal cavity, in the rostral wall of the maxillary sinus, or within the maxillary sinus. The root of the fourth upper cheek tooth (M1) generally projects into the rostral compartment of the maxillary sinus, the fifth (M2) in the region of the septum dividing rostral and caudal compartments, and the sixth (M3) into the caudal compartment of the maxillary sinus. Considerable variations exist between paranasal sinus anatomy and teeth location. The length of teeth change with age and wear, and sinus partitions vary in location and degree of development. Dental root disease is recognized radiographically by loss of continuity of the lamina dura, lysis of the tooth root, and/or surrounding bone with abscessation or fistulation within the bone and new bone production (Figs. 15–112 through 15–115).

TREATMENT

Instruments used in dental surgery are illustrated in Figure 15–116.

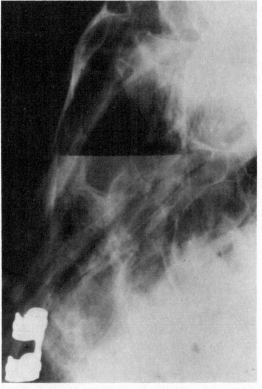

Figure 15–111 Radiograph showing fluid line in maxillary sinus associated with sinusitis secondary to a diseased maxillary tooth.

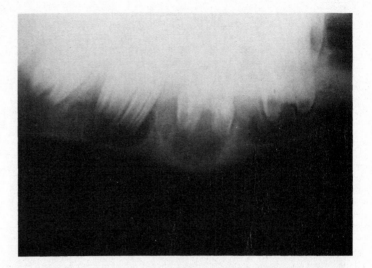

Figure 15–112 Radiograph of diseased mandibular premolar showing resorption of apical tooth root, loss of lamina dura, and sclerosis of mandibular bone. (Courtesy of Dr. W. A. Aanes.)

Cheek tooth removal is generally indicated in the following situations (Scott 1982):

1. Dental fistula originating from the root of an infected cheek tooth;

2. Sinusitis associated with diseased maxillary cheek tooth;

3. Fractured teeth with septic alveolar periostitis and osteomyelitis;

4. Neoplasia, abscesses, or fractures of the mandible or maxilla that affect the viability of a cheek tooth;

5. Prior dental surgery with persistent drainage and fistula formation attributable to incomplete removal of alveolar bone.

Cheek tooth removal is rather unsophisticated and the aftercare problematic, but there is generally no other choice for elimination of the clinical problem. However, drilling out of an open infundibulum, removal of the associated necrotic tooth and root debris, and prosthetic filling of the defect with cement has been successfully performed (Swanstrom and Wolford 1977) and could offer a satisfying alternative in appropriate cases.

In some situations cheek teeth can be extracted through the mouth, but the more usual situation calls for repulsion.

Tooth Extraction. Direct extraction of teeth is usually precluded by their length and generally firm attachment in the alveolus. Even with severe dental disease there is still a wide area of healthy alveolar attachment. In some advanced disease situations or in old horses, some loosening may have occurred and oral extraction may be feasible.

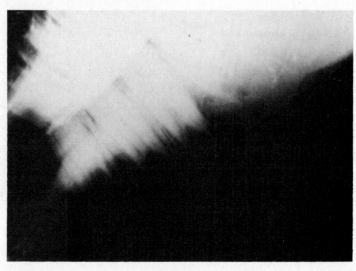

Figure 15–113 Radiograph showing marked loss of tooth substance (fourth mandibular cheek teeth).

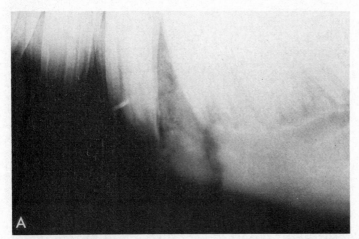

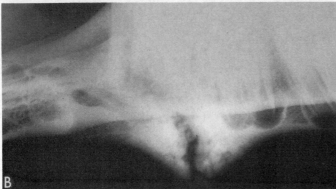

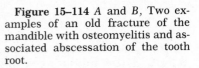

Figure 15–114 A and B, Two examples of an old fracture of the mandible with osteomyelitis and associated abscessation of the tooth root.

Figure 15–115 Follicular cyst formation at the level of the third mandibular cheek tooth.

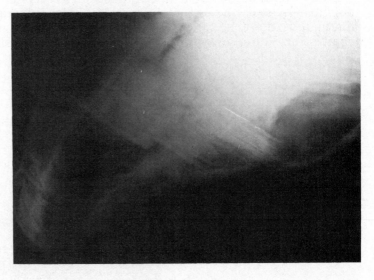

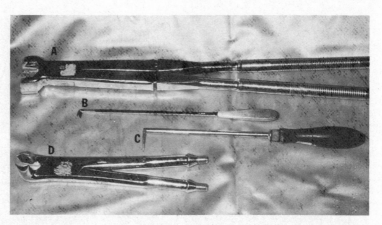

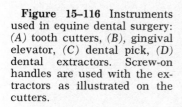

Figure 15–116 Instruments used in equine dental surgery: (A) tooth cutters, (B), gingival elevator, (C) dental pick, (D) dental extractors. Screw-on handles are used with the extractors as illustrated on the cutters.

General anesthesia and a mouth speculum are used. A dental extractor is placed on the tooth and lateral to medial motion applied. Excessive force may cause fracturing of the alveolar bone. When the tooth loosens in the alveolus, there is a sucking noise, and rotary motion may then be used to help elevate the tooth. To remove some teeth from the socket the crown may need to be cut down using molar cutters. Following removal, any debris should be removed from the socket, but the clot is left undisturbed. The cavity is flushed and a gauze pack inserted. This may be replaced with dental wax or some other material to prevent food from packing in the alveolar space as granulation occurs (this is discussed more fully in the next section).

Trephination and Tooth Repulsion. This is indicated whenever a tooth cannot be extracted. General anesthesia is used. A mouth speculum is placed and the site for trephination determined. Tooth repulsion is illustrated in Figure 15–117. The overlying skin is incised (15–117A) and muscles and blood vessels dissected free of the trephine site. The center bit of the trephine is extended 2 mm to fix it to the bone. The trephine is then turned in a back-and-forth rotary motion until it has cut a distinct groove in the bone (Fig. 15–117B). The center bit is then retracted and trephining continued until a disc of bone is detached. Alternatively, a window may be cut in the bone using an osteotome (Fig. 15–117C).

To locate the trephine sites for maxillary cheek teeth, a line is drawn from the medial canthus of the eye to the infraorbital canal and is continued rostrad past the roots of the front cheek tooth. This is the line of maximum height at which trephining may be done for repulsion of maxillary cheek teeth. This line marks the course of the osseous lacrimal canal. Trephine openings for all maxillary cheek teeth should be placed just below this line, except in older horses, in which case the tooth is grown out and the trephine site can be nearer the facial crest. For the first cheek tooth (PM2), the trephination point is placed directly above the center of the table surface of the tooth because this tooth is straight. With the second, third, fourth, and fifth cheek teeth the trephine is centered over the caudal margin of the table surface to allow for the curvature of the teeth. The position and height of the tooth root can also be defined by radiographs. For repulsion of the sixth maxillary cheek tooth, it is necessary to trephine through the frontal sinus 3 cm lateral to midline on a transverse line between the rostral margins of the orbits. A curved dental punch is carried through the frontomaxillary opening into the maxillary sinus to repel the tooth. This is difficult, particularly in young horses in which the apex of the tooth projects caudad beneath the orbit. Fortunately, repulsion of this tooth is rarely indicated.

Trephine sites for the first five mandibular cheek teeth are over the ventrolateral border of the mandible. The trephine site for the first cheek tooth should be directly below the center of the table surface. For the second to fifth teeth the trephine site is centered over the caudal border of the table surface of the tooth to be removed in horses less than nine years old (more towards the center if the horse is older). Exposure of the trephine sites

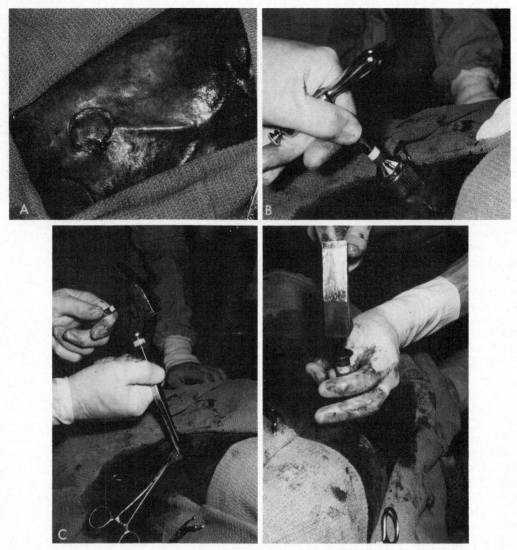

Figure 15–117 Repulsion of maxillary cheek teeth from horse in Figure 15–110. *A,* Skin incision. *B,* Trephination. *C,* Using an osteotome to make a hole in the bone for dental punch. *D,* Repulsion of tooth.
Illustration continued on opposite page

for the fourth and fifth cheek teeth is complicated by the parotid duct and external maxillary artery and vein. For the fourth tooth, the structures are retracted caudally, and for the fifth they are retracted cranially. As with the upper jaw, repulsion of the sixth mandibular cheek tooth presents special problems. A lateral incision is made midway between the table surface of the tooth and the greater curvature of the mandible. The masseter muscle fibers are separated until the bone is reached. The ventral aspect of the tooth is located by identifying the bulge of the root; trephination is performed at this site. Cutting off the crown

is required to repel the tooth in this location.

If a dental fistula is present, the trephine is centered over the fistula, since it usually occurs over the center of the alveolus.

Prior to repelling the tooth, the gum is separated from the tooth crown so that the mucous membrane is not torn. The punch is then positioned over the root of the tooth and tapped while a finger on the table surface ascertains that the procedure is being performed on the correct tooth (Fig. 15–117D). The tooth is then tapped until it loosens. When the punch is firmly seated on the tooth, the hammer

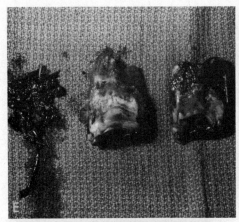

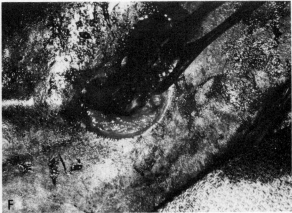

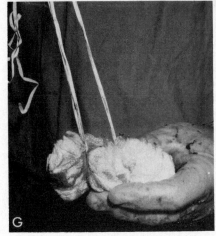

Figure 15–117 *Continued E*, Cheek teeth removed. Note the short roots (horse was 20 years old). *F*, Removal of necrotic material from maxillary sinus (there was chronic empyema in association with the tooth problem). *G*, Preparation of gauze roll to pack socket.

produces a ringing sound, compared with a duller sound and springiness when punching alveolar bone. It is important to maintain the punch in line with the long axis of the tooth. If the tooth is too long to come out without hitting the opposite arcade, the portion projecting beyond the gum line is cut off and removed.

After repulsion of the tooth (15–117E), the socket is examined and any particles or slivers removed (Fig. 15–117F). It is then necessary to insert some form of plug in the socket to prevent packing of foreign material within the cavity while it fills with granulation tissue. One traditional method is to pack the hole initially with a roll of gauze. Umbilical tape is tied around the center of the pack and is used to tie the pack in place (Fig. 15–117G). During the first few days the pack is changed daily and the hole flushed with mild antiseptic solution. After this a more permanent pack is instilled. Ma-

terials that have been used for this purpose include dental wax or dental acrylic. Maintaining these packs in position is problematical. More recently the use of a methylmethacrylate or hoof acrylic pack on a wire lattice has been used and seems superior. The pack is placed at the time of tooth repulsion. Wire is placed around the teeth craniad and caudad and a cross strut incorporated across the loop. Methylmethacrylate is then prepared and placed in the defect between the teeth and extending about 1 cm beyond the gingival margin. This prevents feed from entering the deeper socket but does not prevent the socket from closing via granulation.

Complications of tooth repulsion include penetrating the hard palate or breaking down interalveolar bone plates of adjacent teeth, which can lead to alveolar periostitis and tooth problems. In removal of mandibular teeth where there has been extensive alveolar periostitis and new bone formation, it is recommended that the strip of bone over the lateral surface of the tooth be removed before attempting to repel the tooth (Wheat 1973).

Drainage of Paranasal Sinuses. In certain cases it is necessary to provide drainage to the sinus or perform surgical debridement of the sinus in addition to removing teeth. In chronic sinusitis, debridement of pyogenic membrane from the sinus or removal of soft tissue masses may be necessary. In such cases, the alternative to selective trephination with subsequent enlargement of the opening is to use a bone flap that will allow surgical exposure of both cranial and caudal compartments of the maxillary sinus simultaneously. A U-shaped incision is made through the bone with an oscillating saw (small holes are predrilled to secure the flap back in position but fixation of the bone on closure is not essential), and the flap is elevated. The flap is left attached at the ventral border (Fig. 15–118). As with trephine holes, careful attention to anatomy is necessary in addition to attention to tooth position depending on age.

Effective drainage of an empyematous sinus requires a surgical opening in a dependent position. If the sinusitis is not severe and the contents are fluid, flushing through the trephine hole and/or other small holes with the fluid passing out the normal orifices in the nose may be satisfactory. However, in chronic situations, in addition to debridement other openings may be necessary for drainage.

An effective way to enhance drainage of the cranial maxillary sinus into the nasal cavity is to pass a large, curved, blunt instrument medially over the infraorbital canal and force it gently through the ventral turbinate into the ventral meatus. Setons or drains may be passed into the nasal cavity and exit at the nostril. These may be used to enhance drainage and delay closure of the fenestration site. As mentioned previously, the presence of pyogenic membrane, soft tissue masses (cysts and tumors), and foreign material requires augmentative debridement. Irrigation of the sinus with sterile solution containing dilute povidone-iodine is performed regularly until the problem is considered

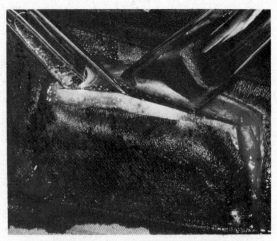

Figure 15–118 Elevation of bone flap over maxillary sinus.

resolved. Exercise and feeding from the floor will assist in promoting drainage.

When there is involvement of the frontal sinus or caudal compartment of the maxillary sinus, dependent drainage may occur into the cranial maxillary sinus, but trephine openings may need to be made over these specific locations. These can be made with knowledge of the normal anatomical boundaries. The conchal portion of the frontal sinus, or conchofrontal sinus (turbinate extension of the frontal sinus), may present a special drainage problem because it is a rostrally placed blind compartment (Scott 1982). To drain this area, a hole is made 3 cm cranial to a line drawn between the medial canthus of the eyes and off the midline. This will provide access to the turbinate extension of the frontal sinus. A mare's catheter is introduced up the nasal passages and is pushed through the cranial border of the dorsal nasal concha. Setons or drains can be placed through the hole (Scott 1982). Hemorrhage can be anticipated.

Dental Tumors

There is some confusion in the nomenclature of dental tumors. The tumors have been classically divided into odontomas, ameloblastomas, and adamantinomas. By definition, the term *odontoma* refers to any tumor of odontogenic origin, but by usage it refers to a tumor in which both epithelial and mesenchymal cells

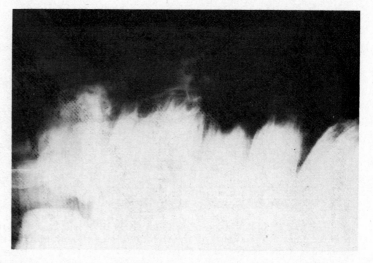

Figure 15–119 Abnormal second maxillary premolar with deformity and irregularity of the germinal area. Note that the tooth has not erupted properly. This was considered to be a benign neoplastic process involving the germinal plate. (Courtesy of Dr. A. S. Turner.)

produce functional ameloblasts and odontoblasts (and therefore enamel and dentin within the tumor) (Baker 1972). Dental tumors are rare and are usually found in young animals. Two instances of ameloblastic odontomas have been described in foals (Lingand and Crawford 1970; Peter, Myers, and Ramsey 1968). They were characterized by the presence of actively proliferating ameloblastic epithelium and mineralized odontoid structures in the same tissue (Peter, Myers, and Ramsey 1968). The tumors continued to enlarge, causing distension of the jaw, face, and/or sinuses. Surgery, if practical, involves curettage of the neoplastic tissue.

Adamantinomas have been defined as tumors arising from the ameloblasts in the enamel region. Although they form enamel, the tumor is normally soft. They are typically locally invasive. Successful surgical removal of an adamantinoma in the horse has been reported (Frank 1964).

Benign neoplastic growths may also be seen occasionally in association with the germinal tooth root; these can affect the development of the tooth. Figure 15–119 is a radiograph of an abnormal second premolar with deformity and irregularity of the germinal area. An aberrant incisor was found in association with the root of this premolar when it was removed.

Dentigerous Cysts

A dentigerous cyst represents a special form of dental teratoma characterized by the presence of dental tissue at the base of a draining tract. The lesion appears as a fluctuant swelling at the base of the ear in a young horse, often accompanied by a discharging fistula (Fig. 15–120). The tooth is usually associated with the temporal bone of the skull. Although the cyst is at the base of the ear, the fistula may open some distance up the margin of the pinna. The condition clinically appears very similar to a conchal cyst or sinus (this condition is not associated with aberrant dental tissue). Radiographs can be used to ascertain the presence of a tooth and its position.

The treatment for a dentigerous cyst is surgery. The tract and cyst are completely removed (Fig. 15–121). The tooth is attached to the temporal bone and the attachments need to be cut or broken.

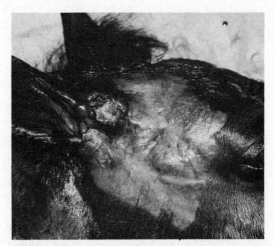

Figure 15–120 External appearance of a dentigerous cyst with a draining tract at the base of the ear.

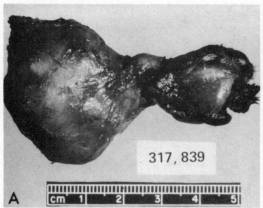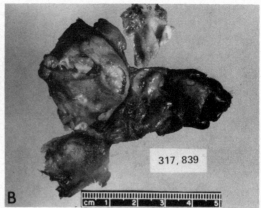

Figure 15–121 Appearance of a dentigerous cyst following removal. *A,* The cyst is unopened. The drainage point at the skin is on the right and the sac containing dental tissue is on the left. *B,* The cyst has been opened to reveal dental tissue.

This should be performed carefully, as the attachment can be very firm and fracture of the temporal bone is possible. A conchal cyst is similarly removed by dissection, ensuring that all secretory tissue is removed.

Surgical Problems of the Salivary Glands

TRAUMA

Fresh wounds involving the salivary glands can be sutured. When suturing is not practical, healing by granulation occurs and permanent salivary leakage is not normally a problem. However, a permanent fistula may develop following trauma to a salivary duct. The fistula is surgically removed down to the duct. Repair of the duct has been described by placing a polyethylene tube into the duct and suturing the distal end into the mouth to facilitate healing of the defect in the duct (Hofmeyr 1974).

SIALOLITHS

These usually occur in Stensen's duct and can achieve considerable size. The calculi consist mainly of calcium carbonate and are considered to require a nidus (small foreign body or inflammatory process) for deposition of the calcium salts (Hofmeyr 1974). Enlargement due to the calculus is the usual clinical feature. Radiographs can be used to confirm the presence of sialolith (Fig. 15–122). The problem is treated by surgical re-

moval (Fig. 15–123). The duct can be left to close by second intention.

SALIVARY CYSTS

These usually arise owing to rupture of a duct and leakage of saliva into the surrounding tissue (Hofmeyr 1974). The cysts present as a soft fluctuant swelling, and saliva is aspirated on needle puncture. The differential diagnosis includes thyroglossal cysts.

The surgical treatment of choice is to attempt to create a fistula from the cyst into the mouth. This can be done by placing a Penrose drain from the cyst into the mouth. If this fails, radical excision of the cyst and associated salivary gland can be considered.

ESOPHAGUS

Anatomy

The esophagus of the adult horse is 125 to 150 cm in length and can be divided into cervical, thoracic, and abdominal portions (Getty 1975). The cervical portion is 10 to 15 cm longer than the thoracic part and thus represents over 50 per cent of the total length of the esophagus. The abdominal portion is only 2 to 3 cm long. The esophagus begins in the median plane above the cranial border of the cricoid cartilage of the larynx. It is positioned dorsal to the trachea until it reaches the fourth cervical vertebra, where it descends obliquely

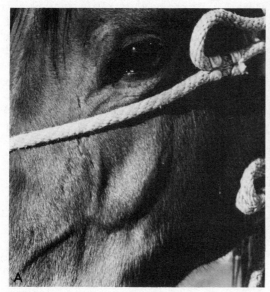

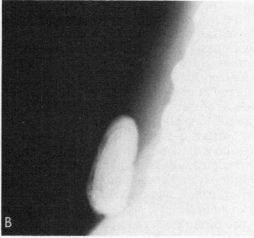

Figure 15–122 Facial swelling (*A*) associated with and radiograph (*B*) of a salivary calculus in the parotid duct. (Courtesy of Dr. T. S. Stashak.)

across the left side of the trachea. It usually reaches the median plane ventral to the trachea at the caudal aspect of the sixth cervical vertebra and enters the thorax in this position. The cervical portion of the esophagus is the most accessible (and therefore of primary importance surgically). Within the thorax, the esophagus re-assumes a position dorsal to the trachea and passes right and then left again to the esophageal hiatus of the diaphragm and terminates at the cardiac orifice of the stomach, slightly to the left of the median plane.

The principal relations of the esophagus at its origin are the cricoid cartilage and dorsal cricoarytenoid muscles ventrally, the guttural pouches and ventral straight muscles dorsally, and the carotid arteries laterally. In the middle of the neck, the relations are the left longus colli muscle dorsally; the trachea medially; and the left carotid artery, vagosympathetic trunk, and recurrent laryngeal nerve dorsolaterally. Near the thoracic inlet the esophagus is usually in contact with the left jugular vein for a short distance. At its entrance into the thorax the trachea is on its medial side, and the first rib and roots of the brachial plexus are lateral. After the esophagus reaches the dorsal surface of the trachea, the aorta lies to the left, and the azygos vein and right vagus nerve are to the right. As the esophagus passes through the

caudal mediastinum, the esophageal branches of the vagus nerve lie above and below the esophagus.

The esophageal wall is composed of four layers: a fibrous sheath (tunica adventitia); a muscular layer (tunica muscularis); submucosa (tela submucosa); and a mucous membrane (tunica mu-

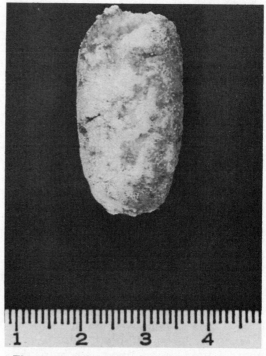

Figure 15–123 Salivary calculus following removal (courtesy of Dr. T. S. Stashak).

cosa). The muscular layer consists of striated muscle from the pharynx to the base of the heart, where it changes to smooth muscle. The muscular layer also becomes thicker as the esophagus progresses caudad. Except at each end of the esophagus, the tunica muscularis chiefly consists of two layers of fibers arranged spirally or elliptically, and these intercross dorsally and ventrally. The mucosa, which provides the greatest tensile strength upon closure of an esophageal incision, is pale and covered with stratified squamous epithelium. It lies in longitudinal folds, which obliterate the lumen except during deglutition. The mucosa is loosely attached to the muscular coat by an abundant submucosa, and these two layers show distinct separation from the relatively inelastic muscularis and adventitia on surgical incision.

The arterial blood supply to the cervical part of the esophagus originates from the carotid arteries. The thoracic and abdominal parts are supplied by the bronchoesophageal and gastric arteries. The vascular pattern is arcuate, but segmental and collateral circulation is minimal. The nerve supply comes from the glossopharyngeal (IX) and vagus (X) nerves and the sympathetic trunk and the myenteric plexus within the muscle layers. The myenteric plexus is considered to be present only when smooth muscle supplants striated muscle in the esophageal wall (DeBoom 1975).

Physiology

The esophagus is quiet at rest and contracts during swallowing. The proximal esophagus is closed by a functional sphincter (the upper esophageal sphincter). The musculature producing this sphincter effect is thought to derive from caudal fibers of the thyropharyngeus muscles, the cricopharyngeus muscle, and the cranial fibers of the longitudinal muscle layer of the esophagus. Swallowing is a combined reflux-voluntary mechanism (O'Brien, Harvey, and Brodey 1980). The upper esophageal sphincter relaxes in coordination with pharyngeal contraction to accommodate a bolus during swallowing. A swallowed bolus initiates a primary peristaltic wave, and this is propagated throughout the length of the esophagus. Esophageal distension may elicit a secondary peristaltic wave that can commence at the area of distension anywhere along the length of the esophagus. Reverse peristaltic waves and large numbers of tertiary waves, or spontaneous contractions, are abnormal (O'Brien, Harvey, and Brodey 1980).

A lower esophageal sphincter at the terminal esophagus can also be identified by manometry. This sphincter prevents reflux of ingesta from the stomach. In coordination with the passage of a bolus into the terminal esophagus, the pressure in the lower esophageal sphincter drops and then elevates to complete peristalsis before returning to resting levels.

At rest, thoracic esophageal pressures are subatmospheric and approximate intrathoracic pressures, whereas cervical esophageal pressures are near atmospheric pressure (Derksen and Robinson 1980). Peristalsis produces a wave of increased intraluminal pressure (80 mm Hg above resting cervical esophageal pressure) that travels rapidly for the first 90 cm and slowly for the terminal 30 cm of the esophagus, corresponding to the areas of striated and smooth muscle, respectively (Derksen and Robinson 1980). The time interval from the initiation of swallowing until the bolus reaches the stomach is approximately 12 to 16 seconds.

Diagnosis of Esophageal Disorders

Choke is the general manifestation of esophageal disturbances and has been defined as an inability to swallow as a sequela to partial or complete obstruction of the esophagus (Alexander 1967). Causes of such obstruction include foreign bodies, wounds, stricture or narrowing, diverticulum, dilation, and esophageal spasm. These various entities will be discussed separately.

Diagnostic evaluation of a horse with an esophageal problem includes clinical examination, radiology, and endoscopy. Most esophageal problems in the horse are associated with an anatomical problem such as a foreign body obstruction, stricture, or diverticulum, but functional disorders also occur occasionally. In these latter instances, manometric, cineradiographic, and electromyographic studies may be appropriate.

CLINICAL MANIFESTATIONS AND PHYSICAL EXAMINATION

Clinical signs associated with obstruction of the esophagus include ptyalism, dysphagia, coughing, and regurgitation of food, water, and saliva from the mouth and nostrils. Some horses will show considerable distress with anxiety and sweating. Attempts at ingestion often result in painful attempts at swallowing (odynophagia) with repeated extension of the head and neck. The animal may be anorectic if the problem causes severe pain. The time interval from swallowing until pain or regurgitation is observed depends on the location of the obstruction within the esophagus. Signs will usually be immediate with obstruction in the upper esophagus, but with obstruction of the lower esophagus, odynophagia and retching may occur 10 to 12 seconds after swallowing (Stick 1982).

The rate of onset of the disease is also important. An acute onset is typical of a foreign body obstruction, whereas a gradually developing obstruction is more typical of a stricture. Nonobstructive conditions may have intermittent episodes of the previously mentioned signs interspersed with periods of relief as ingesta builds up secondary to the functional problem and is then passed.

In the patient with an obstruction of the cervical esophagus, the distended esophagus can usually be palpated and/or visualized. If there is evidence of cellulitis in the area, loss of integrity in the wall of the esophagus should be considered. The possibility of disease of the oropharynx, including oral foreign bodies, dental disease, cleft palate, and inflammatory or neoplastic disease, should be eliminated by careful oral examination. Pharyngeal paralysis will cause dysphagia, manifested principally as nasal regurgitation of food and water, and must be eliminated. Pharyngeal causes of dyphagia are discussed in the previous section.

The passage of a nasogastric tube will often confirm the presence of an esophageal obstruction and will also localize the problem. If there is an ingesta obstruction, lavage through the tube may enable clearance of the obstruction. If this occurs, endoscopic examination will determine the presence or degree of damage to the esophageal mucosa (to assess the potential for stricture formation and re-obstruction).

Clinical evaluation to assess the possible presence of concurrent respiratory disease should be performed. Aspiration pneumonia is a common secondary complication of esophageal obstruction. Dehydration and electrolyte imbalances should also be assessed, particularly with obstruction of some duration.

RADIOGRAPHIC EXAMINATION OF THE ESOPHAGUS

Radiographic examination of the cervical esophagus is frequently useful in diagnosing and defining the extent of an obstruction (Fig. 15–124). A plain radiograph is made initially (Fig. 15–125A); some lesions will be demonstrable with this alone. Contrast radiography may then be performed (Fig. 15–125B); three different techniques are suggested for a complete study (Stick 1982). Positive contrast material administered orally will outline the mucosal folds of the esophagus with the lumen undistended. Liquid barium administered under pressure through a nasogastric tube with an inflatable cuff to prevent reflux into the pharynx enables evaluation of the distensibility of the esophagus and provides demonstration of strictures and fistulae. The use of a 10-mm OD nasogastric tube with an inflatable cuff* has been described (Stick, Derksen, and Scott 1981). Liquid barium followed with air through the nasogastric tube provides a double contrast study and allows examination of the nasal folds with the esophagus distended. A diagnosis will commonly be made without using all three of these contrast techniques. However, each technique can demonstrate lesions that may be missed with the other two techniques. Therefore, all three contrast

*Inflatable cuff with pilot balloon (9.5 mm ID), Veterinary Specialties Inc., Cedar Rapids, IA.

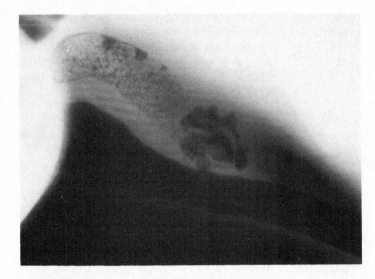

Figure 15–124 Radiograph of obstruction of the esophagus with feed material.

techniques are necessary before a study can be considered complete in the case of a difficult diagnosis. The paste and liquid contrast media can be made by mixing barium sulfate powder* and 30% barium gastric suspension† (paste = 3 g powder/ml suspension, liquid = 2 g powder/ml suspension (Stick 1982).

False signs of stricture formation can be produced by swallowing during a contrast radiography study. Therefore, attempts should be made to obtain contrast radiographs with the entire cervical esophagus fully distended. Xylazine ad-

*Veri-O-Pake, General Electric Company, Detroit, MI.

†Redi-Paque, Burns-Biotec Laboratories, Omaha, NB.

ministered intravenously five minutes previous to a barium-pressure or contrast study helps eliminate swallowing artifacts by decreasing secondary peristaltic waves associated with esophageal distension (Stick 1982). It has been suggested that if an obstruction is high in the upper cervical region, it is safer to use an iodinated organic compound not exceeding 5 ml (Alexander 1967).

Positive contrast radiography of the cervical esophagus, properly performed, will provide a better evaluation of esophageal problems than negative contrast radiography. Radiographic evaluation of the thoracic esophagus is problematical in the horse owing to the size of the patient's thorax and the need for high-

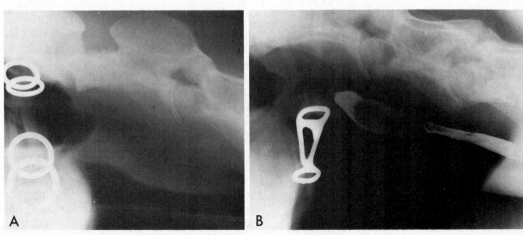

Figure 15–125 *A*, Plain radiograph of obstruction of the esophagus with feed material. *B*, Contrast radiograph of the same obstruction.

capacity equipment. Fortunately, thoracic esophageal problems are much less common than cervical problems.

ENDOSCOPIC EXAMINATION OF THE ESOPHAGUS

Endoscopic examination of the esophagus is indicated when the clinical and radiographic findings are inconclusive or when esophageal lesions have been diagnosed and the clinician wishes to further define their size and severity. Examination with a flexible fiberoptic endoscope is safe and convenient and can be performed in the standing animal. Contraindications to the technique are few but include acute corrosive or necrotizing esophagitis (perforation could occur through the friable esophagus).

For effective examination the clinician must be aware of the normal endoscopic anatomy and its variations. The normal longitudinal folds of esophageal mucosa can be observed when the endoscope is retracted retrograde (toward the head). These folds can be flattened with air insufflation. Transverse folds in the mucosa can be produced by advancing the endoscope toward the stomach. Swallowing obstructs the view through the endoscope and can cause changes in the lumen of the esophagus that may resemble diverticuli or sclerotic rings. The best diagnostic assessment can be made by fully inserting the endoscope and slowly pulling it retrograde while insufflating the esophagus. Irrigation may be necessary after a swallowing wave. If complete examination of the thoracic esophagus is desired, it may be necessary to create a cervical esophagostomy because of limitations in endoscope length (Freeman and Naylor 1978).

The physical examination, including nasogastric tube passage, esophageal lavage, and radiography, will provide a diagnosis in most instances. Endoscopy may provide better definition of the actual lesion. If available, manometry, cineradiography, and electromyography could be considered when anatomic disease cannot be demonstrated and a physiologic disorder is suspected (Bowman et al. 1978).

Food or Foreign Body Obstruction

Impaction of the esophagus with feed is the most common cause of esophageal obstruction. The animals involved are often greedy feeders. Horses with bad teeth are also prone, as are Shetland ponies, which have a relatively narrow esophagus (Hofmeyr 1974; Kindrey and Lundvall 1972). However, such predisposing causes are not always identified. Obstruction with feed material may also be caused by pre-existing esophageal disease, and this must be recognized. Other foreign bodies may also lodge in the esophagus; anthelmintic boluses have been a classic cause in the past (Kindrey and Lundvall 1972), but their use has declined in recent years (Fig. 15–126).

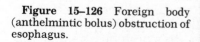

Figure 15–126 Foreign body (anthelmintic bolus) obstruction of esophagus.

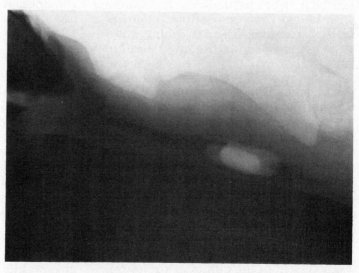

The horse will show variable amounts of distress, with arching and extension of the neck. Saliva will run from the mouth or nostrils and often contains feed particles. The other clinical signs have been described previously. The presence of an obstruction and its position are confirmed by passage of a stomach tube. Plain radiographs will typically demonstrate foreign material in the esophagus causing esophageal distension, gas accumulation between the walls of the esophagus, and the impaction and ventral deviation of the trachea. Gas in the soft tissues adjacent to the esophagus is indicative of esophageal perforation or fistula formation (Alexander 1967). Contrast radiology is indicated to demonstrate nonradiopaque foreign bodies and define esophageal damage (following removal of the foreign body).

Treatment of esophageal obstruction can involve medical, manipulative, and surgical methods; a fixed protocol is not appropriate. Many cases of obstruction with feed material will resolve themselves spontaneously or with simple medical support. Tranquilizers can be useful. The use of smooth muscle relaxants is not indicated for obstructions of the cervical esophagus (this is composed of striated muscle in the horse). Some clinicians prefer the previously mentioned method of treatment of ingesta obstructions in the initial stages rather than performing repeated nasogastric tube passages and inflicting further trauma on the esophagus.

However, gentle manipulation with a stomach tube, particularly if combined with lavage, can be useful in clearing a feed obstruction. Regular tubing and lavage can help soften the mass and facilitate saliva penetration, but gentleness is paramount. In all instances, there are drawbacks. The presence of any impaction for too long can cause pressure necrosis of the esophageal mucosa and subsequent stricture formation; overzealous manipulations can have similar effects. Good clinical judgement is important. If there is a hard- or rough-surfaced foreign body present, early removal is essential to avoid permanent damage.

In many instances, permanent esophageal damage due to prolonged obstruction with or without tube manipulation is the result of the clinician's reluctance to perform an esophagotomy. This reluctance is not without foundation; the difficulties and complications associated with esophageal surgery are well known and will be discussed; however, timely and competent surgical intervention is a necessary part of the management of esophageal obstruction.

If the results of conservative management techniques are not successful there are some other alternatives prior to performing an esophagotomy. Many obstructions are just distal to the pharynx, and clearance may be possible under general anesthesia using a person with a small hand. Long forceps can sometimes be useful here also. Lavage can sometimes be better performed under anesthesia. Probing with a pneumatic cuff (Thygesen extractor) may also be helpful in securing a foreign body (Hofmeyr 1974). Such instruments do carry an added risk of damaging the esophageal wall.

The next step is to surgically expose the esophagus (using the same approach as that described for esophagotomy) and manipulate the mass externally. Manipulation through the pharynx and lavage can also be performed simultaneously. If this is unsuccessful, esophagotomy is indicated. The surgeon should always remember that a well-performed esophagotomy is less traumatic than prolonged pressure and bruising to the esophageal wall. The same applies to the use of forceps and damage to the esophageal mucosa. In special circumstances it may be possible to remove a foreign body under fiberoptic visualization using grasping forceps (Traver, Egger, and Moore 1978).

ESOPHAGOTOMY

The esophagus has properties quite distinct from the remainder of the gastrointestinal tract, and these are important surgically. The esophagus is not covered by serosa (this promotes a rapid seal due to exudation of fibrin following intestinal surgery). The musculature of the esophagus is weak and holds sutures poorly, but the mucosa is *relatively* strong (in the remainder of the gastrointestinal tract the mucosa is weak and the submucosa is the strongest layer). Nonabsorbable suture material is used to close the mucosa rather than catgut, which is absorbed too quickly. The esophagus can be distended considerably but has little stretch longitudinally. Short blood vessels require care and limitations in mobilizing the esophagus. Gentleness is used in handling the esophagus, and crushing clamps are not used. These principles must be borne in mind when operating on the esophagus.

The major complications in healing of an esophageal wound are leakage and dehiscence, and contributing factors include the lack of serosa, the easily disrupted segmental blood supply, and constant motion of the esophagus.

Additional complications of esophageal surgery include extension of infection into surrounding tissues, stricture, fistula, diverticula, and dilatation. Longitudinal esophagotomy with primary closure of the incision results in minimal complications when performed in an area of normal esophagus (Stick et al. 1981). Sutured esophagotomies heal significantly faster than nonsutured esophagotomies; the latter group develop traction diverticula (Stick et al. 1981).

Esophagotomy for removal of an obstruction in the cervical esophagus is conveniently performed using a ventral midline approach (Fig. 15–127). General

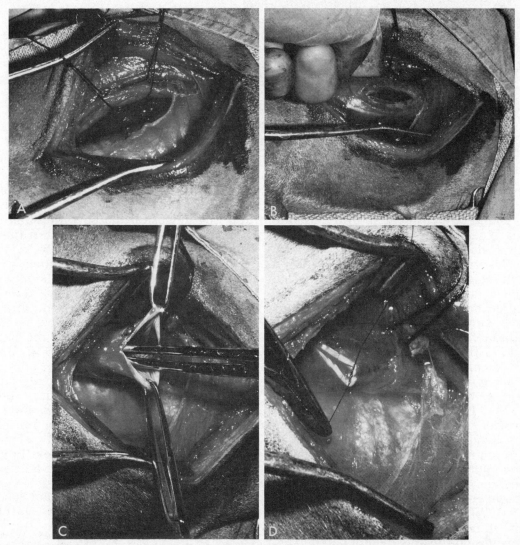

Figure 15–127 Esophagotomy. *A*, Division of ventral neck musculature and retraction of carotid sheath to expose ventral aspect of esophagus. *B*, Incision through musculature and mucosa of esophagus. *C*, Removal of foreign body with forceps. *D*, Closure of esophageal mucosa with simple interrupted sutures tied in the lumen.

Illustration continued on following page

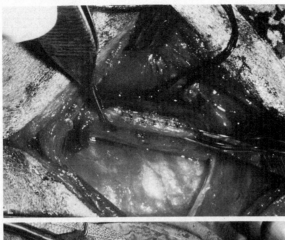

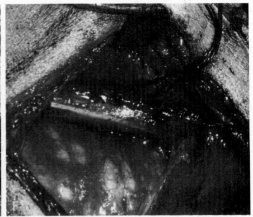

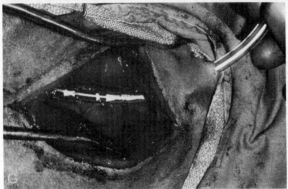

Figure 15–127 *Continued E,* Completed closure of esophageal mucosa. *F,* Closure of esophageal musculature. *G,* Placement of fenestrated suction drain prior to closure of muscle and fascia.

anesthesia is used, and a nasogastric tube is placed as far as the foreign body to facilitate identification of the esophagus. The patient is placed in dorsal recumbency and the ventral aspect of the neck surgically prepared. An 8- to 10-cm skin incision is made on the ventral midline over the area of obstruction. The paired sternothyroideus, sternohyoideus, and omohyoideus muscles are divided to expose the trachea. The fascia on the left side is then bluntly dissected to locate the esophagus. The ventral wall of the esophagus is exposed with careful dissection of adventitial tissue (Fig. 15–127A). Elevation of the esophagus is avoided to minimize interference with the blood supply. The left carotid sheath containing the carotid artery and vagus and recurrent laryngeal nerves is identified and retracted laterally. The esophagotomy is performed using a scalpel (Fig. 15–127B). The surgeon attempts to incise in normal esophageal wall, but this depends on the site, mobility, and extent of the obstruction.

Following removal of the foreign body

(Fig. 15–127C), the mucosa of the esophagus is examined, and, if it appears normal, the mucosa is closed with 2-0 or 3-0 polypropylene* in a simple interrupted or continuous pattern (Fig. 15–127D). The knots are tied within the lumen (Fig. 15–127E). The musculature is closed with 2-0 polypropylene or polyglactin 910† (Fig. 15–127F). A 1/4-in. fenestrated suction drain‡ is placed beside the esophagus and exits through the skin caudal to the skin incision (Fig. 15–127G). It is maintained for 48 hours to remove serum and blood from the surgery site. Retention of the drain beyond this period is contraindicated unless there is salivary leakage. The muscle and fascia of the neck incision are closed with polyglactin 910 in a simple interrupted pattern. The skin is closed with nonabsorable material.

Extraoral alimentation is not used postoperatively when a primary closure

*Prolene, Ethicon, Inc., Somerville, NJ.
†Vicryl, Ethicon, Inc., Somerville, NJ.
‡Redi-Vacette, perforated tubing 1/4 in. (64 mm) OD, Orthopedic Equipment, Bourbon, IN.

on healthy esophagus has been performed. Food is withheld for 48 hours, and then small quantities of pelleted feed in a slurry are given. Normal feeding is resumed in 8 to 10 days.

If the esophagotomy has been performed through a compromised esophagus, a system for extraoral alimentation is recommended postoperatively. Either the incision may be closed and an esophagostomy tube placed through a separate incision distally, or an esophagostomy tube is placed directly into the initial esophagotomy incision. Cervical esophagostomy has been documented as a safe and convenient means of tube feeding in the horse (Freeman and Naylor 1978; Stick, Derksen, and Scott 1981) and is preferred over the use of a nasogastric tube or pharyngostomy.

CERVICAL ESOPHAGOSTOMY

Cervical esophagostomy can be conveniently created at the level of the fifth cervical vertebra, where the esophagus is readily accessible and has minimal contact with major structures. At this point the esophagus inclines to the left in most horses, and the carotid sheath is dorsolateral to the esophagus (Freeman and Naylor 1978). If not being performed in conjunction with other esophageal surgery, the esophagostomy may be created in the standing animal using sedation and local analgesia. A 6- to 8-cm incision is made on the ventral midline of the neck at the junction of the middle and lower thirds and is continued between the paired sternothyrohyoideus and sternohyoideus muscles. The trachea is identified and retracted to the right to expose the esophagus (a tube is present within the lumen to facilitate identification). With gentle traction and fascial dissection, the esophagus is drawn ventrad away from the carotid sheath.

Alternatively, a ventrolateral approach can be made ventral to the left jugular vein. The sternocephalicus and brachiocephalicus muscles are separated and retracted. The deep cervical fascia is incised to expose the esophagus (it may also be necessary to go through omohyoideus or cutaneous colli musculature, depending on the exact site of the incision). This technique probably provides better access to the esophagus while avoiding impingement of the feeding tube against the trachea.

A 1- to 2-cm incision is made in the muscle layer on the ventral or ventrolateral aspect of the esophagus. The mucosa is grasped to evert it through the incision in the muscular layer. A transverse incision is then made through the mucosa of sufficient size to admit the tube (the nasogastric tube is previously removed). The esophagostomy tube is passed in until its end is in the stomach. Large-diameter tubes are preferred to avoid plugging with ingesta when feed is administered. The mucosa is then sutured tightly around the tube using simple interrupted sutures of 2-0 catgut (this measure still does not preclude salivary leakage). The caudal half of the incision in the neck muscles and fascia is closed with 2-0 absorbable suture and the skin closed with nonabsorbable sutures. The tube is then secured using butterfly tape bandages sutured to the skin on the side of the neck and an elastic tape bandage. A cork is placed in the tubes between feedings, and the tubes are flushed with water at the end of feeding to maintain patency.

Some salivary loss around the tube is anticipated. Wounds need to be cleaned daily. Localized infection around the wound occurs, and there is initial swelling, which regresses. All sutures except those securing the tube to the skin are removed at 10 days. The use of a complete pelleted diet (7 g/kg in 5 L water three times a day) is satisfactory (Stick, Derksen, and Scott 1981).

Ten days of extraoral alimentation will be sufficient in most esophageal surgery cases. The tubes are removed and the stoma left to close. The duration of tube feeding has a significant influence on the healing time of the surgical esophagostomy following removal of the feeding tube (Stick et al. 1981). Traction diverticula develop in association with stomal healing by second intention, but they do not seem to be of clinical consequence (Freeman and Naylor 1978; Stick et al. 1981). They are wide necked and therefore do not entrap food material (Freeman and Naylor 1978). The placement of the end of the tube in the thoracic esophagus minimizes reflux of food around the tube, but there is a risk of tube dislodgement and replacement is difficult and risky.

Blood electrolyte and acid-base changes associated with salivary depletion will occur in horses with cervical esophagostomies (Stick, Robinson, and Krehbiel 1981). Despite lack of mastication, copious salivation can still occur and has been associated with stimulation of salivary secretion by the indwelling tube, esophageal distension, and the decreased roughage in the pelleted ration (Stick, Robinson, and Krehbiel 1981). Significant hyponatremia and hypochloremia and marginal hypocalemia occur in conjunction with metabolic alkalosis (Stick, Robinson, and Krehbiel 1981). These changes can be easily managed by the administration of oral sodium chloride.

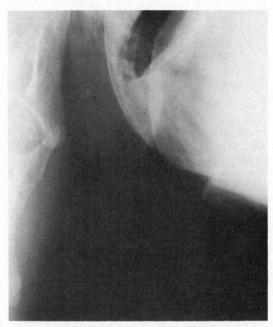

Figure 15–128 Perforation of esophagus with a piece of wire. Gas accumulation can be seen proximal to the wire.

Perforation or Rupture of the Esophagus

Breakdown in the esophageal wall can occur secondarily in long-standing obstruction, foreign body perforation, external trauma to the cervical area, or extension of infection (Fig. 15–128) (DeMoor et al. 1979; Raker and Sayers 1958). If there is no drainage to the outside, the leakage of saliva and ingesta into the tissues of the neck causes severe cellulitis and phlegmon development. Defects that drain through the skin will be less likely to cause associated tissue problems and septicemia. The presence of a ruptured cervical esophagus will therefore manifest as a wound draining saliva and ingesta or a severe swelling and cellulitis in the neck. A ruptured thoracic esophagus will cause a septic mediastinitis and pleuritis and is not generally compatible with life.

Early establishment of ventral drainage in rupture of the cervical esophagus is important to avoid dissecting cellulitis (which can extend to mediastinitis and pleuritis) and septicemia. If a perforation is recognized within 12 hours and there is minimal damage to the esophageal wall, primary closure of the defect as described for esophagotomy may be appropriate. When there is severe damage to the esophageal wall and/or significant infection of the surrounding tissue, it is better to leave the defect to heal spontaneously while providing adequate drainage and placing an esophagostomy tube aboral to the defect. The animal is fed through the tube as described previously. In some instances of severe generalized tissue infection it may be preferable to place a tube through the initial defect, treat the tissue infection, and, when this is resolved, perform an esophagostomy to allow repair of the defect.

Esophageal ruptures can heal spontaneously without any specific treatment in some instances. However, even with careful extraoral feeding and fastidious management of tissue infection, stricture or fistula formation may still result. In some instances, resection of a portion of esophagus and anastomosis may be the only feasible method of treatment.

Esophageal Stricture

Simple strictures have been classified as annular and tubular (Fretz 1972). Stricture formation in the horse is usually an annular lesion. These lesions, in turn, have been classified into three types depending on the esophageal wall layers involved in the induration and fibrosis (Stick 1982): mural lesions that involve only the adventitia and muscularis; rings or webs involving only the mucosa and submucosa; and annular stenosis that involves all layers of the esophageal wall.

Esophageal strictures may follow external or internal trauma to the esophageal wall, local pressure necrosis of the mucosa, esophagotomy or perforation, severe esophagitis due to caustic anthelmintics, or any other inflammatory process involving the esophageal wall. The typical sequence when necrosis of the esophageal mucosa occurs (for whatever reason) is as follows (Fretz 1972). During the first seven days the necrotic area becomes inflamed and the mucosa sloughs, leaving an ulcer. During the next seven days granulation tissue fills the defect; this subsequently organizes into fibrous tissue. The fibrous tissue will then begin to contract, ultimately resulting in stricture formation (Fig. 15–129). This scarring process may continue for several months, depending on the severity of the original injury. It is to be noted that mucosal ulceration does not always lead to stricture formation.

Patients manifest typical signs of esophageal obstruction. The stricture usually impedes passage of a nasogastric tube; in some instances a narrow tube

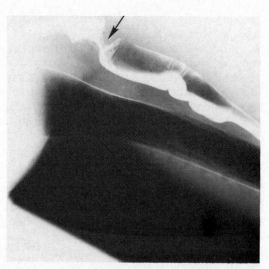

Figure 15–130 Positive contrast radiograph of annular stricture in proximal cervical esophagus (arrow).

might pass, but a normal-sized tube will not. The lesion can be demonstrated by a positive-pressure contrast esophagram (Fig. 15–130). The lesion may also be demonstrated on endoscopy in some instances. The outcome in cases of esophageal strictures in horses is frequently poor, with aspiration pneumonia, inanition, and dehydration as sequelae. Diverticulum formation and esophagotracheal fistulization have been reported as sequelae to esophageal stenosis in the horse (Tvedten and Keahey 1974).

Conservative therapy for esophageal stricture is aimed at dilation of the stenotic segment of esophagus. It may be possible to dilate early postsurgical stricture formation by feeding small, frequent quantities of soft food (soaked horse pellets) over several weeks (if prestenotic dilation does not occur). (Stick 1982). Strictures are usually too firm by the time of diagnosis for such a practice to be of benefit. The use of bougienage to dilate annular lesions is well documented in man, and the response to treatment is usually good, especially if the fibrosis is confined to the superficial layers (Fretz 1972). The prognosis becomes less favorable as the stricture widens or the fibrous ring becomes denser. In the one report in horses, bougienage was unsuccessfully performed for 21 days on an annular lesion in the thoracic esophagus, with bougienage becoming

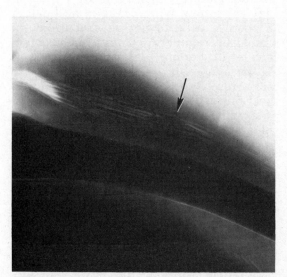

Figure 15–129 Loss of normal mucosal structures with contrast esophagram in an area of mucosal scarring (arrow).

progressively more difficult (Freeman and Naylor 1978).

The only feasible methods of handling most esophageal strictures are surgical. Methods available include esophagomyotomy, partial resection, complete resection and anastomosis, and esophagoplasty with muscle or synthetic patch grafting.

ESOPHAGOMYOTOMY

This procedure can be useful in cases in which the strictures are mural in origin (Stick 1982). Poor results have been documented in the literature (Fretz 1972; Lowe 1964), and such results can be anticipated if mucosa is involved.

The surgery is performed with the horse under general anesthesia with a nasogastric tube preplaced and the esophagus approached in the same manner as that described for esophagotomy. The esophagus is incised longitudinally to the level of the mucosa, with the incision extending 1 cm proximad and distad to the stricture. The nasogastric tube is then passed through the stenotic area (if this is not possible a satisfactory result from myotomy cannot be anticipated). The muscularis is then dissected from the mucosa around the circumference of the esophagus. The myotomy is not sutured, and the neck incision is closed and a drain inserted as described for esophagotomy.

Small quantities of soft feed are fed if there is any evidence of prestenotic dilation of the esophagus (Stick 1982). If there is no dilation or when it resolves, normal feeding is instituted. As with all surgeries for stricture, restricture can occur weeks or months later. A recurrent obstruction may resolve with a change in diet roughage to completely pelleted feed. Otherwise, another myotomy or some other surgical procedure is the only alternative.

PARTIAL RESECTION

This technique involves the previously described esophagomyotomy combined with mucosal resection (Stick 1982). The procedure is indicated when the stricture involves the mucosa and prevents nasogastric tube passage following myotomy (Stick 1982).

An esophagomyotomy is performed as previously described. The mucosa is then incised longitudinally to identify the pathologic section of mucosa. The mucosal scar is then separated from the muscle and removed utilizing circumferential incisions proximad and distad to the lesion. The muscular tube of the esophagus is thus left intact. If the cut edges of the mucosa can be apposed without undue tension, they are closed with simple interrupted sutures of 3-0 or 2-0 polypropylene with the knots in the lumen. The myotomy incision is sutured closed if mucosal scarring was the sole source of the stricture; if the problem was an annular stenosis involving the entire esophageal wall, the myotomy incision is left unsutured. Closure of the neck is as described previously.

Following this surgery, if feasible, an esophagostomy is made distal to the surgery site and a feeding tube placed. When this is not possible, frequent feeding of small quantities of soft food is commenced 48 hours after surgery and is continued 10 days before normal feed is offered to the patient. If the stricture recurs following this procedure, complete resection or patch grafting is indicated.

COMPLETE RESECTION

Resection of the esophagus is indicated in cases of esophageal rupture with wall devitalization, when there is no healthy muscular tube to act as a scaffold for mucosal regeneration, or for problem cases of esophageal stricture (Lowe 1964; Vaughan and Hoffer 1966). With ruptures of the esophagus requiring resection, cellulitis of the surrounding tissue will be present and delay of surgery is appropriate until some of the acute inflammation has subsided. At the same time it is appropriate to train the animal to tolerate a standing martingale. This measure is warranted in all candidates for esophageal resection, as it is used postoperatively to prevent elevation of the head and tension on the esophageal anastomosis.

The esophagus is surgically exposed as previously described for esophagotomy. The necessary amount of esophagus is immobilized. Rubber tubing clamped with hemostats is used to occlude the

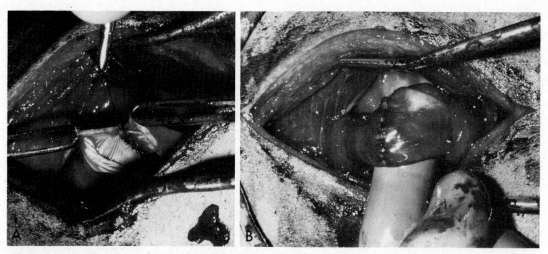

Figure 15–131 Esophageal resection and anastomosis. *A*, Anastomosis of mucosa using simple interrupted sutures with the knots tied in the lumen. *B*, Completion of mucosal layer closure. Note how the muscularis has retracted.

esophageal lumen (to avoid the use of crushing clamps). The diseased segment of esophagus is removed using two circumferential incisions in healthy tissue. The mucosa is apposed using simple interrupted sutures of 2-0 polypropylene with the knots tied in the lumen (Fig. 15–131). The muscular layer is closed with mattress sutures of 2-0 polyglactin 910 or polypropylene. Other cases documented in the literature have utilized mattress sutures in the mucosal closure (Lowe 1964; Vaughan and Hoffer 1966). There have been no comparative studies, but it is suggested that asepsis, lack of tension on the anastomosis, and appropriate postoperative management are more critical factors with regard to successful results. The limitations with regard to how much esophagus can be removed have not been accurately defined; 3 cm is the largest length documented in the literature (Vaughan and Hoffer 1966). The muscle layer is the limiting layer of elasticity, and, if considered necessary, a relief incision (circular myotomy) 4 to 5 cm proximal or distal to the surgery site can be made to decrease tension on the anastomotic site (Stick 1982). A suction drain is placed adjacent to the esophagus and the neck incision closed as previously described.

Postoperatively, cervical esophagotomy distal to the anastomosis and tube feeding are preferable. The placement of a tube proximally so that it passes through the anastomotic site is contrain-dicated because of motion at the anastomotic site. If extraoral alimentation is not used, soft foods (only after 48 hours) are given until primary healing is evident based on endoscopic or radiographic examination.

ESOPHAGEAL RESECTION AND REPLACEMENT WITH OTHER TISSUES

Various organ substitutes have been used successfully to replace resected portions of esophagus in man. The indications (usually esophageal neoplasia) are more frequent in man, but in the horse the possibility should be considered when the surgeon is faced with resecting an amount of esophagus incompatible with simple re-anastomosis. Jejunal grafts with the vascular pedicle retained are used in man and are feasible for thoracic esophageal defects in dogs (Reed 1974). Gastric grafts have also been used. In man, right or left colon is also used as a replacement (retaining vascular pedicle as with jejunum), and it is possible to anastomose up to the level of the pharynx (Sabiston 1981). Such pedicle grafts have limited application in the horse, but free graft with re-anastomosis of the blood supply is potentially feasible. Free grafts using stomach and colon with re-anastomosis to the subclavian artery have been used to replace cervical esophagus in man. A jejunal graft has been placed in the cervical esophagus of a horse with reanastomosis to the carotid and jugular vessels (Gideon 1979). Skin tubes have also been used in man. Such techniques need consideration in a case in which our normal techniques will not accomplish the task.

ESOPHAGEAL RESECTION AND REPLACEMENT WITH A PROSTHESIS

The potential usefulness of a tubular prosthesis to replace a segment of resected esophagus is obvious. However, despite many attempts, consistently successful results have not been obtained (Mark and Briggs 1964; Salama 1975). Earlier problems with leakage at the anastomotic site have been overcome, but migration of the prosthesis followed by stricture continues to be a problem (Salama 1975).

MUSCULAR PATCH GRAFTING

When the size of an esophageal stricture precludes resection and anastomosis because of excessive tension on the suture line (and partial resection techniques are also not feasible), the alternative is a patch graft using the sternocephalicus muscle (Hoffer et al. 1977). In this technique, the left sternocephalicus muscle is incorporated into the esophageal closure, thus widening the esophageal lumen (Hoffer et al. 1977).

The patient is operated on under general anesthesia with a nasogastric tube in place; a ventral incision is made as described for esophagotomy. The left belly of the sternocephalicus muscle is reflected laterally and the deep fascia separated to expose the esophagus. A longitudinal incision is made through the tunica muscularis and extends 3 cm proximad and distad to the lesion. The esophageal submucosa and mucosa are then incised. The left side of the mucosal defect is sutured to the body of the sternocephalicus muscle with through-and-through mattress sutures of 2-0 polypropylene. These are preplaced through the mucosa and left side of the muscle belly. Care should be taken to bridge the ends of the mucosal incision with a mattress suture, as this area is considered most vulnerable to leakage. The tunica muscularis on the left side is then sutured to the sternocephalicus with simple interrupted sutures of polypropylene.

The right side of the mucosal defect is then closed in the same fashion as the left side using preplaced mattress sutures. The tunica muscularis is then sutured to the right edge of the sternocephalicus to complete the patch graft. A suction drain is placed next to the esophagus and the incision in the neck closed. Preoperative antibiotics are used and the drain removed in 48 hours.

External alimentation with an esophagostomy aborally for 10 days is the preferred postoperative regimen (if the location of the stricture permits).

Alternatively, a lateral approach to the esophagus may be made and the brachiocephalicus muscle used for the patch graft (Stick 1982).

Narrowing of the Esophagus

This section covers narrowing of the esophagus caused by other than fibrous tissue formation in the wall of the esophagus itself, including neoplasia and abscessation of the wall of the esophagus or extra-esophageal lesions such as abscesses, neoplasia, or goiter (Fig. 15–132) (Aanes 1975; Hofmeyr 1974). These problems are differentiated from strictures within the esophagus by clinical, radiological, and endoscopic examination. Neoplasia is usually not treated. Abscesses are treated in conventional fashion.

Esophageal Fistula

Esophageal fistulae result from the same causes as those discussed for esophageal perforation and rupture. They may also occur as a sequela to esophageal surgery. Large fistulae with drainage to the exterior are obvious clinically. However, a small fistula without drainage to the outside is more difficult to diagnose. There may be dysphagia and cervical swelling but normal stomach tube passage. Contrast studies under pressure are the best means of diagnosing the problem; barium swallow esophagrams may be normal (Stick 1982).

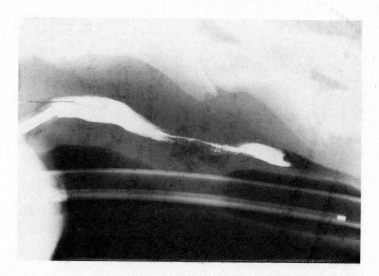

Figure 15–132 Positive contrast radiograph of narrowing in cervical esophagus associated with abscessation.

Many fistulae will heal spontaneously; the establishment of ventral drainage is the only treatment requirement. If a fistula does not heal, surgical excision of the fistulous tract and closure of the esophageal defect should be performed.

Esophageal Diverticulum

There are two types of esophageal diverticula (Aanes 1975; Hackett, Dyer, and Hoffer 1978). Traction diverticula result when contraction of periesophageal fibrous scar tissue causes outward traction and tenting of all layers of the esophageal wall. They commonly develop at the site of a healed esophagostomy or following spontaneous healing of an esophageal wound or fistula (Freeman and Naylor 1978; Stick, Derksen, and Scott 1981). Traction diverticula have a wide neck or opening and are of little clinical significance to the horse. A pulsion diverticulum is a local protrusion of mucosa through the esophageal musculature. Although two mechanisms described for the development of a pulsion diverticulum are fluctuations in esophageal intraluminal pressure and overstretch damage to esophageal muscle fibers by impacted feedstuffs, external trauma has been implicated in equine cases (Aanes 1975; Hackett, Dyer, and Hoffer 1978). A pulsion diverticulum is spherical or flask-like in appearance radiographically. It has a tendency to enlarge progressively with time, so the risk of obstruction or impaction with perforation increases. Surgical repair is therefore indicated.

A diverticulum of the cervical esophagus will typically present with an enlargement in the neck that results in dysphagia or choke. The swelling may increase in size in association with swallowing. The diagnosis may be confirmed with contrast radiology (Fig. 15–133). The defect may also be noted with endoscopy (Hackett, Dyer, and Hoffer 1978).

The two options available for repair of a pulsion diverticulum are diverticulectomy (resection of the mucosal sac and reconstruction of esophageal mucosal and muscular layers) and mucosal inversion (inversion of the mucosal sac with reconstruction of the muscular layer). The technique of mucosal inversion is favored in the horse since the esophageal mucosa is left intact, minimizing the risk of postoperative leakage, infection, or fistula formation (Aanes 1975; Hackett, Dyer, and Hoffer 1978). Inverted mucosa may predispose to postoperative obstruction, but this is not generally a problem. Diverticulectomy could be considered with a large diverticulum.

MUCOSAL INVERSION OF ESOPHAGEAL DIVERTICULUM

The esophagus is exposed and the diverticulum identified. The edges of the ruptured tunica muscularis are dissected from the mucosa, being careful to avoid

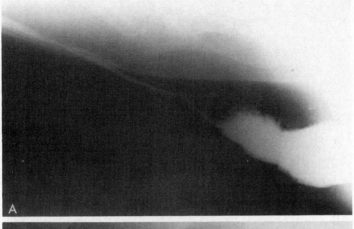

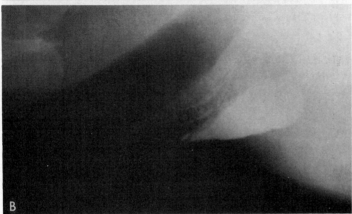

Figure 15–133 *A* and *B*, Contrast radiographs of esophageal diverticula. (Courtesy of Dr. W. A. Aanes.)

penetration of the mucosa. The mucosal sac is inverted and the debrided edges of the tunica muscularis sutured together with simple interrupted sutures of 3-0 polypropylene. A suction drain is inserted and the neck incision closed. Feed is withheld for 24 to 48 hours, and then a diet of soaked horse pellets is fed for at least another five days.

Intramural Esophageal Cyst

There have been only two reported cases of intramural esophageal cysts in the horse (Scott et al. 1977; Stick, Boles, and Scott 1977). In both cases the cysts were classified histologically as keratinizing squamous epithelial inclusion cysts, and they were considered to be congenital in origin.

Clinical findings include dysphagia and regurgitation, a palpable soft tissue mass in the neck, and resistance to nasogastric tube passage at the site of the cyst. A filling defect is observed on contrast radiography.

The cyst can be removed using a ventral approach to the esophagus and a longitudinal incision through the tunica adventitia and tunica muscularis to enucleate the cyst. Redundant mucosa may be inverted or excised; the defect is closed in the same fashion as with esophagotomy.

Developmental Anomalies

Two other developmental anomalies of the esophagus have been reported in the horse. Although neither was amenable to surgery, they should be noted, as both presented with typical signs of esophageal obstruction. Reduplication of the esophageal lumen was found in a 12-month-old filly that presented with signs of dysphagia, regurgitation, and inanition (Swanstrom and Dade 1979). Congenital esophageal dilation or ectasia was diagnosed in a four-month-old colt with a history of intermittent milk regurgitation since birth (Rohrbach and Rooney 1980). The esophageal ectasia was related to developmental defects of both neural and muscular elements of the esophageal wall (see also Megaesophagus).

Esophageal Neoplasia

Neoplasia in the equine esophagus is rare and is usually squamous cell carcinoma (Moore and Kintner 1976; Roberts and Kelly 1979). A localized stenotic lesion may occur in the cervical esophagus, but the validity of surgical resection is to be questioned. When esophageal involvement stems from neoplasia in the stomach there is no treatment (Moore and Kintner 1976).

Esophagitis and Mucosal Ulceration

The role of nonspecific esophagitis in causing esophageal dysfunction in the horse is poorly defined. Esophagismus or spasm of the esophagus has been described as an entity in the horse, and esophagitis has been listed as a cause (Alexander 1967; Hofmeyr 1974). Another author described five cases of recurrent choke as being caused by esophageal spasm brought on by injury and irritation to the esophageal mucosa (Fig. 15–134) (Hoffman 1965). However, there was never direct examination of the areas of stricture observed with contrast studies. These cases were treated with "esophageal rest" that included nasogastric intubation. The use of anti-inflammatory drugs and spasmolytics may be useful in some cases.

Mucosal ulcerations usually occur secondary to long-standing impactions and can be identified with contrast radiography and/or endoscopy. Although some of these mucosal ulcers may proceed to strictures as previously described, spontaneous healing can occur with conservative management (antibiotics, anti-inflammatory medication, and soft foods) (Stick 1982).

Spasm of the esophagus has also been described as a primary entity in nervous, highly bred horses (Hofmeyr 1974). Treatment of acute cases with antispasmodic analgesics (morphine or meperidine) or sodium or potassium bromide for habitual esophagismus has been suggested (Hofmeyr 1974).

Megaesophagus

There has only been one clinical case reported of megaesophagus, or dilatation of the esophagus resulting from hypomotility unassociated with an anatomical lesion or obstruction (Bowman et al. 1978). The authors suspected that the problem was achalasia (a generalized neuromuscular dysfunction and enlargement of the esophagus with narrowing of the distal portion). The patient was a six-month-old colt that presented with a

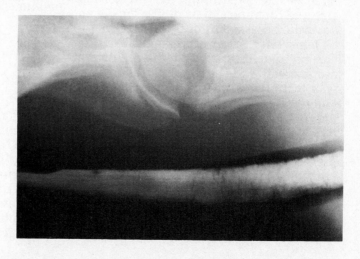

Figure 15–134 Roughening of the mucosa as evidenced by a contrast radiograph in a case of esophagitis. (Courtesy of Dr. J. L. Lebel.)

history of recurrent esophageal obstruction. Megaesophagus was confirmed by radiography. Suspected achalasia could not be demonstrated without fluoroscopy or serial radiography. A modified Heller's esophagomyotomy was performed using a thoracotomy approach to the distal esophagus and cardia. The colt died of acute pulmonary edema on the third postoperative day. No abnormalities were observed in the esophageal tissue. The myenteric and submucosal plexuses appeared normal, which correlated with similar observations in the esophagus of dogs and cats with hypomotility of the esophagus and resultant achalasia (Bowman et al. 1978). Quantitation of cell numbers in the dorsal motor nucleus (a feature of achalasia in man) was not performed. There was no evidence of muscular abnormalities, which distinguishes this case from the case of esophageal ectasia discussed previously (Rohrbach and Rooney 1980).

Complications of Esophageal Surgery

The problems associated with esophageal surgery have been inferred as each surgical condition of the esophagus has been discussed. However, these problems should not cause the clinician to hesitate in instituting the correct treatment of a given esophageal condition. The three clinical objectives of an esophageal surgeon have been listed as (1) obtain leak-proof healing of a primary anastomosis or incision, (2) dilate a restricted aperture, and (3) return the dilated or disrupted esophagus to normal size and function (Stick 1982). This is an accurate assessment of the situation.

Dehiscence of an esophageal incision can be related to poor conditions of the esophageal wall, adjacent infection, or poor technique. In some instances, problems can develop despite careful technique. Early recognition of breakdown is important. The suction drain placed near the esophagus at the time of surgery provides a method of detecting early salivary leakage as well as evacuating serum and blood. Aspiration of saliva could be an indication for retaining the drain longer than 48 hours. Esophageal incisions that leak saliva will not necessarily dehisce if saliva is removed from the periesophageal tissues (Stick 1982). If complete dehiscence occurs, the establishment of ventral drainage and lavaging of the area should be instituted. Nutrition is maintained by esophagostomy and tube placement distal to the surgery site if possible. The patient is permitted to drink. Electrolyte imbalances associated with salivary loss have been discussed in the section on esophagostomy.

Restricture of the esophagus is the fear of any surgeon and can only be prevented by early and correct management of the initial problem. The management of stricture has been discussed elsewhere. Return to normal function following surgery can be facilitated by the correct aftercare, which is discussed under the individual conditions.

One other complication that occurs with surgery on the cervical esophagus is laryngeal hemiplegia. The surgeon needs to avoid any trauma to the adjacent recurrent laryngeal and vagus nerves when operating on the esophagus.

Hiatal Hernia

This condition is included here, as the typical manifestations are referable to the esophagus. The condition is uncommon in the horse. The author is familiar with one case that was presented as a choke. On radiographs, herniation of a proximal portion of the stomach through the diaphragm was diagnosed (Fig. 15–135). Since the diagnosis, the horse has been fed with front legs elevated and has had no clinical recurrences.

STOMACH

Anatomy

Externally, the equine stomach is similar to that of other animals; differences include the expanded left sac, the *saccus caecus*, and a short, sharply angled lesser curvature. The gastric mucosa is divided into two parts. The part that lines the greater part of the left sac resembles the esophageal mucosa and is termed the esophageal part, or *pars esophagea*. It is

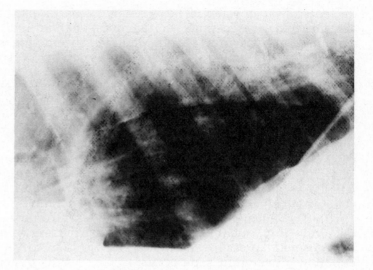

Figure 15–135 Protrusion of a portion of the stomach (spherical gas density) through diaphragm in a case diagnosed as a hiatal hernia. (Courtesy of Dr. W. A. Aanes.)

white, devoid of glands, and covered with a thick, squamous, stratified epithelium. At the cardiac (esophageal) orifice there are numerous folds that occlude the opening (Getty 1975). This peculiar arrangement at the cardia prevents retrograde movement of fluid, gas, or ingesta through the cardia and into the esophagus. The pars esophagea terminates abruptly, forming an irregular, raised edge, termed the *margo plicatus* (Getty 1975). Beyond this is the glandular part (*pars glandularis*). This portion is divided into a narrow cardiac gland region along the margo plicatus and the larger fundic and pyloric gland regions. The capacity of the equine stomach is 8 to 15 liters.

The stomach is located behind the diaphragm and liver, mainly to the left of the median plane. Along the stomach's greater curvature the spleen is interposed between stomach and left body wall (DeBoom 1975). The caudal aspect of the stomach is related dorsally to the transverse colon, and the greater curvature is normally in contact with the left dorsal colon.

The stomach is held in position mainly by the pressure of the surrounding viscera and by the esophagus. The following peritoneal folds connect the stomach to other viscera.

1. The *gastrophrenic ligament* connects the greater curvature, from the cardia to the left extremity, to the diaphragm.

2. The *lesser omentum* connects the lesser curvature and proximal duodenum to the liver.

3. The *gastrosplenic omentum* passes from the left part of the greater curvature to the hilus of the spleen and is continuous ventrally with the greater omentum. This structure can be involved in small intestinal incarceration.

4. The *greater omentum* connects the ventral part of the greater curvature of the stomach and the first curve of the duodenum with the distal large colon and proximal small colon, forming a large sac.

5. The *gastropancreatic* fold, which extends from the left sac above the cardia to the duodenum, is attached dorsally to the liver and vena cava and ventrally to the pancreas.

Physiology

The peculiar anatomy of the cardiac region generally precludes regurgitation or vomition, and excessive gastric distension often results in gastric rupture. The stomach selectively retains contents until they undergo a degree of digestion and reach a critical size for removal. Particles are retained according to size (Argenzio 1980). Most of the reflexes controlling gastric emptying are inhibitory, except for distension, which stimulates gastric mechanoreceptors. The primary inhibitory control of gastric emptying is the enterogastric reflex. These reflexes are initiated by receptors in the duodenum. Emptying may be inhibited by osmolarity, acid, lipid, protein, and carbohydrate content of the ingesta (Argenzio 1980). Various gastrointestinal hormones have been incriminated, but the role of some is still not defined.

The mean osmotic pressure of stomach contents is considerably higher than plasma over a 12-hour period. Values of up to 700 mOsm/kg have been measured four hours after feeding a conventional pelleted hay–grain ration (Argenzio 1975). The normal stomach mucosa is relatively impermeable, and, although large osmotic pressure gradients exist, bulk flow of water does not occur.

The pathophysiology of complete failure of stomach emptying has not been studied in any controlled manner, but the effect of complete obstruction (ligation) of the duodenum has been reported (Datt and Usenik 1975). Five of six horses died of ruptured stomachs, and the mean survival time was 18.52 hours. About two hours prior to death the horses exhibited severe colic. There was an initial rise in blood pH (coinciding with increased HCO_3) six hours after obstruction, followed by a continuous fall. There was a slight decrease in Na^+ up to 12 hours and a rise at 18 hours; K^+ rose to almost twice the pre-obstruction value in association with the progressive acidosis, and Cl^- decreased sharply. Severe hemoconcentration developed.

Gastric Dilation

Dilation of the stomach may be a primary condition associated with physical obstruction or a functional disturbance. The condition is also commonly observed in association with obstruction further down the intestinal tract. The most common cause of acute primary gastric dilation is overingestion of grain. Large amounts of dietary starch are not natural in the diet of horses. Gastric fluid is absorbed by the grain mass, and swelling occurs. Shock and metabolic acidosis develop rapidly.

The consumption of a large quantity of cold water by an animal soon after exertion may result in pyloric spasm and accompanying gastric dilation. This type of dilation is usually transient. It has also been suggested that a horse offered hay or straw soon after a race while still "blowing out" may swallow air, and, in the presence of gastric hypomotility, gastric dilation would result (Owen 1975). Dilation may also be associated with pyloric stenosis. A crib-biting horse may swallow a considerable quantity of air, and this can cause a chronic gastric dilation. Impaction of the stomach with dry feed contents may also occur occasionally.

Primary gastric dilation will typically present as an acute colic. Because of the stomach's position within the deep rib cage, abdominal distension is not a feature, but dyspnea may be evident owing to pressure on the diaphragm. Hypovolemic shock may develop with dilation associated with grain overload. Otherwise, the horses, despite pain, are in good systemic condition. A definitive diagnosis of gastric dilation is made by stomach tube passage. Reflux of fluid and gas is typical of primary dilations except grain engorgement and secondary dilations. In grain overload, stomach tube passage may only yield a small amount of fluid and some grain. Any cause of a dilation distal to the stomach needs to be ascertained. The presence of acute pain with stable systemic signs (healthy mucous membranes), acid pH of reflux contents, marked response to stomach decompression, and/or instillation of 50 to 60 ml 2% lidocaine is an indication of a primary gastric dilation. Severe pain with rapid intoxication, alkaline stomach contents, and an equivocal or temporary response to stomach tube passage are indications of an intestinal problem.

Primary gastric dilations not due to grain engorgement respond immediately to decompression by stomach tube. Medical treatment is indicated in all cases of grain engorgement; this includes decompression (when possible), judicious use of lavage and mineral oil, analgesia, maintenance of systemic circulation, and attention to the common sequela of laminitis. Surgical relief of a gastric impaction has been described (Clayton-Jones 1974). In this case the stomach could be emptied using a tube inserted through a stab incision and lavage. Un-

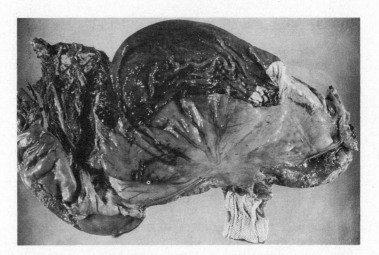

Figure 15–136 Rupture of the stomach along greater curvature.

less tube evacuation is possible, surgery is considered generally futile and unwarranted because of inaccessibility of the stomach and resultant peritoneal contamination.

Gastric Rupture

As discussed previously, gastric rupture commonly occurs in association with excess distension of the stomach. Immediate decompression is indicated whenever stomach distension occurs. Based on experience with relieving dilation secondary to intestinal ileus, decompression of the stomach can be difficult, and lavage, air distension, or suction needs to be used. Despite regular attempts to evacuate the stomach, rupture has still been seen in some instances. Rupture usually occurs along the greater curvature in the fundic area (Fig. 15–136), an area where the wall is considered relatively inelastic (Jubb and Kennedy 1963).

Sudden cessation of signs of pain followed by progressive systemic deterioration is the usual sign of gastric rupture. In some instances when intestinal problems and endotoxic shock are already present, occurrence of a rupture may not be recognized until necropsy. There is no treatment.

Gastritis and Gastric Ulceration

Severe infestations of *Gastrophilus* larvae can produce gastritis and ulcera-

tion in the mucosa. Consequent alterations in stomach motility and pyloric spasm could cause gastric dilation. Damage from the larvae can also potentially cause gastric perforation and pyloric blockage (Fig. 15–137). Stomach ulceration has also been associated with *Habronema megastoma* larvae. Chronic gastritis with severe mucosal thickening has also been observed in racehorses and is possibly associated with prolonged administration of phenylbutazone. The author has had one case that presented as an acute abdomen; exploratory laparotomy revealed pyloric stenosis.

Perforating gastric ulcers may be located at the esophageal or pyloric gland regions (Rooney 1964). The lesions in the esophageal region have been related to mechanical damage due to *G. intestinalis* larvae or stones or other sharp crystalline material (Rooney 1964). Perfora-

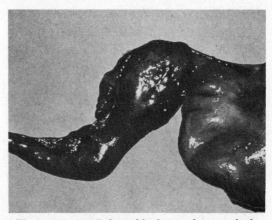

Figure 15–137 Pyloric blockage of stomach due to *Gasterophilus* larvae.

tion always occurred at the margo plicatus. The pyloric lesions have been attributed to long-term stress and drug therapy (Robertson 1982; Rooney 1964). Another author recorded three cases of perforating ulcers (one in the esophageal portion and two in the pyloric region), and these were all associated with heavy stress due to other neonatal disease problems (Valdez 1979).

Gastric ulcers can potentially be diagnosed by an appropriately long endoscope. Medical treatment could include the use of antacids. Up to now, most ulcers have been diagnosed at necropsy. No surgical treatment of gastric ulcers has been described. Gastric ulceration has also been incriminated as a cause of recurrent colic in adults. The presence of occult blood in gastric lavage solution may be a useful diagnostic aid for this condition.

Gastric Stenosis

Gastric stenosis has only been reported once in the horse. The cause was uncertain but was considered to be some form of local chronic irritation (Peterson, Donawick, and Merritt 1972). The patient presented with clinical signs of recurrent abdominal pain, salivation, and regurgitation of small quantities of ingesta. Fluoroscopic examination revealed a dilated esophagus and a stricture in the proximal portion of the stomach. The tissue causing the stricture in the cardia was excised using a left thoracotomy approach to the stomach, but the horse died of fibrinous pleuritis 20 days following surgery.

Pyloric Stenosis

Congenital pyloric stenosis is rare but has been reported (Barth, Barber, and McKenzie 1980; Crowhurst et al. 1975). Signs include abdominal pain, salivation, and teeth grinding. In one instance signs developed immediately after suckling (Crowhurst et al. 1975), whereas clinical signs in another case developed at six weeks of age when the foal started to eat significant amounts of solid feed (Barth, Barber, and McKenzie 1980). The condition has been treated by Ramstedt's pyloromyotomy (Crowhurst et al. 1975) and Weinberg's modification of the Heineke-Mikulicz pyloroplasty (Barth, Barber, and McKenzie 1980) through a ventral midline laparotomy approach. Sectioning of the hepatoduodenal ligament facilitates the presentation of the pylorus at the abdominal incision.

Pyloric stenosis may possibly occur secondary to chronic gastritis. The author has seen only one case but it is well documented in other species. Direct surgical access to the pylorus and proximal duodenum in adult horses is not feasible as it is in foals. An alternative method of surgical treatment for pyloric stenosis is gastroduodenostomy. This has been performed in one case (Donawick 1980). Because of short-term follow-up in this case and lack of other reports, it is not known if the potential complication of stagnant loop syndrome presents a problem.

Gastric Neoplasia

Squamous cell carcinoma is the most common equine stomach tumor but is of low prevalence. The tumor develops in the esophageal part of the stomach, is seen in older horses, and produces a clinical picture of anorexia and progressive weight loss (Meagher et al. 1974). Specific clinical signs are generally lacking. There may be extensive metastases in the abdominal and thoracic cavities. Rectal examination, abdominal paracentesis, gastric washings, endoscopy, and laparotomy may be used to establish a diagnosis. Biopsy is used to confirm a diagnosis. Some cases may present with pleural effusion and respiratory distress (Smith 1977; Wrigley et al. 1981). There is no treatment. The occurrence of a pedunculated mass of granulation tissue in the stomach has also been described (MacKay, Iverson, and Merritt 1981). Because of the problems with exposure in the adult, surgical intervention does not seem to be a practical alternative in such a case.

SMALL INTESTINE

Anatomy

The small intestine is about 22 meters long. The duodenum is about 1 meter long. The first part is directed right from the pylorus and forms an S-shaped curve (sigmoid or *ansa sigmoidea*). The convexity of the first part is dorsal and, of the second part, ventral. The first part of the duodenum is in contact with the middle and right lobes of the liver, and the pancreas is attached to the concavity of the second curve (Getty 1975). The second part of the duodenum passes dorsocaudad, skirting the right lobe of the liver and the right dorsal colon and, on reaching the right kidney and base of the cecum, curves medially, opposite the last rib. The third part of the duodenum passes behind the attachment of the base of the cecum, crosses the median plane behind the root of the small intestinal mesentery, and turns craniad to become continuous with the jejunum ventral to the left kidney. The duodenum thus forms a wreath around the base of the cecum (DeBoom 1975). The duodenum is suspended in the abdominal cavity by a short peritoneal fold termed the *mesoduodenum*. Because of this, the duodenum is fixed in position, and mobilization and visualization at surgery are not feasible. Depending on position, the duodenum is fixed to the liver, right dorsal colon, base of cecum and right kidney, sublumbar muscles, terminal large colon, and proximal small colon. The latter attachment is described as the *duodenocolic fold* and is present at the duodenojejunal flexure.

The jejunum and ileum are collectively termed the *mesenteric part of the small intestine*. With the exception of the origin and termination, this part of the small intestine is very mobile and lies in numerous coils, mingled with those of the small colon mainly in the dorsal part of the left side of the abdomen between the stomach and pelvis. The ileum is characterized by its antimesenteric border, which continues into the ileocecal fold. The ileum also has a thicker wall. The jejunum and ileum are attached to the dorsal abdominal wall by the *great mesentery*, which consists of two layers of peritoneum between which the vessels and nerves reach the bowel. The *root of the mesentery* is attached to a small area around the cranial mesenteric artery under the first and second lumbar vertebrae. The mesentery is short in the proximal jejunum but becomes longer distally (up to 50 cm), sufficiently long to allow coils of intestine to reach the abdominal floor, pelvic cavity, and inguinal canals. Such mobility facilitates the various displacements of clinical importance that are encountered.

The intestinal wall has four layers: serosa, muscular layer (external longitudinal and inner circular layers), submucosa, and mucosa. The arteries of the small intestine come from the celiac and cranial mesenteric arteries; the veins go to the portal vein. The numerous lymph vessels drain into the mesenteric lymph nodes and then into the cisterna chyli. The nerves are derived from the vagus and sympathetic nerves through the celiac plexus.

The peritoneum consists of a single layer of mesothelial cells covering the abdominal organs (visceral peritoneum) and body wall (parietal peritoneum). Connecting folds are termed omenta, mesenteries, ligaments, or folds and contain a varying quantity of connective tissue, fat, and lymph glands. An omentum is a fold that passes from the stomach to other viscera. There are three in the horse: lesser omentum, greater omentum, and gastrosplenic omentum. These have been discussed in the stomach section. A concept of clinical importance is that of considering the parietal peritoneum as one sac and the visceral peritoneum as another smaller sac. These two sacs communicate by a relatively narrow passage called the *epiploic foramen* (Fig. 15–138). This opening is situated on the visceral surface of the liver dorsal to the portal fissure. It can be entered by passing the finger along the caudate lobe of the liver toward its root. Its dorsal wall is formed by the caudate lobe and caudal vena cava; its ventral wall consists of pancreas, gastropancreatic fold, and portal vein. The walls are normally in contact, so it should be considered a potential space, but with age and caudate lobe atrophy the space increases in size. The foramen is about 10 cm long and 2.5 to 3 cm wide at the lateral extremity (narrowest point). If the finger is passed into the foramen from right to left, it enters the cavity of the lesser sac or visceral peritoneum. This cavity is contained by the greater omentum and is termed the *omental bursa* (see Fig. 15–138). The greater omentum

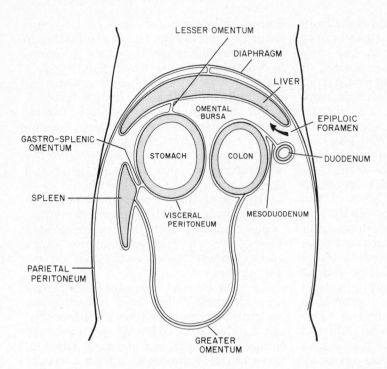

LESSER OMENTUM
DIAPHRAGM
LIVER
OMENTAL BURSA
EPIPLOIC FORAMEN
GASTRO-SPLENIC OMENTUM
STOMACH
COLON
DUODENUM
SPLEEN
VISCERAL PERITONEUM
MESODUODENUM
PARIETAL PERITONEUM
GREATER OMENTUM

Figure 15–138 Diagrammatic horizontal section of peritoneal cavity demonstrating epiploic foramen and the omental bursa.

is relatively small and insignificant in the horse. It is generally folded up in the space between the visceral surface of the stomach and the intestine.

Physiology

Motility of the small intestine permits two actions: mixing of the ingesta by segmental contraction to facilitate absorption, and movement of ingesta toward the large intestine by peristaltic contractions. Movement of ingesta through the small intestine is rapid (60 to 70 per cent of the liquid phase of a meal reaches the cecum in two hours, and this retention is primarily in the stomach [Argenzio 1980]), and the ileocecal junction is only a minor barrier to flow and cannot discriminate against particulate matter, as can the pylorus. The basic control system for small intestinal motility is the electrical slow wave or basic electrical rhythm (Argenzio 1980). The frequency of the slow wave decreases distally, so that peristaltic activity is more prevalent in the upper small intestine; contractile waves, which travel short distances or not at all (segmentation), are characteristic of the distal small intestine.

The autonomic nervous system and endocrine and prostaglandin systems modulate the inherent motility of the small intestine. Intrinsic and extrinsic innervations may increase or decrease the excitability of the smooth muscle. The peristaltic reflex is the most important nervous reflex of the small intestine. Distension of one segment initiates activity proximad and inhibition distad (Argenzio 1980). Extrinsic reflexes are significant in motility inhibition. Handling or distension of a portion of bowel may reflexly inhibit motility of the entire small intestine (intestino-intestinal inhibitory reflex). Both afferent and efferent pathways appear to travel through the splanchnic nerves. Stimulation of the peritoneum reflexly inhibits small intestinal motility, and this seems primarily sympathetic. Vagal afferents conduct stimuli from mechanoreceptors, and these reflexes are primarily excitatory. Cholecystokinin stimulates jejunal contractions, whereas secretin inhibits them, and these hormones may be involved in the physiological control of motility. Prostaglandin E usually relaxes or inhibits contraction of the circular muscle layer and stimulates the longitudinal layer in the small intestine (Bennett, Eley, and Scholes 1968). It is believed that prostaglandins released in the gut wall rather than those systemically circulating are the primary factors involved.

The small intestine is an important organ for both digestion and water and electrolyte movements, so that any abnormality will have a marked effect on the systemic status of the patient. The principal digestive and absorptive mechanisms of carbohydrate, fat, and protein are in the proximal small intestine. There are luminal and mucosal phases to digestion. Secretion of electrolytes, water, and digestive enzymes is an active process controlled by the neuroendocrine system. The pancreas secretes large quantities of buffer to neutralize the acid pH of the inflowing gastric contents. The concentration of bicarbonate in equine pancreatic secretion is less than that in other species (never exceeding 60 to 70 mEq/L at high rates of flow), but it is profuse and continuous and can increase fivefold with vagal stimulation (Argenzio 1980). The bile ducts also contribute buffer to the duodenum by secreting an HCO_3^--rich fluid. In the horse, bile is secreted continuously into the duodenum. There is also an exchange of luminal chloride for extraluminal bicarbonate in the distal small intestine, and this seems to be of major importance in the horse. This permits the absorption of Cl^- without the accompanying absorption of water, and the cecum receives large volumes of fluid rich in HCO_3^-. Most of the Cl^- secreted into the stomach is effectively re-absorbed by the time the ingesta reaches the terminal small intestine. The Na^+ concentration in small bowel contents approximates that in plasma. The gastric contents are hypertonic. The small intestine equilibrates the osmolality of its contents with the blood owing to absorption of ions and secretion of isotonic fluids, so the ileum and cecum are presented with an isotonic fluid.

The volume of fluid secreted into the small intestine is immense. In a 100-kg pony, the sum of parotid, biliary, and pancreatic secretions is approximately 30 liters (1.5 times extracellular volume) (Argenzio 1980). To this must be added unknown amounts of gastric and small intestinal secretions. Fourteen liters of fluid are presented to the large intestine from the ileum. This fluid is efficiently absorbed in the large intestine. One of the prime functions of the distal small intestine and colon, apart from digestion and absorption of nutrients, is the re-absorption of isotonic secretions delivered to the small intestine. Large quantities continue to be secreted during fasting, and their re-absorption by the distal intestine is critical in maintaining extracellular fluid volume.

The normal microbial flora is vitally important to intestinal function. It influences mucosal cell structure and promotes the establishment of local tissue defense mechanisms (which aid or stimulate the formation of lymphatic cells and activate the reticuloendothelial system) in the newborn. The normal microbial flora acts as a defense barrier either by making the target cell unavailable to the pathogen (attachment to this is the first step in producing disease in most instances) or by creating an environment detrimental to the pathogen (Hirsh 1980). The small intestine and cecum contain relatively large numbers of Enterobacteriaceae (mainly *E. coli*), enterococci, and *Lactobacillus* species (Hirsh 1980). In addition to the microbial barrier, a chemical barrier consisting of acid hydrolases, secretory IgA, and lysozyme is present. This barrier minimizes the absorption of bacteria and bacterial endotoxins in normal intestine.

A brief mention of the peritoneum is a necessary prelude to a discussion of conditions of the small intestine. The peritoneum has an important function in providing frictionless movement between one surface and the other. Interest in this mesothelial layer is primarily related to its role in various pathological conditions. It reacts to noxious stimuli, and these reactions are manifested in changes in peritoneal fluid samples. Normally, the peritoneal fluid acts as a filtrate of plasma. The peritoneal membranes are also capable of absorbing fluids and solutes. The ability of peritoneum to heal (with or without adhesions) is also important in abdominal surgery.

The visceral peritoneum receives its blood supply from the cranial mesenteric artery, and venous drainage is into the portal vein. The parietal peritoneum receives its arterial supply from the underlying muscles of the abdominal wall, and venous drainage is directly into the systemic circulation. The lymphatic drainage of both visceral and parietal surfaces is into the thoracic duct. The importance of this circulation pattern when bacterial endotoxins enter the peritoneal cavity and are absorbed directly into the systemic circulation has been emphasized (White and Moore 1982).

Pathophysiology as related to various surgical problems of the small intestine is discussed in the sections hereafter.

Specific Surgical Conditions of the Small Intestine

The various surgical conditions of the small intestine will be discussed under three major headings: simple obstruction, strangulating obstruction, and non-strangulating infarction. This system of classification is appropriate when considering pathophysiology. However, it should be emphasized that some problems (e.g., pedunculated lipoma) can cause a single or strangulated obstruction in different cases; such overlap needs to be kept in mind.

SIMPLE OBSTRUCTION

Pathophysiology

Simple obstruction is an obstruction of the small intestinal lumen without (at least initially) vascular compromise. Initially, the integrity of the mucosal barrier remains intact. Obstruction leads to sequestration of fluid and electrolytes, causing bowel distension and pain. In the initial stages of a complete obstruction or in a partial obstruction, absorption in the intestine continues, and it may be some time before signs of dehydration are evident. With time, dehydration and hemoconcentration develop, necessitating intravenous fluid replacement. As well as causing pain, distension of the bowel (whether caused by tympany or fluid accumulation) causes reduction in intestinal blood flow and initiates net fluid secretion rather than absorption (Bury, McClure, and Wright 1974; Shields 1965). The venous congestion and low flow state associated with

persistent distension may result in mucosal degeneration and, ultimately, necrosis. Intraluminal pressure will also quickly exceed capillary pressure. Such degeneration results in passage of bacteria and endotoxins into the peritoneal cavity and systemic circulation.

The severity of clinical signs associated with a simple obstruction of the small intestine depends on the degree of obstruction (complete or incomplete) and the level of the obstruction (proximal or distal). Complete obstruction shows more dramatic clinical signs, with rapid onset of pain owing to bowel distension, and faster development of hypovolemia. Proximal obstruction shows a more intense clinical picture owing to rapid proximal sequestration of fluid. Stomach rupture is an anticipated sequela in the untreated case (Datt and Usenik 1975). A minimal area of intestine is available for re-absorption proximal to the obstruction, and hemoconcentration develops.

With experimental complete obstruction at the level of the duodenum the blood pH increases for the first six hours in association with an increase in HCO_3^-; this can be related to lack of HCl sequestration and continued ability to absorb HCO_3^-. After six hours, progressive acidosis develops, presumably owing to intestinal wall compromise and failure of HCO_3^- re-absorption. With more distal obstruction of the small intestine, there is no initial rise in HCO_3^- and acidosis is continuously developing; this can be related to the increased proportion of alkaline intestinal fluid in the proximal segment where re-absorption is compromised. The clinical signs of simple obstruction can include abdominal pain, development of signs of hemoconcentration and acidosis, distended small intestine on rectal examination, and a peritoneal fluid that is unimpressive but that shows progressive deterioration with bowel compromise.

Ascarid Impaction

Ascarid impaction of the small intestine can occur in young horses up to one year of age with heavy burdens of *Parascaris equorum*. Obstruction usually occurs shortly after anthelmintic treatment. Partial or complete obstruction of the small intestine may occur. Rupture

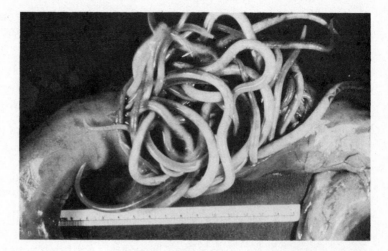

Figure 15–139 Ascarid impaction with rupture of small intestine.

of the intestine can result in severe cases (Fig. 15–139).

The intensity of clinical signs depends on the degree of obstruction. Complete obstruction produces severe pain and gastric reflux, which may contain ascarids. In addition to eventual hemoconcentration associated wtih fluid sequestration, it has been suggested that dead ascarids cause a toxic or allergic effect, which may exacerbate any systemic deterioration (Robertson 1982).

Surgical relief of the obstruction through enterotomy is indicated for complete obstruction or any obstruction that has not responded to administration of mineral oil.

Adhesions

Adhesions are common sequelae to peritonitis or abdominal surgery. Fibrinous exudate is produced by inflamed peritoneum, and subsequent organization can lead to a nonelastic band or stricture (Figs. 15–140 and 15–141). Such lesions cause compromise of the lumen of the bowel. Previous abdominal surgery is the most common cause of clinical adhesions. Adhesions can also result from acute *Strongylus vulgaris* infection (Drudge 1979). Adhesions may also lead to a strangulating obstruction.

Simple obstructions associated with adhesions are commonly partial and may present with a history of recurrent colic. In some instances a patient with a history of several episodes of "medical" colic presents with severe, persistent colic. Small intestinal distension and

fluid reflux are common findings. Signs of active peritonitis are not usually present. A diagnosis of small intestinal obstruction associated with adhesion formation should be considered in any horse with recurrent colic that has a previous history of peritonitis or abdominal surgery.

The treatment of intestinal adhesions is either separation or cutting of the adhesions so that a patent lumen and normal bowel configuration are re-established or intestinal resection and anastomosis (in some cases a side-to-side anastomosis leaving the strictured bowel in situ is more appropriate). Any severed or

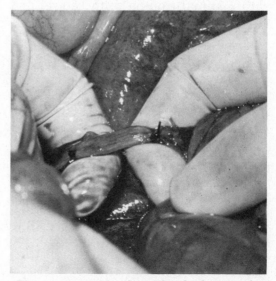

Figure 15–140 Nonelastic band of tissue that caused obstruction of the jejunum.

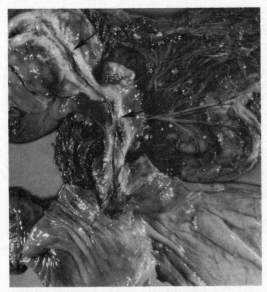

Figure 15–141 A fibrous tract (arrows) in the greater omentum (considered to arise from perforation of the jejunum) that led to obstruction of jejunum.

separated surfaces need to be oversewn to minimize adhesion re-formation. The prognosis is fair to good for a single or localized adhesion. The prognosis is poor for multiple adhesions; re-formation of adhesions is anticipated. With extensive adhesion formation, euthanasia is advised. Because adhesion formation is most commonly a complication of abdominal surgery, prevention is the key; this involves fast, competent surgery with minimal trauma to the bowel and peritoneal cavity.

Pedunculated Lipoma

Pedunculated lipomas of the mesentery may cause simple obstruction in a fashion similar to that causing adhesions (Figs. 15–142 and 15–143). They commonly cause a strangulating obstruction. They are a problem of older horses, with the youngest reported case in a 12-year-old horse (Meagher 1974b).

Horses with pedunculated lipomas will typically present with a history of recurrent colic and signs of small intestinal obstruction. Laparotomy is needed to confirm the diagnosis. Distension of the small intestine proximal to the obstruction has commonly been present for some time, and normal motility may not return to such a segment following removal of

the obstruction. In these cases, resection and anastomosis are recommended, if feasible.

Muscular Hypertrophy of the Ileum

Muscular hypertrophy of the muscles of the distal ileum (at the ileocecal valve) may cause intestinal obstruction (Fig. 15–144). The condition has been associated with stenosis of the ileum secondary to a mucosal lesion, strongyle larval migration, and neurogenic stenosis with prolonged closure of the ileocecal valve. The condition has also been seen in association with ileocecal intussusception (Horney and Funk 1971). There is some confusion between this condition and similar conditions that involve initial inflammatory and proliferative changes in mucosa followed by secondary hypertrophy, such as terminal ileitis in pigs (Schneider, Leipold, and Kennedy 1972). A condition similar to that observed in the horse has been described in pigs (Nielson 1955), and the pathogenesis was suggested as either a primary idiopathic muscular hypertrophy or a secondary hypertrophy associated with a functional neurogenic disturbance resulting in spasm of the ileocecal valve (an analogous condition is present in pyloric spasm in man) (Rooney and Jeffcott 1968). No anatomical stenosis of the ileocecal valve was evident (Rooney and Jeffcott 1968). The condition may be

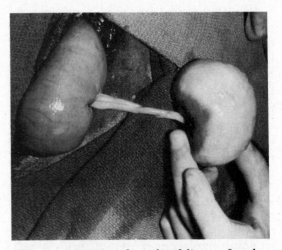

Figure 15–142 A pedunculated lipoma found as an incidental finding during abdominal exploration. The potential for this structure to cause obstruction is obvious.

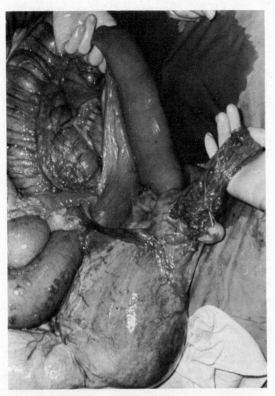

Figure 15–143 Simple obstruction of the jejunum caused by a pedunculated lipoma. The chronically dilated intestine proximal to the obstruction can be seen in the lower part of the photograph. Omentum is also attached to the pedunculated lipoma.

classified as primary idiopathic hypertrophy when predisposing lesions cannot be found at necropsy (Lindsay, Confer, and Ochoa 1981). A case of more diffuse hypertrophy in which maximal hypertrophy was 10 cm cranial to the ileocecal valve

has also been reported (Schneider, Leipold, and Kennedy 1972).

The obstruction will progress from incomplete to complete, with the clinical signs varying accordingly. Diagnosis is confirmed at laparotomy. Cases have been treated by ileal myotomy (Horney and Funk 1971) and ileocecal anastomosis (Donawick, Christie, and Stewart 1971). Rupture of the affected area has also been reported (Lindsay, Confer, and Ochoa 1981).

Abdominal Abscesses

Abdominal abscesses may produce compression or stricture of a portion of the small intestine (Figs. 15–145 through 15–147). Systemic spread from respiratory infections is considered the most common cause of abdominal abscesses; *Streptococcus equi, S. zooepidemicus,* and *Corynebacterium pseudotuberculosis* are the most common isolates (Rumbaugh, Smith, and Carlson 1978). Abdominal abscesses have also been associated with umbilical infection (Mason et al. 1970). The majority of abdominal abscesses involve the mesentery (Rumbaugh, Smith, and Carlson 1978).

Internal abdominal abscessation typically presents with intermittent, prolonged colic or chronic weight loss (Rumbaugh, Smith, and Carlson 1978). Horses with intermittent or prolonged colic do not respond to the usual medical treatments. Marked depression and anorexia are consistent features. Gut motility is decreased frequently, and most horses show some degree of dehydration. In a

Figure 15–144 Ileocecal junction area from a case of muscular hypertrophy of the ileum. Cecum is on the left and ileum to the right. Note the dilatation of the ileum and the thickening of the ileal wall at the constricting portion. (Courtesy of Dr. T. S. Stashak.)

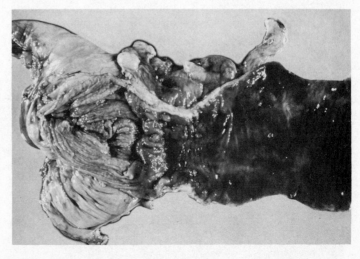

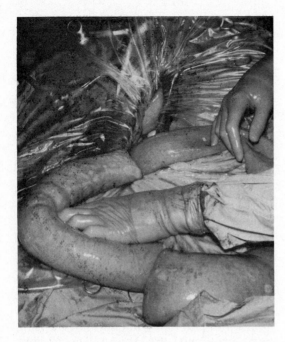

Figure 15–145 Distended jejunum due to obstruction associated with an abscess.

Figure 15–146 Abscess that involved jejunum and caused an obstruction.

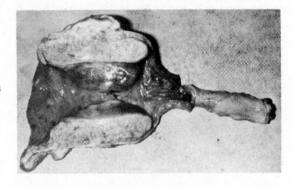

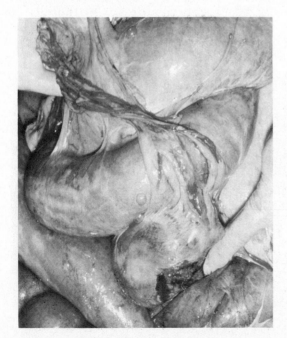

Figure 15–147 Diffuse compromise to small intestine due to abscessation and adhesion formation.

good proportion of cases, a mass can be palpated on rectal examination. Clinicopathological findings include a neutrophilia with a marked left shift, an increased plasma fibrinogen (normal 500 mg/dl), and hypergammaglobulinemia. Peritoneal fluid samples can generally be classified as exudates based on gross appearance, specific gravity (>1.017), protein content (> 2.5 g/dl), and WBC counts (>10,000). Culture results from peritoneal fluid are generally negative.

Long-term penicillin administration has been used successfully in the treatment of internal abdominal abscessation. In one report involving 13 cases, the usual dose was 40,000 U/kg/day (Rumbaugh, Smith, and Carlson 1978). Rectal palpation, repeated abdominal paracenteses, and CBCs are used to assess response to treatment. Treatment periods vary from two weeks to five and one-half months.

Surgical treatment is indicated in some instances if abscesses can be drained intraoperatively or marsupialized without peritoneal contamination. Intestinal resection and anastomosis and abscess removal can be appropriate in selected cases of localized obstruction associated with abscessation (Valdez et al. 1979). Prophylactically, antibiotic treatment of respiratory infection should be continued 10 days beyond disappearance of clinical signs.

Neoplasia

Apart from pedunculated lipomas, neoplasms of the intestine are uncommon. Lymphosarcoma may be seen involving the abdomen, particularly the mesenteric lymph nodes. Cases may present with chronic colic. Other clinical signs include weight loss, diarrhea, ascites, and change in appetite (Pearson et al. 1975). Masses may be palpated per rectum, and diagnosis can be confirmed using a flank laparotomy (Fig. 15–148). In two cases experienced by the author abdominal paracentesis was not diagnostic. Jejunal intussusception at the site of tumor development has also been reported (Pearson et al. 1975).

A case of fibroma in the abdomen has been reported; this case presented as colic and showed signs consistent with simple intestinal obstruction. There was fluid reflux on stomach tubing. The tumor caused a partial intestinal obstruction (Wilson and Sykes 1981). Squamous cell carcinoma can metastasize throughout the abdomen (Fig. 15–149), but colic may not be the primary sign (Meagher et al. 1974). With the exception of lipomas, surgical correction of abdominal neoplasia is not generally feasible.

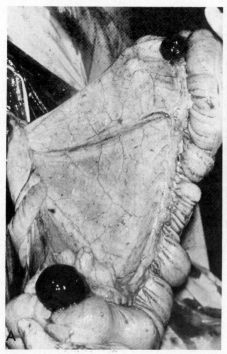
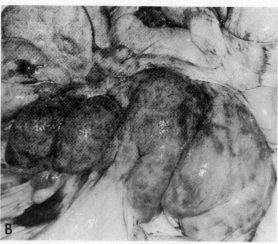

Figure 15–148 *A,* Lymphosarcomatous nodules in small intestinal mesentery demonstrated at flank laparotomy. *B,* A larger mass at the base of the mesentery demonstrated at necropsy.

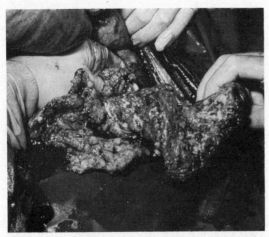

Figure 15–149 Squamous cell carcinoma at exploratory laparotomy.

Duodenitis Syndrome

This disease entity was first recognized in Europe (Huskamp and Boening 1981) and has been observed in the U.S. The horses present with clinical signs of a simple proximal obstruction of the small intestine. There is voluminous reflux of fluid on stomach tubing and hemoconcentration. Rectal findings are often negative but a distended transverse duodenum can sometimes be palpated. It is difficult to distinguish the condition from other causes of intestinal obstruction. Laparotomy reveals thickened edematous duodenum. Duodenocecostomy has been used in an attempt to provide drainage of accumulating fluid into the cecum (Huskamp and Boening 1981). The technique is performed using a right lateral approach to the abdomen, removing the last rib to provide access to both the duodenum and the base of the cecum. The initial responses to this treatment have been dramatic. However, in two cases in which this procedure was performed, subsequent examination showed no glucose absorption even though food material was present in the small intestine (White 1981b). Some cases will respond to conservative management.

Duodenal Stenosis

Duodenal stenosis is an uncommon condition that has been reported in foals four months and younger (McIntosh and Shupe 1981; Wagner, Grant, and Schmidt 1979). In all cases the strictures have been reported in the area of the *ansa sigmoidea*, and two of three cases involved the normal stricture between the two dilated portions of the sigmoid (ampulla duodeni and ampulla hepatopancreatica). The etiology of the stenosis is unknown. Both congenital and traumatic etiologies have been proposed.

The clinical signs of duodenal stenosis are similar to those of pyloric stenosis and include recurrent dysphagia and regurgitation, salivation, mild intermittent colic, metabolic alkalosis, depression, anorexia, and unthriftiness. Esophagitis in the lower half of the esophagus has been reported and is related to acidic reflux (McIntosh and Shupe 1981; Wagner, Grant, and Schmidt 1979). Surgical correction of a case has been performed. A longitudinal enterotomy was performed and was closed in a transverse fashion (McIntosh and Shupe 1981). Surgical exposure of the site is difficult but is possible in a foal. The enterotomy technique is inadequate for a longer stenotic segment, and an alternative procedure such as duodenal myotomy or gastroduodenostomy should be considered. In another case, the duodenal stricture could not be palpated at laparotomy (Wagner, Grant, and Schmidt 1979).

STRANGULATING OBSTRUCTION

Pathophysiology

A strangulating obstruction of the intestine is characterized by simultaneous interference of the intestinal blood supply and blockage of the intestinal lumen (White, Moore, and Trim 1980). Examples of strangulating obstructions of the equine small intestine include incarceration, volvulus, and intussusception and represent a common cause of acute abdominal crisis. Strangulating obstruction of the small intestine occurs more frequently than does simple obstruction (Tennant 1976). Because vascular compromise of the intestine is present at the outset of the condition, the pathophysiological changes associated with this problem are more acute and severe than those associated with simple obstruction. The mortality rate of surgical cases with strangulating obstruction is high (Tennant 1976).

The interruption of blood flow (ischemia) produces rapid spastic contractions of the intestine (Moore et al. 1980), followed subsequently by flaccidity and distension with fluid and/or gas. A typical strangulating lesion will cause venous occlusion before arterial occlusion with consequent venous congestion. The intestinal wall becomes congested and edematous. As the ischemic intestine distends with gas, the consequent increase in intraluminal pressure causes a reversal of net absorption to net secretion of fluid and electrolytes from the circulation to the bowel lumen as previously described. This results in bicarbonate-rich fluid sequestration in the small intestine and stomach, systemic hypovolemia, and metabolic acidosis. In addition, the bowel distension stimulates visceral pain receptors in the intestinal wall and exacerbates the circulatory compromise of the intestinal mucosa. Strangulating obstruction results in more severe abdominal pain than occurs with a simple obstruction.

The intestinal ischemia quickly leads to mucosal degeneration. It has been shown experimentally that the mucosa at the tip of the villus is the first to be affected (White, Moore, and Trim 1980). Degeneration of mucosa continues from the villus tip to the base; this is followed by degeneration of the lamina propria. With experimental ischemia, progressive mucosal degeneration continues after release of the ligature and evidence of re-established perfusion and motility is seen (White, Moore, and Trim 1980). This degeneration has been related to increased countercurrent exchange or shunting of oxygen between arterial and venous segments of capillaries in the villus (Lundgren and Haglund 1978). The apical portion of the villus is thus deprived of oxygen. The administration of gaseous oxygen intraluminally can prevent the sequential mucosal degeneration if the villus lesion has not progressed beyond the stage of loss of epithelial cells from the tip of the villus and minimal hemorrhage into the lamina propria (Moore et al. 1980).

Mucosal degeneration allows the passage of bacteria or bacterial endotoxins into the circulation via mesenteric veins, lymphatics, or transmural routes (through intestinal wall and into peritoneal cavity), and this leads to endotoxemia and shock. The poor perfusion resulting from endotoxic shock may further perpetuate the mucosal degeneration.

Shock is an important feature of acute abdominal crises in the horse, particularly with strangulating or infarctive lesions, and deserves discussion. Shock is a systemic state characterized by capillary perfusion insufficient to maintain cellular function (Nelson 1976). The pathogenesis of shock in the acute abdominal patient can be related to a combination of hypovolemia and endotoxemia. Hypovolemia occurs owing to fluid loss from the extracellular fluid space and circulation in association with lack of fluid intake, obligatory fluid losses, and the net secretion of fluid into the lumen of the bowel. Severe hypovolemia alone may reduce the intestinal blood supply sufficiently to produce mucosal ischemia and degeneration (White and Moore 1982). The absorbed bacteria and endotoxins will cause further compromise of the circulatory system and cellular metabolism.

Endotoxin is a biologically toxic component of the outer cell wall of a number of gram-negative bacteria (e.g., *E. coli*, *Salmonella* spp., *Klebsiella* spp., *Proteus* spp., and *Pseudomonas* spp.) (Moore, Garner, and Shapland 1981). It is composed primarily of lipopolysaccharide, and the lipid A portion is associated with most of the toxic and lethal effects (Burrows 1981). Endotoxin is released into the surrounding medium upon bacterial death or during extremely rapid bacterial growth phases, and therefore normally exists in the intestinal lumen. Two mechanisms exist to protect an animal against the development of systemic endotoxemia. First, the mucosal cell barrier limits the transmural movement of bacteria and bacterial endotoxin. As described previously, this mucosal barrier breaks down with intestinal ischemia. The second protective mechanism is the hepatic reticuloendothelial system (Kupffer cells). These cells remove absorbed endotoxin from the portal blood and systemic circulation (Moore, Garner, and Shapland 1981). In a normal animal this clearance mechanism has been shown to be fast and effective (Berg, Nausley, and Riegle 1979), but its efficiency during stress, hypovolemia, and acidosis is unknown.

Experimental administration of endotoxin in the horse results in arterial hypoxemia, reduced arterial blood pressure, increased central venous pressure, poor capillary refill, hemoconcentration, leukopenia, colic, diarrhea, systemic lactic acidosis, tachypnea, and dyspnea (Burrows and Cannon 1968; Moore et al. 1980). The essential feature of endotoxic shock is the inadequate perfusion or stagnant hypoxia of vital organs that it causes. This does not differ from the result of hypovolemic shock.

The mechanisms by which endotoxin exerts deleterious effects are numerous. The endotoxin binds to cell membranes including those of the reticuloendothelial system (Burrows 1981). Neutrophils and platelets are sequestered in the capillary beds of the lungs, liver, and spleen, with subsequent disintegration and systemic release of serotonin, histamine, and lysosomal enzymes. There is an increase in epinephrine and norepinephrine levels, the terminal complement system is activated, and there are increases in kinins, prostaglandins, endogenous pyrogen, interferon, pancreatic myocardial depressant polypeptide, and macrophage derived–glucocorticoid antagonizing factor in the circulation (Burrows 1981). The significant role of arachidonic acid release, with cellular damage and subsequent synthesis of prostaglandins, in endotoxemia has been recently emphasized (Moore, Garner, and Shapland 1981). Intense vasoconstriction is mediated by PGF_2 and thromboxane A2, vasodilation by PGE and PGI_2, and abdominal pain (colic) and diarrhea by PGE (Moore et al. 1981). Arachidonic acid metabolism can be blocked pharmacologically by the nonsteroidal anti-inflammatory agents that inhibit the action of cyclo-oxygenase. A potent cyclo-oxygenase inhibitor, flunixin meglumine, has been shown to prevent the deleterious effects of injected endotoxin (Moore et al. 1981). It has been suggested that endotoxin-mediated endothelial damage releases arachidonic acid from cell membranes, initiates platelet adhesion to exposed collagen, and stimulates the formation of vasoactive metabolites, which mediate arterial hypoxemia, lactic acidosis, colic, and diarrhea.

Disseminated intravascular coagulation (DIC) will also occur as a generally terminal event in association with the endotoxic shock of strangulating obstruction (McClure, McClure, and Usenik 1979). (See Chapter 7.)

Clinical Signs of Strangulating Obstruction

The clinical picture is acute. Pain is moderate to severe and continuous, with no or only temporary relief from analgesics. The rate of systemic deterioration depends on the site of the obstruction and the degree of strangulation. The pulse rate may increase to levels of 80 to 100 beats/min or greater, and pulse quality deteriorates. Mucous membranes become congested, and capillary refill increases. There is a progressive increase in packed cell volume (PCV) and total protein (TP), and there is concurrent development of metabolic acidosis. The respiratory rate increases in response to pain and metabolic acidosis. The clinical course is rapid, and most horses with an untreated strangulating obstruction of the small intestine will die within 24 to 36 hours of the onset of disease. In experimental strangulating obstruction of the ileum the mean survival time was 21.16 hours, with a range of 16.5 to 29 hours (Datt and Usenik 1975).

Small intestinal sounds are reduced or absent. Multiple distended loops of small intestine may be palpated on rectal examination. If the strangulated portion of bowel can be palpated, the wall will be thickened and the lumen fluid filled. There will be vasogastric reflux of fluid, the volume of which depends on how proximal the obstruction is.

Peritoneal fluid changes are relatively rapid. The fluid changes to amber or red with some turbidity within six hours. With time the color progresses to a dark red. The protein increases, and a marked neutrophilia as well as an increase in RBCs will be seen. With further progression of the disease there is toxic degeneration of the neutrophils. With devitalization of the bowel wall, bacteria may be seen.

Intussusception

An intussusception is the invagination of a segment of intestine (intussusceptum) and its mesentery into the adjacent distal segment of bowel (intussuscipiens). The small intestine is the most common site of occurrence for this condition, involving the jejunum, ileum, or terminal ileum (ileocecal intussusception). The condition occurs more frequently in young horses (Rooney 1965; Tennant 1976) but is not confined exclusively to the young. A pathogenetic hypothesis based on a concept of segmental atony and hyperperistalsis has been advanced (Rooney 1965) (Fig. 15–150). Any factors that alter intestinal motility could, therefore, lead to the development of the condition. These factors could include heavy ascarid infection, sudden dietary changes, enteritis, mesenteric arteritis, simple obstructions, or previous enterotomy (Lowe 1968; Rooney 1965). The ileal artery runs along the mesenteric border of the ileum, and there is no collateral blood supply. This results in increased susceptibility of the ileum to vascular compromise. This would render it more liable to peristaltic arrest and atony following partial or complete oc-

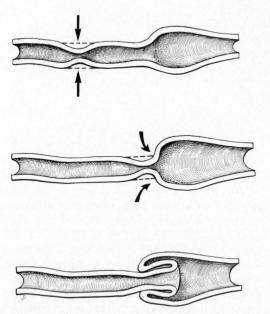

Figure 15–150 Pathogenetic concept of intussusception as developed by Rooney (1965). The area of peristalsis (arrows) hits the dilated area of segmental atony at right and pushes into the dilated portion.

clusion of the ileal artery (Rooney 1965). This may explain the tendency for the condition to occur in this area.

Small intestinal or ileocecal intussusception is usually characterized by signs of complete obstruction. There are reduced or no gut sounds. Some dark, blood-stained mucus may be present in the rectum. Rectal examination may not be feasible in the young patient. If rectal examination is possible, distended loops of small intestine may be palpated and the actual intussusception may sometimes be palpated (thickened and sensitive). The peritoneal fluid will undergo changes but may not accurately reflect the degree of bowel ischemia and necrosis owing to the devitalized segment of gut being contained within the intussuscipiens. Systemic deterioration of the patient is not as acute as with a volvulus, and the condition can run a course of two to three days.

Subacute intussusception as a sequela to diarrhea has been reported in foals (Crowhurst et al. 1975). The obstruction is incomplete, and the clinical signs include anorexia, depression, intermittent moderate abdominal pain, and unthriftiness (Crowhurst et al. 1975; Mason et al. 1970). It is not a commonly recognized condition.

Intussusception is easily recognized at laparotomy, with systematic exploration of the small intestine starting at the ileocecal valve (Fig. 15–151A). Reduction of the intussusception may be possible (Fig. 15–151B) but may be precluded by excessive swelling of the intussuscipiens or serosal adhesions. Some intussusceptions have been treated by reduction alone (Pearson et al. 1975), but resection of all intussusceptions should be a general consideration. Even with an apparently viable intussuscipiens, progressive mucosal degeneration can still develop (Owen et al. 1975). Serosal color is a poor indicator of potential bowel viability. Because of its vulnerable vascularity, this point applies particularly to the ileum. For intussusception involving the ileum, a jejunocecal anastomosis is performed. This procedure is preferred over ileocecal anastomosis (Donawick, Christie, and Stewart 1971; Owen et al. 1975) because it is considered safer to resect all ileum and perform an anastomosis of the ter-

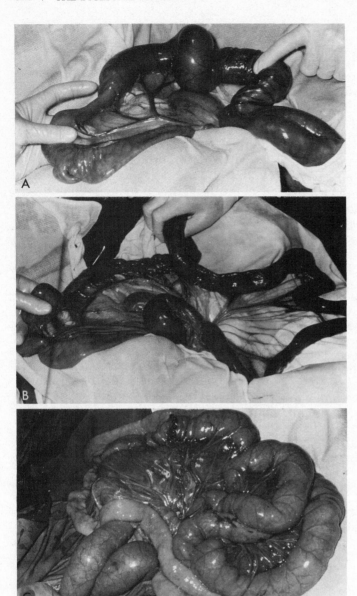

Figure 15–151 Intussusception of jejunum at laparotomy. *A,* Prior to reduction. *B,* Following reduction. Note the devitalized intussusception at right. *C,* Following resection and end-to-end anastomosis.

minal jejunum to the cecum (Donawick, Christie, and Stewart 1971). Jejunal cecal anastomosis is usually performed as an end-to-side technique. Postoperative edema in the area of the stoma has been reported by one author, who proposes the use of a side-to-side technique (Huskamp 1977). When staples are used for the anastomosis, a side-to-side technique is performed. If the intussusception involves the jejunum, resection and end-to-end anastomosis are performed (Fig. 15–151C).

Volvulus

Volvulus is produced by a 180° or greater rotation of a segment of jejunum or ileum about the long axis of the mesentery (Nieberle and Cohrs 1967). Rotations of up to 180° may occur physiologically without producing disturbances. Volvulus may occur as a primary displacement or may be secondary to a preexisting lesion such as an incarceration in mesentery, epiploic foramen, gastrosplenic omentum, mesodiverticular bands, Meckel's diverticulum, adhesions, or infarctions. In such cases it is thought that such an obstruction or area of decreased motility provides a fixed axis for the bowel to twist around (Nieberle and Cohrs 1967). When a peristaltic wave in the proximal segment strikes an atonic segment, it is postulated that the intestine loops around this fixed axis. Obstruction of this portion of bowel is now present and distension occurs. Eventually, reversal of the twist becomes impossible. Continued twisting around the atonic focus can occur.

When an obvious primary lesion is not present, segmental atony of the bowel may be the initiating cause, as described with intussusception. Ascarid impaction, strongyle migration, and dietary changes have been implicated in foals (Crowhurst et al. 1975; Rooney 1965). The ileum is commonly involved; the reason for this has been given as the fixed nature of the ileocecal valve and terminal ileum. However, it could also be related to an increased tendency for vascular compromise and consequent hypomotility.

There is no particular direction in which volvulus occurs. The length of small intestine incorporated into a volvulus will vary. It is considered that the strangulation primarily affects the veins so that the ischemic state is characterized by venous congestion (Nieberle and Cohrs 1967). Experimental work has shown venous occlusion to be a more effective means of producing intestinal

infarction than arterial occlusion (Adams 1979).

Patients present with signs typical of severe strangulating obstruction of the small intestine; volvulus is probably the most acute and severest of the strangulating obstructions. There is loss of gut motility proceeding to complete ileus; gas distension in the intestine, which may cause visible abdominal distension in foals; and intense pain, which can diminish or decrease as bowel necrosis develops. Rectal examination will reveal distended thickened loops of bowel. Systemic compromise occurs quickly, with a rapid and weakening pulse, peripheral perfusion deterioration, hypovolemia, and acidosis. The PCV may reach 60 or greater. Peritoneal fluid samples become sanguineous in appearance.

Treatment of volvulus involves surgical reduction and intestinal evacuation. At laparotomy, the discolored, thickened, and distended loops of bowel are usually found at the incision (Fig. 15–152A). The direction of the volvulus is ascertained by palpating the mesentery. The mesentery is twisted in a cordlike spiral at the mesenteric root in a severe volvulus (Fig. 15–152B). The presence of another primary lesion needs to be ascertained. Volvulus may occur around an incarceration (most commonly) or, alternatively, in the incarcerated segment itself. Which malposition is corrected first depends on the individ-

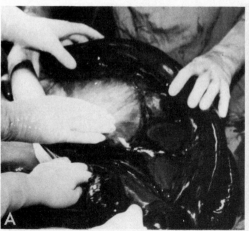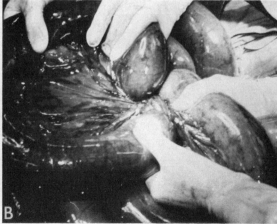

Figure 15–152 Volvulus of the small intestine. *A,* Discolored, thickened, and distended loops of small intestine. *B,* The twisted segment of bowel needs to be followed into the abdomen.

ual case. Correction of the volvulus is performed by rotating all affected loops together in the appropriate direction. Cases of volvulus as well as mesenteric herniation can be very difficult to correct because the greater the degree of involvement, the shorter the mesentery. Care is needed because of friability of both intestinal wall and mesentery. Prior evacuation of the intestine may be necessary but can be very difficult. In some instances transecting the bowel proximal and distal to the obstruction is appropriate. Following reduction, nonviable bowel is resected if feasible. Resection of greater than 50 per cent of small intestine is not indicated, and the patient should be destroyed (Tate 1981). Following resection, an end-to-end or jejunocecal anastomosis is performed, depending on the bowel resected.

The prognosis in cases of volvulus is generally poor because of the rapid deterioration of the patient and, in many instances, involvement of excessive lengths of intestine.

Internal Hernias

An internal hernia is a displacement of organs through a normal or pathological opening within the abdominal cavity (Nieberle and Cohrs 1967). There is generally no hernial sac. Internal herniation of small intestine usually results in incarceration. The epiploic foramen represents the normal opening through which internal herniation of small intestine may occur. Internal herniation through pathological openings is more common and includes mesenteric defects (acquired or congenital); tears in the greater, lesser, or gastrosplenic omenta; and defects in the broad ligament and through foramina formed by fibrous bands or adhesions. The signs are generally typical of strangulating obstruction of the small intestine. In some instances strangulation has not yet occurred and the intestine is still viable.

EPIPLOIC FORAMEN INCARCERATION. The anatomy of the epiploic foramen has been described previously. The youngest horse in which this condition has been reported was seven years of age (Meagher 1974). In older horses, the epiploic foramen enlarges in association with atrophy of the right lobe of the liver. Herniation usually occurs by a loop of intestine passing from the peritoneal cavity through the epiploic foramen into the omental bursa (right to left or antegrade [Huskamp 1977]) (Fig. 15–153), but it occasionally occurs in the opposite direction (left to right or retrograde). The latter problem will involve herniations through the omentum or pushing the omentum ahead of it. Distension of the incarcerated portion of bowel occurs.

The condition is confirmed at laparotomy during systematic exploration of the small intestine or routine palpation of the epiploic foramen. The epiploic fora-

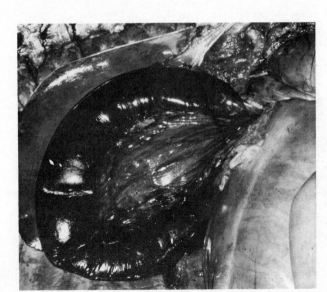

Figure 15–153 Necropsy specimen of incarceration of portion of small intestine through the epiploic foramen. The herniation was from right to left. Omentum has been removed from the area. (Courtesy of Dr. A. S. Turner.)

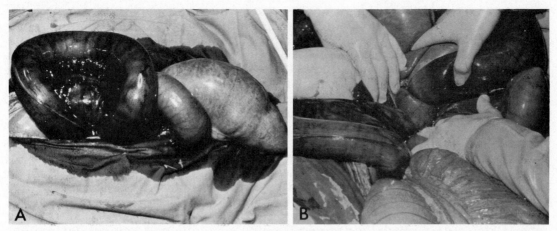

Figure 15–154 Two views of mesenteric incarceration of the small intestine. *A*, A loop of black ileum is presented when the abdomen is opened. *B*, Deeper exploration reveals both a herniation through the mesentery (right) and a volvulus.

men is located by standing on the patient's left side and passing the left hand down and forward into the right hypochondriacal area. The pylorus and sigmoid flexure of the duodenum are located. As one grasps the duodenum with the left hand and positions the back of the hand against the caudate lobe of the liver, the fingers will encounter the foramen. Reduction of the hernia can usually be accomplished following the decompression of the loop of incarcerated intestine and using gentle traction with cautious manipulation of the foramen. Manual enlargement of the foramen is dangerous. Prior decompression is not always needed. In some cases the previously mentioned techniques are not successful owing to intestinal swelling. In these cases the intestine should be sectioned and oversewn proximal and distal to the obstruction and each stump drawn through separately. Resection and anastomosis are usually necessary. Closure of the epiploic foramen is not practical. The prognosis is fair to good.

MESENTERIC DEFECTS. Incarceration through an acquired rent in the mesentery usually occurs through the ileal mesentery. In most cases the rent occurs at the same time as the incarceration. A pathogenesis similar to that of intussusception and volvulus has been proposed (Rooney 1965). A hyperperistaltic wave strikes a segment of atonic bowel and with a whip-like action bursts through the mesentery. Hyperperistalsis alone,

with a wave striking the ileocecal junction, could similarly cause the intestine to burst through the ileal mesentery (Rooney 1965).

Mesenteric incarceration can also occur in association with an anomalous mesodiverticular band, which is formed by a persistent vitelline artery and its embryonic mesentery. A pocket is thus formed between the mesentery and the antimesenteric border of the intestine, and a piece of intestine can be caught and then rupture through the adjacent mesentery (Freeman, Koch, and Boles 1979). Intestine may also become incarcerated within inflammatory bands and adhesions that are associated with the mesentery.

In any of the previously mentioned instances the herniated piece of intestine can become incarcerated and strangulated by the hernial ring (Fig. 15–154). Volvulus may occur secondarily. Signs are typical of strangulation obstruction of the small intestine. They will generally be more severe if there is an associated volvulus.

If volvulus of the herniated segment of bowel is found at laparotomy, it should be corrected first. Reduction of the mesenteric hernia may require prior evacuation of the herniated portion of intestine as well as enlargement of the hernial ring. The strangulated jejunum and/or ileum is resected and an end-to-end or jejunocecal anastomosis performed. Effective closure of the mesenteric rent may not always be possible, and care must be taken to avoid damaging mesenteric vessels. If complete obliteration of a mesenteric defect is not possible or if later breakdown is anticipated, it is better to leave a large defect than a small one. This will hopefully minimize the chance of incarceration and strangulation of a piece of bowel if it does pass through the defect.

OMENTAL DEFECTS. Herniation of small intestine through a rent in the greater omentum or a window formed by an omental adhesion (Norrie and Heistand 1975) may occur rarely. Herniation of small intestine through the gastrosplenic omentum (also called gastrosplenic mesentery) can occur (Tennant 1976). Clinical signs and surgical management are similar to those for other internal hernias. Defects in the greater omentum are best handled by removal of the offending portion of omentum. Obliteration of a defect in the gastrosplenic omentum is not feasible.

BROAD LIGAMENT (MESOMETRIUM). Herniation of small intestine through the mesometrium has been reported but is uncommon (Becht and McIlwraith 1980). In the reported case, the mare was pregnant. The incarcerated intestine was viable and resection was not necessary. The defect in the mesometrium could not be closed (Becht and McIlwraith 1980).

PEDUNCULATED LIPOMA. Pedunculated lipoma has been previously discussed. In some instances, in addition to obstructing bowel, strangulations will occur. Pedunculated lipomas are considered a common cause of small intestinal strangulation in older horses (Tennant 1976). The incarceration of intestine through a ring created by the pedicle of the lipoma may be considered a form of internal hernia. Treatment involves pedicle severance, lipoma removal, and intestinal resection and anastomosis.

External Hernias

An external hernia is a displacement of abdominal contents beyond the abdominal cavity. Examples include inguinal hernias, umbilical hernias, ventral abdominal hernias, and diaphragmatic hernias. With the exception of diaphragmatic hernias, hernias can be noted with external examination. In these instances the hernia is regarded as consisting of a hernial sac formed by the invaginated peritoneum, accessory hernial coverings formed by the overlying soft tissues that vary with the site of the hernia, the hernial orifice or hernial ring, and the hernial contents (Nieberle and Cohrs 1967).

INGUINAL OR SCROTAL HERNIA. The term *inguinal* is used if hernial contents descend into the inguinal canal; if the contents descend into the scrotum the term *scrotal hernia* is appropriate (Nieberle and Cohrs 1967). The term *inguinal hernia* is often used to mean either condition. Acquired inguinal hernia is a problem in stallions. Scrotal hernia is rare in Thoroughbred foals but more common in heavier breeds (Crowhurst 1970). There is a predisposition in Standardbreds (Sembrat 1975). Inguinal hernias in newborn foals rarely become strangulated and usually disappear spontaneously within a few weeks. Acquired inguinal hernias in stallions are usually unilateral and almost always produce acute strangulating obstruction of the jejunum or ileum. The vaginal ring forms the hernial orifice, and the tunica vaginalis forms the hernial sac. There has been one report of rupture through the tunic also. Herniation may be caused by breeding, abdominal trauma, strenuous work, or any other event that could increase intra-abdominal pressure. Inguinal herniation may also occur occasionally as a sequela to normal or cryptorchid castration.

The hernia is usually apparent on examination of the scrotum and inguinal area. The small intestine passing down through the vaginal ring can be detected on rectal examination.

Surgery is performed using an inguinal approach over the neck of the scrotum. The common vaginal tunic is exposed by blunt dissection. The tunic is opened and the bowel examined. If the intestine is considered viable it is returned to the abdominal cavity. Enlargement of the vaginal ring may be necessary. With strangulated jejunum, resection and end-to-end anastomosis are performed through the inguinal incision. If the ileum is involved, a ventral midline or paramedian laparotomy is necessary to perform a jejunocecal anastomosis.

Castration on the affected side is preferred to minimize the chance of recurrence of the hernia and is performed in most cases. A transfixion suture is placed to ligate the cord, and it is severed distal to the ligature. The inguinal canal may be packed with gauze, but suturing of the external inguinal ring is preferred using simple interrupted sutures. If salvage of the testis is desired, a purse-string suture is placed around the tunica vaginalis as close to the vaginal ring as possible to reduce the diameter of the tunica vaginalis. It is placed in such a fashion as to exclude the spermatic cord. The caudal end of the external inguinal ring is left open to allow unobstructed passage of the spermatic cord.

UMBILICAL HERNIAS. Incarceration through an umbilical hernia is rare but occasionally occurs. Most hernias are reducible and produce no problems. If an incarceration recurs, the hernia is surgically reduced (the hernial ring may need to be enlarged to do this) and resection and anastomosis performed if appropriate. Umbilical herniorrhaphy is then performed.

VENTRAL HERNIAS. Acquired hernias occur in the ventral or ventrolateral abdominal wall secondary to abdominal trauma, the stress of parturition, or previous abdominal surgery. As with umbilical hernias, acute incarceration is uncommon but some abdominal discomfort can occur. Surgery is generally elective and delayed until acute inflammation and infection are controlled and the hernial ring is sufficiently fibrosed. Intestinal incarceration requires immediate surgery. The surrounding tissue is often friable at this stage, and hernial repair can be difficult. Surgical mesh may be necessary in the repair of some of these hernias.

DIAPHRAGMATIC HERNIA. Diaphragmatic hernias are rare. Most diaphragmatic defects are acquired and may be associated with thoracic trauma or sudden increases in intra-abdominal pressure, but congenital hernias do occur (Fig. 15–155) (Crowhurst et al. 1975; Firth 1976; Pearson et al. 1977; Wimberly, Andrews, and Haschek 1977). Acquired rents may occur in various locations in the diaphragm (Wimberly, Andrews, and Haschek 1977). The majority of lesions occur in the tendinous portion of the diaphragm, most commonly where the centrum tendineum blends into the pars costalis, which is a logical point of weakness between the more pliable muscle and the rigid tendinous portions of the diaphragm (Wimberly, Andrews, and Haschek 1977). Chronic lesions with acute exacerbations were the most common situation in one series of 18 cases (Wimberly, Andrews, and Haschek 1977). Congenital defects occur less frequently and are a result of incomplete fusion of the pleuroperitoneal folds (Spiers and Reynolds 1976). Therefore, most congenital defects are in the dorsal tendinous portion of the diaphragm and represent an enlargement of the esophageal hiatus. Small and/or large intestine can herniate through a diaphragmatic hernia.

A peritoneopericardial hernia in a

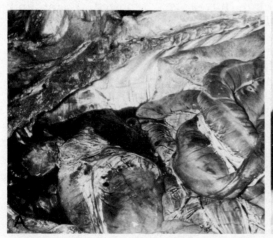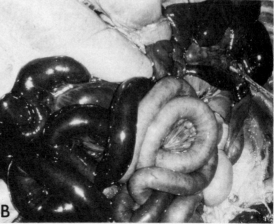

Figure 15–155 A, Diaphragmatic hernia in a newborn foal with both small and large intestines in the thorax. B, Strangulating obstruction of small intestine due to a diaphragmatic hernia in an adult.

three-year-old Standardbred stallion has been recently reported (Orsini, Koch, and Stewart 1981). This is the first report of a hernia into the pericardium in a horse. Colon was herniated through the defect. It was also noted that there is no direct communication between the peritoneal and pericardial cavities during embryogenesis; therefore, peritoneopericardial communication must arise as a secondary phenomenon in the development of the diaphragm (Orsini, Koch, and Stewart 1981).

The clinical signs associated with diaphragmatic hernia are variable and nonspecific and depend on the size of the hernial orifice and the amount of herniated viscera. Signs of abdominal pain can be related to excessive tension on the mesentery due to displacement or intestinal obstruction (which may be simple or strangulated). The tear itself and tension on the pleura may also cause pain. Signs of respiratory compromise may also be present. In 17 of 18 cases in one series, the animals demonstrated one or all of the following: tachypnea, painful respirations, and forced respirations (Wimberly, Andrews, and Haschek 1977). Auscultation of the thorax may reveal an absence of lung sounds ventrally or increased intestinal sounds. The assessment is difficult, as referred intestinal sounds are commonly heard over the lung field of a normal horse. Dullness on percussion of the ventral thorax may be detected owing to viscera or pleural fluid. Most cases of diaphragmatic hernia have been definitively diagnosed at laparotomy or necropsy. A definitive clinical diagnosis is possible by thoracic radiography (i.e., demonstration of gas-filled loops of intestine, ventral thoracic density, and discontinuity or loss of diaphragmatic shadow).

Successful surgical correction of non-strangulating diaphragmatic hernia has been reported in one foal (Spiers and Reynolds 1976) and one mare (Scott and Fishback 1976). A ventral midline laparotomy approach was used in each case. A mesh implant was used to repair the diaphragmatic defect in the mare (Scott and Fishback 1976). Positive-pressure ventilation is obviously needed for these repairs. The prognosis for surgical repair of a diaphragmatic hernia in an adult horse is generally poor owing to inaccessibility of the dorsal diaphragmatic rents and inability to retract the viscera as well as friability of the damaged diaphragmatic tissue.

The recently reported case of peritoneopericardial hernia was sucessfully managed by laparotomy and replacement of the colon in the abdominal cavity. The hernial defect was not closed, and the horse was normal at the one-year follow-up (Orsini, Koch, and Stewart 1981).

Embryonic Anomalies

As mentioned previously, there are two embryonic abnormalities that may lead to small intestinal obstructive conditions: Meckel's diverticulum and meso-diverticular bands.

MECKEL'S DIVERTICULUM. Meckel's diverticulum results from persistence of a portion of the omphalomesenteric (vitelline) duct, which is usually obliterated and disappears (Nieberle and Cohrs 1967). The nature of the persistent duct varies. In cases reported in the horse the persistent duct has presented as a finger-like Meckel's diverticulum 2 cm in diameter and 4 to 6 cm long projecting from the antimesenteric surface of the ileum with a fibrous band (obliterated duct) connecting the diverticulum to the abdominal wall in the area of the umbilicus (Grant and Tennant 1973) (Fig. 15–156). The lumen of the diverticulum communicates with the lumen of the ileum.

Two cases of volvulus of the small intestine secondary to Meckel's diverticulum have been reported (Grant and Tennant 1973). The fibrous band had served as an axis for the volvulus. Severing the band facilitated correction of the volvulus. Other forms of simple or strangulating intestinal obstruction are potentially possible with this anomaly. Meckel's diverticulum may also cause recurrent colic because of impaction of the diverticulum or fatal peritonitis due to rupture of the diverticulum (Nieberle and Cohrs 1967). A case of an impacted diverticulum that was presumed to be a Meckel's diverticulum is illustrated in Figure 15–157. This case was handled by resection and jejunocecal anastomosis. Diverticulitis is a syndrome reported

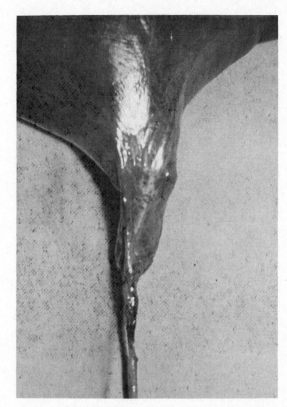

Figure 15–156 A Meckel's diverticulum with its associated fibrous band. (Courtesy Dr. T. S. Stashak.)

in man, but it has not been recognized in the horse. Recently, a case of a Meckel's diverticulum within an umbilical hernia has been described (Hilbert, Jacobs, and Cullen 1981). The filly was asymptomatic until the diverticulum became impacted with ingesta.

MESODIVERTICULAR BANDS. A mesodiverticular band is formed by persistence of a distal segment of a vitelline artery and its associated embryonic mesentery. The band extends from one side of the small intestinal mesentery to the antimesenteric surface of the intestine (usually jejunum) (Figs. 15–158 and 15–159). A triangular hiatus is formed between the mesodiverticular band, jejunal mesentery, and jejunum. Entrap-

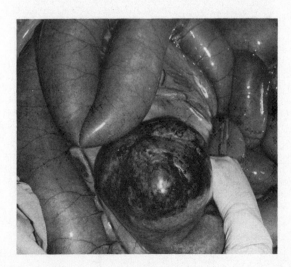

Figure 15–157 An impacted diverticulum at the junction of jejunum and ileum which was presumed to be a Meckel's diverticulum.

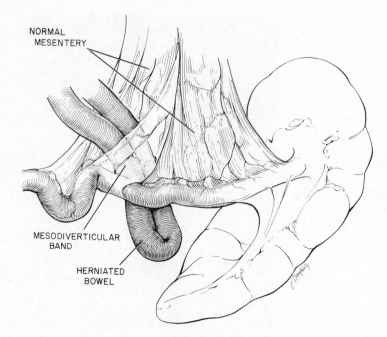

NORMAL
MESENTERY

MESODIVERTICULAR
BAND

HERNIATED
BOWEL

Figure 15–158 Diagram of mesodiverticular band showing bowel that has entrapped between the band and the mesentery and then herniated through the mesentery.

ment of intestine in this hiatus can cause herniation of intestine through jejunal mesentery and secondary volvulus (Freeman, Koch, and Boles 1979). Treatment consists of reduction of the strangulation and volvulus and intestinal resection and anastomosis.

NONSTRANGULATING INFARCTION

The term *nonstrangulating infarction* is used to classify infarction of the intestine that is unassociated with stran-

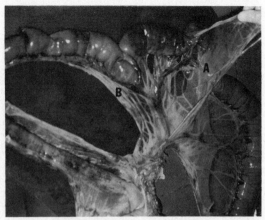

Figure 15–159 A case of mesodiverticular band (*A*) with an associated rent (*B*) in the mesentery that caused intestinal incarceration. (Courtesy of Dr. P. B. Fretz.)

gulation. This condition has usually been classified as thromboembolic colic, but for reasons discussed hereafter this is not the most appropriate term. Although there may be different types of disease involved, different pathogenetic factors and their relative importance are still not well defined. Most horses suffer some arterial damage during their lives (Wright 1972), but few progress to a final clinical picture of infarction. Nonstrangulating infarction will be discussed here as a single entity, but the various theories as to its pathogenesis will be reviewed.

Pathophysiology

The actual pathophysiology of this condition is poorly defined, and there are several possibilities regarding the development of the infarctive lesion. Thrombotic disease in the mesenteric vasculature has been associated with *Strongylus vulgaris* larval migration or the resulting arteritis. *S. vulgaris* larvae have been considered to predispose to colic in several ways.

1. Thrombotic lesions completely blocking the ileocecocolic artery with acute infarction.

2. Severe thromboembolic lesions in which blood may pass through the ileocecocolic artery but major branches,

such as dorsal or ventral colon, are blocked by thrombosis or embolism, leading to bowel stasis with impaction, intussusception, or volvulus.

3. Mild thromboembolic lesions. This was considered the common reaction. Emboli were thought to pass from thrombi in the cranial mesenteric and ileocecocolic arteries and block smaller branches, leading to temporary cessation of motility.

4. Enlargement of the cranial mesenteric artery and its major branches, resulting in pressure on the coeliacomesenteric ganglion and plexus with resultant interference with nerve supply to the intestine (Ottway and Bingham 1946). Histologic examination of nerves has not substantiated this theory (Rooney 1970).

The association of *S. vulgaris* arteritis and thrombotic disease is not disputed, but terminology and pathogenetic concepts require definition. The classical concept of thromboembolism or peripheral embolization of thrombi should be questioned based on both experimental and clinical data. The results of experimental infection of foals with *S. vulgaris* larvae indicate death within 13 to 21 days owing to intestinal infarction (Drudge 1979; Georgi 1973); the infarction occurs in the terminal ileum, cecum, and ventral colon owing to thrombosis of small arterioles. However, it was noted that the thrombosis develops from the endothelial damage caused by migrating fourth-stage larvae and not from embolization from the cranial mesenteric artery (Georgi 1973). The third-stage infective larva is swallowed with food by the host. It penetrates the mucosa of the cecum and ventral colon and undergoes a moult within eight days. It then penetrates an arteriole in the submucosa and migrates toward the cranial mesenteric artery, damaging the endothelium. The track of its migration can be recognized by a linear thrombotic deposit on the intima of the vessels (Nieberle and Cohrs 1967). The larvae may cause obliterating endarteritis of the smaller arteries. The lesions of hemomelasma of the ileum (*hemomelasma ilei*) (Fig. 15–160) are hemorrhagic infarcts caused by *S. vulgaris*–induced thrombi in the smaller vessels of the gut wall (Nieberle and Cohrs 1967). The fourth-stage larva ends its migration in the cranial mesenteric artery with some migration proximad and distad along the aorta. Studies of 18 naturally occurring cases of intestinal infarction associated with thrombosis of the mesenteric vasculature did not support gross peripheral embolization of thrombi as the predominant cause of nonstrangulated bowel infarction (White 1981a).

Nonstrangulated bowel infarction seems to be definitely associated with lesions in the cranial mesenteric artery or its immediate branches. In 18 cases studied, nine horses had a lesion in the

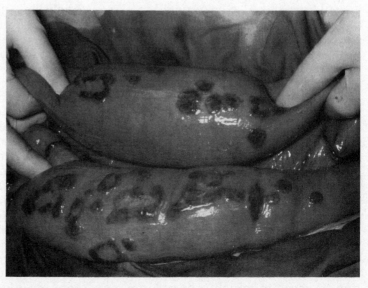

Figure 15–160 Hemomelasma ilei of the small intestine.

ileocecocolic artery and five horses had multi-arterial lesions involving both the cranial mesenteric and ileocecocolic arteries (White 1981a). Arterial lesions included wall thickening, ragged thrombus formation, and dilatation of the arterial lumen. Peripheral mesenteric vascular blockage was only seen in two cases. In summary, it would seem that nonstrangulating infarction of intestine in the horse is primarily associated with thrombotic lesions of the cranial mesenteric and/or its ileocecocolic branch. More peripheral vascular occlusion would not seem to be an important cause of infarction, but this does not preclude its playing a significant role in temporary spasmodic colic that resolves either spontaneously or with medical therapy, is related to temporary ischemia with subsequent collateral revascularization, and does not result in infarction. No matter what the cause (and it is again stressed that it does not seem thromboembolic in nature), peripheral occlusion of small visceral arteries usually produces minimal ischemic changes with transient alteration in motility.

Having accepted thrombosis of the cranial mesenteric and ileocecocolic arteries as the primary cause of nonstrangulating infarction, the factors that cause critical infarction are still unclear. Infarction of small or large intestine is difficult to produce experimentally by ligating the arterial supply in the small (Adams 1979) or large (Nelson and Adams 1966) intestine. Patent collateral vasculature has also been noted in association with infarcted segments in clinical cases (White 1981a). These findings imply that more than simple vessel occlusion is involved in the production of an infarct. It is possible that nonocclusive vascular disease may be involved in some instances of equine intestinal infection. In man, this has been associated with a low flow state, which can be associated with shock or low cardiac output. Low blood flow has not been reported in an equine mesenteric artery, but it has been implied by angiographic studies in experimentally produced S. vulgaris arteritis (Slocombe et al. 1977). This low flow mechanism with subsequent hypoxia could explain initiation of a mucosal lesion with subsequent infarction in cases in which a completely occlusive lesion is not found or in which collateral vessels appear patent (White 1981a). However, as mentioned before with experimental arterial ligation, the bowel does not seem very sensitive to ischemic hypoxia and other factors would seem necessary.

It is also possible that the release of a vasoactive prostaglandin from platelets may be involved in the development of a low flow state. Platelet aggregation has been observed histologically around intimal damage caused by fourth stage S. vulgaris larvae migrating up the arterial tree. Platelets are capable of elaborating and releasing thromboxane, a vasoconstrictive prostaglandin. If the thromboxane is not inactivated in the arterial tree, then its vasoconstrictive properties may be involved in the initiation of a low flow state. However, intimal damage associated with fourth stage larval migration is common. Why some horses would be susceptible and others not is unknown. Peripheral DIC may also be involved.

Finally, it is noted that although an anemic infarct may be anticipated following arterial occlusion, the condition is generally one of hemorrhagic infarction (Nieberle and Cohrs 1967). Simultaneous occlusion of arterial and venous mesenteric vasculature results in anemic infarction with pale, nonthickened intestinal wall (Adams 1979). The observation of hemorrhagic infarction has been explained in terms of decreased blood flow causing ischemic damage to capillaries, which increases permeability (Nieberle and Cohrs 1967). Blood is then introduced through small anastomoses into these dilated and permeable capillaries. The blood flow is determined by back flow of venous blood (Nieberle and Cohrs 1967). Venous occlusion is more predictable in experimental production of infarction than is arterial occlusion. It has been recognized that primary mesenteric venous occlusion can occur as a separate entity from primary arterial occlusion in man (Nanson 1960). It is frequently secondary to inflammatory and neoplastic disease or intestinal displacements but can also recur as an idiopathic primary mesenteric venous thrombosis (Nanson 1960).

Nonstrangulating infarction may also be associated with vascular spasm (causes unidentified) or increased pressure in the intestinal wall secondary to obstructive lesions.

Pathology and Distribution of Lesions

The areas of infarction subsequently undergo necrosis and gangrene (Nieberle and Cohrs 1967). Color changes range from blue-black through greenish-brown to pale yellow. There may be extensive thickening. In earlier cases preinfarctive ischemic changes may be found at laparotomy.

Although this disease has been considered one predominantly of large intestine, a recent study of 18 cases showed small intestinal infarction in 10 horses, infarction of the colon in 6, and cecal infarction in 4 (one horse had combined cecal and colic infarction and another had small intestinal-cecal involvement) (White 1981a). Intestinal lesions were both diffuse and focal (White 1981a). In another report of 82 exploratory laparotomies, 24 (29 per cent) were related to verminous arteritis based on the finding of thrombosis or aneurysm formation in the cranial mesenteric trunk (Moore et al. 1980). Cases included intestinal ischemia and infarction (12), intussusception (4), hemorrhagic nodules with or without peritonitis (6), impaction of small colon (1), and abscessation and invagination of the cecum (1) (Moore et al. 1980). These associations, although accepted by many clinicians, still require proof.

Clinical Signs

With no obstruction to the intestinal lumen, distension is slower to develop and pain is usually less intense. Clinical signs are highly variable (White 1981a). Signs of colic range from no evidence of pain through mild and moderate pain to severe pain. The degree of pain cannot be related to the site of infarction or the amount of intestine involved. Most horses have minimal bowel distension. Gastric reflux and palpation of small intestinal distension on rectal examination are the most useful indications but still do not correlate that well with severity and site of disease. Palpation of the mesenteric artery is of no value in diagnosing mesenteric artery disease. Heart rate

and clinicopathological changes are equally variable. Peritoneal fluid changes and blood parameters are not very useful in making a diagnosis or prognosis. In one series the peritoneal fluid was yellow-orange in one-half of the horses just prior to surgical or necropsy diagnosis of intestinal infarction (White 1981a). Although such findings may help rule out a strangulation (serosanguineous fluid), it will not confirm nonstrangulating infarction.

Treatment

Intestinal resection and anastomosis is the only effective treatment with infarcted intestine, and this is limited to a localized lesion. The disease is usually multifocal and progressive, with postoperative infarction of bowel that is apparently viable at laparotomy being a major problem. Similar problems and low survival rate also exist in man.

In some cases the author has operated on horses with acute abdomens that showed vascular compromise at surgery; the abdomens were closed and the animals subsequently survived. These cases should obviously be classified as temporary ischemia rather than infarction but underscore the justification for recovery of the animal when viability is questionable. Aggressive supportive treatment with fluids as well as corticosteroids or flunixin meglumine is indicated.

The adjunctive use of antithrombotic drug therapy warrants investigation. The use of low-molecular-weight dextran (dextran 70) in the treatment of "verminous aneurysm" in the horse has been reported as successful (Greatorex 1977), but these cases were clinical diagnoses, and the lack of definition of the actual problems needs to be recognized. A discussion of the use of larval anthelmintic treatment of cases of "thromboembolic colic" is not considered appropriate. The reader is referred to another publication (Drudge 1979).

Postoperative Small Intestinal Problems

Paralytic ileus is a common complication following intestinal surgery. To minimize such problems requires timely surgical intervention for the original problem; competent, fast surgery with attention to minimal trauma to the bowel; avoidance of irritation to the peritoneal cavity; and aseptic technique (Huskamp 1977). Details on these aspects are reviewed in Equine Colic Surgery.

LARGE INTESTINE

Anatomy

By definition, the large intestine extends from the ileocecal junction to the anus and therefore includes the cecum, large colon, small colon, and rectum (Getty 1975). However, for our purposes the rectum will be considered separately, and this section will discuss conditions of the cecum and colon.

The cecum is a large comma-shaped cul-de-sac, approximately 1.25 m long, with a capacity of 25 to 30 liters. It is situated chiefly to the right of midline, extending from the right iliac and sublumbar regions to the abdominal floor behind the xiphoid cartilage. It consists of a base, body, and apex (Fig. 15–161). The base is attached dorsally by connective tissue and peritoneum to the ventral

surface of the pancreas and right kidney and a small area of the abdominal wall behind these; it is attached medially to the terminal part of the large colon and ventrally to the origin of the small colon. The body is attached dorsolaterally to the large colon by the cecocolic fold. The apex is free and can therefore vary in position.

The cecum has four longitudinal bands or teniae (dorsal, ventral, lateral, and medial), which cause four rows of sacculations. The dorsal band begins at the apex of the cecum and continues into the ileocecal fold. The medial band extends to the apex and bears the medial cecal vessels. The ventral band joins the medial band near the apex. The lateral band, bearing the lateral cecal vessels, continues into the cecocolic fold. The lateral band may not extend to the apex of the cecum (DeBoom 1975). The ileocecal orifice is located on the lesser curvature (medial aspect) of the base of the cecum. The cecocolic orifice is approximately 5 cm caudolateral to the ileocecal orifice, and the two orifices are separated by a large intervening fold. The cecocolic orifice is oval and approximately 5 cm in diameter.

The large colon is more than twice the

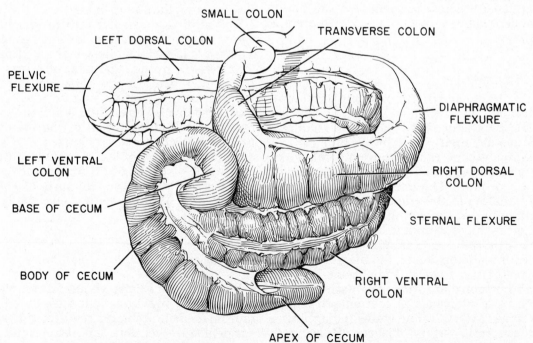

Figure 15–161 Diagram of cecum and large colon of the horse.

size of the cecum. It is attached to the body wall at the origin of the right ventral colon and the termination of the right dorsal colon, the remainder of the large colon forming a free loop interconnected by mesocolon. The large colon commences at the cecocolic orifice as the right ventral colon, passing forward to the sternal flexure, where it becomes the left ventral colon (see Fig. 15–161). Both these parts are 20 to 25 cm wide, have four bands, and are sacculated. The two dorsal bands are covered by mesocolon. The left ventral colon runs caudad and narrows to 6 to 10 cm at the pelvic flexure, after which it becomes the left dorsal colon. The left dorsal colon is smooth and nonsacculated and has one band, which is covered by mesocolon. As it proceeds craniad from the pelvis it widens gradually to the diaphragmatic flexure, and there is a further increase in width in the right dorsal colon (30 to 50 cm wide). The right dorsal colon has three bands, one of which is covered by mesocolon. On reaching the medial surface of the base of the cecum, the right dorsal colon turns left behind the left sac of the stomach and becomes constricted to 8 to 10 cm in diameter (transverse colon) and joins the small colon below the left kidney. The transverse colon is closely attached to the dorsal body wall cranial to the root of the cranial mesenteric artery. Partial situs inversus of the cecum and colon, an almost complete

mirror image of normal position of the cecum and colon, is a rare anomaly that departs from this normal anatomy (Vitums and Kainer 1953).

The small colon is 3 to 4 m long and has a consistent diameter of 7.5 to 10 cm. It normally lies in coils in the left dorsal quadrant of the abdomen. It is attached to the sublumbar region by the colic mesentery and to the terminal duodenum by the duodenocolic fold. The small colon has two bands. One is covered by mesocolon and one is distinctly sacculated and in an antimesenteric position. The small colon becomes the rectum at the pelvic inlet.

The serosa of the large cecum and colon does not cover the opposed surfaces of cecum and colon, which are between the layers of the cecocolic fold and mesocolon, nor the areas of parietal attachment of the cecum and colon. The muscular layer consists of longitudinal and circular fibers. The bulk of the longitudinal muscle comprises the bands of the cecum and colon, but the amount varies. The bands of the cecum and the ventral part of the large colon are largely composed of elastic tissue. The bands of the dorsal part of the large colon are largely muscular, and those of the small colon are almost entirely muscular (Getty 1975).

The blood supply to the cecum and colon is derived from the cranial and caudal mesenteric arteries (Fig. 15–162)

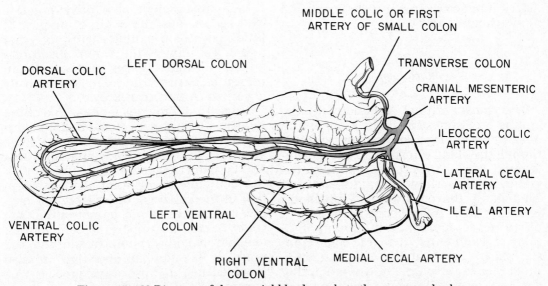

Figure 15–162 Diagram of the arterial blood supply to the cecum and colon.

(Getty 1975). The cranial mesenteric artery has three main branches: left, right, and cranial. The left gives rise to the mesenteric vessels of the jejunum. The right, or ileocecocolic artery, gives off the ileal artery (which goes to the terminal ileum and unites with the most caudal of the mesenteric vessels), the lateral and medial cecal arteries (in the lateral and medial bands), and the ventral colic artery. The last-named supplies the ventral parts of the large colon and sends a branch to the base of the cecum. The cranial branch of the cranial mesenteric artery divides into the dorsal colic artery, which supplies the dorsal colon, and the middle colic artery or first artery of the small colon, a smaller supplier, which goes to the origin of the small colon (Getty 1975). The dorsal and ventral colic arteries meet at the pelvic flexure and also anastomose through numerous branches between the right ventral and dorsal colon (see Fig. 15–162).

The caudal mesenteric artery arises from the aorta 12 to 15 cm behind the origin of the cranial mesenteric artery. It is much smaller than the cranial mesenteric artery and supplies the greater part of the small colon and rectum. It descends in the colic mesentery and divides into two branches. The caudal branch gives off three or four arteries, which divide and form anastomotic arches to the small colon. The most cranial branch joins the middle colic branch of the cranial mesenteric artery. The caudal branch of the caudal mesenteric artery supplies the rectum as the cranial hemorrhoidal artery.

Physiology

The most critical function of the equine large intestine is the storage and absorption of large amounts of fluid. Although the small intestine absorbs a substantial part of secreted and ingested water, studies show that 19.4 liters of fluid enter the cecum from the ileum each day in a 160-kg pony (Argenzio et al. 1974). In addition, a minimum of 10 liters of water enters the large colon from the plasma, so that the large intestine must recover a volume of water equal to the total extracellular fluid volume during a 24-hour period. A second function of the cecum and colon is that of microbial digestion. At least one-half of the animal's energy requirement is furnished by nutrients absorbed by the cecum and colon (Argenzio 1975). To achieve the previously mentioned functions, mechanisms are required to limit the rate of passage of contents, provide optimal conditions for microbial digestion, and efficiently transport solutes and water.

The transit time of liquid and particulate matter through the cecum is relatively short compared with that of the large colon (Argenzio 1975). Ingesta is retained for a longer period of time. There is homogeneous mixing within the cecum and ventral, dorsal, and small colons but no retrograde flow between them. Resistance to flow at the various junctions increases distally, so that the transverse colon provides the greatest resistance. Retardation of flow at the pelvic flexure and transverse colon would appear necessary to provide time for microbial digestion and the subsequent absorption of nutrients, inorganic electrolytes, and water. The dorsal colon selectively retains particles to a greater degree than the ventral colon (Argenzio et al. 1974). Distension of the large colon, as well as outlet resistance, accounts for ingesta retention (Argenzio 1980).

The large colon has considerably more fluid reabsorptive capacity than the small intestine, not only because of its large volume capacity but also because of a more efficient absorptive process. The cecum absorbs a large amount of fluid. The colon exhibits both secretion and absorption, with a net absorption effect. Normally, 95 per cent of the fluid presented to the large colon is effectively absorbed (Argenzio 1980).

Table 15–3 provides an example of the relative importance of each area with reference to fluid fluxes. These values are averages from a study and apply to a 160-kg pony (Argenzio et al. 1974).

A complete description of ion absorption in the colon is not possible nor necessary here. It should be noted that the colon makes an important contribution to electrolyte absorption. In addition, the products of microbial digestion are also involved in this absorptive process (Argenzio 1980).

Table 15–3 FLUID FLUX WITHIN THE LARGE INTESTINE

Part of Large Intestine	Liters Entering	Liters Secreted	Liters Absorbed
Cecum	19.4	0.9	13.5
Ventral large colon	6.8	5.3	9.6
Dorsal large colon	2.5	5.2	4.4
Small colon	3.3	0.5	2.3

Specific Surgical Conditions of the Large Intestine

SIMPLE OBSTRUCTION

Large intestinal obstructions can be divided into the same three categories as those of small intestinal obstructions, and the pathophysiological principles are generally the same.

Pathophysiology

Simple obstructions include impaction, obstruction by foreign bodies or enteroliths, and entrapments or displacements in which strangulation does not occur. Simple obstructions may be partial or complete.

In general, the clinical signs or rate of systemic deterioration is much less dramatic in simple obstruction of the large intestine compared with simple obstruction of the small intestine. In experimental obstruction of the small colon, for instance, signs of colic are intermittent and mild compared with those of higher obstructions, and changes in pulse, hydration, and acid-base status are slow to develop (Datt and Usenik 1975). However, there is considerable variation depending on whether the obstruction is partial or complete, the site of the obstruction, and the pain tolerance of the patient. With complete obstruction there is more severe and continuous pain, with gaseous distension of the large colon and more rapid systemic deterioration. As was discussed with the small intestine, obstructive pressure can produce ischemia of the bowel wall and can complicate the picture as the condition progresses. It should also be noted that even if such ischemia does not lead to infarction, irreversible compromise to motility may develop.

Clinical Signs and Diagnosis

Diagnosis of simple obstruction of the large intestine is based on history, clinical signs, rectal examination, and laboratory determinations. Relevant points of history include the presence of any causative factors, such as feed changes, water deprivation, exposure to and ingestion of unusual materials, any diet or management changes, parasite exposure and control; the progression of clinical signs; and immediate feed intake and fecal output.

Systemic signs are often normal in simple obstruction, and it is the results of *repeated* examinations that may be the critical diagnostic factors and the important indicators for surgery. Motility will vary depending on the stage of the condition. Increased spasmodic motility may be noted with minor or early conditions. Depressed motility is common in many obstructions, and complete ileus can be anticipated as complete obstruction progresses. Tympany of the cecum and colon can be detected with auscultation and percussion and will also manifest as abdominal distension. It should also be noted that a number of complete obstructions will cause a significant accumulation of fluid in the stomach. This is usually due to tension on the duodenocolic ligament, which causes some degree of duodenal obstruction or direct pressure on the duodenum from a distended cecum or large colon.

Rectal examination is a most important diagnostic parameter with simple obstruction of the large intestine. The operator needs to be familiar with normal anatomy, including normal position, and should not attempt rectal examination without having this prerequisite. The small colon is easily identified as a chain of fecal balls. The pelvic flexure can usually be palpated in front of the pelvic brim and may be left or right of the midline. The cecum is palpated on the right side; it will be flaccid in the normal state, but a band is palpable. The clinician should also be able to recognize the caudal border of the spleen and its normal position, the left kidney, the reproductive organs, the bladder, the aorta, the iliac ateries, and the inguinal rings. The rectal findings with specific conditions are discussed with each condition.

In many instances of obstruction by impaction or foreign body, definitive diagnosis by rectal examination is not possible. This applies particularly to obstructions in the right dorsal and transverse colon. The administration of 4-mm particulate markers has been described to determine the presence and degree of obstruction and assist in the assessment of the need for surgery (Moore, Traver, and Johnson 1978). Complete retention of markers at 36 to 48 hours was an indication for surgical intervention (Moore, Traver, and Johnson 1978).

Tympanites of the Cecum and Colon

Primary tympanites of the cecum is rare. It usually occurs secondary to ileus or complete obstruction of the large intestine. Acute colic develops with moderate pain. The distended cecum can be percussed and palpated on the right side with rectal examination. Systemic parameters are usually normal.

Primary cecal tympanites can be treated by percutaneous trocarization. Trocarization is a valid treatment technique if not abused. The usual clinical situation for its use is cecal and/or accompanying colonic distension; the operator uses trocarization to relieve abdominal distension and respiratory compromise. The patient will respond in a primary tympanites. If distension recurs, the tympanites is secondary and surgical intervention is indicated. Trocarization is performed in the right paralumbar fossa following appropriate skin preparation using a cecal trocar or a 10- to 12-gauge, 3- to 4-in needle or an intravenous catheter. Neither repeated trocarization nor multiple trocarizations, if the initial one is nonproductive, should be performed. Rectal localization of the cecum while trocarization is being performed (Gruber and Langner 1971) can aid in correct positioning of the trocar.

It should be noted that the white cell count rises dramatically following trocarization (up to 200,000/mm^3). Although it is not a cause for alarm, it will affect the diagnostic value of paracentesis in recognizing other conditions. On a one-time basis, trocarization can generally be considered innocuous, but tearing of bowel and consequent peritoneal contamination have been observed and can be obviated by good technique.

As with cecal tympanites, primary tympanites of the colon is relatively uncommon. The condition is characterized by abdominal distension and is diagnosed on rectal examination. The condition will often represent a surgical obstruction, but in a patient with normal vital signs, medical treatment (see Impaction) or trocarization has been used. Trocarization may not be as effective for primary tympanites of the colon as it is with the cecal condition owing to the colon's size and the gaseous entrapment within segments; in such unresponsive cases, laparotomy and decompression are indicated.

Impaction with Ingesta

Impaction of the large intestine is a common cause of intestinal obstruction. In one series of 453 cases of intestinal obstruction, impaction was the cause in 112 cases (Tennant 1975). Of these 112 cases, there were 5 cases of primary impaction of the cecum, 65 cases of impaction of the large colon, and 42 cases of impaction of the small colon. Impaction with ingesta or sand is discussed here; obstruction and impaction associated with foreign bodies will be considered separately.

IMPACTION OF THE CECUM. This condition is uncommon. Impaction of the cecum is typically insidious in onset, and predisposing factors are vague. It has been suggested that the condition is more often secondary to a distal obstruction or a pathological problem of the cecocolic orifice (Foerner 1982).

The course of this condition is one of intermittent colic for a week or more. Since the cecum is a blind sac, fluid and some ingesta can bypass the obstruction (Meagher 1974). It is the only form of large intestinal impaction in which there is continued fecal production. Generally the horse will continue to eat some food and will pass reduced amounts of feces (which can be diarrheic). Normal gut motility persists. Diagnosis of the condition is based on rectal examination, during which the hard, impacted cecum can be palpated on the right side of the abdominal cavity. Differential diagnosis includes abdominal abscesses and neoplasia.

If the impaction is unresponsive to medical treatment, surgical intervention is indicated. Surgical treatment consists of the injection of saline and dioctyl sodium sulfosuccinate (DSS) directly into the impacted mass. Manual massage is performed to break up the impacted mass and distribute the injected fluids. This procedure may be performed through a standing flank laparotomy. Manual evacuation of the cecum is only performed as a last resort.

The prognosis should be guarded with cecal impactions. Normal motility may not return; this is related to how long the condition has been present. In addition, the base of the cecum may rupture in association with devitalization of the bowel wall. The use of a side-to-side anastomosis between an area of cecum toward the apex and the right ventral colon may be considered to facilitate emptying of the apex of the cecum.

IMPACTION OF THE LARGE COLON. This is a frequent cause of simple obstruction of the large colon. Ingesta impactions usually occur at the pelvic flexure or the right dorsal colon–transverse colon area of narrowing of the large colon. Functionally, the pelvic flexure has been identified as an area of resistance to aboral flow (Sellers, Lowe, and Brondum 1979) and is a probable pacemaker area. Selective retention of large particles occurs in the right dorsal colon, and the transverse colon provides more resistance to flow than the pelvic flexure (Argenzio 1980). Factors that may precipitate impaction include poor quality feed, decreased water intake and dehydration, and parasite damage.

Sand impactions occur in the right dorsal or ventral colon. They have a geographical distribution and are associated with availability of sand or gravel and feeding of the animals off the ground. Some horses will persist in eating sand even when abundant high quality feed is provided away from the sand.

Typically there is a gradual onset of moderate abdominal pain. The intensity of colic signs varies between horses based on their pain tolerance. Abdominal signs may decrease in frequency and intensity but usually persist. It has been shown that episodes of pain in pelvic flexure impaction are associated with longer, louder sounds on auscultation and multiple contractions (closely grouped series lasting three to five minutes) of greater than 40 mm Hg intraluminal pressure (Lowe, Sellers, and Brondum 1980). Fecal production can persist for a period but eventually ceases with complete impaction. An impaction in the right dorsal colon may cause gastric reflux owing to tension on the duodenocolic fold or presssure on the duodenum. Pelvic flexure impactions can be readily palpated on rectal examination. The pelvic flexure is distended with material, which varies from doughy to hard. Impactions of the right dorsal colon and transverse colon are commonly nonpalpable, and diagnosis is based on continued monitoring and response to treatment. Sand impactions may be palpated in the ventral abdomen but are often out of reach. The presence of appreciable sand in the manure or on paracentesis (the ventral colon lies on the ventral body wall) is a strong indication for sand impaction. The differential diagnosis includes enteroliths and foreign bodies.

Most ingesta impactions respond to conservative medical mangement, which includes the administration of mineral oil and/or DSS together with oral and intravenous fluids if necessary. Medication is used for pain control. It has been shown that xylazine diminishes intraluminal pressure (pressure changes cease for 30 minutes following administration). Flunixin meglumine relieves signs of colic, but there is no evidence of change in intraluminal pressure (Lowe, Sellers, and Brondum 1980). Whether its effect is one of analgesia (directly by inhibiting sensory nerves or indirectly by suppressing prostaglandin production) or some other mechanism is not known (Lowe, Sellers, and Brondum 1980). If the problem persists for three to five days or if there is systemic deterioration or the development of refractory pain, surgical intervention is indicated. Although unnecessary surgery is not desired, prolonged hesitation can leave the surgeon with a devitalized large colon.

At surgery the impactions may be injected and massaged as described for cecal impaction, or evacuation of the bowel can be performed. Which method is used depends on the individual case. Injection and massage are appropriate if the mass can be easily broken up and the bowel is healthy. It is better to remove larger impactions when motility is depressed. The pelvic flexure is exteriorized and an enterotomy performed. Warm water is flushed into the bowel to facilitate atraumatic breakdown and removal of the contents. This technique is considerably better than manually milking out the dry ingesta, particularly for left dorsal–transverse colon impactions. Manipulations of these impactions when they are advanced may result in rupture of the colon (Fig. 15–163). The prognosis is generally good with ingesta impactions.

Sand impactions represent a more difficult problem. Some cases will respond to conservative treatment. In addition to the use of mineral oil or DSS, the natural fiber laxative psyllium hydrophilic mucilloid (Metamucil, Searle) can be most helpful in some cases. Surgical intervention is necessary if there is no response to medical treatment. Although the prognosis is generally poor, results can be improved using the combined lavage-evacuation technique. Very large amounts of sand can accumulate. In cases that are surgically treated, loss of colonic motility and recurrence of the conditions are potential problems.

IMPACTION OF THE SMALL COLON. Ingesta impactions can also occur in the small colon. Their occurrence has been related to sudden unrelenting spasm of the musculature on one side of the bowel, particularly in a tenia (Foerner, Phillips, and Barclay 1981). A predisposition in ponies for small colon impaction has been reported (Tennant 1975). Impacted contents in the small colon can become inspissated and hard and are then referred to by some as fecaliths. Treatment of impactions in the small colon can be by injection into the bowel and massage, retrograde flushing and massage with a hose inserted per rectum (Taylor et al. 1979), or evacuation through an enterotomy. If an enterotomy is performed in the small colon the teniae should be avoided; the high muscular content is not conducive to good wound healing. Rupture of the small colon with containment of the contents within the mesentery has also been reported (Merritt, Pickering, and Bergerin 1975). Impactions of the small colon are more commonly associated with ingestion of foreign material.

It should always be remembered that impaction can result secondarily whenever bowel stasis develops. Whenever an impaction is identified at surgery, a complete exploration should be performed to ensure that there is no other obstruction.

Foreign Body Impaction

Impactions may occur in association with the ingestion of nondigestible foreign materials, such as baling twine, braided materials, and rubber or nylon products. This is typically observed in foals and young horses (Boles and Khon 1981; Gay, Spiers, and Christie 1971). A particular problem has been experienced in association with the ingestion of rubberized fencing material (Boles and Kohn 1981) or nylon-based cording from tires (DeGroot 1971). The impacting material consists of a firm concretion of ingesta surrounding a core of foreign fibrous strands. Long periods between exposure to the material and development of a clinical problem indicate that strands of cording may be present in the bowel lumen for a long time (up to five

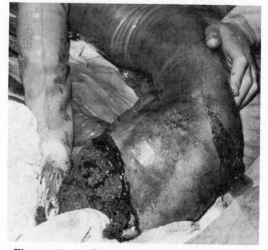

Figure 15–163 Rupture of right dorsal colon associated with advanced ingesta impaction.

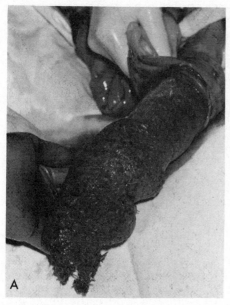

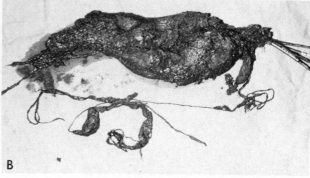

Figure 15–164 Foreign body impaction of the small colon. *A*, Removal of an impaction due to volleyball netting. *B*, Another impacted mass due to baling twine.

years) before amalgamating to cause an obstruction (DeGroot 1971).

The presenting signs are similar to those of impaction. However, owing to the nondegradable nature of the impacting mass, medical treatment is of no value. Surgical removal of the offending material is necessary. The obstruction typically occurs in the small colon and/or transverse colon, but the material may extend into the right dorsal colon. Surgical exteriorization of the right dorsal colon, transverse colon, or immediate proximal colon is not possible. An enterotomy is made in a portion of the right dorsal colon that can be exteriorized or through the small colon distal to the obstruction. Removal of a foreign body obstruction through the small colon is illustrated in Figure 15–164. In some instances removal may not be possible. Bowel wall devitalization can also lead to rupture during surgical manipulation. The overall prognosis is good if bowel is healthy and if removal can be performed without problems.

Enteroliths

Enteroliths are concretions composed primarily of ammonium magnesium phosphate (Blue 1979). They form by the deposition of salts in concentric layers about a central nidus. The central nidus can be a metal fragment, a small stone, or some other foreign material. The fac-

tors that cause precipitates of salts and enterolith formation are still uncertain. Excessive amounts of magnesium phosphate and ammonia have been associated with defective absorption of magnesium phosphate and excessive production of ammonia, respectively (Blue 1979; Nieberle and Cohrs 1967). High concentrations of magnesium in the drinking water have been implicated in one report (Blue and Wittkopp 1981). The natural relative hypomotility of the large colon may also be conducive to mineral concretion.

Enteroliths occur in the large intestine and can remain there for long periods unassociated with signs of clinical disease unless they become impacted in a narrower part of the digestive tract. Small enteroliths may be passed in feces without clinical signs (Blue and Wittkopp 1981). They may cause obstruction in the right dorsal colon, but the most common site of obstruction is in the proximal small colon (Blue 1979). Larger enteroliths are characteristic of the right dorsal colon (Ferraro 1973). Enteroliths are not found in horses younger than 5 years of age and are most common in horses 5 to 10 years of age. The enteroliths are generally spherical or tetrahedral in shape. When multiple stones are present they are usually tetrahedral, whereas a single enterolith (the most common finding) is usually spherical.

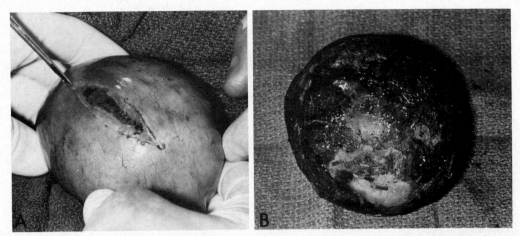

Figure 15–165 *A*, Removal of enterolith lodged in small colon. *B*, Enterolith after removal. Radiographs revealed a small piece of wire as the central nidus.

Horses typically present with recurrent mild colic, which may range from 12 hours to a week in duration (there may be a history of abdominal discomfort prior to this time also). Inappetence, gaseous distension of the large colon, and decreased intestinal motility are other clinical features. If the enterolith causes an incomplete blockage, the colic is similar to an impaction. Gas, fluid, and mineral oil can still be passed, but there is little solid fecal material. A complete obstruction will cause a colic that increases in intensity and is typically more severe than an impaction. The development of severe abdominal pain is associated with severe tympany of the colon. Rectal examination reveals large colon distension, but a definitive presurgical diagnosis is uncommon with enteroliths.

At surgery there is distension of bowel proximal to the enterolith, and the small colon is empty distal to the obstruction. If the enterolith is present in a portion of the bowel that can be exteriorized, an enterotomy is performed and concretion removed (Fig. 15–165). Commonly the enterolith is present in bowel that cannot be exteriorized (proximal small colon or distal right dorsal colon). In this instance the enterolith is moved retrograde until it is positioned in a portion of the dorsal colon that can be exteriorized for enterotomy. Retrograde flushing with water using a hose inserted up the small colon is a useful adjunctive technique (Taylor et al. 1979), but caution should be exercised because of weakened bowel wall

owing to ischemia where the enterolith is lodged. Intraluminal manipulation with a hand introduced through an enterotomy (as used with foreign body impactions) may be indicated in some instances. The prognosis is fair (47 per cent success rate in one report of 30 cases [Blue 1979]). Success depends on removal of the enterolith prior to bowel devitalization, as bowel rupture associated with removal of the enterolith is not uncommon. In addition, contamination of the abdominal cavity should be avoided.

Displacement or Nonstrangulating Torsion

This category includes various conditions that have been generally classified as torsions, which are characterized by abnormal large colon position without strangulation of the blood supply. They are surgical conditions, but because of the lack of bowel strangulation the patient shows slow systemic deterioration and the success rate with timely surgical intervention is good. A number of malpositions can occur. The most common displacement involves the pelvic flexure being located in the cranial aspect of the abdomen (Fig. 15–166). This type of malposition may be complicated by a torsion as well. European equine surgeons have classified these displacements as right dorsal displacements of the large colon (Huskamp and Boening 1981). In other instances, the pelvic flexure may be in a normal position, but the left dorsal and

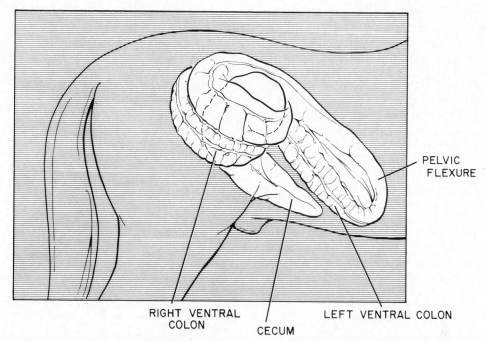

PELVIC
FLEXURE

RIGHT VENTRAL
COLON

CECUM

LEFT VENTRAL COLON

Figure 15–166 Diagram of displacement of large colon with pelvic flexure positioned in the cranial part of the abdomen.

left ventral colon rotates 180° around the sternal and diaphragmatic flexure (Fig. 15–167). This is considered to be a torsion but is not generally strangulating. Rotations of 90° or less are nonclinical and are only incidental findings at surgery. The essential feature of these conditions is blockage to the passage of ingesta, but the vascularity is not compromised. With progression of time, or

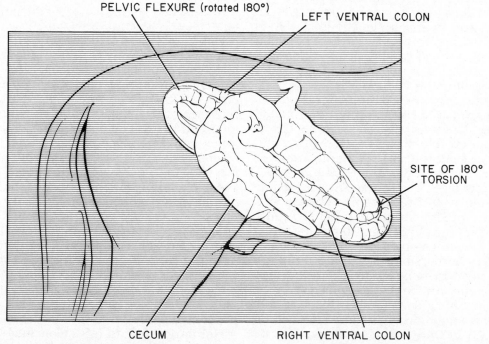

PELVIC FLEXURE (rotated 180°)

LEFT VENTRAL COLON

SITE OF 180°
TORSION

CECUM

RIGHT VENTRAL COLON

Figure 15–167 Diagram of a 180° torsion of the large colon around the sternal and diaphragmatic flexures.

with severe torsions, the condition is a strangulating one.

These patients present with moderately painful colic due to large colon distension. The large bowel has decreased motility and tympany. Rectal examination reveals a distended large colon. A distended pelvic flexure will be palpated with a 180° torsion; the clinician cannot identify this stricture in cases of cranial displacement of the pelvic flexure.

The condition is identified at surgery by recognition of abnormal positioning; the displacement is corrected and the colon decompressed. The prognosis is generally good in these cases because surgical intervention generally precedes any permanent changes in the intestinal wall or severe systemic deterioration.

Left Dorsal Displacement or Nephrosplenic Entrapment of Large Colon

This condition is characterized by displacement of the left dorsal and left ventral colon between the dorsal body wall and the suspensory ligament of the spleen (nephrosplenic ligament) (Milner, Tarr, and Lochner 1977) (Fig. 15–168). The diaphragmatic and sternal flexures of the large colon are positioned between the stomach and the left lobe of the liver. The cause of the condition is uncertain, but it has been related to splenic contraction at a time when the left colon is filled with gas (Evans 1981). The colon displaces dorsally, and, as the spleen refills, the base of the spleen hooks under the colon and traps it.

Patients present with moderate to severe pain that can be intermittent and respond temporarily to xylazine but is ultimately unresponsive. Heart rate will increase but the horse generally remains systemically stable. There is some loss of gut motility. Rectal findings can include an impacted or gas-distended pelvic flexure in a more cranial position or failure to locate the pelvic flexure but detection of a distended colon. In some instances it may be possible to palpate teniae of the colon running up in a dorsocraniad direction. Although the spleen may be displaced caudomedially, this is not a pathognomonic sign, as any stomach dilation will cause splenic rotation. Gastric reflux may be present and is considered

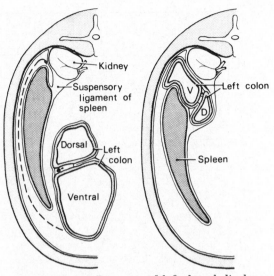

Figure 15–168 Diagram of left dorsal displacement of the large colon. The colon moves dorsad lateral to the spleen to become positioned over the supsensory ligament of the spleen (nephrosplenic ligament).

to be due to tension on the duodenocolic ligament. Attempts at paracentesis will frequently result in a bloody sample because of the changed position of the spleen. Because of the intermittent colic signs and slow rate of deterioration, surgical intervention sometimes does not take place until a relatively long period of time has elapsed (Milne, Tarr, and Lochner 1977).

At surgery an impacted or distended left colon is encountered and it is not possible to exteriorize as much of the colon as usual (Fig. 15–169A). The colon is followed under the spleen. The displacement is corrected by passing a hand between the spleen and body wall and retracting the spleen medially as the colon is lifted up. The colon is then repositioned on the visceral surface of the spleen (Fig. 15–169B). Generally, compromise to the bowel is minimal, but some blanching at the entrapment site can be observed occasionally. The prognosis is generally good; the author has encountered two cases in which there was measurable compromise to the colon at the site of entrapment. Although spontaneous correction of a left dorsal displacement has been recognized, immediate surgical intervention is still advocated.

Herniation of the left colon may also occur through the gastrosplenic omen-

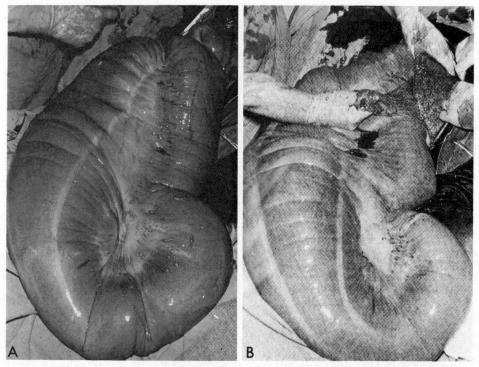

Figure 15–169 Left dorsal displacement of large colon at surgery. *A,* Prior to reduction when less than the usual amount of colon can be exteriorized. *B,* Following reduction with the colon now repositioned medial to the spleen and omentum.

tum (described previously). Signs are similar to those of left dorsal displacement. The treatment involves reduction of the hernia.

Intramural Hematoma

This is an uncommon cause of obstruction of the small colon (Pearson et al. 1971; Spiers et al. 1981). It has been associated with chronic ulceration, iatrogenic rectal damage, and unknown causes. The horse shows severe pain, in excess of that normally seen with obstruction of the small colon. This has been associated with the tight distension in the intestinal wall associated with the hematoma. Treatment involves resection and anastomosis of the affected portion of the small colon.

Congenital Atresia of the Colon

This is also a rare condition. It is classically encountered as one of the abnormalities in lethal white foals, resulting from breeding an overo (color pattern where white is continuous over the body) paint to another overo paint (Schneider and Leipold 1978). Atresia of the intes-

tine may occur at the level of the colon or rectum. Atresia coli may also occur in other breeds, and the causative factors are uncertain. In a recent report a foal with congenital atresia of the left dorsal colon was repaired surgically by resection and anastomosis (Schneider et al. 1981).

Abscessation, Adhesions, and Neoplasia

Internal abdominal abscesses, adhesions, and neoplasia can cause simple obstruction of the large intestine in the same fashion as that previously described for the small intestine (Fig. 15–170). The treatment principles and prognosis are the same. However, it should be noted that if intestinal resection is indicated it is more difficult (and often impossible) in the large intestine. A side-to-side anastomosis may be appropriate to bypass a strictured pelvic flexure.

STRANGULATING OBSTRUCTION

Strangulating obstructions of the large intestine include intussusception (cecum or colon), torsion and volvulus of the

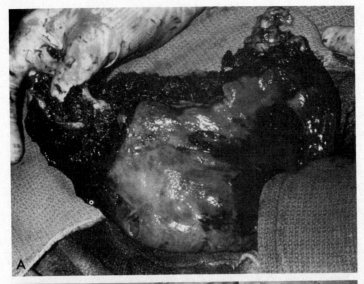

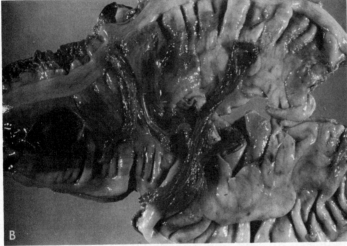

Figure 15–170 Abscessation and adhesions of the colon. *A*, At laparotomy following rupture when attempting to free pelvic flexure from adhesion to pelvic wall. *B*, A necropsy specimen showing adhesions between adjacent parts of the small colon.

large colon, and incarceration or volvulus of the small colon. With the exception of torsion and volvulus of the large colon and cecum, these conditions are rare and much less common than their counterparts in the small intestine.

The pathophysiology of strangulating obstruction of the large intestine is the same as that previously described in the small intestine, but there are some points of variance. The rate of systemic deterioration can vary markedly between a cecocecal intussusception and a large colon volvulus, for instance. In addition, the marked distension of the colon in large colon volvulus has severe physiological implications in itself; respiratory compromise to the point of death can occur.

Intussusception

Intussusception of the cecum may occur as cecocecal or cecocolic intussusception (Allison 1977; Cowles, Bunch, and Flynn 1977; Pearson et al. 1975; Robertson and Johnson 1980). The cause is uncertain, but predisposing factors that have been implicated include verminous arteritis, intramural abscessation of the wall of the cecum (Pearson, Messervy, and Pinsent 1971; Robertson and Johnson 1980), abnormal motility following deworming with an organophosphate compound (Cowles, Bunch, and Flynn 1977), and tapeworm infestation (Barclay, Phillips, and Foerner 1982).

Horses typically present with subacute colic of several days' duration, but there is considerable variation. Total cecocolic intussusception may cause persistent and severe colic or may be manifested as subacute colic followed by chronic weight loss and the passage of scant amounts of soft feces (Allison 1977). Animals may show anorexia and depression. Rectal examination may reveal a large mass in the right dorsal quadrant of the abdomen. Serosanguineous fluid may be obtained on paracentesis.

At surgery the cecum cannot be located. The intussusception will be identified by examination of the right ventral colon. Treatment involves reduction of the intussusception (the colon may have to be opened) and partial typhlectomy if necessary. This latter treatment has been successful in cases up to 10 days in duration (Robertson and Johnson 1980).

One case of intussusception of the colon at the pelvic flexure has been reported. This case was successfully corrected by manual reduction alone (Meagher and Stirk 1974).

Torsion of the Cecum

Torsion of the cecum alone is rare (most commonly associated with torsion of the colon). Incidental displacements of the cecum routinely encountered during surgery are commonly classified as torsions (usually 90° torsions) but are not considered pathological problems. If true cecal torsion does occur, it presents as an acute colic with right-sided abdominal distension. A distended cecum will be palpable on rectal examination, but the large colon will be normal. Paracentesis may reveal serosanguineous fluid,

and systemic deterioration can occur at a rate comparable to that of small intestinal strangulation.

At surgery, a discolored, distended cecal apex will be found, and exploration will reveal the torsion. Following decompression, the torsion is reduced. Resection of the cecum can be performed if feasible. In addition to partial typhlectomy, a technique for complete typhlectomy and ileocolic anastomosis has been described (Huskamp 1977). The latter procedure requires flank laparotomy. The prognosis depends on the amount of compromised cecum.

Torsion and Volvulus of the Large Colon

It has been suggested that the left dorsal colon moving medially or laterally and downward initiates the torsion (Meagher 1974a; Wheat 1975). As mentioned previously with displacements, torsions vary in degree and may be "physiological," nonstrangulating, or strangulating. Rotations of 90° or less are probably frequent. They are considered incidental findings at laparotomy and are not thought to cause any problem. Torsions of 180 to 270° will stop the passage of ingesta and can potentially compromise the blood supply (Fig. 15–171). Torsions of 360° or greater are strangulating obstructions, and ischemic necrosis develops rapidly.

Torsion is most commonly clockwise (viewed from the back of the standing horse). Torsions may occur spontaneously and have been considered to occur with rolling or struggling to rise or secondary to milder colics and impac-

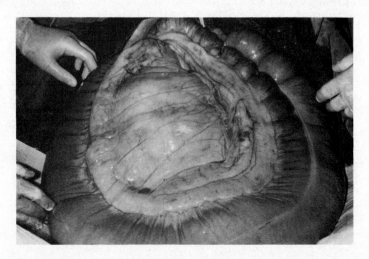

Figure 15–171 A 180° torsion of the left ventral and left dorsal colon at laparotomy. Note the edema in the mesocolon, which suggests early compromise to the venous return.

tion. Disproportionate amounts of gas or ingesta in various parts of the colon have been incriminated. The weight of an impaction could influence the development of a torsion. A tendency for torsion of the colon to occur in older horses has been noted (Sembrat 1975; Tennant 1975). Torsion of the large colon at the sternal and diaphragmatic flexure has been reported in a three-day-old foal (Crowhurst et al. 1975).

As discussed previously, nonstrangulating torsions present with signs similar to those seen with impactions. However, strangulating torsion or volvulus of the large colon constitutes the most severe and rapidly fatal acute abdominal crisis in the horse. Most strangulating torsions are 360° or greater and occur either at the origin of the large intestine and involve the cecum or cranial to the cecum in the right colon so that the cecum is not involved. Because these torsions occur near the attachment of the large colon to the body wall, strangulation of the blood supply results in a condition similar to strangulation of the mesenteric root in small intestinal volvulus; hence, this condition is commonly referred to as volvulus of the large colon. Torsions may only involve the pelvic flexure or the left dorsal and ventral colons; the majority of these are nonstrangulating. Most strangulating torsions involve the entire large colon. In 25 cases of large colon volvulus, the twist occurred at the base of the cecum or the origin of the transverse colon (Barclay, Foerner, and Phillips 1980).

Patients with strangulating torsion present with severe, unrelenting abdominal pain. Systemic deterioration is rapid, with a rapid weak pulse, poor peripheral perfusion, and a high PCV. Patients can manifest signs of severe shock within a few hours of torsion. There is marked abdominal distension, and the distended large colon is easily palpable per rectum, usually forced back into the pelvic cavity. Gastric reflux may be present in association with tension on the duodenocolic ligament or pressure on the duodenum. A peritoneal sample may be obtained. However, a recent review of peritoneal fluid analysis in 21 cases of volvulus of the colon revealed poor correlation between the color, white blood cell count, and protein content of peritoneal fluid and devitalization of the colon (Koch 1981).

Rapid entry into the abdomen following anesthetic induction is paramount in many of these cases because of respiratory compromise. With 360° volvulus, the colon presents as grossly distended but typically appears in a normal position because of the complete 360° twist. The color of the serosa varies from white to blue to black and the wall will be edematous (Fig. 15–172). The large colon is evacuated prior to detorsion. This removes endotoxin that can be potentially absorbed following detorsion and also decreases distension prior to further manipulation. The bowel is evacuated by exteriorizing the pelvic flexure, making an enterotomy, and performing lavage-evacuation as previously described. At this time, the stage of ischemic necrosis of the colon is also assessed, based on the appearance of the mucosa. The appearance of the mucous membrane may range from normal thickness and pink (good prognosis) through dark red to markedly thickened and black (poor prognosis) (Fig. 15–173). Dark, bloody fluid contents at evacuation is another feature of necrosing mucosa (Fig. 15–174).

The direction of the torsion is then evaluated. Viewing the horse in the ventral surgical position, most torsions at the base of the colon are counterclockwise. With the torsed portion of the colon exteriorized, it is rotated in a clockwise

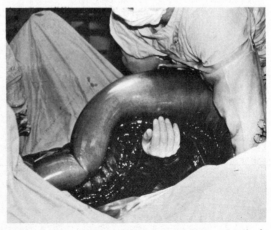

Figure 15–172 Exteriorization of 360° torsion (volvulus) of large colon. The bowel wall and mesentery in this case were purple-black.

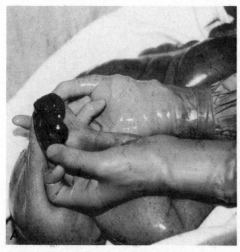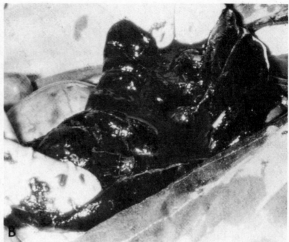

Figure 15–173 Examination of mucosa to assess stage of necrosis with volvulus of the large colon. *A*, Dark red mucosa. *B*, Markedly thickened and black mucosa.

direction to correct the torsion. It should be noted that if the colon is positioned in its normal U shape and one position is used as a constant reference point (e.g., the front), the desired direction of rotation changes from counterclockwise to clockwise as one goes from left to right colon.

The serosal surface color typically improves following detorsion. Mucosal evaluation is a more important criterion for assessing potential viability. The use of oxygen insufflation may be attempted; experimental findings indicate that the typical necrotic mucosa is beyond reversibility (Moore et al. 1980).

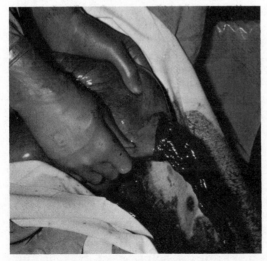

Figure 15–174 Evacuation of the large colon using lavage. The dark, bloody fluid is indicative of mucosal necrosis of the colon.

The survival rate is low. All horses with necrotic mucosa die presumably because of endotoxin release and loss of mucosal integrity. In gastric volvulus in dogs, mucosal sloughing can occur and animals can still survive. It seems that the amount of necrotic mucosa in horses is incompatible with survival; however, improved attempts to medically support the animal and combat massive endotoxemia may offer some potential for increased survival (Moore et al. 1981). Horses need to be operated on very early to survive. The presence of thick, blackened mucosa is probably sufficient grounds for euthanasia, but attempts to develop improved methods of support should not be neglected. With a localized strangulating torsion of the pelvic flexure, resection and anastomosis can be performed, but resection is obviously not feasible with the typical volvulus at the root of the colon.

Incarceration and Volvulus of the Small Colon

Although the small colon has a long mesentery, both incarceration and volvulus are rare (Adams and McIlwraith 1978; Foerner 1982). Incarceration can occur through a mesenteric rent or in association with a pedunculated lipoma (Fig. 15–175). Clinically, the systemic manifestations are relatively acute, as with any strangulating obstruction. Motility is depressed. There is no fecal production from an early stage, and gastric

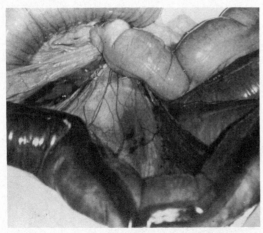

Figure 15–175 Incarceration of the small colon that was amenable to resection and anastomosis.

reflux is unusual. The distended small colon will be palpable on rectal examination.

The cases are managed surgically in the same fashion as the equivalent conditions in the small intestine. However, healing following resection and anastomosis in the small colon can be more complicated compared with that of the small intestine; the muscular activity of the bowel is higher, the bacterial count is increased, the material passing through it is harder, and there are increased concentrations of collagenase.

Diaphragmatic Hernias

Diaphragmatic hernias may cause nonstrangulating or strangulating obstruction of large as well as small intestine. The pathophysiology, diagnosis, and treatment of diaphragmatic hernias are discussed in the section on conditions of the small intestine.

NONSTRANGULATING INFARCTION

Nonstrangulating infarction represents a significant problem of both small and large intestine. In one series of 18 cases, small intestinal infarction was seen in 10 horses, infarction of the colon was found in 6 horses, and cecal infarction was found in 4 horses (1 horse had cecal and large colon involvement and 1 had cecal and small intestinal involvement) (White 1981). The pathogenesis and pathophysiology of this condition (previously described as thromboembolic colic) were presented in the section on the small intestine and will not be repeated here.

As noted previously, a definitive diagnosis can be difficult and conventional parameters are of limited use (White 1981). Animals may show a variable clinical picture ranging from depression with minimal pain to violent acute pain. In experimental infarction of the colon by venous ligation, intense pain was not a feature (Turner and McIlwraith 1980). The degree of pain cannot be related to the site of the lesion or the amount of intestine involved. Heart rate and clinicopathological data similarly vary widely. Intestinal lesions can be diffuse or focal. Color changes range from blue-black to greenish-brown, and the intestinal wall may or may not be thickened (Fig. 15–176).

The only treatment for infarction is resection and anastomosis. Partial typhlectomy may be feasible if there is localized infarction of the cecum. Complete typhlectomy with ileocolostomy has been described (Huskamp 1977). This operation requires a right lateral approach and resection of the eighteenth rib. Malabsorption problems have not been observed after total typhlectomy. Diffuse involvement of the colon is untreatable. When localized involvement indicates the need for resection, the case can still be complicated by further progressive ischemia and infarction. Localized infarction of the small colon has also been observed by the author.

In some instances, a preinfarctive ischemia or "low flow" state may be encountered at surgery. In these instances the animal should be recovered and vigorous support therapy instituted. Apparently, viability of the bowel may be retained as some cases survive.

RUPTURE OF THE LARGE INTESTINE

Rupture can occur as a sequela to conditions described previously owing to tension and decreased viability of the bowel wall. There is no treatment once gross contamination of the peritoneal cavity has occurred. Prevention calls for rapid but careful resolution of the primary problem.

Rupture of the cecum or colon has also

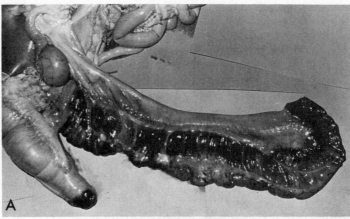

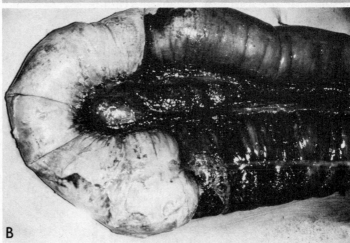

Figure 15–176 *A* and *B*, Nonstrangulating infarction of the large colon.

been reported in association with parturition (Voss 1969). Factors involved include recent feeding with a colon full of ingesta and a large foal with the pressure of labor compressing fluid within the ileocecocolic area. It was suggested that feeding large amounts of feed prior to parturition could be detrimental (Voss 1969).

RECTUM

Anatomy

The rectum of the horse extends from the pelvic inlet to the anus, a distance of approximately 30 cm (Getty 1975). The cranial segment is covered in peritoneum; it is anatomically similar to the small colon and is suspended by a continuation of the mesocolon termed the *mesorectum*. The caudal portion is retroperitoneal and forms a flask-shaped dilation termed the *ampulla recti*. This portion is attached to surrounding structures by connective tissue and muscular bands (Getty 1975). Near the pelvic inlet the two muscular bands typical of the small colon fan out to form thick bundles of loosely bound smooth muscle over the ampulla recti.

The position of the peritoneal reflection over the rectum (about the level of the fourth or fifth sacral segment) is an important anatomical consideration with reference to rectal tears. There is a dorsal pararectal fossa and a ventral rectogenital pouch that extends well into the pelvic cavity; the distance between the peritoneum and anus is short. In an adult 1000-lb horse this distance is approximately 15 to 20 cm (Arnold, Meagher, and Lohse 1978). The distance will be greater in an older fat horse than in a younger thin one.

The blood supply to the terminal small colon and rectum consists of the cranial hemorrhoidal (rectal) branch of the caudal mesenteric artery and the middle and caudal hemorrhoidal branches of the internal pudendal artery. There are anastomoses between the branches.

Rectal Tears

INCIDENCE AND PATHOGENESIS

Rectal tears are a relatively common accident and are typically iatrogenic in association with rectal examination. The survival rate is low (36 per cent in one series of 42 clinical cases [Arnold, Meagher, and Lohse 1978]), and they are the most common cause of malpractice claims (Stanffer 1981).

The tears occur most commonly in the dorsal aspect of the rectum, between the positions at 10 and 12 o'clock, and are typically longitudinal. Most occur near the pelvic inlet 25 to 30 cm from the anus (i.e., peritoneal).

There is a high incidence of tears in young horses. This is considered to reflect nervousness, resentment to palpation, and increased straining before they become used to rectal examination. Some older horses may also have some predisposing weakness in the rectal wall due to degeneration in association with disease or previous rectal injury. There is an increased incidence of injuries in the Arabian breed, and this has been related to increased resistance to palpation, straining, and decreased size of the rectum and anus (Arnold, Meagher, and Lohse 1978). Stallions and geldings also sustain more rectal tears in relation to the relative infrequency of rectal palpation in males compared with mares. This can be related to the patient's unfamiliarity with the technique as well as the deeper palpation usually involved (diagnosing abdominal disorders or abdominal cryptorchidism rather than routine reproductive palpation in most mares). Most tears are associated with rectal examination, and failure of the rectal wall to relax is properly the primary etiological factor. Persistence in palpating against a taut rectal wall is the primary human error involved. Appropriate restraint and drugs should be used when necessary.

Rectal perforations may also occur from accidental entry of the stallion's penis into the rectum of the mare. They may also occur with dystocia or with forceps removal of meconium (Spiers, Christie, and Van Veenendaal 1980). Spontaneous rupture may occasionally occur in association with rectal impaction, infarction, and neoplasia (particularly melanomas) (Arnold, Meagher, and Lohse 1978).

Most tears occur near the pelvic inlet and in a dorsal longitudinal direction, and this has been related to a number of factors. This is the common site for palpation of the reproductive organs, and there is narrowing and downward deflection of the rectum-small colon in this area. The rectal wall is often stretched forward as palpation occurs, and this reduces the pliability of the wall (the latter factor can be obviated by introducing the hand cranial to the area of palpation and then retracting it). In addition it is speculated that there is predisposing wall weakness dorsally in this area lateral to the dorsal band where blood vessels penetrate the muscular layer (Arnold, Meagher, and Lohse 1978).

CLASSIFICATION OF RECTAL TEARS AND THEIR CONSEQUENCES

The consequences of a rectal tear depend on its size and position, the tissue layers penetrated, and the time between injury and the initiation of treatment. Also, cellulitis and tissue plane dissection can occur in association with straining and fecal contamination so that minor perforations may progress to more serious situations. Rectal tears have been classified according to the tissue layers penetrated at the time of injury (Arnold and Meagher 1978).

Grade 1. Tears involving the mucosa or submucosa. These will usually heal without serious complications. Occasionally, extension of involvement into deeper layers may result.

Grade 2. The muscular layers are ruptured, whereas the mucosa, submucosa, and serosa remain intact. These tears are really theoretical, but most grade 3 and 4 tears probably heal with this situation as an end result.

Grade 3. Tears that involve mucosa, submucosa, and muscular layers, including tears that extend into the mesentery (in these instances rectal contents are retained within the layers of the mesorectum). These tears are life threatening, and serious complications frequently develop. Tears into the retroperitoneal portion of the rectum have a better prognosis than tears in the peritoneal region, but cellulitis and abscessation can still develop. If abscessation is positioned near the peritoneal pouches, contamination of the peritoneal cavity can potentially occur. Dissecting abscessation or cellulitis in the retroperitoneal area can spread into the fascial planes of the thigh and cause gas gangrene. Localized abscessation can lead to fistulization, stricture formation, or diverticulum formation. A grade 3 tear in the peritoneal region can lead to acute peritonitis. This may result in diffuse peritonitis and death or localized peritonitis with abdominal abscessation or stricture and adhesion formation.

Grade 4. Tears that perforate all layers and extend into the peritoneal cavity. These produce immediate contamination and acute peritonitis. Unless there is immediate surgical treatment, endotoxic shock and death usually result.

DIAGNOSIS

The presence of fresh blood on a glove or on the feces is good evidence of a rectal tear. A sudden relaxation of the rectal wall while palpating, especially if there is concurrent straining, is another sign of a serious rupture. Often the palpator is unaware of any problem until the hand is withdrawn from the rectum and blood is observed. If none of these indicators are noted but a horse develops sweating and discomfort within two hours following rectal examination or any other rectal insult, a perforated rectum should be considered. Some horses will remain stable for longer than two hours, but systemic signs eventually develop. Sweating, pain, depression, and intestinal ileus are usual features. Signs of endotoxic shock appear at a rate that varies with the severity of the perforation. If there is any suspicion of a rectal tear, the owner should be informed and further evaluation performed.

An abdominal paracentesis is used to assess the degree of peritonitis present. Peritonitis develops quickly, and gross changes in the fluid are usually seen. Color ranges from amber through red to brown, and fibrin clots may be present. Particles of ingesta may be seen if there is gross peritoneal contamination. Serial taps are used to monitor the progression of the peritonitis. Even with incomplete tears, severe peritoneal inflammation can occur with purulent peritoneal fluid and high white cell counts. Table 15–4 illustrates the profound peritoneal reaction to a rectal tear. Although very high neutrophil counts develop, toxic changes in the neutrophils themselves are minimal. The rise and fall in protein plus cellular levels can be observed as the problem is resolved.

Manual evaluation of the rectal tear is a necessary procedure, but care is needed to avoid further damage. Epidural analgesics or irrigation of the rectum with local analgesic solution is preferred to the use of parasympatholytics to reduce straining. Pharmacological reduction in peristalsis is considered undesirable in patients in whom peritonitis and some degree of ileus are the usual features. The tear is carefully palpated using a well-lubricated surgical glove. This is the primary means by which the treatment plan is assessed. Palpation of an undermined flap is probably indicative of a grade 1 tear; however, thickening of such a flap can give the impression of a deeper tear and can cause confusion between grades 1 and 3 tears. A deep cavity with a membrane that prevents complete passage of the fingers into the rectum is indicative of a grade 3 perforation. Fecal balls are commonly retained in the cavity; they should be removed if this can be done easily. If the fingers can be passed completely through the tear, this usually signifies a grade 4 tear. An exception includes passage up into a dissected channel within the mesorectum. In grade 4 tears, one might palpate the roughened serosal surface of other viscera.

TREATMENT

Whatever grade of tear is present, if treatment is going to be attempted, immediate institution of antibiotic and

Table 15–4 SERIAL PERITONEAL FLUID SAMPLES*

Days after Tear	Color	Appearance	Total Protein	White Cell Count	Neutrophils
1	Pink/yellow	Cloudy	4.9	190,800	88% Healthy
2	Orange/yellow	Very cloudy	6.1	267,600	93% Doehle bodies
3	Yellow	Cloudy	5.8	88,800	93% Healthy
5	Yellow	Cloudy	5.3	37,000	82% Healthy
7	Yellow	Cloudy	4.4	31,000	86% Healthy
8	Yellow	Cloudy	3.9	14,800	69% Healthy

*From mare with a 12 × 4-inch incomplete rectal tear treated conservatively with peritoneal drainage.

other supportive therapy is important. Broad spectrum antibiotic therapy such as procaine penicillin (25,000 U/kg b.i.d.) and kanamycin sulfate (5 mg/kg t.i.d.) is indicated. Intravenous fluid therapy should be administered as necessary. The administration of flunixin meglumine (1 mg/kg) is also advocated for its beneficial effects in endotoxemia (Moore et al. 1981).

Other treatment principles are based on the type and extent of the tear.

Grade 1 Rectal Tears

Tears close to the anus may sometimes be sutured through the anus with epidural analgesia. Retractors or a Caslick speculum is needed, and the procedure is difficult. Synthetic absorbable suture (0 to 1) is used in a continuous pattern. Grade 1 tears that cannot be sutured easily without causing additional damage should be treated conservatively. The patient is placed on antibiotics, and mineral oil is administered to soften the feces. Pasture is preferable as a feed, otherwise alfalfa is satisfactory. Repalpation of the tear is avoided for at least a month.

Grade 3 Rectal Tears

Surgery is generally indicated for grade 3 tears if the cases are seen early enough. However, the decision to perform surgery can be difficult. The list of surgical procedures includes suturing of the tear (via laparotomy, per rectum, or utilizing prolapse of the rectum) and colostomy. However, direct suturing of the rectum is difficult and often impossible, and colostomy may result in postoperative problems. In most instances colostomy will be used if any surgery is performed. Incomplete tears do not always result in death, and in certain situations, particularly if the horse is seen some time after injury and is stable systemically, the conservative route may be chosen. If gross fecal contamination of the peritoneal cavity is evident either on clinical examination or at laparotomy, euthanasia is indicated.

SUTURING TEAR THROUGH LAPAROTOMY. This technique should only be considered if the tear is greater than 25 cm cranial to the anus and in a ventral position. If this technique is considered possible, the horse is anesthetized and placed in dorsal recumbency with the hind quarters slightly elevated to facilitate exposure of the rectum. A ventral midline approach is used, with the incision extending caudally between the mammary glands in mares. In males a paramedian incision is used and is extended caudally as far as possible (exposure is not as good in the male as in the female).

A short glass speculum is passed up by the rectum and is positioned so that the tear is over the glass tube (Arnold and Meagher 1978). This technique will facilitate visualization of the tear and its suturing. Absorbable or nonabsorbable suture material can be used, but, based on findings that there is increased collagenase activity in wounds of the distal alimentary tract, there is reasonable argument for the use of nonabsorbable or synthetic absorbable materials. A two-layer inverting closure is recommended. If possible, suturing the tear transversely rather than longitudinally can minimize any reduction in diameter of the rectal lumen. The abdomen is lavaged with sterile polyionic solution and the laparotomy incision closed.

This approach is not appropriate for dorsal tears in the area of the mesorectum. Some of these may be amenable to suturing through a rectal approach.

SUTURING TEAR THROUGH RECTUM. Laparotomy is still required for this approach. A Caslick speculum is inserted into the rectum, and an assistant intraabdominally telescopes the bowel over the speculum. When the tear is visualized, stay sutures are placed to retain the tear in position. However, mucosal folds still tend to obstruct visualization of the defect and the technique is difficult. A simple continuous suture pattern through all layers is used for convenience. Suture materials with excessive drag (synthetic absorbable materials) have disadvantages in this procedure. Although not the ideal material to use in an area of marked collagenolytic activity, catgut is easy to handle and has good knot security and may be the best choice. As much fecal material as possible should be removed from the defect before closure to minimize intramural abscess formation. A flank or ventral midline approach can be used for suturing a tear through the rectum. Although difficult, this technique has been successful in a number of cases (Arnold and Meagher 1978) and obviates the possible sequelae of a colostomy. If suturing is not successful with this approach, the surgeon may proceed with a colostomy.

SUTURING TEAR UTILIZING PROLAPSE OF THE RECTUM. The successful use of this technique has been reported in one experimental animal (Arnold and Meagher 1978). The distal small colon is intussuscepted into itself and the bowel exteriorized out the anus, which allows visualization of the tear from the mucosal side. An assistant, working intraabdominally, initiates the intussusception by pushing the sponge into the surgeon's fingers that are within the rectum, allowing the surgeon to retract the bowel.

The usefulness of the technique in clinical cases has yet to be established. It may only be appropriate in young thin horses. There is usually considerable fat in the mesentery and retroperitoneum, which may preclude the induction of the prolapse. Prolonged exteriorization of the bowel under tension could also cause tearing or thrombosis of the mesenteric vessels. The technique would also not be appropriate on a tear of any duration because of edema and thickening in the area.

PULL-THROUGH PROCEDURE. The use of a pull-through operation on the colon after resection of the rectum has been attempted in two instances but was unsuccessful (Spiers, Christie, and Van Veenendaal 1980). Even if the technique were technically feasible, problems are anticipated because of the tension and displacement in the mesocolon with consequent infarction. The use of colostomy is preferred.

COLOSTOMY. Temporary colostomy is used to divert fecal material from the rectal tear until it is healed sufficiently for normal continuity of the bowel to be re-established. The technique has been used with moderate success in most reports (Azzie 1975; Herthel 1975; Spiers, Christie, and Van Veenendaal 1980; Stashak and Knight 1978). The procedure does have complications and may indeed cause the demise of the patient. Comparisons of success rates between conservative treatment and colostomy are invalid because the severity of the tears in the two groups is quite different. For severe rectal tears, colostomy is the only technique that offers a chance of survival. In addition, with experience, the technique has been improved to help obviate some of the complications (Shires 1981). If the tear cannot be directly sutured or if suturing is feasible but there is devitalization of the wound edges, colostomy is indicated.

Both end colostomies (transection of the small colon with closure of the distal segment) (Herthel 1975; Stashak and Knight 1978) and loop colostomies (continuity of colon maintained with diversion through a stoma on the antimesenteric aspect of the small colon) (Azzie 1975; Shires 1981; Spiers, Christie, and Van Veenendaal 1980) have been used. End colostomy has been proposed as the better technique in that it ensures complete diversion of feces from the distal colon (Stashak and Knight 1978). However, marked atrophy of the distal segment occurs, requiring special techniques for reanastomosis. Shortening of the distal segment can also make reanastomosis difficult. The loop colostomy retains the distal segment at the colostomy site, and size and partial function can be retained. At the same time, the colostomy effectively diverts fecal material from the distal segment. Both creation of the colostomy and its later closure can be conveniently performed through a flank incision (Shires 1981).

Lower flank (Herthel 1975; Stashak and Knight 1978) and ventral abdominal sites (Azzie 1975; Spiers, Christie, and Van Veenendaal 1980) have been used. Herniation or intussusception of the small colon out through the colostomy is a well-recognized problem, and it is possible that its occurrence is more likely with a ventrally located colostomy. A ventrally located colostomy can also cause problems in closing the abdominal wall defect when colon continuity is reestablished. Finally, the tight fascial bands ventrally can potentially cause problems with stricture of the colostomy.

A loop colostomy in the left flank region (Shires 1981) can obviate some of these problems and has some other advantages. The procedure can be performed in the standing animal (the pain associated with peritonitis may preclude this [Herthel 1975]). This eliminates the insult of general anesthesia on a toxic patient and allows placement of the colostomy with the tissue layers in normal position. Closure of the colostomy is similarly convenient.

A left flank incision is made with the standing patient under mild sedation using a local analgesic block (line block or inverted "L" block). A vertical incision is made through skin, subcutaneous tissue, and external abdominal oblique muscle (primarily fascia in this location). The internal abdominal oblique and transversus abdominis muscles are divided in the direction of their fibers. The retroperitoneal fat and peritoneum are divided and the laceration manually examined. A loop of small colon immediately cranial to the tear is exteriorized and placed vertically in the ventral aspect of the incision with the antimesen-

teric band lateral (Fig. 15–177A). The dorsal part of the incision in the external abdominal oblique fascia that does not enclose the loop of colon is sutured using simple interrupted sutures of 1 polyglactin 910 (Vicryl). The loop of small colon is then sutured to the edges of the external abdominal oblique fascia using 0 polyglactin material in a simple interrupted or continuous pattern (Fig. 15–177B). These sutures do not penetrate the lumen of the colon. The subcutaneous tissue and skin dorsal to the loop of colon are then closed. A 10-cm incision is made into the lumen along the antimesenteric band and the mucosa sutured to the skin incision using nonabsorbable suture material. Simple interrupted sutures or mattress sutures between skin edge and mucosa can be used (Fig. 15–177C).

Vaseline is applied ventral to the colostomy to prevent scalding. The rectum and distal segment of small colon are flushed daily with dilute povidone-iodine solution to help keep the distal segment clean as well as functional (this procedure is not essential). Broad spectrum systemic antibiotics are also used, the horse is maintained on a laxative diet, and the colostomy site is kept clean.

Possible complications include detachment, prolapse, herniation, retraction, and stenosis (Herthel 1975). Although the use of retention sutures has been proposed to prevent prolapse of the small colon through the incision (Azzie 1975), there is an accompanying risk of the sutures causing obstruction of the colostomy. The colostomy should be regularly monitored so that any problem is observed early. A two-week healing time is sufficient for many tears (Shires 1981), and early closure of the colostomy obviates some of the complications.

The use of general anesthesia may be preferred for closure of the colostomy. Separation of the colonic loop and closure of the stoma in the colon have been described (Shires 1981). In some instances (if the colostomy site is traumatized), resection and anastomosis of the colon may be preferred to eliminate any deformities. An end-to-end anastomosis using a simple crushing or Gambee pattern can be used. It is possible to exteriorize the colon sufficiently through the flank incision to perform the anastomo-

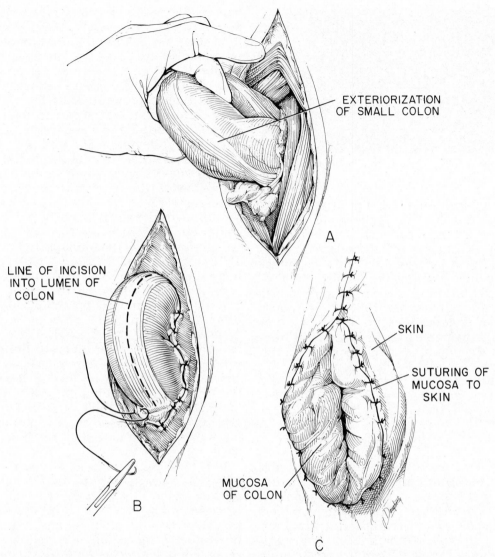

EXTERIORIZATION
OF SMALL COLON

A

LINE OF INCISION
INTO LUMEN OF
COLON

B

SKIN

SUTURING OF
MUCOSA TO
SKIN

MUCOSA
OF COLON

C

Figure 15–177 Technique of loop colostomy in the left flank region. *A*, Exteriorization of a loop of small colon through flank laparotomy incision. *B*, Positioning of colon in flank incision and suturing it to the edges of the external abdominal oblique fascia. The position of the incision into the colon is marked by the dotted line. *C*, Mucosa has been incised and its edges sutured to the skin. The subcutaneous tissue and skin have been closed dorsally.

sis. The muscle layers in the flank are closed. The defect in the external abdominal oblique fascia and skin may preclude a complete primary closure. Normal diet can be resumed gradually over the following two weeks.

Grade 4 Rectal Tears

Surgical intervention (colostomy) for grade 4 tears is indicated if the tear is small and treatment is instituted early enough before gross contamination of the peritoneal cavity has occurred. Euthanasia is commonly indicated.

Rectal Prolapse

CLASSIFICATION

Rectal prolapses may be classified into four categories: (1) mucosal prolapse; (2) complete prolapse; (3) complete prolapse with invagination of the colon; and (4) intussusception of the peritoneal rectum or colon through the anus (Turner and Fessler 1980). Either of the first two is usual. These conditions are differentiated by palpation. Mucosal prolapse usually presents as a circular swelling at the anus resulting from the submucosa

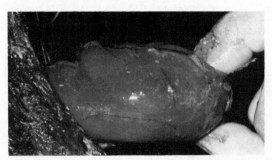

Figure 15–178 Complete rectal prolapse in a foal.

and mucous membrane protruding caudally. A complete prolapse is usually larger and more cylindrical and involves all or a portion of the ampulla recti (Fig. 15–178). If invagination of the colon accompanies a complete prolapse, the prolapsed portion will be firmer and thicker (Turner and Fessler 1980). The fourth type of prolapse presents as a protrusion with a palpable trench within the rectum, the depth of which depends on the length of the intussusception.

With all types of rectal prolapse, the exposed mucosa can become inflamed, desiccated, traumatized, or necrotic.

PATHOGENESIS

A rectal prolapse can be caused by any condition that causes tenesmus including constipation, diarrhea, enteritis, proctitis, intestinal parasitism, rectal foreign body, dystocia, urethral obstruction, colic, or local irritation from *Gastrophilus* larvae. Foals with diarrhea probably represent the most common situation. Although predisposing factors, including loss of anal sphincter tone, loose attachments of the rectum to the muscular coat of the rectum, and loose attachments of the rectum to perirectal tissues, have been cited, such conditions have not been actually demonstrated.

TREATMENT

If a prolapse is encountered, early conservative treatment may be used. This may include epidural anesthesia to prevent further straining, manual reduction of the prolapse, and the use of a purse-string suture in the anus to maintain retention. If changes in the mucosa are minimal and the cause of the prolapse can be alleviated, this conservative therapy may be successful. However, horses tend to strain against the anal irritation produced by the purse-string suture, and equine feces are formed and dry and do not pass through a restricted anus easily. In addition, reprolapse after the purse-string suture is removed can occur (Levine 1978; Turner and Fessler 1980). For permanent alleviation of a prolapse, surgical intervention is recommended; if tissues are devitalized or if the animal continues to strain, such intervention is necessary.

Submucosal resection is the surgical treatment of choice for the first three categories of rectal prolapse (Levine 1978; Turner and Fessler 1980). This technique has several advantages over complete amputation: (1) the adventitia is not exposed and the possibility of peritonitis or pararectal abscess is decreased; (2) the rectal arteries are not involved; (3) postoperative straining is reduced; (4) the rectal lumen is less constricted; (5) there is no loss of healthy tissue; and (6) healing is more rapid (Johnson 1943). Viability of the serosal and adventitial tissue is not usually a problem, and amputation is unnecessary.

In some type 3 prolapses, a laparotomy may also be necessary to reduce the intussusception. The fourth type of prolapse involving small colon intussusception is a special problem and requires laparotomy. Infarction may follow correction of the intussusception with resection and anastomosis because of vascular compromise due to excessive tension on the mesocolon. The possibility of such compromise increases with the length of the intussusception. The use of colostomy may be a feasible approach in some cases (Turner and Fessler 1980).

Submucosal Resection. The tail is wrapped and the hair around the anus clipped. The area is aseptically prepared. Epidural anesthesia is used unless the animal's disposition suggests using general anesthesia. Two 18-gauge, 6-in. needles are placed through the anal sphincter and rectal tissue to maintain the prolapse while dissection is performed (Fig. 15–179A). Circumferential incisions are made through the mucosa at the junction of healthy and nonviable

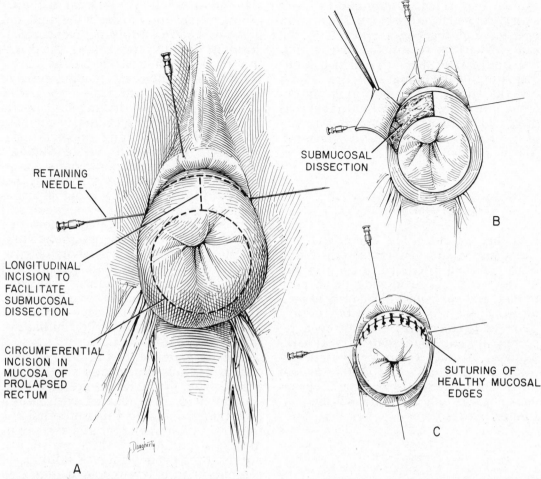

Figure 15–179 Submucosal resection for treatment of a prolapsed rectum. *A*, Needles placed in prolapse and incision lines demarcated. *B*, Elevation of mucosa to be removed. *C*, Suturing of healthy mucosal edges.

mucosa at both the reflection of the prolapse and the apex. A longitudinal incision is also made to facilitate the submucosal dissection. Excessive hemorrhage is controlled with ligation or electrocautery. The mucosa is dissected free by following the cleavage plane in the submucosa (Fig. 15–179B). After dissection is complete the healthy mucosal edges are apposed using simple interrupted sutures of 2 catgut or 2/0 synthetic absorbable suture (Fig. 15–179C). A submucosal layer of sutures is optional. The transfixion needles are then removed and the prolapse stump manually replaced. Whether a purse-string suture is maintained postoperatively depends on the individual (not used by the author). Antibiotics are used, and mineral oil is administered.

Strangulation of the Rectum

One case of strangulation of the rectum by a pedunculated lipoma has been reported (Mason 1978). The animal presented with colic, and constriction of the rectum was diagnosed clinically. The mare was operated on under epidural analgesia and the constricting lipoma removed through an incision in the dorsolateral aspect of the vagina (Mason 1978).

Atresia Ani and Atresia Recti

Atresia ani is rare in the foal. Straining at defecation is the presenting sign, and the condition is easily diagnosed by physical examination. Surgical treatment can be performed. A circular piece of skin is excised over the bulge, the rectum opened, and the edges sutured to the skin. When the rectum is absent, outward bulging of the skin can still occur owing to the abdominal pressure.

If the end of the colon cannot be located in the pelvic cavity, euthanasia is indicated. If there is only partial atresia of the rectum, anastomosis to the exterior may be possible.

MISCELLANEOUS CONDITIONS OF THE ABDOMINAL CAVITY

In this section, a few conditions that can cause acute abdominal crises and have not been discussed previously will be reviewed. These include ileus, peritonitis, and splenomegaly. Surgical conditions of the accessory digestive organs (liver and pancreas) have not been reported, although pancreatitis is often diagnosed (usually as an incidental finding) at necropsy. Hepatitis is an important medical disease, and liver biopsy is often indicated and will be considered here.

Ileus

Ileus can be defined as a functional intestinal obstruction in which there is ineffective or absent peristaltic activity and intestinal tone. It may present as the primary cause of an acute abdominal crisis or it may follow medication (atropine sulfate is the best example) but is most commonly observed as a complication of abdominal surgery or concurrent with peritonitis.

Patients may have signs typical of an acute abdomen. There is gastric reflux of fluid on stomach tubing, intestinal motility is markedly reduced or absent, and distended loops of the small intestine can be palpated on rectal examination. The presence and degree of peritonitis can also be assessed with clinical examination and clinocopathological tests. The important feature to note when assessing a case of ileus is whether an actual anatomical obstruction is present.

The treatment of ileus initially is conservative. The presence of bowel disten-

sion promotes ileus. Regular stomach tubing is necessary to drain the fluid and prevent gastric rupture. Nonsurgical drainage of fluid farther down the digestive tract is not possible in the horse. Walking may help by causing passive motion to the inert intestines. The use of analgesics is often indicated. Various drugs have been advocated to promote gut motility including dexpanthenol (Panacol), neostigmine sulfate (Stiglyn), and even the cholinergic agents carbamylcholine chloride and bethanechol (McIlwraith 1979). The exact pharmacological events leading to ileus are still controversial. In man, attention has been drawn to excess sympathetic stimulation caused by hyperactivity of sympathetic nerve endings in the gut and high levels of circulating catecholamines. The use of the sympatholytic drug phentolamine has been advocated (Neeley and Catchpole 1971) but has not been evaluated in the horse.

If ileus is refractory to conservative treatment, laparotomy and surgical decompression of the bowel are indicated. Gas and fluid are evacuated, with careful attention given to inflicting minimal further trauma to the bowel and exacerbating the condition. Needles and suction are used for evacuating gas. Milking of contents with enterotomies as indicated is used for fluid removal.

Prevention of ileus is based on fast, effective, and atraumatic abdominal surgery and selection of medications that do not decrease intestinal motility or cause irritation to the peritoneal surface.

Peritonitis

Peritonitis is an inflammation of the parietal and visceral peritoneum that causes ileus, severe abdominal pain, and hypovolemic and endotoxic shock. Its inclusion in this text as a surgical disease pertains to its potential importance in the postoperative abdominal patient and the role of surgical intervention in the treatment of some cases.

ETIOLOGY AND PATHOGENESIS

Etiological factors include external penetrating wounds to the abdominal wall, iatrogenic trauma (liver biopsy can cause hemorrhage or bile leakage, and blind installation of abdominal drains has caused colonic perforation [Vaughan 1980]), bowel rupture, and transmural passage of bacteria across ischemic or devitalized bowel wall. Migrating *Strongylus* larvae can cause a chronic low-grade peritonitis. Peritonitis is most commonly found as a complication of surgery and may be associated with poor technique (contamination, excess trauma, introduction of irritant materials into peritoneal cavity) or uncontrolled sepsis (virulent organism, insensitivity to treatment regimen, continued bowel devitalization). Abdominal abscesses in the horse represent a special entity in which the infection is believed to usually arise from previous respiratory infection and specific pathogens are involved (Rumbaugh, Smith, and Carlson 1978).

Note should be made that, following abdominal surgery, peritonitis per se regularly occurs because inflammation is present, but this "normal" peritoneal inflammation usually resolves spontaneously. Clinical peritonitis in the horse normally refers to clinically significant peritoneal inflammation of bacterial etiology that causes serious clinical disease.

The infections are typically considered to be multimicrobial, with both aerobes and anaerobes of significance. There are limited data in the horse, but cecal samples have been taken in experimentally induced colic. Average bacterial levels increased, and alpha staphylococci, streptococci, and anaerobes were particularly prominent (Linerode and Goode 1971). Studies are needed to recognize the relative role of different bacteria in clinical peritonitis. Anaerobic isolation techniques have been performed infrequently in the past. Synergistic bacterial mechanisms have been recognized as important in the pathogenesis of human peritonitis, and different organisms may account for different types or stages of disease. In experimental studies, for instance, it has been shown that coliforms such as *E. coli* and *Proteus* may account for early death in acute bacterial peritonitis but that an important later stage, characterized by persistent intra-abdominal abscesses, is associated with anaerobic infection (Weinstein et al. 1975).

PATHOPHYSIOLOGY

The peritoneum typically reacts to insult with an inflammatory reaction characterized by hyperemia, edema, and peritoneal effusion. There are chemotactic phagocytosis and suppuration in response to bacterial infection. A fibrin deposit soon forms on the peritoneal surface. The inflamed peritoneum is more permeable, and extensive absorption of toxins is possible.

The extent of this reaction depends on the nature of the infection, the degree of contamination, and the effectiveness of treatment. If not controlled quickly there is considerable loss of fluid and electrolytes into the third space (this consists of three compartments including peritoneal cavity, extraperitoneal tissues [mainly edema], and the intestinal lumen). Both hypovolemic and endotoxic components are significant in the shock that ensues.

DIAGNOSIS

Peritonitis in the horse manifests as an ileus with superimposed signs of systemic illness and shock. As with ileus, there are abdominal pain, loss of motility, distended intestines on rectal examination, and gastric reflux. Diarrhea can sometimes occur. Parietal pain rather than visceral pain may be more prominent. The horse will be febrile and depressed, with varying degrees of circulating deficits manifested as a fast weak pulse, poor peripheral perfusion, and hemoconcentration. Protein loss may be evidenced by decreased total plasma protein despite a persistently high or increasing PCV. Leukopenia commonly occurs.

Paracentesis is used to obtain a definitive diagnosis. There will be a marked increase in the leukocytes (normal $<9000/mm^3$), with an increase in the proportion of neutrophils (Bach and Ricketts 1974). The protein will be typically greater than 2.5 mg/dl. Cytological examination may reveal degenerate changes in the neutrophils including nuclear hypersegmentation, pyknosis or karyolysis, cytoplasmic vacuolation, and basophilia (Adams, Fessler, and Rebar 1980). Extracellular bacteria may be observed. Samples should be cultured (aerobically and anaerobically) to identify both the bacteria and its antibiotic sensitivity.

TREATMENT

The choice of antibiotics is difficult, and theoretical considerations and actual clinical results are often at variance. Potent broad spectrum therapy is the rule in man. In one report there was progression from penicillin and chloramphenicol to cephalothin and kanamycin and then, more recently, cephalothin-gentamicin-clindamycin. Objections to the use of such heavy artillery in horses include expense and the risk of promoting bacterial resistance problems and consequent nosocomial infections. Regimens that are useful in the horse include penicillin (22,000 IU/kg b.i.d.) and kanamycin (5 gm/kg t.i.d.) in combination and sodium ampicillin (11 mg/kg q.i.d.). Although chloramphenicol is supposedly more effective than penicillin and kanamycin for anaerobes, it seems to be of questionable value in the horse (McIlwraith 1979). In man, the antibiotics that are generally used in the treatment of equine peritonitis, i.e., penicillin and aminogylcosides, are ineffective against anaerobes (Lorber and Swenson 1975). Anaerobic infection is present in the majority of cases of human peritonitis, and specific attention is critical (Lorber and Swenson 1975); however, routine anaerobic culture is needed in equine peritonitis to identify the relative importance of anaerobic infection. Prolonged treatment with penicillin alone is appropriate for intra-abdominal abscesses (Rumbaugh, Smith, and Carlson 1978). In another clinical report in man, aerobic gram-positive and gram-negative organisms were considered as the important pathogens, and the authors reported good results with penicillin or ampicillin combined with an aminoglycoside (Gerding, Hall, and Schierl 1977).

Surgical management of peritonitis in the horse has been generally restricted to drainage and lavage. Although the use of drainage of inflammatory fluid is log-ical, the question of how effectively the peritoneal cavity can be drained is uncertain. However, with acute peritonitis drainage is recommended and the use of a sump drain is advocated (Fig. 15–180). The adjunctive use of peritoneal lavage may be worthwhile when an animal does not respond quickly to antibiotic therapy and drainage, but its use should be qualified. Ingress and egress through a ventral drain (Valdez, Scrutchfield, and Taylor 1979) is of questionable usefulness. The fluid should be instilled through the flank, but it is still not known how effectively this technique lavages the entire abdomen. In addition, lavage may induce severe hypoproteinemia in the patient. Lavage should be performed with sterile polyionic fluids. Although the use of dilute povidone-iodine has been recommended (Valdez, Scrutchfield, and Taylor 1979), there is research to indicate that this agent has a deleterious rather than a beneficial effect in peritonitis (Lagarde, Bolton, and Cohn 1978; Lores, Ortiz, and Rossello 1981). Until this is clarified, the use of sterile solutions along with systemic antibiotics is recommended. The additional use of heparin (100 U/kg intraperitoneally or subcutaneously) has been recommended to prevent the apposition of fibrin and render the bacteria more susceptible to cellular and noncellular cleaning mechanisms (Hau and Simmons 1978). Subsequent work showed that whereas a dose rate of 250 U/kg intraperitoneally increased survival and decreased adhesions and abscesses in experimental per-

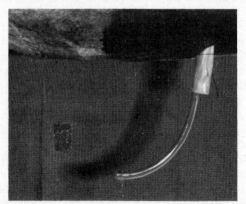

Figure 15–180 Sump drainage of the abdomen in the treatment of peritonitis. To make the drain, a Penrose drain is placed outside a fenestrated tube drain.

itonitis in rabbits, a dose rate of 150 U/kg was not effective (Davidson, Cardenas, and Busuttil 1981).

Radical surgical debridement has been proposed as the most consistently successful procedure in the treatment of advanced generalized bacterial peritonitis in man (Hudspeth 1975). It is proposed to prevent residual abscess formation and allow the peritoneum to clear infection by breaking down inflammatory adhesions, removing necrotic tissue, eliminating any possible anaerobic condition, and reducing the bacterial count to a minimum. This method of treatment is not considered a practical alternative in the horse; at present the use of lavage seems our only method of debriding the peritoneum. The usefulness of low-frequency sound therapy to induce micromotion of the abdominal organs and limit adhesion formation has been recently documented in rats (Colasante et al. 1981).

Inadequacies of current treatments are reflected in continued deaths from generalized peritonitis in horses. In one report of five operative cases of peritonitis the survival rate was zero (Sembrat 1975). In addition, apparently successful management of acute peritonitis can still result in a problem of generalized and untreatable adhesions at a later time (Fig. 15–181).

Splenomegaly

Although the spleen is not a digestive organ, its close anatomical relationship with the stomach and the potential for splenomegaly to produce recurrent colic (Varra and Nelson 1976) warrant its consideration in this section.

Primary splenomegaly due to hyperactivity or congestion is rare in the horse but has been reported (Varra and Nelson 1976). Clinical features include a history of recurrent colic, low PCV, and rectal palpation of an enlarged spleen. Splenectomy through a left lateral approach (removing the seventeenth rib and displacing the sixteenth and eighteenth ribs) was successfully performed (Varra and Nelson 1976). The enlarged spleen had displaced the left kidney owing to tension on the nephrosplenic ligament. The nephrosplenic ligament was incised and the splenic and gastrosplenic vessels ligated and transected as the spleen was removed.

Splenomegaly in association with infarction of the spleen has been reported (Scott, Trapp, and Derksen 1978). This case was treated medically and the horse died three weeks after presenting with acute clinical signs of depression, fever, anemia, a PCV of 10, bloody paracentesis, and splenomegaly (on rectal examination).

Splenic rupture also occurs in the horse but is rapidly fatal. Patients can be anticipated to present dead or in hemorrhagic shock. The problem appears unassociated with trauma, and the cause is undefined (Steiner 1981).

Liver Biopsy

This diagnostic test is the only surgical procedure performed on the equine liver.

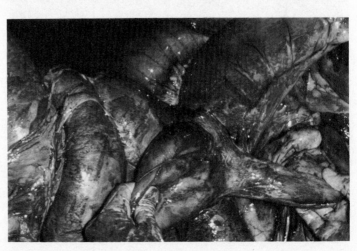

Figure 15–181 Severe adhesions in an abdomen following apparently successful treatment of peritonitis some time previously.

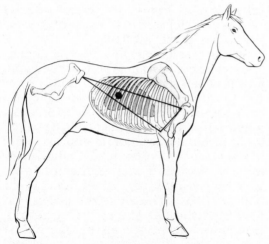

Figure 15–182 Diagram to demonstrate the site of liver biopsy in the horse.

Histological examination of the biopsy specimen can potentially provide the specificity in the diagnosis of hepatic disease that is not possible with clinical and biochemical tests alone (Tennant, Evans, and Schwartz 1973).

The biopsy is performed in the twelfth or thirteenth intercostal space on the right side. The site is determined by drawing an imaginary line from the tuber coxa to the point of the olecranon (Fig. 15–182). Following aseptic preparation, a stab incision is made in the intercostal space and the biopsy needle inserted. When the needle penetrates the diaphragm, it will move backward and forward as the horse breathes. The needle is then advanced into the liver and the biopsy taken.

The technique is considered safe. Post-biopsy hemorrhage has been reported in 1 of 27 cases in one report (Tennant, Evans, and Schwartz 1973). Delayed coagulation is a contraindication for the technique. The correlation between the biopsy findings and later necropsy findings has been reported as excellent (Tennant, Evans, and Schwartz 1973).

Pancreatitis

The importance of pancreatitis as a cause of acute abdominal disease in the horse is poorly defined. However, it does exist as a differential diagnosis in the acute abdomen (Baker 1978). Diagnosis is based on the measurement of serum and peritoneal fluid amylase levels. If diagnosed, the treatment is medical. Surgical disease of the pancreas is an unknown and unexplored entity.

Cholelithiasis

Cholelithiasis is an uncommon occurrence in the horse but should be considered as a differential diagnosis in some colic cases (Fig. 15–183). Typically, there will be signs of abdominal pain but gut motility and fecal passage continue. Elevated alkaline phosphatase and direct bilirubin levels can be useful diag-

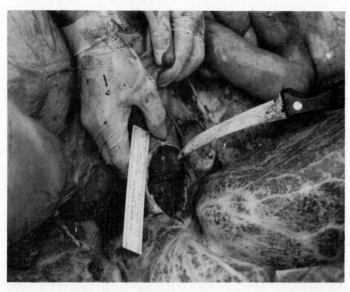

Figure 15–183 Necropsy specimen of choleliths in the common bile duct.

nostic parameters. At this stage the condition cannot be considered as a surgical one owing to diffuse cholelithiasis of the biliary tree and associated hepatic fibrosis.

REFERENCES

Aanes, W. A.: The diagnosis and surgical repair of diverticulum of the esophagus. Proceedings of the American Association of Equine Practitioners:211, 1975.

Adams, S. B.: Unpublished data, 1979.

Adams, S. B., and Becht, J. L.: Surgical repair of a severe laceration in a horse's tongue. VM/SAC 73:1394, 1978.

Adams, S. B., Fessler, J. F., and Rebar, A. H.: Cytologic interpretation of peritoneal fluid in the evaluation of abdominal crises. Cornell Vet. 70:232, 1980.

Adams, S. B., and McIlwraith, C. W.: Abdominal crisis in the horse: a comparison of presurgical evaluation with surgical findings and results. Vet. Surg. 7:63, 1978.

Alexander, F., and Hickson, J. C. D.: The salivary and pancreatic secretions of the horse. In Physiology of Digestion and Metabolism in the Ruminant. Phillipson, A. T. (ed.). England: Oriel Press, 1970, p. 375.

Alexander, J, E.: Radiologic findings in equine choke. JAVMA 151:47, 1967.

Allison, C. J.: Invagination of the caecum into the colon in a Welsh pony. Equine Vet. J. 9:84, 1977.

Argenzio, R. A.: Comparative physiology of the gastrointestinal system. In Veterinary Gastroenterology. Anderson, N. V. (ed.). Philadelphia: Lea & Febiger, 1980, pp. 172–198.

Argenzio, R. A.: Functions of the equine large intestine and their interrelationship in disease. Cornell Vet. 65:303, 1975.

Argenzio, R. A., Lowe, J. E., Pickard, D. W., et al.: Digesta passage and water exchange in the equine large intestine. Am. J. Physiol. 226:1035, 1974.

Arnold, J. S., and Meagher, D. M.: Management of rectal tears in the horse. J. Equine Med. Surg. 2:64, 1978.

Arnold, J. S., Meagher, D. M., and Lohse, C. L.: Rectal tears in the horse. J. Equine Med. Surg. 2:55, 1978.

Azzie, M. A. J.: Temporary colostomy in the management of rectal tears in the horse. J. S. Afr. Vet. Assoc. 46:121, 1975.

Bach, L. G., and Ricketts, S. W.: Paracentesis as an aid to the diagnosis of abdominal disease in the horse. Equine Vet. J. 6:116, 1974.

Baker, G. J.: Surgery of the head and neck. In Equine Medicine and Surgery, 2nd ed. Catcott, E. J., and Smithcors, J. F. (eds.). Wheaton, IL: American Veterinary Publications, Inc., 1972. pp. 752–791.

Baker, G. J.: Some aspects of equine dental radiology. Equine Vet. J. 3:46, 1971.

Baker, G. J.: Some aspects of equine dental disease. Equine Vet. J. 2:105, 1970.

Baker, R. H.: Acute necrotizing pancreatitis in a horse. JAVMA 172:268, 1978.

Barclay, W. P., Foerner, J. J., and Phillips, T. N.: Volvulus of the large colon in the horse. JAVMA 177:629, 1980.

Barclay, W. P., Phillips, J. N., and Foerner, J. J.: Intussusception associated with Anoplocephala perfoliata in 5 horses. JAVMA 180:752, 1982.

Barth, A. D., Barber, S. M., and McKenzie, N. T.: Pyloric stenosis in a foal. Can. Vet. J. 21:234, 1980.

Batstone, J. H. F.: Cleft palate in the horse. Br. J. Plast. Surg. 19:327, 1966.

Becht, J. L., and McIlwraith, C. W.: Jejunal displacement through the mesometrium in a pregnant mare. JAVMA 177:435, 1980.

Bennett, A., Eley, K. G., and Scholes, G. B.: Effects of prostaglandin E1 and E2 on intestinal motility in the guinea pig and rat. Br. J. Pharmacol. 34:638, 1968.

Bennett, D. G.: Predisposition to abdominal crisis in the horse. JAVMA 161:1189, 1972.

Berg, J. N., Nausley, C. A., and Riegle, L.: Heat extraction of animal plasma in preparation for endotoxin testing with the limulus amebocyte lysate test. Am. J. Vet. Res. 40:1048, 1979.

Blue, M. G.: Enteroliths in horses—a retrospective study of 30 cases. Equine Vet. J. 111:76, 1979.

Blue, M. G., and Wittkopp, R. W.: Clinical and structural features of equine enteroliths. JAVMA 179:79, 1981.

Boles, C. L., and Kohn, C. W.: Fibrous foreign body impaction colic in young horses. JAVMA 179:193, 1981.

Bowman, K. F., Tate, L. P., Evans, L. H., and Donawick, W. J.: Complications of cleft palate repair in large animals. JAVMA 180:652, 1982.

Bowman, K. F., Vaughan, J. T., Quick, C. B., et al.: Megaesophagus in a colt. JAVMA 172:334, 1978.

Burrows, G. E.: Endotoxemia in the horse. Equine Vet. J. 13:89, 1981.

Burrows, G. E., and Cannon, J.: Endotoxemia induced by rapid intravenous injection of Escherichia coli in anesthetized ponies. Am. J. Vet. Res. 31:1967, 1968.

Bury, K. D., McClure, R. L., and Wright, H. K.: Reversal of colonic net absorption to net secretion with increased intraluminal pressure. Arch. Surg. 108:854, 1974.

Cannon, J. H., Grant, B. D., and Sande, R. D.: Diagnosis and surgical treatment of cyst-like lesions of the equine paranasal sinuses. JAVMA 169:610, 1976.

Clayton-Jones, D. G.: Gastric impaction in a pony: relief via laparotomy. Equine Vet. J. 4:98, 1972.

Coffman, J. R.: Diagnosis of disease of the teeth and sinuses of the horse. VM/SAC 64:497, 1969.

Colasante, D. A., Au, F. C., Sell, H. W., et al.: Prophylaxis of adhesions with low frequency sound. Surg. Gynecol. Obstet. 153:357, 1981.

Cowles, R. R., Jr., Bunch, S. E., and Flynn, D. V.: Cecal inversion in a horse. VM/SAC 72:1346, 1977.

Crowhurst, R. C.: Abdominal surgery in the foal. Equine Vet, J. 2:22, 1970.

Crowhurst, R. C., Simpson, D. J., McEnery, R. J., et al.: Intestinal surgery in the foal. J. S. Afr. Vet. Assoc. 46:59, 1975.

Datt, S. C., and Usenik, E. A.: Intestinal obstruction in the horse. Physical signs and blood chemistry. Cornell Vet. 65:152, 1975.

Davidson, R. K., Cardenas, A., and Busuttil, R. W.: The effects of heparin and low molecular weight dextran on survival after fibrinopurulent peritonitis. Surg. Gynecol. Obstet. 153:327, 1981.

DeBoom, H. P. A.: Functional anatomy and nervous control of the equine alimentary tract. J. S. Afr. Vet. Assoc. 46:5, 1975.

DeGroot, A.: The significance of low packed cell volume in relation to the early diagnosis of intestinal obstruction in the horse, based on field observations. Proceedings of the American Association of Equine Practitioners:309, 1971.

DeMoor, A., Wouters, L., Mouens, Y., et al.: Surgical treatment of a traumatic oesophageal rupture in a foal. Equine Vet. J. 11:265, 1979.

Derksen, F. J., and Robinson, N. E.: Esophageal and intrapleural pressures in the healthy conscious pony. Am. J. Vet. Res. 41:1756, 1980.

Donawick, W. J.: Techniques in equine gastrointestinal surgery. Paper presented at the 8th Annual Veterinary Surgical Forum, Chicago, 1980.

Donawick, W. J., Christie, B. A., and Stewart, J. V.: Resection of the diseased ileum in the horse. JAVMA 159:1146, 1971.

Drudge, J. H.: Clinical aspects of Strongylus vulgaris infection in the horse. Emphasis on diagnosis, chemotherapy, and prophylaxis. Vet. Clin. North Am. Large Anim. Pract. 1:251, 1979.

Evans, L.: Personal communication, 1981 (cited by J. Foerner).

Ferraro, G. L., Evans, D. R., Trunk, D. A., et al.: Medical and surgical management of enteroliths in equidae. JAVMA 162:208, 1973.

Firth, E. C.: Diaphragmatic hernia in horses. Cornell Vet. 66:353, 1976.

Fletcher, J. R., Ramwell, P. W., and Herman, C. M.: Prostaglandins and the hemodynamic course of endotoxic shock. J. Surg. Res. 20:589, 1976.

Foerner, J. J.: Differential diagnosis and surgical management of diseases of the large intestine. Vet. Clin. North Am. Large Anim. Pract. 4:129, 1982.

Foerner, J. J., Phillips, T. N., and Barclay, W. P.: Surgical diseases of the large intestine. Proceedings of the American Association of Equine Practitioners:231, 1981.

Frank, E. R.: Veterinary Surgery, 7th ed. Minneapolis: Burgess Publishing Company, 1964.

Freeman, D. E., Koch, D. B., and Boles, C. L.: Mesodiverticular bands as a cause of small intestinal strangulation and volvulus in the horse. JAVMA 175:1089, 1979.

Freeman, D. E., and Naylor, J. N.: Cervical esophagostomy to permit extraoral feeding of the horse. JAVMA 172:314, 1978.

Fretz, P. B.: Repair of esophageal stricture in a horse. Mod. Vet. Pract. 53:31, 1972.

Gabel, A. A.: A method of surgical repair of the fractured mandible in the horse. JAVMA 155:1831, 1969.

Gay, C. C., Spiers, V. C., and Christie, B. A.: Foreign body obstruction of the small colon in six horses. Equine Vet. J. 11:60, 1979.

Georgi, J. R.: The Kikuchi-Enigk model of Strongylus vulgaris migrations in the horse. Cornell Vet. 63:220, 1973.

Gerding, D. N., Hall, W. H., and Schierl, E. A.: Antibiotic concentrations in ascitic fluid of patients with ascites and bacterial peritonitis. Ann. Intern. Med. 86:708, 1977.

Getty, R.: Sisson and Grossman's The Anatomy of the Domestic Animals, 5th ed. Philadelphia: W. B. Saunders, 1975.

Gideon, L.: Surgery of the esophagus. Paper presented at A.C.V.S., Surgical Forum Chicago, 1979.

Grant, B. D., and Tennant, B.: Volvulus associated with Meckel's diverticulum in the horse. JAVMA 162:550, 1973.

Greatorex, J. C.: Diagnosis and treatment of "verminous aneurysm" formation in the horse. Vet. Rec. 101:184, 1977.

Gruber, J., and Langner, P.: Trocarization of the horse. JAVMA 159:1036, 1971.

Hackett, R. P., Dyer, R. M., and Hoffer, R. E.: Surgical correction of esophageal diverticulum in a horse. JAVMA 173:998, 1978.

Hau, T., and Simmons, R. L.: Heparin in the treatment of experimental peritonitis. Ann. Surg. 187:294, 1978.

Haynes, P. F., and Qualls, C. W., Jr.: Cleft soft palate, nasal septum deviation, and epiglottic entrapment in a Thoroughbred filly. JAVMA 179:910, 1981.

Herthel, D. J.: Colostomy in the mare. Proceedings of the American Association of Equine Practitioners:187, 1975.

Hilbert, B. J., Jacobs, K. V., and Cullen, L.K.: Umbilical hernia of a diverticulum of the vitelline duct in a horse. Austr. Vet. J. 57:190, 1981.

Hirsh, D. C.: Microflora, mucosa and immunity. In Veterinary Gastroenterology. Anderson, N. V. (ed.). Philadelphia: Lea & Febiger, 1980, pp. 199–219.

Hoffer, R. E., Barber, S. M., Kallfelz, F. A., et al.: Esophageal patch grafting as a treatment for esophageal stricture in a horse. JAVMA 171:350, 1977.

Hoffman, P. E.: Practice tips. Proceedings of the American Association of Equine Practitioners:16, 1965.

Hofmeyr, C. F. B.: The digestive system. In Textbook of Large Animal Surgery. Oehme, F. W., and Prier, J. E. (eds.). Baltimore: Williams & Wilkins, 1974.

Hofmeyr, C. F. B.: Comparative dental pathology (with particular reference to caries and paradontal disease in the horse and dog). J. S. Afr. Vet. Assoc. 31:471, 1960.

Horney, F. D., and Funk, K. A.: Ileal myotomy in the horse. Mod. Vet. Pract. 52:49, 1971.

Howard, D. R., Davis, D. G., Merkley, D. F., Krahwinkel, D. J., Schirmer, R. G., and Brinker, W. O.: Mucoperiosteal flap technique for cleft palate repair in dogs. JAVMA 165:352, 1974.

Hudspeth, A. S.: Radical surgical debridement in the treatment of advanced generalized bacterial peritonitis. Arch. Surg. 110:1233, 1975.

Huskamp, B.: Some problems associated with intestinal surgery in the horse. Equine Vet. J. 9:111, 1977.

Huskamp, B., and Boening, J.: Unpublished data, 1981.

Jackson, L. L., Blevins, W. E., and Wiggers, K.: Radiographic diagnosis of alveolar periostitis in the molar tooth of a horse. JAVMA 158:511, 1971.

Johnson, H. W.: Submucus resection, surgical correction and prolapse of the rectum. JAVMA 102:113, 1943.

Jones, R. S., Maisels, D. O., de Geus, J. J., and Lovius, B. B. J.: Surgical repair of cleft palate in the horse. Equine Vet. J. 7:86, 1975.

Jubb, K. V. E., and Kennedy, P. C.: Pathology of Domestic Animals. New York: Academic Press, 1963, p. 94.

Kendrick, W. J.: Cleft palate in a horse. Cornell Vet. 40:188, 1950.

Kindrey, B. W., and Lundvall, R. L.: Oral and esophageal conditions. In Equine Medicine and Surgery, 2nd ed. Wheaton, IL: American Veterinary Publications, 1972, pp. 252–257.

Knight, A. P.: Dysphagia resulting from unilateral rupture of the rectus capitis ventralis muscles in a horse. JAVMA 170:735, 1977.

Koch, C.: The diagnosis and medical management of obstructive diseases of the large colon. Proceedings of the American Association of Equine Practitioners:221, 1981.

Kral, F.: Equine sinusitis—a new therapeutic approach to equine sinusitis. JAVMA 124:373, 1954.

Lagarde, M. C., Bolton, J. S., and Cohn, I., Jr.: Intraperitoneal povidone-iodine in experimental peritonitis. Ann. Surg. 187:613, 1978.

Levine, S. B.: Surgical treatment of recurrent rectal prolapse in a horse. J. Equine Med. Surg. 2:248,255, 1978.

Lindsay, W. A., Confer, A. W., and Ochoa, R.: Ileal smooth muscle hypertrophy and rupture in a horse. Equine Vet. J. 13:66, 1981.

Linerode, P. A., and Goode, R. L.: The effects of colic on the microbial activity of the equine large intestine. Proceedings of the American Association of Equine Practitioners:321, 1971.

Lingand, D. R., and Crawford, T. B.: Congenital ameloblastic odontoma in a foal. Am. J. Vet. Res. 31:801, 1970.

Lorber, B., and Swenson, R. M.: The bacteriology of intra-abdominal infections. Surg. Clin. North Am. 55:1349, 1975.

Lores, M. E., Ortiz, J. R., and Rossello, P. J.: Peritoneal lavage with povidone-iodine solution in experimentally induced peritonitis. Surg. Gynecol. Obstet. 153:33, 1981.

Lowe, J. E.: Intussusception in three ponies following experimental enterotomy. Cornell Vet. 58:288, 1968.

Lowe, J. E.: Esophageal anastomosis in the horse. Cornell Vet. 54:636, 1964.

Lowe, J. E., Sellers, A. F., and Brondum, J.: Equine pelvic flexure impaction. A model used to evaluate motor events and compare drug response. Cornell Vet. 70:401, 1980.

Lundgren, O., and Haglund, V.: The pathophysiology of the intestinal countercurrent exchanger. Life Sci. 23:1411, 1978.

MacKay, R. J., Iverson, W. O., and Merritt, A. M.: Exuberant granulation tissue in the stomach of a horse. Equine Vet. J. 13:119, 1981.

Mark, J. B. D., and Briggs, H. C.: Segmental replacement of the thoracic esophagus with woven teflon. J. Surg. Res. 4:400, 1964.

Mason, B. J. E.: Empyema of the equine paranasal sinuses. JAVMA 167:727, 1975.

Mason, T. A.: Strangulation of the rectum of a horse by the pedicle of a mesenteric lipoma. Equine Vet. J. 10:269, 1978.

Mason, T. A., Johnson, D. E., Wallace, C. E., et al.: Laparotomy in equine colic: a report of thirteen clinical cases. Austr. Vet. J. 46:349, 1970.

Mason, T. A., Speirs, V. C., McLean, A. A., and Smyth, G. B.: Surgical repair of cleft soft palate in the horse. Vet. Rec. 100:6, 1977.

McClure, J. R., McClure, J. J., and Usenik, E. A.: Disseminated intravascular coagulation in ponies with surgically induced strangulation obstruction of the small intestine. Vet. Surg. 8:78, 1979.

McIlwraith, C. W.: Postoperative management of the acute abdominal patient and complications. Vet. Clin. North Am. Large Anim. Pract. 4:167, 1982.

McIlwraith, C. W.: Complications of laparotomy incisions in the horse. Proceedings of the American Association of Equine Practitioners:209, 1979.

McIntosh, S. C., and Shupe, J. R.: Surgical correction of duodenal stenosis in the foal. Equine Pract. 3:17, 1981.

McLaughlin, G. B., and Doige, L. E.: Congenital musculoskeletal lesions and hyperplastic goiter in foals. Can. Vet. J. 22:130, 1981.

Meagher, D. M.: Intestinal strangulation in the horse. Arch. A.C.V.S. 4:59, 1975.

Meagher, D. M.: Surgery of the large intestine in the horse. Arch. A.C.V.S. 3:9, 1974a.

Meagher, D. M.: Surgery of the small intestine in the horse. Arch. A.C.V.S. 3:3, 1974b.

Meagher, D. M., and Stirk, J. A.: Intussusception in the colon of a filly. Mod. Vet. Pract. 55:951, 1974.

Meagher, D. M., Wheat, J. D., Tennant, B., et al.: Squamous cell carcinoma of the equine stomach. JAVMA 164:81, 1974.

Merritt, F. D., Pickering, L. A., and Bergerin, J. D.: Small colon impaction and rupture into the colic mesentery in a horse. VM/SAC 70:1097, 1975.

Milne, D. W., Tarr, M. J., and Lochner, F. K.: Left dorsal displacement of the colon in a horse. J. Equine Med. Surg. 1:47, 1977.

Moore, J. N., Garner, H. E., and Shapland, J. E.: Equine endotoxemia: an insight into cause and treatment. JAVMA 179:473, 1981.

Moore, J. N., Garner, H. E., Shapland, J. E., and Hatfield, D. G.: Prevention of endotoxin-induced arterial hypoxaemia and lactic acidosis with flunixin meglumine in the conscious pony. Equine Vet. J. 13:95, 1981.

Moore, J. N., Garner, H. E., Shapland, J. E., et al.: Lactic acidosis and arterial hypoxemia during sublethal endotoxemia in conscious ponies. Am. J. Vet. Res. 41:1696, 1980.

Moore, J. N., Johnson, J. H., Garner, H. E., et al.: A case report of inguinal herniorrhaphy in a stallion. Equine Vet. J. 1:391, 1977.

Moore, J. N., and Kintner, L. D.: Recurrent oesophageal obstruction due to squamous cell carcinoma in a horse. Cornell Vet. 66:589, 1976.

Moore, J. N., Traver, D. S., and Johnson, J. H.: Particulate fecal markers in the diagnosis of large intestinal obstruction. J. Equine Med. Surg. 2:541, 1978.

Moore, J. N., White, N. A., Trim, C. M., et al.: Effect of intraluminal oxygen in intestinal strangulation obstruction in ponies. Am. J. Vet. Res. 41:1615, 1980.

Myers, V. S., and Gordon, G. W.: Ruptured common digital extensor tendons associated with contracted flexor tendons in foals. Proceedings of the American Association of Equine Practitioners:67, 1975.

Nanson, E. M.: Vascular lesions producing the "acute abdomen." Surg. Clin. North Am. 40:1241, 1960.

Neeley, J., and Catchpole, B.: Ileus: the restoration of alimentary tract motility by pharmacological means. Br. J. Surg. 58:21, 1971.

Nelson, A. W.: The unified concept of shock. Vet. Clin. North Am. 6:173, 1976.

Nelson, A. W., and Adams, O. R.: Intestinal infarction in the horse: acute colic arterial occlusion. Am. J. Vet. Res. 27:707, 1966.

Nelson, A. W., Curley, B. M., and Kainer, R. A.: Mandibular symphysiotomy to provide adequate exposure for intraoral surgery in the horse. JAVMA 159:1025, 1971.

Nieberle, K., and Cohrs, P.: Textbook of Special Pathological Anatomy of Domestic Animals. Oxford: Pergamon Press, 1967.

Nielson, S. W.: Muscular hypertrophy of the ileum in relation to "terminal ileitis" in pigs—a preliminary report. JAVMA 127:437, 1955.

Norrie, R. D., and Heistand, D. L.: Chronic colic due to an omental adhesion in a mare. JAVMA 167:54, 1975.

O'Brien, J. A., Harvey, C. E., and Brodey, R. S.: The esophagus. In Veterinary Gastroenterology. Anderson, N. V. (ed.). Philadelphia: Lea & Febiger, 1980.

Olivet, R. T., and Payne, W. S.: Congenital H-type tracheoesophageal fistula complicated by achalasia in an adult. Mayo Clinic Proc. 50:464, 1975.

Orsini, J. A., Koch, C., and Stewart, B.: Peritoneopericardial hernia in a horse. JAVMA 179:907, 1981.

Ottaway, C. W., and Bingham, M. L.: Further observations on the incidence of parasitic aneurysm in the horse. Vet. Rec. 58:155, 1946.

Owen, R. R.: Illness after racing: acute gastric dilatation? Vet. Rec. 96:437, 1975.

Owen, R. R., Physick-Sheard, D. W., Hilbert, B. J., et al.: Jejuno- or ileocecal anastomosis performed in seven horses exhibiting colic. Can. Vet. J. 16:164, 1975.

Pass, M. A.: Surgical repair of esophageal defects. JAVMA 159:1453, 1971.

Pearson, H., Messervy, A., and Pinsent, P. J. N.: Surgical treatment of abdominal disorders in the horse. JAVMA 159:1344, 1971.

Pearson, H., Pinsent, P. J. N., Denny, H. R., et al.: The indications for equine laparotomy—an analysis of 140 cases. Equine Vet. J. 7:131, 1975.

Pearson, H., Pinsent, P. J. N., Polley, L. R., et al.: Rupture of the diaphragm in the horse. Equine Vet. J. 9:32, 1977.

Peter, C. P., Myers, V. S., and Ramsey, F. K.: Ameloblastic odontoma in a pony. Am. J. Vet. Res. 29:1495, 1968.

Peterson, F. B., Donawick, W. J., and Merritt, A. M.: Gastric stenosis in a horse. JAVMA 160:328, 1972.

Raker, C. W., and Sayers, A.: Esophageal rupture in a Standardbred mare. JAVMA 133:371, 1958.

Reed, J. H.: Esophageal surgery. In Canine Surgery, 2nd ed. Archibald, J. (ed.). Wheaton, IL.: American Veterinary Publications, 1974, p. 498.

Roberts, M. C., and Kelly, W. R.: Squamous cell carcinoma of the lower cervical esophagus in a pony. Equine Vet. J. 11:199, 1979.

Robertson, J. T.: Differential diagnosis and surgical management of conditions of the stomach and small intestine. Vet. Clin. North Am. Large Anim. Pract. 4:105, 1982.

Robertson, J. T., and Johnson, F. M.: Surgical correction of cecocolic intussusception in a horse. JAVMA 176:223, 1980.

Rohrbach, B. W., and Rooney, J. R.: Congenital esophageal ectasia in a Thoroughbred foal. JAVMA 177:65, 1980.

Rooney, J. R.: Autospy of the Horse. Baltimore: Williams & Wilkins, 1970, pp. 83–86.

Rooney, J. R.: Volvulus, strangulation and intussusception in the horse. Cornell Vet. 55:644, 1965.

Rooney, J. R.: Gastric ulceration in foals. Pathol. Vet. 1:497, 1964.

Rooney, J. R., and Jeffcott, L. B.: Muscular hypertrophy of the ileum in a horse. Vet. Rec. 83:217, 1968.

Rumbaugh, G. E., Smith, B. P., and Carlson, G. P.: Internal abdominal abscesses in the horse: a study of 25 cases. JAVMA 172:304, 1978.

Sabiston, D. C.: Textbook of Surgery, 12th ed. Philadelphia: W.B. Saunders, 1981.

Salama, F. D.: Prosthetic replacement of the esophagus. J. Thorac. Cardiovasc. Surg. 70:739, 1975.

Schneider, J. E., and Leipold, H. W.: Recessive lethal white in two foals. J. Equine Med. Surg. 2:479, 1978.

Schneider, J. E., Leipold, H. W., and Kennedy, G.: Muscular hypertrophy of the small intestine in a horse. J. Eq. Med. Surg. 3:226, 1972.

Schneider, J. E., Leipold, H. W., White, S. L., et al.: Repair of congenital atresia of the colon in a foal. J. Equine Vet. Sci. 1:121, 1981.

Scott, E. A.: Surgery of the equine oral cavity. Vet. Pract. North Am. Large Anim. Pract. 4:3, 1982.

Scott, E. A.: Cervical abscess and pharyngeal fistula in a horse. JAVMA 166:775, 1975.

Scott, E. A., and Fishback, W. A.: Surgical repair of diaphragmatic hernia in a horse. JAVMA 168:45, 1976.

Scott, E. A., Gallagher, K., Boles, C. L., Beasley, R. D., and Reed, S. M.: Dental disease in the horse: five case reports. J. Equine Med. Surg. 1:301, 1977.

Scott, E. A., Snoy, P., Prasse, K. W., et al.: Intramural esophageal cyst in a horse. JAVMA 171:652, 1977.

Scott, E. A., Trapp, A. L., and Derksen, F. J.: Splenomegaly and splenic infarction in a Standardbred colt. VM/SAC 73:1549, 1978.

Sellers, A. F., Lowe, J. E., and Brondum, J.: Motor events in equine large colon. Am. J. Physiol. 237:E457, 1979.

Sembrat, R. F.: The acute abdomen in the horse—epidemiologic considerations. Arch. A.C.V.S. 4:34, 1975.

Shields, R.: The absorption and secretion of fluid and electrolytes by the obstructed bowel. Br. J. Surg. 52:774, 1965.

Shires, G.M.H.: Palatoplasty in the horse. Proceedings of the Annual Meeting of the American College of Veterinary Surgeons, Knoxville, 1980.

Shires, M.: A temporary diverting colostomy for the management of rectal tears. Proceedings of the Annual Meeting of the American College of Veterinary Surgeons, New Orleans, 1981.

Shuttleworth, A. C.: Dental disease of the horse. Vet. Rec. 60:564, 1948.

Slocombe, J. O. D., Owen, R., Pennock, P. W., et al.: Arteriographic presentation of the early development of vascular lesions in ponies infected with Strongylus vulgaris. Proceedings of the American Association of Equine Practitioners:305, 1977.

Smith, B. P.: Pleuritis and pleural effusion in the horse. A study of 33 cases. JAVMA 170:208, 1977.

Spiers, V. C., Christie, B. A., and Van Veenendaal, J. C.: The management of rectal tears in horses. Austr. Vet. J. 56:313, 1980.

Spiers, V. C., Hilbert, B. J., and Blood, D. C.: Dorsal displacement of the left ventral and dorsal colon in two horses. Austr. Vet. J. 55:542, 1979.

Spiers, V. C., and Reynolds, W. T.: Successful repair of a diaphragmatic hernia in a foal. Equine Vet. J. 8:170, 1976.

Spiers, V. C., Van Veenendaal. J. C., Christie, B. A., et al.: Obstruction of the small colon by intramural haematoma in three horses. Austr. Vet. J. 57:88, 1981.

Stanffer, V. D.: Equine rectal tears—a malpractice problem. JAVMA 178:798, 1981.

Stashak, T. S., and Knight, A. P.: Temporary diverting colostomy for the management of small colon tears in the horse: a case report. J. Equine Med. Surg. 2:196, 1978.

Steiner, J. V.: Splenic rupture in the horse. Equine Pract. 3:37, 1981.

Stick, J. A.: Surgery of the equine esophagus. Vet. Clin. North Am. Large Anim. Pract. 4:33, 1982.

Stick, J. A., Boles, C. L., and Scott, E. A.: Esophageal intramural cyst in a horse. Letter to the Editor. JAVMA 171:1133, 1977.

Stick, J. A., Derksen, F. J., and Scott, E. A.: Equine cervical esophagostomy. Complications associated with duration and location of feeding tubes. Am. J. Vet. Res. 42:727, 1981.

Stick, J. A., Krehbiel, J. D., Kunze, D. J., et al.: Esophageal healing in the pony: Comparison of sutured vs. nonsutured esophagotomy. Am. J. Vet. Res. 42:1506, 1981.

Stick, J. A., Robinson, N. E., and Krehbiel, J. D.:Acid-base and electrolyte alterations associated with salivary loss in the pony. Am. J. Vet. Res. 42:733, 1981.

Stick, J. A., Slocombe, R. G., and Derkson, F. J.: The effects of feed type on healing of esophagotomies in the pony. Unpublished data, 1982.

Stickle, R. L., Goble, D. O., and Braden, T. D.: Surgical repair of cleft soft palate in a foal. VM/SAC 68:159, 1973.

Swanstrom, O. G., and Dade, A. A.: Reduplication of the esophageal lumen in a Quarter Horse filly. VM/SAC 74:75, 1979.

Swanstrom, O. G., and Wolford, H. A.: Prosthetic filling of a cement defect in premolar tooth necrosis in a horse. VM/SAC 72:1475, 1977.

Swanwick, R. A., and Wilkinson, J. S.: A clinical evaluation of abdominal paracentesis in the horse. Austr. Vet. J. 52:109, 1976.

Tate, L. P.: Effects of extensive small intestinal resection in the pony. Proceedings of the Annual Meeting of the American College of Veterinary Surgeons, New Orleans, 1981.

Taylor, T. S., Valdez, H., Norwood, G. W., et al.: Retrograde flushing for relief of obstructions of the transverse colon in the horse. Equine Pract. 1:22, 1979.

Tennant, B.: Intestinal obstruction in the horse. Some aspects of differential diagnosis in equine colic. Proceedings of the American Association of Equine Practitioners:426, 1976.

Tennant, B., Evans, C. D., and Schwartz, L. W.: Equine hepatic insufficiency. Vet Clin. North Am. 3:279, 1973.

Thoday, K. L., Charlton, D. A., Graham-Jones, O., Frost, P. L., and Pullen-Warner, E.: The successful use of a prosthesis in the correction of a palatal defect in a dog. J. Small Anim. Pract. 16:487, 1975.

Tolksdorff, E.: Surgical approach to cleft palate. Proceedings of the American Association of Equine Practitioners:41, 1966.

Traver, D. S., Egger, E., and Moore, J. N.: Retrieval of an esophageal foreign body in a horse. VM/SAC 73:783, 1978.

Turner, A. S., and McIlwraith, C. W.: Unpublished data, 1980.

Turner, T. A., and Fessler, J. F.: Rectal prolapse in the horse. JAVMA 177:1028, 1980.

Tvedten, H. W., and Keahey, K. K.: Esophagotracheal fistulation after esophageal stenosis in a horse. VM/SAC 69:868, 1974.

Valdez, H.: Perforating gastrointestinal ulcers in three foals. Equine Pract. 1:44, 1979.

Valdez, H., McLaughlin, S. A., and Taylor, T. S.: A case of colic due to an abscess of the jejunum and its mesentery. J. Equine Med. Surg. 3:36, 1979.

Valdez, H., Scrutchfield, W. L., and Taylor, T. S.: Peritoneal lavage in the horse. JAVMA 175:388, 1979.

Varra, D. L., and Nelson, A. W.: Primary splenomegaly in a horse. JAVMA 168:608, 1976.

Vaughan, J. T.: Peritonitis and acute abdominal diseases. In Veterinary Gastroenterology. Anderson, N. V. (ed.). Philadelphia: Lea & Febiger, 1980, pp. 651–673.

Vaughan, J. T., and Hoffer, R. E.: An approach to correction of cervical esophageal stricture in the equine. Auburn Vet. 19:63, 1963.

Vitums, A., and Kainer, R. A.: A partial situs inversus of the large intestine of a horse. Cornell Vet. 42:20, 1953.

Voss, J. L.: Rupture of the cecum and ventral colon of mares during parturition. JAVMA 155:745, 1969.

Wagner, P. C., Grant, B. D., and Schmidt, J. M.: Duodenal stricture in a foal. Equine Pract. 1:29, 1979.

Weinstein, W. M., Onderdonk, A. B., Bartlett, J. G.,

et al.: Antimicrobial therapy of experimental intra-abdominal sepsis. J. Infect. Dis. *132*:282, 1975.

Wheat, J. D.: Causes of colic and types requiring surgical intervention. J. S. Afr. Vet. Assoc. *46*:95, 1975.

Wheat, J. D.: Sinus drainage tooth repulsion in the horse. Proceedings of the American Association of Equine Practitioners:171, 1973.

White, N. A.: Intestinal infarction associated with mesenteric vascular thrombotic disease in the horse. JAVMA *178*:259, 1981.

White, N. A.: Personal communication, 1981b.

White, N. A., and Moore, J. N.: The pathophysiology and preoperative management of the acute abdomen. Vet. Clin. North Am. Large Anim. Pract. 4:61, 1982.

White, N. A., Moore, J. N., and Trim, C. M.: Mucosal alterations in experimentally induced small intestinal strangulation obstruction in ponies. Am. J. Vet. Res. *41*:193, 1980.

Wilson, T. D., and Sykes, G. D.: Fibroma in the abdomen of a horse. Vet. Rec. *108*:334, 1981.

Wimberly, H. C., Andrews, E. J., and Haschek, W. M.: Diaphragmatic hernias in the horse: a review of the literature and an analysis of six additional cases. JAVMA *170*:1404, 1977.

Wright, A. I.: Verminous arteritis as a cause of colic in the horse. Equine Vet. J. 4:169, 1972.

Wrigley, R. H., Gay, C. C., Lording, P., et al.: Pleural effusion associated with squamous cell carcinoma of the stomach of a horse. Equine Vet. J. *13*:99, 1981.

EQUINE COLIC SURGERY

G. MICHAEL SHIRES, M.R.C.V.S.

The horse has a marked tendency toward gastrointestinal disturbances (Bennett 1972), most of which are grouped together under the heading of *colic*. In the horse this term refers to a myriad of problems presenting with a host of clinical signs and prognoses. The word colic probably originates from the Greek word *kolikos* meaning "suffering in the colon," but today colic refers to nonspecific abdominal pain of varying severity. The horse is quick to evidence pain, particularly abdominal, and thus the word has become synonymous with any abdominal pain, some of which may not stem from the gastrointestinal tract and is properly referred to as "false colic."

In this surgical text it would be out of place to expound on the predisposing causes and manifestations of equine colic or to include a full discussion of its medical treatment, all of which have been exhaustively documented elsewhere (Alexander 1972; Delahanty 1965; Donawick 1975a; 1975b; Leeds 1974; Meagher 1975; Seckington 1972; Wright 1972). However, an accurate diagnosis is an essential prelude to an intelligent decision regarding the advisability of surgical intervention. Where they relate to this choice, the clinical signs and diagnostic procedures will be alluded to briefly.

PRELIMINARY EVALUATION

It is not very often that even the most astute clinician is absolutely certain of what will be revealed after celiotomy and location of the etiological lesion in horses with colic. A plethora of clinical and ancillary observations may be required to enable the conscientious clinician to decide on surgical intervention in preference to the more conservative medical therapy in any particular equine colic patient.

Not the least of the preliminary evaluations is a complete history evaluation and thorough clinical examination (Meagher 1974a). Evaluation of the cardiovascular system via well-defined clinical indices including auscultation, heart rate, capillary refill time, color, pulse frequency and quality, and presence of any pulse deficit must be included, especially if the patient may be subjected to anesthesia. As far as certain environmental influences affecting any particular type of colic, factors such as the weather or time of year should be considered (Rollins and Clement 1979).

Gastrointestinal motility, or lack of it, must be carefully investigated by thorough auscultation over the complete abdomen. Normal abdominal borborygmi are not consistent with major pathological tissue changes (Coffman and Garner 1972). The absence of any borborygmi must be considered a grave sign, and if clinical symptoms and vital signs support this, surgical exploration of the abdomen would be indicated unless the prognosis were hopeless. It should always be remembered that some drugs like atropine may have been administered before the examination and may have precipitated the cessation of intestinal motility. Hence the importance of a complete history in each case. The presence of easily discernible borborygmi could support a decision for delaying surgery if ancillary findings were supportive. It must be clear, however, that any delay in initiating surgery, when called for, will most likely adversely affect the prognosis in most cases.

The quality and severity of pain and its response to drug therapy is another indicator to be utilized in overall patient evaluation (Greatorex 1972). In general, the more unrelenting, acute, and refractory the pain, the more likely the need for surgical intervention.

Any signs that could be used to estimate the presence or likelihood of shock developing would alert the surgeon to the necessity for supportive therapy. Devitalization of the intestine allows for transmural passage of bacteria and endotoxins, which hasten shock (White, Moore, and Trim 1980).

Assessment of the state of hydration as well as of the acid-base status of the patient is a necessary prelude to rational treatment. Blood values should include the following: packed cell volume (PCV), bicarbonate or total CO_2, total protein (TP), osmolarity, complete blood count (CBC), and a selection of relevant enzyme values. It has not been necessary to invest heavily in equipment, such as a blood gas machine, to estimate the animal's acid-base values since the advent of a small and inexpensive kit* for CO_2 determination. This apparatus has been demonstrated to perform with the recurring accuracy and consistency found in much more expensive and sophisticated equipment (Gentry and Black 1975). Other common laboratory tests that could assist the clinician in making a diagnosis and prognosis include blood pH, serum electrolytes, serum lactate levels, plasminogen/fibrin degradation products, and fecal culture (Adams and McIlwraith 1978; Byars and White 1977; Donawick et al. 1976; Linerode and Goode 1970; McClure, McClure, and Usenik 1979; Moore, Owen, and Lumsden 1976). Clinical pathological data are subject to error, especially those that are derived rather than measured; the experienced clinician realizes this and should confirm any values that may be at variance with the clinical picture. It is the author's opinion that these laboratory values are seldom pathognomonic and should be used only as support in reaching a diagnosis after weighing all the findings.

Passage of a nasogastric tube into the stomach should be used as a diagnostic aid; it provides useful information pertaining to the status of the stomach and its contents. Dilation of the stomach may be indicative of failure of the stomach to empty, as occurs in cases of obstruction high in the gastrointestinal tract. Decompression of the dilated stomach not only aids the cardiovascular and respiratory functions but reduces the risk of rupturing this distended organ during tabling.

Abdominal paracentesis is a relatively simple procedure that may provide a

---

*Harleco CO_2 Apparatus, Harleco, Philadelphia, PA.

wealth of information concerning the intra-abdominal status of the patient. Collection of peritoneal fluid via a needle, teat cannula, or catheter has been well described and is a standard procedure in a proper clinical examination of the colic patient that may be a candidate for surgery (Adams, Fessler, and Rebar 1980; Hamilton and Hardenbrook 1973; Loomis 1975; Shires 1977). This fluid can be collected in a sterile tube and evaluated grossly before sending it to the laboratory for detailed examination. Macroscopic examination should note the turbidity, clotting properties, presence of debris or fecal matter, and amount of sediment. A quick gram stain and CBC should reveal any gram-negative organisms or other bacteria and should provide valuable information regarding peritonitis and the integrity of the bowel wall. Other laboratory tests should include total protein, specific gravity, evidence of toxicity in the cells, and culture of the specimen.

The rate of intoxication relative to the toxic by-products of degenerative changes occurring in the intestinal wall as well as the bacterial toxins will give some indication of the magnitude of the condition with respect to irreversible changes in the intestinal tract (Coffman 1970).

The quantity and location of any abdominal distension may assist in defining the problem. The small intestines do not comprise a large volume and the stomach is confined within the rib cage, whereas the large intestines do have a large volume, so that any obstruction of the latter organs would tend to produce more noticeable abdominal distension (Tennant 1975).

Rectal Examination

Not the least of the patient evaluation procedures is a thorough and careful rectal examination and palpation (Vaughan 1970). In the author's opinion, routine rectal examination on every horse you are called upon to treat for colic is unnecessary unless the clinical evidence demands this procedure such as in a stallion with colic, in which case it is mandatory to examine the inguinal ca-

nals. In light of the frequency of litigation coupled with the unfavorable outcome following rupture of the rectal wall, even the most experienced clinician should hestitate before performing a rectal examination without due cause. In any colic patient in which the rectal examination and palpation will assist in making a diagnosis or in cases in which conservative therapy has failed to resolve the problem, this procedure should be included in the examination.

To glean relevant clinical information from a rectal examination in the horse, the examiner must be familiar with the normal anatomy and anatomical relationships of the abdominal organs. Familiarization with the normal anatomy and consistency of abdominal viscera via the rectal examination is a sine qua non for any intelligent and informative examination. A review of relevant texts on this subject coupled with every available opportunity to examine the normal animal should be the aim of every clinician who might be required to make a diagnosis via rectal examination in equine colic patients.

Unfortunately in many cases, even the most experienced clinician is unable to make any positive conclusions from a rectal examination. If the findings from the extensive clinical and pathological examinations indicate that surgical intervention is the procedure of choice, the sooner this is performed the better likelihood there is of a successful outcome.

EXPLORATORY CELIOTOMY

Impaction or obturation obstructions are most often found in the large intestine (colon or cecum) with its many alterations in lumen size and volume together with its frequent directional changes and slow flow of contents (Downs and Lundvall 1972). Digestion, mastication, and diet play a role in obstructive colic as well as in other types of abdominal disorders. The large colon may be completely obstructed with large amounts of sand owing to persistent feeding in sandy conditions (Ferraro 1973). However, ingesta impaction of the large intestine of the horse can usually be managed by conservative, patient, and intensive medical therapy (Meagher 1974a).

Foreign bodies can be expected anywhere in the gastrointestinal tract; however, certain contributory factors should be taken into account. Horses that are kept on premises that are fenced with rubber material as well as patients with a history of fence biting would have a good chance of obstruction caused by an enterolith. These obstructions are usually located in the small colon or terminal large colon (Blue 1979; Gay et al. 1979; Getty et al. 1976; Robertson 1980). The presence of polyhedral enteroliths indicates that others must have been present owing to the pattern of wear. Thus, if found during enterotomy, care should be taken to make a thorough search for all of these objects. Because access to the transverse colon is severely limited owing to its short attachment, an intraoperative enema may assist in retrograde flushing of these foreign bodies to within the surgeon's grasp.

Displacements of the large intestine are most commonly found involving the left colon because of its greater maneuverability than the right colon, which has several ligamentous attachments stabilizing it and the surrounding organs (Figs. 15–184 and 15–185). Several cases have been reported of volvulus of the large colon, either at the base of the cecum or at the origin of the transverse colon, in contradistinction to the free colon (Barclay, Foerner, and Phillips 1980). Displacements include left dorsal displacement of the large colon (Milne et al. 1970); torsion of the large colon (usually left) (Johnson 1970); and torsion of the large colon along its long axis, to mention only the commonest probabilities. The small intestines may also be displaced and strangulated over the nephrosplenic ligament; entrapped in the epiploic foramen (usually in adult horses); or displaced via tears or holes in the mesentery or omentum.

Volvulus or strangulation and vascular occlusion may be caused by a variety of factors and most frequently involve the small intestines. Volvulus of the fixed portion of the large colon is seen (Barclay, Foerner, and Phillips 1980) and volvulus of the terminal ileum has been reported (Rooney 1965). Vascular occlusion may also be seen in strangulation or entrapment of the bowel in hernias—inguinal, umbilical, incisional, diaphragmatic (Meagher 1975)—or in entrapment in the epiploic foramen.

Congenital anomalies may be responsible for strangulations, mainly of the small intestines. The two anomalies most commonly described are Meckel's diverticulum and mesodiverticular bands (Freeman, Koch, and Boles 1977; Grant and Tennant 1973).

Angiopathies reducing flood flow of a sufficient magnitude to cause tissue necrosis may result in acute colic. These vascular obstructions may be intravascular, from trauma or obstruction owing

Figure 15–184 Schematic representation of equine cecum and its ligamentous attachments. 1 = Ileocecal fold; 2 = cecocolic fold; L.V. = left ventral colon; R.V. = right ventral colon.

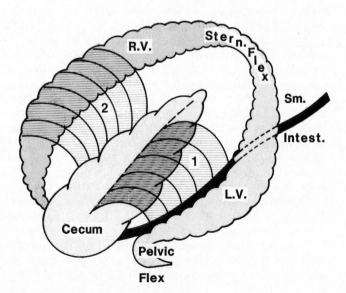

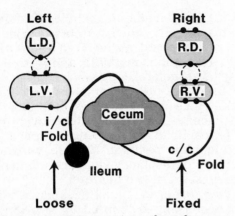

Figure 15–185 Cross section through cecum in the horse showing relationships between intestines and their attachments. Ileocecal fold is on dorsal surface of cecum and ileum. Cecocolic fold is on ventral cecum to right ventral colon. L.D. = Left dorsal colon; L.V. = left ventral colon; i/c = ileocecal fold; R.D. = right dorsal colon; R.V. = right ventral colon; cc = cecocolic fold.

to migrating strongylid larvae, or extravascular, from pressure of strangulation or obstruction (Nelson, Collier, and Griner, 1968; Nelson 1964).

Intussusception of the small intestine is more common in younger horses but may be seen in animals of any age. An intussusception that may be seen is that of the terminal ileum into the cecum at their juncture. The cecum has been reported to intussuscept on itself (Donawick and Stewart 1971).

Neoplasms may cause occlusion of the intestinal lumen, resulting in colic. Pedunculated lipomas have been found causing strangulation of sections of the small intestine in horses older than 11 years (Meagher 1974b).

Inflammatory lesions resulting from localized peritonitis or abscessation may cause adhesions or may directly obstruct the bowel. Horses with a history of recurrent bouts of colic, especially if they have had abdominal surgery previously, may have intestinal obstructions owing to adhesions from previous surgery.

Miscellaneous causes of colic may include the following conditions: muscular hypertrophy of the small intestine (Schneider, Kennedy, and Leipold 1979), torsion of the uterus (Barber 1979), gastric stenosis (Peterson et al. 1972), and hematoma of the broad ligament. These and other problems may require celiotomy for diagnosis or correction. In the

foal and weanling, other causes of colic that may demand surgical intervention include atresia coli, ascarid impaction, and ruptured bladder (Johnson 1970).

To summarize, general indications for celiotomy in the horse in cases of colic are (1) when the diagnosis of physical displacement is made and surgery offers the best possible choice for a successful recovery; (2) when no diagnosis can be made but unrelenting pain and lack of response to medical treatment result in a deterioration in the patient's condition; and (3) when chronic or subacute colic occurs; surgical intervention should only be pursued after patient medical treatment and thorough clinical examination reveals this to be the only satisfactory solution.

EXPLORATORY SURGERY

Advances in surgical technique, equipment, vital signs monitoring, patient supportive treatment, pharmaceuticals, and anesthesia have enabled the veterinary surgeon to regard intra-abdominal exploratory surgery in the horse as, if not an everyday procedure, at least an acceptable choice.

Preoperative Preparation

Once surgery has been selected, preparation of the patient in all its various facets should commence without any delay. Careful analysis of and attention to any fluid deficit, electrolyte imbalances, acid-base changes, or signs of shock should be vigorously and fully undertaken. Concomitant with the required medical patient support should be the preparation for surgery.

Proper antibiotic therapy should be initiated as soon as possible, keeping in mind the possibility of abdominal contamination. Antitetanus immunization must be given unless the patient's status is beyond question. If even the most skilled surgeon is to be encouraged by successful postsurgical recovery, careful attention must be paid to vigorous and complete life-supporting adjunctive therapy, pre-, intra-, and postsurgically. The therapy of the patient does not cease with recovery from the surgery but continues in the stall and for several days thereafter. This is not the place for a complete discussion on all the aspects of medical support for the severely compromised surgical patient. However, as many a surgeon has been bitterly disappointed by losing a patient after a technically perfect surgical procedure, a brief outline of the support of the celiotomy patient is included.

The most important aspect is to monitor and support the cardiovascular system for maintenance of adequate tissue perfusion and cellular oxygenation. Acceptable arterial blood pressure is paramount. Fluids are the backbone of this support, as is the judicious use of selected pharmaceuticals such as corticosteroids (Bowen 1980) and perhaps flunixin meglumine, especially if endotoxic shock is a possibility. Shock and its devastating finality hang above the surgeon's head like the legendary sword of Damocles.

If feasible, some form of monitoring the cardiovascular system should be employed to alert the clinician to any change in the patient's status. Regular blood sampling for sequential PCV, blood gas, or other acid-base measuring system should be the minimum amount of intraoperative patient monitoring. Evaluation of central venous pressure (CVP) will give some indication of the effectiveness of fluid administration. A simple and inexpensive intravenous water manometer can be set up to give continuous evaluation of CVP changes. Arterial blood pressure is a better method of measuring cardiac output and can be measured by direct invasive methods via the femoral or other arteries or by indirect noninvasive methods. An inexpensive Doppler device,* using ultrasonic technique, may be used with acceptable accuracy (Kvart 1979). Regardless of how simple the device, it is to the surgeon's advantage to be kept cognizant of any changes in the patient's status.

Meticulous attention to adequate ventilation and oxygenation not only during surgery but during the recovery and early postrecovery phases is important. Post-

operative administration of oxygen via a demand valve should increase pulmonary pressure and Pao_2 levels in an attempt to hasten reoxygenation and minimize cell damage due to anoxia.

Reduction of gastric pressure before placing the animal on the table is very important; this should be done via a nasogastric tube and suction. Any evidence of an enlarged, overfull bladder should initiate passage of a urethral catheter and reduction in pressure before dropping the horse.

Preparation of the surgical site involves standard procedures, i.e., a wide clip over the selected site and careful shave if this is preferred, followed by at least three alternating 70% alcohol and povidone-iodine scrubs.

For the severely compromised colic patient that probably has metabolic acidosis and cardiovascular incompetence, the choice of anesthetic for induction is very important. In the author's opinion, the "crash" induction method using an intravenous bolus of thiobarbiturates is contraindicated under these and most other circumstances. The hypotensive and apneic potential of this anesthetic agent will do nothing but burden the cardiovascular system further, worsen the anoxia, and probably hasten the patient's demise. Light doses of anesthetic agents such as ketamine hydrochloride, xylazine, and/or guaiafenesin are much more suitable for controlled induction and relaxed endotracheal intubation for inhalant anesthesia. As soon as the patient is intubated, halothane should be administered at low levels until the desired plane of anesthesia is reached. With thiobarbiturates, the patient has to be quickly intubated and higher levels of inhalant agents administered so that the patient remains anesthetized.

The surgical site selected should provide the best access to the probable site of the lesion but at the same time be in a suitable anatomical location for secure closure and wound healing. It is not always possible to meet these criteria with respect to celiotomy in the horse with colic. The wisest choice affords the best access and greatest exposure of the objective organ, while at the same time allowing for secure reconstruction (Vaughan 1979). Some points of entry

---

*Parks 811, Parks Electronic, Beaverton, OR.

may obviously follow natural openings, such as the inguinal ring or umbilicus, and hence the incisional site is predetermined in these cases.

Technique

For greatest exposure and access to most abdominal viscera in the equine, the ventral midline incision should be the incision of choice. This approach is quick, and well-defined landmarks are obvious to the careful surgeon. A longitudinal skin incision should be made over the linea alba and generally from the umbilicus anteriorly for 15 to 30 cm. This incision can be enlarged, if necessary, both cranially and caudally for better exposure, although caudal extension in the male may involve the prepuce and, in the gravid mare, the udder. The linea alba is a narrow fibrous raphe extending from the xiphoid to the pubis, and care must be taken to keep within this structure. This avoids the muscle belly of the rectus abdominis, reducing hemorrhage, and, therefore, time and trauma.

The incision is extended through the superficial fascia and fat that lies over the peritoneum. Careful puncture and incision of the peritoneum is most desirable owing to the proximity of the underlying organs, which may be pressed tightly against the visceral surface of the peritoneum owing to their enlargement by gas. Routine quarter and fenestrated laparotomy drapes should have been placed before making the skin incision. These drapes should be of an impervious material and should be large enough to include the hocks as well as any abdominal contents that may have to be exteriorized. Once the incision is completed, a laparotomy sheet with pliable ring fenestration is a most useful addendum to the drapes. Not only does this serve as an extra barrier between the abdominal wall and visceral contents, but it minimizes contamination of the cut edges of the incision. All the drapes should be large enough and strong enough to provide a supportive sling for any exteriorized bowel.

An alternate choice to the ventral midline approach is the ventral paramedian approach (Marcenac 1950), which may be made on the left or right of the midline if so desired. With this approach, the common tendon of the external abdominal oblique muscle is incised in the same plane as the skin, exposing the rectus muscle. This muscle is split longitudinally in the direction of its fibers, and any branches of the caudal epigastric vessels should be ligated as they are encountered. The deep sheath of the rectus muscle, which is the aponeurosis of the transverse abdominal muscle, is then exposed and can be split transversely in the direction of its fibers or, for better exposure, can be incised in the same plane as the laparotomy incision, bearing in mind that this aponeurosis supplies little extra strength to the closure. The fatty tissue under the deep sheath is more prevalent than on the midline and may be trimmed before incising the peritoneum if necessary.

Not all abdominal approaches need to be performed on the recumbent animal. For diagnostic, economical, or logical anatomical reasons, the surgeon may select a lateral or flank approach (Johnson 1970). These approaches are usually performed under sedation and local anesthetic block in the standing animal. Muscle dissection is most often done along the planes of their fibers. With this grid or modified grid approach, greater security of closure is assured, but very limited exposure is allowed. The flank approach has been advocated for diagnostic confirmation in patients suspected of having a hopeless prognosis, thus greatly reducing the expense and effort as well as the animal's suffering (Meagher 1974b). It must be remembered that specific organs can be reached and even partially exteriorized via a flank incision—the cecum on the right side and the pelvic flexure on the left, for example (Johnson 1970).

The surgeon must be cognizant of the fact that unless the indications for flank approaches are absolute, it may be necessary to close the flank incision and reenter the abdomen via the ventral midline to gain access to the lesion. The flank approach also requires a cooperative patient that will remain standing throughout the operation.

For the flank incision, a 15- to 20-cm

vertical skin incision is made midway between the tuber coxae and the last rib. A modified grid approach is made whereby the only muscle fibers incised are those of the external oblique muscle. The internal oblique and transverse abdominal muscles are split along the plane of their fibers. This allows for slightly better exposure than a complete grid approach without sacrificing closure security. Incisions may be in the mid or low flank, offering greater exposure than the paralumbar approach, or high to avoid the muscle belly of the internal oblique muscle. The site chosen is to a greater or lesser extent dependent on the surgeon's preferences, but all lateral approaches enjoy the advantages of the grid technique of speed and closure security and the disadvantages of limited exposure and little physical control of the patient.

Closure of the flank approach usually consists of two or three layers of absorbable sutures reconstructing the individual muscle layers. Simple interrupted sutures placed in the superficial abdominal fascia immediately under the skin will lessen wound tension, reduce dead space, and contribute to support of the closure. Contrary to skin closure in some other animals, skin sutures in the horse should be tense enough to fully appose the cut edges with a slight bulge. Skin closure suture patterns may be chosen according to the surgeon's personal preference, but, since speed is a necessary element, the Ford interlocking suture pattern using nonabsorbable material is a good choice.

Should the surgeon decide to lavage the abdominal cavity in the standing patient with some antiseptic/antibiotic solution, great care must be taken to select only solutions that are nonirritating to the peritoneum to prevent a violent, painful reaction, causing the standing patient to collapse with an open laparotomy incision.

Some indications for a lateral approach include exploratory diagnostic or prognostic procedures, biopsy, ovariectomy, unilateral abdominal cryptorchidectomy, enterotomy for certain conditions of the small colon and cecum, obstruction of the pelvic flexure, colostomy, and uterine torsion.

Exploration

It is certainly advisable to have some preoperative idea of what to expect when entering the abdomen and where to find it, but the surgeon must refrain from plunging into the abdomen immediately on opening the peritoneum. A moment studying the pattern and composition of the bowel distension may help locate the problem. In general, acute distensions due to obstructions of the small intestines are fluid filled and often result in gastric reflux and distension, whereas obstruction of the large bowel causes mostly gaseous distension.

Having ensured that the suction apparatus is ready and available, the first step is to reduce the amount of distension in the bowel. Tension through stretching not only causes most of the visceral pain but results in ischemia of the bowel wall, anoxia, and ileus. Deflation of the distended loops of the bowel therefore not only improves the viability of the bowel wall but allows much greater ease of manipulation of the viscera and therefore improves exposure (Milne 1961, Scott 1977). If the distension is from gas only, a medium-gauge needle attached to the suction pump is introduced into the bowel lumen through the antimesenteric border or through one of the bands. Should the enlargement be caused by fluid, a small stab incision is made in healthy bowel and a larger bore tube attached to the suction used to empty the distended bowel. If only part of the small intestine is distended, there is probably a volvulus or entrapment of a section of bowel. If all of the small intestine is distended but none of the large, then the ileocecal area should be checked for evidence of obstruction, usually intussusception. Secretion of gastric juice in the horse is continuous and only slightly affected by starvation or feeding, a fact of considerable importance in cases of obstruction in which cessation of food and water intake will not prevent the accumulation of gastric secretion anterior to the obstruction (Littlejohn 1965).

If distension of the large colon extends only to the left ventral colon, the problem is most likely at the pelvic flexure. If both dorsal and ventral limbs of the left colon are distended, a torsion or entrapment should be anticipated. If distension of the right dorsal colon exists, then enteroliths or impaction in the transverse colon may be present.

In addition to noting the obvious distension, the surgeon should note any discoloration of the bowel wall that could be related to pathological changes in the blood circulation. This is of importance not only in demarcating the affected section of bowel but in evaluating the viability of this section, once the obstruction has been corrected, for possible resection. If resection is to be performed, it is simple to use one end of the resected section to siphon off the toxic contents before completing the resection. By this means it is easy to empty a reasonable section anterior and posterior to the resection area far away from the abdominal cavity into a bucket on the floor, for instance, and reduce the chances of contamination.

If the surgeon has no immediate indication of the site of the lesion, it is quicker and less traumatic to the viscera to examine the bowel with some logical plan from distal to proximal (Vaughan 1977). To do this, a point of reference is needed, and the easiest one to use is the terminal ileum, which is located by lifting the tip of the cecum back to reveal the dorsal band of the ileocecal fold. Follow this down to the lesser curvature of the cecum, and the ileum should be reached and can be exteriorized almost to its termination in the cecum. The ileum is easily identified by the unique antimesenteric fold and segmental blood supply. If your clinical observations coupled with the pattern of distension suggest a distal small intestinal problem, this end of the organ can be carefully examined by tracing cranially from the ileum. The small intestine of the adult horse is some 20 meters in length, and precious time can be needlessly lost in tracing the entire length of this organ. Should examination of the terminal ileum and jejunum prove negative, it is probably quicker to select and examine those sites most likely to be problematical in the small intestine of that particular horse. These include the inguinal rings in the male; uterus or mesovarium in the female; nephrosplenic ligament; Meckel's diverticulum and mesenteric bands; and duodenum and epiploic foramen in the older animal.

As the examination progresses, careful manipulation and anatomical replacement of organs should be followed, with attention paid to minimal tension on the mesentery and vasculature. Aimless pawing and exteriorization of section after section of bowel will occupy a great deal of precious time and will further compromise the patient. If any obvious lesion is visible on opening the peritoneum, the diagnosis should be clear; however, the diligent observer will take care to ensure that this is the only lesion present. In most cases, the lesion or lesions are not that obvious, and careful exploration of the abdominal contents is required. A common error is to encounter an extensive mass of dry ingesta in the large colon and mistakenly identify this as the primary lesion. The ingesta will most often become dry and hard as a result of decreased peristalsis and reduced fluid from a higher blockage. The presence of distended gas-filled loops of large intestine should, after deflation, encourage the surgeon to direct the initial examination at the large bowel; unless discoloration of segments leads the surgeon directly to the area in question, a quick check of the most likely trouble spots can be made. The pelvic flexure, left colon, ileocecal-cecal area, and transverse colon are the most likely sites for lesions. The transverse colon is best located by following the small colon proximally from the left caudal abdomen. Careful and thorough examination of all the clinical observations both before and after entering the abdomen should direct the astute clinician to the lesion without undue delay.

While exploring the abdomen, any ancillary information concerning the state of the peritoneal cavity and its contents should be noted and evaluated for its influence on the problem at hand. Fecal matter, fibrinous tags, and inflamed peritoneal surfaces should alert the observer to the probability of ruptured bowel, gross peritoneal contamination, and a poor prognosis. Heroic resection and anastomosis of necrotic bowel in the face of highly unfavorable complications may not be in the best interests of patient and owner. Constant observation·of the intra-abdominal conditions coupled with patient monitoring of vital signs should be automatically evaluated by the surgeon continuously. No surgeon likes to finish before the last skin suture has been properly placed, but, on the other hand, needless and costly procedures should be terminated once the prognosis has become hopeless.

Corrective Measures

Once the section of bowel responsible for the problem has been located, it should, if possible, be carefully exteriorized and examined. Evaluation in each case should determine if resection of the bowel is necessary or possible or if correction of a strangulation will permit the vasculature to perfuse the area sufficiently for revitalization of the bowel wall. When the pressure has been released, a short period of time should be allowed to elapse to observe if the color is returning, if pulsations are seen in the mesenteric vessels, and if any signs of peristalsis occur in the section in question. In some early cases the bowel will be minimally devitalized and, as soon as the circulation has been restored, will quickly return to normal. Significant guides to bowel viability in the dog are electromyographical patterns of acidotic or normal serosal pH in the range of 7.3 to 7.8 (Katz et al. 1974).

If enterotomy has to be performed, the incision should not be made into devitalized tissue; attempts should be made to move the offending obstruction and remove it via an incision in healthy tissue.

Careful examination of the mesenteric blood vessels is required for evaluation of tissue perfusion and must be done before planning any resection and anastomosis of bowel. The ends to be anastomosed must have a healthy and abundant blood supply for optimum wound healing, and a careful consideration of this has to be made prior to determining the resection site. Double ligation is desired for the mesenteric vessels when resecting bowel, and some form of gentle but secure clamping must be placed over each end of the cut bowel to prevent contamination. Any tears or holes in the mesentery should be repaired or removed to prevent strangulation of bowel.

If bowel is to be resected, a generous amount of healthy tissue should be allowed on each side of the devitalized tissue. Careful and leakproof anastomotic technique must be employed to allow a quick fibrin seal over the junction. The suture pattern and material for the anastomosis depend on the surgeon's preference; however, a few basic surgical principles apply. When lumen size is not a critical factor, it is preferable to suture with a double layer of inverting sutures. These inverting patterns can best be utilized in the large bowel in the horse and can be placed quickly without real concern for restriction of the lumen. When technically feasible, end-to-end anastomosis is the simplest and most physiologically compatible method. Everting suture patterns may encourage leakage, bacterial contamination, adhesions, and anastomotic failure (Reinertson 1976). The modified Gambee suture pattern and the "crushing" end-on suture pattern have recently gained favor, especially when lumen size is critical (Abramowitz and Butcher 1971; Poth and Gold 1968). Whatever suture pattern is chosen, it is essential to appose the cut surfaces as anatomically correctly as possible and at the same time secure the anastomosis from leakage. The most likely area of leakage in an end-to-end anastomosis is at the mesenteric border, and extra care must be exercised when closing this area. The material used for suturing is commonly one of the absorbable types and may be catgut or synthetic. Many surgeons still prefer to use silk for bowel anastomosis owing to its ease of knot tying and secure closure.

Lesions caused by fibrous bands, anatomical anomalies, or pedunculated lipomas may have to be freed by severing the restricting tissue.

Any bowel exteriorized during surgery must be kept moist with warm sterile solutions and covered with saturated laparotomy cloths as often as possible. Surgical sites should be carefully washed with warm solutions before returning the bowel to the abdomen. Any soiled drapes should be discarded and surgical gloves changed before closure of the abdominal incision.

In any area where the site of the lesion cannot be exteriorized, alternate plans must be made. Two inaccessible sites where lesions do occur are the transverse colon (enteroliths) and the ileocecal area (intussusception). To remove enteroliths from the transverse colon, access must be made via an accessible part of the bowel and the surgeon's arm passed through its lumen into the transverse colon. The left dorsal colon can be opened and the arm passed via the diaphragmatic flexure into the transverse colon. In some cases, retrograde deep enemas via the rectum may flush the enterolith into a more accessible site.

The terminal ileum may intussuscept into the cecum; in such cases it is usually necessary to resect the ileum about 15 to 30 cm from the ileocecal junction, which cannot be exteriorized. The remaining stump of the terminal ileum is closed with the Parker-Kerr technique. Patency is recreated by anastomosing the healthy proximal section to an incision made in the base of the cecum about 20 cm ventral to the natural ileocecal junction (Donawick and Stewart 1971; Peterson and Stewart 1978).

Large quantities of sand may accumulate in the large intestines of the horse, and ingesta will continue to pass over it until sufficient sand is collected to obstruct the flow. It is extremely difficult to exteriorize the sand-filled colon owing to its size, weight, and viability; therefore, great care must be exercised in exteriorizing and evacuating the distended bowel. In most cases patient and vigorous medical treatment will eventually loosen the sand and obviate surgery.

Following any surgery in which the mesentery has been incised or herniated, attempts should be made to suture all rents to prevent them from becoming sites for future strangulations. In cases in which bowel is strangulated through hernia rings, such as the inguinal ring canal, it may not be possible to return the bowel to the abdominal cavity without resection owing to edema, inflammation, and necrosis. When incisions have been made over these lesions, it might be necessary to make a second incision into the abdominal cavity to facilitate resection of the diseased section and anastomosis of the healthy segments.

When celiotomy reveals that thromboembolism of sufficient magnitude has caused ischemic necrosis of sections of bowel, resection may not be possible owing to the extent of the circulatory impairment. In some cases of limited infarction, resection of the affected area may be feasible such as in cases of the apex of the cecum. Generally, resection and anastomosis of the large bowel does not offer as good a prognosis as that of the small intestine.

Celiotomy is indicated for creation of a colostomy in cases in which it is necessary to divert the fecal flow either temporarily or permanently. In the management of rectal tears, a temporary diverting colostomy via enterectomy of the descending colon and reanastomosis at a later date may be utilized (Arnold and Meagher 1978; Stashak and Knight 1978), or, using another technique, a temporary diverting loop colostomy may be created (Shires 1981).

With the compromised abdominal crisis patient, the shorter the time that the animal has to be kept under anesthesia the better. Paralytic ileus and shock parallel operative time, trauma, hemorrhage, and contamination (Vaughan 1977). To aid in reducing the time taken in performing a variety of bowel resection and anastomosis techniques, mechanical stapling equipment has been designed for the human patient and has been utilized in the horse (Gideon 1975) as well as in other animals. Considerable debate has surrounded the use of this equipment owing not only to its expense but to the fact that its use creates an everting anastomosis in at least two-thirds of the anastomotic circumference. A newer stapler, the E.E.A. Stapler,* permits the creation of an inverted circular anastomosis held by a double, staggered row of staples. This instrument is used in the human patient mainly for construction of a colorectal anastomosis (Adloff, Arnaud, and Beehary 198) but may have application in the horse.

One way to reduce the postoperative complications of peritonitis and its cohort ileus is through careful and meticulous attention to minimizing contami-

---

*E.E.A. Stapler, United States Surgical Corporation, New York, NY.

nation of the operative site and abdomen. Careful rinsing of the intestine with sterile solutions before replacement with, perhaps, the addition of an antibiotic suitable for intra-abdominal instillation should be selected by the surgeon as the minimal effort to reduce the chances of peritonitis. It must be kept in mind that members of the aminoglycoside family of antibiotics, coupled with some inhalant anesthetics, may precipitate neuromuscular blockade. Peritoneal lavage via a Foley catheter using Ringer's lactate, kanamycin, and povidone-iodine has been reported beneficial in the horse (Valdez, Scrutchfield, and Taylor 1979). Excessive peritoneal lavage may be responsible for electrolyte imbalances and/or protein losses. The peritoneum of the horse does not appear to be particularly susceptible to peritonitis; however, the normal defense mechanisms of the compromised patient should be considered to be weaker than those of a normal horse (Littlejohn 1965).

Wound Closure

Having adhered to the general surgical principles of minimal tissue trauma, sharp dissection, careful hemostasis, scrupulous attention to aseptic techniques, and speedy but careful resolution of the problem, the final surgical challenge is quick and secure wound closure. Probably the most critical challenge related to wound security in the horse is the immediate postoperative recovery period, when enormous tensions are placed on suture lines, especially during a stormy recovery and until the animal is fully conscious and able to stand unaided (Milne 1972).

Immediately before commencing closure, check briefly for any foreign bodies, such as sponges or instruments, that may have been left in the abdomen. It is also an excellent idea to deflate any distended bowel not only to facilitate closure but to reduce the chance of postoperative ileus.

In the closure, the surgeon should attempt to eliminate all pockets of dead space to reduce postoperative seroma formation and unnecessary wound tension.

It is not essential to close the peritoneum, but if this can be managed quickly and easily some apposition of the peritoneal lining may facilitate closure by holding the abdominal viscera out of the incision during closure. In the ventral incision, the linea alba is carefully closed with a suture material and pattern of the surgeon's choice. Simple interrupted sutures using absorbable material offer easy closure and, while this pattern may take longer than a continuous pattern, does offer good security. Many surgeons prefer nonabsorbable suture materials, which should be properly sterilized prior to use to reduce the formation of suture fistulae or abscesses. Suture patterns that are recognized for strength are the modified Mayo mattress (vest-over-pants) and pulley (near far–far near) suture patterns. Whatever suture material and pattern are selected, the same attention to suture placement and knot tying is required. Knots should be tightened sufficiently to appose cut edges firmly but not tight enough to compromise blood circulation to the healing edges.

When gross contamination has occurred or peritonitis is to be expected, it has been suggested that drains be placed in the peritoneal cavity alongside the incision just prior to closure (Meagher 1974). The use of intra-abdominal drains has enjoyed varying degrees of popularity, but it must be realized that without care and maintenance coupled with careful removal they may serve as a source of infection. The use of Penrose drains is not advocated. Fenestrated tube drains appear to function better in the abdominal cavity. Drains in the peritoneal cavity should usually be removed within 24 to 48 hours postoperatively (McIlwraith 1980).

Following closure of the linea alba, the subcutaneous musculature and tissue are closed with a simple continuous pattern of absorbable suture material. Subcuticular sutures may be placed in selected cases where necessary. Skin is closed with either a Ford interlocking continuous pattern using nonabsorbable material or any pattern providing a quick and secure skin closure. Metal skin staples have been used with excellent results. If the chief surgeon is tired, it may improve the wound healing process if another surgeon is allowed to close.

In the paramedian and flank approaches, the peritoneum and deep sheath of the rectus muscle are usually closed together. In the paramedian approach, the superficial sheath of the rectus muscle is closed in the same manner as in the linea alba, ensuring intimate contact of fascia to fascia. Any fat or muscle between this apposition will greatly weaken the repair. Closure of the fascial layers and muscles in the flank incision is routine using a continuous pattern of absorbable sutures. A subcutaneous drain may be placed between the internal and external abdominal oblique muscles to reduce seroma formation. Skin is closed with a continuous pattern using nonabsorbable material. Care must be taken in inverting suture knot ends in subcutaneous tissue so that they do not protrude through the apposed skin edges.

Postoperative Care

The use of some form of abdominal support during the recovery phase and immediate postoperative period has been advocated to provide added wound support during the time of extra tension and to reduce postoperative wound edema, especially for incisions in the ventral midline (Coffman et al. 1969).

During the immediate postoperative phase, the patient should be allowed to recover as quickly as possible but should not be encouraged to stand before it is able to do so. Placement in a warm, well-ventilated, quiet, padded, and dimly lit recovery stall with observation windows is an excellent way to allow the patient to recover. While in the recovery room, the horse should be supplied with oxygen at flow rates of 6 to 10 liters/min via either a demand valve or an intranasal tube. It has been theorized that a demand valve will increase the Pao_2 levels beyond those obtained with an intranasal tube owing to increased pulmonary pressure when using the demand valve. Once the horse is up, a nasal tube can still be attached with high flow rates to offer the best possibility of good tissue oxygenation.

As soon as the animal is recovered and out of the recovery room, blood samples should be taken for acid-base determination as well as for PCV values. Fluids may well have to be continued in the stall after recovery, and bicarbonate may also be required. Continuance of other supportive therapy such as antibiotics should be as scheduled.

Once the patient is returned to its stall and in a suitable state, a nasogastric tube should be passed to deflate the stomach if any distension exists. After adequate recovery, limited controlled hand walking often brightens the horse and may help to counteract postoperative intestinal ileus.

In most cases, postoperative analgesics are not indicated, but if they are, phenylbutazone or flunixin meglumine would be good choices and the latter especially so if any possibility of endotoxic shock exists.

Careful monitoring of the patient's status for 48 hours postsurgery is essential. Feed may have to be withheld for 48 hours or longer. If it is eager to drink, offer limited amounts of water at frequent intervals until the patient's thirst is satisfied, after which water ad lib can be supplied. Electrolytes can be added to the drinking water. However, some horses will refuse to drink supplemented water and should be given fresh water rather than be allowed to dehydrate. Electrolyte imbalances may occur, and sodium, potassium, and chloride levels should be monitored for the first few days, although normally, once the patient has eaten a little hay, these imbalances, especially potassium, quickly disappear. Overexuberant administration of sodium-containing fluids may result in hypernatremia. To avoid this, it is suggested that these solutions be diluted to reduce the sodium content by 50 per cent. Hypokalemia is often present postoperatively owing to a multitude of metabolic and dietary factors and is aggravated by the administration of sodium or glucose. If administration of potassium is to be done intravenously, it should be done slowly and carefully owing to its effect on the myocardium. Since the great majority of potassium is absorbed via the gastrointestinal tract and hay is rich in this element, as soon as the horse starts to eat good quality hay the potassium level should return to normal. Daily blood counts should be made for any indications of an inflammatory or infectious process. A precipitous drop in leukocytes should also be noted, as this may herald a calamitous *Salmonella* infection. Other blood values of interest are total protein and the albumin:globulin ratio (Evans 1977; 1976; 1974). Note should be made of frequency and quantity of urine voided as well as any defecation of the patient.

It goes without saying that a meticulous and sequential record should be maintained of all the indices, treatments, and findings for the patient from the time of admission until discharge. Not only will this show the patient's progress, but it will be very useful in the unfortunate event of any litigation.

Sutures can be removed in 7 to 18 days postoperatively and should not be left in too long, causing suture fistulae or abscesses.

Among the commonest complications following celiotomy in the horse are incisional herniation, peritonitis, wound dehiscence, diarrhea, adhesions, laminitis, rhabdomyolysis, suture abscessation or fistulation, and death. These complications are greatly influenced by any of the following:

1. *Time*. How quickly the diagnosis was made and the correct treatment initiated greatly influences the outcome. How quickly the actual surgical procedure was performed also has a bearing on the prognosis.

2. *Skill*. A team of competent professionals is required if any encouraging results from abdominal surgery in the horse are to be expected.

3. *Asepsis*. Contamination both before and during surgery greatly affects the prognosis.

4. *Trauma*. Careful atraumatic tissue handling enhances wound healing.

5. *Equipment*. Although it is not essential to have a huge armamentarium of equipment, it will improve the prognosis to have suitable facilities and to be able to do some basic monitoring of the vital signs as well as to be able to reverse any fluid deficit, shock, or acid-base problems that may be present. Adequate ventilation is also an integral part of a successful outcome.

6. *Monitoring*. Postoperative vigilance pays handsome dividends.

7. *Exercise*. Controlled postoperative exercise will hasten the return to normal.

8. *Drugs*. Administration of medicaments to encourage peristalsis may be attempted; dexpanthenol has been useful, and the stronger cholinergic drugs may be indicated following surgery of the bowel.

9. *Pain*. Some postoperative pain may need to be controlled and, if so, may be done via phenylbutazone, flunixin meglumine, or xylazine in light doses.

10. *Diet*. Laxative feeds should be recommended for the immediate postsurgical period. Wheaten bran is an excellent mild laxative and should be included in the diet for a while. It is not a bad idea to offer bran to any horse on a regular basis to keep the ingesta from becoming too hard and dry.

11. *Rhabdomyolysis*. Myositis may be a problem, especially when horses have had extended periods of recumbency. Careful attention must be paid to adequate padding between the horse and the supports. Although this problem is very closely related to the time taken for surgery, other factors also play a role—ventilation, anoxia, acidosis, tissue perfusion, blood pressure, venous return, and support for the hind legs. During any lengthy recumbency in the equine patient, the upper hind leg should be supported during lateral recumbency and the hind legs should not be fixed in extension during dorsal recumbency, thus compromising the femoral nerve. In any recumbent animal, the legs should be moved and repositioned from time to time during a lengthy procedure.

12. *Sutures*. Prompt and complete removal of all nonabsorbable sutures will reduce wound problems.

13. *Housing*. Careful control of patient admissions and rigid cleaning and antisepsis should lessen the risk of postoperative infections from the environment.

14. *Recovery*. A violent recovery following weaning from the anesthetic machine places a tremendous stress on both the wound sutures and the patient's metabolic reserves. Often this stormy period is potentiated by hypoxemia, which may be aggravated by slowed drug degradation from hepatitis, release of endotoxin into the circulation, acidosis, and muscle ischemia due to body position (Garner et al. 1977). Careful intra- and postoperative oxygenation, ventilation, and perfu-

Table 15–5 OUTLINE OF PROTOCOL FOR EQUINE COLIC SURGERY CASES

History

Owner and any other handlers fully describe symptoms; any prior attacks; any previous treatment (if so, what and how did this work); any other veterinarians involved (if yes, consult them)

Feed and feeding regimen—feed on floor, recent changes, etc.

Vices

Housing and environs—sandy area, rubber fencing; weather

Exercise program and any recent changes

Teeth floated recently—quidding

Frequency, quality, and nature of feces and urine

Any other horses in the same stable showing similar symptoms

Other related facts—stallion just been breeding, recently returned from show, etc.

Physical Exam
  General
    Evidence, type, and magnitude of pain; any unusual posture or acts of horse—looking at flank, rolling, stretching, straining, depressed, trembling, sweating; any evidence of contusions
    Hydration—skin elasticity, sunken eyes, PCV, TP, osmolarity
    Temperature—take rectally and feel extremities
    Mucous membranes—color, injected, icterus, refill time < 3 secs
    Urine—amount, color, pH, consistency
    Blood—CBC, WBC, differential count, gram stain, electrolytes, acid-base balance, pH, enzymes, lactate
  Cardiovascular
    Heart rate, character, any pulse deficit (linguofacial), murmurs, arrhythmias, digital pulse (laminitis)
    Any evidence of shock or impending shock
  Gastrointestinal
    Auscultate entire abdomen on both sides
    Insert nasogastric tube for decompression—check volume, pH, nature, abdominal distension
    Abdominal paracentesis—gross and microscopic evaluation
    Rectal examination—thorough and careful palpation including bladder, uterus, broad ligament, inguinal rings

Procedure
  Anesthesia
    Decompress stomach
    Evaluate fluid, electrolyte, acid-base statuses
    Prep surgical site
    Ready suitable induction and inhalant anesthetic; padding and positioning
    EKG evaluation
    Ventilation
    Careful monitoring of vital signs
  Surgery
    Perform skillfully and quickly
  Recovery
    Oxygenation—careful weaning from ventilator for quiet, controlled, and uneventful recovery
    Support wound, if necessary
  Postoperative
    Oxygenate
    Provide water, feed, electrolytes; laxative diet; regulated, controlled exercise; antibiotics
    Monitor carefully
    Control pain

---

sion should reduce this problem. Sudden disconnection of the patient from the respirator may cause severe hypoxemia and should be avoided. Oxygen insufflation must begin immediately after disconnection to be of value.

15. *Hernias.* Incisional herniation is not usually an emergency problem and thus can usually be handled on an elective basis. Some support provided to the wound in the form of an abdominal bandage, at least during the recovery stage, may help. Extensive hernias may have to be repaired with the assistance of synthetic mesh implants to reduce the deficit (Scott 1979).

With the knowledge, equipment, drugs, and skill available to every veterinary surgeon, abdominal surgery in the horse is a rational and proper treatment choice if indicated by the correct diagnosis. It is hoped that this incomplete discussion will stimulate further thought and will encourage the competent and adventurous surgeon to regard celiotomy in the horse as a routine procedure.

In Table 15–5, a protocol for admitting horses with abdominal problems is offered as a skeleton on which to construct a methodical and logical diagnosis and treatment regimen for equine colic surgery patients in veterinary practice.

REFERENCES

Abramowitz, H. B., and Butcher, H. R., Jr.: Everting and inverting anastomoses: An experimental study of comparative safety. Am. J. Surg. 121:52, 1971.

Adams, S. B., Fessler, J. F., and Rebar, A. H.: Cytologic interpretation of peritoneal fluid in the evaluation of equine abdominal crises. Cornell Vet. 70(3):232, 1980.

Adams, S. B., and McIlwraith, C. W.: Abdominal crisis in the horse: A comparison of pre-surgical evaluation with surgical findings and results. Vet. Surg. 7:63, 1978.

Adloff, M., Arnaud, J.-P., and Beehary, S.: Stapled vs. sutured colorectal anastomosis. Arch. Surg. 115:1436, 1980.

Alexander, F.: Certain aspects of the physiology and pharmacology of the horse's digestive tract. Equine Vet. J. 4:166, 1972.

Arnold, J. S., and Meagher, D. M.: Management of rectal tears in the horse. J. Equine Med. Surg. 2:64, 1978.

Barber, S. M.: Case report: Torsion of the uterus—a cause of colic in the mare. Can. Vet. J. 20:165, 1979.

Barclay, W. P., Foerner, J. J., and Phillips, T. N.: Volvulus of the large colon in the horse. JAVMA 171(7):629, 1980.

Bennett, D. G.: Predisposition to abdominal crisis in the horse. JAVMA 161(11):1189, 1972.

Blue, M. G.: Enteroliths in horses—a retrospective study of 30 cases. Equine Vet. J. 11(2):76, 1979.

Bowen, J. M.: Are corticosteroids useful in shock therapy? JAVMA 177(5):453, 1980.

Byars, T. D., and White, N. A.: Plasminogen/fibrin degradation products in normal horses: Diagnostic relevance to the equine abdominal crisis. Abstract. Research proposal, University of Georgia, 1977.

Coffman, J. R.: Diagnosis and management of acute abdominal diseases in the horse (Part 1). VM/SAC 65:669, 1970.

Coffman, J. R., Fishburn, F. J., Finocchio, E. J., and Johnson, J. H.: An abdominal support for horses. VM/SAC 64:780, 1969.

Coffman, J. R., and Garner, H. E.: Acute abdominal diseases of the horse. JAVMA 161(11):1195, 1972.

Delahanty, D. D.: Colics. Paper presented to the Arizona Veterinary Medical Association, Mesa, Arizona, December 1965.

Donawick, W. J.: Metabolic management of the horse with acute abdominal crisis. Arch. A.C.V.S. IV:39, 1975a.

Donawick, W. J.: Pre-operative diagnosis, evaluation and initial treatment of equine gastrointestinal obstructive disease. In Gastrointestinal

Proceedings of the A.C.V.S. Annual Forum, October 1975b.

Donawick, W. J., Ramberg, C. F., Paul, S. R., and Hiza, M. A.: The diagnostic and prognostic value of lactate determinations in horses with acute abdominal crisis. J. South Afr. Vet Assoc. 46(1):127, 1975.

Donawick, W. J., and Stewart, J. V.: Resection of diseased ileum in the horse. JAVMA 159(9):1146, 1971.

Downs, D. W., and Lundvall, R. L.: A review of colic in the equine arising from impaction of the cecum. Senior Paper, Iowa State University, 1972.

Evans, L. H.: Postoperative patient care following abdominal colic surgery. A.C.V.S. Fifth Surgical Forum, October 1977.

Evans, L. H.: Closure of the abdomen and postoperative patient care following abdominal colic surgery. A.C.V.S. Fourth Surgical Forum, October 1976.

Evans, L. H.: Postoperative patient care following abdominal colic surgery. A.C.V.S. Second Surgical Forum, October 1974.

Ferraro, G. L.: Diagnosis and treatment of sand colic in the horse. VM/SAC 68:736, 1973.

Freeman, D. E., Koch, D. B., and Boles, C. L.: Mesodiverticular bands as a cause of small intestinal strangulation and volvulus in the horse. JAVMA 175(10):1089, 1977.

Garner, H. E., Moore, J. N., Amend, J. T., Johnson, J. H., Tritschler, L. G., Traver, D. S., and Coffman, J. R.: Post-operative management of hypoxia in the equine abdominal crisis. In Proceedings of the American Association of Equine Practitioners:177, 1977.

Gay, C. C., Speirs, V. C., Christie, B. A., Smyth, B., and Parry, B.: Foreign body obstruction of the small colon in six horses. Equine Vet. J. 11(1):60, 1979.

Gentry, P. A., and Black, W. D.: Evaluation of Harleco CO_2 apparatus: Comparison with the Van Slyke method. JAVMA 167(2):156, 1975.

Getty, S. M., Ellis, D. J., Krenhbiel, J. D., and Whitenack, D. L.: Rubberized fencing as a gastrointestinal obstruction in a young horse. VM/SAC 71:221, 1976.

Gideon, L. A.: Staple sutures for bowel surgery in the horse (a film presentation). In Proceedings of the American Association of Equine Practitioners:127, 1975.

Grant, B. D., and Tennant, B.: Volvulus associated with Meckel's diverticulum in the horse. JAVMA 162(7):550, 1973.

Greatorex, J. C.: The clinical diagnosis of colic in the horse. Equine Vet. J. 4:182, 1972.

Hamilton, D. P., and Hardenbrook, H. J.: Abdominal paracentesis in the horse. VM/SAC 68:519, 1973.

Johnson, J. H.: Surgical considerations of the abdomen: Newborn foals. VM/SAC 65:614, 1970a.

Johnson, J. H.: Surgical approaches to the abdomen in the horse. VM/SAC 65:836, 1970b.

Katz, S., Wahab, A., Murray, W., and Williams, L. F.: New parameters of viability in ischemic-bowel disease. Am. J. Surg. 127:136, 1974.

Kvart, C.: An ultrasonic method for indirect blood pressure measurement in the horse. J. Equine Med. Surg. 3:16, 1979.

Leeds, E. B.: The evaluation of the abdomen of the trauma patient. In Proceedings of the A.C.V.S. Forum, Shock and Trauma, 1974.

Linerode, P. A., and Goode, R. L.: The effects of colic on the microbial activity of the equine large intestine. In Proceedings of the American Association of Equine Practitioners, 1970.

Littlejohn, A.: The surgical relief of intestinal obstruction in horses: A review. II. The effects of intestinal obstruction. Br. Vet. J. 121:568, 1965.

Loomis, W. K.: The practitioner's approach to the handling of the acute abdominal crisis. In Proceedings of the American Association of Equine Practitioners, 1975.

Marcenac, N.: Laparotomie chez les equides. Rec. Med. Vet. 126:129, 1950.

McClure, J. R., McClure, J. J., and Usenik, E. A.: Disseminated intravascular coagulation in ponies with surgically induced strangulation obstruction of the small intestine. Vet. Surg. 8:78, 1979.

McIlwraith, C. W.: Surgical approaches to the equine abdomen. A.C.V.S. Annual Forum, October 1980.

Meagher, D. M.: Intestinal strangulations in the horse. Arch. A.C.V.S. 4:59, 1975.

Meagher, D. M.: Surgery of the large intestine in the horse. Arch. A.C.V.S. 3:9, 1974a.

Meagher, D. M.: Surgery of the small intestine in the horse. Arch. A.C.V.S. 3:3, 1974b.

Merritt, A. M.: Normal and abnormal function of the equine gastrointestinal tract. In Proceedings of the 7th Annual Forum, A.V.C.S., Gastrointestinal Section, 1979.

Milne, D. W., Tarr, M. J., Lochner, F. K., McAllister, E. S., Muir, W. W., and Skarda, R. T.: Left dorsal displacement of the colon in the horse. J. Equine Med. Surg. 1:47, 1977.

Milne, F. J.: Equine abdominal surgery—in retrospect. Equine Vet. J. 4:175, 1972.

Milne, F. J.: Equine abdominal surgery technics. In Proceedings of the American Association of Equine Practitioners, 1961.

Moore, J. N., Owen, R. R., and Lumsden, J. H.: Clinical evaluation of blood lactate levels in equine colic. Equine Vet. J. 8(2):49, 1976.

Nelson, A.: Intestinal infarction. In Proceedings of the American Association of Equine Practitioners:35, 1964.

Nelson, A. W., Collier, J. R., and Griner, L. A.: Acute surgical colonic infarction in the horse. Am. J. Vet. Res. 29(2):315, 1968.

Peterson, F. B., Donawick, W. J., Merritt, A. M., Raker, C. W., Reid, C. F., and Rooney, J. R.: Gastric stenosis in a horse. JAVMA 160(3):328, 1972.

Peterson, F. B., and Stewart, J. V.: Experimental ileocecal anastomosis in the horse. J. Equine Med. Surg. 2:461, 1978.

Poth, E. J., and Gold, D.: Intestinal anastomosis: A unique technic. Am. J. Surg. 116:643, 1968.

Reinertson, E. L.: Comparison of three techniques for intestinal anastomosis in Equidae. JAVMA 169(2):208, 1976.

Robertson, J. T.: Evaluation—medical or surgical colic. A.C.V.S. Annual Forum, October 1980.

Rollins, J. B., and Clement, T. H.: Observations on incidence of equine colic in a private practice. Equine Prac. 1(5):39, 1979.

Rooney, J. R.: Volvulus, strangulation, and intussusception in the horse. Cornell Vet. 55(4):644, 1965.

Schneider, J. E., Kennedy, G. A., and Leipold, H. W.: Muscular hypertrophy of the small intestine in a horse. J. Equine Med. Surg. 3:226, 1979.

Scott, E. A.: Repair of incisional hernias in the horse. JAVMA 11:1203, 1979.

Scott, E. A.: Surgery of the equine cecum and colon. A.C.V.S. Annual Forum, October 1977.

Seckington, I. M.: Treatment of colic from a practitioner's point of view. Equine Vet. J. 4:188, 1972.

Shires, G. M. H.: A temporary diverting loop colostomy for management of rectal tears. In Proceedings of the Annual Meeting of A.C.V.S., February 1981.

Shires, G. M. H.: An overview of equine abdominal disorders—colic. A.C.V.S. Annual Forum, 1977.

Stashak, T. S., and Knight, A. P.: Temporary diverting colostomy for the management of small colon tears in the horse: A case report. J. Equine Med. Surg. 2:196, 1978.

Tennant, B. C.: Equine gastroenterology. In Proceedings of the A.C.V.S. Annual Forum, Gastrointestinal Section, 1975.

Valdez, H., Scrutchfield, W. L., and Taylor, T. S.: Peritoneal lavage in the horse. JAVMA 175(4):388, 1979.

Vaughan, J. T.: Surgical approaches, exploration and closures of the horse's abdomen. A.C.V.S. Annual Forum, 1979.

Vaughan, J. T.: Exploratory laparotomy. ACVS Annual Forum, 1977.

Vaughan, J. T.: Digestive disturbances in the horse: Diagnostics and indications for surgical intervention. In Proceedings of the American Association of Equine Practitioners:294, 1970.

White, N. A., Moore, J. N., and Trim, C. A.: Mucosal alterations in experimentally induced small intestinal strangulation obstruction in ponies. Am. J. Vet. Res. 41(2):193, 1980.

Wright, A. I.: Verminous arteritis as a cause of colic in the horse. Equine Vet. J. 4:169, 1972.

DIGESTIVE SURGERY IN THE SHEEP AND GOAT

DON E. BAILEY, D.V.M.

RECTAL PROLAPSES

Rectal prolapses occur frequently in the ovine species, most commonly in fattened lambs. Some of the etiological causes are irritation due to coccidiosis with mucosal ulceration, short tail docking, coughing due to dust and pneumonia, fly strike, heavy concentration of pelvic fat, and use of growth-promoting implants.

Surgical repair of rectal prolapse is not economically feasible in readying a lamb for market. The most practical procedure is to send lambs with rectal prolapse to slaughter if they are of market weight and are otherwise healthy.

A simple rectal prolapse usually involves only the mucosal layer of the rectum and terminal colon. A local infusion of anesthetic can be injected, with a purse-string suture of nonirritating suture material used after replacing the rectum. The anal opening should be left open enough to allow fecal passage but restrict the prolapse.

Complete prolapse of the rectum involving 4 to 24 inches of colon requires amputation of the prolapse. A caudal epidural anesthetic is preferred to general anesthesia.

A caudal epidural is rather difficult to perform in ovine and caprine species. A 1-in, 20-gauge needle is inserted between the last sacral and first coccygeal vertebrae or between the first and second coccygeal vertebrae. The needle is pointed cranially and inserted almost horizontally, with the point slightly lowered.

A lumbosacral epidural is much easier to perform, but the danger of shock due to pooling of the blood in the viscera is greater. With this technique, the front and hind legs are tied together to open the lumbosacral space. Care must be taken not to inject the local anesthetic into the subarachnoid space. A 1½- to 2-in., 18-gauge needle is used to inject 3 to 4 ml of 2% lidocaine.

Amputation of the rectum in cases of advanced rectal prolapse with lacerations and necrosis is done by first suturing with interrupted mattress suture around the two mucosal layers or by using rectal rings.

Commercial plastic rectal rings, homemade plastic, hard rubber, or plastic syringe cases are inserted into the lumen of the prolapse. The ligation sutures or elastrator bands are secured around the outside of the prolapse and up close to the body of the lamb. The ligation should fit into the groove of the ring or pipe. The distal portion of the prolapse sloughs in a few days, along with the ring.

Topical treatment of the simple mucosal prolapse consists of tannic acid, powdered alum, or granulated sugar. These compounds cause constriction and shrinking of the edematous mucosa. Long-term alcohol epidural blocks are sometimes used.

PORCINE DIGESTIVE SURGERY

BRUCE L. HULL, D.V.M.

With the exception of experimental surgery, very little is recorded concerning porcine digestive surgery. This is probably owing to the difficulty in diagnosis and the economic value of the majority of the population. Some valuable individuals do, however, warrant gastrointestinal surgery.

BLEEDING ULCERS

Ulcers are one of the most common digestive diseases of pigs. These are probably stress related. The earliest signs of ulcers in pigs are usually either brown-black tarry feces or pallor of the mucous membranes. The pig usually exhibits rapid shallow respirations at this time and becomes completely anorectic and gaunt. Temperature is rarely elevated and is more likely normal or subnormal. Bleeding ulcers may cause acute death with no premonitory signs.

It is impossible to tell if the ulcers are single or multiple on the basis of clinical evaluation. Multiple ulcers can cover the entire glandless area of the cardia. If the value of the pig makes surgery feasible, a blood transfusion (if available) or a transfusion of plasma extenders should be started before surgery. Inhalation anesthesia with halothane is the anesthesia of choice.

A ventral midline incision from the xiphoid caudal provides the best exposure to the stomach. The serosal surface should be evaluated for changes in texture or appearance, which could indicate the location of the ulcer. If the ulcerated area can be located, it is elevated with bowel clamps or stay sutures and the abdomen is packed off. The stomach should then be gently emptied, avoiding abdominal contamination, and the mucosal surface inspected for any additional ulcers. If the ulceration is profuse or generalized, there is very little that can be done. Solitary ulcers can be surgically dissected, the edges cauterized, and the defect in the wall closed with an inverting suture of 0 chromic catgut. If, because of location, the ulcer is impossible to dissect, it may be coagulated with electrocautery. The wall of the stomach is then closed with two layers of an inverting suture. The abdomen is then closed in a routine manner.

INTESTINAL OBSTRUCTIONS

Intestinal obstruction caused by foreign bodies, intussusceptions, and volvulus does occur in pigs but is rarely diagnosed in the live animal. Incarcerated hernias do occur and are more easily diagnosed. Signs of intestinal obstruction include vomiting, decrease in amount of feces, abdominal distension, and depression. Blood and diptheritic membranes may be passed in the feces in the case of intussusception. Again, economic value often precludes surgery.

If, however, surgery is indicated, it will usually be in the nature of an exploratory laparotomy to achieve a definitive diagnosis. The ventral midline approach with the pig restrained in dorsal recumbency is ideal for this. Once a definitive diagnosis is achieved, intestinal surgery for relief of the condition would be as described for the other species.

ATRESIA ANI (Figure 15–186)

Atresia ani is probably the most important cause of intestinal obstruction in the porcine. Atresia ani is more prevalent in pigs than in other domestic animals. As the pig vomits easily, it will often not

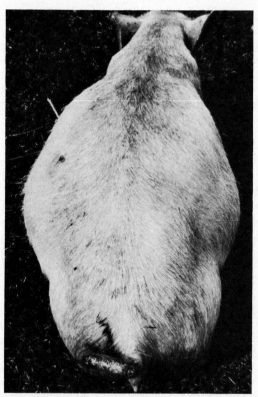

Figure 15–186 Atresia ani in a pig.

show signs of atresia until it is three to four weeks of age. The signs include abdominal distension and a slower growth rate than the littermates. The most significant finding on examination is the absence of an anal opening.

Pigs older than one month of age but showing similar signs should be suspected of having a rectal stricture. These pigs usually have an anal opening; however, this opening comes to a blind end at a variable distance in from the anus. The blind end can usually be confirmed by taking the animal's temperature or by digital examination. Most cases of rectal stricture occur secondary to a rectal prolapse that has constricted after repair or slough, but a possible infectious rectal stricture has been reported (Lillie, Olander, and Gallina 1973). Rectal stricture may respond to surgical procedures similar to those used for atresia ani. Therefore, the two entities will be discussed together.

In cases of atresia ani, there may be a bulge beneath the tail or, in the female, there may be a rectovaginal fistula allowing the feces to come out through the vagina. With local anesthetic infiltration, a ring of skin is removed over the bulging rectum. At this point the rectum can be crudely lanced, or it may be sutured to the skin and gently opened to create a new anal opening. If there is no bulge in the skin over the rectum, deep pelvic dissection may be attempted. However, the rectum, as well as the anus, is often atretic, and the distended rectum cannot be located and exteriorized. In these cases, abdominal surgery and a colostomy can be performed, but the economic benefits of such procedures are doubtful.

The rectal stricture can often be manually dilated. If this is accomplished, one must remember to redilate the rectum at least every other day for 10 to 14 days to assure continued patency. If the stricture is too extensive or too firm for dilation, one should attempt retraction and resection of the strictured portion with suturing of the viable rectum to the skin at the anus. Again, a colostomy can be considered, but the economic benefits are doubtful.

RECTAL PROLAPSE

Rectal prolapse is probably the most common gastrointestinal procedure in the porcine. The etiology of rectal prolapse may well be multifactorial. Diarrhea is probably the most implicated cause, but diet, cough, and piling up in cold weather have also been implicated.

The simplest procedure for rectal prolapse is replacement and retention with a purse-string suture. This procedure should only be used when the rectal mucosa seems to be viable. The edematous rectum is gently massaged and forced back through the anal sphincter. A finger is used to be sure that the rectum is completely back into the normal position. The purse-string suture should then be placed outside the anal sphincter. A general rule of thumb in the porcine is to leave a one-finger opening into the rectum. This is large enough to permit fecal passage but is usually small enough to prevent prolapse. Nonabsorbable suture should be used for the purse-string, and it should be left in place for four to five days.

If the mucosa is too necrotic to replace

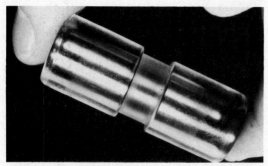

Figure 15–187 The prolapse ring, used for complete amputation of the rectum.

and suture, one should perform a submucosal resection. Two circumferential incisions through the mucosa are made: one at the proximal portion of the prolapse and one at the distal portion of the prolapse. A longitudinal incision is used to connect these two circumferential incisions, and the mucosa is peeled off, revealing the white fibrous submucosa. The proximal and distal portions of normal mucosa can then be sutured together with interrupted sutures of 0 chromic catgut. However, this step is usually not performed in the porcine. The rectum is gently replaced, and a purse-string suture is placed for four to five days.

Complete amputation of the rectum should probably be reserved for cases of severe laceration, which precludes replacement. Complete amputation leads to a higher incidence of rectal stricture than do other methods of correction. In complete amputation, a finger is placed into the rectal lumen and horizontal mattress sutures of nonabsorbable suture are placed at the proximal edge (anal sphincter) of the prolapse. These sutures start at the skin, go to the lumen (touch finger in the rectum), and return to the skin at the rectal sphincter, where they are firmly tied. These horizontal mattress sutures must be placed close together and an adequate number must be employed to completely circumvent the prolapse. After all the horizontal mattress sutures are placed and tied tightly to control hemorrhage, the prolapse is amputated just distal to the sutures.

An alternative method of complete amputation is to use the prolapse ring (Fig. 15–187), syringe case, or PVC tubing. This open tube is placed into the rectum

and a broad ligature, such as umbilical tape, is placed around the prolapse and pulled tightly down. The tube maintains the rectal lumen while the suture causes the prolapsed portion to slough. Instead of a suture, an elastrator ring can be used around the prolapse.

UMBILICAL HERNIA (Fig. 15–188)

When considering the etiology of umbilical hernias in the pig, one must consider heredity, although many porcine umbilical hernias are secondary to a navel infection and/or umbilical abscess. As with many other porcine surgical procedures, the cost of effective treatment may preclude surgical correction.

General anesthesia is preferred for repair of an umbilical hernia; however, a ring block around the hernia will provide the necessary anesthesia. In the male pig the penis, prepuce, and preputial diverticulum must be elevated from the hernial sac and reflected either posteriorly or to one side. In doing this, care must be exercised to avoid the penis and preputial diverticulum. The preputial diverticulum is a very thin-walled, bilobed dorsal outpouching of the prepuce and is located just posterior to the end of the sheath. As the diverticulum is thin walled, it is often difficult to locate. Therefore, in dissecting it free from the hernial sac, it is wise to dissect close to the hernial sac, which is more readily identifiable.

Once the prepuce has been reflected, dissection of the connective tissue is carried down to the hernial ring. At this

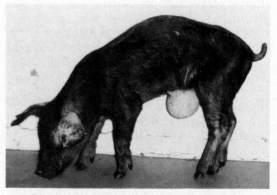

Figure 15–188 Umbilical hernia in a pig.

point the hernial sac can be removed or inverted, intact, into the abdomen. In either case the abdominal defect should be closed with an overlapping suture pattern of heavy chromic catgut or a nonabsorbable suture that has been heat sterilized. The prepuce, diverticulum, and penis are brought back into normal anatomical position and are tacked into place with absorbable sutures. After removing any excess skin, the skin wound is closed with nonabsorbable suture.

Surgical correction of umbilical hernia in the female is similar to that of the male. An elliptical incision is made around the hernial sac to remove any excess skin that might become dependent and edematous. This dissection is then carried into the hernial ring. The rest of the procedure is as is described for the male.

REFERENCE

Lillie, L. E., Olander, J. H., and Gallina, A. M.: Rectal stricture of swine. JAVMA 164(4):358, 1973.

INDEX

Note: Page numbers in italics refer to illustrations; those followed by (t) refer to tables.

Ascarid, in intestinal impaction, 606–607
Ascending reticular activating system (ARAS), 76
Ascites, cardiac impulse and, 20
Aseptic technique
electrocautery and, 781
in orthopedic surgery, 780–782
operative site draping for, 780–781
skin sterilization in, 780
suction machine use in, 781–782
Aspergillus, 1184
Aspergillus fumigatus, guttural pouch mycosis due to, 1036
Aspergillus nidulans, guttural pouch mycosis due to, 1036
Aspiration, transtracheal complications of, 471–472
instruments for, 471
Aspirin, 1196
Ataxia, 86–87, 95
in cattle, 10
in cervical vertebral malformations, 1026
Atelectasis, after surgery, 383, 384
Atlanto–occipital malformation, in horses, 721
ATP (adenosine triphosphate), 160
Atresia ani
in horses, 653–654
in swine, 682–683
Atresia recti, in horses, 653–654
Atropine sulfate, 1182, 1194
in brain surgery, 988
in keratoplasty, 1189
in shock therapy, 174–175
tumor therapy and, 1088
Auditory tube
in horses, 328
in ruminants, 346
pharyngeal opening to, 328
Auriculopalpebral nerve
facial paralysis and, 1012
in horses, 1151–1152, *1152*
Auscultation, of cardiovascular system, 22–24
Autograft, 316
Axonotmesis, and equine facial paralysis, 1013
Ayrshire cow, growth curve of, 34

Bacillaceae, 133–137
Bacillus(i)
for sarcoids, 1170
in tumor therapy, 1987
Bacillus anthracis, 133, 134(t)
Bacillus Calmette-Guérin (BCG), for sarcoids, 1170

Bacillus cereus, 133–134, 134(t)
Bacillus megaterium, 134(t)
Bacillus subtilis, 134(t)
Bacitracin, 157
and cell wall synthesis, 151(t)
Bacteria. See also specific type.
drug-resistant, 157–158
gram-negative. See *Gram-negative bacteria*.
gram-positive. See *Gram-positive bacteria*.
Bacteroidaceae, 138–139, 140–141
biochemical characteristics of, 141(t)
Bacteroides, 140
Bacteroides amylophilus, 141, 141(t)
Bacteroides clostridiiformis, 141(t)
Bacteroides nodosus, 141, 141(t)
Bacteroides putredinis, 141(t)
Bacteroides ruminicola, 141(t)
Bacteroides succinogenes, 141(t)
Balanitis
in cattle, 8
in horses, 1084
Bandage
Esmarch's, 782, 783, 784
Robert-Jones, 770–771
indications for, 771
Barbiturates, in combination anesthesia, 1093
Base
deficit of, 122
excess of, 122
loss of, metabolic acidosis and, 125
Basilar artery, in horse, 986, *987*
Basophil, 53
age factors and, 59
in goats, 69(t)
in sheep, 67(t)
stippling of, 63
in cattle, 65
BCG (bacillus Calmette-Guérin) for sarcoids, 1170
Bearing retainer, 1119
Behavior, examination of, 75–76
Bellowing, in cattle, 76
Benzocaine, 1187
Berge, nerve block technique of, 1153
Beta hemolysis, 132
due to streptococcus, 149
Beta rays, 1190
Beta-aminopropionitrile, 291
Beta-toxin, 130
Bicarbonate(s)
measurement of, 121
precursors of, 126

Bicarbonate(s) (*Continued*)
replacement therapy with, 119–120
Biceps, reflex of, 90
Biceps brachii, bilateral ossification of, 944
Biceps femoris muscle, rupture of, 944
Bile duct, carcinoma of, 236–237
Biliary tract, surgical needles for, 1230(t)
Bilirubin, of plasma, in horses, 61
Biocidal suture, 143
Biopsy
of liver, in cattle, 543
in horses, 657–658
Robson-Heggers, 148
synovial, 741–743
Black disease, 135
Bladder, urinary. See also *Urogenital system*.
in cattle, formation of stones in, 1074
neoplastic diseases of, 237
paralysis of, 1073
repair of, 1079–1080
rupture of, 1074
vaginal prolapse and, 1109–1110
paresis of, 95
prolapse of, in mare, 1136–1137
sutures for, 1227
healing, 1232
Bleeding. See *Hemorrhage*.
Blepharoplasty, 1174–1175, *1176–1178*, 1179
Blepharospasm, due to IBK, 1183
Blindfolding, of horses, 1208
Blindness, night, of Appaloosas, 77
Blink response, 77
Blinking, in equine facial paralysis, 1011
Bloat, as postoperative complication, 208
Bloat whistle, 521–522
Blood
carbon dioxide tension of, in shock, 167
cells of, examination of, 47–49
coagulation of, abnormalities of, 62
in cattle, 67
in DIC. See *Disseminated intravascular coagulation (DIC)*.
in horses, 62
crossmatching of, 55
EDTA preservation of, 48
filtration of, in lung, 371
flow of, and ventilation, 364

Calcium borogluconate, 1145
Calculi. See *Stone(s)*.
Calf(ves). See also *Cattle*.
  abomasum of, surgical
    condition of, 523
  arthrogryposis in, 501
  brachygnathism in, *498*, 501,
    501
  bull, 8
  cannon bone fractures in, 817
  cleft palate in, 501
  colonic atresia in, 551
  diaphragmatic herniation in,
    523
  erythrocyte values for, 62(t),
    62–63
  femur fractures in, 867, *868*,
    868–869, 872–873
  fibrinogen values of, 65
  foreign body ingestion by,
    541–542
  gastric resection in, 542
  humerus fractures in, 799–
    800
  in utero infection of, 76
  leukocyte values for, 64(t)
  limb deformities in, 769
  luxations in, coxofemoral,
    899
    lateral patellar, 900–901
    of stifle joint, 901–902
    of tarsal joint, 902
  monitoring of, 164–166
  omphalophlebitis of, 7
  orthopedic surgery in, 793–
    794
  plasma protein in, *39*, 65
  pyloromyotomy in, 541–542
  spiral colon in, 548, *549*
  tendons of, suturing of, 920
  tibia fractures in, 887, *888*,
    889
    prognosis for, 891
    temporary immobilization
      of, 886–887
    transfixation pinning of, 887
  umbilical herniation in, 551
Calf knee. See *Carpal bone,
  fracture of*.
Calmette-Guérin bacillus (BCG),
  in tumor therapy, 1087
Calvarium
  malformation of, 96
  radiography of, 98
Calving
  nutrition and, *29*, 29
  paresis following, 9
Canal, vertebral
  in stabilization of cervical
    spine, *1031*
  malformations of, 1024
Cancer. See *Neoplasm(s)*;
  Carcinoma.
Candida, 1184, 1186
Cannon bone, fractures of, 817–
  818
Capillary
  gas exchange in, 359

Capillary (*Continued*)
  refill time of, 20
Carbenicillin, 152(t), 156(t)
  administration of, 154(t)
Carbon dioxide
  diffusion of, 362
  exchange of, 359–362
  transport of, mechanism of,
    374
Carbon dioxide pressure,
  arterial, 365–366
Carbon dioxide tension, 121
Carcina, location of, in horse,
  340
Carcinoma. See also
  Neoplasm(s).
  and equine facial paralysis,
    1012
  basal cell, of eyelid, in horse,
    1170
  intraocular, 1196
  squamous cell, and ocular
    habronemiasis, 1171
    anesthetic techniques and,
      200
    enucleation and, 258, 260
    exophthalmos due to, 1156
    in cattle, 233, 235, 236,
      241–242
    in goats, 247–248
    in horses, 223–224, 228–
      229, *230*, 232–233, 1189–
      1190, *1191*
    in sheep, 243–247
    of abdomen, 611, *612*
    of conjunctiva, 1180
    of cornea, *1188*
    of esophagus, 597
    of eye, 232–233, 241–242,
      247
      cryosurgery for, 1192–
        1193
      hyperthermia for, 1193–
        1194
      in cattle, 1191–1192
      radiotherapy for, 1194
    of genital tract, in mares,
      1123
    of penis and prepuce in
      horse, 1086
      management of, 1087–
        1088
      surgery for, 1088–1092
    of stomach, 228–229,
      602
    vs. dermoids, 1182
Cardiac. See *Heart*.
Cardiopulmonary system
  anesthetic effects on, 356
  function in, 371–374
  organs of, 357, *358*
  species differences in, 385–
    386
  surgical problems and, 384–
    385
Cardiovascular system
  after surgery, 384
  auscultation of, 22–24

Cardiovascular system
  (*Continued*)
  cuneiform cartilage in, 329
  diseases of, 488–492
  during surgery, 386
  in cattle, 5–6
  in shock, 161, 162
  palpation of, 20
  percussion of, 20–21
  prior to surgery, 986, 988
Carotid artery
  angiogram of, *457*
  in guttural pouch mycosis,
    1035, 1036
  in horse, 986, *987*
  ligation of, 464, 465
Carotid body, 376. 378
Carotid sheath, in pigs, 354
Carotid sinus, baroreceptor in,
  373
Carpal bone
  abnormalities of, in horses,
    719
  accessory, fractures of, 813–
    814
  degenerative joint disease of,
    732
  fracture of, in horses, 719
  slab fractures of, 810–813
    carpitis-associated, 810
    postoperative treatment of,
      812–813
    radiographic examination
      of, 811, 812
    reduction of, 812
  tenosynovitis in, 935–936
Carpal canal syndrome
  clinical signs of, 934–935
  surgical treatment of, 935
Carpal joint
  arthrocentesis of, 748
  carpitis of, 807–808
  chip fractures of, 808–810
  flexural deformities of, 968–
    971
  hygroma of, 815–816
  luxation of, 814
  osteochondrosis dissecans of,
    814–815
  subchondral bone cyst of,
    814–815
Carpitis
  carpal fracture and, 810
  clinical signs of, 807
  treatment of, 807–808
Cartilage. See also specific
    types, e.g. *Cricoid cartilage*.
  articular, aging of, 708–710
    anatomy of, 691–692
    biomechanics of, 710–712
    calcified layer of, 694
    chondrocytes of, 693, 694
    collagen in, 694–695
    compressive stiffness of,
      710
    deep layer of, 694
    degenerative process in,
      729–731

Conjunctivitis (*Continued*)
  in horses, 1180
Connective tissue, tumor of, in
  sheep, 243
Contracted foal syndrome, 1016.
  See also *Foal.*
  scoliosis and, 1018
Contracted tendon. See
  Flexural deformity(ies).
Convulsions, hypomagnesemia
  and, 117
Coordination, examination of,
  76
Cornea
  carcinoma of, *1188*
  changes in, due to
    exophthalmos, 1157
  dermoids of, in cattle, 1182
    in horses, 1182
  foreign bodies in, 1182–1183
  implants and, 1158–1159
  in equine facial paralysis,
    1012, 1013
  in IBK, 1183–1184
  keratectomy of, 1187–1188
  lacerations of, 1182–1183
    repair of, *1183*
  lesions of, in horse, treatment
    for, 1187
  medication tubing and, 1153–
    1154, *1154*
  protection of, and
    tarsorrhaphy, 1166, *1167*
  sutures for, 1227
  transplantation of, in horses,
    1188–1189, *1189*
  trauma to, by vibrissae
    in cattle, 1173–1174
    in horses, 1171–1173, *1172,
      1173*
    in sheep, 1173
  ulceration of, and nictitating
    membrane, 1180
    in horses, 1180, 1184,
      1186–1187, *1187*
Corpuscles, mean volume of, 50
Corticospinal tract, anatomy of,
  997, 998
Corticosteroid(s)
  effects of, 753–754
  horse racing and, 753–754
  in cerebral edema, 988
  in degenerative joint disease
    therapy, 753–756
    beneficial effects of, 754
    detrimental effects of, 754–
      755, 756
    dosage in, 755–756
  in evaluating ataxia, 1026
  in habronemiasis, 1171
  in horses, 14–15
  in shock therapy, 172–173
  in spinal cord trauma, 1023
Corynebacterium, 138
  characteristics of, 139(t)
Corynebacterium diphtheriae,
  138

Corynebacterium equi, 138,
  139(t)
  vertebral abscess due to, 1014
*Corynebacterium pseudo-
  tuberculosis*, 129(t), 138,
  139(t), 609
  vertebral abscess due to, 1014
Corynebacterium pyogenes, 78,
  129(t), 138, 139(t), 911, 912
  vertebral abscess due to, 1014
Corynebacterium renale, 138,
  139(t)
Cosmetic surgery, 262–263. See
  also surgical site and
  specific procedure, e.g.
  Blepharoplasty.
  in cows, 1115, 1118
Costochondrial articulation,
  species differences of, 329–
  330
Cotton, sutures of, 1221(t),
  1221–1222
  construction of, 1222
  strength of, 1226
  uses of, 1225(t)
Cough, 370
Cow(s). See also *Cattle*, and
  specific breeds.
  acquired injuries in, 1111–
    1113
  cesarean section in, 1113–
    1114
  dairy. See *Dairy cow(s).*
  episiotomy in, 1115, 1118
  genital tract in
    anatomy of, 1109
    physiology of, 1109–1110
    surgical conditions of,
      1110
  Hereford, growth curve of, *34*
  Holstein Swiss, growth curve
    of, *34*
  mammary glands of, 263–271
  surgery in, restraint for, 1110
  teats of, amputation of, 270–
    271
    cannula for, 267, *268*
    contracted sphincters of,
      267
    fistula of, 269
    imperforate, 267
    lacerations of, 269, *270*
    leaking, 267
    mastitis of, 133, 270–271
    traumatic injuries to, 267–
      269
  twinning in, and freemartin
    syndrome, 1111
  urethroplasty in, 1118
  urinary tract in
    anatomy of, 1109
    physiology of, 1109–1110
    surgical conditions of, 1110
  uterine prolapse in, 1115
  vaginal prolapse in, *1114,*
    1114–1115, *1115, 1116,
    1117*

CPBA (competitive protein-
  binding assay), 1097
Cradle, in physical restraint
  of horses, 1208, *1209*
  of swine, 1217, *1218*
Cranial nerve(s), *1035*
  I, 77
  II, infection of, 78
    vitamin A deficiency and,
      77
  III, examination of, 78–81
    Horner's syndrome and, 79
    in equine facial paralysis,
      1012
    injury to, 78
    strabismus of, 79
  IV, examination of, 79–81
    in equine facial paralysis,
      1012
  V, examination of, 81–82
  VI, examination of, 79–81
    in equine facial paralysis,
      1012
  VII, anatomy of, 1010
    examination of, 82–83
  VIII, anatomy of, 1010
    examination of, 83–84
  IX, examination of, 84–85
  X, examination of, 84–85
  XI, examination of, 84–85
  XII, examination of, 85–86
  examination of, 77–86
  gluteal, paralysis of, 94
  paralysis of, 80
Craniectomy
  care following, 994
  techniques for, 990
Craniotomy
  care following, 994
  for coenurosis, 1010
  for gid, 1010
  techniques for, 990, *991–992,*
    993–994
    in horses, 993
Cranium
  anatomy of, 984, *985*
  fractures of
    classification of, 1006–1007,
      1007
    clinical findings in, 1006
    site of, 1005–1006
    treatment for, 1008
  injury to, 78
  necrosis of, 78
  surgery of, 983
Cricoid cartilage, 328
  anatomy of, in horse larynx,
    337, *337*
    in pig larynx, 353
    in ruminants, 347
Cricothyroid ligament, 328
  attachment of, in horse
    larynx, 336
  in ruminants, 347
Cricotracheal membrane,
  eversion of
    clinical signs of, 454

Fracture(s) *(Continued)*
of phalanx, of extensor process
of, 860–861
periosteal proliferation in,
850
postoperative care of, 852
radiographic evaluation of,
846, *849*
sagittal, 861–863
surgical complications of,
845–846
surgical treatment of, 845
temporary immobilization
of, 846, 854
transfixation pin use in,
850–851
wing, 861–863
of premaxilla, 896
in horses, 565–566
of proximal phalanx, 844–852
of radius, 804–807
bone grafting for, 806–807
causes of, 804
compression plating of, 805
diagnosis of, 805
full limb cast for, 806
in adult patients, 804–805
in young patients, 806
transfixation pins for, 806
of scapula, as draining
wounds, 796
in young animals, 795
occurrence of, 794–795
of body of, 795
of neck of, 795
radiographic analysis of,
795
symptoms of, 794–795
treatment of, 795–796
of second phalanx, 852–858
of sesamoid, 835–844
apical, 835–837
bilateral, 835, 840, 844
cancellous bone grafts for,
838
causes of, 835
clinical signs of, 835
of midportion of, 837–838,
839, 840
postoperative care of, 837
surgical treatment of, 835–
838, *839*, 840–844
of sustentaculum talus, 886
of tarsal bones, 884–886
fibular, 884–885
slab, 885–886
of tibia, 886–891
causes of, 886
compression plating of,
888–891
conservative management
of, 886
diagnosis of, 887
external coaptation of, 887–
888
in young animals, 886, 887,
888, 889

Fracture(s) *(Continued)*
of tibia, incomplete, 886
prognosis for, 891
temporary immobilization
of, 886–887
through proximal growth
plate, 887
transfixation pinning of, 887
of trachea, 473
slab, of tarsal bones, 885–886
spinal cord injuries and,
1021–1022
spiral, of metacarpal bones,
826–827
of metatarsal bones, 826–
827
stress, of metacarpal bones,
827–828
in horses, 720
Freemartin syndrome, 9, 1111
Frontal nerve
in cattle, *1155*
in horses, 1151, *1151*
Frontal sinus, 328
in cattle, 345
in horses, 333, *334*
in pigs, 352, *352*
FSP (fibrinogen split product),
56
Fungus, and corneal ulcers,
1184, 1186–1187
Furacin (nitrofurazone), 1050,
1052, 1059
Furosemide (Lasix), in cerebral
edema, 988
Fusiformis necrophorus, 141(t)
Fusobacterium, 140
Fusobacterium fusiforme,
antimicrobials for, 156(t)
Fusobacterium necrophorum,
141, 141(t)
vertebral abscess due to, 1014

Gag reflex, 84
Gait
abnormalities of, grading of,
87–88
ataxia of, 86–87
cranial nerve VII and, 83
dysmetria of, 87
spasticity of, 87
stringhalt-like, 93
tibial paralysis and, 93–94
weakness of, 86
Gallbladder, in cattle, anatomy
of, 542
surgery of, 543
Gamma-glutamyl transferase,
16
Ganglioneuroma, intraocular,
1196
Gangrene, of limbs, 141
Garamycin. See *Gentamycin
sulfate.*

Gas, exchange of, and
respiratory reflex, 375
in fibrotic lung, 361
in tissues, 374
in veins and arteries, 361
mechanics of, in lung, 359
regional differences of, 363,
364, 364
Gas mixture, and surgical
recovery, 383
Gastritis
Gastrophilus larvae and, 601
pyloric stenosis and, in horses,
602
traumatic, case history of,
513–514
complications of, 514–515
diagnosis of, 513
in cattle, 513–514, 515
nonsurgical treatment of,
515
symptoms of, 513
treatment of, 514, 515
Gastrocentesis, 538–539
Gastrocnemius muscle
lacerations of, 928, 929
ruptures of, 928, 929
Gastroenteropathy,
phenylbutazone and, 14
Gastrointestinal tract. See
Digestive tract. See also
specific organs, e.g., *Small
intestine.*
Gastrophilus, 652
Gastrophilus intestinalis, 601
Gelatin sponge(s)
in cranial fractures, 1008
in laminectomy procedures,
1026
in neurosurgery, 989, 993
Gelding, of horses, 16
General anesthetic, 202–204.
See also *Anesthesia.*
for ovine cesarean section,
1120
in combination anesthesia,
1093
Genital tract. See also
Urogenital system and
associated organs.
neoplastic disease of, 230, 239
of cows, anatomy of, 1109
physiology of, 1109–1110
surgery of, 1110
sutures for, 1227
Gentamycin sulfate (garamycin), 152(t), 155, 156(t),
157
administration of, 154(t)
inactivation of, 155
Gid
diagnosis of, 1009–1010
treatment for, 1010
Gingivitis, in horses, 1012
Glaucoma
in cattle, 1199
in horses, 1198–1199

Hernia(s) (*Continued*)
  inguinal, in pigs, repair of,
    1081
  inguinal-scrotal, in cattle, 552
  internal, broad ligament in,
    620
    definition of, 618
    epiploic foramen
      incarceration in, 618–619
    in horses, 618–620
    mesenteric defects in, 619–
      620
    omental defects in, 620
    pedunculated lipoma in, 620
  of abdomen, in cattle, 551–
    552
  peritoneopericardial, 621–622
  scrotal, 620–621
    in cattle, 1070
  surgery for. See
    Herniorrhaphy.
  surgical mesh for, 1232
  umbilical, 621
    in calves, 551
    in foal, 1146
    in swine, 684–685
  ventral, 621
Herniorrhaphy
  castration and, 1101–1102
  in horse, 1101–1102
  inguinal, in cattle, 1066–1069
    diagnosis of, 1066, 1067,
      1066
    procedure for, 1067, *1068*,
      1069
    types of, 1066
Herpes virus, type I, in horses. 95
Hetrazan (diethylcarbamazine
  citrate), 1195
High ringbone, 858–860
Hilus, of lung, in horses, 341
Hind limb
  angular deformities of, 961–
    968
    diaphyseal dysplasia as, 963
    due to hypoplasia, 961
    due to inadequate cuboidal
      bone ossification, 961
    epiphyseal dysplasia as, 963
    femur fractures and, 964,
      966
    growth plate injuries and,
      963, 964–965, *967*, 968
    metaphyseal dysplasia as,
      961–963
    pelvic fractures and, 963,
      964
    slipped capital femoral
      epiphysis and, 963–964
  examination of, 91–94
  femur fractures of, 867–873
  hock joint of, 878–886
  orthopedic conditions of, 866–
    893
  patella fractures of, 866–867
  pelvis, fractures and, 891–893

Hind limb (*Continued*)
  stifle joint, fractures and,
    873–878
  tarsal bones, fractures and,
    883–886
  tibia, fractures and, 886–890
Hip, innervation of, 703
Hip dysplasia, in horses, 722
Histamines, deactivation of, 371
Hobble, for restraint
  of cattle, 1213, *1213*
  of horses, 1205, *1205*, 1208
  of swine, 1217
Hock, flexion of, 93–94
Hock joint, 878–882
  bone spavin of, 878–880
  cunean tendon bursitis-tarsitis
    syndrome of, 880
  fractures of, 882–883
  osteochondrosis dissecans of,
    880–882
    clinical signs of, 880
    pathogenesis of, 882
    surgical treatment of, 881–
      882
  sustenaculum talus fractures
    in, 886
  tarsal bone collapse in, 883–
    884
    clinical signs of, 883–884
    treatment of, 884
  tarsal bone fractures in, 884–
    886
    fibular, 884–885
    slab-type, 885–886
Holstein cow
  body condition of, *31*
  feeding of, 39
  hematological values for, 63(t)
Holstein Swiss cow, growth
  curve of, *34*
Honda, for restraint
  of cattle, 1211
  of swine, 1215
Hoof disease, lameness due to,
  in cattle, 536
Hormone(s)
  cryptorchidism and, 1096,
    1097
  HCG test for, 1097–1098
  influence of, in cervical
    vertebral malformation,
    1024
Horn(s)
  anesthetic block of, 200
  removal of. See *Dehorning.*
Horner's syndrome
  differential diagnosis of, 1012
  in cattle, 79
  in guttural pouch mycosis,
    1036
  in horses, 79
Horse(s). See also *Mare(s);
  Foal*; and specific breeds.
  abscess in, of abdomen, 609–
    611, 639

Horses(s) (*Continued*)
  anemia of, 61
  anesthesia for, 177
    administration equipment
      for, 198–199
    anesthetic agents for, 178–
      183
    anesthetic concentrations
      for, 181
    anesthetic maintenance in,
      190–191
    circulatory system effects
      of, 179, 181
    delivery apparatus for, 183–
      187
    delivery of, 187–188
    general principles of, 188–
      192
    inhalation, 177–194
    intravenous, 194–199
    patient evaluation in, 188–
      189
    postanesthetic period and,
      191–192
    preanesthetic period and,
      188–189
    respiratory system effects
      of, 181–182
    side effects of, 182–183
    tracheal intubation in,
      190
  angular deformities in, 964,
    966
  anorexia of, 34, 61
  Arabian, 57
  arteritis in, 624, 625
  arthritis in, traumatic, 716–
    717
  arthrogryposis in, 688, *689*
  arthus-mediated immunity of,
    28
  arytenoid chondritis in, 450–
    454
  atlanto-occipital malformation
    in, 721
  atresia ani in, 653–654
  atresia recti in, 653–654
  auditory tube of, 328
  bilateral ossification of biceps
    brachii in, 944
  bilirubin in, *35*
  blood coagulation of, 62
  brachycardia in, 23
  brachygnathism in, 558, 560
  bucked shins of, 827–828
  cannon bones of, fractures of,
    817–818, 820
  cardiovascular disease in,
    congenital, 488
  carpal bone fractures in, 810–
    813
    chip, 808–810
  carpal bone of, abnormalities
    of, 719
  carpal canal syndrome in,
    934–935

Joint(s) (*Continued*)
  synovial, anatomy of, 995
  traumatic injury to, in horses,
    718–719
Jugular vein, engorgement of,
  in cattle, 5, 6

Kanamycin, 151(t), 152(t),
    156(t)
  in brain surgery, 988
  in vertebral osteomyelitis,
    1015
Kebsis, of dairy cows, 37
Keith's bundle, surgical needles
    for, 1230(t)
Keratectomy, 1192
  and dermoids, 1182
  in fungal infections, 1186
  superficial, 1187–1188
Keratitis
  due to fungus, 1184
  exposure, 1156
Keratitis sicca, in equine facial
    paralysis, 1012
Keratoconjunctivitis, in horses,
    1180
Keratoplasty, in horses, 1188–
    1189, *1189*
Ketamine, 196–197, 198
  for caprine cesarean section,
    1121
Ketamine hydrochloride, in
    combination anesthesia,
    1093, 1094
Ketonemia, 26
Ketosis, in digestive tract
    diseases, in cattle, 498
Kidney(s)
  and pH regulation, 366
  neoplastic disease of, in
    cattle, 237
  removal of, 1080, 1110
  surgical needles for, 1229
Kirby-Bauer susceptibility
    method, 151
Kirschner-Ehmer splint, 794,
    896
Klebsiella pneumoniae, 139–
    140
  antimicrobials for, 156(t)
Kligers iron agar, biochemical
    reactions on, 139(t)
Knots, surgical, security of,
    1223
Knowles forceps, 1137, 1138
Kyphoscoliosis
  definition of, 1016
  occurrence of, 1018–1019
Kyphosis
  definition of, 1016
  due to trauma, 88
  occurrence of, 1018–1019
  of spinal cord, 92

Laboratory report form, 47–48

Laceration(s)
  in cattle, 257–258
  of cornea, 1182–1183, *1183*
  of tongue, 501
Lacrimal gland
  hyperactivity of. See
    Epiphora.
  in horses, acquired conditions
    of, 1164–1165
  anatomy of, 1160–1163
  congenital obstructions of,
    1163–1164
  evaluation of, 1161–1162,
    1162
  worms in, in cattle, 1180,
    1182
  in horses, 1180, 1182
Lacrimal nerve, in horses,
    1152
Lacrimal punctum, in horses,
    stenosis of, 1164, *1164*
Lacrimal sinus, 328
  in pigs, 352–353
Lacrimation, 82
  and facial paralysis, in horses,
    1012
  excess of. See *Epiphora.*
Lactation, and leukocyte
    response, 52
Lactic acid, shock and, 121
Lactic acidosis, 126
Lamb
  suckling of, 39
  vertebral abscesses in, 1014
Lambert suture, 1133, 1147
Lameness
  bovine. See *Spastic paresis.*
  diagnosis of, 9
  in DJD, conformational
    effects and, 719
    severity of, 735
  in goats, 19
  in sheep, 19
  muscle fatigue in, in horses,
    719–720
  obesity and, 29
  of hind limb, in horses, 13
Lamina propria, 330
Lamina transversalis, 351
Laminectomy
  for spinal trauma, 1001
  Funquist type B, 1026
  subtotal, in cervical vertebral
    malformations, 1025–
    1026
  operative procedure in,
    1026–1029, *1027, 1028,
    1029*
  postoperative care in, 1029–
    1030
  preoperative considerations
    in, 1026
Laminitis, 1147
  of horses, 42, 43
  postoperative, 218
Laparotomy
  exploratory, in horses, 13

Laparotomy (*Continued*)
  in cattle, guidelines for, 509–
    510
  in mare, detorsion of uterus
    per, 1143–1145
  ovariectomy per, 1141–
    1143, *1142*
  in stomach penetration, 505,
    506
Large intestine. See also
    Cecum; Colon.
  anatomy of, in cattle, 543–544
  in horses, 628–630
  displacement of, and colic,
    667
  location of, in horses, 628
  nonstrangulating infarction
    of, in horses, 644
  physiology of, in cattle, 544
  in horses, 630, 631(t)
  rupture of, in horses, 644–
    645
  simple obstruction of, by
    abscess, 639, *640*
    by adhesions, 639, *640*
    by enterolith, 635–636
    by foreign bodies, 634–635
    by ingesta impaction, 632–
      634
    by neoplasia, 639
    by torsion, 636–638
    by tympanites, 632
    clinical signs in, 631
    diagnosis of, 631–632
    in horses, 631–639
    pathophysiology of, 631
    rectal examination of, 631–
      632
  strangulating obstruction of
    by diaphragmatic hernia,
      644
    by torsion, 641–643
    by volvulus, 642, 643–644
    in horses, 639–644
    intussusception in, 640–641
    pathophysiology of, 640
  surgical conditions of, in
    cattle, 547–551
    considerations of, 544–
      545
Laryngeal nerve, remyelination
    of, 85
Laryngoplasty, prosthetic, 439–
    444
  complications of, 444
  cricoid cartilage penetration
    in, 443
  hemorrhage control in, 439,
    444
  prosthesis in, 442–443
  suture placement in, 442,
    445
  ventriculectomy with, 439
Laryngotomy, ventral, 415–417,
    419
  epiglottic entrapment,
    resection by, 448–449

Neoplasm(s) *(Continued)*
  connective tissue tumors as,
    in sheep, 243
  cutaneous papillomatosis as,
    224, 233, 247
  dental, in horses, 578–579
  embryonal nephroma as, 250–
    251
  ethmoturbinate tumor, 245
  exophthalmos due to, 1156
  fibroma as, 234
  granulosa cell tumor as, 238
  hemangioma as, 234
  in wound healing, 291
  incidence of, 221–222
  intestinal obstruction by, 608,
    611, *612*, 639
  lymphosarcomas as, in cattle,
    234–235
    in goats, 248
    in horses, 226–227
    in swine, 250
  mastocytoma as, 226
  melanomas as, in cattle, 234
    in goats, 248
    in horses, 224–225
    in swine, 249
  neurofibromas as, in cattle,
    239–240, *240*
  neurological signs of, 96
  of adrenal cortex, 240–241,
    247
  of bladder, in cattle, 237
  of caudal tract, in mares,
    1139
  of conjunctiva, in cattle, 1180
    in horses, 1180
  of digestive tract, in cattle,
    235–236
    in horses, 228–229
    in sheep, 246
  of endocrine system, in cattle,
    240–241
    in horses, 231–232
    in sheep, 247
  of esophagus, 235–236
    in horses, 597
  of eyelid, blepharoplasty for,
    1174–1175, *1176–1178*,
    1179
  of genital tract, in mare,
    1123
  of hematopoietic organs, in
    sheep, 244–245
  of kidneys, in cattle, 237
  of liver, in cattle, 236–237
    in sheep, 246–247
  of lung, in goats, 248
  of lymphoid organs, in cattle,
    234–235
    in goats, 248
    in horses, 226–227
    in sheep, 244–245
  of musculoskeletal system, in
    horses, 226
    in sheep, 243–244
  of nasal cavity, 227–228

Neoplasm(s) *(Continued)*
  of nervous system, in cattle,
    239–240
    in horses, 230–231
  of nictitating membrane, in
    cattle, 1180, *1181*
    in horses, 1180, *1181*
  of paranasal sinuses, 410–411
  of penis, in horses, 1086
    management of, 1087–1088
    surgery for, 1088–1092
  of pharynx, in cattle, 500, *500*
  of reproductive tract, in cattle,
    238–239
    in horses, 229–230
  of respiratory tract, in cattle,
    235
    in horses, 227–228
    in sheep, 245–246
  of skin and soft tissues, in
    cattle, 233–234, 258–260
    in goats, 247–248
    in horses, 222–226
    in sheep, 242
    in swine, 249–250
  of stomach, in horses, 602
  of testes, in horses, 1103
  of urinary tract, in cattle, 237
  of uterus, in mare, 1123
  osteochondromas as, 226
  osteomas as, 226
  osteosarcomas as, 226
  papillomas as, in sheep, 243
    in swine, 249–250
  pheochromocytomas as, 241,
    247
  pulmonary adenomatosis as,
    245–246
  sarcoids as, 222–223
  species specificity of, 221
  squamous cell carcinoma as,
    in cattle, 233, 235, 236
    in goats, 247–248
    in horses, 223–224, 228–
      229, *230*, 232–233
    in sheep, 243, 247
  thymomas as, in cattle, 235
    in goats, 248
  types of, 221
Nephrectomy, in cattle, 1080
Nephritis
  drug-induced, in horses, 15
  urolithiasis due to, in cattle,
    1073
Nephroblastoma, 250–251
Nephroma, embryonal, 250–251
Nerve(s). See also specific
  nerves.
  auriculopalpebra, and equine
    facial paralysis, 1012
  blocks. See also *Anesthesia.*
    in bovine ophthalmic
      surgery, 1154–1156
    in equine ophthalmic
      surgery, 1151–1153, *1152*
  buccal, and equine facial
    paralysis, 1012–1013

Nerve(s) *(Continued)*
  control mechanisms of, 379
  cranial. See *Cranial nerve(s).*
  femoral, injury to, *10*
  frontal, in cattle, *1155*
    in horses, 1151, *1151*
  glossopharyngeal,
    examination of, 84–85
    in guttural pouch mycosis,
      1035, 1036
  of equine face, anatomy of,
    1010–1011
    paralysis and, 1011–1013,
      1011
  of larynx, 336
  of respiratory control, 375,
    377, *376*
  of ruminant larynx, 347
  petrosal, and equine facial
    paralysis, 1012
  spinal, anatomy of, 996
  suprascapular, paralysis of,
    1019–1021
  surgical needles for, 1230(t)
  tibial, neurectomy of, 1034–
    1035
  to equine eye, 1151, *1151*
  to pleura, 330
  vagus, in guttural pouch
    mycosis, *1035*, 1036
Nerve sheath, tumor of,
  231
Nervous system
  examination of, 75–95
  in cattle, 10–11
  neoplastic disease of
    in cattle, 239–240
    in horses, 230–231
Neurapraxia, and equine facial
    paralysis, 1013
Neurectomy, of tibial nerve,
    1034–1035
Neuritis, and equine facial
    paralysis, 1012
Neurofibroma(s)
  in cattle, 239–240, *240*
  intraocular, 1196
Neurosurgery. See also
    Craniotomy; Craniectomy.
  care following, 994
  controlling hemorrhage in,
    989–990
  objectives of, 990
  preoperative medication for,
    988
Neurotmesis, and equine facial
    paralysis, 1013
Neutropenia, 52
Neutrophils, 52
  in cattle, 64–65
  in goats, 69(t)
  in sheep, 67(t)
  morphology of, 56
  persistent hypersegmented, in
    horses, 59
Neutrophilia, 53
Newberry knife, 1062, *1062*

Orthopedic surgery *(Continued)*
internal fixation techniques
in, 784–794
bone plating as, 789–791
compression plating as,
784–787
intramedullary nailing and
pinning, 791–793
screws in, 786, 787–789
transfixation pins, 793–794
postoperative care of, 213, 219
requirements for, 780–784
tourniquet use in, 782–784
Osmotic pressure, 100–101
Ossification, bilateral, 944
Osteitis, 906–908
clinical signs of, 907
postoperative care in, 908
treatment of, 907–908
by antibiotic therapy, 908
by sequestrectomy, 908
Osteoarthritis. See also
*Degenerative joint disease
(DJD).*
definition of, 716
hereditary, 721
of vertebrae, clinical findings
in, 1014–1015
occurrence of, 1013–1014
treatment of, 1015–1016
Osteochondromas, in horses,
226
Osteochondrosis dissecans, in
horses, 719, 724
nutrition and, 723
of carpal joint, 814–815
of fetlock, 834–835
of hock joint, 880–882
of scapulohumeral joint,
797–798
of stifle joint, 873, 876–878
surgical treatment of, 877–
878
Osteodystrophy fibrosis, spinal
cord injury and, 1021
Osteomas, in horses, 226
Osteomyelitis, 98
hematogenous, 908–911
clinical signs of, 909
following internal fixation,
910–911
in newborn animals, 908
treatment of, 909–910,
911
of distal phalanx, 864
of maxillary sinus, in cattle,
499
of vertebrae, clinical findings
in, 1014–1015
occurrence of, 1013–1014
treatment of, 1015–1016
Osteoporosis, due to splints, 770
Osteosarcomas, in horses, 226
Osteotomy
for femur fracture, 872
in DJD, 761

Otitis media, 80
and equine facial paralysis,
1012
Ovariectomy, in mares, 1100,
1124
per colpotomy, 1140–1141,
1141
per laparotomy, 1141–1143,
1142
Ovariohysterectomy, in mares,
1147–1148
Ovary(ies)
excision of, in mares, 1140–
1143, *1141, 1142,* 1147–
1148
neoplastic disease of, in
cattle, 238
stromal tumors of, 229–230
Overfeeding, 37, 723
adverse effects of, 29
cervical vertebral
malformation and, 1024
Ox. See also *Ruminants.*
lung size of, 350
thoracic inlet of, 349
Oxacillin, 152(t), 156(t)
administration of, 154(t)
Oxalates, bovine urolithiasis
due to, 1073, 1074
Oxygen
consumption of, in shock, 163
delivery of, and hypoxemia,
367(t)
diffusion of, 359–360
dissociation curve of, *361,* 372
exchange of, in lung, 359–362
hemoglobin saturation of, *361,*
372, 372
levels of, in blood, 371–372
partial pressure of, 121–122
toxicity of, 383
transport of, in blood, 371–
374
Oxygen tension, 121–122
Oxyhemoglobin, formation of,
361–362
Oxymorphome, in postoperative
care, 994
Oxyphenylbutazone, in
postoperative care, 994
Oxytocin, 1120, 1145
following cesarean section,
1147

PaCO$_2$, 359, 360
PaO$_2$, 359–360
determination of, in
hypoxemia, 368, 368(t)
Pachymeninges, anatomy of,
995, *996*
Packed cell volume
determination of, 49
in cattle, 63
in goats, 69(t)

Packed cell volume *(Continued)*
in Holstein cattle, 63(t)
in horses, 16
in sheep, 67(t)
Pain, postoperative, 212–213,
213(t)
Palate, soft, in ruminants, 346–
347
Palatine sinus, 328
Palatoglossal arch, of horses,
334
Palatopharyngeal arch
anatomy of, in ruminants,
346, *346*
displacement of, 431
of horses, 334
rostral displacement of, 430–
431
endoscopic evaluation of,
430–431
exercise intolerance and,
430
Palatoplasty, 564–565
Palatoschisis. See *Cleft palate.*
Palpebral nerve, in horses,
1153
Pancreas, in cattle
anatomy of, 542
surgical conditions of, 543
Pancreatitis, in horses, 658
Pancytopenia, neutropenia and,
52
Panton-Valentine leukocidin,
130
Papilloma
in cattle, 235–236, 1052
in sheep, 243
in swine, 249–250
keratinized, 516, *517*
of conjunctiva, 1180
of esophagus, 235–236
of penis, 1086
Papillomatosis, cutaneous, 224,
233, 247
Papovavirus, fibropapillomas
due to, 1052
Paracentesis
of abdomen, in horses, 15
technique of, 1194
Paralumbar fossa, anesthetic
block of, 200–201
Paralysis
bovine spastic, 10, 1032–1035
clinical findings in, 1032–
1034, *1033*
surgical therapy for, 1034–
1035
congenital, 10, *10*
due to impact injuries, 999–
1000
of face, in horses, 1010–1013
clinical findings in, 1011–
1013, *1011*
differential diagnosis of,
1012
treatment for, 1013

Physical restraint, See *Restraint, physical.*
Physical therapy, postoperative applications of, 213–215
Pia mater
anatomy of, 984, *985,* 995, *996*
Pig(s). See also *Swine.*
anemia of, 71
castration of, 1080–1082
costochondrial articulation of, 330
erythrocyte values for, 69–71, 70(t)
hematological values for, 69, 70(t)
inguinal hernia repair in, 1081
leukocyte values of, 70(t), 71
leukopenia of, 71
lower airway of, 354–355, *355*
penis of, lateral deviation of, 1082
persistent frenulum in, 1082
plasma proteins of, 71
platelets of, 71
prepuce of, resection of, 1082
respiratory system in, anatomy of, 350–355
restraint of, chemical, 1217
physical, 1214–1217
safety in, 1214
salt poisoning in, 84
upper airway of, 350–354
larynx of, 353–354, *353*
nasal cavity of, 351–352
nasopharynx of, 353
paranasal sinuses of, 352–353, *352*
trachea of, 354, *354*
vasectomy in, 1082
wound microorganisms of, 129(t)
Pimaricin, 1184
Pin
Steinmann, 1023
transfixation, in phalanx fracture, 850–851
in radial fracture, 806
in tibial fracture, 887
Pituitary gland, abscess of, 81
Plank method, for detorsion of equine uterus, 1144
Plasma, protein in
clinical significance of, 101–102
in cattle, 65
in horses, 61
in pigs, 71
in sheep, 68
Plaster cast(s), 771–779
casting techniques for, 772, 774–777
anesthesia use in, 774
wound care in, 774

Plaster cast(s) *(Continued)*
convalescent care and, 777–779
fiber glass and, 773, 774–777
for fracture immobilization, 772
for newborn animals, 773
full limb, 776–777
hospitalization and, 777
inspection of, 777–778
plaster of Paris and, 773
removal of, 779
Plastic surgery, 153. See also site and specific procedures, e.g. *Blepharoplasty.*
Platelets, 53–54
in cattle, 65
in goats, 69, 69(t)
in pigs, 71
in sheep, 68
presurgical screening of, 62
Plesiotherapy, 1190
Pleura
anatomy of, 330–331
in horses, 340
in pigs, 349, 354, 355
blood supply of, in horses, 340
effusion of, 20
parietal, 330–331
surgical needles for, 1230(t)
Pleuritis
fibrinous, in cattle, *514*
water loss in, 106
Pneumonia
in cattle, 4
inhalation, in lambs, 40
lordosis and, 1019
Pneumothorax, 381
Pneumovagina, due to parturition, 1126
Podophyllin, in tumor therapy, 1087
Podophyllum, 1169
Poisoning
by fluoride, 724
by lead, 76, 724
in horses, 85
by salt, in pigs, 84
by zinc, 724
due to forage, 36
yellow star thistle, 85
Polyamide, sutures of, 1221(t), 1221–1222
Polycythemia, 61
Polydactyly, 687
Polydioxanone (PDS), sutures of, 1221, 1221(t)
construction of, 1222
types of, 1224(t)
Polyester
surgical mesh of, 1232
sutures of, 1221(t), 1221–1222
construction of, 1222–1223
strength of, 1226
Polyglactin, sutures of, 910, 1221, 1221(t)
construction of, 1222

Polyglactin *(Continued)*
sutures of, strength of, 1226
types of, 1224(t)
Polyglycolic, sutures of, strength of, 1226
Polyglycolic acid, sutures of, 1221, 1222(t)
construction of, 1222
Polymerase, DNA and, 151, 151(t)
Polymyxin B, 151(t), 151, 152(t)
bone grafts and, 1030
Polyneuritis equi, and facial paralysis, 1012
Polyolefin, sutures of, 1221(t), 1221–1222
Polyp(s)
nasal, 402
pharyngeal, in cattle, *500*
Polypropylene
surgical mesh of, 1232
sutures of, 1221(t), 1221–1222
and infection, 1226
construction of, 1223
Pony
crossbred, differential cell counts of, 60(t)
leukocyte counts of, 60(t)
erythrocyte values of, 57
hypertriglyceridemia of, 26
shock in, anti-inflammatory drug therapy for, 174
due to gram-negative bacteria, 161
experimental observations of, 161–164
Porcine. See *Pig(s); Swine.*
Porcine stress syndrome, 18
Posthetomy, partial, in horses, 1088–1090, *1089*
Posthioplasty, of prepuce, in horses, 1088–1090, *1089*
Posthitis, acute, of equine penis, 1084
Postoperative care, 205–220
active exercise in, 213–214
diathermy in, 214
faradism in, 214
hydrotherapy in, 214, *214*
in implant removal, 219–220
objectives of, 205
of bloat, 208
of disseminated intravascular coagulation, 216–217
of enteritis, 217
of hemorrhage, 219
of ileus, 217–218
of intraruminal pressure, 211–212
of laminitis, 218
of myopathy, 218
of peritonitis, 219
of postoperative complications, 208, 211–212, 215–218
of wound dehiscence, 216
of wound infection, 215–216

Sedative-hypnotics, 195
Sedimentation rate, 55
  in cattle, 64
Seeds, in radiotherapy, 1190
Selenium
  and acquired torticollis, 1017
  deficiency of, 71
  poisoning by, 724
Semicoma, 76
Semilunar valve, 23
Seminoma, of testes, 1103
Sepsis, and arterial blood gases,
  19
Septicemia, 133
  colostrum and, 38
  of colibacillosis, 10
Septum
  nasal, 328
    in horses, 332
    in ruminants, 343
  of maxillary sinus, 333
Seroma(s)
  following hematoma surgery,
    1046
  in wound healing, 292
  of uterus, in mare, 1123
  of vagina, in mare, 1123
Serratia marcescens, 139(t)
  biochemical differentiation of,
    140(t)
Sertoli cell, tumor of, in equine
  testis, 1103
Sesamoid bone
  dehiscence of, 840, *841*
    treatment of, 841–848
  fractures of, 835–844
    apical, 835–837
    bilateral, 835, 840, *844*
    cancellous bone graft for, 838
    clinical signs of, 835
    postoperative care of, 837
    surgical treatment of, 835–
      838, *839*, 840–844
  sesamoiditis of, 835
Setaria, infection due to, in
  equine penis, 1086
Setaria igitata, 1195
Shackle, in porcine restraint,
  1216–1217, *1217*
Shanks, halter and chain, 1204
Sheep. See also *Ruminants*.
  adrenal cortex neoplasms in,
    247
  anesthesia for, 203
  arthrogryposis in, 688
  castration of, 18, 1106–1107
  cerebrospinal nematodiasis of,
    82–83
  cesarean section in, *1120*,
    1120–1121
  chondrosarcoma in, 243–244
  connective tissue tumors in, 243
    costochondral articulation
      of, 330
  embryological joint ankylosis
    in, 687
  endotoxemia of, 41

Sheep (*Continued*)
  entropion of, 1173
  erythrocyte values for, 67–68
  ethmoturbinate tumors in,
    245
  femur fractures in, 873
  fertility of, 28
  gid in, clinical findings of,
    1009–1010
    treatment for, 1010
  hematological values for, 67(t)
  Horner's syndrome of, 79
  infectious arthritis in,
    treatment of, 912
  in adrenal cortex neoplasm,
    247
  inhalation pneumonia of, 40
  intestinal tissue of, for
    sutures, 1222
  Johnes' disease of, 34
  ketonemia of, 26
  leukocytes, value of, 67(t), 68
  lungworm infestation of, 4
  lymphosarcomas in, 244–245
  nasolacrimal system in, 1165
  neoplastic disease in, 242–247
    gastric resection in, 542
    incidence of, 242–243
    of digestive tract, 246
    of endocrine system, 247
    of hematopoietic organs,
      244–245
    of liver, 246–247
    of lymphoid organs, 244–
      245
    of musculoskeletal system,
      243–244
    of respiratory tract, 245–246
    of skin and soft tissues, 243
    pulmonary adenomatosis as,
      245–246
  nostrils of, 342, *342*
  obesity of, 29
  ocular carcinoma in, 1194
  papillomas in, 243
  paranasal sinuses of, 343, *344*
  PCV of, 67(t)
  pheochromocytomas in, 247
  pituitary abscess of, 81
  plasma proteins of, 68
  platelets of, 68
  postoperative care of, 207–208
  preoperative examination of,
    18–19
  rectal prolapse in, 681
  restraint of, chemical, 1219
    physical, 1218–1219
    safety in, 1217
  reticulocytes of, 68
  splints for, Kirschner Ehmer
    type, 794
  squamous cell carcinoma in,
    243, 247
  tracheal cartilage of, *349*
  uterine prolapse in, 1120
  vaginal prolapse in, 1119–
    1120

Sheep (*Continued*)
  vasectomy in, 1107–1108,
    1107
  wound microorganisms of,
    129(t)
Shigella, 139
Shirodkar technique, 1138
Shock
  antibiotic therapy in, 168–169
  atropine in, 174–175
  blood carbon dioxide tension
    in, 167
  blood chemistry in, 163, 164
  blood-gas abnormalities in,
    163
  cardiac output in, 165–166
  cardiogenic, 160–161
  cardiovascular response in,
    162
  central venous pressure in,
    165
  classification of, 160–161
  clinical management of, 166–
    175
  clinical signs of, 162
  corticosteroids in, 172–173
  definition of, 160
  due to surgery, 382
  endotoxic, 613–614
  gram-negative bacterial, 161
  hematological alterations in,
    162–163
  hemorrhagic, 160, 161
  heparin in, 174
  hypovolemic, 160
  in acute abdominal crises, 613
  in colic surgery, 665
  intravascular fluid volume in,
    167
  intravenous solution use in,
    167–168
  lidocaine in, 175
  management of, 160–176
  mean arterial blood pressure
    in, 165
  metabolic factors in, 160
  metabolic acidosis in, 169,
    172
  monitoring of, 164–166
  nonsteroidal anti-inflam-
    matory drugs in, 173–174
  oxygenation in, 166–167
  pathological changes in, 164
  pathophysiology of, 161
  plasma chemical values in,
    163–164
  pulmonary artery pressure in,
    166
  pulmonary capillary wedge
    pressure in, 166
  respiratory abnormalities in,
    163
  symptoms of, 161
  traumatic, 160, 161
  vasodilator therapy in, 175
  ventilation in, 166–167
  volume replacement in, 168

Soft palate (*Continued*)
dorsal displacement of,
definition of, 423
diagnosis of, 424, 425
endoscopic evaluation of,
424–425
epiglottic entrapment with,
446, 447, 448, 449
epiglottis shortening in,
425–426
etiology of, 424
functional pharyngeal
obstruction in, 424
in arytenoid chondritis, 452
management of, 426–427
partial resection of, 427–428
postoperative, 449
radiographic evaluation of,
425
sternothyrohyoideus muscle
resection in, 428
symptoms of, 423
surgical correction of, 434
Sorbital dehydrogenase, 16
Sores
pressure, and splint, 769, 770
due to plaster cast, 778–779
summer, 1171
Space, epidural. See *Epidural
space.*
Spastic lameness. See *Spastic
paresis.*
Spastic paresis, 10, 1032–1035
clinical findings in, 1032–
1034, *1033*
surgical therapy for, 1034–
1035
Spasticity, of gait, 87
Spatula needle, 1229, *1229*
Spavin, 763
etiology of, in horses, 719
Spectrophotometry
of erythrocytes, 55
of hemoglobin, 49
Spermatic cord, in horses,
infection of, 1095
Spina bifida, 91
Spinal cord
anatomy of, 995, *996*, 996–
998, *997*
blood supply to, *998*, 998–999
coenurosis of, diagnosis of,
1009–1010
treatment for, 1010
compression of, 88, 91
compressive injuries to, 1000
examination of, 74
impact injuries to, 999–1000
injury to, 1021–2023
etiology of, 1021–1022
pathology of, 1022
postoperative care for, 1023
treatment for, 1022–1023
lesions of, 96
lymphosarcoma of, 96
nerves to, 996

Spinal cord (*Continued*)
surgery to, 994–995
trauma to, treatment for,
1000–1001
Spine
abscess of, clinical findings
in, 1014–1015
occurrence of, 1013–1014
treatment of, 1015–1016
cervical. See *Cervical spine.*
Spinocerebellar tract, anatomy
of, *997*, 997–998
Spirochetes, infection due to, in
equine penis, 1086
Splanchnoptosis, 1126, 1132
in mares, 1122, 1124
relief of, 1133
Spleen
contraction of, and packed
cell volume, 49
rupture of, in horses, 657
Splint(s)
construction of, 768
Kirschner Ehmer, 794
orthopedic use of, 768–770
in newborns, 768–769
plaster casts vs., 768
pressure sores and, 769, 770
Thomas, 770
Sponges
collagen, in neurosurgery, 993
gelatin, in cranial fractures,
1008
in laminectomy procedures,
1026
in neurosurgery, 989, 993
Spore, "drum stick," 137
Spore former
aerobic, 133–134
anaerobic, 134–137
Squeeze, commercial, in
restraint of swine, 1217
Stabilization procedure, for
large animals, 1001
Stanchion bar, and elbow
abduction, 6
Standardbred horse, growth
curve of, *34*
Staphylectomy, 427–428
Staphylococcosis, of cervix, in
mare, 1124, 1139
of spermatic cord, 1095
Staphylococcus, 911, 912
species differences of, 130(t)
Staphylococcus aureus, 129(t),
130–131, 152
antimicrobials for, 156(t), 157
drug resistance of, 157
vertebral abscess due to, 1014
Staphylococcus epidermidis,
130–131
drug resistance of, 157
Staphylococcus pyogenes,
vertebral abscess due to, 1014
Staphylococcus saprophyticus,
130

Stapling, surgical instruments
for, 1242–1244
Steel
stainless, surgical mesh of,
1232
sutures of, 1221(t), 1221–1222
and infection, 1226
construction of, 1223
uses of, 1225(t)
Steinmann pin, stabilization
with, 1023
Stenosis
duodenal, in horses, 612
gastric, in horses, 602
in cerebral vertebrae
malformations, 1024–1025
of lacrimal punctum in
horses, 1164, *1164*
pyloric, congenital, 602
gastric dilation–associated,
600
in cattle, 535
surgical treatment of, 602
tracheal, 476
Stent bandage, 1030
Step mouth, 568
Sternal recumbent position, and
respiratory function, 380
Sternothyrohyoideus muscle,
resection of, 428–430
Steroids
for parturition, 38
in postoperative care, 994
wound healing effects of,
292–293
Stifle joint, 873–876
arthritis of, 873
chondromalacia in, 874
clinical signs of, 874
treatment of, 875
blood-borne infections in,
874
clinical signs in, 874–875
cruciate ligament rupture in,
873, 874, 875
innervation of, 703
luxation of, 901–902
meniscal injuries in, 874,
875–876
osteochondrosis dissecans of,
873, 876–878
subchondral bone cyst in,
876
surgical treatment of, 877–
878
radiographic analysis of, 875
vasculature of, 702
Stomach
abomasum of. See
Abomasum.
anatomy of, in cattle, 505, 506
in horses, 598–599
dilation of, etiology of, 600
in horses, 600–601
foreign body penetration of, in
cattle, 505